The Principles and Practicability
OF
BOENNINGHAUSEN'S THERAPEUTIC POCKET BOOK
FOR
HOMOEOPATHIC PHYSICIANS
TO USE
AT THE BESIDE AND IN THE STUDY
OF THE
MATERIA MEDICA

T. F. Allen

B. JAIN PUBLISHERS PVT. LTD

> **Note from the Publishers**
>
> *Any information given in this book is not intended to be taken as a replacement for medical advice. Any person with a condition requiring medical attention should consult a qualified practitioner or therapeutist.*

Reprint Edition: 2003

All rights are reserved. No part of this book may be reproduced, stored in a retrieval system or transmitted, in any form or by any means, mechanical, photocopying, recording or otherwise, without any prior written permission of the publisher.

© Copyright with the Publishers

Price: Rs.90.00.

Published by Kuldeep Jain for

B. Jain Publishers (P) Ltd.

1921, Street No. 10, Chuna Mandi,
Paharganj, New Delhi 110 055.(INDIA)
Phones: 2358 0800, 2358 1100, 2358 1300, 2358 3100
Fax: 011-2358 0471; *Email:* bjain@vsnl.com
Website: www.bjainbooks.com

Printed in India by
J.J. Offset Printers
522, FIE, Patpar Ganj, Delhi - 110 092

ISBN 81-7021-010-0
BOOK CODE BA-2009

BOENNINGHAUSEN'S THERAPEUTIC POCKET BOOK

PART I

INTRODUCTION
by

H.A. ROBERTS
ANNIE C. WILSON

PREFACE

Bœnninghausen's *Therapeutic Pocket Book* has been used for more than a century by many masters of homœopathic practice. If it has fallen into comparative disuse during the past few years it is because few of the younger generation of homœopathic physicians have had a knowledge of its philosophic background and practical principles. It is not our purpose to set forth the superiority of any one general repertory over another; but it is our desire to demonstrate the sound philosophy and practical application of this work to such states as the physician meets in everyday practice. It is as nearly fool-proof as any repertory can be, once its principles are assimilated. In the following pages the statement is made that the book is not perfected; it has not grown to its full possibilities of usefulness; but the principles upon which it is based are sound and will allow further development and expansion without endangering those basic principles or distorting their balanced importance.

Let us utilize all the means at our disposal to insure to each patient the *simillimum*, which is his only hope of cure, and let us do so with the fullest possible comprehension of natural laws, and the application of those laws in practical form as they appear in our homœopathic literature. Let us not forget that every man who has labored constructively for homœopathy has built upon some law or definite guiding principle; if we will utilize these works we shall see the wisdom of the past flowering in the healing of the present.

Derby, Conn.
August, 1935.

BŒNNINGHAUSEN (1785-1864)

Baron Clemens Maria Franz von Bœnninghausen was born in the Netherlands on a family estate of his father. The family traced its lineage through Westphalian and Austrian ancestry, one ancestor having been appointed as Field Marshal by Ferdinand II of Austria in 1632. Since for centuries the family had devoted themselves to military careers the family fortunes were but moderate.

His early life was spent in the open, and he entered rather late upon his education, but after once starting, his progress was rapid. He graduated from the Dutch university at Gröningen with the degree of Doctor of Civil and Criminal Law, and thereafter for several years he filled increasingly influential and arduous positions at the court of Louis Napoleon, King of Holland, remaining in the Dutch Civil Service until the resignation of the king in 1810, when Bœnninghausen too retired from the Dutch service. In 1812 he married and went to one of the family estates in what later became western Prussia. He devoted much thought to developing the state agriculturally, and became greatly interested in agriculture and allied sciences, particularly botany. Through his interest in the development of agricultural resources he came in touch with the most prominent agriculturists of Germany, and he formed the first agricultural society in the western part of Germany. At the reorganization of the Prussian provinces of Rhineland and Westphalia in 1816 he was offered the position of President of the Provincial Court of Justice for the Westphalia district. As a part of these duties he was called upon to act as the sole Judicial President in the evaluation of land in the two provinces, because of his technical knowledge of agriculture and land values. This work necessitated much traveling, and later his appointment as one of the

General Commissioners kept him traveling throughout the provinces almost constantly.

Bœnninghausen made diligent use of these opportunities to study the flora of the provinces, and he published a book covering the abundant flora in these districts which called to him the attention of some of the best botanists of Europe; these botanists came into even closer touch with him upon his appointment, at about this time, as Director of the Botanical Gardens at Münster. His agricultural and botanical writings brought him the honor of diplomas in many learned societies and two prominent botanists of that day each named a genus of plants after him.

In 1827 he suffered a derangement of health, which had hitherto been excellent. Two of the most celebrated physicians obtainable declared this to be purulent tuberculosis. His health continued to decline until the spring of 1828, when all hope of his recovery was given up. At this time he wrote a farewell letter to his close botanical friend, A. Weihe, M. D., who was the first homœopathic physician in the province of Rhineland and Westphalia, though Bœnninghausen was ignorant of the fact, their whole correspondence having touched on botanical, not medical, subjects. Weihe was deeply moved by the news and answered Bœnninghausen's letter immediately, requesting a detailed account of his symptoms and expressing the hope that by means of the newly found curative method he might be able to save a friend whom he valued so highly. In response to the reply which Bœnninghausen sent to this letter, Weihe sent some *Pulsatilla* which Bœnninghausen took according to the directions, following also the course of advice which Weihe gave him regarding hygienic measures. Bœnninghausen's recovery was gradual but constant, so that by the end of the summer he was considered as cured.

This event bred in Bœnninghausen a firm belief in the results of homœopathic treatment, and he looked well into the matter. He became thoroughly interested in the principles of the new method of healing, and did his best to create an interest in homœopathy among the physicians

INTRODUCTION TO THE THERAPEUTIC POCKET BOOK

with whom he came in contact, as he himself was one of the founders of the medical society at Münster; but they were deaf to his arguments, and he himself set out to master the subject through such books as he could procure. In his university days he had had some medical lore, although he was not an approved physician. Two of the most aged physicians eventually became interested in the subject of homœopathy through Bœnninghausen's cures of some of their stubborn cases, and they remained faithful to homœopathy during the remainder of their lives. By this time Bœnninghausen's fame had spread to France, Holland and America, and he had gained many converts to the new doctrine of healing among physicians in these lands, by correspondence and literary efforts. During this time, not being an approved physician, he had practiced but little but devoted himself to furthering the cause by his literary efforts, which were extended in the effort of making the work of practicing homœopathy easier. At this time, you will remember, there was no short way to approach the study of homœopathy. No repertories, save a brief one in Latin by Samuel Hahnemann himself, had been published as an index to point the way to the indicated homœopathic remedy, and many hours must have been devoted to the study of remedy after remedy before the true picture was seen. Jahr did not publish his first repertory until 1834, and in his fourth edition he writes a preface in which he gives Bœnninghausen credit for the system of evaluating the remedies which he (Jahr) had only then begun to use; this fourth edition was published in 1851.

King Friedrich Wilhelm IV, under date of July 11, 1843, issued to Bœnninghausen a document empowering him to practice medicine without any restraint.

From 1830 Bœnninghausen was in close touch with Hahnemann, until the close of Hahnemann's life, and as long as Bœnninghausen lived he kept in close touch with all those practicing homœopathy. However, his literary work was much hampered by the permission to practice freely, and he did not publish his books as frequently after that event, although he spent much time at that labor. It is interesting to note that his earliest works found instant circulation among those interested in the new doctrine, and almost every practicing homœopath had Bœnninghausen's works in his library. Bœnninghausen's works in the order of their appearance are listed here:

The Cure of Cholera and Its Preventatives (according to Hahnemann's latest communication to the author). 1831.

Repertory of the Antipsoric Medicines, with a preface by Hahnemann. 1832.

Summary View of the Chief Sphere of Operation of the Antipsoric Remedies and of their Characteristic Peculiarities, as an Appendix to their Repertory. 1833.

An Attempt at a Homœopathic Therapy of Intermittent Fever. 1833.

Contributions to a Knowledge of the Peculiarities of Homœopathic Remedies. 1833.

Homœopathic Diet and a Complete Image of a Disease. (For the non-professional public.) 1833.

Homœopathy, a Manual for the Non-Medical Public. 1834.

Repertory of the Medicines which are not Antipsoric. 1835.

Attempt at Showing the Relative Kinship of Homœopathic Medicines. 1836.

Therapeutic Manual for Homœopathic Physicians, for use at the sickbed and in the study of the Materia Medica Pura. 1846.

Brief Instructions for Non-Physicians as to the Prevention and Cure of Cholera. 1849.

The Two Sides of the Human Body and Relationships. Homœopathic Studies. 1853.

The Hom. Domestic Physician in Brief Therapeutic Diagnoses. An Attempt. 1853.

The Homœopathic Treatment of Whooping Cough in its Various Forms. 1860.

The Aphorisms of Hippocrates, with Notes by a Homœopath. 1863.

Attempt at a Homœopathic Therapy of Intermittent and Other Fevers, especially for would-be homœopaths. Second augmented and revised edition. Part I. *The Pyrexy.* 1864.

After the proclamation empowering him to practice medicine, Bœnninghausen founded the society for homœopathic physicians in Westphalia, which flourished for many years under the interest which was roused in the homœopaths whom Bœnninghausen drew about him.

Bœnninghausen was a close friend of Adolph Lippe, and also of Carroll Dunham. Both of these men expressed their appreciation of the work Bœnninghausen had accomplished, in Vol. 4 of the *American Homœopathic Review*. Lippe mentions particularly the repertorial work of Bœnninghausen and its accuracy, and one wonders if it was not this which fired his interest in repertorial work, which Lippe's son brought forth in a completed form.

Lippe gives the year of Bœnninghausen's birth as 1777. It is not a matter for controversy, since Bœnninghausen devoted all the time he had to the promulgation of the work which he held so dear.

Of his seven sons the two eldest chose homœopathic medicine as their profession, which was a great joy to him. The elder of these sons practiced for a time in the neighborhood of his boyhood home, later going to Paris where he married the adopted daughter of Hahnemann's widow. He lived with Madame Hahnemann and her daughter, and had access to Hahnemann's library and manuscripts.

REPERTORY USES

The intelligent use of a repertory implies that we understand the scope of a repertory as well as the purpose of a repertory. We may ask: *What is a repertory?* To which the reply might be: *A repertory is an index of symptoms, arranged systematically*. The system of arrangement may be founded in turn upon definite guiding principles; or it may be alphabetical or schematic.

Again we may ask: *What is the purpose of a repertory?* Our answer may be: A repertory has two definite purposes: 1. To serve as a reference and guide in looking up a particular symptom that may indicate the *simillimum*, or that may make the necessary distinction between two or more similar remedies in any given case; 2. For careful study of all the symptoms that may appear in a chronic case.

The repertory is not meant for use in those cases where there are clear indications for the *simillimum*. In those cases the additional symptoms that might be secured from the patient, under pressure of questioning, possibly would confuse a case that already stands out clearly; or if the repertory is used here, it might be used in the manner of a quick reference, to verify the leading indications for the remedy, or if some slight doubt were felt, to differentiate between those seemingly indicated. In clearly cut cases, even if the repertorization verified the picture, for the student of materia medica this would have been a waste of time.

On the other hand, we must take into consideration those physicians who have not gained a thorough knowledge of the materia medica; or to be considered still more, those chronic cases where several remedies emerge only in shadowy outlines from a background that is a network of chronic symptoms ever more intricately woven. There are many such cases that come to the homœopathic physician, cases that have suffered many things of many doctors; cases with mismanagement after mismanagement superimposed upon circumstantial stress and that again upon hereditary tendencies. These cases rarely show a clear picture of a single indicated remedy, and very often show no related group of remedies. Often it is impossible to see any remedy-likeness in such a symptom group without careful repertorization, but with that analysis we may see not only the single indicated remedy, but we may trace the probable sequence of remedies that may be necessary to bring the case to the desired cure, for it is possible to envision the probable sequence of remedies, at times, just as we can look back over a chronic history and see the indications for various remedies at various periods in the patient's past life.

The value of any repertory depends upon several elements:

I. *The art of the physician in taking the case.*
II. *A knowledge of the repertory one attempts to use:*
    (a) Its philosophic background
    (b) Its construction
    (c) Its limitations
    (d) Its adaptability
III. *Intelligent use of the resulting analysis.*

THE ART OF THE PHYSICIAN IN TAKING THE CASE

This embraces the art of the physician in securing the confidence of the patient and in drawing out from him those subjective symptoms, of mind, body and spirit, that are an integral part of the difficulty for which he seeks help; it embraces also the art of observation of those observable symptoms, plus the general atmosphere radiated by the patient, that go to make up the objective symptoms in their widest sense. This combination of the subjective and objective symptoms comprises what we term *the case*. Still further, the art of the physician in taking the case must so record it that we may glean from this record those elements that may be translated intelligently into the rubrics of the repertory, or that may be left aside for later comparison with the materia medica after the bulk of the symptoms has been translated into, and used as, rubrics in the repertory analysis.

However, we often find that it is impossible to secure from the patient a clear-cut picture of his difficulties, in spite of the best art the physician may exercise.

Bœnninghausen himself recognized that with the best possible case taking the record is often left in an incomplete or fragmentary state. In some instances the localities or parts affected are not clearly stated. In others the sensation or affection is not indicated or described in an intelligible manner. Most frequently the conditions of aggravation and amelioration of particular symptoms, or of the patient's general condition, could not be stated because of the patient's lack of observation. Perhaps the patient could not state what relations the symptoms had to each other as to time, place and circumstances, if there were alternating symptom groups.

In these modifications of symptoms, such as conditions of aggravation and amelioration, lie the keys that unlock the similitude of remedies to the individual case; and in quite as great a degree do we find the interrelationship of symptoms of value.

Bœnninghausen comprehended the difficulties encountered by the physician in securing a complete picture of the case, and his comparisons of his case records and the records of provers convinced him that the same lack of observation existed in the provers as existed in patients.

Noting these deficiencies in the materia medica, therefore, and realizing the importance of these auxiliary modifying and concomitant symptoms of disease, Bœnninghausen for many years diligently observed and collected all such symptoms as they appeared in the cases which came to him for treatment. Every case was examined symptomatically with this purpose always in view, *viz.*, to make every symptom as complete in itself as possible, covering the specific points of locality, sensation, conditions of aggravation and amelioration, and the concomitance or co-existence of other symptoms under the same circumstances.

He soon learned that symptoms which existed in an incomplete state in some part of a given case could be reliably completed by *analogy,* by observing the conditions of other parts of the case. If, for instance, it was not possible by questioning a patient to decide what aggravated or ameliorated a particular symptom of the case, the patient would readily express a condition of amelioration of some other symptom. It did not take long to discover that conditions of aggravation or amelioration are not confined to this or that particular symptom; but that, like the red thread in the cordage of the British Navy, they apply to all the symptoms of the case.

Bœnninghausen tells us in his *Preface,* page ix:

From one point of view the indicated conditions of aggravation or amelioration have a far more signficant relation to the totality of the case and to its single symptoms than is usually supposed; they are never confined exclusively to one or another symptom, but on the contrary, a correct choice of the suitable remedy depends very often chiefly upon them.

In reality, then, they are the general characteristics. By observing them and applying this principle he was enabled to complete many symptoms from clinical observation; and experience has borne out the truth and reliability of his method.

The *Totality of the Symptoms* and its corresponding *simillimum* which the homœopathic prescriber seeks are both based on the same idea. In examining a case, he gets what appears to the novice to be a heterogeneous lot of symptoms, or fragments of symptoms. Possibly there may not appear to be one complete symptom in the record. He will find a clearly expressed sensation in some part, but no condition of aggravation or amelioration. In another part, a clearly expressed condition of aggravation or amelioration, but an indefinite sensation; or perhaps the patient will simply give a condition of aggravation or amelioration which he refers simply to himself in general. He says, "*I* feel worse" under such and such conditions.

In reality the patient is not expressing many symptoms, but only parts of a very few complete symptoms, which the examiner must bring together and complete. Bœnninghausen so designed his *Pocket Book* that it would enable the physician to bring the symptoms together and complete one part by another.

The perceptible symptoms of disease are often broken up and scattered through the different parts of a patient's organism in much the same way that symptoms are dispersed in the ordinary repertories. The scattered parts must be found and brought together in harmonious relation according to the typical form.

Bœnninghausen proceeds upon the Hahnemannian theory that it is the *patient* who is sick—not his head, nor his eye, nor his heart. Every symptom that refers to a part may be predicated of the whole man. If there is a stitching pain felt in the eye it belongs to the man, and stitching pain is noted as a characteristic of his complaint in general. If motion of the legs, as in walking, increases the pain in the eyes, < from motion is noted as referring to the totality—the man himself. If he has at the same time chilliness on moving, and nausea with retching, these are noted as concomitant symptoms, parts which go to make up the whole of the grand or typical symptom called the *totality*. Really, the *totality* is simply the complete picture of the disease. *The totality is to the disease what the man, the ego, is to his organism. It is that which gives individuality and personality.*

Just as each particular symptom is made up of locality, sensation, and conditions of aggravation and amelioration, so the *totality* is made up of general characteristics of the particular symptoms PLUS the condition (that cannot be referred to a part) under the same general divisions of locality, sensations and conditions.

For a brief and comprehensive classification of the homœopathic symptomatology for therapeutic purposes no plan has ever been devised superior, or equal, to that of Bœnninghausen in his *Therapeutic Pocket Book*. The plan is fundamental, and probably final, because it is founded upon the principles of logic, and has been verified by the experience of a century.

Certain portions of Bœnninghausen's plan have been criticized, notably by Hering, who objects that Bœnninghausen makes too broad an application of the principles of concomitance or association. Bœnninghausen's avowed object was to open, as he put it, "a way into the wide field of combinations." In other words, his *Pocket Book* was to serve as an index to the similar remedies, and the carefully trained mind of the physician would find among these remedies the most similar.

The symptoms of the materia medica, like the symptoms appearing in sickness, may be reduced to certain fundamental forms, corresponding to the genera and species of biological science, or the generals and particulars of logic. These Bœnninghausen called *primary* and *secondary* symptoms. These are the elements of symptomatology. In like manner, each particular symptom, pri mary or secondary, may be reduced to its elements of location, sensation and condition.

These primary and secondary symptoms were not related to time so much as to their relation to the case; in other words, those symptoms which seemed to have a direct bearing on the complaint, and the other group of almost equal importance, the concomitant symptoms.

Symptoms appear in constantly varying combinations, in proving and in sickness. The form which symptoms may take in any given case is governed by the peculiarities of the individual. In the grouping of symptoms, therefore, the *personal equation* rules in every individual case. All cases of rheumatism, for instance, will present certain symptoms in common—the diagnostic symptoms; but besides these common symptoms each case will present what Hahnemann calls *uncommon, peculiar, (characteristic) symptoms,* symptoms which represent the individual factor in the case, symptoms which differentiate it from the other cases of its class. These symptoms vary in every case.

The Hahnemannian doctrine is that these symptoms really represent that which is curable in each case of disease, and they are therefore the basis of the homœopathic prescription. It is for these *peculiar symptoms* that the similar remedy must be found, rather than for those general symptoms which appear commonly in almost every case.

This free, one might be tempted to say lawless, grouping of symptoms has always been the great stumbling block for therapeutics. It has led to the arbitrary grouping of symptoms and the erection of so-called typical forms to which names have been assigned, as if they were real entities. Moreover, such artificial forms or entities have been made the object of treatment, and the search for specifics goes on without ceasing. Very naturally such a search is futile, and the treatment is a failure, for the simple reason that the typical forms as they appear in the textbook are never found in practice, since they lack in the textbook those *uncommon, peculiar, characteristic* symptoms which give individuality to each case met in practice. In every case we find a few *typical* symptoms plus many atypical symptoms—symptoms which belong to the individual, the concomitants of the disease symptoms *per se*.

Bœnninghausen applies the principles of concomitance when, in an obscure case, he brings order out of chaos by combining the scattered fragments of symptoms into one or more typical symptoms by fixing a locality in one part, taking the character of the sensations from the symptoms expressed by the patient in relation to other parts, and the conditions of aggravation and amelioration perhaps from an affection of some other part, or perhaps from a consideration of all the parts affected. It is to be remembered, however, that these symptoms are not chosen at random; they must all bear a definite relationship to each other in the matter of time and circumstance even though they have a seeming irregularity in grouping. By a wider application of the principle he gathers all the affected localities, all the sensations and all the conditions, *each in its proper place,* and thus erects the totality, which at the same time reveals both the remedy and the disease. The system is unique and extremely logical; like fitting together many pieces of a puzzle we find every symptom or part of a symptom, however seemingly irrelevant or illogical, fitting smoothly into its place.

The totality is related equally to the remedy and to the disease. The symptoms of the remedy must correspond perfectly to the symptoms of the disease. They are counterparts; they may even be considered as identical as to origin and nature in the last analysis. A group or totality of symptoms may as well be called *Pulsatilla* as Measles in homœopathic practice. Under certain conditions, *viz.,* the state of symptom similarity, they are practically identical. For the sake of the conventions of general medicine we distinguish between them, since common usage and diagnosis have given us names for certain symptom groups; but as students of the *Law of Similars* we recognize the value of the totality in our consideration of the patient, and we recognize equally of how little value the diagnosis is as an aid to a comprehension of the symptom totality.

It is the business of the physician accurately to observe, faithfully record, and scientifically classify the phenomena of disease for the purpose of discovering and applying the curative remedy. This is equally incumbent upon him, whether he is engaged in the conduct of a proving where a disease is artificially engendered, the study of an epidemic, studies in the natural history of a single disease, or in the treatment of an individual patient. Precisely the same principles should govern in all these departments.

The typical form of any disease is discovered only by observing many patients and collating their symptoms in such a manner as to bring out its personality, just as the sphere of action of the remedy is discovered by assembling under one schema all the symptoms of many provers. Not all the symptoms that a remedy is capable of producing can be elicited from any one prover. Several, or many, provers of both sexes are required to bring out the entire range of symptoms of any drug. The symptoms of the many provers, by the Hahnemannian method, are all collated, classified, and arranged under a schema based on the anatomical divisions of the body. The resulting typical form, which we call the *totality*, is an abstract form or image, comprising all that can be known of the artificial disease, so arranged as to have an individuality of its own.

In a similar way the discovery of an epidemic remedy in any epidemic disease depends upon the study of many cases for the purpose of observing and collating all the symptoms that form its totality. An epidemic might be considered as a gigantic, involuntary proving of some noxious element, germ or miasm, affecting a large number of persons at the same time under certain peculiar conditions. To find the antidote to the poison that is making the people sick, or in other words, the epidemic remedy, many patients must be observed, their symptoms recorded and the remedy that corresponds to the totality found by the Hahnemannian method of comparison.

When we come to deal with the sick individual we find that just as not all the symptoms of a disease as classified in the textbooks can be found in any given case of that disease, so all the symptoms of a remedy as observed in the provings cannot be found in any one case.

Each typical group or totality, whether arising clinically or in a patient, contains many lesser, but none the less characteristic, groups of symptoms.

The symptoms as first elicited from the patient or prover may be, and usually are, scattered, fragmentary, often apparently unrelated. It is the business of the therapeutic artist to piece these fragments together in a definite and symmetrical form; to give them their true form and individuality; to erect the totality, which at the same time indicates both the disease and the remedy. This he must do according to some preconceived plan and form. He must have a framework or skeleton upon which and around which to build his symptom structure, if it is to have coherency or consistency. He must be able to see through the confused and scattered symptoms and fragments of the symptoms the outline, at least, of the remedy; and he must find means also to fill up the vacancies, supplying the missing links, and combine these fragments so as to make one harmonious whole.

When all the symptoms of a case have been gathered, and the totality has been found, we have all that can be known of the disease. It exists then in a form to which other different general names have been applied, as *the symptom picture, the case, the individuality of the case,* and so on. Confusion always arises when the attempt is made to make the true totality conform to the terms and classifications of theoretical pathology. There is no necessity for making such an attempt. The homœopathic ideal will have been attained when such individual true totality is simply called by the name of the drug which corresponds to it. Simplicity demands this, and the better our understanding of homœopathic philosophy and our materia medica the more clearly we comprehend the truly scientific background for such a recognition of the individual diagnosis, both of the case and of the remedy.

The totality, in homœopathic practice, is the true diagnosis of the disease, and at the same time the diagnosis of the remedy. The totality eliminates all the theoretical elements and speculations of traditional medicine and deals only with the actually manifest facts. These facts it assembles, not according to some arbitrary or imaginary form, but according to a natural order. The same principles of classification that govern the botanist or zoologist in their classification of plant and animal life should govern the physician in his classification of the phenomena of disease.

In the note at the close of the preface to the first edition of his *Repertory of the Antipsorics*, Bœnninghausen voiced his concept of the orderly classification of symptoms under Hahnemann's system in this glowing tribute to the genius of Hahnemann:

> Hereafter, like the botanists, all the world's physicians will understand each other, and also prescribe with safety one and the same remedy for *identical morbid symptoms*, and not for *identical names of diseases*.

THE PHILOSOPHIC BACKGROUND

The intimate knowledge of the repertory is our study at this time, but in order to get a comprehensive view of the repertory and its potentialities for the chronic case we must regard it as a means to an end, never an end in itself. It is often the bridge of knowledge between the physician and the chronic patient; it is across the structure of the repertory that the physician may reach and treat the patient suffering from any obscure disease condition, but particularly the obscure chronic condition, and by means of which the physician may return again and again, if necessary, to a consideration of the case and its progress. From the structure of the repertory the physician gains the best outlook into the patient's past condition, his present symptomatology and his probable future development. To one who has not studied the general repertory carefully its possibilities are lost in the mists of half-knowledge. "Truth rises more clearly from error than from half-truth," and to one who knows a little it is often difficult to teach the full comprehension. Therefore, in studying Bœnninghausen's *Therapeutic Pocket Book* we shall glance briefly at the state of homœopathic literature at the time Boenninghausen composed his repertories.

After Hahnemann's *Materia Medica Pura* was written, it became more and more apparent that some method should be devised that would make it possible to find the *simillimum* more easily and quickly. By this time the records of symptoms developed through provings had reached bulky proportions, yet the only method of referring to the records of proven symptoms was the tedious perusal of page after page of materia medica. Hahnemann, who had watched carefully all the provings and who had proved many remedies under his own personal observation, had in all probability the least trouble in identifying the symptoms of any individual remedy; yet the letters from patients who visited him during his later years record the fact that he often searched through pages of manuscript before administering a remedy. Further evidence that identifying symptoms had become a stupendous task, even to Hahnemann, is the fact that he himself compiled a short repertory of some of the leading symptoms; this was printed in Latin. Later he developed the repertory idea still further, but these later repertories are still in manuscript form, never having been published. (Dr. Richard Haehl speaks of these in his *Life of Hahnemann*.)

Boenninghausen was a close friend and student of Hahnemann, and it was with the encouragement of Hahnemann that Boenninghausen developed his first repertory, *Repertory of the Antipsorics,* published in 1832. This contained a preface by Hahnemann himself, and was undoubtedly one of the very earliest published repertories.

In 1835 Boenninghausen published his *Repertory of the Medicines which are not Antipsoric;* in 1836 his *Attempt at Showing the Relative Kinship of Homœopathic Medicines*. Ten years later he published his *Therapeutic Manual for Homœopathic Physicians,* and this volume contained the principles and general method of construction set forth in the former volumes, much amplified and perfected as the fruit of his constant observations over a period of several years, and yet so compactly constructed that it avoided the cumbersome features of Jahr's and other early repertories.

In constructing his *Therapeutic Pocket Book* Bœnninghausen based his grouping of symptoms on Hahnemann's teaching that it is imperative that the homœopathic physician prescribe on the *totality of the case*. He proceeded on the hypothesis that this *totality* was not only the sum total of the symptoms, but was in itself one grand symptom—the symptom of the patient; and that whether the individual parts of the symptom were considered or the grand symptom—the totality itself—three factors must be present: 1. *Locality* the part, organs or tissues involved in the disease process. 2. *Sensation:* the kind of pain, sensation, functional or organic change characterizing the morbid process. 3. *Conditions of Aggravation or Amelioration* of the symptoms: the circumstances causing, exciting, increasing, or otherwise affording modification or relief of the suffering.

Bœnninghausen recognized that symptoms naturally occur in groups, some of which are marked and prominent and some of which are subsidiary. These appear in every chronic case, and often to a marked degree. These are always leading symptoms, and these may be defined as those symptoms for which there is clear pathological foundation; or the symptoms that are most prominent and clearly recognizable; or the symptoms which first attract the attention of the patient or physician; or which cause the most suffering; or which indicate definitely the seat and nature of the morbid process; which form the "warp of the fabric," as it has been expressed. In the leading symptoms alone, however, there is nothing particularly characteristic from the standpoint of the prescriber.

For instance, we have 150 remedies which produce cerebral congestion; thirty-six which produce inflamed liver; ninety-six produce inflamed lungs; fifty-four produce inflamed ovaries; the same number produce inflammation of the uterus. Any one of these may become a *leading symptom,* yet the inflammation of any organ is not a fact of any great value in leading the prescriber to the *simillimum.*

In any of these conditions we have a location, if we properly diagnose the case, but unless we can qualify the *location* by the *sensations* and *conditions of aggravation and amelioration,* we have no alternative except to proceed empirically in the selection of the remedy.

It was because of this that Hahnemann insisted on the necessity for considering the *totality of the case.* Bœnninghausen, in the plan of his repertory, emphasized the value of the completed symptom (by locality, sensations and conditions of aggravation and amelioration) but added a fourth requirement, equally imperative to the first three, and yet in itself often divisible into those three divisions. This was the *concomitant symptom,* and has led to the statement that his repertory is founded on the *doctrine of concomitants.* We should say; *the doctrine of the totality of the case, which must include the concomitants.*

The word *concomitant* means *existing or occurring together; attendant;* the noun means *attendant circumstance.*

We have spoken of the peculiar usefulness of the repertory analysis in obscure chronic cases with many symptom groups, where no single symptom group stands forth with sufficient clarity to warrant a prescription. Here the penetrative powers of the *Pocket Book* come into play, for it was with a consideration of these cases in mind, together with Hahnemann's instructions for the considerations of the case, that Bœnninghausen developed this repertory.

No matter how many symptom groups appear, if they are co-existent, or if they appear in some relation of time to the outstanding symptom group, such as alternating summer and winter symptoms, these may all be taken into consideration through this method.

We may go further and say that in nearly every case we may find one or more concomitant symptoms, and we often find that the concomitant symptoms are not only co-existent, but they are those symptoms that seemingly have no relation to the leading symptoms from the standpoint of theoretical pathology. They are often symptoms for which we can find no reason for their existence in the individual under consideration. We might almost term them *unreasonable attendants* of the case in hand; yet they have an actual relationship in that they exist at the same time, in the same patient. They must not be overlooked nor under-valued because they cannot be made to conform with the theories of traditional medicine nor with our own ideas of their peculiar unrelatedness.

Nevertheless, this seemingly erratic grouping of symptoms in individuals *is governed by a principle,* and it was the discovery of this principle which led Bœnninghausen to devise the plan upon which the repertory is based.

It is conceivable that one could prescribe successfully upon one symptom by following the plan laid down in the *Pocket Book, provided that one symptom was complete.* Given simply a pain of a certain definite character, in a definite locality or organ, a condition of aggravation or amelioration, and a differentiating factor—the so-called concomitant or accompanying symptom—and the remedy can be found. (Very often the condition of aggravation or amelioration is itself the differentiating factor.) If in a page of fragmentary symptoms these four elements can be found and brought together to make one complete symptom, there is hope of finding the remedy. The location, sensation and condition are not enough; the concomitant must be added, that peculiar or accidental feature which always exists in every totality, in both patient and remedy, by which it is differentiated from every other case or remedy.

The concomitant symptom is to the Totality what the condition of aggravation or amelioration is to the single symptom. It is the differentiating factor.

That portion of a symptom that cannot be completed in the part itself may be completed in some other part, as the concomitant or associated symptom; and as has been indicated before, this concomitant frequently is a condition of aggravation or amelioration.

It is not necessary that the condition of aggravation or amelioration should be actually found in relation with the local or particular symptom. Very often it is not possible to find this. The larger view of the case, which recognizes that every symptom or part of a symptom belongs to the case as a whole, enables us, by Bœnninghausen's plan, to complete partial symptoms by combining separated fragments as a whole. Experience bears out the truth of Bœnninghausen's doctrine of the importance of concomitant symptoms.

Let us put this another way. Bœnninghausen proceeds upon the Hahnemannian theory that it is the man who is sick, and that all the discomforts which have laid hold upon him are a part of his condition, and are therefore to be considered in the attempt to free him from his discomforts and bring him to a perfect cure.

In his essay on the *Treatment of Intermittent Fevers*, Bœnninghausen says:

It is well known that the most striking characteristic of intermittent fevers is a series of attacks of chills, heat and sweat, these various symptoms either succeeding each other, or appearing simultaneously, or else alternating in various ways. These symptoms, *which ought to be regarded as one,* are generally so prominent, that all the other accompanying symptoms are either left out of consideration, or else are so much obscured, as it were, by the former, that they are either deemed unworthy of note, or are summed up in the vague denomination of an intermittent fever in disguise. But next to the character of the fever paroxysm itself, *it is precisely those accompanying or secondary symptoms which ought to decide the selection* of the remedy. This is so true that a drug which has been chosen in accordance with the *totality of the symptoms observed during the apyrexia,* affects a certain cure of the fever, although it may never before have been employed for that purpose.

In the selection of the drug, the moral symptoms of the patient ought to be strictly considered of course. Experience has abundantly shown that the safest indication of a remedy is the totality of the symptoms existing during the apyrexia, in other words, the concomitant symptoms given. . . . These ought to be considered exclusively and *even in contradiction to the symptoms of the paroxysms,* until a drug shall have been discovered, in the course of our provings upon healthy men, which shall correspond to both these orders of symptoms. It is such remedies as these alone which will speedily effect a certain and permanent cure. . . .

Several of the remedies which will be found indicated hereafter exhibit a striking analogy of symptoms. *This analogy may be looked upon as a thread which unites them into one family in spite of their differences.* This analogy is found in the accessory symptoms as well as in the symptoms of the paroxysm. *Experience teaches that this analogy is extremely important in the selection of the remedy.* This analogy may guide the physician in the selection of the remedy, especially for those cases of intermittent fever which have been imperfectly described to him by patients living at a distance.

Referring to epidemics, he says:

> The various symptoms which appear in different patients may all be grouped together, and this group will indicate the remedy which will be homœopathic to the cure.

The human organism is like a great complicated machine, composed of many parts assembled according to a definite plan or idea. There must be a storehouse for the parts. The repertory is like a stockroom of a factory, for orderly storage of parts, each on its own shelf. The workmen select the parts necessary to form the machine, and assemble according to the plan.

The parts lying loose on the shelves, on the floor, on the workman's bench are not the machine, but only the parts. There must be the parts plus the plan or idea. Combined, they give individuality, form, utility, efficiency. The *Therapeutic Pocket Book* of Bœnninghausen furnishes both the plan and the parts.

The foundation of Bœnninghausen's *Pocket Book* is the doctrine of concomitance. It is that which gives the book its peculiar value. The group is of more importance than the single symptom, no matter how peculiar the single symptom may appear to be. This is only another way of saying that the totality must govern.

The single peculiar symptom sometimes gives individuality to the group, as some personal peculiarity distinguishes each member of a family who may otherwise strongly resemble each other; but the individualizing feature is more often found in some modality common to all the symptoms of the group.

CONSTRUCTION OF THE REPERTORY

Bœnninghausen, in the construction of his *Therapeutic Pocket Book,* embodied several original features. In fact, at that time the repertory was a new adventure in homœopathic literature, developed because of the pressure of necessity in indexing the many provings that had accumulated. Bœnninghausen's legal mind seized upon several salient features in the cumbersome provings, by means of which he was able to devise and perfect a repertory that was much more convenient, much more elaborate, and at the same time compact, comprehensive and easy to use.

One of the outstanding differences in repertory construction that Bœnninghausen embodied in his earliest repertories was the variation in sizes of type, signifying the varying importance of the symptom-rubric to the various drugs listed.

Even in his first repertory Bœnninghausen used the five variations in type that indicated the individual evaluation of each remedy to the given symptom or rubric. In the early editions we find these denoted by italics with each letter separated from the next by a blank space, italics, ordinary type spaced, ordinary type, and ordinary type in parentheses.

Jahr published the first edition of his repertory in 1834, two years later, but it was very cumbersome and Jahr made no attempt to evaluate symptoms until his fourth edition, prepared in 1851. In the preface to this edition he writes: "In imitation of Bœnninghausen, I have adopted in my repertory four different kinds of print . . ." It is obvious that he failed to recognize the fifth evaluation given by Bœnninghausen.

In his *Preface,* page vi, Bœnninghausen says:

INTRODUCTION TO THE THERAPEUTIC POCKET BOOK

The scope of this *Pocket Book,* as given in its title, is double, *viz.:* on the one hand, to aid the memory of the physician at the bedside in the selection of a remedy, and on the other, to act as a guide in the study of the *Materia Medica Pura,* by means of which one may be able to find his way and to judge of the greater or less value of each symptom, and to make the whole more complete and sharply defined.

On account of the large number of remedies, under nearly every rubric, it has been thought indispensable, on account of both the above-mentioned objects, to distinguish their relative values by means of various types, as I have done in my former repertories, and which Hahnemann has repeatedly shown to be necessary.

In Allen's edition we find these ranks distinguished by CAPITALS (5), **bold face** (4), *italics* (3), roman (2) and (roman in parenthesis) (1). This last evaluation is seldom used in the body of the book but is more often found under the section on *Relationships.* Of this evaluation Bœnninghausen says *(Preface,* page vii):

"The fifth place, the last of all, contains the doubtful remedies, which require critical study, and which occur most seldom. . . ." In other words, these are the remedies that have been found to have that symptom but rarely, or to have had it verified in clinical work only.

Of this work of evaluation of the remedies, Bœnninghausen tells us *(Preface,* page viii):

I could not even intimate the greater or less leaning to the higher or lower rank, but I could only go so far that the mistake should be less than half an interval. Without having the assurance to maintain that everywhere within these limits accuracy has been attained, I can say with certainty that no industry, care nor circumspection has been wanting on my part to avoid errors as far as possible . . .

While this evaluation of symptoms was a unique feature in Bœnninghausen's repertory construction, it was not comparable to the actual method of construction which he employed, of which the evaluation was but one item. Before viewing closely the actual construction, let us glance again briefly at the repertorial background of his time.

The existing repertories were especially defective in

that they were largely constructed upon the concordance plan, which breaks every sentence or idea up into component words or parts and scatters them throughout the work in their alphabetical order. Once scattered, according to this plan, they can never be brought together again. Some plan had to be devised by which the symptoms of the then rapidly increasing materia medica could be arranged and classified, so that they could be found easily and brought together in consistent and logical form without separating or breaking them up too much. They must be separated, but only in such a manner as would not destroy their individuality nor restrict their integrity. That which was separated must be capable of being reassembled at will. The plan must be elastic enough to allow the separated parts of a remedy or a symptom to be brought together in such form as would correspond to any group of symptoms that might arise in practice. As Nature combined the elements of disease in ever-varying forms, so may Art combine the elements of materia medica to meet Nature's forms.

The problem was a difficult one, but the fine analytical mind of the Sage of Münster solved it. He conceived the figure of a great all-inclusive *Symptom Totality*, made up of the cardinal points of *location, sensation, conditions of aggravation and amelioration,* and *concomitance,* under which all the symptoms of the materia medica, and all the symptoms of the disease as well, should be covered.

Now to consider the actual plan of construction we must study the earliest available editions, for it is a foregone conclusion that any book that has gone through as many editions as the *Pocket Book* must have departed in some particulars from the original text, and the general outlines may well have suffered in consequence as the work was handed on from one edition to another.

About two years after Bœnninghausen first published his *Pocket Book* an English edition was published in Münster. No translator's name has been given for this edition, but the translation was done, Bœnninghausen tells us on page vii of his *Preface*, "by one of the most eminent German homœopathic physicians, who is perfectly acquainted with the English language and literature, but who does not care to be known." In spite of typographical errors and obsolete phrasing, then, we may assume that it conveys an excellent picture of the author's thought.

Only a short time afterward, Hempel translated the book, which was published in this country, and he keeps to the same general outlines. We find these early editions divided into seven parts:

1. *Mind and Intellect.* (The oldest editions give it as *Mind and Soul.*)
2. *Parts of the Body and Organs.*
3. *Sensations and Complaints*
    I. *in general*
    II. *of glands*
    III. *of bones*
    IV. *of skin*
4. *Sleep and Dreams*
5. *Fever*
    I. *Circulation of Blood*
    II. *Cold Stage*
    III. *Coldness*
    IV. *Heat*
    V. *Perspiration*
    VI. *Compound Fevers*
    VII. *Concomitant Complaints*
6. *Alterations of the State of Health*
    I. *Aggravations according to time*
    II. *Aggravations according to situations and circumstances*
    III. *Amelioration by positions and circumstances*
7. *Relationship of Remedies*

PART 1

MIND AND INTELLECT

We find comparatively few rubrics under the section *Mind*. Bœnninghausen was a follower of Hahnemann and in close correspondence with him for many years; he had turned his legal mind to homœopathic problems with great sincerity and purpose, and we may ask ourselves why he gave so few mental symptoms when Hahnemann taught that the measure of a man's personality and his deviations from normal lay largely in his mental and spiritual reactions.

Because they failed to grasp the concept of the *Pocket Book* many competent Hahnemannians have criticised the lack of mental symptoms listed therein. It must be remembered that Bœnninghausen based his work on the concept of the *whole man*, placing the balance of the emphasis on the value of the concomitant symptoms and the modalities; it was not his intention to reflect the picture of the whole man through his mental reactions, because he realized how warped a view even the most careful observer must have at times; or through any other predominant group of symptoms, no matter how important. It was his stand that the solid basis of the four-square foundation was the only method of securing the totality of the case. In considering the value of the mental symptoms in relation to the *Pocket Book,* Bœnninghausen meets this criticism in his *Preface:*

> It is necessary to observe with regard to the first section that our *Materia Medica Pura* contains nowhere more consecutive effects than amongst the symptoms of the mind and that on the other hand most of the tyroes are apt to make mistakes, or very often overlook this part of a complete picture of the disease. I have therefore deemed it advisable to give here only the most essential and predominant points under as few rubrics as possible, in order to make it more easy to find them out.

This was therefore not an oversight on Bœnninghausen's part, but a deliberate attempt to clarify the use of the book for those beginning the study of homœopathy.

On the other hand, before leaving the consideration of the somewhat rudimentary material under the section *Mind*, it is worth while to turn to the section *Aggravations* and follow through the seventeen rubrics devoted to *Emotional Excitement*. Hahnemann held that the emotional cause of disturbed functions was an important factor in reestablishing a state of equilibrium; Bœnninghausen's experience led him to the same conclusions. They believed that the disturbed emotional sphere might manifest itself in a long and varied train of symptoms, varying according to many and varied circumstances and conditions of environment, training and convention; but that the consequences of these disturbed states, while often so deep that they appear to be permanent, do not always manifest themselves clearly in the mental sphere, and therefore the homœopathic physician, in solving one of these difficult problems, would find it of inestimable value to take into consideration the symptom of initial emotional disturbance.

Therefore we may reasonably assume that these rubrics under *Aggravations* that deal with emotional causes of functional disturbances are closely related to that part dealing with mental and emotional symptoms.

Bœnninghausen's explanation of his section on *Intellect* was much the same as that on the *Mind:* in order to clarify the use of the book he simplified the number of rubrics as far as possible, leaving it to later authors to give, if they would, more rubrics and more particular rubrics.

PART 2

PARTS OF THE BODY AND ORGANS

This section of the book follows, in general, the anatomical schema used by Hahnemann—in fact, used by all students of the human anatomy since earliest medical history, beginning with the upper parts (head) and proceeding downward to the mouth, then following the alimentary tract downward; next considering the urinary organs and functions, then sexual organs and functions, then respiratory organs (from above downward) then external chest, heart, neck, back, upper and lower limbs.

This work has run through many editions, as has been stated before, and in many of these, translations have been necessary. Hempel, Okie, Boger and T. F. Allen, among others, have given of their time and genius in attempting to perfect this little work. Probably T. F. Allen has left a more lasting impression upon the *Pocket Book* than any other one editor, because it was he who added many of the eye symptoms, and it was he who conceived the idea of combining Bœnninghausen's *Repertory of the Sides of the Body* with the original *Pocket Book*. In spite of the many mistakes that crept in through clumsy translations and assembling, this has added vastly to the value of the work, but in order to make the best possible use of this work we must understand the mistakes and how to avoid them; this we shall consider at a later time.

This section on the parts of the body and organs runs from page 24 to page 142, following the general schema outlined previously, and begins with a chapter on *Internal Head*, to be followed by one on *External Head* and then by brief chapters on the *Sides of the Head*.

Next we come to a chapter on *Eyes*, and we must note in this connection that this chapter, that deals with the various locations in the eye, is followed by a chapter on *Vision*. In other words, in dealing with any location that has a definite function, especially of the senses, we find first the location with its modifications, then immediately following, a section devoted to symptoms of the function. It is unnecessary to go into this in greater detail, since it holds true in general throughout this part of the book.

Under the chapter *Face*, however, we find first the objective symptoms that may be observed in the face, and then following this, a section devoted to *Face. Locations of Sensations in.*

Again, we find the rubrics devoted to locations in the abdomen are followed by chapters on *Flatulence* and *Stool;* the chapter on *Urinary Organs* by one on *Urine,* and that again by one dealing with the symptoms arising from urination. The section on *Sexual Organs* is followed by a chapter on *Menstruation* and that by a chapter on *Leucorrhœa.*

When we consider *Respiration,* however, we find the symptoms of respiration are given first consideration; this chapter is followed by one on *Cough* and expectoration, and that by one on the *Air-Passages,* containing two specific locations, one or two conditions, and the voice rubrics.

It is important to note that under these chapters devoted to *Parts of the Body and Organs* we find also a few aggravations, and an occasional rubric that might have been listed under *Sensations and Complaints.*

The following rubrics may logically be considered as aggravations:

Troubles Before Stool 90
  —*During Stool* 91
  —*After Stool* 91
Troubles Before Micturition 100
  —*At Beginning of Micturition* 101
  —*During Micturition* 101
  —*At Close of Micturition* 101
  —*After Micturition* 101
Before Menstruation 109
At Beginning of Menstruation 110
During Menstruation 110
After Menstruation 110

Rubrics that might have been listed under the chapter on *Sensations and Complaints* are:

Stopped Feeling in Ears 44
Toothache 59
Heartburn 72

Flatulent Pain 84
Labor-Like Pains 104 (*cf. Labor-Like Pains* 166)

With these few exceptions, and those rubrics dealing with *labor* and *tenesmus,* there are no subjective symptoms to be found in this second part of the book.

There is another group of symptoms that may be considered, as one of the original features introduced by Bœnninghausen, and one that has made this repertory both brief and comprehensive. These are the *concomitant* rubrics. Of these Bœnninghausen writes in his *Preface,* page vii:

. . . Convinced of the importance of symptoms which occur simultaneously, and therewith form symptom-groups, I have been adding for many years to the concomitant symptoms which are found in the *Materia Medica Pura* whatever belonging to them the experience of myself and others could offer, and their number increased so incredibly that I have been able to deduce general rules. From these it is certain that some remedies, more than others, incline to concomitant symptoms, and that these do not consist exclusively of particular symptoms, but in general of every sort of complaint which lies within the sphere of the remedy, though indeed the characteristics may be found more frequently among them than elsewhere. This discovery, tested by long experience, led me to place the *Concomitant Symptoms* together under each section. . . .

Thus we find the following:

Drugs which have Concomitants of Mental Symptoms 23
Accompanying Symptoms of Nasal Discharges 49
Accompanying Troubles of Leucorrhœa 111
Accompanying Troubles of Respiration 114
Troubles Associated with Cough 120

We may also place in this group those already mentioned for consideration in the group of aggravations:

Troubles Before, During and After Stool; Before, During and After Micturition; Before, During and After Menstruation, etc.

These rubrics, when their value is fully comprehended, prove extremely useful both for analysis of a case or for quick reference.

PART 3

SENSATIONS AND COMPLAINTS

As we shall see under the section devoted to limitations of this repertory, this title should read: *Sensations and Complaints* rather than merely *Sensations*, as the Allen edition puts it. Even casual observation reveals that this section contains not only subjective symptoms in the way of true sensations, but many complaints (or conditions) and many objective symptoms as well, and a few locations.

Under the subjective symptoms, we find many descriptions of discomfort, as well as the following rubrics: *Desire for Open Air; Aversion to Open Air; Intolerance of Clothing; Inclination to Lie Down; Aversion to Motion; Desire for Motion; Restlessness; Sensitiveness to Pain; Inclination to Sit; Illusions of Touch; Dread of Washing; Dread of Water, etc.*

The symptoms of location are generalized or directional, as follows: *Symptoms on One Side; Left Side; Right Side; Crosswise, Left Upper and Right Lower; Crosswise, Left Lower and Right Upper, etc.*

The symptoms covering complaints are such as: *Apoplexy, Consumption, Convulsions, Dropsy, Emaciation, Tendency to Take Cold, Nervous Excitement, Hæmorrhage, Frozen Limbs, Apparent Death (Asphyxia), Indurations, Inflammations, Paralysis, etc.* These are by no means all those that appear under this general classification.

We find under truly objective symptoms: *Blackness externally; Carphology; Clumsiness; Cracking of Joints: Cyanosis, etc.*

These are not divided sectionally, but follow alphabetically throughout that part of the work devoted to *Sensations and Complaints*. By following this plan Bœnninghausen succeeded in condensing the cumbersome features of a repertory and at the same time sacrificed nothing necessary to its comprehensiveness. This is a vital part of the book and bears frequent study, for it yields in proportion to the cultivation it receives.

It has just been stated that this part of the book is not divided sectionally, but this is meant to refer only to the general symptom groupings just mentioned. In the Allen edition there is a single heading for this general section, which we have just considered covering the symptoms of the patient in general, without reference to special parts except as are mentioned in following chapters. In the older editions these four chapters comprised one great section of the book, with the main section and three sub-sections; in the Allen edition the general headings have been removed so that to a casual glance these chapters now seem to be disassociated and we would expect to locate them more truly under PART 2, *Parts of the Body and Organs*.

These must be thought of as follows: *Sensations and Complaints, In General;* (1) *of the Glands;* (2) *of the Bones;* (3) *of the Skin*. Now we have a more accurate estimate of their scope of usefulness, for these sections have the alphabetical grouping of subjective and objective symptoms, and can be applied readily to the symptom-grouping as expressed by the patient.

PART 4

SLEEP AND DREAMS

This part of the book is fairly obvious, except for some poor judgment in assembling; this we shall discuss later.

This covers such symptoms as *Yawning, Sleepiness, Sleeplessness,* with their various modifications; *Positions in Sleep; Dreams*.

PART 5

FEVER

In the old editions there were seven sub-sections in this part of the book. In this edition the sub-heads have been removed but the same general outline is followed, with a single exception which will be noted. The original outline is given:

I. *Circulation of the Blood*
II. *Cold Stage*
III. *Coldness*
IV. *Heat*
V. *Perspiration*
VI. *Compound Fevers*
VII. *Concomitant Complaints*

The first division in this part of the book has to do with conditions of the blood as *Anæmia, Congestion, etc.;* objective and subjective symptoms of the blood vessels; pulse symptoms.

The second division, formerly called *Cold Stage,* is what we may term the chilly stage, as these rubrics are several modifications of chilliness.

In the Allen edition the third and fourth divisions have been reversed, and we find the variations of the symptoms of the fever following immediately after the chilly stage. The cold symptoms follow the heat, and the symptoms covering shivering follow the coldness rather than the cold stage (chilliness).

The rubrics devoted to perspiration follow in the old order, with their modifications, and we come to the rubrics dealing with *Compound Fever.* These rubrics cover certain variations in the onset of chill, heat and sweat, and their alternations. The old seventh division, *Concomitant Complaints,* are scattered more or less throughout the part, immediately following the old divisions. Thus we find: *Heat with Associated Symptoms,* 259; *Sweat with Associated Symptoms,* 265; *Before Fever, During Fever, After Fever,* 268; etc. The three last mentioned may also be used as aggravations.

PART 6

ALTERATIONS OF THE STATE OF HEALTH

I. *Aggravations According to Time*
II. *Aggravations According to Situations and Circumstances*
III. *Amelioration by Position and Circumstances*

As in some of the former sections, Allen has removed the headings of the sub-sections and has left but two, *Aggravations* and *Ameliorations*. However, under *Aggravations* we find the same general arrangement as in the old editions, the time aggravations coming first, and then alphabetically, those aggravations according to "situations and circumstances".

The section *Aggravations* covers a number of conditions, while the section devoted to *Ameliorations* is comparatively small. Aggravations are much more often reported by the patient than ameliorations; they were much more apt to be reported by the provers of the remedies because they were much stronger, therefore more noticeable. Aggravations that were produced by the remedy were a reaction of the remedy and therefore reported as such; amelioration of a condition was sought when the comfort of the prover was so greatly disturbed as to necessitate relief, and was not so often reported as having a definite relationship to the remedy being proven. However, we are often forced to make use of the contrary condition in selecting our rubrics from the Allen edition, for while Bœnninghausen, in his early editions, had more rubrics under *Ameliorations*, Allen often deleted these and put them in under *Aggravations* of the contrary state; thus the rubric $>$ *Heat* has been rendered $<$ *Cold*. In some cases it was necessary to enlarge the rubric and make it more general by the addition of more remedies in order to cover both modalities comprehensively.

While Bœnninghausen reasoned in this way to some

INTRODUCTION TO THE THERAPEUTIC POCKET BOOK

extent, it was Allen's idea to make the book even less cumbersome by this means.

PART 7

RELATIONSHIPS OF REMEDIES

In his *Preface,* Bœnninghausen speaks of his publishing in 1836 a work on *Relationships of Remedies* which he later found to contain a number of errors and omissions, and which he then discarded. In the earlier editions of the *Pocket Book* he refers to this chapter as *Concordance of Remedies* but Allen returns to the earlier and more easily comprehended title for this chapter.

To the majority of homœopathic physicians the last chapter in the *Pocket Book, Relationships,* has been a complete mystery. Even though the physician has a fair knowledge of the general use of the rest of the book this section was practically useless to him, except for occasional reference at the bedside.

It must be remembered, in any consideration of this masterpiece of Bœnninghausen's, that his was the trained mind of the lawyer. With this training he was able to weigh comparative values, first, the value of homœopathy as compared to orthodox medicine, and then later, the comparative value of remedies in relation to particular symptom groups. He tells us in his *Preface* something of his method in gathering data; how he kept notes for years on various symptoms, their relationship to each other, and the relationship of remedies to symptom groups. From these accumulated data he devised the *Pocket Book*. With this background we cannot believe that any part of the book would be for merely casual use; it was the accumulation of practical knowledge of many years' experience. Let us then look at this chapter with a view to securing some knowledge of its practical value to us.

We find that the chapter on *Relationships* is divided into sections, each section being devoted to a remedy, in alphabetical order. Each of these remedy-sections is subdivided into rubrics, as are all the general sections in the book, but in this chapter we find the rubrics are not particularized as symptoms, but are generalized symptom groups, as it were, such as form the subject-matter of the sections in the first chapters in the book. For instance, we find the first rubric in each remedy-section to be *Mind;* the second *Localities;* the third *Sensations;* then *Glands, Bones, Skin; Sleep and Dreams; Blood, Circulation and Fever; Aggravations.* SO FAR WE FIND THAT EACH RUBRIC IN THIS CHAPTER OF THE BOOK CORRESPONDS TO A GENERAL SECTION HEADING IN THE FIRST PART OF THE BOOK. To this is added one, two or three additional rubrics, as the case may be. The one that is always present bears the title: *Other Remedies.* This might better be translated: *The general relationship of remedies* (other than the one heading this particular section of the chapter on *Relationships*) *to the remedy heading this particular section.* This means, then, that while specific symptoms grouped under a general schematic section such as *Mind, Localities,* etc., are given in their respective relationship to the remedy under consideration, there are some symptoms that do not fall entirely within this section-grouping, and this rubric, *Other Remedies,* covers all those symptoms which do not fall into such regular groups. This means, then, that the rank of the remedies in this rubric represents a general relationship of these remedies in the unclassified symptom groups, to the remedy under consideration.

Of the other two rubrics which occasionally appear, *Antidotes* and *Injurious,* these are easily comprehended.

So much for the physical make-up of this chapter. Let us look at its reason for being, the thought behind Bœnninghausen's concept of the value of such a work as this.

Each remedy partakes to some extent of the attributes of every other remedy. It would hardly be possible to select two remedies so different from each other that they would not touch at some point. They will have some symptoms in common. Look over any remedy in Bœnninghausen's chapter on the *Relationships of Remedies* where he compares it in each of its divisions according to this schema with the remedies in the corresponding subdivisions of the repertory, and note how into the comparison of nearly every remedy is brought the greater part of the remedies contained in the earlier editions of the book, and so far studied for their relationships to other remedies. Even a casual study of the remedies listed in this chapter shows conclusively that the work on this section of the book is very far from being as complete as the other chapters.

In Allen's *Preface* to the American edition, he says:

> The *Relationships* (Chapter VII) of a part only of the new remedies have been added, and this work has been underdone rather than overdone, for much remains to be determined, and it must be confessed that most of our new symptomatologies have not borne the searching light of clinical experience so well as those left us by Hahnemann. In this chapter we need more help from critical students of materia medica and homœopathic therapeutics.

It is a task that takes fine discrimination and much careful study, but so far as it goes it is complete. If the other remedies listed in the other sections of the book could be carefully weighed in their respective relationships, this very valuable section of the book would have a much wider usefulness.

The pathogenesis of every remedy seems to be made up of symptoms that touch closely upon those of other remedies. Herein lies one of the dangers in key-note prescribing. It is as if the remedies had all evolved from one common original substance, becoming modified and individualized and therefore differentiated in varying proportions, so that when they become activated by potentization their effects are exhibited as in a varying scale through that complicated and exceedingly delicate laboratory of the living man. Here we can see the symptoms held in general by a number of remedies—the original symptoms, as it were—as well as their individually developed personalities. One of the best illustrations of this is *Pulsatilla*, which has a strong individuality of its own, yet which is so closely allied by evolution to *Silica* and *Kali sulph.*, that it bears a strong family likeness to both of these substances.

Some remedies are in harmony with others, some neutral, some inimical. The most similar ones, as a rule, are complementary; they antidote each other's bad effects, follow each other well and often make up for the deficiencies of the others. Others with a lesser degree of similarity may be used at a greater interval of time and finish up the work started by the other remedy. In other words, they have a much lower ratio of similarity.

We may use here the illustration of the concentric circles of similarity, as suggested by Joslin. The nearer the center the smaller the circle and the higher the ratio of similarity. As the circle widens the complementary qualities of the remedies occupying the outward curves lessen until their similarity to the *simillimum*, or their complementary relationship to the *simillimum*, is very slight. Every mineral or chemical element has grouped closely about it a little circle of closely related vegetable remedies, which are complements of each other.

LIMITATIONS OF THE REPERTORY

Many criticisms have been made of Bœnninghausen's *Pocket Book*.

Bœnninghausen was the first to discover that the governing influence of the characteristic modalities was not limited to the particular symptoms with which they were found associated or with which they might have been recorded in the provings, but that they might be accepted as having a modifying relationship to any or all of the symptoms. Hering criticized this stand as leading into too wide a field of seemingly similar remedies. This might be true if it were not for the consideration of the whole case, including concomitants, for here many of the remedies are ruled out simply because of the latitude in selecting rubrics of aggravation and amelioration, which naturally restricts the possibility of a great number of remedies coming through, *if the case be well and thoroughly taken.*

Thus we find that one of the strongest criticisms is overcome by careful case taking, and by giving attention to the philosophic construction of the book.

Bœnninghausen's work was carefully done and thoroughly tested. It is reasonable to suppose that any work that has gone through several editions, and especially one that has been translated into foreign languages, must have suffered many changes in text. Bœnninghausen tells us that the first English translation was "made by one of the most eminent German homœopathic physicians, who is perfectly acquainted with the English language and literature, but who does not care to be known". This edition is not practical for present-day use because the translator used many phrases now obsolete.

Hempel has been sharply criticized for his careless

translations of such works as Hahnemann's *Chronic Diseases,* but a careful comparison of several editions, and comparisons with the materia medica, must convince us that of the older editions Hempel's translation is more nearly correct in its original form and more practical than any other of the early editions available at this time.

Allen's edition has suffered from faulty translation to a marked degree, and these mistakes in translation plus his rearrangement of the headings, has marred the usefulness of what should have been the most valuable edition of the work. It must be remembered that T. F. Allen, indefatigable worker that he was, was unable to attend to all the details of all the work he undertook, and it must be recognized that work delegated to others often suffers in some way from lack of personal supervision. It is seldom possible to have assistants who take the same viewpoint and feel the same sense of responsibility and evince the same degree of capability as the one who conceives the plan. Therefore we cannot hold Allen culpable for any shortcoming graver than that he undertook more than he personally could compass.

It is only just to give Allen the credit for the work he did, and if he had been spared longer it is probable that this work would have been perfected, but it is not always given to an individual to perfect what he has taken to be his task.

Bœnninghausen had 126 remedies in his original work. Allen dropped four remedies that appeared in Bœnninghausen's editions: *Angustura,* because of the difficulty at that time in securing the true bark and because the false had been sold for the true to such a degree that severe poisonings had occurred from the use of the crude form and Germany had forbidden its sale. Allen felt some question about the authenticity of the provings and so left it out of his edition. He dropped the three magnetic remedies also: *Magnetis poli ambo, Magnetis polus arcticus* and *Magnetis polus australis*. Allen added some 220 remedies, so that the number now appearing in the Allen edition is about 342.

the *external* abdomen, and then the two sides of the *external* abdomen follow.

The rubrics covering the sides of the sexual organs, chest, back, upper and lower extremities, are embodied properly in the proper chapters at the end of the other rubrics.

Mention has been made of the mistake in heading the section on *Sensations,* which should read *Sensations and Complaints;* and the student should never forget that the chapters on *Glands, Bones* and *Skin* should be considered as sub-heads of the chapter on *Sensations and Complaints.*

It may be out of order to mention here the complete inadequacy of the index. It is not only incomplete but incorrect in certain details, and in order to get the fullest possible use of the repertory it is advisable to learn the book itself; then it will not be necessary to turn to the index. A little study of the plan of the book and the general headings will give the physician facility in the use of the book and this knowledge will grow rapidly in detail as it is in daily use.

Now we pass to a consideration of the translation of rubrics. Unfortunately it has been impossible to secure an original German copy of the *Pocket Book,* therefore comparisons have been made by the tedious method of comparing the text in Allen's edition, rubric by rubric, with those in Hempel's translation, and where there has been question, these have been compared with other available editions and the remedies therein taken to the materia medica as well for differentiation of meanings. This work has been completed so far as the comparison of the repertories is concerned; it has not been possible at this time to carry all questionable rubrics to the materia medica for verification. Therefore, we trust that the physician will follow the same guide-post in using the questionable rubrics that have not been verified as he must follow in selecting the *simillimum* from the similar remedies; that guide-post reads: GO TO THE MATERIA MEDICA. Some of these rubrics are noted where there is a close analogy, in order to give to the rubric the broadest possible mean-

The remedies that Allen added appear in comparatively few rubrics, and careful observation will convince the student that they appear much more frequently in locational rubrics or those dealing with functional symptoms, than in the subjective or modifying symptoms. It is in this particular that we are convinced that Allen did not consider his work complete, but that the edition went to press with the idea of giving it to the homœopathic profession in the state it had reached at that time rather than as a perfected edition.

Let us examine further some of the errors that appear to be most flagrant.

It has been said that Allen combined two volumes in one, while keeping the work in small size, Bœnninghausen's *Therapeutic Pocket Book* and his repertory, *Sides of the Body*. The work of combination has not been smoothly done, and unless the physician watches for these irregularities he may lose the value of the second involution. For instance, we find the chapter on *Internal Head* has as its last rubric (page 26) *One-sided in General*, and we have reason to assume that this finishes the chapter, since a chapter on *External Head* begins on page 27. However, on page 29 we find another heading, *Internal Head*, but this contains only two rubrics, one pertaining to the left and one to the right side. Following this again we find the heading *External Head* once more, and this too covers the two sides.

Under the chapters devoted to *Eyes, Ears, Nose, Face, Teeth*, we find the rubrics for the two sides incorporated at the end of but within the chapter. However, for the chapter on *Mouth* we do not find the side rubrics, but pass at once to *Throat*, and following that section find another heading, *Mouth and Fauces*, having just those two rubrics (page 65). The chapters on *Internal* and *External Abdomen* follow each other immediately, without being rounded out by the two rubrics for left and right sides; here the same mistake was made as in assembling the head rubrics, for the rubrics for the two sides of the *internal* abdomen follow the general location rubrics of

INTRODUCTION TO THE THERAPEUTIC POCKET BOOK 45

ing. Wherever there is definite reason for the choice of one rubric over another, this is indicated by a star. It is suggested that where a rubric has been found incorrect in its title, the correction be made in the book.

page	ALLEN'S EDITION	CORRECTIONS
	MIND	
18	Avarice	Covetousness
	Boldness	Daring
	Despair	Hopelessness
	Excitement	*Irritability
	Fretfulness	Peevishness
19	Gentleness	*Mildness
	Joyfulness	*Gayety
	Mischievousness	*Maliciousness
	INTELLECT	
20	Activity	*Excitement
21	Confusion	*Dullness (as is experienced with cold in the head, or after intoxication)
	Imaginations	Fantastic Illusions
	Impaired	Affections of the Mind in General
	VISION	
36	Flickering	Vibrations of light before the eyes
	Dark	*Illusions of vision in relation to colors in general
37	Distorted	(Inability to judge distances from objects, moving about of objects before vision, *etc.*)
	Distorted Features and Making Faces	(in an attempt to focus the vision)

Fiery	*Illusions, fiery: stars, *etc.*
38 Mist	*Mistiness or gauze before the eyes
Tremulousness	Tremulous vibrations before eyes
Vanishing	Momentary loss of sight as from fainting, *etc.*

HEARING

43 Ringing	(and Tinkling)
Roaring	(and Humming)

NOSE

45 Back	*Bridge

SMELL

50 Illusions of smell, Bituminous	Illusions of smell, as of pitch

FACE

51 Color Coppery	*Color copperish (acne rosacea)
53 Drawn	*Distortions of the Face: Risus sardonicus, *etc.*

FACE, LOCATIONS

57 Malar Bone	*Zygomatic and malar bone

MOUTH

62 Mouth in General	Buccal cavity in general

HUNGER AND THIRST

67 Aversion to Cereals	Aversion to dishes of meal and flour
68 — to soup	— and broth
69 Desire for liquid food	— soups
— — Tonics	*Cold drinks, juicy things and refreshing things

ERUCTATIONS

75 Uprisings	*Risings into the throat
Waterbrash	*Confluence of water in the mouth

NAUSEA AND VOMITING

75 Retching	Empty retching (gagging)

INTRODUCTION TO THE THERAPEUTIC POCKET BOOK 47

STOOL
87 Constipation on Account of Inactivity (of the bowels)

URINE
96 Profuse — Urine too frequent
97 Suppressed — or too scanty
100 Involuntary at night — involuntary in bed

MENSTRUATION
107 Hæmorrhage, not at Menstrual Times. — *Discharges of blood before the proper period (the establishment of menstruation at too early an age)

Menstruation Beginning. Delayed in girls. — *Delay of the first menses

RESPIRATION
112 Loud — *Breath loud (without mucous rattle)

AIR-PASSAGES
122 Voice Shrieking (and Squeaking) — *Voice shrill and screeching

CHEST
126 Palpitation Anxious — *Palpitation of the heart with anguish

SENSATIONS — *SENSATIONS AND COMPLAINTS

145 Biting — *Biting Pain (pungent) (in children)
147 Carried, desire to be
Clamp, Sensation of an Iron — As if parts were compressed with an iron band
Clamp-like pains — Squeezing pains
148 Coat of skin drawn over inner parts, Sensation of — *As if covered with fur in inner parts
150 Contractions (after Inflammation) — Strictures after inflammation
Contractions of Extremities — Limbs drawn together crookedly

153 Crushing Sensation	Contusions
154 Dead Feeling	(in single parts)
Death, Apparent	Appearance as if dying Asphyxia (these rubrics are identical)
Debility	Lassitude
155 Dilated Sensation	Sensation as if distended, enlarged
Dislocations	*Sprains
Dislocation Easy	*Disposition to spraining
Drawing Inward of Soft Parts	Retraction
156 Dryness of Internal Parts	(usually moist)
158 Faintness	Fainting
Falling Easily	Inclination to tumble
159 Forcings	Pushing
Formication	Tingling
Gout-like pains (arthritic)	(... in the joints)
162 Hardened (Muscles)	Muscles, induration of
166 Knotted Sensation	Sensation as of a lump
167 Loose Feeling in Joints	Sensation as if joints were disjointed
169 Obesity	Tendency to get fat
171 Pinching	Dragging
172 Plucking, Sensation of	*Twitching and pulling
173 Pressing, Deep, Inward, with Instruments	*Deep pressure marks from holding violin, scissors, etc.
174 Pressing sticking ...	Pressing with stinging ...
176 Reeling	Staggering when walking
Retraction of soft parts	Shrinking (wasting) of soft parts
Shortened Muscles	(being actually shortened)
179 Shuddering	*Concussion
182 Sprain from lifting	Disposition to *strain* a part by lifting things
186 Sticking ...	Pricking ...

INTRODUCTION TO THE THERAPEUTIC POCKET BOOK 49

	Stopped Feeling internally	Sensation as if inner parts were obstructed
	Strangling Pain (Constriction)	Stifling (strangulating pain)
	Surging (in Body)	(Erethism)
192	Thrusts (Pushing Pain)	Pain as if from shocks
193	Twistings	Turning (twisting, writhing)
	Twitchings	Quivering
	Twitching of Muscles	Convulsive motions of the muscles (subsultus tendinum)
194	Vibrations	Dull tingling
196	Weakness, Paralytic	Weakness as if paralyzed
	Wind, Cold	Sensation as if touched by a current of cold air
	Wringing Pain	Twisting together (rolling up)

BONES

*SENSATIONS AND COMPLAINTS OF THE BONES

201	Jerking Pain	Darting pain
	Loosened from Flesh, Feeling as if	As if flesh were beaten off the bones
202	Softening	(and bending)
203	Sticking ...	Pricking ...

SKIN

*SENSATIONS AND COMPLAINTS OF THE SKIN

204	Biting	Biting (stinging)
	Chilblains, Crawling in	Chilblains tingling
207	Cracks	Rhagades (chapping)
	Dryness	Dryness, want of sweat (except the head)
208	Eruptions on Hairy parts	
	— Biting	(stinging)
210	— Gooseflesh (in the house)	See also for larger rubric: Chilliness with Gooseflesh, page 255
211	— Itch, Suppressed	Scabies suppressed,

50 INTRODUCTION TO THE THERAPEUTIC POCKET BOOK

	driven in by mismanagement
	(See also: Suppressed with Mercury and Sulphur)
228, 229, 230 Tetter	(Eczema)
SLEEP	
241 Arms on Back	*Lying on the Back
242 Head Hanging Low Down	*Lying with head low
243 Sleep Comatose	Drowsiness
— Intoxicated with	Somnolency
244 Sleep Sound	Sleep deep
— Stupid	Sleep like a stupor
247 Dreams of Difficulty	Dreams with feeling of embarrassment
— of Bad Luck	— about fatal accidents
248 — Confused, continued	— continuing a long while
— Confused, after Waking	— continuing after waking
— Continuation of Former Ideas	— continuation of the thoughts of the day
— of excelling in Mental Work	— with reflection
— of Gold	— of money
— Joyful	— merry
— of Love	— amorous
— Disgusting	— disagreeable and disgusting
— with Illusions of Hope	— about blasted hopes
— of Sick People	— about injuries received
— with Strivings	— busy
FEVER	
261 Shivering in General (Note the error in	Shuddering

INTRODUCTION TO THE THERAPEUTIC POCKET BOOK 51

    indentation in the text. This is not a subhead of *Coldness* but a new heading)

264 Sweat easy	Great inclination to perspire
Sweat, Odorous, of Elderberries	Perspiration smelling like lilacs
265 — — of Mush (typographical error)	— — of Musk
— — Sulphuretted Hydrogen	— — like rotten eggs
268 Shivering then Chill	Shuddering followed by chilliness
AGGRAVATIONS	
273 Clear Weather	(Bœnninghausen's was a much larger rubric than this of Allen's)
274 Cloudy Weather	(and foggy)
Clutching Anything	From taking hold of anything
276 Cold, Becoming Cold	
After Becoming Cold	*After taking cold

(The first of these two rubrics is given to point the likeness in the rubric headings as they appear in Allen, but the difference in meaning is obvious after comparison with older editions.) The two following rubrics should read:

	After taking cold in the head
	After taking cold in the (or through the) feet
283 Food, Beans and Peas	Vegetables with husks
284 — Pork	Pork, fat, and the smell of
285 —Vegetables (green)	Vegetables without husks

	Grasping Anything Tightly	From holding fast to anything (compare exertion)
286	Hiccough	From sobbing or hiccoughing
287	Jar	Concussion
289	After Lying Down	*After lying down and having risen again
289	— in Bed	While lying in bed
292	Motion, False	(Misstep, *etc.*)
	Narrating Her Symptoms	Stories, from exciting
294	Organ, Playing the	(or hearing it played)
295	Pustule, Malignant	From the poison of anthrax
	Raising Affected Limb	(or part affected)
296	Riding One Leg over the Other	From crossing the limbs (compare Touch and Pressure)
297	After Rising from a Seat	(compare Beginning to move)
299	Sleep, at Beginning of	During the first hours of sleep
301	Society	In company
	Stooping	(Bending)
302	Stumbling	On knocking a part against anything
305	Vaults (Cellars, *etc.*)	(In vaulted places, churches, cellars)
307	Walking over Water	Walking beside or across a river
309	Wet, Getting Feet	From the feet getting wet; also, After a footbath

AMELIORATION

| 311 | Attention, Paying (this is identical with | Attending to, or thinking of, the pain |

INTRODUCTION TO THE THERAPEUTIC POCKET BOOK 53

  Thinking of something
   else, page 304)
314 Grasping   Touching anything
  Hæmorrhage   After bleeding of the af-
            fected part
  Inspiration   (while talking)
318 Shrugging Shoulders From drawing the shoul-
            ders back

Another limitation, or what might be termed a limitation, is the fact that a number of rubrics appear under *Aggravations* that might appear under *Sensations and Complaints* to even better advantage. One wonders, for instance, why *Apparent Death (Asphyxia)* is so different in its thought from (conditions arising from the effects of) *Arsenic Fumes*, and the latter is found under *Aggravations*. The appended list is to be thought of as suitable for use in the same way as if they were listed in *Sensations and Complaints*, and may be used so at the discretion of the repertory analyst. Of course, in some instances they may be thought of also in the light of true aggravations.

Arsenic Fumes, 271
Burns, 273
Children Especially, Remedies for, 274
Copper, Fumes of, 276
Cuts, For, 276
Disordered Stomach, 277
Drinkers, for Hard (Old Topers), 277
Eruptions, after Suppression of, 279
Injuries (Blows, Falls, and Bruises), 286
—Bleeding Profusely, 286
—with Extravasations, 286
—of Soft Parts, 286
Intoxication, After, 287
Jar (should read Concussion), **287**
Lying-in Women, 291
Mercury, Abuse of, 291
—Fumes of, 291
Narcotics, 293

Nasal Discharges, Suppression of, 293
Onanism, 293
Pregnancy, 294
Quinine, Abuse of, 295
Scarlet Fever, After, 298
Splinters, 301
Stone Cutters, for (Masons), 301
Women, For, 310

The greatest limitation in the use of any repertory is lack of comprehension in the one who attempts to use it. Therefore too much emphasis cannot be placed on the value of constant use: thumb the pages over and become acquainted with the general outlines and the particular rubrics. Only in this way can you learn to locate them promptly. As in all repertories where there are rubrics covering a symptom in the widest possible sense, and with modifying subheads, we find some seeming confusion in arrangement. As an illustration let us note those under *Skin,* such large symptom groups as *Eruptions,* covering some eight pages. Under this heading come the various forms of rashes, chicken-pox, measles, scarlet fever, smallpox; also scabies, hives, abscesses, carbuncles, and many variations in the subjective and objective symptoms of the eruption.

In a broad sense we may use the rubrics listed as *Tetter* to cover the eczematous eruptions.

It is well to bear in mind and compare the sections on *Eruptions, Excrescences,* and *Tetter,* when searching for certain symptoms. We find *Salt-Rheum,* for instance, listed under the section on *Ulcers.*

If we take the time to understand this little work, we shall find in it a wealth of material, based soundly on the rock of homœopathic philosophy, in spite of the mistakes that have crept in from time to time to mar the perfect concept.

ADAPTABILITY

The *Pocket Book* would have been of comparatively little use as a general repertory if it had not had the adaptability by means of which the general principles laid down by Bœnninghausen's keen analytical mind could be made to cover the widest possible range of symptomatology.

Let us consider first the adaptability of that little-known chapter on *Relationships of Remedies*. We find it of use in the acute case, and again in the chronic case.

Suppose, in an acute case, we have symptoms that seemingly lead us to a remedy, yet we are not quite satisfied that one remedy is sufficiently clear-cut in its indications. It is possible to select one or two leading rubrics, discarding those remedies that are obviously not indicated in the case, and run against the leading rubrics one or two governing the modalities, or some other outstanding peculiarity of the case. This can be done very quickly at the bedside, and with excellent results.

Again, suppose we are called in on a case following the initial acute stage. Here is a case that seemed to be a simple cold in a child of three years, and in the hands of a good Hahnemannian prescriber the condition apparently cleared under *Belladonna;* but *Belladonna* failed to hold, and the child was running a daily maximum temperature of 105°. The glands of the throat were involved, sore and swollen. In the meantime another physician had been on the case. It still seemed as if *Belladonna* might be indicated, yet there were a few symptoms that seemed to contraindicate it.

After the child was looked over carefully and no definite outstanding indications were secured, the case was analyzed by the chapter on *Relationships*, under the remedy

56 INTRODUCTION TO THE THERAPEUTIC POCKET BOOK

Belladonna. Only the remedies ranking 3, 4 and 5 under the rubric *Mind* were taken (with the exception of *Chamomilla*, because of its peculiar adaptability to child life) and the other rubrics under *Belladonna* were checked against them. The workout is given here:

Belladonna

	Mind	Localities	Sensations	Glands	Bones	Skin	Sleep and Dreams	Blood, Circulation & Fever	Aggravations	Other Relationships	
Apis	4	5	4	.	.	+	1	2	3	5	8/28
Bapt.	4	4	3	.	.	.	1	1	1		7/18
Bry.	3	4	4	4	.	3	2	4	5	4	9/33
Can. i.	5	3	3	.	.	2		1	4		6/18
Cham.	2	3	3	.	.	2	3	4	3		7/20
Lyc.	4	4	4	5	3	4	2	.	3	4	9/33
Op.	4	3	3	.	.	.	.	.	3		
Puls.	3	5	5	4	4	5	5	5	5	5	10/46
Rhus	4	3	4	.	.	5	2	4	4	4	8/30
Sul.	3	5	5	4	2	4	4	4	4	4	10/39

Suppose we had taken first the rubric *Glands* and selected therefrom those remedies related to *Belladonna* in glandular affections. We should have found (in the 4's and 5's) *Arnica, Bryonia, Lycopodium, Mercurius, Phosphorus, Pulsatilla* and *Sulphur*. Checking these through all ten rubrics we should have found *Arnica* ruled out; *Mercurius* 9/37 and *Phosphorus* 10/34 would have been added to our group coming through in sufficient degree for consideration, but even with these additions *Pulsatilla* holds the lead over all others.

A casual study of *Pulsatilla* verified this brief analysis, and the remedy was given. In three days the temperature was normal, having fallen gradually in the interval, the glands were normal in size and sensations, and the child was rapidly gaining strength and his normal lively interest in the world.

This was particularly pleasing in that one of the specialists at a well-known Eastern university had given a prognosis of an eight to ten weeks' run of fever inasmuch as "nothing could be done" for these cases.

In a case where the outstanding complaint of the patient was related to the *Bones,* or the *Skin,* we might select our remedies from those rubrics, under the remedy that had served well at first in the acute state.

Or when we have worked out a chronic case, and all possible benefit has been secured from the remedy selected as the *simillimum,* we sometimes have occasion to consider a related group of remedies that will carry the patient to a complete cure. Remember, we are speaking now of longstanding chronic cases, often those hopelessly muddled by wrong living conditions and everything that scientific medicine, so-called, has been able to do for them. We cannot expect every one of these to respond 100% to the most carefully selected remedy; or perhaps because of the incompleteness of the materia medica, or our incomplete knowledge of it or imperfect case-taking, we have been unable to select the *simillimum,* but a remedy with a fairly close degree of similarity. In such cases, because of some definite lack of available knowledge, we often zigzag a case toward cure. Again, in some serious conditions such as advanced tuberculosis, we dare not give the indicated remedy because it is too deeply active, and we must give a remedy that will meet the conditions of the patient but not stir too deeply the enfeebled vital energy. Here the complementary remedy is often called into play and may be so renovating in its action as to put the patient into a condition where he can tolerate the deeper acting remedy, and respond favorably to it.

After we have worked such a complicated case, and have judged the ability of the patient to react, we are in a position to consider the relationship of the remedy we select as the *simillimum* and those that have come through the analysis in a correspondingly high rank.

In considering the adaptability of this little work, we must first know the contents of the book, the rubrics to be found there; then we must be able to translate the symptoms of the patient into repertory language. Suppose the patient complains of feeling as if there were a weight on the chest. We will not find this rubric in the book, but we find *Pressing as from a Load* and *Heaviness*. If a patient complains that she is sensitive to noises, we must differentiate between < *Noises,* and *Hearing, Sensitive,* or *Hearing Acute.*

The patient has a swelling of the upper lip. We do not need to find a location plus the condition in this case if we know the adaptability of the repertory; we turn to page 56 and find *Swelling, Upper Lip.* So with eruptions in any given location on the face, we need not look for the major rubric covering *Eruptions in General,* under *Skin,* but can find the locational part of the symptom under the section devoted to *Face,* such as: *Eruptions in Eyebrows, etc.*

Under the adaptability of the repertory we must consider also the rubrics covering sensations and conditions of the glands, of the bones and of the skin, as well as the larger rubrics found under *Sensations (and Complaints)* in general.

In any case where there are confusing symptoms, whether they be many or few, or where the remedy likeness is veiled, we can so adapt the *Pocket Book* as to bring order out of chaos and the remedy will stand revealed, IF we do not ask that the repertory in itself make the decision for us.

INTRODUCTION TO THE THERAPEUTIC POCKET BOOK

In considering its adaptability, let us glance briefly at the records of a few cases.

CASE I. This case offered comparatively few symptoms, but those few so clearly cut that we find them illustrative of the four necessary elements which we must have to use as foundations for our perfect case.

This man suffered terribly with tic douloureux, the intense spasms coming at about five-minute intervals. There was acute pulling pain in the left trigeminus nerve, accompanied with marked flushing of the face, with profuse sweat on head and chest. The upper jaw and cheek were very tender and painful. The conditions were greatly < by touch, excitement or talking; < wet weather; < at night; > by rubbing. With this condition there was ravenous hunger which always came on with the attacks.

His history divulged the fact that he had had for years a discharge from the ear, which had been stopped eight years ago by an ear specialist. Since then he had suffered from these attacks, which were increasing in frequency and violence.

Now let us see what a well rounded repertory analysis can make of this case.

1. LOCATION: Left side of face, page 59
    Cheeks, page 57
    Upper Jaw, page 57
2. SENSATION: Pulling Sensation, page 175
3. CONDITIONS OF AGGRAVATION AND AMELIORATION:
    < touch, page 304
    < talking, page 303
    < night, page 270
    < excitement, page 279
    < wet weather, page 309
    > rubbing, page 318
4. CONCOMITANTS: Ravenous hunger, page 66
    Sweat, upper parts, 262
    Heat in flushes, 258
    Ear, discharge, 41

The concomitant symptom of ravenous hunger is one which seemingly has no relationship to the case, but it actually occurs in distinct relationship to the case and is a most interesting concomitant.

The symptom of discharge from the ear might seem to have no relationship to the case, but since we find no rubric in Bœnninghausen's *Pocket Book* relating to the suppression of ear discharges, and since it was one of the first symptoms present in the chronic constitutional condition of this patient, we are certainly justified in using it in our analysis.

From these fourteen rubrics, then, we worked this case. Let us consider those remedies which came through these rubrics, having twelve or more symptoms. They were: *Ars.* 12/41; *Bry.* 14/45; *Calc. c.* 12/47; *Caust.* 12/36; *Chin.* 12/42; *Kali c.* 13/38; *Merc.* 13/46; *Nit. ac.* 12/38; *Nux vom.* 13/47; *Phos.* 13/47; *Puls.* 13/50; *Rhus* 13/51; *Sep.* 13/47; *Sil.* 12/45; *Spig.* 13/44; *Stann.* 13/39; *Staph.* 12/40; *Sulph.* 14/58.

Calc. carb., Caust., Merc., Phos. and *Rhus* all lacked the characteristic sweating (note the difference here between the *sweat of upper parts* and *sweat of anterior parts* for *Calc. carb.*). *Caust.* lacked the < wet weather. The trembling and twitching of the chronic *Merc.* case was absent; neither did this patient have the general constitutional symptoms of *Phos.* or *Rhus tox.*

The characteristic pulling sensation was absent from *Ars., Calc. carb., Chin., Kali carb., Nit. ac.* and *Sil. Ars.* lacked also the < wet weather; *China* lacked the relationship to discharges from the ear; *Nit. ac.* lacked the < talking; *Puls., Sep.* and *Sil.* lacked the > rubbing. *Nux vom.* and *Stann.* have no relationship noted to discharging ears. *Spig.* lacked the < excitement.

In *Bry.* 14/45 and *Sulph.* 15/58 we find every symptom present. The family attested to the fact that this man showed marked irritability during the attacks. Both *Bry.* and *Sulph.* have marked irritability, so we cannot use this as a means of differentiation. We might have used this as a rubric in analyzing the case. For further means of differentiation let us consider the depth of the disorder, and the fact that, while the ear was not discharging at this time, we must consider the significance of these symptoms coming on after the ear discharges were suppressed. *Sulphur* is one of those deep-acting remedies that have the power to unlock suppressions and to open up masked conditions, and it has also the power in itself to carry the case on, many times, to a complete cure.

This consideration confirmed our decision to give this patient *Sulphur*. It is no part of this exposition of Bœnninghausen's *Pocket Book* to consider the question of potencies, but it may be remarked here that *Sulphur* 1M., one dose, was given this patient. There was a slight aggravation during the first few hours, then amelioration. *As amelioration took place the discharge from the ear returned.* Occasional doses of the remedy over a period of time—three doses in a period of some eighteen months—not only cured the recurrence of these attacks but the ear discharge as well. The ear discharge, being the earliest obtainable symptom in the man's chronic case, and a matter of several years' priority to the other symptoms, was the last symptom noted to disappear, as we have been taught to expect, thus demonstrating once more the accuracy of the law of the direction of cure.

The criticism has been made that the remedies coming through repertory analyses by this method may remove symptoms by suppressing them. This case offers evidence of the reëstablishment of a suppressed discharge, that later was removed through the continued action of the *simillimum*—the remedy revealed by the analysis. Although this case was repertorized several years ago, the man has attained and maintained excellent health.

* * * *

CASE. II. This acute case was a peculiarly interesting one, as it had received the prescriptions of two able prescribers of the homœopathic school without any help—rather, the patient continued to grow worse. The case had the further merit of being checked by laboratory analysis.

The patient, a woman 65 years of age, complained of a pain which began as a soreness in the epigastrium and right hypochondrium, increasing to a sore pain. The pain was > while sitting, > belching; < lying on the back, markedly < lying on right side; < on motion, especially on turning over in bed. There was a constant sensation of pulling in the right hypochondrium, < lying on the right side. The pain causes sweating. There is pain as of repeated blows in the region of the right scapula. The mouth is exceedingly dry. There is a great aversion to food or drink, and the odor of food, or any other strong odors, are very offensive and cause nausea. The patient vomits as soon as water becomes warm in the stomach; there is no thirst. Although there is much flatus, none passes. The urine has an offensive odor.

It may seem strange that two of our ablest prescribers failed to see the outstanding characteristics of the remedy, possibly because this patient was not the characteristic "type" of the *simillimum,* which was found by this repertorization. At this time the white blood count was 19,000. Let us consider the case further.

This case presents the four points so necessary in making a repertory analysis:

LOCATION: Epigastrium, page 79
Hypochondrium, right, page 82

SENSATION: Pulling, page 175
Hammering, page 162
Sore Pain, Internally, page 181

CONDITIONS OF AGGRAVATION AND AMELIORATION:
< Lying on back, page 290
< Lying on right side, page 290
< Motion of affected part, page 292
< Turning over in bed, page 304
< Strong odors, page 293
> Sitting, while, page 319
> Belching (eructations), page 313

CONCOMITANTS:
Sweat with associated symptoms, page 265
Thirstless, page 66

Mouth in general, page 62
Dryness internally (of parts usually moist), page 156
Incarcerated flatus, page 85
Urine offensive, page 95

Since Bœnninghausen has no rubric covering the concomitant symptom, *vomiting as soon as water becomes warm in the stomach,* this was reserved for reference to the materia medica.

The case was repertorized on the eighteen symptoms noted above, with the following results: *Sulph.* 18/71; *Phos.* 18/68; *Nux vom.* 16/71; *Puls.* 16/63; *Bry.* 15/58; *Acon.* 15/57.

In spite of the considerable difference in numerical totality between *Sulphur* and *Phosphorus,* it was a simple matter to differentiate between the *simillimum* and the similar.

Phosphorus 1M. was administered; the patient became more comfortable and two days later the white blood count had dropped to 11,200. Improvement continued and the whole condition cleared completely within a few days.

It is almost unnecessary to point out that the symptom, *vomiting as soon as water becomes warm in the stomach,* served as the differentiating factor in the case. With a knowledge of our materia medica it would seem unnecessary to repertorize a case so clearly marked, yet after the failure of two outstanding homœopathic prescribers one might hesitate to undertake to select the *simillimum* without a thorough analysis of the case. The result warranted the time taken.

* * * *

CASE III. A young man, 25 years of age, gave the following history:

As a child he was very stout, and as a small child he had asthmatic attacks. At 11 years of age he was exposed to the weather, soaked through with rain and thoroughly chilled; rheumatic fever that settled in his knees followed. He later (following the rheumatic fever) became very thin, and developed chorea to the point of clonic convulsions. He was sent to a camp in Maine where the regular hours and the out-door life entirely relieved his condition and he began to gain in weight.

In 1919 he developed eczema on his arms; this was suppressed by local applications. The eczema itched to the point of agony; it was < nights, < warmth of the bed, < sweating. He could not endure being covered at night as it caused sweating and this in turn < the itching.

In 1930 he contracted a cold that was thought to be tubercular; he was sent to an institution but was discharged at the end of six months. In 1932 he had scabies "cured" by external applications, and a return of asthmatic attacks. These attacks waken him from sleep at night. There is copious expectoration, gray, green or yellow. Attacks come on also or are < from wind, < winter, < wet weather, < dust. He is still nervous; he craves candy and sweets.

The following rubrics were chosen:
1. Oppressed respiration, page 113
2. < wind, page 309
3. < wet weather, page 309
4. < winter, page 310
5. Symptoms causing sleeplessness, page 246
6. Expectoration gray, page 118
7. Expectoration green, page 118
8. Expectoration yellow, page 119
9. Sweat with associated symptoms, page 265
10. Scabies suppressed with mercury and sulphur, page 211
11. < warm wraps, page 308 (cannot endure being covered)
12. Tetter itching, page 229
13. < night, page 270
14. < warmth of bed, page 308
15. Nervous excitement, page 157
16. Convulsions clonic, page 150
17. Arthritic pains (in the joints), page 161
18. < getting wet, page 309
19. Desires sweets, page 69

INTRODUCTION TO THE THERAPEUTIC POCKET BOOK

The following remedies came through in sufficient rank for consideration:

Calc. carb. 19/66 has every symptom. *Puls.* 17/69 lacks 7 and 19; *Sep.* 17/69 lacks 2 and 19; *Sulph.* 17/66 lacks 7 and 10; *Phos.* 17/61 lacks 10 and 19; *Lyc.* 17/65 lacks 10 and 15; *Nux vom.* 17/56 lacks 10 and 18; *Carb. veg.* 17/51 lacks 7 and 15; *Ars.* 16/59 lacks 14, 15 and 19.

Without any question *Calc. carb.* not only met every symptom but was his constitutional remedy—the remedy he should have had in childhood. Fortunately, it was still indicated.

Calc. carb. 1M. was given with amelioration of the asthmatic attacks but return of the eczema, to the patient's disgust. He returned at long intervals for a period of two years, but distrusted the remedy because of the skin aggravation that he twice suffered. The asthmatic attacks disappeared except for an occasional very mild reminder of the difficulty, and the eczematous condition steadily improved until it, too, practically disappeared. The patient was so much better he stopped coming, and the last reports were that he was in good health and gaining weight, although there was some itching at times.

* * * *

CASE IV. A young woman, 17 years of age, had suffered from hay fever for fifteen years. Her appearance was one of the worst it has been our lot to see; she looked quite a sodden mess. Her symptoms were as follows:

Attacks begin in April and last until frost. Itching of the eyes when the attacks start, then profuse lachrymation, and later, a sensation as if pins were sticking in the eyes. Raising the eyes to look upward is painful; for relief she pulls the lids away from the eyes. Conjunctiva very red; worse in the left eye, but this condition alternates from side to side. She wants to shut the eyes often. Stopped nose, which is > upon first rising in the morning; there is some discharge, white, watery and profuse at times. Considerable sneezing < toward night. Quantities of mucus in the throat in the morning, thick and yellow, which she must cough to raise. All the above conditions are < nights, < dry weather, > rainy days, < light and < reading. There is swelling of the cheeks with these attacks and pimply eruptions on the face.

It is hard to get to sleep because of the stuffy nose and her sleep is restless.

She takes cold easily, and has frequent attacks of bronchitis in winter.

She always wants warm clothing, and there is no sweating. Menstrual periods are three weeks late but there are no other menstrual symptoms.

She has had measles, scarlet fever, whooping cough. Vaccinated at 11 years; injections four years ago and allergic treatments with mixed pollens.

The case was repertorized on the following symptoms:
1. Lachrymation, page 32
2. Conjunctiva, page 31
3. Itching, page 165
   (Mucous surfaces being *internal* surfaces in essence)
4. Inflammation mucous membrane, page 164
5. < pressure, page 294
6. < opening eyes, page 294
7. < looking upward, page 288
8. < light, page 287
9. < reading, page 295
10. Swelling of cheeks, page 55
11. Eruptions on face, page 53
12. Becomes chilled easily, page 255
13. Tendency to take cold, page 148
14. Mucous secretions increased, page 168
15. Falling asleep prevented by symptoms, page 240
16. Sleep restless, page 244
17. < evening, page 270
18. < dry weather, page 278
19. Stopped coryza, page 47
20. Nasal discharge watery, page 48
21. Sneezing, page 49
22. Internal throat, page 64
23. Cough with expectoration, page 115
24. Expectoration yellow, page 119

25. Menses late, page 108
26. Skin dry (want of sweat), page 207
27. Internal chest, page 124
28. > rising from bed, page 317

The following remedies ranked:

Sil. 27/113 lacked 28 (but it has > change of position); *Sep.* 27/109 lacked 6; *Puls.* 26/115 lacked 6 and 18; *Phos.* 26/110 lacked 18 and 28; *Sulph.* 26/109 lacked 6 and 7; *Nux vom.* 26/103 lacked 7 and 28; *Bry.* 26/102 lacked 7 and 28; *Ars.* 26/97 lacked 3 and 6; *Caust.* 26/78 lacked 6 and 20.

At first glance this girl appeared to be a *Pulsatilla* case, but a repertorization and closer study demonstrated that *Silica* was the correct choice, since it had the modalities that *Puls.* lacked. After *Sil.* 1M. there was a sharp but very brief aggravation and steady and rapid improvement and but one very mild return of the symptoms, that was quickly cleared by a second powder of the same potency.

* * * *

CASE V. A young woman, 35 years of age, was brought n by her family physician who felt he needed help on the case. She was greatly depressed, cried a great deal, and felt so unlike her cheerful self that she "felt frightened at herself." She has a "mad desire to walk" although she is averse to any work, mental or physical. She "faces the day with dread"; feels as if alone in the world; music, of which she has been very fond, is now extremely distasteful. She admits there is no reason why she should not be happy and content, since she has pulled through some hard times and now the road has been smoothed out. She has not slept for several days. Previously, she would awaken from sleep with a general quivering, especially in the pit of the stomach. She feels "weak in the knees" and has an "all-gone" sensation which is better after 4 p. m. She has developed an aversion to being with people, especially crowds.

There is a great deal of headache, dull pain that comes and goes across the forehead, < in the morning; it becomes throbbing on stooping. There is a ringing in the left ear and sense of pressure in the ears as if they were stopped. Her tonsils are enlarged.

She is eating poorly and has recently lost 15 pounds. She sweats all over. Her feet blister, and sweat. The nails are brittle.

The following rubrics were used:
Disposition generally affected, page 17
Sadness, page 19
Desire for motion, page 167
Epigastrium, page 79
Trembling internally, page 193
Waking in distress, page 240
Sleeplessness, page 245
Nervous weakness, page 195
Sensation of emptiness, page 157
< music, page 293
Pain dull, page 169
Forehead, page 24
Sweat easy, page 264
Sweat, special parts, page 262
Stopped sensation in ears, page 44
Ringing in ears, page 43
Throbbing internally, page 191
< stooping, page 301
Emaciation, page 157 (Tendency to lose weight)
< morning, page 269
Eruptions, blisters, page 214
Feet, page 138
Nails brittle, page 223
Tonsils, page 64

Of the 24 rubrics used the following remedies ranked: *Sepia* 23/92 (lacks *Tonsils*); *Puls.* 22/90 (lacks *Tonsils, Nails brittle*); *Merc.* 22/86 (lacks *Waking in distress, < music*); *Calc. carb.* 22/84 (lacks *Waking in distress, Tonsils*); *Sul.* 21/91; *Bry.* 21/86; *Lyc.* 21/76.

Reference to the materia medica showed that *Sepia* reflected the likeness of the patient, and the remedy was administered. There was a decided aggravation and later amelioration, but it was necessary to repeat the potency within a few days and later to raise the potency, which held the patient in a satisfactory manner.

USE OF THE ANALYSIS

The objection has been made that the Bœnninghausen process of analysis takes too long for a busy physician. One might well ask: HOW LONG DO YOU SPEND IN STUDY OVER A REFRACTORY CHRONIC CASE? If an hour or two spent in repertorizing the case will bring before your mind the similars, from which you can easily select the *simillimum*, is this a waste of time?

We have spoken of the method of reaching the totality, from the numerical point of view, in the repertory analysis. Supposing that several remedies come through with high totalities but one or two symptoms are lacking. Need we always select the remedy that has all the symptoms and the highest totality? Not by any means; while experience teaches us that we most often find this the *simillimum*, because of the careful work done in assembling the repertory and in giving the remedies their proper evaluation under every symptom-rubric, we occasionally find remedies lacking one or more symptoms which actually are of very similar relationship to the disease condition, while the one having the highest totality may not be the *simillimum*.

Any repertory analysis is sure only when it meets the picture we find in the materia medica. The most careful repertory analysis avails us nothing if the case is poorly taken; so also while the repertory analysis may be the final basis of remedy selection, without reference to the materia medica, we may here distort the picture. Reference to the materia medica may reveal that the one symptom missing in the repertory actually appears in the materia medica in some form although perhaps not in sufficiently high rank to include it in the repertory.

On the other hand, when you find a symptom given you by your patient which has no counterpart in the repertory, do not say that you cannot work the case. Leave this aside and work the other symptoms, then carry the analysis to the materia medica, plus the symptom not found in the repertory, and you will find this symptom is a part of one of your similar remedies.

Bœnninghausen, by his use of the doctrine of concomitance and the principle of analogy, assumes that when an aggravation of one symptom has occurred in the proving it may be, and frequently is, to be found in relation to other symptoms. *This is not to be taken to mean a direct opposite of such symptoms as have been proven,* however, *or such remedies as have been found to have contrary modalities in different parts,* such as the general aggravation of *Arsenicum* by cold, with the exception of the headache, which is relieved by cold; *Phosphorus,* with its coldness in special parts and its pains, cough and diarrhœa aggravated by cold while the head symptoms are ameliorated by cold.

This is a matter for intelligent use of the repertory analysis; therefore, the more complete the analysis the more quickly the physician can sift the ranking remedies on the basis of the true relationship of the remedies to the individual case.

The repertory analysis can do no more for you than to point the way to a group of remedies that are similars, among which you will find the *simillimum*. The value of our repertory analysis is that in difficult cases where the *simillimum* has seemed obscure, we almost invariably find that the repertory analysis clears our vision and points us to the remedy that will cure the patient.

Such a case is cited here.

A very attractive young woman, a brunette, came to me complaining of the following symptoms:

She disliked the cold weather because she felt the cold so severely. She was generally cold, but especially her hands and feet. When she became cold her hands, and especially her fingers, felt numb and lifeless, and her fingers became colorless. She had a sensation as of a band about her. There was hiccough and belching, < when hungry.

Further questioning brought forth the fact that her sleep was restless; she could not sleep unless heavily covered; she had many pleasant dreams, and she wakened frequently. She found it difficult to get to sleep unless she lay flat on her stomach. She moaned and talked in her sleep. There was some puffiness of the face, especially of the cheeks. She was continually taking cold. The family indicated that there were fits of temper, and that she frequently went into tantrums.

The following rubrics were selected:
Irritability, page 18
Coldness in general, page 260
Coldness of special parts, page 260
Sensation of a band, page 144
Hiccough, page 73
Belching, page 72
< when hungry (see < before eating, page 278)
Dreams pleasant, page 248
Sleep restless, page 244
Lies on abdomen, page 241
Waking frequently at night, page 241
Wants much clothing (Becomes chilled easily, page 255)
Whiteness of parts, page 196
Dead feeling (in single parts), page 154
Fingers, page 132
< becoming cold, page 276
Tendency to take cold, page 148
Swelling of cheeks, page 55

Out of the eighteen rubrics, *Calc. carb.* 18/64 was the only remedy having every symptom. The following remedies lacked the rubric, *Lies on abdomen: Nux vom.* 17/70, *Sulph.* 17/68; *Phos.* 17/67; *Merc.* 17/62; *Caust.* 17/50. *Puls.* 17/67 lacked < *becoming cold. Bry.* 16/58, *Nit. ac.* 16/58 and *Ars.* 16/57 all lacked the rubric, *Lies on abdomen*; in addition *Bry.* lacked *Whiteness of parts, Nit. ac.* lacked *Hiccough* and *Ars.* lacked *Dead feeling in parts. Bell.* lacked the last mentioned symptom and *Whiteness of parts.*

It was possible to eliminate rapidly some of the ranking

remedies; knowledge of the materia medica and knowledge of the patient help greatly in discarding some of the remedies where a number come through an analysis, because of the difference in grouping in the patient and in the remedy, and taking into consideration also that symptom of personality as a whole. The remedies seriously considered for materia medica study and differentiation were *Merc., Nux vom., Phos., Sulph.* and *Nit. ac. Sepia* was also considered, although it lacked three symptoms in the repertory analysis. Of these remedies only *Nit. ac.* met the requirements, and we find the missing symptoms in the materia medica. We also find *Sleep, anxious, with sobbing; restless, unrefreshing, etc.* (Bœnninghausen has no rubric for *moaning in sleep*.) Clarke's *Dictionary* and Allen's *Encyclopædia* reveal this: *Fingers feel as if dead in cold air*.

Thus we find that the materia medica reveals what the repertory fails to complete. In addition, the physician's personal knowledge of the dyscrasia acquired by the father when a young man complemented the repertory analysis and materia medica study and more insistently indicated the selection of *Nit. ac.* as the *simillimum*.

Time has demonstrated the value of this selection, for this patient has required repetition of the remedy only at long, and ever-lengthening, intervals. Her health is excellent and the tendency for repeated colds has been eliminated.

Too much emphasis cannot be placed on the axiom, that must never be forgotten in any case: THE FINAL DECISION, IN THE SELECTION OF ANY REMEDY, MUST REST WITH THE MATERIA MEDICA, in the likeness of the individual remedy to the individual case. As has been so aptly stated, the remedy must speak like the patient; in its essence it must have the characteristics of the patient, although it may vary in some of its individual symptoms. The repertory is not, and was not meant to be, more than a systematic arrangement of symptoms, so that confusing items might be arranged in such a form as to show clearly the symptomatic trend of the patient, which must be diagnostic of both the disease and of the remedy. This holds true in studying the relationships of remedies in their relation to the case just as much as it does in the first selection of the remedy.

The criticism has been made that in repertorizing a case by the Bœnninghausen method only the polychrests come through. This is true to a certain extent, and is partly due to the physical limitations of the *Pocket Book;* it has not grown to its full stature. Allen attempted to add remedies to the rubrics but the work was not carried far enough to make them really useful in working a large case.

Another and more potent reason for the polychrests appearing so frequently in long chronic cases is given by Bœnninghausen in his *Preface,* page v:

> ... Since the polychrests, which are rich in symptoms, as is natural, present the most points of contact, so an intimate acquaintance with these points will enable him to use these drugs easily and to the greatest advantage.

If the repertory is rounded out by the completion of those remedies already added in part, its usefulness will be greatly increased; yet even then the polychrests will outrank all others in the complex chronic cases.

It is well to reiterate that the mathematical results are not in themselves an end; they are near the end, but through them we may reach the art of prescribing the *simillimum,* or if not the ultimate *simillimum,* we may so unlock the case that by sequence we may reach the *simillimum*. This embraces the intelligent use of the mathematical results of our analysis and the intelligent comparison of these results with the materia medica.

Our homœopathic philosophy enters the picture in our taking of the case; it is there while we consider the results of our analysis and it comes into play even more definitely upon the consideration of the patient and the remedy, our final comparison, if you will; and we still depend upon it after administration of the remedy.

The homœopathic materia medica has a pathology of its own. The symptom which the pathologist would exclude as accidental and meaningless is usually the symtom which decides the choice of the homœopathic remedy. It actually has a vital relation to the case. This is only one reason for placing great emphasis on that axiom: IN THE FINAL ANALYSIS WE MUST GO TO THE MATERIA MEDICA.

Two important points in studying and examining a case by Bœnninghausen's method must not be overlooked: 1. To see that no contradictory symptom is admitted into the final synthesis. Let us comprehend clearly what we mean by contradictory symptoms. No symptoms are contradictory if they actually occur in a patient and are true; what we must avoid as contradictory symptoms are those symptoms that a patient may report in one breath, to refute in the next. Or we may find that the symptoms reported when the patient tells his story are contradicted in a review of the case. It may be that we will find seemingly contradictory symptoms through a lack of concept of the relationship of the various elements, or through your failure to interpret the case clearly. Thus a patient may complain that she is worse out of doors, yet her coryza is better out of doors. What she may mean is that her coryza is better out of doors, but her rheumatic complaints are worse out of doors. This may be because of the various relationships of locations, sensations and aggravations, or it may be that she is better from being where it is warm or where her body is warmly clothed, and her pride prevents her from the wearing of a necessary amount of clothes; it may not be a question of open air at all. It may be that a patient will report a dry mouth, and an excess of saliva. These are not necessarily contradictory symptoms; they may be manifestations of an alternation of symptoms that are not contradictory, but actually valuable concomitants of the case.

It is well to note that Bœnninghausen himself warns against confusing the issue in selecting the remedy by allowing our judgment to be swayed by what we may think is a condition of aggravation or amelioration, but is really an alternation of symptoms. We find his admonition on page viii of the *Preface:*

INTRODUCTION TO THE THERAPEUTIC POCKET BOOK   75

In particular, one must avoid considering as an aggravation what is merely the alternating action of the remedy, even though in other ways there should be recognized an aggravation of the general condition. . . . Such symptoms, which we call in provings secondary or alternating effects, are even met with in the course of natural diseases, in which there may be a condition opposite to that of the original trouble, but none the less morbid, and which may easily lead the unskilful to the choice of the wrong drug.

This is something we are not always in a position to judge when we are selecting the rubrics for a repertory analysis; it is a matter of judgment in selecting the remedy from the similar group brought out for analysis. This is one more reason for the axiom that must never be forgotten in repertory work: CARRY THE RESULTS TO THE MATERIA MEDICA. The repertory is a means to an end, never an end in itself.

The problem in every case is to find, among many similars, the *most similar;* and so the symptoms of the patient are collected and pieced together, and compared with the symptoms of remedies under the general type or figure common to all remedies until an image is built up, feature by feature, in which an individuality stands forth. It matters not that the symptoms as grouped in the particular case were never grouped in exactly the same manner in the provings of the single drug. All the symptoms of all the drugs taken and combined under one grand totality, as they are in Bœnninghausen's *Pocket Book,* give us a proving in which the symptoms of any individual case of disease can be found.

Just as all the symptoms of many provers of a drug are combined in one scheme, and all the symptoms of many patients are put together to delineate the typical disease in the textbook on practice, or as all the symptoms of many cases are assembled in finding the epidemic remedy, so Bœnninghausen in his *Pocket Book,* carrying the principle a step farther in its logical development, arranges all the symptoms of all the drugs in the form of one universal and all-inclusive drug. He combines all the lesser totalities into one grand Totality. He organizes all the individuals into a community, all his communities into a state, all the states into a nation!

Bœnninghausen's *Therapeutic Pocket Book* is the result of his long years of indefatigable labor, the full fruition of all his profound studies, the sum total of all his vast experience, a perfected type of the mechanism by which the principles of homœopathy are made practical of application. When we understand it as well, and are able to make good use of it as he did, we shall indeed be masters of the healing art.

BŒNNINGHAUSEN'S

THERAPEUTIC POCKET BOOK,

FOR

HOMŒOPATHIC PHYSICIANS,

TO USE

AT THE BEDSIDE AND IN THE STUDY

OF THE

MATERIA MEDICA.

A

Fifth American Edition,

BY

DR. TIMOTHY FIELD ALLEN.

B. Jain Publishers Pvt. Ltd.
NEW DELHI-110055

BOENNINGHAUSEN'S

Therapeutic Pocket Book

FOR

HOMOEOPATHIC PHYSICIANS,

TO USE

AT THE BEDSIDE AND IN THE STUDY

THE

MATERIA MEDICA.

With a German Edition.

2000

Publishers : **B. Jain Publishers (P) Ltd.**
1921, Chuna Mandi, 10th Street,
New Delhi-110055 (INDIA)

PREFACE

TO THE

NEW AMERICAN EDITION

BŒNNINGHAUSEN'S POCKET BOOK has proved so invaluable to all conscientious homœopathists, that every edition has been exhausted and the need of a new one is pressing. In preparing this, new remedies have been added, to bring the book up to the present time. These additions really represent the advance of homœopathy since Hahnemann's period. The additions surpass in number the remedies contained in the original. Many, indeed, are not excelled in importance by any of the older ones. In making these additions, clinical experience has been consulted freely and our symptomatologies have been scrutinized by the light of this experience.

The list of drugs, under the various rubrics of the original, have not been altered, except in some cases to elevate the rank of the remedies, a proceeding amply justified by their increased usefulness. For example, under "Orbits," rhus has been elevated to the very highest rank.

The Relationships (Chapter VII) of a part only of the new remedies have been added, and this work has been underdone rather than overdone, for much remains to be determined, and it must be confessed that most of our new symptomatologies have not borne the searching light of clinical experience so well as those left us by Hahnemann. In this chapter we need more help from critical students of Materia Medica and homœopathic therapeutics.

It is confidently expected that this little book will serve to give an impetus to a closer study of symptomatology, from which alone the most successful results at the bedside are to be obtained.

It must be borne in mind constantly that this is intended only as a guide to the proper remedy and in no way should be used to supersede the materia medica.

In this edition, the drugs are divided, as in Bœnninghausen's Original, into five ranks; as follows:

    CAPITALS.
    Antique.
    Italic.
    Roman.
    Roman in parentheses (rarely used).

BŒNNINGHAUSEN'S
ORIGINAL PREFACE

More than fifteen years ago, I first issued a repertory which verified its usefulness by enjoying a wide circulation, either in my original editions, or in that of the industrious Jahr, which was prepared according to my model, essentially unchanged. Its uninterrupted use during this period has amply sufficed to judge of its advantages, as well as its defects, and the appearance and ready sale of similar works, even up to the present time, clearly demonstrate that the need of them has not yet been satisfied.

There is no doubt that a diligent and comprehensive study of the pure materia medica cannot be thoroughly accomplished by the use of any repertory whatever. I have not intended to dispense with such a study, but rather have considered all works of such intent positively injurious. Still, it is not to be denied that a homœopathic physician can only devote himself to such studies in his leisure hours (which are, indeed, few enough), and that he needs in his practice, to aid his memory, a work which is abridged, easily consulted, and which contains the characteristic symptoms and their combinations, to enable him, in any individual case of sickness, to select from the remedies generally indicated the one suitable and homœopathic, without a too great loss of time.

The defects of the repertories hitherto published, lie chiefly, in my opinion, in their being limited to the material given in the *Materia Medica Pura*, joined to the carefully-tested cases in practice, but these have never been combined so as to furnish the means of judging the value of each symptom, of completing those which were incomplete and of filling the numerous vacancies constantly met with by every practitioner.

If many symptoms are incomplete, either because the part of the body or the kind of sensation is not clearly indicated, or, what is most frequent, because the aggravations or ameliorations, according to time or circumstances, are omitted, the difficulties of correct apprehension and the judgment of the value of such symptoms for the necessities of curing are greatly increased, for the *characteristic* never shows itself in a single symptom, however complete it may be, since the individuality of the prover exercises an influence over the proving which easily misleads and since also secondary symptoms creep in together with alternate effects of inferior worth, and since in general the worth or worthlessness of most symptoms can be ascertained only by means of pains-taking comparisons of the whole, never from the *Materia Medica Pura* just at the moment it is required without previous study.

PREFACE

An inevitable result of this has been that, on account of the old arrangement of the repertories, on the one hand more or less important symptoms have been scattered among different rubrics and the comprehension of the totality rendered difficult, or on the other, numerous gaps have occurred, for the filling of which there has been no basis, such as analogy might have furnished.

This uncertainty and incompleteness, together with all the prolixity which is known to every homœopathist, induced me several years ago, to seek an arrangement which should remedy the above-mentioned defects, at least so far as the present state of our science makes it possible, and I must thankfully remember my late honored teacher and friend, Hahnemann, for his invaluable support and advice throughout an uninterrupted correspondence.

Fearing to divide symptoms more than has been done hitherto, and which has been deprecated many times, it was my first intention to retain the form and arrangement of my original repertory, which Hahnemann repeatedly assured me he preferred to all others, and to condense it into one volume, making it clearer in every part, as well as more complete from analogy as well as from experience. But, after finishing about half of the manuscript, I found it had increased on my hands beyond all expectation to such a size that, at last, I gave it up, as I saw it was extremely probable that a similar object might be attained in a more simple and satisfactory manner, if, by bringing out the peculiarities and characteristics of the remedies according to their various relations, I opened a way into the wide fields of combinations which hitherto had not been trodden.

In order to avoid increasing homœopathic literature with a useless book, experience was first to be consulted, and, as after using a similar arrangement confined to the polychrests, the most satisfactory results were attained, and the late honored founder of the new school pronounced my idea "excellent and eminently desirable," so I had no more misgivings about finishing the work, which I now present to the homœopathic public in the form of the present Pocket-book, with the hope of a friendly reception and of leniency towards its unavoidable defects and errors.

The scope of this Pocket-book, as given in its title, is double, viz.: on the one hand, to aid the memory of the physician at the bedside in the selection of a remedy, and on the other, to act as a guide in the study of the *Materia Medica Pura*, by means of which one may be able to find his way and to judge of the greater or less value of each symptom, and to make the whole more complete and sharply defined.

On account of the large number of remedies, under nearly every rubric, it has been thought indispensable, on account of both the above-mentioned objects, to distinguish their relative values by means of various types, as I have done in my former repertories, and which Hahnemann has repeatedly shown to be necessary. So, throughout the whole work, there will be found five classes distinguished by the type, of which the four most essential ones are in the first division, Mind and Disposition, under the rubric "Covetousness," which may serve as an example. The word *Puls,* in spaced Italics, occupies the highest, most prominent place. After this follow, in descending order, in simple Italics, *Ars.* and *Lyc.,* as less important, but still especially distinguished by the characteristics of the remedies as well as by practice. Of a still lower order are the spaced Roman letters in N a t r. and S e p., and in the last rank will be found Calc., printed in Roman letters not spaced. The fifth place, the last of all, contains the doubtful remedies, which require critical study, and which occur most seldom; these are enclosed in parentheses.*

It is evident that the estimation and limitation of these classes, to increase the number of which seemed neither important, useful, nor easily accomplished, could not be fixed with mathematical accuracy; I could not even intimate the greater or less leaning to the higher or lower rank, but I could only go so far that the mistake should be less than half an interval. Without having the assurance to maintain that everywhere within these limits accuracy has been attained, I can say with certainty that no industry, care, nor circumspection has been wanting on my part to avoid errors as far as possible. I therefore took upon myself the tedious task of correcting the proof-sheets, and also prepared both an English and French translation, so that, wherever the types permitted, it would be necessary to change only the name of the rubrics, retaining, stereotyped, the carefully revised texts of the rest. The English translation was made by one of the most eminent German homœopathic physicians, who is perfectly acquainted with the English language and literature, but who does not care to be known. The French translation I made myself, and if in the latter, particularly, there are, here and there, mistakes in regard to the genius of the language, which seems not to be very rich in words, I hope, as a foreigner, to meet with indulgence. The correction of the proof-sheets has been extremely difficult, how much so the sixth form may show, which, on account of a necessary journey, was consigned to another person to correct, and in which many letters will be found misplaced, which, however, leave no doubt as to the meaning. The few misleading typographical errors and omissions of whole words are given at the end of the book.

It is easy to comprehend the arrangement of the work, and but few explanations and remarks will be required. It falls into seven distinct parts, in each of which, in order to facilitate the use of the book, as far as possible, a systematic order has been united with an alphabetical arrangement. Although each section may be considered by itself a complete whole, yet each one gives but one portion of a symptom, which can be completed only in one or several other parts. In toothache, for example, the seat of the pain is found in the second section, the kind of pain in the third, the

* NOTE.—The type used in this edition is different. See page 10.

aggravation or amelioration according to time or circumstances in the sixth, and whatever concomitant symptoms are necessary to complete the picture and select the remedy, are also to be found in the various sections.

In regard to the first section, it must be especially observed that our *Materia Medica Pura* contains nowhere more secondary symptoms than under The Mind and Disposition, and, on the other hand, most beginners in homœopathy are liable to overlook this part of the picture of the disease or to make mistakes. Therefore, I have considered it wise to give here only what is essential and prominent, under as few rubrics as possible, in order to facilitate reference. The rubric "Intellect," I have been able to simplify very greatly, since any symptoms, as, for example, "Insanity," by means of the different moods, have been clearly defined in other places.

In the second section, "Parts of the Body and Organs," there is as much condensation as possible, because the tendency of the whole work is to have one part examined critically by the others; however there will be found in this section symptoms (for example, face, cough) which would be vainly looked for in other works. Besides, this part of the work serves particularly to point out the medicines which, in the higher or lower degrees, act upon the various parts and organs of the body; in the case of certain organs, a few other symptoms have been added, and which are confined to these, and for which no other suitable place could be found.

The third section contains an alphabetical arrangement of all the sensations and complaints; (1) in general, then specially; (2) of the glands; (3) of the bones; and (4) of the skin and exterior parts; and also shows the more or less characteristic complaint of each sort in the same way as the preceding section, pointing out the various parts of the body.

The fourth section treats of sleep and dreams; the fifth of fevers: but both only according to essential and clearly defined peculiarities.

In regard to the second, fourth and fifth sections, an explanation must be made concerning the rubric "Concomitant Complaints." Convinced of the importance of the symptoms which occur simultaneously, and therewith form symptom-groups, I have been adding for many years to the concomitant symptoms which are found in the *Materia Medica Pura* whatever belonging to them the experience of myself and others could offer, and their number increased so incredibly that I have been able to deduce general rules. From these it is certain that some remedies, more than others, incline to concomitant symptoms, and that these do not consist exclusively of particular symptoms, but, in general, of every sort of complaint which lies within the sphere of the remedy, though indeed the characteristics may be found more frequently among them than elsewhere. This discovery, tested by long experience, led me to place the "Concomitant Symptoms" together under each section, in which I have again pointed out the varying values of the remedies by means of different type; and when they are taken into account they must be looked for under the peculiarities of those remedies which are more or less concomitant.

The sixth section, which comprises the changes in the symptoms due to time and circumstances, does not fall behind the preceding sections in importance, but in application it needs the greatest circumspection. In particular, one must avoid considering as an aggravation what is merely the alternating action of the remedy, even though in other ways there should be recognized an aggravation of the general condition. For example, diarrhœa which appears only in the morning may often be cured by Bryonia, although constipation and an evening aggravation belong to the most peculiar primary action of this remedy. Such symptoms, which we call in provings secondary or alternating effects, are even met with during the course of natural diseases, in which there may be a condition opposite to that of the original trouble, but none the less morbid, and which may easily lead the unskilful to the choice of the wrong drug. From one point of view the indicated conditions of aggravation or amelioration have a far more significant relation to the totality of the case and to its single symptoms than is usually supposed; they are never confined exclusively to one or another symptom but, on the contrary, a correct choice of the suitable remedy depends very often chiefly upon them. So, to give an example, my friend, Dr. Luterbeck, took charge of one of my patients in my absence, to whom, under such circumstances, I always transfer my patients; this one I had cured of a very deeply seated tubercular phthisis; but on account of some symptoms still remaining, particularly a disagreeable smoothness of the teeth, which were covered with much mucus, always much worse for two days after shaving, he prescribed carbo animalis 30 with the most decided and permanent result, although the only skin symptom of the face which had been observed by Dr. Adams was not present, and in general the symptom of this aggravation had not once been completely observed. The experienced homœopathist will easily find that I have bestowed particular care upon this section, and have given in it many results of my own experience, which will be sought for in vain in the *Materia Medica Pura* or elsewhere.

The seventh and last section, under the rubric "Concordance," presents the results of the comparative action of the various remedies mentioned in the work; firstly, in regard to the preceding sections noted with corresponding numbers, and finally, under the figure VII, according to each particular remedy, everywhere with reference to their value in rank, indicated in the same manner as in the preceding sections. This laborious and time-taking work (which, indeed, has broadened and rectified my knowledge of the *Materia Medica Pura*) will supply the place of the "Relationships" which were published in 1836, and which were acknowledged to be very imperfect, yet my critic, contradicting himself, acknowledged their utility by copying them literally in his handbook of Homœopathic Materia Medica (Leipzig, Schumann), with all their faults and errors, and with a few, for the most part faulty, additions, without giving the source from which he had obtained them, although before his book was published he had ridiculed them. I therefore hope that no one will consider this section useless and superfluous in this improved, and, as far as possible, corrected form. For myself, who for the past fifteen years have made the *Materia Medica Pura* my chief study as one of the most indispensable works of homœopathy, this concordance has been of extreme importance, not only for the recognition of the genius of the remedy, but also for testing and making sure of its choice, and for judging of the sequence of the various remedies, especially in chronic diseases. It is freely granted that one must be tolerably conversant with the *Materia Medica Pura*, but it is made easier for the beginner by the use of this concordance, since the polychrests, which are rich in symptoms, as is natural, present the most points of contact, so an intimate acquaintance with these points will enable him to use these drugs easily and to the greatest advantage. At the conclusion I have given the antidotes that are known, and also the noxious drugs under the word *(Nox.)*. I may also remark that the same reason which caused me in 1835 to omit osmium and several other drugs still holds, and I will not willingly mix what is sure and tested with what is doubtful and uncertain.

For the benefit of beginners in homœopathy, for whom the pocket-book is chiefly intended, it may be judicious to say a few words concerning its use, especially with reference to its two-fold object according to the above-mentioned scheme.

In studying the *Materia Medica Pura* I have found it the most simple and profitable way to underline with a pencil, according to the order of this pocket-book, all of those characteristic symptoms which have been indicated by the explanatory type used, either in the original or in one of my repertories or in those of others, and to add those which are wanting; this costs but little time and trouble and affords an easy review, which may be made complete by means of greater experience. In such a manner one may acquire not only a fundamental knowledge of the most important symptoms and of the genius of each remedy, but also an enduring written collection of what is most valuable, which by means of this preparation becomes deeply fixed in the memory, and afterwards may be reviewed in difficult cases, and frequently will be found of the greatest service in the right choice of the remedy.

In using this book at the bedside much depends upon whether one is entirely a beginner, or is already somewhat skilled in homœopathy. But he who knows nothing whatever must, indeed, make a most careful search for everything without exception. The more he knows the less he has to look for, and, finally, only to use it here and there to help his memory. This may be best shown by an example: This I have taken for the purpose from my most recent practice, wherein the choice of the remedy was not

PREFACE

difficult and at first seemed very easy, though through lack of attention a mistake might easily have been made. This case may serve for the beginner in homœopathy to try his own skill.

E. N., of L., a man of about 50 years, of a blooming, almost florid complexion, usually cheerful, but during his more violent paroxysms inclined to outbreaks of anger with decided nervous excitement, had suffered for a few months with a peculiar kind of violent pain in the right leg after the previous dispersion allopathically of a so-called rheumatic pain in the right orbit by external remedies, which could not be found out; this last pain attacked the muscles of the posterior part of the leg, especially from the calf down to the heel, but did not involve the knee or ankle-joint. The pain itself he described as extremely acute, cramping, jerking, tearing, frequently interrupted by stitches extending from within outward; but in the morning hours, when the pain was generally more endurable, it was a dull burrowing with a bruised feeling. The pain became worse towards evening and during rest, especially after previous motion, while sitting and standing, particularly if he did it during a walk in the open air. While walking the pain often jumped suddenly from the right calf into the left upper arm if he put his hand into his coat-pocket or his breast and kept the arm quiet, but it was relieved while moving the arm, and then the pain suddenly jumped back again into the right calf. The greatest relief was experienced while walking up and down the room and rubbing the affected part. The concomitant symptoms were sleeplessness before midnight, frequently recurring attacks in the evening of sudden flushes of heat with thirst without previous chill, a disagreeable fatty taste in the mouth with nausea in the throat, and an almost constant pressing pain in the lower part of the chest and pit of the stomach as if something there were forcing itself outward.

No skilful homœopathist, who is perfectly familiar with the action of his remedies, will long remain in doubt as to the correct remedy in this case, with so complete and accurate a picture of the disease, for all these symptoms together correspond to a single one, which is thoroughly homœopathic; but the beginner will be obliged to look for nearly every symptom and only after long search will he find the one most fit among the concurrent remedies. Between these two extremes of knowing and not knowing, lie many degrees of partial knowledge, which require a more or less frequent consultation of the book.

One person, for example, knows that the pains repeatedly changing from place to place, worse towards evening and during rest, together with the fatty taste in the mouth, the sleeplessness before midnight and others of the symptoms mentioned, belong especially to the action of *pulsatilla,* but he is not sure whether the remaining symptoms also belong to it, and he will not, if he acts conscientiously, spare the trouble to compare these latter; but he will soon see that *pulsatilla* is not the correct homœopathic remedy, because, in addition to the mental symptoms, there are others which are not similar, but, indeed, are directly, contradictory to it.

Another person who has studied more the peculiarities of the pains and distinctly remembers that *china* corresponds to the paralytic and bruised pains as well as to the jerking tearings and the stitches from within outward and to the pains jumping from place to place. In addition, he believes that also symptoms, like sleeplessness before midnight, the aggravation during rest, as well as the relief from motion and rubbing, together with the flushes of heat with thirst, correspond to this drug, but because he does not know he also must consult the books; so he will soon meet with contradictions, just as the previous one did, and he will see clearly the unfitness of *china* for the case.

Neither of these two, however, will think of administering to the patient a remedy whose curative power in this case is so improbable, but as conscientious homœopathic physicians, they will look farther and compare, and by the help of this hand-book they will soon find, without great difficulty, the only really homœopathically indicated remedy.

But even a third physician, educated in homœopathy, one who recognizes the contra-indications of *pulsatilla, china* and other concurrent remedies, does not know sufficiently that *valeriana* corresponds to the chief symptoms, and in order to be perfectly sure about this rather infrequently used remedy, he will quickly look up the few doubtful symptoms, and convince himself that this drug, among all the known medicines, is the best adapted to this case, as was proved in the result; for, after a single very small dose exhibited in a high potency in water, the whole trouble, with all the concomitant symptoms, was completely removed within three days. The half-educated physician, however, who consults only the original sources and discards every sort of repertory will not easily think of looking for this drug, which is seldom used for similar complaints, in the second volume of the *Archiv.*, and before doing it, he will expend much time and trouble, which might have been more usefully employed, in comparing other and more frequently used remedies; and if, at last, he should consult it, he will even here meet with difficulties and doubts, which are not easily overcome by the unskilled without other help, since most of the symptoms which must be considered here, must be more or less completed by the characteristics of the remedy, in order to be found suitable, and besides many errors in the notes, many secondary effects which are not marked as such and hence are not easily recognized, increase the uncertainty.

It is by far more difficult for the inexperienced homœopathist to cure patients even with a few symptoms without a repertory, because many remedies seem to correspond. For example, at present there is in this region a pernicious whooping-cough among children which, in the beginning, in only exceptional cases, presents the well-known indications of drosera, never those of the other remedies usually indicated in whooping-cough. However, tne sick children were characterized by a remarkable puffiness and swelling, not so much of the whole face as especially above the eyes, between the lids and the brows, which was frequently like a thick little sac, a symptom which, hitherto, has been observed only in kali carb., and in fact from the beginning of the epidemic, this has been the only quick and permanently curative medicine. Only in the latter period of the disease, there appeared another form characterized by cold sweat on the forehead during vomiting, which called for *veratrum alb*.

This is not the place to say anything about the size and repetition of the dose, concerning which opinions do not yet coincide. However, I cannot refrain from calling attention to what I have already said in the *New Archivs.* for homœopathy, and from giving the assurance that my experience has been most pronounced for the high potencies, of long continued action and against the repetition of the dose, without intercurrent remedies, even in diseases of the bones, for example, in curvature of the spine and protrusion of the shoulders and hips. I have seen more cures follow in a much shorter time after the high than I had ever experienced before from the lower dynamizations. I can, therefore, from my own extended practice only reiterate what our true Hahnemannian adherents have communicated, and I am far better satisfied with my results of the past two years (in which I have used almost exclusively the high potencies) than formerly, although the far larger proportion of my patients have come from the hands of the allopaths.

In conclusion, I recommend this little work as the fruit of almost three years' labor to the thoroughly unprejudiced, yet friendly, criticism of all those who, like myself, wish only for what is best and who have made the firm resolution to devote the rest of their lives to homœopathy and to suffering humanity.

BŒNNINGHAUSEN'S
THERAPEUTIC POCKET BOOK

PART II

Therapeutic Pocket Book.

Mind.

Disposition generally affected.—*Abrot.*, **Acon.**, Agar., Agn., *Aloe*, Alum., Ambr., *Am. carb.*, Am. m., Anac., *Ant. cr.*, Ant. t., **Arn.**, **Ars.**, Asaf., Asar., **AUR.**, *Bar. c.*, **BELL.**, Bism., Bor., *Bov.*, **Bry.**, Cact., Calad., **Calc. c.**, *Calc. ph.*, Camph., **Cannab. i.**, *Cannab. s.*, **Canth.**, **Caps.**, *Carb. an.*, *Carb. v.*, *Carb. sul.*, **Caust.**, **Cham.**, Chel., *Chin.*, *Cic.*, *Cina.*, *Cinnab.*, Clem., **Cocc.**, *Coff.*, Colch., Coloc., **Con.**, *Croc.* Cup., *Cyc.*, *Dig.*, Dros., Dulc., Euphorb., Euphr., *Fer.*, *Gel.*, **Graph.**, Guai., Hell., *Hep.*, **Hyos.**, **IGN.**, *Iod.*, *Ip.*, K. carb., K. nit., Kre., Lach., Laur., Led., **LIL. T.**, **LYC.**, Mag. c., Mag. m., Mang., Mar., *Meli.*, *Meny.*, **Merc.**, Mez., Mos., Mur. ac., **NAT. C.**, **NAT. M.**, *Nit. ac.*, Nux m., **NUX. V.**, Oleand., **Op.**, Oxyt., Par., Petrol., **PHOS.**, *Pho. ac.*, Pic. ac., **PLAT.**, Pb., *Pso.*, **PULS.**, Ran. b., Ran. s., Rheum, Rhodo., **Rhus**, Ruta, Saba., Sabi., Samb., Sars., Sec. c., Sele., Seneg., **Sep.**, **Sil.**, Spig., *Spo.*, Squ., Stan., **Staph.**, **Stram.**, Stro., **SUL.**, *Sul. ac.*, Tar., Thuj., *Valer.*, **VERAT. A.**, Verb., *Vio. o.*, *Vio. t.*, Zinc.

Absence of Mind.—Acon., *Agn.*, Alum, **Am. carb.**, Anac., **Arn.**, Aur., **Bar. c.**, *Bell.*, **Bov.**, Calad., Calc. c., **CANNAB. I.**, *Canab. s.*, *Carb. sul.*, **CAUST.**, **CHAM.**, *Chin.*, *Cic.*, **Cocc.**, Colch., *Croc.*, Cyc., Dulc., *Graph.*, Hell., Hep., Ign., *K. br.*, *K. carb.*, Lach., Led., **Lyc.**, **Mang.**, **Merc.**, **Mez.**, Mos., Nat. c., *Nat. m.*, Nit. ac., **Nux m.**, Nux v., *Oleand.*, **Op.**, Petrol., Phos., *Pho. ac.*, Plat., **PULS.**, Rhodo., Rhus, **SEP.**, *Sil.*, Spig., **Stan.**, Stram., **Sul.**, Sul. ac., *Thuj.*, **VERAT. A.**, Verb., Vio. o., Vio. t.

Alternating Moods.—*Agn.*, Acon., **ALUM.**, Ant. t., Arn., *Asaf.*, Asar., **Aur.**, **Bar. ac.**, **Bar. c.**, *Bell.*, *Bism.*, Bov., Cannab. s., **Caps.**, **Carb. an.**, **Caust.**, *Con.*, **Croc.**, Cup., *Cyc.*, Dros., **FER.**, **Graph.**, *Hyos.*, **IGN.**, *Iod.*, *Lyc.*, Merc., **Naj.**, Nat. c., *Nat. m.*, **Nux m.**, Op., *Phos.*, **PLAT.**, **Puls.**, Sars., **Stan.**, Stram., *Sul.*, **SUL. AC.**, *Tarent.*, *Valer.*, **ZINC.**

Amativeness.—Acon., **Ant. cr., Apis,** Bell., Calad., *Calc. c., Calc. ph.,* CANNAB. I., Cannab. s., CANTH., Carb. v., *Chin.,* Coff., *Coloc., Con.,* Croc., Dulc., Graph., HYOS., Ign., K. carb., LACH., Lyc., Meny., *Merc., Mos., Nat. c.,* **Nat. m.,** Nux m., **Nux v.,** Op., PHOS., PLAT., Pb., **Puls.,** Rhus, Ruta, *Sabi.,* Sele., **Sil., Staph.,** Stram., Sul., Thuj., VERAT. A., Verb., *Zinc.*

Anxiety.—ACON., Acon. f., *Agar.,* Agn., All. c., *Alum.,* Ambr., *Am. carb.,* Am. m., *Amyl.,* Anac., Ant. cr., **Ant. t.,** Arn., ARS., AUR., Bar. c., **BELL.,** Bor., BRY., *Cact.,* Calad., *Calc. ac.,* CALC. C, *Calc. ph., Camph.,* CANNAB. I., Canth., *Caps., Carb. an.,* **Carb. v.,** *Caust.,* Cham., Chel., *Chin.,* Cic., *Clem.,* Cocc., *Coff.,* Coloc., *Con.,* Cup., *Cyc.,* DIG., Dros., Fer., Graph., Hell., Hep., *Hyos.,* Ign., K. carb., *K. iod., K. nit.,* Lach., Lyc., Meny., **Merc.,** Merc. c., Mur. ac., *Nat. c.,* **Nit. ac.,** Nux v., Op., *Ox. ac., Petrol.,* PHOS., Pho. ac., *Plat.,* Pso., PULS., Raph., RHUS, Ruta, Saba., **Sabi.,** *Samb.,* SEC. C., **Sep.,** Sil., *Spig.,* Spo., Stan., Stram., Stro., Sul., *Thea.,* Thuj., Valer., VERAT. A., Zinc.

Avarice.—ARS., Calc. c., Lyc., *Nat. c.,* PULS., Sep.

Boldness.—Acon., Ant. t., Bov., *Calad.,* IGN., Mez., Nat. c., OP., *Puls.,* Squ., Tar., Verat. a.

Despair.—*Acon.,* Agn., Ambr., Am. m., *Ant. t.,* ARS., AUR., *Bar. c.,* **Bell.,** *Bry.,* Calc. c., Camph., **Cannab. i.,** Canth., Carb. an., Carb. v., Caust., Cham., *Chin.,* Coff., Colch., **Con.,** Dig., Graph., *Hep.,* IGN., Iod., Lyc., *Merc.,* **Nat. c., Nat. m.,** Nit. ac., Nux v., Phos., Pho. ac., Pb., Pso., Puls., Rhus, Ruta, Sep., *Sil.,* Spig., *Stan.,* Sul., Sul. ac., Thuj., Verat. a., Verb.

Excitement.—*Abrot.,* ACON., Ambr., Am. m., *Anac.,* Ant. cr., *Arn., Ars.,* AUR., *Bar. c.,* Bell., Bor., Bry., *Calc. c., Calc. ph.,* Camph., *Cannab. i.,* Canth., Carb. an., *Carb. v.,* Caust., Ced., CHAM., Chin., Cic., *Cina.,* Cocc., COFF., Croc., Cup., Dulc., Fer., *Hep.,* **Hyos.,** *Ign.,* Iod., *Ip.,* Kre., *Lach., Laur.,* Lyc., *Mar., Merc.,* **Nat. c., Nat. m.,** Nit. ac., NUX V., Oleand., Op., *Ox. ac., Petrol.,* **Phos.,** Pho. ac., Puls., Ran. b., *Seneg.,* Sep., *Sil.,* Stan., *Stram., Stro.,* Sul., Sul. ac., **Thea.,** *Valer.,* **Verat. a.,** Zinc.

Fretfulness.—*Ab. c., Abrot.,* ACON., Aesc., *Agar.,* Aloe, Alum., *Am. carb., Am. m.,* Anac., Ant. cr., Arn., Ars., Ars. iod., Asaf., Asar., AUR., BELL., Bism., Bor., *Bor.,* Bry., *Calc ac.,* CALC. C, *Calc. ph., Cannab. i., Cannab. s.,* Canth., *Caps.,* **Carb. ac.,** Carb. v., Caust., Cham., *Chel., Chin., Cic.,* Cina., *Cinnab., Clem., Cocc., Coff., Colch.,* Coloc., **Con.,** Croc., *Crot. tig.,* Cup., Cyc., Dios., Dros., Dulc., Fer.,

MIND.

Gran., *Graph.*, Guai., **Hep.**, *Hyos.*, Ign., Iod., Ip., K. carb., Kre., *Lach.*, Laur., *Led.*, LYC., Mag. c., *Mag. m.*, Mang., Mar., **Meli.**, Meny., **Merc.**, Merc. c., Mez., Mur. ac., Nat. c., Nat. m., NIT. AC., NUX V., Op., Petrol., Phos., Pho. ac., *Phys.*, Plat., *Pso.*, PULS., RAN. B., **Rhus**, Ruta, Sabi., Samb., Sars., Seneg., Sep., SIL., *Spo.*, Squ., *Stan.*, Staph., Stram., Stro., SUL., Sul. ac., *Thea.*, THUJ., **Verat. a.**, VERAT. V., Verb., Vio. t., Zinc.

Gentleness.—Acon., *Ambr.*, Anac., ARN., ARS., Asar., Aur., BOR., Bov., Cact., Calad., Cannab. i., *Caps.*, Carb. an., Caust., *Ced.*, *Chel.*, *Cic.*, **Cina**, *Clem.*, Cocc., *Con.*, Croc., **Cup.**, Euphorb., Euphr., Hell., *Ign.*, Iod., Lil. t., Lyc., Mag. m., Mang., Mur. ac., Nat. c., NAT. M., Nit. ac., Op., Phos., Pho. ac., Pb., PULS., RHUS, Sep., SIL., **Spo.**, *Stan.*, Stram., *Sul.*, *Thuj.*, Verat. a., Zinc.

Haughtiness.—Anac., Arn., Aur., *Caust.*, Chin., Cic., Cup., Dulc., *Fer.*, Guai., *Hyos.*, Ign., Ip., *Lach.*, LYC., Merc., Nux v., Par., *Phos.*, PLAT., Stram., VERAT. A.

Indifference.—Agar., Agn., Alum., Am. m., *Anac.*, Apis, *Arn.*, *Ars.*, Asaf., Asar., *Bell.*, Calc. c., *Calc. i.*, *Cannab. i.*, Caust., *Cham.*, **Chel.**, Chin., Cic., Clem., Cocc., **Con.**, *Cyc.*, *Dig.*, *Euphr.*, Graph., *Hell.*, **Gel.**, Ign., Ip., Lach., Laur., Lyc., Meli., Meny., Merc., Mez., *Mur. ac.*, **Nat. m.**, Nit. ac., Nux v., Oleand., *Op.* PHOS., PHO. AC., *Phyt.*, **Pic. ac.**, Plat., PULS., Rheum, Rhodo., SEP., Sil., *Squ.*, *Staph.*, Stram., Sul., Vio. t., *Zinc.*

Joyfulness.—*Agar.*, Alum., Ant. t., Aur., Bell., CANNAB. I. Cannab. s., Caps., **Carb. an.**, *Cic.*, COFF., Con., CROC., *Cup.*, *Oyc.*, *Dig.*, *Fer.*, HYOS., *Ign.*, *Iod.*, LACH., Laur., *Lyc.*, *Meny.*, NAT. C. Nat. m., **Nux m.**, OP., **Phos.**, Pho. ac., **Plat.**, Pb., Saba., Sars., Seneg., Spig., **Spo.**, Stram., Tar., *Thea.*, *Valer.*, Verat. a., *Verb.*, Zinc.

Mischievousness.—Acon., Agar., Am. carb., Am. m., ANAC., Arn., Ars., Aur., *Bell.*, Bor., *Caps.*, Caust., Chin., Cic., Coloc., **Cup.**, *Guai.*, Hyos., Ign., *Lach.*, Led., *Lyc.*, Mang., *Nat. c.*, *Nat. m.*, *Nit. ac.*, NUX V., *Par.*, Phos., *Plat.*, Sec. c., Squ., Stram., Verat. a.

Mistrust.—*Abs.*, ACON., **Anac.**, *Ant. cr.*, *Apis*, Arn., *Arg. n.*, ARS., Aur., Bap., *Bar. ac.*, BAR. C., Bell., Bor., BRY., Cact., Calc. c., *Calc. ph.*, *Camph.*, CANNAB. I., CAUST., Cham., CIC., *Cinric.*, Cocc., Con., Cup., DIG., Dros., *Dub.*, *Gel.*, *Glon.*, Hell., Hyos., *K. br.*, *Lach.*, *Lil. t.*, LYC., *Meny.*, **Merc.**, Nat. c., Nit. ac., Op., Phos., **Pb.**, *Pso.*, PULS., RHUS, Ruta, Sep., SEC. C., *Sil.*, Stan., Staph., STILL., STRAM., SUL., Sul. ac., *Thea.*, *Valer.*, Verat. a.

Sadness.—*Abrot.*, ACON., *Aesc.*, *Agar.*, **Agn.**, *Aloe*, Ambr., Am.

carb., **Anac.**, **Arg. n.**, ARS., Asar., **AUR.**, **Bell.**, Bov., *Bry.*, **Cact.**, *Calc. ac.*, **Calc. c.**, *Calc. f.*, *Calc. ph.*, Camph., *Cannab. i.*, **Caps.**, Carb. an., Caust., Cham., *Chel.*, *Chin.*, *Cic.*, CIMIC., Cina., *Cinnab.*, Cocc., *Coff.*, *Colch.*, *Con.*, Corn. c., Croc., Cup., Cyc., **Dig.**, Dros., *Fer.*, **Gel.**, **Graph.**, *Hell.*, *Helo.*, Hep., Hyos., IGN., Iod., **Ip.**, **K. carb.**, *K. br.*, *K. iod.*, Kre., *Lach.*, Laur., LIL. T., **Lyc.**, **Meli.**, Meny., **Merc.**, *Merc. c.*, MEZ., **Naj.**, NAT. C., NAT. M., NIT. AC., **Nux v.**, Oxyt., Petrol, Phos., Pho. ac., **Phyt.**, **Plat.**, PSO., **Puls.**, Ran. s., Rheum, RHUS, **Sabi.**, Sep., Sil., Spig., Spo., STAN., *Staph.*, Still., **Stram.**, SUL., Sul. ac., THUJ., **Verat. a.**, Vio. o., Vio. t., *Zinc.*

Seriousness.—*Alum.*, Ambr., *Am. carb.*, Am. m., Anac., Ant. cr., Ars., Aur., *Bar. c.*, Bov., *Cannab. s.*, Caust., Cham., Cina., Cocc., *Con.*, Cyc., Euphorb., Ign., Iod., **Led.**, *Lyc.*, *Merc.*, *Nat. c.*, Nux m., Oleand., Pho. ac., *Plat.*, Pb., Puls., Rhus, Seneg., *Sep.*, Spig., Staph., Sul., **Sul. ac.**, Thuj., Verat. a.

Intellect.

Activity.—Acon., **Agar.**, Alum., Ambr., Am. carb., Anac., *Ant. cr.*, BELL., Cannab. i., Cannab. s., *Chin.*, COFF., *Dig.*, Hyos., LACH., Laur., Lyc., *Mur. ac.*, Nux m., OP., **Phos.**, Plat., Saba., *Stram.*, Sul., **Sul. ac.**, Valer., *Verb.*, Vio. o., Zinc.

Befogged.—Acon., **Agar.**, *Alum.*, *Am. m.*, Ant. t., **Arg.**, Ars., *Asar.*, Aur., BELL., Bov., BRY., **Calc. c.**, Camph., Cannab. s., *Caps.*, *Carb. v.*, *Caust.*, Cham., *Chel.*, Chin., Cic., **Cocc.**, *Coff.*, Con., Croc., Dulc., **Gel.**, Graph., Hell., Hyos., Ign., Ip., **K. carb.**, K. nit., Kre., LAUR., *Lyc.*, **Mag. m.**, Merc., **Mez.**, Mos., Nat. c., *Nat. m.*, *Nux m.*, **Nux v.**, OP., *Petrol.*, *Phos.*, Pho. ac., Puls., Rheum, *Rhodo.*, Rhus, Saba., *Samb.*, Sars., *Sec. c.*, **Sep.**, Sil., Spo., Squ., Stram., Sul., Sul. ac., Tar., *Thuj.*, *Valer.*, Verat. a., ZINC.

Comprehension Difficult.—*Agar.*, **Agn.**, *Alum.*, **Ambr.**, Am. carb., Anac., Ant. cr., *Ars.*, Asaf., *Asar.*, Aur., BAP., *Bar. c.*, **Bell.**, Bor. BRY., *Calc. c.*, Camph., *Cannab. i.*, Cannab. s., Caps., *Carb. sul.*, Carb. v., Caust., Cham., **Chel.**, Chin., Cimic., *Cocc.*, *Colch.*, CON., **Corn. c.**, Crotal., Cup., Cyc., Dig., Dulc., GEL., Hell., Hep., **Hyd. ac.**, *Hyos.*, Ign., *K. bi.*, K. br., Laur., LYC., **Meli.**, Meny., MERC., **Merc. c.**, **Mez.**, Mos., Mur. ac., NAT. C., *Nat. m.*, Nit. ac., NUX M., *Nux v.*, Oleand., OP., *Petrol.*, PIC. AC., PHOS., PHO. AC., Plat., **PB.**, Puls., **Ran. b.**, Rheum, Rhus, *Ruta*, Saba., *Sec. c.*, Sele., SEP., Sil., Spig., *Spo.*, Stan., **Staph.**, Stram., *Sul.*, *Sul. ac.*, Tab., Thuj., *Verat. a.*, Vio. o., Vio. t., **Zinc.**

Comprehension Easy.—Ambr., Bar. c., **Cannab. i.**, Cannab. s.,

INTELLECT. 21

Caust., **COFF.**, **Hyos.**, **Lach.**, **Lyc.**, **OP.**, **Phos.**, *Saba.*, **Sep.** **Sul.**, *Valer.*, *Verat. a.*, **Vio. o.**

Confusion.—Acon., *Agar.*, Alum., Ambr., *Am. carb.*, *Am. m.* **Anac.**, *Ant. t.*, **Apis,** **Arn.**, **Ars.**, *Asaf.*, *Asar.*, **Aur.**, *Bar. c.*, **Bell.**, *Bism.* Bor., Bov., **Bry.**, Calad., **CALC. C.**, Camph., *Cannab. s.*, **Canth.**, **Caps. Carb. an.**, *Carb. v.*, *Carb. sul.*, **Caust.**, *Chel.*, **Chin.**, **Cic.**, Clem., Cocc., **Coff.**, Colch., Coloc., **Con.**, **Croc.**, *Dig.*, Dros., Euphr., **Fer.**, Glon., Graph., Hell., Hep., *Hyos.*, Ign., *Iod.*, *K. br.*, **K. carb.**, *K. nit.*, **Kre.**, **Lach.**, *Laur.*, Led., *Lyc.*, **Mag. c.**, *Magn. m.*, **Mang.**, **Meny.**, **MERC.**, **Mez.**, Mosch., Mur. ac., Nat. c., **NAT. M.**, *Nit. ac.*, **NUX M.**, **NUX V.** Oleand., **OP.**, Par., **PETROL.**, **Phos.**, *Pho. ac.*, *Pb.*, **Puls.**, **Ran. b.**, *Rheum*, Rhodo., **RHUS.**, *Ruta*, **Saba.**, *Sabi.*, Samb., Sars., **Sec. c.**, **Seneg.**, **SEP.**, **SIL.**, Spig., Spo., *Squ.*, **Stan.**, **Staph.**, Stram., Stro., **SUL.**, *Sul. ac.*, Tar., Thuj., Valer., *Verat. a.*, Verb., *Vio. o.*, *Vio. t.* **Zinc.**

Delirium.—*Abrot.*, **Abs.**, Acon., *Acon. f.*, *Act.*, *Agar.*, Am. carb., Anac., Ant. cr., **Ant. t.**, **Apis**, **Arn.**, **ARS.**, **Arum. t.**, **Atrop.**, **Aur.**, Bap., **BELL.**, Bism., **BRY.**, *Buf.*, Calc. c., **Camph.**, **CANNAB. i.**, *Cannab. s.*, **Canth.**, *Carb. sul.*, Cham., *Chel.*, Chin., **Cic.**, *Cimic.*, *Cina*, Cocc., Coloc., Con., Croc., Crotal., Cup., **Dig.**, *Dub.*, *Dulc.*, *Gel.*, *Hell.*, Hyd. ac., **HYOS.**, *Hyper.*, Ign., Iod., **Ip.**, **K. carb.**, *K. br.*, **LACH.**, Lyc., Merc., **Merc. c.**, *Mur. ac.*, Nux m., *Nux v.*, **OP.**, *Par.*, **Petrol.**, Phos., *Pho. ac.*, *Plat.*, Pb., Puls., *Ran. b.*, Rheum, Rhus, Saba., Samb., *Sec. c.*, Spo., **STRAM.**, Sul., Sul. ac., Tar., *Tarent.*, *Ther.*, Valer., **VERAT. A.**, **VERAT. V.**, *Zinc.*

Ecstasy.—ACON., **Agar.**, **Agn.**, **Ant. cr.**, Arn., *Bell.*, Bry., **Cannab. i.**, Cham., *Lach.*, Oleand., **Op.**, **PHOS.**, Pho. ac., Plat., Stan., *Stram.*, Verat. a.

Imaginations.—Acon., *Agar.*, Ambr., Anac., Ant. cr., **Ars.**, **Aur.**, Bap., Bar. c., **BELL.**, *Bry.*, *Calc. c.*, **CANNAB. I.**, *Cannab. s.*, *Canth.*, **Carb. an.**, *Carb. v. Carb. sul.*, *Canst.*, *Chin.*, Cic., **COCC.**, Coff., Con., Croc., Crotal., Cup., *Dub.*, Euphr., **Glon.**, **Hell.**, Hep., **Hyos.**, **IGN.** Iod., *K. bi.* K. carb., Lach., Led. **Lyc.**, Mag. m., Merc., Mur. ac., Nit. ac., *Nux. v.*, **Op.**, PETROL., Phos., **PHO. AC.**, Plat., Pso., Puls., **Rhus**, **SABA.**, Samb., **Sec. c.**, *Sep.*, Sil., Spo, *Stan.* **Staph.**, **STRAM.**, **SUL.**, Ther., Thuj., **Valer.**, *Verat. a.*, Verb., Vio. o.

Imbecility.—*Abs.*, *Agar.*, **ANAC.**, *Ant. cr.*, **Ars.**, Asar., Aur., *Bar. c.*, **BELL.**, Bov., **Bry.**, *Calc. c.*, Cannab. s., *Caps.*, *Carb. sul.*, *Cham.*, **Cocc.**, Coff., *Con.*, Cup., Cyc., *Dulc.*, *Hell.*, **HYOS.**, *Ign.*, Lach., **Laur.**, **Lyc.**, Merc., **Merc. c.**, Mez., Mos., *Mur. ac.*, **NAT. C.**, *Nat. m.*, *Nux. m.*, Nux v., Oleand., **Op.**, Par., Petrol., **Phos.**, **PHO. AC.**, **Pic. ac.**, **Pb.**,

INTELLECT.

Puls., *Ran. b.*, Rheum, Rhus, Ruta, Saba., *Sec. c.*, Sele. Seneg., **Sep.**, Sil., **Spo.**, **Stan.**, **Staph.**, Stram., Sul. ac., Verat. a.

Impaired.—Acon., *Agar.*, Agn., ALOE, Ælum., *Ambr.*, Am. carb., **Anac.**, *Ant. cr.*, **Arn.**, *Ars.*, Asar., Aur., **Bap.**, *Bar. c.*, BELL., Bov., *Bry.*, Calad., **Calc. c.**, *Calc. ph.*, Camph., *Cannab. i.*, **Cannab. s.**, *Canth.*, **Caps.**, Carb. v., *Carb. sul.*, Caust., *Cham.*, Chel., *Chin.*, *Cic.*, Cocc., *Coff.*, Colch., **Con.**, Croc., *Cup.*, Cyc., **Dios.**, *Dul.*, Dulc., Graph., **Hell.**, Hep., HYOS., Hyper., Ign., Iod., K. carb., *K. bi.*, K. br., LACH., Laur., Led., **LYC.**, **Meli.**, Meny., **Merc.**, Mez., Mos., *Mur. ac.*, **Nat. c.**, Nat. m., Nit. ac., *Nux m.*, NUX V., *Oleand.*, OP., **Oxyt.**, Par., Petrol., PIC. AC., **Phos.**, PHO. AC., **Plat.**, **Pb.**, Puls., Ran. b., Rheum., Rhus, Ruta, *Saba.*, **Sabi.**, *Sec. c.*, *Sele.*, SEP., *Sil.*, Spig., Spo., *Stan.*, *Staph.*, STRAM., SUL., Sul. ac., Tar., **Ther.**, Thuj., *Valer.*, VERAT. A., Verb., *Vio. o.*, Zinc.

Insanity.—Acon., Agar., **Anac.**, Ant. cr., Ars., **Aur.**, BELL., Cannab. s., *Canth.*, Caust., *Chel.*, Cic., Cimic., Cocc., Coloc., Con., Croc., **Cup.**, *Dig.*, Dulc., Glon., HYOS., *Ign.*, K. br., *Lach.*, LYC., Merc., *Nat. c.*, Nux m., Nux v., Oleand., *Op.*, Par., *Phos.*, **Plat.**, Pb., Rhus., Sec. c., Sep., Squ., STRAM., Sul., VERAT. A., Zinc.

Memory Active.—Acon., Anac., Aur., BELL., Coff., Croc., Cyc., HYOS., Op., *Phos.*, Seneg., *Vio. o.*

Memory Lost.—*Abs.*, Agn., ANAC., Bar. ac., Bar. c., BELL., *Bry.*, *Calc. ph.*, Camph., **Cannab. i.**, *Carb. sul.*, *Chel.*, *Cocc.*, Con., Cyc., Dig., GLON., *Graph.*, Hell., HYOS., Hyper., K. br., K. carb., **Lyc.**, Meli., **Merc.**, Mez., *Nat. c.*, Nat. m., NUX M., Oleand., Op., Petrol., PHOS., Pho. ac., PB., *Puls.*, Rhus., *Sele.*, Sep., *Sil.*, Spig., Staph., Stram., Sul., Tell., VERAT. A., Zinc.

Memory Weak.—*Acon.*, *Agar.*, Alum., Am. carb., ANAC., Arn., *Ars.*, Aur., **Bap.**, *Bar. c.*, BELL., **Bov.**, Bry., **Calc. c.**, *Carb. sul.*, **Carb. v.**, Caust., Cocc., **Colch.**, **Con.**, **Croc.**, Crotal., **Cup.**, Cyc., Dig., **Graph.**, **Guai.**, Hell., Hep., HYOS., *Ign.*, K. carb., *K. br.*, **Kre.**, Lach., Laur., **LYC.**, MERC., Mez., Mos., **Nat. m.**, Nux m., Oleand., *Op.*, Petrol., Phos., Pho. ac., Plat., Pb., *Puls.*, Rhodo., Rhus., *Sabi.*, Sele., *Sep.*, *Sil.*, Spig., *Staph.*, **Stram.**, Stro., Sul., Sul. ac., VERAT. A., *Verb.*, Vio. o., *Zinc.*

Stupefaction.—Acon., Agar., Alum., *Ant. t.*, APIS, Arg., **Arn.**, **Ars.**, Asar., *Bar. c.*, BELL., Bov., Bry., *Caj.*, Calc. c., Camph., *Cannab. s.*, Caps., Carb. ac., *Carb. sul.*, Caust., *Cham.*, Chel., Chin., Cic., COCC., *Coff.*, Con., *Crotal.*, **Cup.**, Dulc., **Gel.**, Graph., Hell., Hyd. ac., HYOS., Ip., *K. carb.*, **K. nit.**, Lach., **Laur.**, Led., **Lyc.**, **Mag. m.**, Meli., *Merc.*, **Merc.**

INTELLECT.

c., *Mez., Mosch.,* Mur. ac., Nat. c., **Nat. m., Nux m., Nux v.,** *Oleand.,* **OP., PHOS.,** PHO. AC., Pb., **Puls.,** Rheum, *Rhodo.,* **RHUS,** Saba., *Sec. c.,* Sep., **Sil.,** Spig., Stan., **STRAM.,** Sul., Tar., **Ter.,** Thuj., *Valer.,* VERAT. A., Verb., Zinc.

Unconsciousness.—*Abs.,* Acon., *Aconin., Act., Agar.,* Agn., **Ail.,** Alum., Ambr., Am. carb., Anac., Ant. t., **Apis., Arn.,** Ars., Asar., **Bar. c., BELL.,** Bov., *Bry., Calc. c.,* **Camph., CANNAB. I.,** Cannab. s., *Canth., Carb. ac., Carb. sul., Cham.,* Chel., *Chen. a.,* Chin., **Cic., Cina,** Cocc., Colch., *Con., Crotal.,* **Cup.,** Gel., Glon., Guai., **Hell., HYD. AC., HYOS.,** Ip., K. carb., Lach., Laur., *Lyc.,* Merc., Mez., Mos., **Mur. ac.,** Nat. c., **Nat. m.,** *Nit. ac.,* Nux m., *Nux v., Oleand.,* **OP.,** Petrol., **Phos., PHO. AC.,** *Plat., Pb., Puls.,* Ran. b., Rheum, Rhodo., **Rhus,** Ruta, Sec. c., Sele., Sep., **Sil.,** Spig., Stan., Staph., **Stram.,** Sul., *Tar.,* Valer, *Verat. a.,* Vio. o.

Vertigo.—ACON., *Aeth.,* **Agar.,** Agn., *Aloe., Alum.,* Ambr., Am. carb., Am. m., *Anac., Ant. cr.,* Ant. t., APIS., *Arg.,* Arg. n., Arn., Ars., Asaf., Asar., **Aur., Bap.,** Bar. c., BELL., Bism., Bor., *Bov.,* BRY., *Cact.,* Calad., CALC. C., *Calc. i., Calc. ph.,* **Camph., CANNAB. I., Cannab. s., Canth.,** *Caps., Carb. ac., Carb. an., Carb. sul.,* **Carb. v., Caust.,** *Cham.,* **Chel.,** Chin., *Chrom. ac.,* **Cic.,** Cimic., *Coca,* **COCC.,** Coff., Coloc., **CON.,** Croc., *Crotal.,* **Cup.,** Cyc., **Dig.,** Dros., *Dub.,* **Dulc.,** *Eryng., Euphorb.,* Euphr., *Fer.,* GEL., Glon., *Gran., Graph.,* **Hell.,** *Hep.,* Hyd. ac., **Hyos.,** *Ign.,* Iod., *Ip., K. carb.,* K. nit., Kalm., Kre., **Lach.,** Laur., Led., Lob. i., *Lyc.,* Mag. c., Mag. m., Meli., Meny., **Merc.,** *Mez.,* **Mos.,** **Mur. ac.,** *Nat. c.,* **Nat. m.,** Nit. ac., Nux m., **NUX V.,** *Oleand.,* ONOS., **OP.,** *Oxyt., Pall.,* Par., Petrol., **PHOS.** Pho. ac., **Phyt.,** Plat., Pb., **Pso.,** P.ULS., Ran. b., Ran. s., *Rheum, Rhodo.,* **RHUS,** Ruta, *Saba.,* **Sabi., Sal. ac.,** Samb., **SANG.,** Sars., *Sec. c.,* **Sele., Seneg.,** Sep., **Sil.,** Spig., *Spo., Squ.,* Stan., *Staph.,* **Stram.,** Stro., **SUL.,** *Sul. ac.,* **TAB.,** *Tar.,* **Ter.,** Ther., Thuj., Valer., Verat. a., Verat. v., Verb., *Vio. o.,* Zinc.

Drugs which have Concomitants of Mental Symptoms.—ACON., Agar., *Alum.,* Ambr. *Amm. carb.,* Am. m., Anac., *Ant. cr.,* Ant. t., **Arg., Arn., Ars.,** Asaf., **Aur.,** Bar. c., Bell., Bov., *Bry.,* Calad., **CALC. C., Camph.,** *Canth., Carb. an.,* Carb. v., Caust., **Cham.,** Chel., *Chin.,* Cic., Cina, *Cocc.,* Coff., Coloc., Con., *Croc., Cup.,* Dig., Dulc., *Fer.,* **Graph.,** **Hell.,** *Hep.,* **Hyos.,** *Ign.,* Iod., *Ip.,* K. carb., K. nit., **Lach., Laur.,** Led., *Lyc.,* Mag. c., *Mag. m.,* **Merc.,** Mez., Mosch., Nat. c., *Nat. m., Nit. ac., Nux. m.,* **NUX V.,** Oleand., Op., Par., *Petrol.,* **PHOS.,** Pho. ac., **Plat., Pb., PULS., Ran. s., Rhodo.,** *Rhus,* Ruta, *Saba.,* **Sabi.,** Sars. **Sec. c.,**

Sele., Seneg., *Sep.*, Sil., *Spig.*, Spo., Squ., Stan., Staph., STRAM., *Stro.*, *Sul.*, Verat. a., Verb., Zinc.

Internal Head.

In general.—*Abrot.*, ACON., *Aconin.*, *Agn.*, *Agar.*, *All. c.*, *Aloe*, *Alum.*, *Ambr.*, Am. carb., *Am. m.*, *Am. br.*, *Amyl.*, Anac., *Ant. cr.*, *Ant. t.*, Apoc. c., *Arg.*, Arn., *Ars.*, *Asaf.*, *Asar.*, *Aur.*, Bap., *Bar. c.*, BELL., Bism., *Bor.*, *Bov.*, Bry., *Calc. ac.*, Calc. c., *Calc. ph.*, Camph., CANNAB. I., Cannab. s., *Canth.*, Caps., Carb. an., Carb. v., *Carb. sul.*, *Caust.*, Cham., *Chel.*, Chin., *Cic.*, *Cimic.*, *Cina*, Clem., Cocc., *Coc. c.*, *Cod.*, Coff., *Colch.*, Coloc., Con., *Croc. Cup.*, Cyc., *Dig.*, Dros., *Dulc.*, *Elaps.*, *Epiph.*, *Eucal.*, Euphorb., Euph., Fer., *Fer. ph.*, GEL., GLON., Graph., *Guai.*, Hell., Hep., Hyos., *Hyper.*, IGN., Iod., Ip., Iris. v., K. carb., *K. nit.*, Kre., Lach., Laur., Led., Lyc., *Mag. m.*, *Mang.*, Mar., *Meli.*, *Meny.*, MERC., *Merc. c.*, Mez., *Mos.*, *Mur. ac.*, Nat. c., NAT. M., Nit. ac., Nux m., NUX V., *Oleand.*, *Onos.*, *Op.*, *Par.*, PETROL., PHOS., Phos. ac., *Phyt.*, Plat., *Pb.*, Puls., *Ran. b.*, *Ran. s.*, Rheum, Rhodo., *Rhus*, Ruta, SABA., SABI., Samb., SANG., *Sars.*, Sec. c., *Sele.*, *Seneg.*, Sep., SIL., Spig., *Spo.*, Squ., Stan., Staph., Stram., Stro., SUL., *Sul. ac.*, Tar., *Thea*, *Ther.*, Thuj., *Valer.*, Verat. a., *Verat. v.*, VERB., Vio. o., Vio. t., Zinc.

Forehead.—ACON., *Aconin.*, *Aesc.*, *Aeth.*, Agar., *Agn.*, Ail., Aloe, *Alum.*, *Ambr.*, AM. CARB., AM. M., *Anac.*, Antip., Ant. cr., Ant. t., Apis., *Arg.*, Arg. n., *Arn.*, ARS., *Asaf.*, Asar., *Aur.*, *Bar. c.*, BELL., BISM., *Bor.*, *Bov.*, BRY., Calc. c., *Calc. ph.*, Camph., *Cannab i.*, *Cannab. s.*, *Canth.*, CAPS., Carb. ac., *Carb. an.*, *Carb. sul.*, Carb. v., *Caust.*, Ced., *Cham.*, Chel., Chin., *Cic.*, Cina, Cinnab., Clem., COCC., *Coff.*, *Colch.*, *Coloc.*, Con., *Croc.*, *Cup.*, Cyc., Dig., DROS., Dulc., *Euphorb.*, Euphr., Fer., Gel., *Glon.*, *Gran.*, Graph., *Guai.*, *Ham.*, *Hell.*, HEP., HYOS., IGN., *Iod.*, *Ip.*, *Iris v.*, *K. br.*, K. carb., *K. iod.*, *K. nit.*, Kre., Lach., LAUR., Led., *Lyc.*, Mag. c., Mag. m., *Mang.*, Mar., Meny., MERC., *Merc. i. f.*, MEZ., *Mosch.*, *Mur. ac.*, *Naj.*, *Nat. ars.*, NAT. C., NAT. M., Nit. ac., *Nux m.*, NUX V., *Oleand.*, *Onos.*, *Op.*, *Par.*, Petrol., PHOS., Pho. ac., *Phyt.*, Plat., *Pb.*, Puls., Ran. b., Ran. s., Rheum, *Rhodo.*, *Rhus*, *Rumex*, *Ruta*, Saba., Sabi., Samb., *Sang.*, Sars., Sec. c., *Sele.*, *Seneg.*, Sep., SIL., SPIG., Spo., Squ., STAN., Staph., *Stict.*, *Stram.*, Stro., Sul., *Sul. ac.*, *Tar.*, Thuj., *Valer.*, Verat. a., Verb., Vio. o., *Vio. t.*, Zinc.

Temples.—*Abrot.*, *Acon.*, *Aconin.*, *Agn.*, *Agar.*, *All. c.*, Alum., Ambr., Am. Carb., Am. m., ANAC., Ant. cr., Ant. t., ARG., *Arn.*, Ars., *Asaf.*

INTERNAL HEAD.

Asar., Aur., Bar. c., **Bell.**, *Bism.*, Bor., Bov., *Bry.*, *Cact.*, *Calc. ac.*, **Calc. c.**, *Calc. i.*, Camph., *Cannab. i.*, Cannab. s., *Canth.*, *Caps.*, *Carb. ac.*, Carb. an., Carb. v., Caust., Cham., Chel., CHIN., *Cina*, *Clem.*, **Cocc.**, Coff., Colch., *Coloc.*, Con., *Croc.*, *Cup.*, CYC., *Dig.*, Dros., *Dulc.*, Euphorb., Euphr., *Fl. ac.*, Graph., *Guai.*, *Hell.*, Hep., Hyos., Ign., Iod., Ip., K. CARB., K. nit., KRE., *Lach.*, *Laur.*, Led., *Lob. i.* *Lyc.*, **Mag. c.**, Mag. m., **Mang.**, *Mar.*, Meng., **Merc.**, *Merc. cor.*, *Mez.*, Mos., *Mur. ac.*, Nat. c., *Nat. m.*, *Nit. ac.*, NUX M., Nux. v., *Oleand.*, PAR., **Petrol.**, *Phel.*, *Phos.*, **Phos. ac.**, PLAT., Pb., PULS., *Ran. b.*, *Ran. s.*, Rheum, *Rhodo.*, **Rhus**, Ruta, **Saba.**, SABI., *Samb.*, *Sars.*, *Seneg.*, Sep., *Sil.*, *Spig.*, Spo., *Squ.*, **Stan.**, *Staph.*, *Stram.*, *Stro.*, **Sul.**, **Sul. ac.**, *Tar.*, THUJ., *Usn.*, Valer., Verat. a., VERB., *Vio. t.*, Zinc.

Sides of Head.—Acon., *Agar.*, Alum., Am. carb., Am. m., Anac., Ant. t., Arg., *Arg. n.*, Arn., Ars., **Asaf.**, Asar., Aur., *Bar. c.*, Bell., Bor., **Bov.**, Bry., *Cact.*, Calc. c., Camph., Cannab. s., **Canth.**, *Caps.*, Carb. an., Carb. v., Caust., Cham., Chel., Chin., Cic., Cina, *Clem.*, Cocc., Coff., Colch., Coloc., Con., *Croc.*, Cup., Cyc., Dig., Dros., Dulc., Euphorb., Euphr., Fer., *Graph.*, **Guai.**, Hell., Hep., Hyos., Ign., Iod., *K. carb.*, **Kre.**, Lach., **Laur.**, Led., *Lyc.*, *Mag. c.*, *Mag. m.*, *Mang.*, Mar., Meny., Merc., Mez., Mos., Mur. ac., Nat. c., Nat. m., Nit. ac., Nux m., *Nux v.*, Oleand., Par., *Petrol.*, Phos., PHO. AC., *Plat.*, Pb., *Puls.*, Rhodo., Rhus, Ruta, Saba., Sabi., **Sars.**, Sep., Sil., *Spig.*, Spo., Squ., Stan., Staph., Stro., *Sul.*, Sul. ac., Tar., Thuj., Valer., **Verat. a.**, **Verb.**, Vio. t., ZINC.

Vertex.—*Ab. c.*, Acon., Agar., *Agn.*, Alum., *Ambr.*, Am. carb., Am. m., *Anac.*, Ant. cr., Ant. t., Arg., Arn., Ars., Asaf., Asar., Aur., Bar. c., **Bell.**, Bor., Bov., **Bry.**, CACT., Calc. c., **Calc. ph.**, Cannab. s., Canth., Caps., **Carb. an.**, Carb. v., *Caust.*, Chel., *Cimic.*, *Chin.*, Cina, *Cocc.*, Colch., Coloc., *Con.*, Croc., **Cup.**, Cyc., Dig., *Dulc.*, Fer., *Glon.*, Graph., Guai., Hell., *Helo.*, Hep., Hyos., *Hyper.*, Ign., Iod., Ip., *Iris v.*, K. carb., K. nit., *Kre.*, *Lach.*, *Laur.*, *Led.*, Lyc., Mag. c., Mang., **Meny.**, Merc., *Merc. i.f.*, **Merc. i. r.**, *Mez.*, Mos., Mur. ac., *Nat. c.*, *Nat. m.*, Nit. ac., Nux m., Nux v., Oleand., **Pall.**, Par., Petrol., *Phel.*, **Phos.**, *Pho. ac.*, Plat., Puls., Ran. b., RAN. S., Rheum, Rhodo., Rhus, Ruta, *Saba.*, Sabi., Samb., Sars., *Sep.*, **Sil.**, **Spig.**, Spo., Squ., *Stan.*, **Staph.**, *Stict.*, *Stram.*, Stro., **Sul.**, Sul. ac., *Ther.*, **Thuj.**, *Valer.*, VERAT. A., *Verb.*, Vio. t., Zinc.

Occiput.—*Acon.*, *Agar.*, Alum., **Ambr.**, Am. carb., Am. m., *Anac.*, Ant. t., Arg., Arn., Ars., Asaf., Asar., Aur., *Bar. c.*, BELL., *Bism.*, Bor., Bov. (Brom.), BRY., *Calc. c.*, Camph., Cannab. s., Canth., Caps., **Carb. ac.**, Carb. an., CARB. V., Caust., **Chel.**, *Chin.*, Cic., CIMIC., Cina, *Clem.*,

2*

INTERNAL HEAD.

Coca, Cocc., Coff., **Colch.**, Con., *Croc., Crotal.,* Cup., Cyc., Dig., *Dros.*, Dulc., *Euphorb.*, Euphr., *Eup. per.*, **Gel.**, *Graph.*, Guai., *Hell.*, Hep., **Ign.**, Iod., Ip., *Jug. r.*, K. carb., **K.** nit., Kre., Laur., Led., *Lyc.*, *Mag. c.*, **Mag. m.**, *Mang.*, Mar., *Meny.*, *Merc.*, **Mez., Mos** *Mur. ac.*, **Nat. c.**, Nat. m., *Nit. ac.*, Nux m., **Nux v.**, Oleand., *Onos., Op., Par.*, PETROL., *Phos.*, Pho. ac., **Pic. ac.**, Plat., Pb., *Pso.*, **Puls.**, *Ran. b.*, Ran. s., Rhodo., *Rhus*, Ruta, Saba., **Sabi.**, Samb., *Sang., Sars., Sec. c.*, Seneg., **Sep.**, SIL., *Spig., Spo., Squ.*, *Stan.*, Staph., *Stict.*, Stro., **Sul., Sul. ac.**, *Tar.*, Thuj., Valer., Verat. a., **Verb.**, Vio. t., Zinc.

One-sided in General.—Acon., Agar., *Agn.*, ALUM., Ambr., Am. carb., *Am. m.*, ANAC., Ant. cr., *Ant. t.*, **Arg.**, *Arn.*, Ars., ASAF., *Asar.*, Aur., **Bar. c.**, *Bell.*, Bism., Bor., *Bov.*, Bry., **Calc. c.**, Camph., Cannab. s., **Canth.**, Caps., Carb. an., *Carb. v., Caust., Ced.*, Cham., *Chel., Chin.*, Cic., **Cina**, Clem., *Cocc.*, Coff., Colch., *Coloc.*, Con., *Croc.*, Cup., **Cyc.**, Dig., Dros., **Dulc.**, Euphorb., Euphr., Fer., *Graph.*, Guai., *Hell.*, Hep., Hyos., **Ign.**, Iod., K. CARB., K. nit., *Kre.*, Lach., *Laur., Lsd., Lyc.*, *Mag. c., Mag. m.*, **Mang.**, *Mar., Meny., Merc.*, **Mez.**, Mos., **Mur. ac.**, Nat. c., Nat. m., *Nit. ac., Nux m., Nux v.*, **Oleand., Par.**, Petrol., **Phos.**, PHO. AC., PLAT., *Pb., Puls.*, Ran. b., Ran. s., Rheum, *Rhodo.*, Rhus, Ruta, Saba., **Sabi.**, Samb., SARS., Sele., Seneg., Sep., Sil., Spig., *Spo., Squ., Stan.*, Staph., **Stro.**, Sul., SUL. AC., *Tar.*, Thuj., Valer., Verat. a., VERB., Vio. o., Vio. t., Zinc.

External Head.

Motions of Head.—*Agar.*, Agn., Alum., Am. t., Arg., *Asar.*, Aur., BELL., Bry., **Camph.**, Canth., Caust., *Cham.*, Chin., CIC., **Cina**, *Cocc.*, Colch., **CUP.**, Dig., Fer., *Hell.*, Hep., **Hyos.**, **Ign.**, K. carb., Kre., *Lach.*, **Led.**, Lyc., **Merc.**, Nat. m., Nux m., Nux v., Oleand., *Op.*, Par., Phos., **Pho. ac.**, Puls., Rheum, Rhus, **Sep.**, Spig., **Spo.**, Staph., **Stram.**, *Tar.*, Verat. a., Vio. o., Vio. t.

General Sensations in External Head.—Acon., *Agar.*, Agn., **Alum.**, *Ambr.*, Am. ca. ?., *Arg.*, ARN., *Ars.*, Asar., Aur., BAR. C., **BELL.**, Bism., Bor., Bov., *Bry.*, CALC. C., *Cannab. s.*, Canth., Caps., *Carb. an.*, *Carb. v.*, **Caust.**, *Cham.*, Chel., **Chin.**, Cina, Clem., Cocc., *Coc. c.*, Coloc., Cyc., *Dig.*, *Dros.*, Fer., **Graph.**, Guai., *Hell.*, Hep., Hyos., Ign., Iod., *Ip.*, K. carb., *K. nit.*, Kre., Lach., *Laur.*, Led., Lyc., *Mag. m.*, Mang., **Meny.**, **Merc.**, **Mez.**, Mos., *Mur. ac.*, Nat. c., **Nat. m.**, *Nit. ac.*, Nux m., **NUX V.**, OLEAND., Op., **Par.**, *Petrol.*, Phos., *Pho. ac.*, Plat., *Puls.*, *Ran. b.*, *Ran. s.*, Rhodo., RHUS, RUTA, *Saba.*, Sars., *Sele.*, Sep., SIL., Spig., *Spo.*, Stan., STAPH., Sul., Sul. ac., Tar., Thuj., Verat. a., Vio. o., Zinc.

Hair.—*Acon.*, Agar., Alum., Ambr., Am. carb., Ant. cr., *Arg. n.*, *Arn.*, Ars., Asar., Aur., Bar. c., BELL., BOR., Bov., Bry., Calc. c., **Calc. p.**, *Canth.*, Caps., *Carb. an.*, **Carb. v.**, *Caust.*, Chel., **Chin.**, **Cina**, Cocc., Colch., *Con.*, Cyc., Dulc., Fer., *Fl. ac.*, GRAPH., HEP., *Ign.*, *Iod.*, K. CARB., K. nit., *Kre.*, Lach., *Laur.*, LYC., Mag. c., Mag. m., Mang., Meny., **Merc.**, *Mez.*, Mur. ac., Nat. c., NAT. M., **Nit. ac.**, *Nux v.*, *Par.*, **Petrol.**, Phos., *Pho. ac.*, Pb., Puls., Rhus, Saba., Sars., Sec. c., **Sele.**, **Sep.**, **Sil.**, *Spig.*, *Spo.*, Staph., SUL., Sul. ac., Thuj., **Verat. a.**, Zinc.

Dark Hair.—ACON., Ambr., *Am. m.*, **Anac.**, *Ant. cr.*, Arg., **Arn.**, **Ars.**, Asar., *Bell.*, Bry., Calc. c., *Cannab. s.*, Caps., **Carb. v.**, **Caust.**, *Chin.*, Clem., Con., Dros., Dulc., Euphr., *Graph.*, Guai., Hell., Hep., Ign., Iod., Ip., **K. carb.**, Lach., *Led.*, Lyc., Mag. m., Merc., **Mos.**, Mur. ac., *Nat. c.*, **Nat. m.**, NIT. AC., NUX V., *Oleand.*, Petrol., PHOS., **Pho. ac.**, PLAT., *Pb.*, Puls., Rheum, Rhodo, Rhus, Ruta, Sabi., Sars., SEP., Sil, *Stan.*, **Staph.**, **Sul.**, Verat. a., *Verb.*, Zinc.

Light Hair.—Agar., Ambr., Am. m., *Ars.*, Aur., Bar. c., Bell., **Bor.**,

EXTERNAL HEAD.

Bov., Bry., CALC. C., CAPS., Caust., Cham., Cina, **Clem.**, COCC., Coff., Con., *Croc., Cup.*, **Dig.**, Euphorb., Fer., Graph., Hell., **Hep.**, HYOS., Ign., Iod., *Ip.*, K. carb., Lach., Laur., Lyc., *Mag. c.*, Mag. m., **Merc., Mez.**, Mos., Mur. ac., *Nat. c.*, Nux v., Op., Petrol., Phos., *Pho. ac.*, Plat., **Puls.**, Rheum, Rhus, Ruta, *Saba.*, **Sele.**, Seneg., Sep., SIL., **Spig.**, Spo., Stan., Staph., *Stram.*, Sul., Sul. ac., Thuj., *Verat. a.*, Vio. o.

Scalp.—*Acon., Agar., Alum.,* Ambr., Anac., Ant. cr., *Ant. t.*, Arg., Arn., ARS., Aur., *Bap.*, Bar. c., Bell., **Bor.**, *Bov., Bry.*, CALC. C., *Canth.,* Caps., Carb. an., *Carb. v., Caust.*, **Chel.**, Chin., Cic., *Clem., Cyc., Dros., Fer.,* Graph., Hell., **Hep.**, *K. carb., Laur., Led., Lyc.*, Mag. c., Mag. m., MERC., *Merc. i. f.*, MEZ., Mos., Mur. ac., **Nat. m.**, *Nit. ac.*, Nux v., OLEAND., *Par.*, Petrol., Phos., *Puls.*, Ran. s., RHUS, **Ruta**, *Saba.*, Sars., Sele., **Sep.**, SIL., *Spig.*, STAPH., *Still.*, SUL., *Sul. ac.*, Thuj., *Vinc., Vio. t.,* Zinc.

Skull.—Agn., Ant. cr., *Arg.*, **Arg. n.**, Ars., **Asaf., AUR.**, Bar. c., **Bell.**, Bry., **Calc. c.**, *Calc. ph., Canth.*, CAPS., Carb. v., Caust., Cham., Chin., *Clem.*, Cocc., *Cup., Fl. ac.*, Graph., *Guai.*, **Hep.**, Ign., *Ip.*, K. nit., Lyc., *Mang.*, MERC., *Merc. c., Mez.*, Nat. m., NIT. AC., Nux v., **Phos., Pho. ac.**, *Puls.*, Rhodo., *Rhus*, RUTA, Saba., *Sabi., Samb.*, Sep., Sil., *Spig.*, Staph., *Still.*, *Sul.*, Thuj., Verat. a., *Vio. t.,* Zinc.

Beard.—*Agar.,* Ambr., **Calc. c.**, Graph., **Mez.**, Nat. c., **Nat. m.**, *Nit. ac.*, Pb., Sil.

Margins of Hair.—Calc. c., **Nat. m.**, *Petrol.,* Sep., *Tell.*

Scalp of Occiput.—*Ambr.*, Am. carb., Am. m., Ant. cr., *Ant. t.*, Ars., Bar. c., Bell., *Bor.*, Bry., **Calc. c.**, *Carb. an.*, CARB. V., *Caust., Chel., Chin.,* Clem., *Cyc.*, Euphorb., *Graph.*, **Hep.**, *Iod.,* Lyc., Merc., Mez., Nat. c., *Nat. m.*, Nit. ac., *Oleand.*, PETROL., Puls., Rhus, *Ruta*, **Sep.**, SIL., Spig., **Staph.**, Sul., *Tell.*, Thuj., *Vio. o.*, Zinc.

Behind the Ears.—*Alum.,* Ambr., Am. carb., Am. m., Anac., Ant. cr., **Arg., Arn.**, Aur., BAR. C., **Bell.**, *Bry.*, **Calc. c.** Cannab. s., **Canth.**, Carb. an., Carb. v., CAUST., Chel., Chin., *Cic.*, Cina, Cocc., **Con.**, Dros., GRAPH., Hell., **Hep.**, *K. carb., K. nit.*, Lach., Lyc., *Meny.*, Merc., **Mez., Mur. ac.**, *Nit. ac.*, Oleand., PETROL., Phos., *Pho. ac., Pso.*, **Puls.**, *Rhus*, Ruta, Saba., Sabi., Sars., Sele., Sep., SIL., Spo., Stan., STAPH., Sul., Tar., Thuj., Verb., **Vio. t.**, Zinc.

On Temples.—*Alum.,* Anac., Ant. cr., **Arg.**, *Asar.*, Bar. c., **Bell.**, Bry., **Calc. c.**, Carb. v., Caust., Chel., **Chin.**, *Cocc., Cyc.*, **Dros.**, Ign., K. carb., Kre., Lach., Lyc., Mang., Merc., Mur. ac., NAT. M., *Nit. ac., Par., Petrol.*, Phos., *Pho. ac.*, Plat., **Puls.**, *Rhus*, Saba., **Sabi.**, Sep., Sil., *Sul. ac.*, **Thuj.**, Zinc.

EXTERNAL HEAD—INTERNAL HEAD. 29

On sides of Head.—Agar., Ambr., Ars., *Bar. c.*, Bov., **Carb. an.**, **Caust.**, Coloc., Dros., **Graph.**, *Guai.*, *K. carb.*, Lyc., Nit. ac., Phos., Pho. ac., *Ruta*, *Sars.*, **Staph.**, Thuj., *Verat. a.*, Vio. t., ZINC.

On Forehead.—Alum., *Ambr.*, *Ant. cr.*, *Aur.*, Bar. c., **Bov.**, Calc. c., **Carb. an.**, **Carb. v.**, Caust., Chel., *Cic.*, **Clem.**, *Con.*, **Dros.**, *Graph.*, HEP., Iod., Kre., LED., *Lyc.*, *Meny.*, **Merc.**, *Mur. ac.*, **Nat. m.**, *Nit. ac.*, Nux v., Par., **Phos.**, PHO. AC., *Pso.*, Rhodo., **Rhus**, Saba., Sars., SEP., *Sil.*, *Spig.*, **Staph.**, SUL., Verat. a., *Vio. o.*, Vio. t., Zinc.

Hairy Sinciput. *Agar.*, Alum., Am. carb., Am. m., *Anac.*, ARS., **Bar. c.**, **Bell.**, Bism., Bry., Calc. c., *Carb. v.*, Cic., *Con.*, Dros., Dulc., **Graph.**, Hep., *K. carb.*, Kre., *Lyc.*, Mag. c., *Mag. m.*, MERC., *Mez.*, *Nat. c.*, **Nat. m.**, Oleand., *Par.*, **Petrol.**, **Phos.**, Plat., *Ran. b.*, *Saba.*, *Sep.*, Sil., Staph., *Sul.*, *Thuj.*, **Vio. t.**, Zinc.

Scalp of Vertex.—Agar., Ars., **Bar. c.**, Bry., **Calc. c.**, **Carb. an.**, **Carb. v.**, *Caust.*, Cup., GRAPH., Hep., Lyc., *Meny.*, *Mez.*, Nit. ac., Par., Phos., Pb., **Ran. s.**, Sele., *Sep.*, **Sil.**, *Spig.*, Spo., Squ., **Staph.**, **Verat. a.**, Zinc.

Internal Head.

Left Side.—Acon., Agar., Agn., Alum., Ambr., *Am. carb.*, Am. m., *Anac.*, **Ant. cr.**, **Ant. t.**, **Apis.**, **Arg.**, *Arg. n.*, **Arn.**, *Ars.*, Asaf., Asar., Aur., Bar. c., **Bell.**, Bism., Bor., **Bov.**, BROM., Bry., Calad., **Calc. c.**, Camph., Cannab. s., **Canth.**, **Caps.**, *Carb. an.*, **Carb. v.**, *Caust.*, Ced., Cham., **Chel.**, *Chin.*, **Cic.**, Cina, *Clem.*, Cocc., Coff., *Colch.*, **Coloc.**, Con., **Croc.**, *Cup.*, **Cyc.**, **Dig.**, *Dios.*, Dros., *Dulc.*, **Euphorb.**, Euphr., *Fer.*, **Fl. ac.**, **Graph.**, Guai., **Hell.**, Hep., Hyos., Ign., **Iod.**, *Ip.*, **K. carb.**, *K. nit.*, Kre., **Lach.**, *Laur.*, Led., Lyc., **Mag. c.**, *Mang.*, Mar., *Meny.*, **Merc.**, **Mez.**, Millef., Mos., *Mur. ac.*, **Nat. c.**, **Nat. m.**, **Nat. s.**, Nit. ac., **Nux m.**, *Nux v.*, Oleand., Op., **Par.**, *Petrol.*, Phos., *Pho. ac.*, **Plat.**, Pb., **Pso.**, **Puls.**, Ran. b., **Ran. s.**, **Rheum**, Rhodo., *Rhus*, Ruta, Saba., *Sabi.*, **Samb.**, **Sang.**, *Sars.*, Sec. c., **Sele.**, Seneg., SEP., Sil., Spig., *Spo.*, Squ., *Stan.*, **Staph.**, Stram., Stro., **Sul.**, *Sul. ac.*, Tar., Thuj., Valer., *Verat. a.*, **Verb.**, Vio. o., Vio. t., **Zinc.**

Right Side.—Acon., *Agar.*, *Agn.*, **Alum.**, Ambr., Am. carb., *Am. cur.*, An. ac., Ant. cr., Ant. t., *Apis.*, Arg., *Arn.*, Ars., *Asaf.*, Asar., Aur., **Bar. c.**, BELL., Bism., Bor., Bov., Brom., Bry., *Calad.*, CALC. C., Camph., *Cannab. s.*, **Canth.**, *Caps.*, Carb. an., CARB. V., **Caust.**, Ced., Cham., **Chel.**, Chin., Cic., **Cina**, Clem., Cocc., Coff., *Colch.*, Coloc., Con., **Croc.**, Cup., Cyc., Dig., *Dros.*, **Dulc.**, Euphorb., Euphr., Fer., **Fl. ac.**, **Graph.**, Guai., *Hell.*, **Hep.**, *Hyos.*, IGN., Iod., K. carb., K. nit., Kre., **Lach.**, Laur., **Led.**, **Lyc.**, *Mag. c.*, Mang., Mar., Meny., Merc., *Merc. i. f.*,

Mez., Millef., Mos., Mur. ac., Nat. c., **Nat. m.**, Nit. ac., *Nux m.,* **Nux v.,** *Oleand.,* Op., Par., Petrol., *Phos., Pho. ac., Plat.,* **Pb.,** *Pru., Pso.,* **Puls., Ran. b.,** *Ran. s., Rheum, Rhodo.,* **Rhus,** *Ruta,* SABA., **Sabi.,** Samb., Sang., Sars., Sec. c., Sele., Seneg., *Sep.,* SIL., *Spig.,* Spo., *Squ.,* Stan., Staph., *Stram., Stro., Sul.,* **Sul. ac.,** Tar., **Thuj., Valer., Verat. a., Verb.,** Vio. o., Vio. t., *Zinc.*

External Head.

Left Side.—*Acon.,* Agar., Alum., *Amne.,* Anac., Ant. cr., *Ant. t.,* **Arg., Ars., Asar.,** Aur., *Bar. c.,* Bell., *Bor.,* Calc. c., Caps., **Carb. an.,** *Carb. v., Caust.,* Cham., Chel., Chin., CLEM., *Cocc.,* Coloc., **Dig.,** Dulc., *Euphorb.,* **Graph.,** *Hep.,* Iod., **K. carb.,** K. nit., Laur., *Lyc.,* **Mag. c.,** Mag. m., **Mang.,** Meny., **Merc.,** *Merc. c.,* Millef., *Mur. ac.,* Nat. c., **Nat. m., Nit. ac.,** *Oleand., Onos.,* Petrol., **Phos.,** *Pho. ac., Plat., Rhodo.,* Rhus, RUTA, Seneg., Sep., *Sil., Spig.,* Staph., Stro. Sul., *Tar.,* **THUJ.,** *Verb.,* Vio. t., Zinc.

Right Side.—Agar., *Agn., Alum., Ambr.,* Am. carb., *Am. m.,* **Anac.,** *Aur., Bell.,* Bor., Brom., **Bry.,** CALC. C., CANTH., Caps., Carb. an., Carb. v., Caust., **Chel.,** Chin., Clem., Coloc., CON., Dig., **Dros.,** Graph., *Guai.,* Hep., **Iod., K. carb.,** *K. nit., Kre.,* Laur., **Led.,** Lyc., Mag. m., *Mang.,* Meny., Merc., *Mez.,* Mur. ac., *Nat. c.,* Nat. m., **Nit. ac.,** Petrol., Phos., Pho. ac., Plat., Pso., **Puls.,** Ran. b., *Ran. s.,* Rhodo., **Rhus,** *Saba.,* Sars., **Sep., Sil.,** Spig., *Spo.,* Stan., **Staph.,** Stro., Thuj., *Verat. a.,* Vio. t., Zinc.

Eyes.

Aqueous Humor.—*Colch.,* **Crotal.,** *Merc.,* Pb.

Eyeballs.—ACON., **Agar.,** Agn., *Alum., Ambr.,* Am. carb., Am. m., Anac., Ant. cr., *Ant. t.,* Arg., **Arn., Ars.,** Asaf., **Asar.,** *Aur.,* **Bad., Bap.,** *Bar. c.,* **BELL.,** Bism., *Bor.,* Bov., **Bry.,** Calad., CALC. C., Camph., Cannab. s., *Canth.,* Caps., Carb. an., *Carb. v.,* **Caust.,** *Ced.,* **Cham.,** Chel., *Chin.,* Cic., **Cimic.,** Cina, **Clem.,** Cocc., Coff., Colch., *Coloc.,* Com., **Con., Croc.,** *Crot. tig.,* Cup., Cyc., **Dig., Dros.,** Dulc., Euphorb., **EUPHR.,** *Eup. per.,* Fer., **Gel., Graph.,** Guai., **Hell., HEP., Hyd. ac., Hyos.** *Ign.,* Iod., **Ip., K. carb.,** K. nit., *Kre.,* Lach., Laur., *L d.* **Lyc.,** *Mag. c.,* Mag. m., Mang., Mar., Meny., **Merc.,** *Mez.,* Mos., Mur. ac., Nat. c., *Nat. m., Nit. ac.,* Nux m., **Nux v.,** Oleand., *Onos.,* Op., *Oz. ac.,* Par., *Petrol.,* **Phos.,** *Pho. ac., Plat.,* Pb., *Pru.,* **Puls.,** Ran. b., *Ran. s., Raph.,* Rheum, Rhodo., Rhus, *Ruta,* Saba., Sabi., Samb., *Sang.,* Sars., Sec. c., **Sele., Seneg.,** Sep., Sil., SPIG., Spo., Squ., **Stan., Staph., Stram.,** Stro., SUL., *Sul. ac.,* Tar., **Thuj.,** Valer., **Verat. a., Verb., Vio. o.,** Vio. t., *Zinc.*

EYES.

Choroid.—Ars., *Gel.*, *Merc.*, *Pso.*

Conjunctiva.—**ACON.**, Agar., Alum., Ambr., Am. carb., *Am. m.*, *Ant. cr.*, **Ant. t.**, **Apis**, Arg., **Arg. n.**, *Arn.*, **Ars.**, **Ars. iod.**, *Asar.*, *Aur.*, *Bar. c.*, **BELL.**, Bism., Bor., **Bry.**, *Calc. c.*, Camph., **CANNAB. I.**, Cannab. s., *Canth.*, Caps., Carb. v., Caust., **Ced.**, *Cham.*, **Chel.**, **Chin.**, Chloral., Cimic., **Clem.**, Cocc., Coff., *Colch.*, Coloc., **Con.**, *Corn. c.*, Croc., *Crotal.*, *Crot. tig.*, Cup., **Dig.**, Dulc., Euphorb., **EUPHR.**, *Fer.*, *Gel.*, *Grind.*, Graph., **Hep.**, *Hydras.*, **Hyos.**, *Ign.*, **Iod.**, *Ip.*, *Iris, v.*, **K. bi.**, *K. carb.*, **K. Iod.**, Lach., *Led.*, **Lyc.**, Mag. c., *Mag. m.*, Mar., **Meli.**, **Merc.**, *Merc. c.*, *Merc. d.*, *Merc. i. f.*, **Merc. i. r.**, *Merc. n.*, *Mez.*, *Naph.*, **NAT. M.**, *Nat. s.*, Nit. ac., **Nux v.**, *Op.*, Petrol., **Phos.**, Pho. ac., **Pic. ac.**, Pb., *Pso.*, **Puls.**, **Ran. b.**, Ran.s., **Rat.**, RHUS, Saba., Samb., **Sars.**, **SEP.**, **Sil.**, *Sin.*, Spig., Stan., Staph., **STRAM.**, Stro., **SUL.**, *Sul. ac.*, Tar., Thuj., **Verat. a.**, *Vesp.*, Vio. o., ZINC.

Cornea.—*Acon.*, Am. carb., Am. m., Ant. t., *Arn.*, **Ars.**, **Ars. iod.**, **Aur.**, Bar. c., *Bell.*, *Bov.*, Bry., **Cad. s.**, CALC. C., *Calc. ph.*, CANNAB. S., Caps., *Carb. sul.*, **Caust.**, *Chel.*, *Chin.*, *Cinnab.*, *Colch.*, CON., *Crotal.*, Cup., *Dig.*, Dulc., Euphorb., **EUPHR.**, Fer., Graph., **Hep.**, *Hydras.*, Hyos., *Ip.*, **K. bi.**, Kre., Lach., Lyc., **Mag. c.**, MERC., *Merc. c.*, **Merc i. f.**, **Merc. i. r.**, Merc. n., Mos., Nat. c., Nat. m., *Nat. s.*, Nit. ac., Nux v. Op., Phos., **Phys.**, **Phyt.**, Pb., **PULS.**, *Rhus*, **Ruta**, Sars., **Seneg.**, Sep. Sil., *Spig.*, Spo., Squ., *Stan.*, Stram., SUL., Tar., *Thuj.*, Valer., Verat. a.

Iris.—*Apis.*, *Asaf.*, *Aur.*, **Bry.**, **Clem.**, *Colch.*, *Coloc.*, *Gel.*, *Grind.*, **Iod.**, *K. bi.*, *Merc. i. f.*, *Nit. ac.*, *Phys.*, *Ran. b.*, Spig., *Ter.*, *Thuj.*

Lachrymal Apparatus.—**Arg. n.**, *Fl. ac.*, *Nat. m.*, *Petrol.*, **Phos.**, Puls., SIL.

Lens (cataract, including gray, green and reticulated cataracts of B).—Acon., Agar., Am. carb., Am. m., Anac., Ant. t., Arn., Ars., Aur., *Bar. c.*, *Bell.*, Bov., Bry., **Calc. c.**, *Calc. fl.*, Cannab. s., Caps., Caust., *Chel.*, *Chin.*, Cina, **Con.**, Croc., *Dig.*, Dulc., Euphorb., **EUPHR.**, **Hep.**, *Hyos.*, Ign., Kre., *Lyc.*, *Mang. c.*, Mang., Merc., Nat. c., *Nat. m.*, *Nit. ac.*, **Op.**, **Phos.**, Pb., **PULS.**, *Rhus*, **Ruta**, Sars., Sec. c., Seneg., Sep., SIL., Spig., Stan., Staph., Stram., **SUL.**, Tar., Valer., Verat. a.

Optic Nerve.—Bell., **Carb. Sul.**, *Dig.*, Lach., *Nux v.*, *Onos.*, Pb.

Adhesions in Pupils.—Calc. c., **Clem.**, *Graph.*, Nit. ac., *Sil.*, *Sul.*

Pupils Contracted.—Acon., *Agar.*, Anac., Ant. t., **Arn.**, *Ars.*, *Aur.*, Bell., Calc. c., Camph., Canth., Caps., Cham., **CHEL.**, **Chin.**, Cic., *Cina*, Clem., COCC., Croc., Dig., Dros., Hell., Hyos., Ign., *Jab.*, *K. br.*, Laur., Led., *Mang.*, Meny., **Mez.**, Mos., Mur. ac., Nux m., Nux v., Oleand., **OP.**, Phos., Pho. ac., Pb., **Puls.**, *Rheum*, Rhodo., (Rhus),

Ruta, Samb., *Sec. c.*, Seneg., SEP., SIL., **Squ.**, *Stan.*, Staph., *Stram.*, SUL., Tar., **Thuj.**, VERAT. A., Vio. o., Vio. t., **Zinc**.

Pupils Dilated.—Acon., *Aconin.*, Agar., Agn., Anac., Apis, Arn., **Ars.**, Asaf., Aur., **BELL.**, CALC. C., Camph., Canth., **Caps.**, *Carb. an.*, Caust., **Chin.**, CIC., *Cimic.*, **Cina**, **Coca**, **Con.**, Croc., Cup., **Cyc.**, **Dig.**, Dros., *Dub.*, **Dulc.**, Euphorb., **Gel.**, *Gran.*, Guai., **Hell.**, **HEP.**, *Hyd. ac.*, HYOS., **Ign.**, **Ip.**, Kre., *Laur.*, **Led.**, **Lyc.**, *Mang.*, (Meny.), **Merc.**, Mez., Mos., Mur. ac., *Nat. c.*, Nit. ac., **Nux v.**, Oleand., OP., Par., *Petrol.*, Phos., *Pho. ac.*, *Pb.*, **Puls.**, Rheum, Rhodo., *Rhus*, *Samb.*, **Sang.**, Sars., **Sec. c.**, SPIG., Squ., Stan., **Staph.**, STRAM., (Tar.), Thuj., Valer., Verat. a., VERAT. V., Verb., **Zinc**.

Pupils Immovable.—Acon., *Apis*, **Bar. c.**, BELL., Cham., Chin., CIC., Cup., **Dig.**, Fer., **Hell.**, Hyos., Laur., **Merc. c.**, **Nit. ac.**, **Op.**, *Pb.*, Ran. b., Seneg., Spig., STRAM.

Retina.—Ars., Bell., *Crotal.*, **Dig.**, Gel., *Kalm.*, Lach., **Merc.**, **Merc. c.**, *Nux v.*, *Onos.*, Phos., **Phys.**, *Sant.*, Sep.

White of Eye (sclerotic).—*Aur.*, **Chel.**, **Clem.**, Merc. c., *Pb.*, **Puls.**, *Sul.*, Ter., **Thuj.**

Vitreous.—*Carb. sul.*, **Gel.**, *Pru.*, Seneg.

Lachrymation.—*Acon.*, Agar., Agn., ALL. C., *Alum.*, Ambr., Am. carb., Am. m., Anac., *Ant. t.*, Apis, Arn, ARS., Asar., **Aur.**, Bar. c., **BELL.**, Bor., Bov., **Bry.**, CALC. C., *Calc. ph.*, Camph., **Canth.**, **Caps.**, *Carb. an.*, **Carb. v.**, *Carb. sul.*, Caust., *Ced.*, **Chel.**, *Cinnab.*, *Chin.*, Cina, **Clem.**, *Coff.*, Colch., **Coloc.**, *Con.*, *Croc.*, **Crot. tig.**, *Dig.*, **Euphorb.**, EUPHR., *Fer.*, *Graph.*, **Hell.**, Hep., **Ign.**, **Iod.**, **K. bi.**, *K. car b.*, **K. iod.**, K. nit., KRE., **Lach.**, Laur., **Led.**, **Lyc.**, Mag. c., *Mar.*, Meny., **Merc.**, Mez., Mos., Mur. ac., *Nat. c.*, NAT. M., *Nat. s.*, **Nit. ac.**, Nux m., Nux v., Oleand., Op., *Osm.*, *Par.*, **Petrol.**, *Phel.*, **Phos.**, *Pho. ac.*, **Plat.**, PULS., Ran. b., Ran. s., Rheum, Rhodo., **Rhus**, RUTA, Saba., Sabi. Sars., Sec. c., **Seneg.**, SEP., SIL., *Sin.*, Spig., Spo., Squ., **Stan.** STAPH., Stram., Stro., SUL., Sul. ac., Tar., TELL., *Thuj.*, Valer. Verat. a., Vio. o., ZINC.

Brows.—Agar., **Agn.**, *Alum.*, Ambr., Am. m., **Arn.**, *Ars.*, *Asaf.*, Bar c., **BELL.**, Bov., Bry., Camph., Cannab. s., Canth., CAUST., Chin., Cina *Cinnab.*, Clem., *Coloc.*, Croc., Cup., *Dig.*, **Dros.**, Euphorb., Guai., **Hell.** Ign., Ip., *Iris v.*, K. CARB., *Laur.*, Mang., Merc., Mos., *Nat. m.*, Nux v., Oleand., *Osm.*, PAR., Petrol., Plat., Pb., *Ran. b.*, Rhodo., *Rhus*, Ruta, SELE., Sep., Sil. *Spig.*, Spo., Stan., Stram., Stro., *Sul.*, Tar., **Thuj.**, Vio. *t.*, Zinc.

Canthi.—Acon., AGAR., **Alum.**, Am. carb., Am. m., Anac., *Ant. cr.*,

EYES.

Amt. t., Arg., *Arg. n.*, Arn., Ars., *Asar.*, **Aur.**, *Bar. c.*, **Bell.**, Bism., **Bor.**, Bov., **Bry.**, CALC. C., Camph., *Carb. an.*, CARB. V., **Caust.**, Cham., *Chel.*, Chin., Cic., *Cina.*, *Clem.*, Coff., Colch., Coloc., *Con.*, Dig., **Euphorb.**, **Euphr.**, *Graph.*, Guai., *Hell.*, Hep., Hyos., *Ign.*, Iod., Ip., *K. carb.*, K. nit., Lach., *Laur.*, Led., Lyc., *Mag. c.*, Mag. m., Mar. Meny., Merc., Mez., Mos., *Mur. ac.*, Nat. c., NAT. M., Nit. ac., NUX V., Oleand., Par., **Petrol.**, PHOS., *Pho. ac.*, Plat., Pb., **PULS.**, **Ran. b.**, *Ran. s.*, Rhodo., Rhus, *Ruta*, Saba., Sars., Seneg., **Sep.**, SIL., Spig. Spo., *Squ.*, **Stan.**, STAPH., *Stro.*, SUL., Sul. ac., Tar., **Thuj.**, Valer., Verat. a., *Zinc.*

Inner Canthus.—Acon., AGAR., **Alum.**, Anac., Ant. cr., **Ant. t.**, *Apis.*, **Arg. n.**, Arn., Asar., **Aur.**, Bar. c., BELL., Bor., *Bry.*, **Calc. c.**, *Calc. ph.*, **Cannab. i.**, *Carb. an.*, **Carb. v.**, **Caust.**, Chel., Cic., Cina, **Clem.**, Coloc., **Con.**, Dig., *Euphr.*, *Gam.*, *Graph.*, *Hell.*, Hyos., *K. bi.*, Lach., *Laur.*, Led., *Lyc.*, **Mag. c.**, Mag. m., Mar., Meny., Merc., Mez., Mos., Mur. ac., Nat. c., *Nat. m.*, Nit. ac., **Nux v.**, *Par.*, **Petrol.**, **Phos.**, *Pho. ac.*, **Puls.**, *Rhodo.*, Rhus, *Ruta*, Sars., *Sep.*, **Sil.**, Spig., **Stan.**, STAPH., Stro., *Sul.*, Sul ac., Tar., *Thuj.*, Valer., Verat. a., ZINC.

Outer Canthus.—Agar., *Alum.*, Anac., Ant. cr., Asar., **Bar. c.**, **Bor.**, *Bry.*, CALC. C., Camph., Carb. an., Carb. v., Cham., Chel., **Chin.**, Cina, Colch., Con., **Euphorb.**, Euphr., GRAPH., Hep., Hyos., *Ign.*, *Ip.*, *K. carb.*, K. nit., Laur., Lyc., Merc., Mos., *Mur. ac.*, Nat. c., **Nat. m.**, Nit. ac., **Nux v.**, Phos., Pho. ac., Puls., RAN. B., Ran. s., Rhus, Ruta, Saba., Sars., Seneg., *Sep.*, Sil., Spig., *Spo.*, **Squ.**, *Stan.*, **Staph.**, Stro., SUL., *Sul. ac.*, Tar., *Thuj.*

Lids.—Acon., *Agar.*, **Agn.**, **Alum.**, *Ambr.*, Am. m., Anac., Ant. cr., Ant. t., APIS, Arg., Arn., **Ars.**, Asaf., Asar., **Aur.**, *Bap.*, Bar. c., BELL., Bor., Bov., **Bry.**, CALC. C., Camph., *Cannab. s.*, Canth., Caps., Carb. an., *Carb.v.*, *Carb. sul.*, CAUST., **Cham.**, *Chel.*, *Chin.*, Cic., Cina, Clem., *Cocaine*, Cocc., *Cod.*, Colch., Coloc., Con., **Croc.**, Cup., *Cyc.*, **Dig.**, Dros., *Dub.*, Dulc., **Euphorb.**, **Euphr.**, *Fer.*, *Fer. ph.*, *Fl. ac.*, GEL., **Graph.**, Guai., Hell., **Hep.**, *Hydras.*, **Hyos.**, **Ign.**, Iod., *Ip.*, *K. carb.*, **K. iod.**, K. nit., *Kre.*, Lach., Laur., Led., **Lyc.**, *Mag. c.*, Mag. m., Mang., **Mar.**, *Meny.*, **Merc.**, *Merc. i.r.*, Mez., Mos., Mur. ac., *Nat. ac.*, NAT. M., Nit. ac., Nux m., **Nux v.**, *Oleand.*, *Onos.*, Op., *Par.*, Petrol., *Phel.*, **Phos.**, **Pho. ac.**, *Phys.*, *Phyt.*, Plat., *Pb.*, **PULS.**, Ran. b., Ran. s., *Raph.*, *Rheum*, *Rhodo.*, RHUS, Ruta, Saba., Sabi., Sars., Sec. c., Sele., *Seneg.*, SEP., Sil., SPIG., *Spo.*, Squ., *Stan.*, **Staph.**, *Stram.*, Stro., SUL., Sul. ac., Tar., Thuj., Valer., **Verat. a.**, Verb., Vio. o., Vio. t., Zinc.

Upper Lids.—Acon., *Agar.*, **Agn.**, **Alum.**, APIS, Arg., Arn., **Ars.**,

EYES.

Asaf., *Asar.,* Aur., Bar. c., **Bell.,** Bor., **Bry.,** **Calc.** c., Camph., *Cannab. s.,* Canth., Carb. an., Carb., v., CAUST., *Cham.,* **Chel.,** Chin., **Cina,** Clem., *Cocaine,* **Cocc.,** Colch., Coloc., *Con.,* **Croc.,** *Cyc.,* *Dulc.,* *Euphorb.,* *Fer.,* GEL., Graph., Hell., **Hep.,** Hyos., Ign., *K. br.,* *K. carb.,* *K. iod.,* **Kre.,** Laur., *Lyc.,* **Mag.** c., Mag. m., *Mang.,* Mar., *Merc.,* Mez., Mos., **Mur.** ac., *Nat. c.,* Nat. m., Nux v., *Oleand.,* Op., *Pœo.,* *Par.,* **Phos.,** *Pho. ac.,* *Pb.,* **Puls.,** Rheum, Rhodo., **Rhus,** Sabi., *Sal. ac., Sang., Seneg.,* SEP., *Sil.,* SPIG., Spo., Squ., *Stan.,* **Staph.,** *Stram.,* **Sul.,** Tar., Thuj., *Ura.,* **Verat. a.,** Vio. o., Zinc.

Lower Lids.—*Agar.,* **Alum.,** *Am. m.,* Arg., **Ars.,** *Ars. iod.,* Asar., Aur., *Bell.,* Bry., CALC. C, *Canth.,* Carb. v., *Caust.,* Cham., Chin., Cic., *Colch.,* Coloc., *Croc.,* **Dig.,** Dros., Euphorb., Euphr., Fer., Graph., Iod., *Lach.,* Laur., Lyc., **Mag.** c., **Merc.,** Mez., Nat. c., **Nat. m.,** Oleand., Petrol., PHO. AC., PULS., *Ran. b.,* **Rhus,** RUTA, Sabi., Sec., c., SENEG., Sep., Sil., Spig., *Stan.,* Sul., Sul. ac., *Zinc.*

Inner Surface of Lids.—Acon., Agar., ARS., **Bell.,** *Bor., Bry., Calc. c.,* Canth., Caust., *Cham., Coc. c., Con.,* Dros., Ign., **K. bi., Merc.,** **Nat. m.,** *Nat. s.,* **Nux v.,** *Par.,* **Phos.,** *Phyt.,* **Puls.,** RHUS, *Sep., Sil.,* Sul.

Margins of Lids.—Acon., *Agar., Ant. cr., Apis, Arg.,* **Arg. n.,** Arn., Ars., *Aur., Bad.,* Bell., BOR., Calc. c., Canth., *Carb. sul.* Cham., *Chel., Cinnab.,* **Clem.,** *Coc. c., Colch.,* **Dig.,** Euphr., Hep., *Hydras., K. bi., Kre.,* Lyc., MERC., *Merc. i. f.,* Mez., **Nat. m.,** Nux v., *Par., Petrol., Pho. ac., Phyt., Pso.,* PULS., Rhus, *Saba., Seneg.,* Sep., *Sil.,* Spig., **Staph.,** *Stram.,* SUL., VALER., *Zinc.*

Orbits.—*Acon.,* Alum., Am. m., *Anac., Ant. cr., Arn., Ars., Arum. t., Asaf.,* Aur., Bar. c., **Bell.,** *Bism., Bov., Bry.,* Calc. c., Camph., Chel., *Chin.,* Cimic., *Cinnab.,* **Clem.,** Cocc., Coloc., Con., *Coral., Cup.,* Dig., *Hell.,* Hep., *Hyos.,* Ign., *Iod., Lach.,* Laur., Led., *Lyc.,* Mag. c., *Meny.,* Merc., Merc. c., Mez., Mur. ac., Nit. ac., Nux m., *Nux. v.,* Oleand., *Osm., Par., Phos.,* Pho. ac., **Plat.,** Pb., **Puls.,** *Rhodo.,* RHUS, Ruta, Sars., *Sele., Seneg.,* Sep., *Sil.,* SPIG., Spo., **Stan.,** Stro., *Sul.,* Sul. ac., VALER., Verat. a., *Verb.,* Zinc.

Squinting.—Alumen., **Bell.,** *Calc. ph., Cannab. i., Cic., Cina,* Gel., Hyos., *Jab., Sal. ac., Stram.,* Zinc.

Staring.—*Acon.,* Am. carb., **Amyl.,** Ant. t., **Arn., Ars.,** *Asar.,* BELL., Bry., *Camph.,* Canth., *Carb. ac.,* Cham., Chin., CIC., Cina, **Cocc., Con., Cup.,** Dig., Glon., *Hell.,* Hep., Hyos., Ign., K. carb., *Laur.,* Merc., Mos., **Mur.** ac., Nux m., *Nux v.,* Op., Pho. ac., *Rhus,* Ruta, SEC. C., *Seneg., Sep.,* Spig., *Spo., Squ.,* STRAM., Sul., **Verat. a.**

Left.—Acon., Agar., All. c., Alum., Ambr., Am. carb., Am. m., Anac., Ant. cr., Ant. t., **Apis,** Arn., Ars., Arum. t., **Asaf., Asar.,** Aur., Bar. c., Bell., Bor., Bov. Brom., **Bry.,** Calad., Calc. c., Camph., Canth., Caps., **Carb. an.,** Carb. v., **Caust.,** Ced., **Chel.,** Chin., Cina, Clem., Colch., Con., Croc., Dros., Euphorb., Euphr., Fer., Fl. ac., Hell., HEP., Ign., Iod., **K. bi.,** K. carb., K. nit., **Lach., Laur.,** Lyc., Mag. c., Mar., Meny., Merc., **Mez.,** Millef., Mur. ac., Nat. m., Nit. ac., Nux v., Oleand., Op., Par., Petrol., Phos., Pho. ac., Plat., **Pb.,** Pso., **Puls.,** Ran. b., Ran. s., Rheum, Rhodo., Rhus, Ruta, Saba., Sabi., Sars., Sele., Seneg., Sep., Sil., **Spig.,** SPO., **Squ., Stan.,** Staph., Stram., Stro., SUL., Sul. ac., **Tar., Thuj.,** Valer., Verat. a., Vio. o., Vio. t., Zinc.

Right.—Acon., Agar., Agn., Alum., Ambr., **Am. carb.,** Am. m., Anac., Ant. cr., Ant. t., **Apis,** Arn., Ars., Asaf., Asar., Aur., Bar. c., BELL., Bism., Bor., Bov., Brom., **Bry.,** Calad., CALC. C., **Camph.,** Cannab. s., **Canth.,** Caps., Carb. an., **Carb. v.,** Caust., Cham., Chel., Chin., **Cic.,** Cina, **Clem.,** Coff., Colch., COLOC., Com., **Con.,** Croc., Cyc., **Dig.,** Dros., Euphorb., **Euphr.,** Fer., **Fl. ac.,** Graph., Guai., Hep., Hyos., Ign., Iod., **K. carb., K. nit.,** Kre., Laur., Led., LYC., Mag. m., **Mang.,** Mar., **Merc.,** Millef., Mur. ac., **Nat. c.,** NAT. M., NIT. AC., Nux m., Nux v., Oleand., **Par.,** PETROL., **Phos.,** Pho. ac., PLAT., **Pb.,** Pru., Pso., Puls., Ran. b., **Ran. s.,** Rheum, Rhodo., RHUS, Ruta, Saba., Sars., Sele., SENEG., SEP., SIL., **Spig.,** Spo., Squ., Stan., **Staph.,** Stram., Sul., Sul. ac., Tar., Thuj., Valer., **Verat. a.,** Vio. t., Zinc.

Vision.

Blindness.—Acon., Am. carb., Anac., Ant. cr., Ant. t., Arn., Ars., **Aur.,** Bar. c., **Bell.,** Calc. c., Cannab. s., Carb. sul., **Caust., Chel.,** Chin., **Cic.,** Cocc., CON., Croc., **Dig.,** Dros., Dulc., Euphorb., Euphr., Fer., **Gel.** Graph., Guai., Helo., Hep., Hyd. ac., HYOS., Iod., K. br., K. carb., K. nit., Kalm., Laur., **Lith.,** Lyc., Mag. c., Merc., Nat. c., **Nat. m.,** Nit. ac., Nux v., Oleand., **Op.,** Petrol., **Phos.,** Pho. ac., Plat., **Pb.,** PULS., Rhus, Ruta, Sars., **Sec. c.,** Seneg., Sep., SIL., Spig., Staph., STRAM., Stro., **Sul.,** Tab., Thuj., Valer., Verat. a., **Verat. v.,** Vio. o., Zinc.

—**Periodical.**—Acon., Am. carb., Anac., Ant. cr., **Ant. t.,** Bar. c., Bell., Cad. s., Calc. c., Caust., **Chel., Chin.,** Con., Croc., Dig., **Euphr.,** Graph., **Hyos.,** K. nit., Lyc., Merc., Nat. c., **Nat. m.,** Nux v., Petrol., **Phos., Pb., Puls.,** Rhus, Ruta, Sec. c., **Sep., Sil.,** Spig., Staph., Stram., **Sul.,** Verat. a.

Dazzling.—Bar. c., **Calc. c.,** Camph., Carb. an., **Caust., Chel., Cic.,**

CON., Dig., **Dros.**, *Euphr.*, Graph., Hyos., Ign., K. CARB., *Lyc.*, Mang., Merc., Nat. c., *Nit. ac.*, *Nux v.*, Oleand., **Phos.**, *Pho. ac.*, **Seneg.**, SIL., Stram., Sul., **Valer.**

Flickering.—*Acon.*, **Agar.**, *Aloe*, *Alum.*, **Am. carb.**, **Ant. t.**, **Aran.**, Ars., **Bell.**, Bor., *Bry.*, Calc. c., *Clem.*, *Carb. v.*, **Caust.**, **Cham.**, *Chel.*, *Chin.*, *Coca*, *Colch.*, *Coloc.*, *Con.*, *Dig.*, Dros., GRAPH., *Hep.*, **Hyos.**, *Ign.*, Iod., LACH., Led., Lyc., Mez., Mur. ac., **Nat. m.**, **Nux v.**, *Oleand.*, *Op.*, Petrol., **Phos.**, Pho. ac., *Plat.*, Puls., Sec. c., **Seneg.**, *Sep.*, **Sil.**, Staph., *Stram.*, Stro., SUL., **Tab.**, Verat. a.

Motions before Vision.—Agar., Aloe, ARG. N., Bell., **Bor.**, *Calc. ph.*, **Cannab. i.**, *Carb. sul.*, **Cic.**, **Con.**, Euphr., Hyos., Ign., **Lach.**, *Laur.*, Lyc., Meny., Merc., *Mos.*, **Nux v.**, Oleand., *Par.*, Petrol., Saba., *Sep.*, *Stram.*

Illusions of Color, Black.—Acon., *Agar.*, Am. m., Aur., Bar. c., **Bell.**, *Calc. c.*, Caps., Carb. v., *Chin.*, *Chloral.*, *Cic.*, **Cimic.**, **Cocc.**, **Con.**, *Dig.*, *Euphr.*, **K. carb.**, **Lach.**, *Lyc.*, **Mag. c.**, Mang., *Merc.*, Mos., Nit. ac., (Nux v.), Petrol., PHOS., Pho. ac., *Phys.*, Ruta, Sec. c., **Sep.**, **Sil.**, *Staph.*, **Stram.**, *Tab.*, Valer., Verat. a,

Bright.—*Aloe*, Alum., *Am. carb.*, **Ant. t.**, Ars., **Aur.**, *Bar. c.*, **Bell.**, Bor., *Bry.*, **Camph.**, **Cannab. s.**, Caust., **Chel.**, *Cic.*, Coloc., **Con.**, **Croc.**, *Dig.*, Dros., Dulc., Euphr., *Fl. ac.*, *Graph.*, **Hyos.**, Ign., *Iod.*, **K. carb.**, Lyc., Mang., Meny., Mez., Nat. m., **Nux v.**, Oleand., Op., Pho. ac., Plat., Puls., Rhus, Sabi., Sec. c., Seneg., *Spig.*, *Stram.*, Stro., **Valer.**, *Verat. a.*, *Vio. o.*, *Zinc.*

Blue.—Bell., *Dig.*, **Lach.**, **Lyc.**, *Stram.*, *Stro.*, Sul., Zinc.

Dark.—Acon., *Agar.*, Ambr., *Am. m.*, **Anac.**, *Arn.*, Ars., Asaf., **Bell.**, **Calc. c.**, Carb. v., *Caust.*, Cham., **Chin.**, Cic., **Cocc.**, **Con.**, Cup., Dig., Dros., Euphr., Fer., *Hep.*, K. carb., Laur., Lyc., *Mag. c.*, Mang., Meny., **Merc.**, *Mosch.*, Mur. ac., *Nat. c.*, *Nat. m.*, **Nit. ac.**, Nux v., Oleand., Op., Petrol., **Phos.**, Pho. ac., Pb., *Ruta*, Saba., Sec. c., **Sep.**, **Sil.**, Squ., **Staph.**, Stram., SUL., Thuj., Verat. a., Verb.

Gray.—*Cic.*, Nit. ac., (Nux v.), Phos., Sep., Sil., *Stram.*

Green.—*Cannab. i.*, *Canth.*, *Carb. sul.*, **Dig.**, *Merc.*, Osm., PHOS., Ruta, *Sep.*, *Stram.*, *Stro.*, Sul., *Zinc.*

Rainbows.—Bell., **Bry.**, *Cic.*, **Con.**, Dig., Euphorb., *K. carb.*, *K. nit.*, Phos., Pho. ac., Stan., *Stram.*, Sul.

Red.—BELL., **Cact.**, Cannab. s., **Con.**, Croc., Dig., Hep., **Hyos.**, Osm., *Phos.*, Saba., Sars., Spig., Stram., *Stro.*, **Sul.**

Striped.—**Am. carb.**, Am. m., *Bell.*, Cham., *Cic.*, **Con.**, *Dig.*, **Iod.**, K. carb., **Nat. m.**, Phos., *Puls.*, **Sep.**

VISION.

Illusions of Color, Variegated.—Bell., Bry., *Coca,* Cic., *Con., Dig.,* Euphorb., *Hyos., K. carb., K. nit., Osm.,* Phos., Pho. ac., Sep., *Stram.,* Sul.

White.—Alum., *Am. carb., Bell.,* Cannab. s., Caust., Chel., *Chloral, Coca, Coloc., Con., Dig.,* K. carb., Pho. ac., Sul.

Yellow.—*Agar.,* Aloe, *Alum., Am. m.,* Ars., Bell., Canth., *Carb. sul., Crotal.,* Dig., *Hyos., K. carb.,* Mang., Osm., Sep., *Sil., Stro.,* Sul., Zinc.

Illusions of Form, Bright.—Camph., Carb. an., Con., Fl. ac., HYOS., *Nux v.,* Valer.

Confused.—*Cina,* Con., GEL., *Graph.,* Iod., *Iris. v.,* Jab., Led., Lil. t., Lyc., Meli., NAT. M., Plat., *Sil., Stram.*

Distorted.—Bell., Bov., *Cimic., Cocaine,* Dig., Euphorb., Hyos., *K. carb.,* Plat., *Stram.*

Double.—*Agar.,* Am. carb., AUR., Bar. c., Bell., *Carb. sul.,* Cham., Cic., *Coca,* Con., Dig., Euphorb., Gel., Graph HYOS., *Iod.* (K. carb.), Led., Lyc., Merc., Nat. m., NIT. AC., Oleand., *Op.,* Petrol., Pb., Puls., Sec. c., Seneg., *Stram.,* Sul. *Tab.,* Verat. a., *Verat. v.*

—**One Eye.**—Cham.

Horizontal.—Oleand., NIT. AC.

Half Vision.—*Aur.,* Calc. c., Caust., Lyc., Mur. ac., Nat. m., *Stram., Zinc.*

—**Horizontal.**—AUR., *Ars.*

—**Vertical.**—Caust., LITH., Lyc., Mur. ac., Nat. m.

Too Large.—*Cannab. i., Euphorb.,* HYOS., *Laur.,* Nat. m., NUX M., *Osm.,* Phos., Staph., Verb.

Too Small.—Hyos., Plat., *Stram.*

Too Near.—Bov., Cic., Stram.

Too Remote.—Anac., *Carb. an.,* Cic., *Nat. m. Nux m.,* Phos., Stan., Stram., *Sul.*

Distorted Features and making Faces.—Acon., Agar., Ambr., Bell., *Bry.,* Calc. c., *Caust.,* Chin., Cocc., *Con.,* Hep., Hyos., Merc., Op., Phos., Pho. ac., *Rhus,* Samb., Sec. c., *Sil.,* Stram., Sul., *Verat. a.*

Fiery.—*Acon., Am. carb.,* Ars., Aur., *Bar. c.,* BELL., Bry., Calc. c., *Calc. ph.,* Cannab. s., Carb. v., Caust., Cham., *Coca, Coloc., Con.,* Croc., *Cup., Dig., Dulc.,* Graph., Hyos., Iod., K. CARB., Lach., Mang., Merc., Mez., Nat. c., Nat. m., Nux v., Oleand., Op., Petrol., Phos., Pho. ac., Pso., Puls., *Sec. c.,* Sep., *Sil.,* SPIG., Staph., *Stram.,* Stro., Sul., Thuj., Valer., *Verat. a., Vio. o.,* Zinc.

Halo about the Light.—Alum., Anac., BELL., Calc. c., *Chloral, Cic., Dig., Euphorb., Hyos.,* K. carb., K. nit., Lach., OSM., PHOS., Pho. ac., Puls., Ruta, *Sars.,* Sep., *Stan.,* Staph., *Stro.,* SUL., Zinc.

VISION.

Lightnings.—Bell., *Croc.*, *Dig.*, *Fl. ac.*, *K. carb.*, **Nat. c.**, **Nux v.**, Oleand., *Op.*, *Phos.*, *Phys.*, *Sant.*, *Sec. c.*, *Sep.*, **Spig.**, Staph., *Stram.*, Zinc.

Mist.—Acon., *Agar.*, *Alum.*, Ambr., Am. m., Anac., *Ant. t.*, Arg., *Arn.*, Ars., *Asaf.*, Aur., *Bar. ac.*, *Bar. c.*, **Bell.**, Bism., Bov., *Bry.*, CALC. C., Cannab. s., Carb. an., *Carb. sul.*, CAUST., Chel., Chin., *Cic.*, Cina, Con., CROC., Crotal., *Crot. tig.*, Cyc., *Dig.*, Dros., Dulc., Euphorb., *Euphr.*, GEL., Graph., Hep., Hyos., *Ign.*, Iod., K. carb., *Kre.*, *Laur.*, **Lyc.**, Mag. c., *Merc.*, *Nat. c.*, **Nat. m.**, *Nit. ac.*, Op., Par., *Petrol.*, PHOS., **Pho. ac.**, Plat., *Pb.*, *Puls.*, Ran. b., Rhodo., Rhus, **Ruta**, *Sabi.*, *Sars.*, **Sec. c.**, Seneg., *Sep.*, *Sil.*, *Spig.*, *Staph.*, *Stram.*, Sul., Thuj., Verb., Vio. t., ZINC.

Muscae Volitantes.—*Acon.*, **Agar.**, *Aloe*, *Am. m.*, Ant. t., *Aur.*, **Bell.**, Calc. c., *Cannab. s.*, Caust., **Chin.**, Cocc., *Coff.*, Con., Dig., *Dulc.*, Hep., *Hyos.*, *Led.*, Mag. c., *Meli.*, **Merc.**, *Nat. c.*, *Nat. m.*, Nit. ac., Op., PHOS., Pb., Puls., Rhus, *Ruta*, Sec. c., **Sep.**, **Sil.**, Spig., **Stram.**, *Sul.*, Zinc.

Spots.—Acon., *Agar.*, Alum., *Am. carb.*, AM. M., *Anac.*, Aur., **Bar. c.**, **Bell.**, **Calc. c.**, Cannab. s., Carb. v., Caust., **Chel.**, Chin., *Chloral*, *Cic.*, Cimic., *Coca*, Cocc., Con., *Dig.*, Dros., *Euphr.*, Hyos., K. CARB., *Lyc.*, **Mag. c.**, Mang., *Merc.*, Mos., *Nat. c.*, **Nat. m.**, Nit. ac., *Petrol.*, PHOS., *Pho. ac.*, *Phys.*, Ruta, *Sec. c.*, Seneg., **Sep.**, SIL., *Stram.*, Stro., SUL., *Tab.*, Thuj., *Valer.*, *Verat. a.*

Dim.—Acon., **Agar.**, *Aloe*, Alum., *Am. carb.*, Am. m., *Anac.*, **Ant. t.**, *Arn.*, *Ars.*, Asaf., Aur., Bar. c., **Bell.**, *Bov.*, Bry., CALC. C., *Calc. ph.*, CANNAB. S., *Canth.*, Caps., Carb. an., *Carb. sul.*, CAUST., Cham., **Chel.**, *Chin.*, Chloral, Cic., *Cimic.*, *Cina*, **Clem.**, **Cocc.**, *Coloc.*, CON., *Croc.*, Crotal., Cup., Cyc., *Dig.*, Dros., *Dulc.*, Euphorb., EUPHR., Fer., GEL., Graph., *Helo.*, HEP., Hyos., *Ign.*, Iod., Ip., **K. bi.**, *K. br.*, **K. iod.**, Kalm., *Kre.*, LACH., Laur., Led., **Lil. t.**, **Lyc.**, **Mag. c.**, Mag. m., *Mang.*, MERC., Mos., *Nat. c.*, **Nat. m.**, NIT. AC., Nux v., **Op.**, *Osm.*, Petrol., PHOS., Pho. ac., Plat., *Pb.*, PULS., Rheum, Rhodo., **Rhus**, **Ruta**, Saba., **Sabi.**, *Sars.*, Sec. c., **Seneg.**, *Sep.*, SIL., **Spig.**, *Stan.*, Staph., **Stram.**, Stro., SUL., Sul. ac., Tar., **Thuj.**, *Valer.*, *Verat. a.*, **Verat. v.**, Verb., Zinc.

Far-sighted.—Alum., Am. carb., *Bell.*, Bry., **Calc. c.**, **Carb. an.**, *Caust.*, **Chel.**, **Con.**, **Dros.**, **Hyos.**, **Lyc.**, Mag. m., Mez., **Nat. m.**, **Nux v.**, Petrol., SEP., SIL., *Spig.*, Sul.

Letters Run Together when Reading.—*Bell.*, Bry., CANNAB. I., Chin., *Chel.*, *Clem.*, Dros., *Fer.*, Graph., Hyos., Lyc., NAT. M., **Seneg.**, Sil., Stram., *Vio. o.*

VISION. 39

Indistinct.—Agar., Alum., Am. carb., Am. m., ANAC., **Apis, Ars.,** *Aur.,* Bar. c., **Bell.,** Bor., Bry., **Calc. c., Cannab. s.,** Canth., *Caps., Carb. n.,* Carb. v., Cham., **Chel.,** *Chin., Chloral., Cic., Cimic., Cina,* Coff., *Com.,* Con., Croc., *Dig.,* **Dros.,** *Dub.,* Dulc., **Euphr.,** *Gel.,* Graph., **Hep.,** *Hyos.,* **Ign.,** *Iod., Jab., K. br., Kre., Lach.,* Laur., **Led.,** *Lil. t.,* **Lyc.,** Mag. c., **Mang.,** Merc., Nat. c., *Nat. m.,* Nit. ac., Par., **Petrol.,** *Phos.,* Pho. ac., *Plat.,* Pb., *Rheum,* Rhodo., Rhus, RUTA, Saba., Sars., Sec. c., SENEG., *Sep.,* **Sil.,** *Spig.,* **Staph., Stram.,** *Stro.,* SUL., Thuj., Verat. a., Verb., Zinc.

Paralysis of Optic Nerve.—Acon., *Agar.,* Alum., Ambr., Am. carb., Am. m., *Anac.,* Ant. cr., Ant. t., Arn., Ars., Asaf., **Aur.,** *Bar. c.,* BELL., Bor., *Bry.,* **Calc. c.,** Camph., Cannab. s., Canth., *Caps.,* Carb. an., Carb. v., **Caust.,** Cham., *Chel.,* **Chin.,** *Cic., Cocc.,* CON., Croc., Cyc., Dig., *Dros.,* Dulc., *Euphr., Fer.,* Graph., Hep., HYOS., Ign., Iod., *K. carb.,* Kre., *Laur.,* Led., **Lyc.,** Mag. c., Mang., **Merc.,** Mez., *Nat. c.,* **Nat. m.,** *Nit. ac.,* Nux v., *Oleand.,* **Op.,** Par., *Petrol.,* PHOS., Pho. ac., *Pb.,* **PULS., Rhus, Ruta,** Saba., Sabi., Sars., SEC. C., Seneg., *Sep.,* SIL., *Spig., Staph.,* STRAM., Stro., SUL., Thuj., **Verat. a.,** Verb., Zinc.

Photomania.—Acon., Am. m., **Bell.,** STRAM.

Photophobia.—ACON., *Agar.,* **Agn.,** *Ail.,* **All. c.,** Alum., *Am. carb., Am. m.,* Anac., *Ant. cr.,* Ant. t., **Apis, Arg. n.,** Arn., ARS., Aur., *Bar. c.,* BELL., Bor., Bry., **Calc. c., Calc. ph.,** Camph., Carb. an., *Carb. sul.,* Caust., Cham., Chin., Cic., *Cimic., Cina, Clem.,* **Coca,** Coff., *Colch.,* Con., Croc., Crotal., *Crot. tig.,* Cup., Dig., *Dros., Dub., Euphorb.,* EUPHR., Graph., *Hell.,* Hep., Hyos., Ign., K. carb., **K. nit.,** Lach., *Laur.,* Lyc., Mag. c., Mang., MERC., *Merc. c., Merc. n.,* Mur. ac., **Nat. c.,** *Nat. m.,* Nit. ac., Nux m., NUX V., *Osm., Pæo., Phel.,* **Phos.,** Pho. ac., Puls., RHUS, *Sang.,* Sars., *Seneg.,* **Sep.,** *Sil., Spig.,* Staph., **Stram.,** SUL., Sul. ac., Tar., *Thuj.,* Verat. v., *Xan.,* Zinc.

Short-sighted.—Agar., Am. carb., *Anac.,* Ant. t., Calc. c., *Carb. v.,* **Chin.,** *Cimic.,* Con., Cyc., *Euphorb.,* **Euphr.,** Graph., **Hep., Hyos.,** Lach., **Lyc.,** *Mang.,* Mez., *Nat. c., Nat. m.,* **Nit. ac.,** Petrol., PHOS., Pho. ac., *Phys., Pb.,* **PULS.,** Ruta, Sele., Spo., **Stram.,** Sul., **Sul. ac.,** Thuj., **Valer.,** Verb., *Vio. o.,* Vio. t.

Tremulousness.—Bell., **Cannab. i.,** Con., *Kalm.,* Led., **Lyc.,** Phos., *Plat.,* Sabi., Seneg., *Stram.,* Thuj., *Vio. o.*

Vanishing.—*Acon.,* **Agar.,** Alum., Ambr., *Anac.,* Ant. t., **Arg.,** *Arn.,* Ars., Asaf., *Asar.,* Aur., BELL., Bor., Bry., **Calc. c.,** Camph., Cannab. s., Caps., Carb. an., **Caust.,** *Cham., Chel.,* Chin., CIC., Cina, Clem., **Con., Croc.,** Cup., Cyc., *Dig.,* **Dros.,** Dulc., *Euphr.,* **Fer.,** *Graph.,* **Hep.,** HYOS.,

Iod., *K. carb.*, **K. nit.**, Lach., Laur., Led., *Lyc.*, Mag. c., Mag. m., **Mang.**, Meny., MERC., Mez., *Mos.*, *Mur. ac.*, NAT. M., Nit. ac., *Nux v.*, OLEAND., *Op.*, Petrol., PHOS., Plat., Pb., PULS., Ran. b., *Ruta*, Saba., *Sabi.*, *Sec. c.*, Seneg., Sep., *Sil.*, Spig., Squ., *Staph.*, STRAM., *Sul.*, Tar., *Thuj.*, Verat. a., Vio. t., *Zinc.*

Ears.

External.—*Acon.*, **Agar.**, ALUM., Ambr., Am. carb., Am. m., **Anac.**, *Ant. cr.*, APIS, **Arg.**, Arn., Ars., Asaf., Asar., Aur., **Bar. c.**, **Bell.**, **Berb.**, Bism., Bor., Bov., Bry., **Calc. c.**, *Calc. ph.*, *Camph.*, *Cannab. s.*, *Canth.*, CAPS., Carb. an., *Carb. v.*, *Carb. sul.*, *Caust.*, Cham., **Chel.**, **Chin.**, Cic., Cina, Clem., Cocc., Coc. c., *Colch.*, *Coloc*, Con., *Crotal*, *Cup.*, *Dig.*, **Dros.**, *Dulc.*, Fer., *Fer. ph.*, Graph., *Guai.*, **Hell.**, *Hep.*, Hyos., Iod., *K. bi.*, **K. CARB.**, *K. m.*, KRE., *Laur.*, *Lyc.*, *Mang.*, Meny., MERC., *Mez.*, *Mur. ac.*, Nat. c., *Nat. m.*, *Nat. s.*, *Nit. ac.*, Nux v., **Oleand.**, Par., **Petrol.**, Phos., PHO. AC., **Plant.**, Plat., *Pb.*, *Pso.*, **Puls.**, *Rhodo.*, *Rhus*, **Ruta**, Saba., *Sabi.*, Sars., **Sep.** Sil., SPIG., Spo., Squ., *Stan.*, Staph., *Sul.*, Tar., TELL., Thuj., *Verat. a.*, Verb., Vio. o., Vio. t., *Zinc.*

Internal.—Acon., Agar., **Alum.**, Ambr., **Anac.**, Ant. cr., Arg., Arn., Ars., Asaf., **Asar.**, Aur., *Bar. c.*, **Bell.**, Bism., Bor., Bov., *Bry.*, CALC. C., Camph., Cannab. s., *Canth.*, Caps., Carb. an., *Carb. v.*, CAUST., Cham., **Chel.**, **Chen.** *a.*, Chin., Cic., Cina, Clem., *Colch.*, Coloc., Con., Croc., Cup., Cyc., Dig., **Dros.**, **Dulc.**, Euphorb., Euphr., Fer., Graph., Guai., Hell., Hyos., *Ign.*, Iod., Ip., K. CARB., **Kre.**, Lach., Laur., LYC., MANG., Mar., *Meny.*, MERC., *Mez.*, *Mur. ac.*, Nat. c., **Nat. m.**, **Nit. ac.**, *Nux v.*, Oleand., Par., Petrol., *Phos.*, Pho. ac., Plat., *Pb.*, PULS., Ran. b., Rheum, Rhus, *Ruta*, Saba., Sabi., Samb., *Sars.*, Seneg., SEP., *Sil.*, SPIG., Spo., Squ., *Stan.*, Staph., Stram., *Sul.*, Sul. ac., Tar., Thuj., Valer., Verat. a., **Verb.**, Vio. o., *Zinc.*

Middle Ear (Confounded with "Internal").—Ars. Iod., *Bell.*, *Cannab. i.*, *Caps.*, *Dulc.*, *Hydras.*, *K. bi.*, *K. m.*, Merc. c., *Mez.*, *Phyt.*, *Sil.*, *Stict.*, *Sul.*, *Thuj.*, *Verat. v.*, *Zinc.*

Eustachian Tube.—*Agar.*, Ars. iod., Bar. m., *Coc. o.*, *Eryng.*, *Fer. ph.*, *Gel.*, *Iod.*, Merc., Nit. ac., Nux v., Petrol., Phos., *Phyt.*, *Sul. ac.*, *Sil.*, Spig., *Stram.*

Before.—*Arg.*, *Bry.*, Calc. c., Carb. v., Mur. ac., Oleand., Sars., **Sep.**, Sil., Verb., Zinc.

Behind Ears.—Acon., Alum., *Ambr.*, Am. carb., *Am. m.*, Anac., Ant. cr., Arg., *Arn.*, Asar., *Aur.*, *Bar. ac.*, BAR. C., *Bell.*, Bor., *Bry.*, **Calc. c.**, *Calc. ph.*, **Cannab. s.**, CANTH., CAPS., Carb. an., Carb. v., CAUST.,

Cham., Chel., Chin., *Cic.*, *Cina*, *Coc. c.*, Colch., Coloc., **Con.**, Dig., Dros., *Fer. ph.*, **GRAPH.**, Hell., **Hep.**, K. carb., *K. nit.*, Lach., Lyc., Mag. c., Mang., Meny., Merc., **Mez.**, Mur. ac., *Nat. m.*, *Nit. ac.*, OLEAND., PETROL., Phos., *Pho. ac.*, Plat., Pb., *Pso.*, **Puls.**, Rhodo., Rhus, *Ruta*, Saba., Sabi., Sars., Sele., *Sep.*, **Sil.**, Spo., Squ., Stan., **STAPH.**, **Sul.**, Tar., Thuj., Verat. a., *Verb.*, Vio. o., Vio. t., *Zinc.*

Beneath Ears.—Alum., *Arg.*, Asar., Aur., BAR. C., **BELL.**, **Calc. c.**, Carb. an., Carb. v., **Chel.**, *Chin.*, Cina, Cocc., Dros., Iod., Mang., Nat. c., *Nit. ac.*, **Oleand.**, **Phos.**, *Puls.*, **Ruta**, *Sars.*, **Sep.**, **Sil.**, **Sul.**, Verat. a., Zinc.

Lobules.—Alum., Ambr., **Arg.**, *Arn.*, BAR. C., *Bry.*, Camph., Carb. v., **CAUST.**, Chel., **CHIN.**, Colch., Graph., Hyos., **K. carb.**, **K. nit.**, KRE., *Mar.*, Merc., **Nat. m.**, *Nit. ac.*, Oleand., Phos., **Pho. ac.**, Plat., *Rhus*, **Saba.**, Sars., **Sep.**, *Stan.*, Verat. a.

Parotid Glands.—*Am. carb.*, Arg., *Arn.*, Aur., *Bar. c.*, **BELL.**, **Bry.**, **Calc. c.**, Caps., **Carb. an.**, **Carb. v.**, Caust., **CHAM.**, *Chin.*, Cocc., **CON.**, Dig., *Dulc.*, Euphorb., Graph., Hep., *Hyos.*, **Ign.**, K. carb., Lyc., Mag c., Mang., **MERC.**, Mez., Nat. c., *Nit. ac.*, Nux m., Petrol., *Phos.*, Pho ac., **Puls.**, **RHUS**, **Saba.**, *Sep.*, **Sil.**, **Staph.**, **Sul.**, Thuj.

Discharges from Ears.—Alum., Am. carb., Am. m., Anac., **Ars.** Asaf., Aur., Bell., Bor., Bov., Bry., **Calc. c.**, *Carb. an.*, **Carb. v.**, Caust., Cic., *Colch.*, **CON.**, Croc., *Crotal.*, *Fl. ac.*, *Graph.*, *Hep.*, *Hydras.*, Iod., K. carb., *Lach.*, **LYC.**, Meny., **MERC.**, Mos., *Nat. m.*, *Nat. s.*, **Nit. ac.**, Petrol., *Phos.*, **PULS.**, *Rhus*, **Sele.**, *Sep.*, **Sil.**, *Spig.*, *Sul.*, **Tell.**, Zinc.

—**Bloody.**—*Bell.*, Bry., **Calc. c.**, *Cic.*, *Con.*, Graph., Lach., *Lyc.*, **MERC.**, Mos., **Nit. ac.**, Petrol., *Phos.*, **Puls.**, Rhus, *Sep.*, *Sil.*, **Sul.**, Zinc.

—**Excoriating.**—**Ars. iod.**, *Calc. ph.*, *Merc.*, **TELL.**

—**Fetid.**—Ars., **Ars. iod.**, *Cub.*, *Elaps.*, MERC., **PSO.**, **TELL.**, *Thuj.*

—**Moist.**—*Asaf.*, **Carb. an.**, **Caust.**, *Colch.*, Kre., *Meny.*, **Merc.**, Nat. m., **Nit. ac.**, Phos., Spig.

—**Mucous.**—Alum., Bell., Bor., **Calc. c.**, *Fer. ph.*, Graph., **Lyc.**, MERC., *Phos.*, **PULS.**, *Sul.*

—**Purulent.**—Alum., **Am. carb.**, **Asaf.**, **Aur.**, Bell., **Bor.**, **Bov.**, **Calc. c.**, Carb. an., *Carb. v.*, *Caust.*, **Con.**, *Fer. ph.*, Graph., *Hep.*, *K. carb.*, Lach., **Lyc.**, MERC., Nat. m., *Nit. ac.*, **Petrol.**, Phos., **PSO.**, **Puls.**, *Rhus*, Sep., **SIL.**, *Sul.*, Zinc.

Ear-wax, Blood-red.—*Con.*

—**Hard.**—*Con.*, *Lach.*

—**Increased.**—*Agar.*, *Petrol.*

Ear-wax, Thin.—Am. m., **Con.**, Iod., *Lach.*, Merc., Mos., *Sele.*, *Sil.*

Left.—*Acon.*, Agar., Agn., Alum., *Ambr.*, **Am. carb.**, Am. m., ANAC., Ant. cr., Apis, Arg., **Arn.**, *Ars.*, ASAF., Asar., Aur., Bar. c., Bell., *Bism.*, BOR., Brom., Bry., Calad., *Calc. c.*, **Camph.**, Cannab. s., Canth., *Caps.*, Carb. an., *Carb. v.*, *Caust.*, Chel., Chin., Cic., Clem., *Coc. c.*, Colch., Coloc., Con., Croc., Cup., Cyc., Dig., Dros., **Dulc.**, Euphorb., Euphr., Fer., Fl. ac., GRAPH., GUAI., Hep., IGN., Iod., K. carb., K. nit., *Kre.*, *Lach.*, Laur., Lyc., Mang., Mar., Meny., **Merc.**, Mez., **Millef.**, *Mur. ac.*, Nat. c., Nat. m., *Nit. ac.*, Nux m., OLEAND., *Par.*, Petrol., Phos., Pho. ac., Plat., **Pb.**, **Pso.**, *Puls.*, Ran. b., Ran. s., Rheum, *Rhodo.*, Rhus, Saba., *Sabi.*, Sars., Sele., Seneg., *Sep.*, Sil., *Spig.*, Spo., Squ., *Stan.*, **Staph.**, *Sul.*, Tar., *Tell.*, Thuj., Valer., Verat. a., **Verb.**, VIO. O., Vio. t., Zinc.

Right.—Acon., *Agar.*, **Alum.**, Ambr., Am. carb., **Am. m.**, Anac., Ant. cr., Apis, Arg., Arn., Ars., Asaf., *Asar.*, *Bar. c.*, BELL., Bor., Bov., Brom., Bry., *Calad.*, **Calc. c.**, *Cannab. s.*, **Canth.**, **Carb. an.**, Carb. v., *Caust.*, *Cham.*, **Chel.**, Chin., *Cic.*, Clem., *Cocc.*, *Colch.*, Coloc., *Con.*, Croc., Cup., *Cyc.*, Dig., Dros. Dulc. Euphorb., Euphr., Fer., FL. AC., Graph., *Hell.*, **Hep.**, *Hyos.*, IOD., *Ip.*, **K. carb.**, K. nit., Kre., *Lach.*, Laur., Led., Lyc., *Mag. c.*, *Mag. m.*, Mang., Mar., Meny., *Merc.*, Mez., Millef., Mur. ac., Nat. c., Nat. m., **Nit. ac.**, *Nux m.*, NUX V., Par., *Petrol.*, Phos., *Pho. ac.*, PLAT., Pb., Pru., Pso., Puls., *Ran. b.*, **Ran. s.** Rheum, Rhodo., Rhus, Ruta, Saba., Sabi., *Samb.*, Sars., Sele., *Seneg.*, Sep., SIL., Spig., SPO., Squ., Stan. Staph., Sul., Sul. ac., Tar., Thuj., *Valer.*, Verat. a., Verb., Zinc.

Hearing.

Acute.—Acon., Agar., Alum., Arn., *Ars.*, **Aur.**, **Bell.**, *Bry.*, Calc. c., Chin., *Coca*, *Cocc.*, COFF., *Colch.*, **Con.**, Cup., **Hep.**, **K. carb.**, Lach., *Lyc.*, *Mur. ac.*, **Nux v.**, Phos., **Plant.**, **Puls.**, Thuj.

Hardness.—Acon., Agar., Agn., Alum., **Ambr.**, *Am. ca b.*, Am. m., An c., *Ant. cr.*, Arg., *Arn.*, *Ars.*, Asaf., *Asar.*, Aur., Bar. c., BELL., *Bor.* Bov., Bry., Calad., CALC. C., *Calc. ph.*, Cannab. s., Canth., **Caps.**, Carb. an., Carb. v., Caust., Cham., *Chel.*, *Chin.*, Cic., Cocc., Coff., Colch., **Con.**, Croc., *Cyc.*, *Dig.*, Dros., *Dulc.*, Euphorb., *Fl. ac.*, Graph., Hep., HYOS., *Ign.*, Iod., Ip., K. carb., K. nit., Kre., Lach., Laur., Led., LYC., Mag. c., *Mag. m.*, Mang., Mar., Meny., Merc., Mez., Mos., Mur. ac., Nat. c., Nat. m., NIT. AC., **Nux. v.**, Oleand., OP., Par., PETROL., PHOS., PHO. AC., Plat., Pb., PULS., Ran. b., Rheum, *Rhodo.*, Rhus, Ruta, *Saba.*, Sabi., **Sal. ac.**, Sars., SEC. C., Sele., **Sep.**,

HEARING.

SIL., *Spig.*, Spo., Squ., Stan., *Staph.*, **Stram.**, **SUL.**, Sul. ac., *Tab.*, **Tar.**, Thuj. Valer., **Verat. a.**, *Verb.*, Vio. o., Zinc.

Fluttering in Ears.—Acon., *Agar.*, Alum., Ant. cr., *Aur.*, *Bar. c.*, **Bell.**, Bor., **Calc. c.**, *Caust.*, Cham., Chin., Cocc., Con., **Cup.**, Dros., Dulc., **Graph.**, Hep., *K. carb.*, Lach., Laur., Mag. c., **Mag. m.**, Meny., *Merc.*, Mos., Nat. m., Nit. ac., Oleand., *Petrol.*, Phos., **Plat.**, **Puls.**, Rheum, Rhodo, *Saba.*, Sep., *Sil.*, SPIG., Spo., Stan., *Sul.*, Zinc.

Loss of Hearing (from Paralysis of Auditory Nerve).—*Acon.*, Agar., Alum., Ambr., Am. carb. **Anac.**, *Ant. cr.*, **Arg. n.**, *Arn.*, *Ars.*, **Ars. iod.**, *Asar.*, *Aur.*, *Bar. c.*, **BELL.**, *Bor.*, *Bry.*, **Calc. c.**, **Cannab. s.**, *Caps.*, Carb. v., *Carb. sul.*, **Caust.**, Cham., **Chel.**, *Chen. a.*, *Chin.*, *Coca*, **Cocc.**, Con., *Crotal.*, Cyc., Dros., **Dulc.**, *Elaps.*, **Gel.**, **Graph.**, *Guai.*, *Hydras.*, **HYOS.**, *Ign.*, *Iod.*, *K. carb.*, *Lach.*, **Led.**, **Lyc.**, *Mag. c.*, Mang., Merc., *Nat. c.*, *Nat. m.*, Nit. ac., **Nux v.**, Oleand., **Op.**, Petrol., Phos., *Pho. ac.*, *Pic. ac.*, **PULS.**, Rhodo., *Rhus*, Ruta, Saba., **Sal. ac.**, **Sec. c.**, Sep., **SIL.**, *Spig.*, Staph., **Stram.**, Sul., *Tell.*, *Ter.*, Verat. a., *Visc.*

Noises in Ears in General.—Acon., *Agar.*, Agn., *Aloe*, Alum., Ambr., *Am. carb.*, Am. m., Anac., Ant. cr., *Arn.*, **Arg. n.**, Ars., Asaf., *Asar.*, **Aur.**, **Bar. c.**, **Bar. m.**, **BELL.**, **Bor.**, Bov., **Bry.**, *Cact.*, **CALC. C.**, *Calc. ph.*, **Cannab. i.**, Cannab. s., Canth., Carb. an., *Carb. v.*, *Carb. sul.*, **CAUST.**, *Ced.*, **Cham.**, **Chel.**, *Chin.*, *Cic.*, *Coca*, **Cocc.**, **Con.**, **Cup.**, Dros., **Dig.**, *Dulc.*, *Elaps.*, Euphorb., *Fer.*, **GRAPH.**, **Hep.**, Hyos., Ign., Iod., **K. carb.**, Kre., *Lach.*, **Led.**, **Lyc.**, *Mag. c.*, Mag. m., Mang., *Mar.* Meny., Merc., Mez., *Mos.*, *Nat. c.*, **Nat. m.**, Nit. ac., Nux v., *Oleand.* Op., Par., Petrol., Phos., Pho. ac., Pic. ac., Plat., **PULS.**, Rheum, Rhodo., *Rhus*, Ruta, Saba., **SANG.**, Sars., Sec. c., Sep., Sil., **SPIG.**, Spo., *Stan.*, *Staph.*, **SUL.**, *Sul. ac.*, Thuj., Valer., Verat. a., Vio. o., Zinc.

Ringing.—Acon., Agar., Agn., Alum., Ambr., Am. carb., Am. m., Ant. cr., Arn., Ars., Asaf., Asar., *Aur.*, **Bar. c.**, **Bell.**, **Bor.**, **Bry.**, **CALC. C.**, Camph., **CANNAB. I.**, Cannab. s., Canth., Carb. an., *Carb. v.*, *Carb. sul.*, **CAUST.**, *Cham.*, **Chel.**, Chin., Cic., Clem., *Coca*, **Con.**, Croc., *Cup.*, Dig., Dulc., Euphorb., *Euphr.*, Fer., Glon., Gran., Graph., **Hep.**, Hyos., Ign., **K. carb.**, K. nit., Kre., *Lach.*, **Led.**, **Lyc.**, *Mag. c.*, Mang., *Mar.*, Meny., Merc., Mez., *Mur. ac.*, **Nat. m.**, Nux v., *Oleand.*, Op., Osm., Par., Petrol., Phos., Pho. ac., *Plat.*, **PULS.**, Rhodo., *Rhus*, Ruta, Saba., **Sal. ac.**, *Sars.*, Sep., **Sil.**, Spig., Spo., *Stan.*, Staph., **Sul.**, **Sul. ac.**, Tar., Thuj., Valer., Verat. a., Vio. o., Zinc.

Roaring.—Acon., *Agar.*, Agn., Alum., Ambr., Am. carb., *Am. m.*, Anac., Ant. cr., Ant. t., *Arn.*, **Ars.**, Asar., Aur., **Bar. c.**, **Bar. m.**, **BELL.**, Bor., Bov., Bry., *Cact.*, **Calc. c.**, **Cannab. s.**, Canth., *Carb.*

ac., *Carb. an.*, *Carb. v.*, *Carb. sul.*, CAUST., *Ced.*, Cham., **Chel.**, **Chen. a.**, Chin., Cic., *Cimic.*, *Coca*, *Cocc.*, Colch., **Coloc.**, **Con.**, Croc., **Cup.**, **Dig.**, Dros., Dulc., *Elaps.*, **Fer.**, *Gel.*, GRAPH., *Hep.*, *Hyos.*, Ign., *Iod.*, *K. br.*, **K. carb.**, Kre., Lach., Laur., *Led.*, **Lyc.**, *Mag. c.*, Mag. m., Mang., **Mar.**, Meny., **Merc.**, Mos., Mur. ac., Nat. c., **Nat. m.**, *Nit. ac.*, NUX V., Oleand., *Op.*, Petrol., Phos., PHO. AC., **Plat.**, PULS., Rheum, **Rhodo.**, Rhus, Ruta, *Saba.*, **Sal. ac.**, *Sang.*, **Sec. c.**, Sep., Sil., SPIG., Spo., Stan., Staph., Stram., Stro., SUL., Sul. ac., Thuj., *Verat. a.*, **Verat. v.**, Vio. o., *Zinc.*

Hearing, Sensitive.—ACON., Alum., Ambr., *Am. carb.*, Am. m., *Anac.*, *Ant. cr.*, **Arn.**, **Ars.**, Asaf., **Asar.**, AUR., *Bar. c.*, **Bell.**, Bor., Bry., Calad., **Calc. c.**, Camph., Cannab. s., *Canth.*, Caps., Carb. an., Carb. v., *Caust.*, **Cham.**, *Chel.*, *Chen. a.*, *Chin.*, Cina, *Cocc.*, COFF., *Colch.*, **Con.**, *Cup.*, Dig., Graph., Hell., Hep., *Hyos.*, Ign., Iod., Ip., *K. carb.*, *Lach.*, Laur., LYC., *Mag. c.*, Mag. m., *Merc.*, **Mur. ac.**, *Nat. c.*, Nit. ac., Nux m., NUX V., Oleand., **Petrol.**, Phos., Pho. ac., **Plant.**, **Puls.**, *Saba.*, Sabi., *Sang.*, Sars., Sele., Seneg., SEP., SIL., SPIG., Squ., Staph., *Sul.*, Thuj., Valer., *Verat. a.*, **Verat. v.**, Vio. o., Zinc.

Stopped Feeling.—*Acon.*, Anac., Arg., Ars., *Asar.*, Bism., Bor., **Bry.**, Calad., *Calc. c.*, *Carb. v.*, *Carb. sul.*, *Caust.*, Cham., **Chel.**, Chin., Colch., CON., *Cyc.*, *Dig.*, Glon., *Graph.*, Guai., **Iod.**, *K. carb.*, *Lach.*, Led., LYC., Mang., Mar., Meny., Merc., Mez., Nat. c., **Nit. ac.**, Nux m., Petrol., Phos., PULS., Rhus, **Sele.**, Sep., SIL., **Spig.**, Spo., Stan., **Sul.**, Sul. ac., **Verat. a.**, Verb.

Nose.

External.—Acon., *Alum.*, Ambr., *Ant. cr.*, *Apis*, Arn., AUR., *Bar. c.*, *Bell.*, Bor., Bov., Bry., **Calc. c.**, Cannab. s., *Canth.*, *Caps.*, Carb. an., *Carb. v.*, CAUST., *Ced.*, Cham., Chel., *Chin.*, Cic., Clem., Coff., Colch., *Con.*, Dros., Dulc., Euphr., *Graph.*, Hell., Hep., Hyos., *Iod.*, K. CARB., *Laur.*, Lyc., Mag. c., Mag. m., Meny., MERC., Mez., NAT. C., **Nat. m.**, Nit. ac., Petrol., *Phos.*, PHO. AC., **Pb.**, PULS., Rheum, Rhodo., RHUS, Ruta, *Samb.*, Sars., Sep., *Sil.*, SPIG., Spo., *Staph.*, *Sul.*, **Sul. ac.**, Tar., Thuj., Verat. a., Vio. o., Vio. t., Zinc.

Internal.—*Aesc.*, Acon., *Agar.*, *Ail.*, **All. c.**, *Alum.*, Ambr., *Am. carb.*, *Am. m.*, Anac., ANT. CR., *Ant. t.*, *Apis*, Arg., *Arg. n.*, Arn., **Ars.**, ARUM. T., Asar., AUR., *Bar. c.*, **Bell.**, Bor., Bov., Brom., Bry., CALC. C., **Camph.**, **Canth.**, *Caps.*, *Caust.*, Cham., Chel., Chin., Cic., *Cimic.*, **Cina**, *Cinnab.*, Clem., *Coca*, Cocc., Coc. c., *Coff.*, **Colch.**, **Coloc.**, Con., **Coral.**, *Crot. tig.*, Cyc., *Dios.*, Dros., *Elaps.*, Euphorb., Euphr., **Fl. ac.**, *Gam.*, GRAPH., Guai., Hep., **Hydras.**, *Hyos.*, **Ign.**, *Iod.*, **Ip.**,

NOSE.

K. BI., K. carb., K. IOD., *K. nit.*, Kre., Lach., Laur., Led., *Lyc.*, Mag. c., Mag. m., Mang., Mar., Meny., MERC., Merc. c., *Merc. i. r.*, Mez., Mur. ac., Naj., *Nat. ars.*, Nat. c., Nat. m., NIT. AC., *Nux v.*, Osm., Petrol., Phos., Pho. ac., *Phyt.*, *Plant.*, Pb., Pod., PULS., Ran. b., Ran. s., *Rhus*, *Rumex*, Ruta, Saba., *Sang. n.*, Sars., *Sec. c.*, *Sele.*, Seneg., Sep., SIL., Sin., SPIG., Squ., Stan., Staph., *Stict.*, SUL., *Ther.*, Thuj., Verat. a., Wye., Zinc.

Back.—*Alum.*, Calc. c., Canth., Chin., Cinnab., Con., *Ham.*, K. bi., Oleand., PHO. AC., Ruta, Samb., *Spig.*, Spo., *Thuj.*

Bones.—Anac., Arn., Asaf., Ars., AUR., *Calc. c.*, Carb. an., Cinnab., *Clem.*, *Colch.*, Con., *Hep.*, Hyos., *K. bi.*, Lach., MERC., *Mez.*, *Nat. m.*, Petrol., *Phos.*, Plat., *Puls.*, Sil., Spo., *Sul.*, Thuj., Verat. a.

Root.—Acon., Agar., Agn., *Am. m.*, Ant. t., *Arn.*, *Arum. t.*, Asar., Bar. c., Bell., Bism., Calc. c., Camph., Cannab. s., Carb. v., Caust., *Cinnab.*, Cina, Colch., *Coloc.*, Con., *Elaps.*, Fer., Hell., Hep., HYOS., Ign., *Iod.*, K. bi., K. carb., *K. iod.*, *Lach.*, Laur., Meny., Merc., *Merc. c.*, *Merc. i. f.*, *Mez.*, Mos., *Nat. ars.*, *Nat. m.*, Nit. ac., *Oleand.*, Petrol., Puls., *Ran. b.*, Rheum, *Rhodo.*, Ruta, *Sang.*, *Sang. n.*, *Sil.*, Staph., *Stict.*, *Thuj.*, Vio. t., *Zinc.*

Septum.—Aur., Bry., Caust., Cina, Colch., Con., *Crot. tig.*, Hydras., Iod., *K. bi.*, *Lyc.*, Merc., Petrol., Ruta, Sil., Sul., Staph.

Tip.—*Apis*, Aur., Bell., *Bor.*, Bry., Calc. c., *Canth.*, CARB. AN., CARB. V., CAUST., Ced., *Chel.*, Clem., Colch., Con., *K. nit.*, Meny., Merc., *Mos.*, Nit. ac., *Pho. ac.*, Rheum, Rhus, Samb., SEP., Sil., *Spo.*, Sul., *Sul. ac.*, Vio. o.

Wings.—Alum., Ambr., Aur., Brom., *Canth.*, Carb. v., *Caust.*, *Coc. c.*, Con., Dulc., *Euphr.*, Hell., K. carb., *Mag. m.*, *Merc.*, Mez., Nat. c., Nat. m., Nux v., *Phos.*, Pb., Puls., *Rhus*, Sil., Spig., *Squ.*, Staph., *Sul.*, THUJ., Vio. t., Zinc.

Nosebleed.—ACON., Agar., *Aloe*, Alum., AMBR., Am. carb., Am. m., Anac., ANT. CR., Ant. t., Ant. s. aur., Arg., Arn., *Ars.*, *Asar.*, Aur., Bar. c., BELL., Bism., Bar., *Bov.*, Bry., Cact., CALC. C., *Calc. ph.*, Cannab. s., Canth., Caps., *Carb. an.*, *Curb. sul.*, CARB. V., Caust., *Cerium.*, Cham., Chin., *Cinnam.*, Cina, Clem., Cocc., Coff., Colch., *Coloc.*, Con., CROC., *Crotal.*, *Cup.*, *Dig.*, *Dros.*, Dulc., *Elaps.*, Euphr., Fer., Graph., HAM., Hep., *Hydras.*, HYOS., *Ign.*, Iod., Ip., *K. carb.*, K. nit., Kre., Lach., *Led.*, *Lyc.*, Mag. c., Mag. m., Meli., MERC., Merc. c., Mez., MILLEF., Mos., *Mur. ac.*, *Nat. c.*, *Nat. m.*, NIT. AC., *Nux m.*, Nux v., Op., Par., Petrol., PHOS., Pho. ac., Plat., Pb., PULS., Ran. b., Rhodo., RHUS, Ruta, *Saba.*, SABI., Samb., Sars., SEC. C., Sele.

NOSE.

Seneg., Sep., Sil., Spo., *Squ.*, Stan., *Staph.*, **Stram.**, Stro., **Sul.**, Sul. ac., Tar., Ter., *Thuj.*, Valer., **Verat. a.**, Vio. o., *Zinc.*

— **Bright Red.**—Am. carb., *Ant. t.*, **Arn.**, Ars., BELL., Bor., Bov., *Bry.*, *Calc. c.*, Canth., *Carb. v.*, Chin., Dig., *Dios.*, Dros., DULC., Fer., Graph., HYOS., *Ip.*, K. nit., Kre., Laur., **Led.**, Mag. m., *Merc.*, Nat. c., Nux m., **Phos.**, *Puls.*, Rhus, *Saba.*, SABI., **Sec. c.**, Sep., Sil., Stram., *Stro.*, Sul., *Zinc.*

—**Clotted.**—*Arn.*, **Bell.**, Bry., *Canth.*, Carb. an., *Caust.*, CHAM., **Chin.**, *Con.*, *Croc.*, Fer., Hyos., Ign., Ip., Kre., *Mag. m.*, *Merc.*, *Nit. ac.*, Nux. v., Pho. ac., **PLAT.**, **Puls.**, RHUS, Sabi., Sec. c., Sep., **Stram.**, *Stro.*

—**Dark.**—Acon., *Am. carb.*, *Ant. cr.*, **Arn.**, **Asar.**, Bell., *Bism.*, *Bry.*, *Canth.*, Carb. v., **Cham.**, *Chin.*, *Cocc.*, Con., CROC., *Cup.*, Dig., Dros., Fer., Graph., *Ign.*, K. nit., **Kre.**, Lach., Led., *Lyc.*, *Mag. c.*, Mag. m., *Nit. ac.*, **Nux m.**, NUX V., Phos., **Pho. ac.**, *Plat.*, **Puls.**, *Sec. c.*, *Sele.*, **Sep.**, Stram., *Sul.*

— **Tenacious, Stringy.**—CROC., Cup., Mag. c., Sec. c.

Blowing Out of Blood.—*Agar.*, Ambr., *Am. carb.*, Am. m., **Ant. cr.**, Arg., Asar., Bar. c., Bor., *Canth.*, Caps., *Caust.*, Cup., *Dros.*, **Fer.**, **Graph.**, Hep., *K. carb.*, *Lach.*, Led., Lyc., Mag. c., Mag. m., *Meny.*, *Merc.*, *Mez.*, Nat. c., *Nat. m.*, **Nit. ac.**, *Nux v.*, *Par.*, Petrol., **PHOS.**, Pho. ac., **Puls.**, Ran. b., *Rhus*, Ruta, *Saba.*, Sep., *Sil.*, Spig., *Stro.*, SUL., *Thuj.*

Odor from Nose.—Alum., Asaf., AUR., Bell., **Calc. c.**, Caust., *Con.*, Dig., *Dios.*, **Elaps.**, Graph., Hep., Lyc., Mag. m., MERC., *Nat. c.*, **Nit. ac.**, *Nux v.*, Phos., Pho. ac., PULS., *Rhus*, Sep., SUL., Thuj.

— **Sweetish.**—Nit. ac.
— **Urinous.**—Graph.

Nasal Catarrh.—Acon., *Aesc.*, *Agar.*, *Aloe*, *Alum.*, Ambr., *Am. carb.*, **Am. m.**, **Ant. s. aur.**, Ant. cr., *Ant. t.*, *Arg.*, **Arg. n.**, ARS., *Asaf.*, Asar., **Arum t.**, *Aur.*, Bar. c., BELL., *Bor.*, *Bov.*, BROM., Bry., Calad., **Calc. c.**, *Calc. ph.*, Camph., *Canth.*, Caps., Carb. an., *Carb. v.*, *Caust.*, *Cham.*, Chel., Chin., *Cic.*, *Cimic.*, *Cina*, Clem., Cocc., Coff., Colch., Coloc., **Con.**, *Crot. tig.*, Cup., Cyc., *Dros.*, *Eup. per.*, Euphorb., **Euphr.**, **Fer.**, *Gel.*, **Graph.**, Guai., Hell., Hep., *Hydras.*, *Ign.*, **Iod.**, *Jal.*, K. BI., *K. carb.*, **K. iod.**, Kre., **Lach.**, Laur., Led., *Lyc.*, Mag. c., **Mag. m.**, Mang., Mar., Meny., MERC., MERC., C., **Merc. i. r.**, *Mez.*, Mos., Mur. ac., *Naj.*, *Nat. ars.*, **Nat. c.**, Nat. m., *Nit. ac.*, NUX V., **Osm.**, Par., Petrol., **Phos.**, Pho. ac., Plat., *Pb.*, PULS., *Ran. b.*, *Ran. s.*, *Rhodo.*, RHUS, **Rumex**, Saba., *Samb.*, Sang., Sars., SELE., Seneg., Sep., Sil., Spig.,

NOSE. 47

Spo., **Squ.**, Stan. *Staph., Stict., Stro.,* SUL., Sul. ac., *Thuj.*, Verat. a., Zinc.

Stopped Coryza.—Acon., Agar., Agn., Alum., *Ambr.*, **Am. carb.**, Am. m., *Anac., Antip., Ant. cr.*, Arg., **Ars.**, ARUM T., Asar., **Aur.**, Bar. c., ***Bell.***, Bov., **BRY.**, **Calad.**, **Calc. c.**, Camph., **Cannab. s.**, Canth., **Caps.**, *Carb. an.*, **Carb. v.**, *Caust., Cham.*, **Chel.**, Chin., Cic., *Cimic.* Cina, Coff., **Con.**, *Cup., Dig.*, Dros., **Dulc.**, *Elaps.*, Euphorb., **Graph.** Guai., *Hep., Hydras.*, Hyos., Ign., Iod., **Ip.**, **K. bi.**, **K. carb.**, **K. iod.** K. nit., *Kre.*, Lach., *Laur.*, **Lyc.**, *Mag. c., Mag. m., Mang.*, **Mar.**, Meny., Merc., Mez., Mos., *Mur. ac.*, **Nat. c.**, **Nat. m.**, NIT. AC., **Nux m.** NUX V., Op., **Par.**, **Petrol.**, **Phos.**, Pho. ac., Plat., Pb., Pso., PULS., **Ran. b.**, Rhodo., *Saba.*, **Sabi.**, **Samb.**, **Sang.**, *Sars.*, Sele., Seneg., **Sep.**, SIL., SIN., **Spig.**, **Spo.**, Squ., **Stan.**, Staph., *Stict., Stram.,* **Sul.**, *Sul. ac.,* Thuj., *Verat. a.*, Verb., **Zinc.**

Nasal Discharges, Acrid.—ALL. C., ALUM., *Am. carb.*, **Am. m.**, *Anac.*, Ant. cr., ARS., **Ars. iod.**, **Arum t.**, *Bor.*, Calc. c., Cannab. s., Canth., Carb. an., *Carb. v. Cham.*, Chin., *Con.*, Euphorb., **Fer.**, Hep., *Ign.*, Iod., K. carb., **K. iod.**, *Kre.*, Lach., *Lyc.*, Mag. c., *Mag. m.*, Mang., MERC., *Merc. c.*, **Mez.**, Mur. ac., *Nat. m., Nit. ac.*, Nux v., **Phos.**, Pho. ac., *Puls., Ran. b.*, **Sang.**, Sep., Sil., **Sin.**, *Spig.*, Squ., *Sul., Sul. ac.*, Thuj.

—**Bloody.**—Acon., Agar., Alum., Ambr., *Am. carb.*, Ant. t., Arg., *Ars.*, **Arum t.**, Bar. c., Bor., *Bry.*, Canth., Caps., Carb. v., *Caust.*, CHIN., *Clem.*, **Cocc.**, Con., Cup., Dros., Euphr., **Fer.**, Graph., Hep., Iod., **Ip.**, **K. bi.**, K. carb., *Kre.*, Lach., *Laur.*, Led., *Lyc.*, Mag. c., Mag. m., Merc., **Mez.**, *Nat. m., Nit. ac.*, Nux m., **Nux v.**, Op., *Par.*, Petrol., **Phos.**, Pho. ac., *Puls.*, Ran. b., Rhus, Saba., Sabi., Sele., **Sep.**, *Sil.*, Spig., Spo., Squ., Stict., Stro., **Sul.**, *Sul. ac.*, Thuj., *Zinc.*

—**Burning.**—ALL. C., Am. m., **Ars.**, **Ars. iod.**, Calad., *Calc. c.*, Canth., Carb. an., *Cina, Con.*, Euphorb., *Iod.*, K. carb., **K. iod.**, *Kre.*, Mez., Mos., PULS., Sul., Sul. ac.

—**Flocculent.**—Am. carb., **Ars.**, Carb. v., Fer., *Puls.*, Sep., *Sil.*, **Sul.**

—**Gray.**—AMBR., Anac., **Ars.**, *Carb. an., Chin.*, K. carb., **Kre.**, LYC., Mang., *Nux v.* Rhus, Seneg., *Sep.*, Thuj.

—**Green.**—*Ars.*, Asaf., Aur., Bor., Bov., Calc. c., Cannab. s., **Carb. an.**, *Carb. v.*, Colch., Dros., *Fer.*, Hyos., Iod., **K. bi.**, K. carb., *Kre.*, **Led.**, Lyc., Mang., *Merc., Nat. c.*, Nit. ac., Nux v., Par., *Phos.*, Pb., PULS., Rhus, Sep., Sil., *Stan.* Stict., Sul., *Ther.*, Thuj.

—**Hardened.**—Agar., Ant. cr., Bor., Bry., **Con.**, Iod., K. BI., Lach., **Nat. c.**, Phos., *Sep., Sil.*, Staph., *Stict., Stro.*, Sul.

—**Offensive.**—Alum., *Ars.*, Asaf., *Aur., Bell.*, CALC. C., **Caust.**, Chin.,

Con., Cub., Elaps., Graph., Guai., Hep., **K. bi.**, *Kre.*, **Led.**, Lyc., *Mag. m.*, **Merc.**, *Merc. c.*, NAT. C., *Nat. s.*, **Nit. ac.**, *Nux v.*, Petrol., Pho. ac., PULS., Rhus, Sabi., **Sep.**, Sil., Stan., **Sul.**, Ther., Thuj.

Discharges, Purulent.—Acon., Am. carb., Arg., Ars., Asaf., Asar., Bell., CALC. C., Cham., Chin., Cic., Cina, Cocc., CON., Dros., Fer., Graph., Guai., Hep., Ign., *Ip.*, **K. carb.**, *K. nit.*, **Kre.**, Lach., **Led.**, **Lyc.**, Mag. c., *Mag. m.*, **Merc.**, **Nat. c.**, Nat. m., *Nit. ac.*, Nux v., Petrol., Phos., Pho. ac., Pb., **Puls.**, **Rhus**, Sabi., **Samb.**, **Sep.**, **Sil.**, Stan., Staph., Stict., **Sul.**, Zinc.

—**Slimy.**—*Acon.*, **Agar.**, **Agn.**, *Alum.*, *Ambr.*, *Am. carb.*, **Am. m.**, Ant. cr., Ant. t., **Arg.**, ARS., Asar., Aur., Bar. c., **Bell.**, BOR., Bov., **Bry.**, Calad., **Calc. c.**, *Cannab. s.*, Canth., Caps., Carb. an., *Carb. v.*, *Caust.*, *Cham.*, CHIN., **Cina**, Clem., Cocc., Coloc., Con., Dig., Dros., Dulc., *Euphr.*, **Fer.**, *Graph.*, Guai., Hep., *Hyos.*, *Iod.*, *Ip.*, **K. Bi.**, K. nit. *Kre.*, Laur., *Lyc.*, **Mag. c.**, Mang., **Merc.**, Merc. i. r., **Mez.**, Mur. ac., **Nat. m.**, Nit. ac., *Nux m.*, **Nux v.**, *Op.*, **Par.**, *Petrol.*, PHOS., *Pho. ac.*, *Pb.*, **Puls.**, Rhodo., Rhus, Sabi., *Samb.*, Sars., *Sele.*, **Seneg.**, SEP., Sil., Spig., *Spo.*, SQU., **Stan.**, **Staph.**, **Sul.**, *Sul. ac.*, *Thuj.*, Verat. a., ZINC.

—**Tenacious.**—Acon., *Agn.*, *Alum.*, Am. m., *Ant. cr.*, *Ant. t.*, **Ars.**, Bar. c., *Bor.*, BOV., Bry., Calc. c., **Cannab. s.**, *Canth.*, Carb. v., *Caust.*, CHAM., Chin., *Cinnab.*, Cocc., Colch., Dulc., Euphr., Graph., *Iod.*, *K. bi.*, *K. carb.*, **Mag. m.**, *Merc. c.*, **Mez.**, Nat. c., Nux v., **Par.**, Petrol., Phos., *Pho. ac.*, *Pb.*, Puls., Ran. b., Saba., Sabi., **Samb.**, *Seneg.*, Sep., Spig., *Spo.*, Squ., STAN., Staph., Verat. a., *Zinc.*

—**Thick.**—*Acon.*, *Alum.*, Ambr., **Am. m.**, Ant. cr., Arg., *Ars*, **Arum t.**, *Aur.*, Bar. c., Bor., Bov., **Calc. c.**, **Carb. v.**, Caust., Dig., Graph., Hydras., Iod., Ip., **K. bi.**, *Kre.*, Lyc., Mag. c., Mag. m., Mang., **Merc.**, Mur. ac., **Nat. c.**, **Nat. m.**, *Nat. s.*, Nit. ac., Op., Par., Phos., PULS., Ran. b., **Saba.**, **Sang. n.**, Sars., *Sele.*, Sep., *Sin.*, *Spo.*, **Stan.**, **Staph.**, **Sul. ac.**, *Thuj.*, Zinc.

—**Watery.**—*Aesc.*, **Agar.**, ALL. C., *Aloe.*, Alum., Ambr., *Am. carb.*, **Am. m.**, Ant. cr., Ant. t., *Antip.*, *Aral.*, Arg., ARS., **Ars. iod.**, ARUM T., Asar., **Bad.**, Bell., Brom., *Bov.*, **Bry.**, *Calc. ph.*, Carb. an., **Carb. v.**, CHAM., Chin., Clem., Coca, Coff., Coloc., Con., Cub., Cup., Dios., Dros., Euphorb., EUPHR., *Fl. ac.*, *Gel.*, GRAPH., *Guai.*, Hydras., Ign., Iod., K. bi., K. iod., K. nit., Kre., Lach., *Mag. c.*, **Mag. m.**, Meny., **Merc.**, Merc. i. r., **Mez.**, Mur. ac., *Naj.*, Naph., Nat. ars., NAT. C., Nat. m., NIT. AC., NUX V., **Osm.**, Par., Petrol., Phos., Phyt., PLANT., *Pb.*, Puls., Ran. b., Ran. s., Rhus, Rumex, Saba., Sang., Seneg., Sep., **Sil.**, *Sin.*, Spig., Squ., Stan., Staph., *Sul.*, *Sul. ac.*, TELL.

NOSE. 49

Yellow.—Acon., Alum., Am. carb., Am. m., Ant. cr., **Ars., Arum t., Aur., Bar. c.,** Bell., Bor., *Bov., Bry.,* **Calc. c.,** Carb. an., Carb. v., Cham., Cic., Con., Dig., Graph., Hep., Hydras., Ign., **Iod.,** *K. carb.,* **Kre., Lyc.,** Mag. c., Mag. m., Mang., Merc., Mez., Mur. ac., **Nat.** c., *Nat. m., Nat. s.,* **Nit. ac., Nux v., Phos.,** Pho. ac., Pb., **PULS.,** Saba., *Sabi.,* **Sang. n.,** *Sele.,* **SEP., Spig.,** Spo., *Stan., Staph.,* **Sul.,** *Sul. ac., Thuj.,* Verat. a.

Sneezing.—*Acon.,* ...sc., **Agar., Agn., All. c.,** Alum., Ambr., Am. carb, **Am. m.,** *Anac., Antip.,* **Ant. cr., Ant. t.,** *Aral.,* **Arg., Arg. n., Arn., Ars.,** Asaf., Asar., **Bad.,** *Bap.,* **Bar. c., Bell.,** Bor., Bov., **Brom., Bry.,** Calad., *Calc. c., Calc. f., Calc. ph.,* **Camph.,** Cannab. s., *Canth.,* **Caps.,** Carb. an., **CARB. V., Caust.,** Chel., **Chin.,** *Cimic.,* **CINA.,** Clem., Coca, Cocc., *Coc. c.,* **Coff.,** *Colch., Con.,* Croc., **Cyc.,** *Dig., Dios.,* **Dros.,** Dulc., *Euphorb.,* Euphr., *Fl. ac.,* **Gam.,** Graph., Hell., *Hep.,* **Hydras., Iod.,** *Ip.,* **K. bi.,** *K. carb.,* **K. iod.,** K. nit., *Kre., Lach.,* Laur., *Lyc.,* Mag. c., Mag. m., Mang., **Mar., Merc.,** *Merc. i. r.,* **Mez.,** Mos., Mur. ac., *Naph.,* **Nat. c.,** *Nat. m., Nit. ac.,* Nux m., **NUX V.,** Oleand., **Osm.,** *Par.,* Petrol., **Phos., Pho. ac.,** Pb., **PULS.,** Ran. s., Rhodo., **RHUS,** Ruta, **SABA.,** *Sal. ac.,* **Sang., SANG. N.,** Sars., *Seneg.,* **Sep., Sil.,** Spig., Spo., Squ., *Stan.* Staph., *Stict.,* Stro., **SUL.,** Sul. ac., **Tar., Thuj.,** Valer., Verat. a., *Zinc.*

Ineffectual Efforts to Sneeze.—Acon., Alum., Canth., **CARB. V.,** *Caust., Cocc., Colch.,* Euphorb., Hell., *Laur.,* Lyc., **Mez.,** Mur. ac., **Nat. m.,** *Nit. ac.,* **Osm.,** *Phos.,* **Plat.,** *Pb.,* Sars., SIL., Sul., *Sul. ac., Zinc.*

Accompanying Symptoms of Nasal Discharges.—Acon., Alum., Ambr., **Am. m.,** Anac., *Ant. t.,* Arn., **ARS.,** Bar. c., *Bell.,* Bor., Bov., Bry., Calad., **Calc. c.,** Camph., Canth., Caps., Carb. an., **Carb. v.,** *Caust.,* **CHAM.,** *Chin.,* Cic., Cina, Cocc., Coff., Cup., Dig., Dulc., Euphorb., *Euphr.,* **Graph.,** *Hell.,* **Hep.,** Ign., Ip., *K. carb.,* K. nit., Kre., Lach., Laur., **Lyc.,** Mag. c., Mag. m., Mang., Mar., **MERC.,** *Mez.,* Mos., Mur. ac., *Nat. c.,* Nat. m., *Nit. ac.,* Nux m., **NUX V.,** Par., Petrol., **Phos.,** Pho. ac., Plat., **PULS.,** *Rhodo., Rhus,* **Saba.,** Samb., Sars., Seneg., **Sep.,** Sil., **Spig.,** Spo., *Squ.,* Stan., *Staph.,* Sul., Sul. ac., Thuj., Verat. a., Zinc.

Left Side.—*Agar.,* **Am. carb.,** *Am. m.,* Anac., Ant. cr., *Apis,* **Ars.,** *Asar.,* **Aur., Bell., Bor.,** Bov., Brom., *Bry., Calc. c.,* Canth., *Caps.,* Carb. an., **CARB. V., Caust.,** Chel., *Chin., Cina,* Cocc., **Coff., Coloc.,** Dros., *Dulc.,* Fl. ac., Graph., *Hell.,* Hep., K. carb., *Lach.,* Laur., Lyc., *Mag. c., Mag. m.,* Mar., **Merc., NAT. M.,** Nit. ac., **Nux m.,** *Nux v.,* Oleand., Petrol., **Phos., Plat.,** Pso., Puls., **RHODO.,** *Rhus,* Sabi., *Sars.,* **SEP., Sil.,** *Sin., Spo.,* Stan., **Staph.,** *Sul.,* **Tar.,** *Thuj.,* Vio. t., Zinc.

Right Side.—Acon., *Agn.,* Alum., *Ambr.,* Am. carb., Am. m., Anac., Ant. cr., *Asaf.,* **Aur.,** Brom., Bry., *Calad.,* **Calc. c.,** *Canth.,* Carb. an.,

Carb. v., Caust., Chel., Cic., Cocc., Colch., CON., Croc., Dros., Fi. ac., Graph., HEP., Iod., K. bi., K. carb., K. nit., Laur., Lyc., Mang., Mar., Merc., Mez., Nat. c., Nat. m., Nit. ac., Nux v., Petrol., Phos., Pho. ac., Plat., Pso., Puls., Ran. b., Ran. s., Rhus, Sabi., Sars., Sep., Sil., SPIG., Stan., Sul., Sul. ac., Tar., Thuj., Verat. a., Viv. o., Vio. t., Zinc.

Smell.

Sensitive.—ACON., Agar., Alum., Am. carb., Anac., Ant. cr., Arn., Ars., Asar., AUR., Bar. c., BELL., Bry., Calc. c., Canth., Cham., Chin., Cina, Cocc., Coff., Colch., Con., Cup., Dig., Graph., Hep., Hyos., Ign., Ip., K. carb., LYC., Mag. c., Nat. c., Nux m., NUX V., Petrol., PHOS., Pho. ac., Pb., Puls., Saba., Sele., SEP., Sil., Spig., Sul., Thuj., Valer., Vio. o., Zinc.

—**Weak or Lost.**—Alum., Am. m., Anac., Ant. t., Argn. n., Aur., BELL., Bry., CALC. C., Caps., Carb. an., Carb. sul., Caust., Chel., Cocc., Con., Cup., Cyc., Elaps., Graph., Hep., HYOS., Ip., K. carb., K. iod., Laur., Lyc., Mag. m., Mang., Mez., Nat. m., Nit. ac., Nux v., Oleand., Op., Phos., PB., PULS., Rhodo., Rhus, Ruta, Sang., Sec. c., SEP., SIL., Stram., Sul., Sul. ac., Verat. a., Zinc.

Illusions of Smell in General.—Agn., Alum., Anac., Ars., Aur., BELL., CALC. C., Canth., Chin., Con., Dig., Graph., Hep., Kre., Laur., Lyc., Meny., Merc., Mez., Nit. ac., Nux v., PAR., Phos., Pho. ac., Pb., Puls., Seneg., Sep., Sil., Sul., Valer., Verat. a.

—**Agreeable.**—Agn., Puls.

—**Bituminous.**—Ars., Con.

—**Blood.**—Nux v., Sil.

—**Burnt.**—Anac., Calc. c., Graph., Nux v., Sul.

—**Earthy.**—Anac., Calc. c., Sul., Verat. a.

—**Foul.**—Anac., Aur., BELL., Calc. c., Canth., Chin., Con., Dig., Graph., Kre., Meny., Merc., Mez., Nit. ac., Nux v., PAR., PHOS., Pho. ac., Pb., Seneg., Sep., Sul., Valer., Verat. a.

—**of Old Catarrh.**—Graph., Merc., PULS., SUL.

—**of Pus.**—Seneg., Sul.

—**Sour.**—Alum., Bell.

—**Sweetish.**—Aur., Nit. ac., Nux v., Sil.

—**Sulphurous.**—Anac., Ars., Calc. c., Graph., Nux v., Pb.

Face.

Color Alternating.—Acon., Agn., Amyl., Alum., Asaf., Aur., BELL., Bism., Bov., Caps., Carb. an., Cham., Chin., Cina, Croc., Cyc., Fer., Graph., Hyos., IGN., Iod., K. carb., Led., Lyc., Mag. e., Mur. ac.

FACE.

Nat. c., Nat. m., Nux v., *Oleand.*, Op., PHOS., Pho. ac., PLAT., *Puls.*, *Squ.*, *Stram.*, Sul., Sul. ac., Valer., Verat. a., Zinc.

—**Bluish.**—*Acon.*, Agar., Ant. t., **Arg. n.**, **Ars.**, Asar., Aur., **Bell.**, Bry., CAMPH., *Canth.*, Carb. ac., Cham., Cic., **Cina.**, CON., *Crotal.*, *Crot. tig.*, CUP., DIG., Dros., *Gel.*, Hep., *Hyd. ac.*, HYOS., Ign., IP., *K. chl.*, Lach., Lyc., Merc., Mez., OP., Phos., Puls., **Samb.**, Spo., **Staph.**, Stram., VERAT. A.

— —**Around Eyes.**—*Anac.*, ARS., *Bism.*, Calc. c., *Canth.*, Cham., CHIN., Cina, **Cocc.**, **Cup.**, *Fer.*, Graph., *Hep.*, Ign., IP., K. carb., K. iod., Lach., Lyc., Merc., *Mez.*, Nat. c., **Nux m.**, *Nux v.*, OLEAND., Phos., Pho. ac., *Pso.*, RHUS, **Saba.**, *Sabi.*, SEC. C., Sep., Spig., Staph., Stram., *Sul.*, *Tab.*, **Verat. a.**

— —**Around Mouth.**—CINA, Cup., *Pho. ac.*

—**Brown.**—*Ars.*, Bap., *Bry.*, Carb. v., *Carb. ac.*, *Crotal.*, *Gel.*, **Hyos.**, Iod., Kre., Nit. ac., *Op.*, *Puls.*, Sec. c., **Sep.**, *Staph.*, *Stram.*, Sul.

—**Coppery.**—Alum., **Ars.**, Calc. c., Cannab. s., **Carb. an.**, *Kre.*, Led., Rhus, Ruta, *Verat. a.*

—**Earthy.**—Ars., Bism., **Bor.**, Bry., *Canth.*, CHIN., Cic., Cocc., Croc., Euphorb., FER., Hyos., **Ign.**, Ip., *Kre.*, Lach., *Laur.*, **Lyc.**, *Mag. c.*, MERC., Mos., **Nat. m.**, **Nit. ac.**, Nux v., *Op.*, Phos., Pb., Samb., Sec. c., *Sep.*, Sil., Zinc.

—**Gray.**—Berb., *Cad. s.*, **Carb. v.**, *Kre.*, **Lach.**, Laur.

—**Greenish.**—*Ars.*, Carb. v., *Dig.*, **Iod.**, Verat. a.

— —**Around Eyes.**—Verat. a.

—**Lead-colored.**—*Arg. n.*, Crotal.

—**Pale.**—Acon., *Agar.*, Alum., Ambr., *Am. carb.*, Am. m., **Anac.**, ANT. T., **Arg.**, Arg. n., Arn., **ARS.**, Bar. c., Bell., Berb., Bism., Bor., Bov., Bry., **Cact.**, Calc. c. Camph., Cannab. s., *Canth.*, Caps., **Carb. ac.**, Carb. an., Carb. v., *Carb. sul.*, *Caust.*, *Cham.*, Chel., CHIN., Cic., CINA, Clem., Cocc., Colch., *Coloc.*, Con., Croc., Cup., Dig., Dros., Dulc., Euphorb., Euphr., Fer., Gel., Graph., Hell., Hep., Hyos., *Ign.*, **Iod.**, Ip., K. bi., *K. br.*, **K. carb.**, K. chl., K. iod., K. nit., Kre., Lach., Laur., **Led.**, Lyc., Mag. c., *Mag. m.*, Mang., *Mar.*, **Merc.**, Merc. c., Mez., Mos., Nat. c., **Nat. m.**, *Nit. ac.*, Nux m., **Nux v.**, Oleand., OP., **Ox. ac.**, Par., *Petrol.*, Phos., PHO. AC., Phyt., Plat., PB., Pso., Puls., Rheum, Rhus, *Sabi.*, Samb., SEC. C., Sele., SEP., Sil., Spig., *Spo.*, **Stan.**, *Staph.*, Stram., SUL., Sul. ac., TAB., **Ter.**, VERAT. A., Zinc.

—**Red.**—ACON., Agar., Agn., Alum., Ambr., *Am. carb.*, Am. m., **Amyl.**, *Anac.*, Ant. cr., Ant. t., **Apis**, Arg., Arn., *Ars.*, Asaf., Asar., Aur., **Bap.**, *Bar. c.*, BELL., Bor., Bov., BRY., Calad., *Calc. c.*, Camph., *Can-*

nab. s., **Canth.**, *Caps.*, Carb. an., Carb. v., *Carb. sul.*, *Caust.*, **CHAM.**,
Chel., **CHIN.**, **CIC.**, **CINA**, *Clem.*, **Cocc.**, **Coff.**, *Coloc.*, *Con.*, **Croc.**,
Crotal., *Cup.*, Cyc., Dig., **Dros.**, *Dulc.*, Euphorb., Euphr., **Fer.**, **Gel.**,
Glon., Graph., Guai., Hell., **Hep.**, *Hyd. ac.*, HYOS., Ign., Ip., *K.*
carb., *K. nit.*, Kre., *Lach.*, *Laur.*, Led., **Lyc.**, Mag. c., Mag. m., **Mang.**,
Mar., **MELI.**, Meny., **Merc.**, **Merc.** c., **MEZ.**, Mos., *Mur. ac.*, *Nat. c.*,
Nat. m., Nit. ac., Nux m., **NUX V.**, *Oleand.*, **OP.**, Par., *Petrol.*, **Phos.**,
Pho. ac., **Plat.**, Pb., **Puls.**, **Ran. b.**, Ran. s., Rheum, Rhodo., **RHUS**,
Ruta, **Saba.**, Sabi., **Sabi.**, **Samb.**, Sars., Sec. c., Sele., Seneg., **Sep.**, **Sil.**, **Spig.**,
Spo., *Squ.*, **Stan.**, **Staph.**, **STRAM.**, *Stro.*, Sul., Sul. ac., **Tar.**, *Thuj.*,
Valer., **Verat. a.**, **VERAT V.**, Vio. o., *Vio. t.*, Zinc.

— —**Bluish.**—Acon., Agar., **Ant. t.**, **Ars.**, Asar., *Aur.*, BELL.,
BRY., *Camph.*, **CANNAB. I.**, *Carb. ac.*, *Cham.*, Cic., Cina, *Con.*, *Coral.*,
CUP., *Dig.*, Dros., *Grind.*, Hep., *Hydr. ac.*, Hyos., Ign., Ip., **K. chl.**,
Lach., **Lyc.**, **Meli.**, *Merc.*, **Op.**, **Ox. ac.**, *Phel.*, Phos., *Puls.*, *Sang.*, **Samb.**,
Spo., Staph., Stram., *Verat. a.*, *Verat v.*

Circumscribed Redness of Cheeks.—*Acon.*, Ars., *Bry.*, Calc. c.,
Carb. v., **CHIN.**, Con., Croc., *Dros.*, Dulc., **FER.**, Hep., **Iod.**, **K. carb.**,
K. nit., Kre., *Lach.*, Laur., *Led.*, LYC., Merc., Nat. m., Nit. ac., Nux v.,
PHOS., Pho. ac., Puls., Seneg., *Sep.*, Sil., Spo., **Stan.**, *Stram.*, SUL.

—**Erysipelatous Redness.**—ACON., Am. carb., *Ars.*, Bar. c., BELL.,
Bor., *Bry.*, Calc. c., *Camph.*, *Canth.*, *Carb. an.*, **Cham.**, Clem., EU-
PHORB., GRAPH., HEP., **Lach.**, Lyc., *Merc.*, Nat. c., Phos., *Puls.*,
RHUS, *Ruta*, Samb., Sep., *Sil.*, *Stram.*, *Sul.*, Thuj.

—**Spotted.**—*Alum.*, *Ambr.*, Am. carb., Ars., *Bell.*, Bry., **Calc. c.**,
Cannab. s., Canth., **CARB. AN.**, *Colch.*, *Croc.*, *Fer.*, Hell., *Kre.*, *Laur.*,
Led., **Lyc.**, Mar., *Merc.*, Mos., **Nat. c.**, Nux m., Nux v., Op., Par.,
Phos., RHUS, *Ruta*, *Saba.*, *Samb.*, Sars. Sec. c., *Sep.*, SIL., *Sul.*, *Verat. a.*,
Zinc.

—**Yellow Spots.**—SEP.

—**Yellow.**—*Acon.*, **Ambr.**, Ant. cr., **Arg.**, *Arn.*, ARS., Asaf., Aur.,
Bell., Bry., *Calc. c.*, Cannab. s., **Canth.**, **Carb. v.**, Caust., Cham., **CHEL.**,
Chin., (Cina), *Clem.*, Cocc., CON., Croc., *Corn. c.*, *Crotal.*, *Crot. tig.*,
Cup., **Dig.**, Dulc., Euphorb., FER., *Gel.*, *Gran.*, Graph., Hell., *Hep.*,
Ign., Iod., *K. br.*, *K. carb.*, *Lach.*, *Laur.*, Lyc., Mag. m., **Merc.**, Nat. c.,
Nat. m., Nit. ac., NUX V., Op., *Petrol.*, Phos., (Pho. ac.), PB., *Puls.*,
Ran. b., Rheum, *Rhus*, Ruta, Saba., Sec. c., SEP., Sil., *Spig.*, Stan., SUL.,
Sul. ac., Tar., *Verat. a.*

— —**Around Eyes.**—Nit. ac., *Nux v.*, **Spig.**
— —**Around Mouth.**—*Nux v.*, **Sep.**

FACE.

— —**Around Nose.**—*Nux v.*, **Sep.**

Yellow Saddle across Upper Part of Cheeks and Nose.—SEP.

Color, Yellow on Temples.—Caust.

Comedones.—*Dig.*, Dros., **Graph.**, **Nat. c.**, **Nit. ac.**, Saba., *Sabi.*, SUL.

Drawn.—Acon., *Ambr.*, Am. carb., ANT. T., Arg. n., ARS., BELL, Bism., *Bry.*, Calc. c., **Camph.**, Cannab. s., *Canth.*, Carb. v., **Caust.**, Cham., *Chel.*, Cic., *Cocc.*, *Colch.*, **Cup.**, Dig., *Dulc.*, *Gel.*, **Graph.**, Guai., Hell., Hep., *Hyd. ac.*, **Hyos.**, **Ign.**, Iod., Ip., K. carb., *Lach.*, Laur., LYC., Merc., **Merc. c.**, Mos., Nat. c., Nux m., *Nux v.*, Oleand., OP., Phos., Pho. ac., **Plat.**, Pb., *Puls.*, *Ran. b.*, Ran. s., Rheum, **Rhus**, Samb., SEC. C., Sep., *Sil.*, *Spig.*, *Spo.*, **Stan.**, Staph., **Squ.**, STRAM., Sul., TAB., VERAT. A.

Emaciation.—*Calc. c.*, Mez., Pso., Sele.

Eruptions.—Agar., Agn., *Alum.*, *Ambr.*, *Am. carb.*, Am. m., ANT. CR., **Ant. s. aur.**, Arg., Arn., *Ars.*, Aur., *Bar. c.*, **Bell.**, Bor., **Bov.**, **Bry.**, Calc. c., *Calc. ph.*, Cannab. s., *Canth.*, Caps., *Carb. an.*, *Curb. v.*, *Carb. sul.*, **Caust.**, *Cham.*, *Chel.*, *Cic.*, Clem., Cocc., **Con.**, *Crotal*, Dig., Dulc., Euphorb., *Gnap.*, *Graph.*, Hell., *Hep.*, Hyos., Ign., K. bi., K. BR., K. carb., K. nit., **KRE.**, **Lach.**, Laur., LED., Lyc., *Mag. c.*, Mag. m., Mang., *Merc.*, MEZ., Mur. ac., *Nat. c.*, **Nat. m.**, *Nit. ac.*, *Nux v.*, Oleand., Par., Petrol., Phos., **Pho. ac.**, Pso., Puls., RHUS, Ruta, Saba., Sabi., Sars., Sele., SEP., **Sil.**, Spo., **Staph.**, *Stram.*, Stro., **Sul.**, Sul. ac., *Tar.*, Thuj., **Verat. a.**, Vio. t., *Zinc.*

—**On Cheeks.**—Agar., *Agn.*, Alum., *Ambr.*, Am. carb., Anac., ANT. CR., Arn., Asaf., Bar. c., **Bell.**, Bor., **Bov.**, **Bry.**, **Calc. c.**, *Canth.*, Carb. v., **Caust.**, *Cham.*, Chel., Cina, **Con.**, Cyc., *Dig.*, Dulc., EUPHORB., Graph., Hep., Hyos., **K. chl.**, K. nit., **KRE.**, **Lach.**, Laur., Mag. m., Merc., Mez., *Nat. c.*, **Nat. m.**, Nit. ac., Nux v., *Oleand.*, Phos., RHUS, Ruta, Saba., Sabi., Sars., **Sep.**, **Sil.**, *Spo.*, STAPH., *Stro.*, *Tar.*, Thuj., Valer., **Verat. a.**, Verb., **Vio. t.**

—**On Chin.**—Agn., Alum., Ambr., Am., carb., Anac., **Ant. cr.**, Bell., Bor., *Calc. c.*, Canth., *Caust.*, Cic., Clem., **Con.**, *Crotal*, *Dig.*, Dros., Dulc., *Graph.*, *Hep.*, Hyos., *K. carb.*, **Kre.**, Laur., **Lyc.**, Mag. c., **Merc.**, *Mez.*, Nat. c., *Nat. m.*, Nit. ac., Nux m., Nux v., Oleand., **Par.**, Phos., **Pho. ac.**, Plat., Puls., RHUS, Sabi., *Sars.*, **Sep.**, **Sil.**, *Spig.*, Spo., Squ., *Stro.*, **Sul.**, Tar., Thuj., *Verat. a.*, Verb., **Zinc.**

—**Around Eyes.**—*Agn.*, **Ars.**, Calc. c., *Con.*, **Hep.**, Ign., **Merc.**, Oleand., Petrol., Sil., Spo., *Staph.*, Sul.

—**In Eyebrows.**—**Ars.**, **Caust.**, Hell., **K. carb.**, *Nat. m.*, *Par.*, Rhus Sele., Sep., Sil., Staph., Sul., Thuj.

FACE.

—On Forehead.—Agar., Agn., Alum., *Ambr.*, Am. carb., Am. m.. Anac., **ANT. CR.**, Arg., Arn., Ars., Aur., Bar. c., *Bell.*, **Bov.**, *Bry.*, *Calc. c.*, Canth., Caps., Carb. an., *Carb. v.*, **Caust.**, *Cham.*, Chel., Cic., *Clem.*, Cocc., *Con.*, Dig., Dulc., Euphorb., Graph., Hell., **Hep.**, K. carb., **KRE.**, Laur., **LED.**, Lyc., Mag. c., Mag. m., Merc., Mez., Mur. ac., Nat. c., **Nat. m.**, Nit. ac., **NUX V.**, Oleand., *Par.*, **Phos.**, **Pho. ac.**, **Pso.** Puls., *Ran. b.*, Rhodo., **RHUS**, Ruta, Saba., Sars., **SEP.**, *Sil.*, *Staph.*, **SUL.**, Sul. ac., Valer., *Verat. a.*, *Vio. t.*, Zinc.

—On Upper Lip.—Acon., Ant. cr., Arn., **ARS.**, Bar. c., *Bell.*, Canth., *Carb. v.*, *Caust.*, Cic., Con., *Graph.*, Hell., Hep., K. **CARB.**, **KRE.**, Lyc., Mag. c., Mag. m., *Merc.*, **Nat. c.**, **Nat. m.**, Nit. ac., **Par.**, Petrol., Plat., **Rhus**, *Saba.*, *Sil.*, Spig., **STAPH.**, SUL., *Thuj.*, *Zinc.*

—On Lower Lip.—Alum., *Bor.*, **BRY.**, **Calc. c.**, *Caust.*, Cham., Clem., Ign., *Mez.*, **Nat. c.**, **Nat. m.**, Phos., *Pho. ac.*, Rhodo., **SEP.**, **Sul.**

—Around Mouth.—Acon., **Agar.**, *Aloe*, *Alum.*, *Am. carb.*, Am. m., Anac., *Ant. cr.*, **ARUM T.**, Arn., **ARS.**, Bar. c., *Bell.*, Bor., **Bov.**, **BRY.**, **Calc. c.**, *Cannab. s.*, Canth., *Caps.*, Carb. an., Carb. v., **Caust.**, Cham., Chin., Cic., Clem., Cocc., Coloc., Con., *Crot. tig.*, Dig., Dulc., *Graph.*, Hell., Hep., *Hyos.*, *Ign.*, Ip., **K. bi.**, **K. carb.**, K. CHL., **KRE.**, *Laur*, Led., *Lyc.*, *Mag. c.*, *Mag. m.*, Mang., *Merc.*, **Merc. c.**, *Mez.*, **Mur. ac.**, **Nat. c.**, **NAT. M.**, Nit. ac., **Nux v.**, **Par.**, *Petrol.*, Phos., *Pho. ac.*, Plat., *Puls.*, Ran. b., Rhodo., **RHUS**, Ruta, Saba., Samb., **SEP.**, **Sil.**, Spig., *Spo.*, Squ., **STAPH.**, SUL., *Tar.*, Thuj., *Verat. a.*, Zinc.

—Corners of Mouth.—Ant. cr., Arn., Bell., Calc. c., *Calc. fl.*, Carb. v., Caust., *Cic.*, Coloc., Cund., *Graph.*, Hell., **Hep.**, *Ign.*, **Kre.**, *Mang.*, **MERC.**, Mez., *Nat. c.*, **Nat. m.**, **NIT. AC.**, *Petrol.*, **Phos.**, Rhodo., **Sep.**, **Sil.**, Verat. a., Zinc.

—On Nose.—Agar., Agn., **Alum.**, Am. carb., Am. m., Anac., *Ant. cr.*, Arn., Ars., Aur., Bar. c., **Bell.**, Bor., *Bov.*, Bry., *Calc. c.*, Cannab. s., Canth., Caps., **Carb. an.**, **Carb. v.**, **CAUST.**, Cham., Chel., Chin., Cina, **Clem.**, Coloc., Con., Dulc., Euphr., *Graph.*, Guai., Hell., Hep., Ign., Iod., **K. carb.**, *K. nit.*, Lach., Laur., **Led.**, Lyc., *Mag. c.*, *Mag. m.*, Mang., **Merc.**, Mez., Mur. ac., **Nat. c.**, *Nat. m.*, **Nit. ac.**, Nux v., Oleand., Petrol., **Phos.**, **PHO. AC.**, Plat., *Pb.*, Puls., Rhodo., **Rhus**, Saba., Sabi., Samb., *Sars.*, *Sele.*, Seneg., **SEP.**, **SIL.**, Spig., Spo., *Staph.*, Stro., **SUL.**, Sul. ac., Tar., *Thuj.*, Verat. a., *Vio. t.*, Zinc.

—Around Nose.—Alum., Am. carb., **Ant. cr.**, Bar. c., *Bor.*, **Calc. c.**, **Caust.**, Dulc., *Eláps.*, Mag. m., *Nat. c.*, Par., **RHUS**, Sep., *Sil.*, *Sul.*, Sul. ac., Tar., Zinc.

—On Temples.—*Alum.*, Ambr., Anac., **Ant. cr.**, *Arg.*, Arn., Bar. c.,

FACE.

Bell., *Bry.*, *Carb. v.*, *Caust.*, Cocc., *Lach.*, **Lyc.**, *Mur. ac.*, **Nat. m.**, Nit. ac., Sabi., Spig., *Sul.*, Thuj.

Expression Altered.—ACON., Alum., Ant. cr., *Arg. n.*, ARS., BELL., *Bism.*, BAR., *Bry.*, Calc. c., **Camph.**, CANNAB. I., *Canth.*, Caust., Cham., *Chel.*, *Chin.*, *Clem.*, **Colch.**, Coloc., *Crotal.*, Cup., *Dig.*, Gel., Gran., *Graph.*, *Hell.*, Hyos., Ign., Iod., Lach., Laur., **Lyc.**, Mag. c., Merc., Merc. c., Nux v., Oleand., Op., Phos., *Pho. ac.*, **Pb.**, *Pso.*, Puls., *Ran. s.*, Rheum, Rhus, *Sec. c.*, Sep., Sil., *Spig.*, Spo., **Stan.**, STRAM., Sul., VERAT. A., Vio. o., Zinc.

Eyes Protruding.—Acon., *Arn.*, Ars., Aur., BELL., Bor., *Canth.*, Caps., *Chin.*, Cic., Cocc., *Com.*, Con., Cup., **Fer.**, Glon., **Guai.**, **Hep.**, *Hyd. ac.*, Hyos., Laur., **Merc.**, Mos., Nux v., **Op.**, *Phos.*; Rhus, Spig., Spo., Squ., *Stan.*, Staph., STRAM., **Verat. a.**

—**Sunken.**—Ambr., Anac., Ars., Calc. c., **Camph.**, *Canth.*, Carb. sul., CHIN., Cic., CINA., Coloc., *Crotal.*, **Cup.**, *Cyc.*, Dros., **Fer.**, Hyos., Iod., *K. br.*, *K. carb.*, *K. iod.*, Lach., **Lyc.**, *Mar.*, Nit. ac., **Nux v.**, *Oleand.*, Op., **Phos.**, Pho. ac., PULS., Sec. c., *Spo.*, *Stan.*, Staph., Sul., *Tab.*, **Verat. a.**

Freckles.—Am. carb., Ant. cr., Ant. t., *Bry.*, **Calc. c.**, Carb. v., Con., *Dros.*, **Dulc.**, Graph., Hyos., Iod., *K. carb.*, Lach., Laur., **Lyc.**, Merc., Mez., Nat. c., Nit. ac., Nux m., Petrol., PHOS., Pb., Puls., Sep., *Sil.*, Stan., SUL., Thuj.

Oily.—Agar., Aur., *Bry.*, *Chin.*, **Mag. c.**, Merc., **Nat. m.**, *Pb.*, **Rhus**, Sele., Stram.

Open Mouth.—Acon., *Ars.*, BELL., Carb. v., *Camph.*, **Gel.**, **Hyos.**, Lyc., **Op.**, Pb., *Puls.*, Samb., **Squ.**

Swelling.—Acon., Aconin., Agar., Alum., Am. carb., Am. m., APIS., Arn., ARS., *Aur.*, Bar. c., BELL., Bor., *Bor.*, **Bry.**, *Calc. c.*, **Canth.**, Caps., Carb. an., Carb. v., Caust., CHAM., Chel., Chin., Cic., Cina, Cocc., Colch., Coloc., *Com.*, Con., Cup., *Dig.*, Dros., **Dulc.**, *Euphorb.*, **Fer.**, Graph., Guai., **Hell.**, **Hep.**, *Hyd. ac.*, **Hyos.**, Iod., Ip., K. CARB., Kre., LACH., Laur., *Led.*, **Lyc.**, Mag. c., Mag. m., Mar., MERC., **Merc. c.**, Mos., Nat. c., Nat. m., *Nit. ac.*, Nux m., **Nux v.**, Oleand., OP., Petrol., **Phos.**, Pho. ac., Pb., *Puls.*, Rheum, RHUS, Ruta, Sabi., Samb., Sec. c., **Sep.**, Sil., Spig., Spo., *Stan.*, Staph., **Stram.**, **Sul.**, Sul. ac., *Verat. a.*, **Verat. v.**

—**Cheeks.**—Am. carb., Am. m., ARN., *Ars.*, Aur., Bar. c., *Bell.*, Bor., *Bor.*, Bry., *Calc. c.*, *Canth.*, Caust., CHAM., *Chin.*, Euphorb., Fer., Graph., *Hep.*, Iod., **K. carb.**, Lach., *Lyc.*, Mag. c., Mag. m., **Merc.**, Nat. c., Nat. m., *Nit. ac.*, Nux v., Petrol., *Phos.*, Pho. ac., PULS., *Rhus*, Samb., Sep., Sil., Spig., *Spo.*, **Stan.**, Staph., *Sul.*

Swelling Around Eyes.—Ars., *Fer.*, **Phos.**, Puls., *Rheum.*
—**Over Eyes.**—Ruta, **Sep.**
—**Under Eyes.**—**Ars.**, *Bry.*, Cham., *Nux v.*, Oleand., PHOS:, *Puls.*
—**Between Lids and Brows.**—K. carb.
—**Lips.**—Acon., *Alum.*, Arg., **Arn.**, **Ars.**, *Asaf.*, *Aur.*, *Bar. c*, **BELL.,** **Bov.**, **Bry.**, **Calc. c.**, **Canth.**, **Caps.**, Carb. an., *Carb. v.*, Caust., Chin., Con., *Crot. tig.*, Dig., Graph., Hell., Hep., *K. carb.*, *Lyc.*, **Merc.**, **MERC. C.**, *Mez.*, Mos., Mur. ac., Nat. c., **NAT. M.**, **Nit. ac.**, Nux m., Oleand., Op., Par., Petrol., *Phos.*, **Pso.**, **Puls.**, Rhus, Sep., *Sil.*, **Staph.**, Stram., *Sul.*, Thuj., Zinc.
—**Upper Lip.**—Arg., *Bar. c*, **Bell.**, *Bov.*, Bry., Calc. c., *Canth.*, Carb. v., Con., Graph., Hep., *K. carb.*, Lyc., **Merc.**, Mez., **Nat. m.**, *Nit. ac.*, Par., Petrol., *Phos.*, PSO., *Rhus*, Sil., **Staph.**, *Sul.*, Thuj., Zinc.
—**Lower Lip.**—Alum., Asaf., Calc. c., Caust., *Lyc.*, *Mez.*, *Mur. ac.*, Nat. m., **Puls.**, **Sep.**, Sil., SUL.
—**Nose.**—*Acon.*, Agn., Alum., Ambr., Am. carb., Am. m., Ant. cr., *Arn.*, **Ars.**, Aur., *Bar. c*, **BELL.**, Bor., Bov., **Bry.**, **Calc. c.**, Cannab. s., **Canth.**, Caps., Carb. an., Carb. v., **CAUST.**, *Cham.*, Chel., *Chin.*, Cic., Cocc., Con., Croc., Dulc., Euphorb., Graph., Hell., **Hep.**, Hyos., Ign., Iod., K. CARB., K. nit., Lach., *Lyc.*, MERC., Mez., NAT. C., *Nat. m.* **Nit. ac.**, **Nux v.**, Petrol., PHOS., PHO. AC., Pb., **PULS.**, *Ran. b.*, Rhodo., RHUS, Ruta, *Saba.*, *Samb.*, SEP., **Sil.**, Spig., *Spo.*, Stan., Staph., *Stram.*, **Sul.**, Thuj., Verat. a., Zinc.
Wrinkles, Deep.—LYC., Sep., *Stram.*
—**On Forehead.**—Am. carb., Bry., *Cham.*, Graph., **Hell.**, **LYC.**, Nux v., *Rheum*, *Rhus*, **Sep.**, **Stram.**, Vio. o.

Location of Sensations.

Forehead.—*Agar.*, **Agn.**, Alum., **Ambr.**, *Am. carb.*, *Am. m.*, Anac., **Ant. cr.**, *Arg.*, **Arn.**, Ars., *Aur.*, *Bar. c*, **Bell.**, **Bov.**, Bry., *Calc. c.*, **Canth.**, *Caps.*, Carb. an., **Carb. v.**, **Caust.**, Cham., *Chel.*, *Chin.*, Cic., **Clem.**, Cocc., Colch., *Coloc.*, *Con.*, Croc., Dig., *Dros.*, Dulc., Euphorb., Graph., *Guai.*, *Hell.*, HEP., Iod., Ip., K. carb., **Kre.**, *Laur.*, **LED.**, *Lyc.*, Mag. c., *Mag. m.*, Mang., Mar., *Meny.*, Merc., Mur. ac., Nat. c., **Nat. m.**, *Nit. ac.*, Nux v., *Oleand.*, **Par.**, **Phos.**, PHO. AC., Puls., *Rheum*, *Rhodo.*, RHUS, *Ruta*, *Saba.*, *Samb.*, Sars., SEP., *Sil.*, *Spig.*, *Squ.*, Staph., SUL., Sul. ac., Valer., *Verat. a.*, *Verb.*, Vio. o., Vio. t., *Zinc.*

Temples.—*Alum.*, Ambr., Anac., Ant. cr., *Arg.*, Arn., Asar., Bar. c., *Bell.*, Bry., *Carb. v.*, Caust., Cocc., Lach., **LYC.**, *Mur. ac.*, *Nat. m.*, Nit. ac., Sabi., Spig., Sul., Thuj., **Verb.**

FACE—LOCATION OF SENSATIONS.

Malar Bone.—Acon., *Agar., Alum.,* Ambr., Am. m., *Anac.,* Ant. cr., *Ant. t.,* **Arg.,** Arn., Ars., **Asaf., Aur.,** Bar. c., **Bell.,** *Bism.,* Bor., **Bry., Calc. c.,** *Calc. ph.,* Cannab. s., Canth., *Caps., Curb. v.,* Caust., **Chel.,** *Chin.,* Cina, *Cocc.,* **Colch., Coloc.,** *Con., Coral.,* **Dig.,** *Dros.,* Fer., Graph., *Guai.,* Hell., Hep., *Ign.,* **K. carb.,** *K. iod.,* **Kalm.,** Laur., Led., *Lyc.,* Mag. c., **Mag. m.,** *Mang.,* Merc., *Mez., Mos.,* Mur. ac., Nat. c, *Nat. m., Nit. ac., Nux. v.,* OLEAND., Par., Phos., *Plat., Pb., Puls.,* Rhus, *Ruta,* Saba., *Sabi., Samb., Sang.,* **Sep., Spig.,** Spo., STAN., STAPH., Stro., *Sul.,* **Sul. ac.,** *Thuj., Valer.,* Verat. a., VERB., **Vio. o.,** *Zinc.*

Cheeks.—*Acon., Agar.,* Agn., *Alum., Ambr.,* Am. carb., Am. m., *Anac.,* Ant. cr., **Arg., Arn.,** Ars., *Asaf., Asar.,* **Aur., Bell., Bor.,** Bov., **Bry., Calc. c.,** Cannab. s., *Canth.,* Carb. an., **Carb. v., CAUST.,** *Cham.,* Chel., *Chin., Cina,* **Clem.,** *Cocc.,* Coloc., *Con.,* Cyc., *Dig., Dros., Dulc., Euphorb.,* Euphr., Fer., *Graph.,* Guai., Hep., Hyos., Ign., Ip., *Iris. v., K. br., K. carb.,* **K. chl.,** K. nit., Kre., *Lach.,* Laur., *Lyc.,* Mag. m., Mang., *Meny.,* Merc., *Mez., Nat. m.,* Nit. ac., **Nux v.,** *Oleand,* Par., *Phos.,* Pho. ac., *Phyt., Plat.,* **Puls.,** RHUS, Ruta, Saba., *Sabi.,* Samb., *Sars.,* Sep., Sil., *Spig.,* Spo., **Stan.,** STAPH., Stro., Sul., Sul. ac., Tar., *Thuj., Valer.,* Verat. a., Verb., Vio. t.

Upper Jaw.—*Acon.,* **Agar., Alum.,** *Ambr.,* AM. CARB., *Am. m.,* Arn., **Ars.,** Asaf., AUR., **Bell.,** Bor., Bov., *Bry.,* **Calc. c., Calc. ph.,** *Canth.,* Carb. an., CARB. V., *Caust., Cham.,* Chel., CHIN., Clem., Coff., Colch., *Coloc.,* Con., Cyc., Dulc., *Euphorb.,* Euphr., Graph., Guai., *Hell.,* Hyos., *K. bi.,* **K. carb.,** *K. nit.,* **Kalm.,** KRE., *Lyc.,* Mag. c., **Mag. m.,** *Many.,* Mar., *Meny.,* Merc., **Mez.,** *Mur. ac.,* Nat. c., **Nat. m., Nit. ac.,** *Nux m.,* Nux v., Phos., *Pho. ac.,* Plat., Puls., Ran. s., Rheum, Rhodo., Rhus, *Saba.,* Samb., Sars., Seneg., *Sep.,* Sil., Spig., **Spo.,** Stan., *Staph.,* Stro., *Sul.,* **Sul. ac.,** Thuj., Verat. a., *Verb.,* ZINC.

Lower Jaw.—*Acon.,* **Agar., Agn.,** *Alum., Ambr.,* **Am. carb.,** Am. m., *Anac.,* Ant. t., Arg., *Arn.,* Asaf., Asar., **Aur.,** *Bar. c.,* BELL., Bor., Bov., **Bry.,** Calc. c., Camph., Cannab. s., CANTH., Caps., *Carb. an.,* **Carb. v.,** CAUST., CHAM., Chel., **Chin.,** Cic., *Cina,* Clem., Cocc., Coff., Colch., Coloc., Con., **Cup.,** Dig., *Dros.,* Dulc., Euphorb., *Euphr., Graph.,* Guai., *Hell.,* Hep., *Hyos.,* Ign., K. carb., K. nit., *Kre.,* LAUR., Led., *Lyc.,* Mag. c., Mag. m., *Mang.,* Mar., Meny., **Merc.,** Mez., *Mur. ac.,* NAT. C, Nat. m., *Nit. ac., Nux m.,* Nux v., Oleand., **Op.,** Par., Petrol., **Phos.,** Pho. ac., *Plat.,* **PB.,** Puls., Ran. b., Ran. s., Rheum, Rhodo., Rhus, Ruta, *Saba., Sabi.,* Sars., Sele., Seneg., *Sep.,* **Sil.,** *Spig.,* Spo., Squ., *Stan.,* STAPH., Stro., *Sul.,* **Sul. ac.,** Thuj., Valer., **Verat. a.,** *Verb.,* Vio. o., Vio. t., ZINC.

Articulation of Jaws.—*Acon., Aconin.,* Alum., Am. carb., **Am. m.,**

FACE—LOCATION OF SENSATIONS.

Arn., **Arum t.**, *Asaf., Asar.,* **BELL.**, **Bry.,** Calc. c., **Camph.,** *Canth., Carb. ac., Caust.,* Cham., **CHEL.,** Cic., *Cocc.,* **Colch.,** *Con., Coral., Cup., Dios.,* Dros., Euphr., Graph., *Hyd. ac.,* Hyos., IGN., K. carb., Lach., *Laur.,* Mang., Meny., MERC., **Merc. c.**, Mur. ac., Nat. c., Nat. m., *Nit. ac.,* Nux m., **Nux v.,** *Op., Petrol.,* Phos., Pho. ac., **Plat.,** Pb., RHUS, *Saba.,* Sabi., Sars., Sec. c., Sep., Sil., **Spig., Spo.,** Stan., *Staph., Stram.,* Sul., Sul. ac., Thuj., *Verat. a., Verb.*

Lips.—Acon., Agar., *Alum., Am. carb., Am. m.,* Ant. cr., **Ant. t.,** *Arn.,* **Ars., ARUM T.,** Asaf., **Bar. c.,** BELL., *Bor., Bov.,* BRY., **Calc. c.,** *Cannab. i.,* Cannab. s., *Canth., Caps.,* Carb. an., *Carb. v.,* Caust., *Cham., Chin.,* Cic., Clem., **Con.,** Croc., Cyc., Dig., *Dulc.,* Graph., Hell., **Hep.,** Hyos., **Ign.,** Ip., **K. carb.,** *Kre.,* Laur., *Lyc.,* Mag. c., Mag. m., **Merc.,** *Merc. c., Merc. i. r.,* **Mez.,** *Mur. ac.,* **Nat. c.** NAT. M., Nit. ac., **Nux v.,** Oleand., Op., *Par.,* **Phos.,** Pho. ac., Plat., **Puls.,** Rhodo., RHUS, **Saba., SEP., Sil.,** Spig., Spo., Squ., **Staph.,** Stram., Stro., SUL., Tar., *Thuj.,* Valer., *Verat. a.,* **Zinc.**

Upper Lip.—*Acon.,* Agar., Am. carb., Am. m., *Ant. cr.,* Arg., *Arn.,* **Ars.,** BAR. C., BELL., Bor., Bov., **Bry.,** Calc. c., **Calc. ph.,** *Canth.,* Caps., **Carb. v.,** *Caust.,* Chel., Chin., *Cic.,* Coff., *Colch.,* **Con.,** *Cyc.,* Dig., Dulc., **Graph.,** *Hell.,* **Hep.,** Ign., K. CARB., **Kre.,** Laur., Led., *Lyc., Mag. c., Mag. m.,* MERC., Mez., Mos., Mur. ac., **Nat. c.,** *Nat. m., Nit. ac.,* Nux v., Oleand., **Par.,** *Petrol.,* Phos., Pho. ac., *Plat.,* Pb., Puls., Rheum, *Rhus,* **Saba.,** Sars., Sele., Seneg., *Sep., Sil., Spig.,* Squ., **Staph., Stro.,** SUL., Sul. ac., Tar., Thuj., Valer., Verat. a., **Zinc.**

Lower Lip.—Agar, *Alum.,* Am. carb., Am. m., Arn., Ars., *Asaf.,* Aur., Bar. c., Bell., **Bor.,** Bov., BRY., **Calc. c.,** Caps., Carb. v., *Caust., Cham.,* Chin., *Clem.,* Con., Dros., Euphorb., Graph., Hep., Hyos., IGN., K. carb., Laur., Lyc., Mag. c., Mang., *Mar.,* Merc., **Mez.,** Mur. ac., *Nat. c., Nat. m.,* Nux v., Oleand., *Op.,* Par., *Phos.,* **Pho. ac.,** Plat., PULS., *Ran. s.,* Rheum, *Rhodo.,* Rhus, Saba., Sabi., Samb., Sars., SEP., Sil., Spig., Spo., *Stan.,* Staph., **Sul.,** *Valer.,* Zinc.

Corners of Lips.—Ambr., Am. m., ANT. CR., *Arn.,* Asaf., Bar. c., BELL., Bov., Bry., **Calc. c.,** Cannab. s., Canth., *Carb. v.,* **Caust.,** Chel., Coloc., *Crot. tig., Cund.,* Dros., **Graph.,** *Hell.,* **Hep.,** Ign., Ip., Laur., Lyc., **Kre., Mang.,** MERC., *Mez., Nat. c., Nat. m.,* NIT. AC., Nux v., Ol nd., Op., Par., **Petrol.,** PHOS., Ran. b., *Ran. s.,* Rheum, *Rhodo.,* Rhus, *Seneg.,* **Sep., Sil.,** Stro., *Sul., Sul. ac.,* Tar., *Verat. a.,* **Zinc.**

Chin.—Agar., Agn., Alum., Ambr., Am. carb., Am. m., *Anac.,* **Ant. cr.,** *Asaf.,* Aur., **Bell.,** Bor., *Bov.,* Bry., Calc. c., Cannab. s., **Canth., Carb. v.,** CAUST., Chel., Cic., *Clem.,* Cocc., Coloc., *Con., Cup.,* Dig.,

FACE—LOCATION OF SENSATIONS—TEETH.

Dros., *Dulc.*, Euph b., *Euphr.*, Graph., **Hep.**, Hyos., *K. carb.*, **Kre.**, **Laur.**, Led., Lyc., *Mag. c.*, Mag. m., *Mang.*, **Merc.**, *Mez.*, Nat. c., *Nat. m.*, Nit. ac., *Nux m.*, Nux v., *Oleand.*, Op., Par., *Phos.*, Pho. ac., **PLAT.**, Pb., Puls., Ran. b., **Rhus**, Sabi., **Sars.**, *Sep.*, SIL., *Spig.*, **Spo.**, Squ., Stan., *Staph.*, Stram., **Stro.**, **Sul.**, Tar., *Thuj.*, **Verat. a.**, *Verb.*, **Zinc.**

Left Side.—Acon., Alum., *Am. carb.*, Anac., *Ant. cr.*, Ant. t., *Apis*, Arg., *Arn.*, Ars., **Asaf.**, *Asar.*, Aur., *Bar. c.*, **Bell.**, *Bor.*, *Bov.*, **Brom.** Bry., *Calc. c.*, **Cannab. s.**, Canth., **Caps.**, **Carb. an.**, *Carb. v.*, *Caust.*, Cham., *Chel.*, Chin., **Cic.**, *Cina*, **Clem.**, Cocc., *Coff.*, Colch., **Coloc.**, **Con.**, Cup., **Dig.**, *Dros.*, *Dulc.*, **Euphorb.**, *Euphr.*, Fl. ac., Graph., Guai., *Hell.*, Hep., **Hyos.**, *Ign.*, Iod., K. carb., *K. chl.*, K. nit., Kre., **Lach.**, Laur., Led., Lyc., Mag. c., Mag. m., Mang., Mar., Meny., **Merc.**, *Mez.*, *Millef.*, Mos., **Mur. ac.**, Nat. c., *Nat. m.*, Nit. ac., Nux m., Nux v., **Oleand.**, .**Par.**, Petrol., Phos., *Pho. ac.*, *Plat.*, Pb., Pso., *Puls.*, Ran. b., **Rhodo.**, *Rhus*, *Ruta*, *Saba.*, *Sabi.*, *Samb.*, *Seneg.*, **Sep.**, Sil., Spig., **Spo.**, Stan., Staph., Stram., Stro., **Sul.**, Sul. ac., Tar., Thuj., Valer., *Verat. a.*, *Verb.*, Vio. o., Vio. t., Zinc.

Right Side.—Acon., *Agar.*, **Agn.**, *Alum.*, Am. carb., **Am. m.**, *Anac.*, Ant. cr., Ant. t., Apis, *Arg.*, Arn., **Ars.**, Asaf., Asar., **Aur.**, *Bar. c.*, **BELL.**, *Bism.*, Bar., Brom., **Bry.**, CALC. C., **Cannab. s.**, CANTH., Caps., Carb. an., Carb. v., **Caust.**, Cham., *Chel.*, **Chin.**, Cina, Cocc., Colch., Coloc., *Con.*, Cup., **Cyc.**, Dig., Dros., *Dulc.*, Euphr., **Fl. ac.**, Graph., Guai., **Hep.**, Hyos., Iod., *K. carb.*, *K. nit.*, **Kalm.**, **Kre.**, *Lach.*, Laur., Led., **LYC.**, *Mag. c.*, Mag. m., *Mang.*, Mar., Meny., **Merc.**, *Mez.*, Millef., *Mos.*, **Nat. c.**, Nat. m., **Nit. ac.**, *Nux m.*, **NUX V.**, Oleand., Par., Petrol., **Phos.**, Pho. ac., Plat., **Pb.**, **Pso.**, **Puls.**, Ran. b., Ran. s., *Rheum*, Rhus, Saba., Sabi., *Sars.*, **Sep.**, **Sil.**, **Spig.**, Spo., Stan., **Staph.**, Stram., Stro., *Sul.*, Sul. ac., Tar., Thuj., *Valer.*, Verat. a., *Verb.*, Zinc.

Teeth.

Toothache, Generally.—*Acon.*, Agar., *Aloe.*, Alum., **Ambr.**, *Am. carb.*, Am. m., Anac., Ant. cr., Ant. t., Arg., *Arn.*, **Ars.**, Asar., Aur., *Bar. c.*, **Bell.**, *Bism.*, **Bor.**, *Bov.*, BRY., Calad., Calc. c., Calc. f., *Calc. ph.*, Canth., Carb. an., **Carb. v.**, *Carb. sul.*, **Caust.**, CHAM., *Chel.*, CHIN., Clem., Cocc., *Coc. c.*, **Coff.**, *Col. h.*, **Coloc.**, Con., Croc., Cyc., *Dios.*, Dros., Dulc., **Euphorb.**, **Fer.**, Fl. ac., **GLON.**, Graph., Guai., Hell., Hep., Hyos., Ign., Iod., Ip., **K. carb.**, K. nit., Kre., **LACH.**, Laur., *Lyc.*, Mag. c., **Mag. m.**, Mang., *Mar.*, MERC., *Merc. c.*, **Mez.**, Mur. ac., NAT. C., Nat. m., Nit. ac., Nux m., Nux v., Oleand., Par., *Petrol.*, **Phos.**, *Pho. ac.*, Plant., *Plat.*, Pb., Pru., **PULS.**, Ran. s., *Raph.*, Rheum,

RHODO., **Rhus**, Ruta, *Saba.*, **Sabi.**, Sars., Sele., Seneg., SEP., *Sil.*, **Spig.**, Spo., Squ., STAPH., *Stro.*, **Sul.**, *Sul. ac.*, *Tab.*, Tar., *Ther.*, *Thuj.*, **Valer.**, *Verat. a.*, Verb., ZINC.

Incisors.—Agar., Alum., *Ambr.*, Am. carb., Am. m., Arg., Asar., Aur., Bell., Bor., Bov., Calc. c., Canth., *Carb. v.*, *Caust.*, Cham., *Chin.*, Cocc., Coff., COLCH., Dros., Ign., Iod., **K. carb.**, *Kre.*, Lyc., Mag. c., **Mag. m.**, *Mar.*, *Merc.*, Mez., Mur. ac., Nat. c., **Nat. m.**, *Nit. ac.*, Nux m., Nux v., *Petrol.*, *Phos.*, Pho. ac., Plat., *Ran. s.*, Rhodo., **Rhus**, Sars., Seneg., **Sep.**, *Sil.*, *Spig.*, Spo., *Staph.*, **Stro.**, **Sul.**, *Sul. ac.*, Tar., Thuj., Zinc.

Eye Teeth.—Am. carb., Anac., Calc. c., Laur., Mag. m., Mur. ac., *Nat. c.*, Petrol., **Rhus**, Sep., Staph., Stro., Sul. ac., Zinc.

Molars.—*Agar.*, *Alum.*, Ambr., **Am. carb.**, Anac., Ant. t., *Arg. n.*, Arn., Asar., *Aur.*, Bar. c., Bell., Bism., Bor., Bov., BRY., Calad., *Calc. c.*, *Canth.*, Carb. an., **Carb. v.**, *Caust.*, Cham., CHIN., *Clem.*, Cocc., Coff., Colch., Coloc., Croc., *Cyc.*, *Euphorb.*, Graph., Guai., *Hell.*, *Hyos.*, Ign., Iod., *K. carb.*, K. nit., KRE., Laur., *Lyc.*, *Mag. c.*, **Mag. m.**, *Mang.*, Mar., *Merc.*, *Mez.*, Mur. ac., **Nat. c.**, *Nit. ac.*, Nux m., Nux v., *Oleand.*, Par., Petrol., **Phos.**, *Pho. ac.*, Plat., Pb., *Puls.*, **Ran. s.**, Rheum, **Rhodo.**, Rhus, *Saba.*, *Sabi.*, Sars., Seneg., *Sep.*, *Sil.*, Spig., Spo., **Staph.**, Stro., Sul., Sul. ac., Thuj., Verat. a., *Verb.*, ZINC.

Hollow Teeth.—Alum., *Ambr.*, Am. carb., Anac., Ant. cr., Asar., **Bar. c.**, BELL., BOR., Bov., Bry., **Calc. c.**, Carb. an., *Carb. v.*, *Carb. sul.*, Caust., **Cham.**, *Chin.*, Clem., Cocc., Coff., Con., Graph., *Hep.*, **Hyos.**, *Ip.*, *K. carb.*, K. nit., *Kre.*, **Lach.**, Lyc., **Mag. c.**, *Mag. m.*, Mang., MERC., MEZ., NAT. C., *Nat. m.*, Nit. ac., Nux v., *Par.*, Petrol., **Phos.**, *Pho. ac.*, Plat., PB., *Puls.*, *Rheum*, Rhodo., **Rhus**, Ruta, *Saba.*, **Sabi.**, *Sele.*, SEP., *Sil.*, Spig., STAPH., *Sul.*, *Sul. ac.*, TAR., *Thuj.*, *Verat a.*, Zinc.

Upper Teeth.—Agar., Alum., *Ambr.*, AM. CARB., *Am. m.*, Arn., Asar., **Aur.**, BELL., Bor., Bov., *Bry.*, **Calc. c.**, *Canth.*, *Carb. an.*, CARB V., *Caust.*, *Cham.*, CHIN., Clem., Coff., Colch., Con., Cyc., *Euphorb.*, Graph., Guai., *Hell.*, Hyos., **K. carb.**, *K. nit.*, KRE., *Lyc.*, Mag. c., **Mag. m.**, *Mang.*, Mar., Merc., **Mez.**, *Mur. ac.*, **Nat. c.**, **Nat. m.**, Nit. ac. *Nux m.*, Nux v., Phos., *Pho. ac.*, Plat., Puls., **Ran. s.**, Rheum, Rhodo., Rhus, *Saba.*, Sars., Seneg., *Sep.*, Sil., Spig., Spo., *Staph.*, *Sul.*, **Sul. ac.**, Thuj., Verat. a., *Verb.*, ZINC.

Lower Teeth.—Agar., *Alum.*, *Ambr.*, **Am. carb.**, Am. m., *Anac.*, Ant. t., Arg., *Arn.*, Asar., **Aur.**, *Bar. c.*, BELL., Bor., *Bov.*, Bry., Calc. c., CANTH., *Carb. an.*, **Carb. v.**, CAUST., CHAM., **Chin.**, Clem., Cocc.,

Coff., Colch., Coloc., Con., *Dros.*, **Euphorb.**, *Graph.*, Guai., *Hell.*, Hep., *Hyos.*, Ign., K. carb., K. nit., *Kre.*, *Lach.*, LAUR., *Lyc.*, *Mag.* c., **Mag. m.**, **Mang.**, Mar., *Merc.*, Mez., *Mur. ac.*, NAT. C., Nat. m., *Nit. ac.*, *Nux m.*, *Nux v.*, Oleand., Par., Petrol., **Phos.**, Pho. ac., *Plat.*, PB., **Puls.**, Ran. s., Rheum, Rhodo., **Rhus**, **Ruta**, *Saba.*, **Sabi.**, **Sars.**, Sele., Seneg., *Sep.*, Sil., *Spig.*, *Spo.*, Squ., STAPH., *Stro.*, *Sul.*, *Sul. ac.*, *Thuj.*, **Verat. a.**, *Verb.*, ZINC.

Teeth, Black.—MERC.

—Gray.—Merc.

—**Grinding.**—Bell., Cannab. i., *Crotal.*, Pod.

—**Loose (and Falling Out).**—Ars.. Bry., MERC., MERC. C., **Nit. ac.**, Pso., Sil.

—**Covered with Mucus.**—Iod.

— — **Sordes.**—Merc. c.

—**Yellow.**—*Coca*, **Iod.**, **Nit. ac.**, *Pho. ac.*

—Yellow Coat.—*Bry.*

Gums.—Alum., *Ambr.*, **Am. carb.**, Am. m., Anac., Ant. cr., **Apis**, Arg., *Arg. n.*, **Arn.**, Ars., Aur., *Bar. c.*, **Bell.**, Bism., BOR., *Bov.*, *Bry.*, **Calc. c.**, *Canth.*, **Caps.**, **Carb. an.**, **Carb. v.**, Caust., Cham., Chin., Cic., *Clem.*, Colch., Con., *Crotal.*, *Crot. tig.*, *Dol.*, *Dulc.*, *Fl. ac.*, **Graph.**, *Ham.*, Hep., Hyos., *Iod.*, *K. carb.*, K. nit., *Kre.*, *Lach.*, *Lyc.*, Mag. c., Mag. m., Mar., MERC., **Merc. c.**, *Mur. ac.*, Nat. c., **Nat. m.**, *Nit. ac.*, Nux m., NUX V., Par., *Petrol.*, **Phos.**, *Pho. ac.*, **PB.**, **Puls.**, Ran. s., Rhodo., *Rhus*, **Ruta**, Saba., *Sabi.*, *Sars.*, Sec. c., **Sep.**, *Sil.*, Spig., Spo., Stan., STAPH., *Stro.*, *Sul.*, Sul. ac., *Thuj.*, Zinc.

Upper Gum.—*Agar.*, Am. carb., *Aur.*, **Bar. c.**, Bell., CALC. C., *Canth.*, Carb. an., Colch., Graph., K. carb., **Kre.**, Lyc., *Mag. m.*, Mur. ac., Nat. m., *Nit. ac.*, RUTA, Sep., *Stro.*

Lower Gum.—Am. carb., Am. m., Anac., Canth., Carb. an., Caust., Laur., Mag. m., *Mar.*, **Nat. c.**, Petrol., Phos., Rhodo., *Sabi.*, SARS., Spo., **Staph.**, *Sul.*, Sul. ac., *Thuj.*, Zinc.

Inner Gum.—Agar., Ambr., Am. carb., Arn., *Graph.*, K. carb., Nat. c., *Nat. m.*, Pho. ac., *Puls.*, Rhus, **Ruta**, Sep., STAPH.

Left.—*Acon.*, **Agar.**, Alum., Ambr., *Am. carb.*, *Am. m.*, Anac., **Apis**, **Arn.**, *Asaf.*, *Asar.*, *Aur.*, **Bar. c.**, Bell., **Bor.**, *Brom.*, *Bry.*, Calc. c., Cannab. s., Canth., **Carb. an.**, **Carb. v.**, CAUST., CHAM., *Chel.*, Chin., CLEM., Coff., *Colch.*, **Con.**, *Croc.*, *Cyc.*, EUPHORB., Fl. ac., Graph., **Guai.**, *Hyos.*, Iod., K. carb., *K. nit.*, *Kre.*, Laur., *Led.*, Lyc., Mar., **Merc.**, MEZ., *Millef.*, Nat. m., **Nux m.**, *Nux v.*, *Oleand.*, **Phos.**, *Plant.*, **Puls., Ran.** s., *Rheum*, **Rhodo.**, **Rhus**, Saba., *Sabi.*, *Samb.*, **Sele.**, Seneg.,

SEP., **Sil.**, **Spig.**, Spo., *Staph.*, Stro., **SUL.**, **THUJ.**, *Verat. a.*, **Verb.**, Zinc.

Right.—Agar., *Agn.*, Alum., *Ambr.*, *Am. carb.* Anac., Apis., *Aur.*, Bar. c., **BELL.**, *Bov.*, Brom., **Bry.**, Calc. c., *Camph.*, *Cannab. s.*, Canth., Carb. an., Carb. v., *Caust.*, **Chel.**, *Chin.*, *Coff.*, Colch., *Coloc.*, Con., **FL. AC.**, *Graph.*, **Hell.**, **Iod.**, K. carb., **Kre.**, Lach., Laur., Lyc., **Mag. c.**, *Mang.*, *Mar.*, **Merc.**, Mez., *Nat. c.*, *Nat. m.*, *Nit. ac.*, Nux. v., Oleand., Petrol., *Pho. ac.*, Pso., *Puls.*, Ran. b., Ran. s., Rhodo., *Rhus*, *Ruta*, Saba., Sars., *Sep.*, *Sil.*, Spig., Spo., **STAPH.**, Stro., Sul., *Tar.*, Thuj., *Valer.*, **Verb.**, Zinc.

Mouth.

Mouth in General.—*Abrot.*, Acon., Agar., Agn., Alum., *Ambr.*, *Am. carb.*, Am. m., Anac., Ant. cr., *Ant. t.*, *Arg.*, Arn., **ARS.**, **Arum t.**, *Asaf.*, Asar., Aur., Bap., **Bar. c.**, **BELL.**, Bism., Bor., Bov., *Bry.*, Calad., **Calc. c.**, Camph., Cannab. s., **Canth.**, **Caps.**, *Carb. ac.*, *Carb. an.*, **Carb. v.**, *Carb. sul.*, *Caust.*, **Cham.**, **Chel.**, Chin., Cic., Cina, *Cocc.*, *Coff.*, Colch., Coloc., Con., *Corn. c*, *Croc.*, *Crot. tig.*, Cup., Cyc., *Dig.*, *Dios.*, *Dros.*, *Dulc.*, Euphorb., Fer., **Fl. ac.**, *Graph.*, Guai., **Hell.**, *Hep.*, *Hydras.*, *Hyos.*, **Ign.**, **Iod.**, *Ip.*, *Iris. v.*, **K. bi.**, *K. carb.*, **K. CHL.**, *K. iod.*, K. nit., *Kre.*, Lach., *Laur.*, Led., *Lyc.*, *Mag. c.*, Mag. m., Mang., Mar., Meny., **MERC.**, **Merc. c.**, **Merc. d.**, Mez., Mos., Mur. ac., *Nat. c.*, *Nat. m.*, **Nit. ac.**, *Nux m.*, **NUX V.**, Oleand., Op., *Par.*, Petrol., **PHOS.**, *Pho. ac.*, *Phyt.*, Plat., *Pb.*, *Pod.*, **Puls.**, Ran. b., Ran. s., Rheum, *Rhodo.*, *Rhus*, Ruta, **Saba.**, Sabi., Samb., *Sars.*, Sec. c., Sele., *Seneg.*, **Sep.**, *Sil.*, *Spig.*, Spo., Squ., Stan., **Staph.**, **Stram.**, *Stro.*, **Sul.**, **Sul. ac.**, *Tub.*, Tar., **Thuj.**, **Valer.**, **Verat. a.**, Vio. o., Zinc.

Odor from Mouth.—Acon., *Agar.*, Alum., *Ambr.*, Am. carb., Anac., Ant. cr., Ant. t., *Arg. n.*, Arn., Ars., Asar., **Aur.**, Bap., Bar. c., *Bell.*, *Bism.*, Bor., **Bry.**, Calc. c., Camph., **Canth.**, **Caps.**, *Carb. ac.*, *Carb. an.*, **CARB. V.**, *Carb. sul.*, **Cham.**, Chin., Cimic., Cocc., *Coff.*, Croc., Cup., Dig., Dros., **Dulc.**, Fer., *Graph.*, Hell., Hep., Hyos., Ign., **Iod.**, *Ip.*, *K. br.*, K. carb., *K. chl.*, *K. iod.*, K. nit., Lach., Laur., Led., Lyc., **MERC.**, *Merc. c.*, **Merc. d.**, Mez., Nat. m., **NIT. AC.**, Nux. m., **Nux v.**, Oleand., Petrol., Phos., Pho. ac., Pod., PB., **Puls.**, Rheum, Rhus, Ruta, Sabi., Sars., **Sec. c.**, Sep., Sil., *Spig.*, Stan., *Stram.*, Stro., **Sul.**, **Sul. ac.**, **Tell.**, Thuj., *Valer.*, Verb., *Zinc.*, Zing.

Breath Cold.—*Camph.*, Carb. v., *Chin.*, *Colch.*, Mur. ac., Rhus, *Ter.*, *Verat. a.*

Breath Hot.—Acon., *Ant. cr.*, Asar., Bell., *Calc. c.*, *Cham.*, Coff., Fer., *Mang.*, **Nat. m.**, *Phos.*, Plat., Rhus, Saba., *Squ.*, Stro., Sul., *Zinc.*

MOUTH. 63

Saliva Diminished.—Acon., Agar., Agn., Alum., *Ambr.*, Am. carb., Am. m., Anac., Ant. cr., Ant. t., Arg., *Arn.*, **Ars.**, *Asaf.*, Asar., Aur., **Bar. c.**, **BELL.**, Bor., Bov., **Bry.**, Calad., **Calc. c.**, Camph., Cannab. s., *Canth.*, Caps., *Carb. an.*, Carb. v., *Caust.*, **Cham.**, Chel., Chin., Cina, Clem., **Cocc.**, Coff., Colch., Con., Croc., Cup., *Cyc.*, *Dulc.*, Euphorb., Fer., Graph., *Hell.*, Hep., **Hyos.**, Ign., Iod., *Ip.*, *K. carb.*, K. nit., **Lach.**, Laur., Led., **Lyc.**, Mag. c., Mag. m., Mang., *Meny.*, **Merc.**, Mez., Mos., *Mur. ac.*, *Nat. c.*, Nat. m., **Nit. ac.**, NUX M., **Nux v.**, Oleand., **Op.**, Par., *Petrol.*, **PHOS.**, *Pho. ac.*, Plat., **Pb.**, **Puls.**, Ran. b., **Ran. s.**, Rheum, Rhodo., *Rhus*, Ruta, *Saba.*, Sabi., Samb., *Sars.*, Sec. c., **Sele.**, **Seneg.**, **Sep.**, Sil. Spig., *Spo.*, Squ., *Stan.*, Staph., **STRAM.**, **Stro.**, **SUL.**, Sul. ac., Tar., *Thuj.*, **VERAT. A.**, *Zinc.*

—**Increased.**—Acon., **Aesc.**, **Agar.**, Alum., Ambr., Am. carb., *Am. m.*, Anac., Ant. cr., Ant. t., **Arg.**, *Arg. n.*, Arn., **Ars.**, Asaf., *Asar.*, Aur., **Bap.**, **Bar. c.**, **BELL.**, Bism., *Bor.*, Bov., **Bry.**, **Calc. c.**, *Camph.*, Cannab. s., **Canth.**, *Caps.*, **Carb. an.**, Carb. v., *Carb. sul.*, **Caust.**, **Cham.**, Chel., **Chin.**, Cic., *Cina*, Clem., **Cocc.**, Coc. c., **Coff.**, Colch., Con., *Croc.*, *Crot. tig.*, *Cucur.*, Crep., Cyc., **Dig.**, Dros., Dulc., *Euphorb.*, Fer., **Gran.**, **Graph.**, Guai., **Hell.**, *Hep.*, **Hyos.**, Ign., IOD., Ip., **IRIS. V.**, **JAB.**, **K. bi.**, **K. carb.**, **K. iod.**, K. nit., Kre., **Lach.**, Laur., Led., **Lyc.**, Mag. c., **Mag. m.**, Mar., Meny., **MERC.**, MERC. C., **Merc. d.**, **Merc. i. r.**, Mez., Mur. ac., **Nat. c.**, **Nat. m.**, **NIT. AC.**, *Nux m.*, **NUX V.**, Oleand., **Op.**, **Ox. ac.**, Par., *Petrol.*, **PHOS.**, Pho. ac., **Phyt.**, *Plat.*, **Pb.**, **PULS.**, Ran. b., Ran. s., Rheum, Rhodo., **RHUS**, Saba., Sabi., Samb., **Sang.**, *Sars.*, Sec. c., **Sele.**, Seneg., Sep., Sil., **Spig.**, Spo., **Squ.**, *Stan.*, **Staph.**, **STRAM.**, Stro., **SUL.**, Sul. ac., TAB., *Tar.*, *Thea.*, Thuj., **Valer.**, Verat. a., Verb., Vio. t., **Wye.**, Zinc.

Tongue.—Acon., *Acon. f*, *Agar.*, **Ail.**, *Aloe.*, Alum., Ambr., Am. carb., **Am. m.**, Anac., Ant. cr., *Ant. t.*, **Apis**, Arg., **ARG. N.**, Arn., **ARS.**, **ARUM. T.**, Asar., **Bar. c.**, **BELL.**, *Bism.*, **Bor.**, Bov., **Bry.**, *Calc. c.*, **Calc. ph.**, *Cannab. i.*, Cannab. s., **Canth.**, Carb. an., Carb. v., *Carb. sul.*, **Caust.**, **Cham.**, Chel., **Chin.**, *Chrom. ac.*, Cic., Cina, Clem., *Cocc.*, Coff., *Colch.*, **Coloc.**, Con., Croc., *Crotal.*, *Crot. tig.*, Cup., Cyc., **Dig.**, Dros., Dulc., Fer., *Gel.*, Graph., *Hell.*, Hep., **Hydras.**, **Hyos.**, *Hyper.*, Ign., Iod., *Ip.*, *Jab.*, **K. BI.**, **K. br.**, K. carb., **K. iod.**, K. nit., Kre., **Lach.**, Laur., Led., **Lyc.**, Mag. c., *Mag. m.*, Mang., Mar., Meny., MERC., **Merc. c.**, **Merc. d.**, **Merc. i. f.**, *Mez.*, Mos., **Mur. ac.**, *Nat. c.*, **NAT. M.**, **NIT. AC.**, *Nux m.* **Nux v.**, Oleand., **Op.**, *Osm.*, *Ox. ac.*, Par., **Petrol.**, **PHOS.**, *Pho. ac.*, Plat., **PB.**, **Pod.**, **PULS.**, *Ran. s.*, Rheum, Rhodo., **Rhus**, Ruta, **Saba.**, Sabi., *Sang.*, Sars., **Sec. c.**, *Sele.*, Seneg., **Sep.**, Sil., **Spig.**, Spo.,

Stan., *Staph.*, **Stram.**, Stro., SUL., *Sul. ac.*, TAR., *Ter.*, *Thuj.*, **Verat. a.**, VERAT. V., **Verb.**, Vio. t., **Zinc.**

—**Coated.**—Acon., *Agar.*, Alum., *Ambr.*, Am. carb., Anac., ANT. CR., **Ant. t.**, *Arg. n.*, **Arn.**, Ars., Asar., **Bap.**, Bar. c., **BELL.**, **Bism.**, Bor., Bov., BRY., Calc. c., *Cannab. i.*, *Cannab. s.*, **Canth.**, Carb. v., *Carb. sul.*, Caust., **Cham.**, *Chel.*, *Chin.*, *Cina*, **Cocc.**, *Colch.*, Coloc., Croc., Cup., Cyc., *Dig.*, *Dios.*, **Eup. per.**, Euphorb., **Gel.**, Graph., Guai., *Hydras.*, *Ign.*, Iod., Ip., K. BI., *K. nit.*, Lach., Laur., Lyc., Mag. c., Mag. m., **Mang.**, MERC., **Merc. c.**, **Merc. i. f.**, Mez., Mur. ac., *Nat. c.*, *Nat. m.*, *Nat. s.*, NIT. AC., Nux m., *Nux v.*, Oleand., *Osm.*, *Ox. ac.*, Par., *Petrol.*, **Phos.**, Pho. ac., **Pb.**, PULS., Ran. b., Ran. s., Rheum, Rhus, **Rumex**, Ruta, **Saba.**, *Sabi.*, Sars., **Sec. c.**, *Sele.*, *Seneg.*, **Sep.**, Sil., Spig., **Stan.**, Staph., *Stro.*, SUL., TAR., Thuj., **Verb.**, Vio. t., *Zinc.*

Hard Palate.—Ambr., Am. carb., Ant. cr., Arn., *Ars.*, *Aur.*, **Bar. c.**, **BELL.**, *Bor.*, Bov., **Calc. c.**, *Camph.*, Cannab. s., *Canth.*, **Caps.**, Carb. v., Caust., Cham., Chin., *Cocc.*, *Coloc.*, *Croc.*, *Crot. tig.*, Dig., Dulc., *Euphorb.*, Hell., Hyos., *Ign.*, Iod., *K. carb.*, Lach., Laur., Led., Mag. c., Mag. m., *Meny.*, Merc., **Mez.**, Mur. ac., Nat. m., **Nit. ac.**, Nux m., NUX V., **Par.**, **Phos.**, Pho. ac., *Puls.*, Ran. b., Ran. s., Rhodo., *Rhus*, Ruta, *Saba.*, *Sang.*, Sep., Sil., *Spo.*, *Spig.*, **Squ.**, Staph., Thuj., Zinc.

Soft Palate.—*Acon.*, Ant. cr., *Arg.*, *Arg. n.*, **Aur.**, *Bell.*, Calc. c., *Canth.*, *Caps.*, **Carb. ac.**, Carb. v., Caust., Cham., Chin., Coc. c., **Coff.**, *Cop.*, *Dig.*, *Dros.*, Dulc., Hell., Hep., *Iod.*, *K. bi.*, K. carb., *K. nit.*, Lach., Led., Mag. c., Meny., MERC., **Merc. c.**, *Mez.*, **Mur. ac.**, **Nat. ars.**, **Nat. m.**, Nit. ac., Nux m., Nux v., Par., **Phos.**, Pho. ac., *Phyt.*, Ran. b., Ran. s., Rhodo., Ruta, *Sars.*, Seneg., Sep., *Sil.*, Staph., **Stram.**, *Sul.*, *Sul. ac.*, Thuj., *Valer.*, *Verat. a.*, Zinc.

Throat.

—**Internal.**—ACON., *Aconin.*, **Aesc.**, *Agar.*, Agn., **Ail.**, *All. c.*, *Aloe.*, **Alum.**, *Alumen.*, *Ambr.*, Am. carb., Am. m., **Amyl.**, Anac., Ant. cr., *Ant. t.*, APIS., **Arg.**, Arg. n., Arn., **Ars.**, ARUM. T., **Asaf.**, *Asar.*, *Atrop.*, Aur., **Bap.**, BAR. C., **Bar. m.**, **BELL.**, Bism., Bor., Bov., **Brom.**, **Bry.**, *Caj.*, Calad., **Calc. c.**, *Calc. fl.*, *Camph.*, Cannab. s., **Canth.**, *Caps.*, **Carb. ac.**, *Carb. an.*, **Carb. v.**, *Carb. Sul.*, Caust., **Cham.**, *Chel.*, *Chin.*, **Chrom. ac.**, Cic., Cina, *Coca*, *Cocc.*, **Coc. c.**, **Coff.**, *Colch.*, Coloc., **Con.**, Croc., CROTAL., *Crot. tig.*, *Cub.*, *Cund.*, **Cup.**, Cyc., *Dig.*, *Dios.*, **Dol.**, **Dros.**, Dulc., *Elaps.*, Euphorb., Fer., *Fl. ac.*, **Gel.**, *Graph.*, Guai., Hell., *Hep.*, **Hydras.**, *Hyd. ac.*, Hyos., Ign., Iod., *Ip.*, **K. bi.**, *K. br.*, *K. carb.*, **K. chl.**, K. nit., *Kre.*, LACH., *Laur.*, Led., *Lyc.*, Mag. c., Mag. m., **Mang.**,

Mar., *Meny.,* MERC., MERC. C., MERC. CY., *Merc. d.,* MERC. I. F., **Merc. i. r., Merc. n.,** *Mez.,* Mos., **Mur. ac.,** *Naj., Nat. Ars.,* **Nat. c., Nat. m., Nit. ac.,** *Nux m.,* NUX V., Oleand., *Op., Pœo., Par., Petrol.,* PHOS., *Pho. ac.,* **Phyt.,** *Plat., Pb., Pso.,* PULS., Ran. b., Ran. s., Rhodo., **Rhus,** *Rumex,* Ruta, Saba., *Sabi., Sal. ac.,* Samb., **Sang.,** *Sang. n.,* Sars., Sec. c., *Sele.,* **Seneg.,** Sep., *Sil.,* Spig., Spo., *Squ.,* **Stan.,** *Staph., Still.,* STRAM., Stro., Sul., *Sul. ac., Sum., Tab.,* Tar., *Thuj., Valer.,* **Verat. a.,** *Verat. v.,* Verb., **Wye.,** *Zinc.*

Tonsils.—Acon., *Ail.,* **Am. m., Ars., Bap.,** BAR. C., *Bar. m., Calc. ph., Crot. tig.,* **Iod., K. Bi.,** MERC., *Merc. cy.,* **Merc. i. f.,** MERC. I. R., *Mur. ac.,* NIT. AC., PHYT., *Ran. s., Saba., Sul., Sul. ac.*

Mouth and Fauces.

Left Side.—Acon., Alum., Ant. cr., *Ant. t., Apis, Arum. t., Aur.,* **Bar. c., BELL.,** Bov., Calc. c., *Carb. an.,* Carb. v., **Caust.,** *Colch., Croc., Cup.,* Dros., *Euphorb.,* Fl. ac., **Graph., Hep.,** Iod., **K. carb.,** Kre., LACH., Lyc., *Mar., Meny.,* **Merc. i. r.,** *Mez.,* Millef., Nat. m., *Nit. ac., Nux m.,* Nux v., Oleand., *Phos.,* Pho. ac., Plat., Pso., **Puls.,** *Rhodo.,* **Rhus,** Saba., *Sabi.,* Seneg., SEP., *Sil.,* Spig., **Sul.,** *Tar., Thuj., Verat. a.,* **Zinc.**

Right Side.—*Alum.,* **Am. carb.,** Ant. cr. *Ars.,* Aur., Bov., *Brom., Calc. c.,* **Carb. v., Caust.,** *Chin., Coloc.,* **Dros.,** Fl. ac., Graph., Iod., **Kre.,** Lach., LYC., Mar., MERC., Merc. i. f., Millef., *Nat. m., Nit. ac., Nux v., Petrol.,* Phyt., Plat., *Pb., Pso.,* Ran. b., Rhus, *Saba., Sang.,* Sep., Sil., *Spig.,* **Stan.,** Sul., *Thuj.,* Zinc.

Hunger and Thirst.

Loss of Appetite.—Ab. n., Acon., *Agar., Alum.,* Ambr., *Am. carb.,* Am. m., Anac., **Ant. cr.,** *Ant. t., Arg.,* **Arn., Ars.,** Asaf., Aur., **Bap., Bar. c., Bell.,** *Bor.,* Bov., **Bry.,** *Cact.,* Calad., **Calc. c.,** Cannab. s., **Canth.,** Caps., **Carb. ac.,** Carb. an., Carb. v., *Carb. sul., Card.,* Caust., *Cham.,* **Chel.,** CHIN., Cic., *Clem.,* **Coca.,** COCC., **Coff.,** Colch., Coloc., **Con.,** Croc., *Crotal., Crot. tig.,* **Cup.,** CYC., DIG., Dros., *Dulc.,* Euphorb., Euphr., **Fer., Fl. ac., Gran.,** Graph., *Guai., Hell.,* Hep., Hyos., **Ign., Iod., Ip.,** K. BI., **K. carb.,** *K. nit.,* Kre., *Lach., Laur.,* Led., **Lyc.,** Mag. c., *Mag. m.,* Mang., Mar., **Merc.,** *Mez.,* Mos., **Mur. ac.,** Nat. c., **Nat. m.,** *Nit. ac.,* Nux m., NUX V., *Oleand., Op.,* **Petrol.,** Phos., Pho. ac., Plat., Pb., **Pso.,** Puls., Ran. b., Ran. s., *Rheum, Rhodo.,* RHUS, *Ruta,* Saba., Sabi., Sars., Sec. c., *Sele.,* Seneg., SEP., SIL., Spig., Spo., *Squ., Stan.,* Staph., Stram., Stro., SUL., *Sul. ac.,* Thuj., Valer., *Verat. a.,* Verb., Vio. t., Zinc.

Hunger.—*Agar.,* Agn., *Aloe, Alum., Am. carb.,* Am. m., Anac., *Ant. cr.,*

Ant. t., **Arg.**, Arh., *Ars.*, Asar., **Aur.**, **Bar. c.**, **Bell.**, Bor., *Bov.*, **Bry.**, Calad., CALC. C., **Calc. ph.**, CANNAB. I., Canth., Caps., Carb. an., *Carb. v.*, *Carb. sul.*, Caust., Cham., *Chel.*, CHIN., Cic., CINA., Cocc., **Coff.**, Colch., Coloc., **Crot. tig.**, Cup., Cyc., Dig., Dulc., Euphorb., Euphr., **Fer.**, **Gran.**, GRAPH., Guai., **Hell.**, *Hyos.*, *Ign.*, *Iod.*, K. carb., K. nit., **Lach.**, Laur., **Lyc.**, Mag. c., Mag. m., Mang., *Mar.*, Meny., **Merc.**, *Mez.*, Mos., *Mur. ac.*, **Myr.**, **Nat. c.**, *Nat. m.*, Nit. ac., Nux m., *Nux v.*, Oleand., **Op.**, *Par.*, **Petrol.**, **Phos.**, *Plat.*, *Pb.*, PULS., Ran. b., Rheum, Rhodo., *Rhus*, Ruta, **Saba.**, *Sars.*, **Sec. c.**, Seneg., Sep., Sil., Spig., Spo., *Squ.*, **Stan.**, **Staph.**, Stram., *Stro.*, SUL., Sul. ac., **Ther.**, Valer., **Verat. a.**, **Verb.**, Zinc.

—**Without Relish.**—Agar., *Alum.*, Ant. cr., Ant. t., **Arg.**, **Ars.**, **Bar. c.**, *Bell.*, Bor., **Bry.**, Calad., *Calc. c.*, Canth., Carb. v., Caust., **Chin.**, *Cic.*, Clem., *Cocc.*, **Coff.**, Colch., Coloc., *Cyc.*, Dig., **Dulc.**, Euphr., Fer., **Hell.**, Hep., *Ign.*, *Iod.*, K. nit., *Lyc.*, Mag. c., **Mag. m.**, *Merc.*, Mez., Nat. c., NAT. M., *Nux v.*, Oleand., OP., Plat., *Puls.*, RHEUM, *Rhodo.*, RHUS Ruta, *Saba.*, **Sil.**, Staph., *Sul.*, Sul. ac., *Thuj.*, Valer., Verat. a., Verb.

—**Ravenous.**—Agar., *Aloe*, Am. carb., Ant. t., Ars., Asaf., **Aur.**, **Bry.**, CALC. C., *Cannab. i.*, *Caps.*, Caust., Cham., CHIN., CINA., Cocc., Coloc., **Con.**, Dros., **Fer.**, Graph., Guai., *Hell.*, Hep., Hyos., Ign., IOD., **K. carb.**, K. nit., Lach., **LYC.**, Mag. c., Mag. m., Meny., *Merc.*, Mur. ac., Nat. c., **Nat. m.**, Nit. ac., Nux m., NUX V., OLEAND., *Op.*, Petrol., **Phos.**, Pho. ac., Plat., **Puls.**, RAT., Rhus, Ruta, Saba., SEC. C., Sep., SIL., Spig., **Stan.**, Staph., *Squ.*, SUL., Sul. ac., *Ura.*, Valer., VERAT. A., Zinc.

Thirst.—ACON., **All. c.**, **Am. carb.**, **Am. m.**, *Anac.*, **Ant. t.**, **Apoc. c.**, **Arn.**, ARS., Aur., **Bar. c.**, **Bell.**, *Bism.*, *Bar.*, *Bov.*, BRY., Calad., CALC. C., *Camph.*, Cannab. s., **Canth.**, CAPS., Carb. an., **Carb. v.**, *Carb. sul.*, *Caust.*, CHAM., **Chel.**, CHIN., Cic., Cina, Cocc., **Coc. c.**, **Coff.**, **Colch.**, **Coloc.**, **Con.**, Croc., *Crotal.*, *Cub.*, Cup., Cyc., DIG., *Dros.*, Dulc., EUP. PER., Fer., *Fl. ac.*, Graph., Guai., **Hell.**, *Helo.*, **Hep.**, **Hyos.**, *Ign.*, IOD., Ip., *Jat.*, *K. carb.*, **K. iod.**, K. nit., Kre., Lach., *Laur.*, Led., Lyc., Mag. c., *Mag. m.*, MERC., **Merc. c.**, *Mez.*, Mur. ac., **Nat. c.**, NAT. M., *Nat. s.*, Nit. ac., Nux v., Op., Petrol., **Phos.**, Pho. ac., Plat., **Pb.**, **Pod.**, *Puls.*, Ran. b., *Ran. s.*, Rheum, Rhodo., **Rhus**, *Ruta*, *Saba.*, Samb., SEC. C., Sele., Seneg., *Sep.*, Sil., Spig., *Spo.*, Squ., *Stan.*, Staph., STRAM., *Stro.*, SUL., *Sul. ac.*, **Ther.**, Thuj., *Ura.*, Valer., VERAT. A., **Verat. v.**, *Verb.*, **Zinc.**

No Thirst.—Agar., **Agn.**, **All. c.**, *Ambra.*, Am. carb., Am. m., Ant. cr., **Ant. t.**, **APIS**, **Apoc. c.**, Arg., **Arn.**, **Ars.**, Asaf., Asar., Aur., **Bell.**, Bov., Bry., *Calad.*, Calc. c., **Camph.**, Cannab. s., *Canth.*, **Caps.**, Carb. v., Caust.,

Chel., Chin., Cina, *Cocc.,* Coff., *Coloc.,* **Con., Cyc.,** Dig., Dros., Dulc., **Euphorb., GEL., HELL.,** Hep., Hyos., Ign., **Ip.,** K. carb., *K. nit.,* Kre., Lach., *Led.,* Lyc., **Mang., MENY.,** Merc., *Mos., Mur. ac.,* Nat. c., Nit. ac., **NUX M.,** *Nux v.,* Oleand., *Op.,* Petrol., *Phos., Pho. ac.,* **Plat., PULS.,** Rheum, Rhodo., *Rhus,* Ruta, SABA., *Sabi.,* **Samb.,** *Sars.,* **Sep., Spig.,** Spo., *Squ.,* **Staph.,** Stram., *Sul., Tar.,* Thuj., Valer., *Verat. a.*

Thirst with Dread of Liquids.—*Agn.,* Arn., **Bell., Canth.,** Caust., Hyos., *Lach.,* Lyc., *Nat. m.,* **Nux v.,** Rhus, Samb., **Stram.**

Desire to Drink Without Thirst.—**Ars.,** *Calad.,* Camph., *Cocc., Coloc.,* Graph., Nux m., Phos.

Aversion to Acids.—**Bell.,** *Cocc.,* **Fer.,** Ign., *Nux v.,* Pho. ac., **Saba., Sul.**

— —**Beer**—Alum., Asaf., Bell., *Bry., Carb. sul.,* Cham., Chin., **Cocc.,** *Crot. tig.,* **Nux v.,** Phos., Rhus, Spig., Spo., **Stan., Sul.**

— —**Brandy.**—Ign., Merc., **Zinc.**

— —**Bread.**—Agar., Con., Ign., K. carb., **Lyc., Mag. c., NAT. M.,** *Nit. ac.,* **Nux v.,** *Phos., Pho. ac.,* **Puls.,** *Rhus,* **Sep.,** *Sul.*

— —**Black Bread.**—*K. carb.,* **Lyc.,** *Nux v.,* **Puls.,** *Sul.*

— —**Cereals.**—Ars., *Phos.*

— —**Cheese.**—Oleand.

— —**Cocoa.**—*Osm.*

— —**Coffee.**—Bell., Bry., Calc. c., Carb. v., **Cham.,** Chin., **Coff.,** Dulc., *K. br., Lyc., Merc., Nat. m.,* **NUX V., Phos.,** *Rhus, Saba.,* Spig., Sul. ac.

— —**Unsweetened Coffee.**—Rheum.

— —**Fat Food (and Butter).**—Ars., Bell., Bry., Calc. c., **Carb. an., Carb. v.,** *Colch.,* Croc., *Cyc.,* Dros., Hell., **Hep., Meny., Merc., Nat. m., PETROL.,** *Phos.,* Puls., Rheum, Rhus, *Sang.,* Sep., *Sul.*

— —**Fish.**—*Graph.,* **Zinc.**

— —**Fruit.**—*Bar. c.*

— —**Hot Food.**—*Merc. c.*

— —**Insipid Food.**—Rheum.

— —**Meat.**—Alum., Am. carb., Arn., *Ars.,* Aur., *Bry.,* Calc. c., *Carb. sul.,* **Carb. v.,** Caust., **Fer., Graph.,** Hell., *Ign.,* K. carb., **Lyc., Mag. c.,** Merc., Mez., **MUR. AC.,** Nat. c., *Nat. m., Nit. ac.,* Nux v., *Op.,* **PETROL.,** Phos., **Plat., Puls.,** Rhus, Saba., Sep., **SIL.,** Stro., **SUL.,** Thuj., **Zinc.**

— —**Milk.**—Am. carb., Ant. t., Arn., Bell., **Bry., Calc. c.,** *Carb. v.,* Cina, Guai., *Ign., Nat. c.,* Nux v., **Phos., Puls.,** Rheum, **Sep., Sil., Stan.,** *Sul.*

— —**Onions and Garlic.**—**Saba.**

Aversion to Rich Food.—*Puls.*

— —**Salt.**—*Carb. v.*, Graph., Sele.

— —**Solid Food.**—*Fer.*, Merc., Staph.

— —**Soup.**—Arn., *Ars.*, Bell., (Cham.), *Graph.*, *Rhus.*

— —**Sweets.**—*Ars.*, **Caust.**, Graph., *Merc.*, Nit. ac., Phos., **Sul.**, Zinc.

— —**Tobacco.**—*Bry.*, NUX V., *Op.*, *Phos.*, **Puls.**, **Sul.**, *Thuj.*

— —**Vegetables.**—Hell., *Mag. c.*

— —**Water.**—*Aloe*, **Bell.**, *Bry.*, **Calad.**, *Canth.*, Caust., Chin., HYOS., Lyc., *Nat. m.*, NUX V., STRAM.

— —**Wine.**—*Ign.*, Lach., **Merc.**, *Rhus*, Saba., Sul., Zinc.

Desire for Acids.—Ant. cr., Ant. t., Arn., **Ars.**, Bor., Bry., Carb. an., **Cham.**, Chin., **Con.**, *Conv.*, Dig., Hep., *Ign.*, *K. carb.*, Kre., *Lach.*, Mag. c., Mang., **Phos.**, *Pod.*, *Puls.*, **Sabi.**, *Sec. c.*, *Sep.*, **Squ.**, Stram., Sul., VERAT. A.

— —**Beer.**—Acon., **Ars.**, Bry., Calad., Calc. c., *Carb. sul.*, *Caust.*, Chin., *Cocc.*, Graph., K. bi., *Lach.*, Mang., **Merc.**, **Mos.**, **Nat. c.**, Nux v., *Op.*, Petrol., *Pho. ac.*, **Puls.**, **Rhus**, Saba., *Spig.*, Spo., **Stro.**, *Sul.*, Zinc.

— —**Bitters.**—*Dig.*, Nat. m.

— —**Brandy.**—*Acon.*, Arg., **Ars.**, **Asar.**, Bov., Bry., Calc. c., Chin., Cic., *Fer. ph.*, Hep., Mos., Mur. ac., Nux v., OP., Puls., **Sele.**, **Sep.**, *Spig.*, Staph., **Sul.**, *Sul. ac.*

— —**Bread.**—*Aloe*, Am. carb., **Ars.**, Bell., Bov., Fer., Hell., Ign., Mag. c., Nat. c., *Nat. m.*, Pb., Puls., Staph., *Stro.*

— —**Bread and Butter.**—Fer., Ign., **Mag. c.**, MERC., (Puls).

— —**Cakes.**—Pb.

— —**Chalk and Lime.**—Nit. ac., Nux. v.

— —**Cheese.**—*Arg. n.*, Ign.

— —**Coal.**—Cic.

— —**Coffee.**—*Ars.*, Aur., Bry., Caps., *Chin.*, Colch., **Con.**, Mos., Nux m., Sele.

— —**Cold Food and Drink.**—ACON., **Ant. t.**, ARS., CANNAB. I., *Ced.*, Croc., EUP. PER., *Merc.*, *Merc. c.*, **Nat. s.**, *Pho. ac.*, RHUS, VERAT. A.

— —**Cucumbers.**—*Ab. c.*, *Ant. cr.*, Verat. a.

— —**Farinaceous Food.**—Saba.

— —**Fat.**—*Ars.*, *Nit. ac.*, Nux v.

— —**Fat of Ham.**—Mez

— —**Fruit.**—*Aloe*, *Alum.*, Ant. t., *Ars.*, Chin., **Ign.**, Mag. c., Puls., Sul. ac., VERAT. A.

HUNGER AND THIRST—TASTE. 69

Desire for German Rolls.—*Aur.*

— —**Herring (and Sardines).**—*Nit. ac.*, **Verat. a.**

— —**Indigestible Things.**—*Calc. ph.*

— —**Juicy Things.**—*Aloe*, **Pho. ac.**, **Saba.**, *Verat. a.*

— —**Liquid Food.**—*Bry.*, *Fer.*, Merc., Staph., Sul.

— —**Many and Different Things (and Indefinite Things).**—CINA, Sang.

— —**Meat.**—*Ab. c.*, Hell., *Mag. c.*, *Meny.*, Sul.

— —**Smoked Meat.**—Caust.

— —**Milk.**—Anac., **Ars.**, **Aur.**, Bov., *Bry.*, **Calc. c.**, **Chel.**, **Mang.**, **Merc.**, Nat. m., Nux v., *Pho. ac.*, RHUS, **Saba.**, *Sabi.*, *Sil.*, Staph., Stro.

— —**Oysters.**—*Bry.*, **Lach.**, *Rhus.*

— —**Salt.**—*Calc. c.*, CARB. V., **Caust.**, Con., *Nit. ac.*, Phos., VERAT. A.

— —**Sour Kraut.**—*Carb. an.*, Cham.

— —**Spiced Food (and Highly-seasoned Food).**—*Fl. ac.*, **Phos.**, Sang.

— —**Sweets.**—Am. carb., Arg. n., Calc. c., Carb. v., CHIN., *Ip.*, K. carb., Lyc., *Mag. m.*, **Nat. c.**, Nux v., Petrol., *Rheum*, Rhus, Saba., *Sul.*

— —**Tobacco Smoking.**—*Calc. ph.*

— —**Tonics.**—*Aloe*, *Carb. ac.*, Carb. an., *Caust.*, **Cocc.**, *Nux v.*, **Phos.**, Pho. ac., Puls., *Rheum*, Sul. ac., **Valer.**

— —**Vegetables.**—*Alum.*, **Mag. c.**

— —**Warm Food.**—*Cup.*, Cyc., **Fer.**, *Lyc.*

— —**Wine.**—*Acon.*, Arg., Bov., Bry., Calc. c., Chin., **Cic.**, **Hep.**, *K. br.*, *Lach.*, Puls., Sele., **Sep.**, *Spig.*, Staph., Sul.

Taste.

Altered in General.—Acon., Agar., Agn., *Alum.*, Am. br., Am. carb., Am. m., Anac., Ant. cr., *Ant. t.*, *Arn.*, **Ars.**, **Asaf.**, Asar., Aur., *Bar. c.*, **Bell.**, Bism., Bor., Bov., **Bry.**, Calad., *Calc. c.*, Camph., Cannab. s., *Canth.*, **Caps.**, *Carb. an.*, *Carb. v.*, *Carb. sul.*, *Caust.*, **Cham.**, Chel., CHIN., **Cocc.**, *Coff.*, Colch., Coloc., Con., *Croc.*, **Cup.**, Cyc., Dig., Dros., Dulc., *Euphorb.*, Euphr., Fer., Graph., Guai., Hell., *Hep.*, Hyos., Ign., *Iod.*, *Ip.*, **K. carb.**, Kre., *Laur.*, Led., **Lob. i.**, **Lyc.**, *Mag. c.*, *Mag. m.*, *Mang.*, Mar., Meny., **Merc.**, Merc. c., *Mez.*, Mos., *Mur. ac.*, **Nat. c.**, **Nat. m.**, Nit. ac., *Nux m.*, **Nux v.**, Oleand., Op., Par., **Petrol.**, **Phos.**, *Pho. ac.*, Plat., Pb, PULS., *Ran. b.*, Ran. s., *Rheum*, Rhodo., RHUS, Ruta, *Saba.*, **Sabi.**, **Sars.**, Sec. c., Sele., Seneg., **Sep.**, *Sil.*, Spig., Spo.,

TASTE.

Squ., *San.*, **Staph.**, Stram., Stro., Sul., Sul. ac., *Tar.*, *Thuj.*, **VALER.**, Verat. a., Verb., Vio. t., *Zinc.*, Zing.

Acid.—*Acon.*, *Aloe.*, *Alum.*, *Ambr.*, Am. carb., Am. m., *Ant. t.*, *Ars.*, Asar., Aur., **Bar. c.**, **BELL.**, Bism., Bor., *Bry.*, **Cact.**, CALC. C, *Calc. ph.*, Canr ab. s., Canth., *Caps.*, *Carb. an.*, *Carb. v.*, *Carb. sul.*, Caust., **Cham.**, CHIN., Cina, *Cocc.*, *Colch.*, *Con.*, Croc., *Crot. tig.*, *Cup.*, Cyc., Dig., Lros., Fer., *Graph.*, *Hep.*, *Hydras.*, Ign., Iod., *Ip.*, K. carb., Kre., Laur., *Lith.*, **Lyc.**, Mag. c., *Mag. m.*, Mang., **Merc.**, Mez., Mur. ac., *Nat. c.*, **Nat. m.**, *Nat. s.*, *Nit. ac.*, **NUX V.**, Oleand., Op., **Ox. ac.**, Par., Petrol., PHOS., Pho. ac., *Pb.*, *Pod.*, PULS., Ran. b., Ran. s., Rheum, Rhodo., *Rhus*, *Rob.*, Saba., *Sahi.*, *Sars.*, Sec. c., *Sep.*, **Sil.**, Spig., Spo., Squ., Stan., Staph., Stram., SUL., Sul. ac., TAR., Thuj., *Verat. a.*, Zinc.

Bad (Foul, Putrid).—Acon., *Agar.*, Anac., Ant. t., ARN., **Ars.**, Asar., **Aur.**, **Bar. c.**, Bell., Bov., *Bry.*, Calc. c., *Canth.*, *Caps.*, *Carb. an.*, **Carb. v.**, *Carb. sul.*, Caust., **Cham.**, Chin., *Cocc.*, *Coff.*, Coloc., **Con.**, *Cup.*, Cyc., *Dros.*, Euphorb., *Fer.*, Graph., Hep., Hyos., Ign., *K. br.*, K. carb., **Kre.**, **Lob. i.**, *Lyc.*, Mag. c., Mag. m., Mar., **Merc.**, Mos., Mur. ac., **Nat. m.**, Nux m., **Nux v.**, Oleand., Petrol., *Phos.*, Pho, ac., *Pso.*, PULS., **Rheum**, **Rhus**, Ruta, Sep., Spig., *Stan.*, *Staph.*, Sul., Sul. ac., Thuj., **Valer.**, *Verat. a.*, Zinc., Zing.

Bitter.—ACON., Aesc., Aloe, *Alum.*, Ambr., Am. carb., *Am. m.*, Anac., Ant. cr., Ant. t., **Arn.**, **Ars.**, *Asaf.*, Asar., **Aur.**, **Bap.**, *Bar. c.*, *Bell.*, Bism., **Bor.**, Bov., BRY., **Calc. c.**, **Calc. ph.**, *Camph.*, *Cannab. s.*, Canth., *Carb. an.*, *Carb. v.*, *Carb. sul.*, Caust., CHAM., CHEL., Chin., Cocc., Coff., *Colch.*, **Coloc.**, Con., Croc., *Crot. tig.*, **Cup.**, Dig., Dios., **Dros.**, Dulc., Euphorb., Euphr., *Fer.*, *Graph.*, Hell., *Hep.*, Hyos., **Ign.**, Iod., *Ip.*, **K. carb.**, Kre., *Laur.*, Led., **Lyc.**, *Mag. c.*, **Mag. m.**, Mang., Mar., Meny., MERC., MERC. C., **Merc. i. r.**, Mez., *Mur. ac.*, **Nat. c.**, NAT. M., *Nit. ac.*, Nux m., **NUX V.**, Oleand., Op., Par., Petrol., Phos., Pho. ac., *Pb.*, **Pso.**, PULS., Ran. b., Rheum, Rhodo., **Rhus**, *Ruta*, **Saba.**, *Sabi.*, *Sang.*, *Sars.*, *Sec. c.*, SEP., *Sil.*, *Spo.*, Squ., **Stan.**, *Staph.*, *Stram.*, Stro., SUL., Sul. ac., **Tar.**, *Thuj.*, Valer., VERAT. A., Verb., Vio. t., *Zinc.*

Burnt.—*Bry.*, *Cyc.*, Laur., *Phos.*, **Puls.**, *Ran. b.*, *Squ.*, *Sul.*

Earthy.—*Aloe*, **Cannab. s.**, Caps., *Chin.*, Fer., Hep., *Ign.*, Merc., **Nux m.**, Phos., Puls.

Fatty.—Alum., Ambr., ASAF., Bar. c., Bry., Carb. v., CAUST., Cham., Euphorb., Ign., Ip., Laur., Lyc., *Mag. m.*, **Mang.**, *Mur. ac.*, **Petrol.**, **Phos.**, Pho. ac., PULS., Ran. s., Rhodo., *Rhus*, Saba., **Sabi.**, *Sil.*, **Thuj.**, VALER.

TASTE.

Herby.—*Calad.*, NUX V., *Pho. ac.*, Puls., *Sars.*, Stan., Verat. a.

Insipid.—Acon., Agar., *Alum.*, Ambr., Am. m., Anac., **Ant. cr.**, Ant. t., Arg., *Arn.*, **Ars.**, Asaf., Asar., *Aur.*, Bar. c., **Bell.**, BRY., Cannab. s., **Caps.**, Carb. an., *Carb. sul.*, Cham., **Chel.**, CHIN., Cocc., *Colch.*, Coloc., *Crot. tig.*, Cup., *Cyc.*, Dig., Dulc., Euphorb., *Euphr.*, Guai., Hell., Hep., IGN., *Ip.*, **K. bi.**, *K. carb.*, Kre., *Lyc.*, Mag. c., *Mag. m.*, Mang., Merc., Mez., *Nat. c.*, **Nat. m.**, *Nux m.*, Nux v., Oleand., Op., Par., **Petrol.**, *Phos.*, *Pho. ac.*, **Plat.**, **Puls.**, Ran. b., *Rheum*, Rhodo., *Rhus*, *Ruta*, Saba., *Sabi.*, Sars., Sec. c., Seneg., Sep., Spig., *Stan.*, STAPH., Stram., *Stro.*, **Sul.**, Sul. ac., *Thuj.*, VALER., Verat. a., **Verb.**

Metallic.—Aesc., Agn., Aloe, Alum., **Bism.**, *Calc. c.*, *Carb. sul.*, **Coc. c.**, Cocc., Coloc., CUP., Hep., *Ip.*, Merc., *Nat. c.*, **Nux v.**, *Phos.*, Pb., Ran. b., RHUS, Sars., Seneg., **Sul.**, Zinc.

Nauseous.—*Aloe*, Agar., Am. m., Anac., Ant. t., Arg., **Ars.**, *Asaf.*, Bell., **Bism.**, BRY., **Calc. c.**, Cannab. s., *Canth.*, Caps., Carb. an., *Carb. sul.*, Caust., Cham., *Chel.*, *Chin.*, *Cina*, *Cocc.*, Croc., *Crot. tig.*, Cup., Cyc., Dig., *Dros.*, Euphorb., Guai., Ign., **Iod.**, *K. carb.*, **Led.**, Mang., **Mar.**, MERC., Mez., Nat. c., *Nat. m.*, **Nux v.**, Par., Petrol., *Phos.*, Pho. ac., Pb., PULS., Rheum, Rhus, *Suba.*, Sabi., *Sars.*, Sec. c., *Sele.*, Seneg., **Sep.**, Sil., Spig., *Squ.*, **Stan.**, Staph., Stram., **Sul.**, Sul. ac., Thuj., **Valer.**, Verat. a., Verb., **Zinc.**

Salty.—*Alum.*, Ambr., *Am. carb.*, Anac., Ant. cr., **Ant. t.**, Arn., ARS., *Bar. c.*, **Bell.**, *Bov.*, Calc. c., Cannab. s., **Carb. v.**, *Carb. sul.*, Caust., **Chin.**, Coff., Croc., Cup., Dig., Dros., *Euphorb.*, *Graph.*, *Hyos.*, **Iod.**, *K. br.*, **Lyc.**, *Mag. c.*, *Mag. m.*, MERC., Mez., **Nat. c.**, *Nux m.*, Nux v., PHOS., PULS., Rhodo., Rhus, SEP., *Stan.*, Stram., **Sul.**, *Sul. ac.*, *Tar*, **Verat. a.**, *Verb.*, Zinc.

Sweetish.—Acon., Agar., Alum., *Am. carb.*, Anac., **Ars.**, *Asar.*, Aur., Bar. c., Bell., Bism., Bov., **Bry.**, *Calc. c.*, *Canth.*, Carb. v., *Carb. s.*, Chin., Cocc., *Coff.*, Croc., *Crot. tig.*, Cup., **Dig.**, *Fer.*, Hep., Hyos., Iod., *Ip.*, K. carb., Kre., *Laur.*, Lyc., Mag. c., MERC., Mez., Mur. ac., Nat. c., Nit. ac., *Nux v.*, PHOS., *Plat.*, **PB.**, PULS., Ran. b., Ran. s., *Rhus*, SABA., Sabi., Samb., *Sars.*, *Sele.*, Sep., Spo., SQU., **Stan.**, **Sul.**, *Sul. ac.*, Thuj., Verat. a., *Zinc.*

Acute.—Acon., Agar., Arn., Aur., *Bar. c.*, **Bell.**, *Camph.*, CHIN., Cocc., COFF., Colch., Con., Hep., Nux v., Thuj.

Dull.—*Alum.*, Am. m., *Anac.*, **Ant. cr.**, Ant. t., Arg., *Ars.*, Bar. c., **Bell.**, Bry., **Calc. c.**, Cannab. s., *Canth.*, **Caps.**, Carb. an., Carb. v., *Carb. sul.*, Caust., Chin., Cic., Cina, *Cocc.*, Colch., Cup., *Cyc.*, Dros., **Fer.**, Hell., Hep., Hyos., Ign., *Ip.*, *K. carb.*, K. nit., Kre., Lyc., Mag. c., *Mag. m.*,

Mang., *Merc.*, Mos., *Nat. c.*, *Nat. m.*, **Nux. v.**, *Oleand.*, Op., **Par.**, Phos., Pho. ac., Pb., PULS., Rheum, **Rhodo.**, *Rhus*, Ruta, *Sang.*, *Sars.*, **Sec. c.**, Seneg., **Sil.**, Spo., Staph., **Squ.**, **Stram.**, Stro., **Sul.**, *Sul. ac.*, Tar., Thuj., *Verat. a.*, Vio. t.

Lost.—*Acon.*, *Alum.*, **Am. m.**, *Anac.*, *Ant. cr.*, *Ant. t.*, *Apis*, **Arg.**, Ars., Aur., Bar. c., **Bell.**, Bry., *Cact.*, **Calc. c.**, Canth., Carb. an., Carb. v., Caust., Cina, Cocc., Hell., Hep., HYOS., *Ip.*, *K. br.*, *K. carb.*, K. nit., Kre., Lyc., *Mag. c.*, **Mag. m.**, *Merc.*, Nat. c., NAT. M., Nux v., *Op.*, *Par.*, Phos., Pho. ac., Pb., PULS., Rheum, **Rhodo.**, Rhus, Ruta, Saba., **Sang.**, Sars., Sec. c., Seneg., *Sep.*, SIL., Spig., Staph., *Stram.*, Stro., *Sul.*, *Sul. ac.*, Thuj., *Verat. a.*

Eructations.

Belching.—*Acon.*, Alum., Am. m., *Ant. cr.*, ANT. T., *Arg.*, ARN., Ars., *Bar. c.*, **Bell.**, BRY., **Calc. c.**, Camph., **Cannab. s.**, Canth., *Carb. ac.*, *Carb. v.*, *Carb. sul.*, Caust., Cham., Chin., Cic., Cina, Coca, Coloc., **Con.**, Cyc., Dig., *Dros.*, Dulc., Fer., **Graph.**, *Hep.*, Ign., K. carb., Lach., Laur., Lyc., Mag. m., **Mar.**, Merc., Mez., Mos., Mur. ac., Nat. c., *Nat. m.*, Nit. ac., NUX V., Oleand., Par., **Petrol.**, PHOS., Plat., **Pb.**, Puls., Rhodo., Rhus, Sabi., *Sal. ac.*, SARS., Sep., Spo., Staph., Stro., Sul., SUL. AC., Thuj., Valer., **Verat. a.**, Verb., *Zinc.*

Eructations in General.—*Abrot.*, Acon., *A~sc.*, Agar., Agn., **Aloe**, Alum., Ambr., Am. carb., *Am. m.*, Anac., **Ant. cr.**, Ant. t., Arg. n., ARN., Ars., *Asaf.*, *Asar.*, **Bar. c.**, BELL., Bism., *Bor.*, BRY., Calad., **Calc. ac.**, **Calc. c.**, Camph., Cannab. s., **Canth.**, *Caps.*, **Carb. ac.**, Carb. an., Carb. v., *Carb. sul.*, **Caust.**, *Cham.*, **Chel.**, **Chen. a.**, Chin., Cic., *Cina*, COCC., *Coc. c.*, *Coff.*, **Colch.**, **Coloc.**, CON., *Conv.*, Croc., **Cup.**, **Cyc.**, Dig., **Dios.**, *Dros.*, **Dulc.**, Euphorb., Euphr., *Fer.*, **Fl. ac.**, **Graph.**, Guai., *Hell.*, **Hep.**, Hyos., **Ign.**, *Iod.*, **Ip.**, *Iris v.*, **K. carb.**, K. nit., Kre., *Lach.*, Laur., Led., **Lyc.**, *Mag c.*, *Mag. m.*, Mang., Mar., Meny., MERC., **Mez.**, *Mos.*, *Mur. ac.*, NAT. C, NAT. M., **Nit. ac.**, Nux m., NUX V., *Oleand.*, Op., **Ox. ac.**, Par., Petrol., PHOS., **Pho. ac.**, Plat., Pb., *Pod.*, PSO., PULS., **Ran. b.**, Ran. s., Rhodo., RHUS, Ruta, Saba., Sabi., **Sars.**, Sec. c., Sele., Seneg., SEP., Sil., *Spig.*, *Spo.*, Squ., **Stan.**, Staph., Stram., Stro., SUL., **Sul. ac.**, Tar., Thuj., **Valer.**, VERAT. A., **Verb.**, Vio. t., *Zinc.*

Heartburn.—Agar., *Alum.*, *Ambr.*, **Am. carb.**, Ant. cr., *Arg.*, Arn., Ars., Asaf., *Asar.*, *Bar. c.*, **Bell.**, Berb., *Bor.*, Bov., *Bry.*, CALC. C., *Canth.*, **Caps.**, **Carb. an.**, Carb. v., *Carb. sul.*, *Caust.*, Cham., Chin., *Cic.*, *Coc. c.*, Coff., CON., CROC., *Crot. tig.*, **Dig.**, *Dulc.*, Euphorb., Fer., *Fer. ph.*, *Graph.*, Guai., *Hell.*, Hep., Hyos., *Ign.*, **Iod.**, *K. carb.*, *K. nit.*, **Lyc.**, Mang.,

ERUCTATIONS—NAUSEA AND VOMITING.

Merc., Mos., Mur. ac., **Nat. c., Nat. m.,** *Nat. s., Nit. ac., Nux m.,* **NUX V.,** Par., *Petrol.,* **Phos.,** *Pho. ac.,* Plat., **PULS.,** Ran. s., *Saba.,* **Sabi.,** Sec. c., **Sep.,** *Sil.,* Squ., *Staph.,* **Sul.,** *Sul. ac.,* Tar., Thuj., **Valer., Verat. a.,** *Zinc.*

Hiccough.—Acon., **Agar.,** Agn., Alum., Ambr., Am. carb., **AM. M.,** Anac., Ant. cr., Ant. t., Arg., Arn., **Ars.,** Asar., *Bar. c.,* **Bell.,** Bor., Bov., **Bry.,** *Caj.,* Calc. c., *Calc. fl., Calc. iod.,* Cannab. s., **Canth.,** Carb. an., Carb. v., Caust., Cham., Chel., CIC., Cina, *Cocc.,* Coff., Colch., Coloc., Con., *Cup.,* CYC., Dig., **Dios.,** *Dros.,* Dulc., Euphorb., Euphr., *Gel.,* Graph., Hep., HYOS., IGN., Iod., *K. br.,* K. carb., Lach., Laur., Led., *Lyc.,* Mag. c., *Mag. m.,* MAR., Meny., **Merc.,** Mur. ac., *Nat. c.,* Nat. m., *Nux m.,* NUX V., **Op.,** *Par.,* Petrol., Phos., Plat., **Plumb., Puls., Ran. b.,** Ran. s., Rhus, Ruta, Saba., Samb., *Sang., Sars.,* Sec. c., Sele., **Sep.,** Sil., **Sin., Spo.,** Stan., *Staph.,* **Stram.,** *Stro., Sul.,* **Sul. ac., Tar.,** Thuj., **Verat. a.,** *Verb.,* Zinc.

Uprisings.—*Acon.,* Alum., Ambr., **ANT. CR., ASAF.,** Asar., **Bell.,** *Bry., Calc. c., Cannab. s.,* **Canth.,** *Carb. v., Carb. sul., Caust.,* Chel., *Chin.,* Cic., Coff., **Con.,** *Croc.,* Cyc., Dulc., **Fer.,** *Hell.,* Hep., *Ign.,* K. carb., Lyc., Mag. m., Mang., **MERC.,** Merc. c., *Nat. c.,* Nit. ac., *Nux m.,* **NUX V., PHOS.,** *Pho. ac.,* **PLAT.,** Pb., **PULS.,** *Ran. b., Rhus, Rob.,* Ruta, *Saba., Sars.,* **Spig., Stan.,** STRAM., *Sul. ac.,* **Valer., Verat. a.**

Waterbrash.—*Acon., Alum.,* Ambr., **Am. carb.,** Am. m., *Anac.,* **Ant. cr., Ant. t.,** Arn., **Ars.,** *Asar.,* **Bar. c.,** Bell., Bov., **BRY., Calc. c., Calc. ph.,** Cannab. s., *Canth.,* Caps., *Carb. an.,* **Carb. v.,** Caust., Chel., *Chin., Cic.,* Cina, Clem., **Cocc.,** Colch., Con., Croc., Cup., *Cyc.,* Dig., **Dros.,** Dulc., *Euphorb.,* Fer., *Graph., Hell., Hep.,* **Ign.,** Iod., Ip., *K. carb.,* Lach., Laur., **Led., LYC.,** Mag. c., *Mag. m.,* Mang., Meny., **Merc.,** MEZ., Mos., Mur. ac., **Nat. c., Nat. m., Nit. ac.,** Nux m., Nux v., *Oleand.,* **PAR., PETROL.,** Phos., Pho. ac., Plat., Pb., **PULS., Ran. b., Ran. s., Rhodo.,** Rhus, SABA., Sabi., SANG., *Sars.,* Seneg., Sep., SIL., Spig., Spo., Squ., Stan., STAPH., SUL., *Sul. ac., Tur.,* Thea., Thuj., *Valer.,* VERAT. A., Verb., Zinc.

Nausea and Vomiting.

Nausea in General.—Acon., Aesc., Aeth., Agar., *Agn., Ail., Aloe, Alum.,* Ambr., *Am. carb.,* Am. m., Anac., Ant. cr., **ANT. T.,** Arg., ARG. N., *Arn.,* ARS., Asaf., Asar., Aur., Bap., Bar. c., **BELL.,** Bism., Bor., Bov., **Bry.,** Calad., **Calc. c.,** *Calc. i., Calc. ph.,* Camph., *Canch., Cannab. s,* **Canth.,** Caps., Carb. ac., Carb. an., **Carb. v.,** *Carb. s d.,* **Card.,** *Caust.,* **Cham.,** *Chel., Chen. a.,* **Chin.,** *Cic.,* **Cimic.,** Cina, Clem.,

COCC., Coc. c., Coff., Colch., Colcc., Con., Croc., Crot. tig., Cup., Cyc., DIG., Dios., Dros., Dulc., Euphorb., Euphr., Eup. per., Fer., Fl. ac., Gam., Gel., Gran., Graph., Guai., Hell., Hep., Hydras., Hyos., Ign., Iod., Ip., Iris. v., K. bi., K. carb., K. chl., K. nit., Kre., Lach., Laur., Led., Lob. i., Lyc., Mag. c., Mag. m., Mang., Mar., Meny., **Merc., Merc. i. f.,** Mez., Mos., Mur. ac., Nat. c., Nat. m., Nit. ac., Nux m., NUX V., Oleand Op., **Ox. ac.,** Par., PETROL., Phos., Pho. ac., Plat., **PB., Pod.,** PULS., Ran. b., Ran. s., Rheum, Rhodo., RHUS, Ruta, Saba., Sabi., **Samb.,** SANG., Sars., Sec. c., Seneg., SEP., SIL., Spig., Spo., **Squ., Stan.,** Staph., Stram., Stro., SUL., Sul. ac., TAB., Tar., **Ther.,** Thuj., VALER., VERAT. A., **Verat. v.,** Vio. t., ZINC., Zing.

Nausea in Throat.—Acon., Anac., Ant. t., Arg., Ars., Asar., Aur., Bell., Cannab. s., Chin., Cocc., Coff., Croc., **Cup.,** CYC., Fer., Merc., Nit. ac., Oleand., PHO. AC., **Puls.,** Rhus, Sars., Spig., **Squ.,** STAN., Staph., Sul., Tar., **Valer.**

— —**Stomach.**—Acon., **Agn.,** Ant. t., Arn., Asar., Aur., Bar. c., Bell., Bism., Bor., Bov., Calc. c., Cannab. s., Canth., Caps., Carb. an., Carb. v., Caust., Cham., Chel., Chin., Cina, Cocc., Coff., Colch., Croc., **Cup.,** Cyc., Dig., Dros., HELL., Ip., K. carb., Laur., Led., **Lyc.,** Mag. c., Mag. m., Mang., Mar., Meny., Merc., Mez., Mos., Mur. ac., Nat. c., Nat. m., Nit. ac., Nux m., **Nux v., Par., Phos.,** Pho. ac., **Plat.,** Pb., **Puls.,** Rheum, Rhus, Ruta, Saba., Sabi., Samb., Sars., Sec. c., Seneg., Sil., Stan., Stro., Squ., **Sul.,** Sul. ac., Thuj., Valer., VERAT. A., Zinc.

— —**Abdomen.**—Agn., Ant. t., Bell., **Bry.,** Cic., Cocc., Croc., Cup., Cyc., Hell., Hep., Ip., Mang., Mar., Nux m., Par., **Puls.,** Rheum, Ruta, Samb., Sil., Stan., Staph., Valer.

— —**Chest.**—Acon., Anac., Arg., Asaf., Bry., Croc., Merc., Nux v., Par., Rhus, Sec. c., Staph.

Qualmishness.—Acon., Ambr., Ant. t., Arg., Arn., ARS., Bar. c., Bell., Bry., Calc. c., Canth., **Caps.,** Carb. an., Carb. v., CAUST., **Cham.,** Chel., Chin., Cic., Cina, Coff., Croc., **Cyc.,** Dig., Euphr., Hep., Ign., Ip., K. carb., Laur., Lyc., Meny., Merc., Mos., NAT. C., Nat. m., Nit. ac., **Nux v.,** Oleand., Petrol., Phos., Plat., Puls., Rhus, Saba., Sabi., Sil., Staph., Stro., SUL., Tar., Thuj., Verat. a., Zinc.

Nausea, with Inclination to Vomit.—Acon., Agar., Alum., Am. carb., Am. m., Anac., Ant. cr., ANT. T., APOMOR., Arg., Arn., Ars., Asaf., Asar., Aur., Bar. c., Bell., Bism., Bor., Bov., **Bry.,** Calc. c., Camph., Cannab. s., Canth., **Caps.,** Carb. an., Carb. v., Caust., CHAM., Chel., Chin., Cina, Cocc., Coff., Colch., Con., Croc., Cup., Cyc., Dig., **Dros.,** Dulc., Euphorb., Fer., Glon., Graph., Hell., Hep., Hyos., Ign., Iod., IP.,

NAUSEA AND VOMITING.

K. carb., K. nit., Kre., Lach., Laur., *Led.*, Lyc., *Mag. c.*, **Mag. m.**, Mang., Mar., Meny., Merc., Mez., Mos., Mur. ac., *Nat. c.*, Nat. m., *Nit. ac.*, Nux m., **Nux v.**, *Oleand.*, Op., *Petrol.*, *Phos.*, *Pho. ac.*, *Plat.*, **Pb.**, **PULS.**, Ran. s., Rheum, Rhodo., **RHUS**, *Ruta*, **Saba.**, Sabi., *Sars.*, Sec. c., Seneg., **SEP.**, *Sil.*, Spig., Spo., *Squ.*, *Stan.*, Staph., Stram., Stro., *Sul.*, *Sul. ac.*, **TAB.**, **Ther.**, Thuj., *Valer.*, **VERAT. A.**, Verb., Zinc.

Retching.—Acon., **Aesc.**, **Aeth.**, Ambr., Anac., *Ant. cr.*, **Ant. t.**, *Apoc. c.*, Arg., *Arg. n.*, **Arn.**, **Ars.**, Asar., Aur., **BELL.**, Bism., **Bry.**, *Canch.*, Cannab. s., *Canth.*, Carb. v., *Chel.*, **Chin.**, Cocc., Colch., *Coloc.*, *Crotal.*, *Cup.*, Dig., Dros., Dulc., Graph., Hell., *Hep.*, *Hyos.*, Ign., Iod., IP., *K. carb.*, K. nit., Kre., Led., *Lob. i.*, Lyc., Mag. c., Merc., Mez., Mos., Nat. m., **Nux v.**, Oleand., *Op.*, Phyt., *Pb.*, **Pod.**, Puls., Rhus, Sabi., Sars., *Sec. c.*, Seneg., **Sep.**, Sil., *Squ.*, Stan., Stram., Stro., **Sul.**, Thuj., **Verat. a.**, Vio. t., Zinc.

Loathing.—*Acon.*, Alum., Am. carb., Anac., **Ant. cr.**, **Ant. t.**, Arg., **Arn.**, **Ars.**, Asaf., Asar., Bar. c., **Bell.**, Bor., **Bry.**, Calc. c., **Canth.**, Carb. v., Caust., *Cham.*, *Chin.*, **COCC.**, *Colch.*, Con., Cup., Cyc., Dig., **Dulc.**, *Euphorb.*, **Fer.**, **Gam.**, *Guai.*, *Hell.*, Hep., Ign., Iod., IP., K. **CARB.**, Lach., Laur., Lyc., Mag. c., Mag. m., Mang., Meny., *Mos.*, Mur. ac., Nat. c., Nat. m., **Nux v.**, Oleand., *Op.*, Petrol., *Phos.*, *Plat.*, **Pb.**, *Pso.*, Puls., *Rheum*, Rhodo., *Rhus*, Ruta, *Sars.*, *Sec. c.*, Seneg., **Sep.**, **Sil.**, Spig., Stan., Stram., Sul., *Sul. ac.*, Thuj., Valer.

Vomiting.—*Ac. ac.*, Acon., Act., Aesc., Aeth., Agar., Am. carb., Am. m., Anac., **Ant. cr.**, **Ant. t.**, **APOMOR.**, Arg., **ARG. N.**, *Arn.*, **ARS.**, **Asar.**, Bar. c., **Bell.**, Bism., *Bor.*, Bov., **BRY.**, *Cad. s.*, **Calc. c.**, *Calc. ph.*, *Camph.*, Cannab. s., **Canth.**, Caps., *Carb. ac.*, Carb. v., Caust., *Cereum.*, **CHAM.**, Chel., Chin., Cic., Cimic., Cina, *Cocc.*, **Coc. c.**, Coff., COLCH., Coloc., Con., *Crot. tig.*, CUP., **Dig.**, **Dros.**, Dulc., **Euphorb.**, *Eup. per.*, FER., *Gam.*, *Glon.*, *Gran.*, Graph., **Grat.**, Hell., *Hep.*, *Hydras.*, **Hyd. ac.**, Hyos., Ign., **Iod.**, IP., *Iris v.*, Jat., K. BI., K. carb., *K. chl.*, K. nit., Kre., *Lach.*, Laur., Led., *Lob. i.*, *Lyc.*, Mag. c., **Merc.**, **Merc. c.**, **Merc. d.**, *Merc. i. f.*, *Mez.*, Nat. c., Nat. m., **Nit. ac.**, *Nux m.*, **NUX V.**, *Oleand.*, **Op.**, **Ox. ac.**, Petrol., Phos., Pho. ac., **Pb.**, **PULS.**, Rhodo., Rhus, Saba., Sabi., **Samb.**, **Sang.**, Sec. c., Seneg., **Sep.**, SIL., Squ., *Stan.*, *Stram.*, SUL., Sul. ac., TAB., **Ter.**, **Thea.**, **Ther.**, Thuj., **Valer.** VERAT. A., VERAT. V., Zinc., *Zing.*

—**Acid.**—Act., *Am. carb.*, Ant. t., **Ars.**, *Asar.*, Bar. c., **Bell.**, *Bry.*, *Calad.*, CALC. C., Caps., Carb. v., *Caust.*, **Cham.**, CHIN., Cocc., Con., *Fer.*, *Graph.*, *Grat.*, Hep., *Ign.*, **Ip.**, Iris v., *K. bi.*, *K. carb.*, LYC., Nat. c., *Nat. m.*, Nit. ac., NUX V., Oleand., Op., Petrol., PHOS., Pho. ac., **Pso.**,

NAUSEA AND VOMITING.

Puls., ROB., Sabi., *Sars.*, Sec. c., *Sep.*, *Stan.*, Stram., SUL., **Tab.**, Thuj., VERAT. A.

—**Acrid.**—*Iris v.*

—**Bilious.**—Acon., *Ant. cr.*, *Ant. t.*, *Arn.*, ARS., Asar., Bell., *Bism.*, Bor., BRY., *Calc. c.*, Camph., *Cannab. s.*, *Canth.*, *Carb. ac.*, Carb. v., CHAM., Chin., Cina, Cocc., *Colch.*, **Coloc.**, **Con.**, **Crotal.**, *Crot. tig.*, Cup., *Dig.*, Dros., Dulc., EUP. PER., **Grat.**, Hell., *Hep.*, Hyos., **Ign.**, Iod., IP., *K. carb.*, Lach., **Lyc.**, Mag. c., MERC., MERC. C., *Mez.*, Mur. ac., *Nat. c.*, *Nat. m.*, Nit. ac., NUX V., *Oleand.*, **Op.**, *Ox. ac.*, Petrol., Phos., Pb., PULS., Rhodo., Rhus, *Saba.*, *Sabi.*, **Sang.**, Sec. c., SEP., *Sil.*, Stan., *Stram.*, Sul., *Thuj.*, Valer., VERAT. A., Zinc.

—**Black (and Brown).**—*Ant. t.*, ARS., Bism., *Cad. s.*, Calc. c., Camph., *Chin.*, Hep., *Hyd. ac.*, *Ip.*, *Lach.*, Laur., *Lyc.*, *Merc. c.*, NUX V., *Op.*, *Ox. ac.*, Petrol., Phos., Pb., Sec. c., Squ., Stram., Sul., *Sul. ac.*, **Verat. a.**

—**Bloody.**—Acon., *Ant. cr.*, *Ant. t.*, ARN., **Ars.**, Asar., *Bell.*, Bor., *Bry.*, **Cact.**, *Calc. c.*, Camph., *Cannab. s.*, **Canth.**, Caps., Carb. v., *Caust.*, *Cham.*, Chin., Cic., Con., *Crotal.*, Cup., *Dig.*, Dros., FER., *Ham.*, Hep., *Hyos.*, Iod., IP., K. nit., Kre., *Led.*, *Lyc.*, *Merc.*, **Merc. c.**, *Mez.*, **Nit. ac.**, Nux v., *Op.*, *Ox. ac.*, PHOS., **Phyt.**, Pb., Puls., *Rhus*, *Sabi.*, **Sec. c.**, Sep., *Sil.*, Stan., Stram., Sul., Sul. ac., Thuj., *Verat. a.*, Zinc.

—**Curdled Milk.**—ÆTH., Ant. cr., *Ant. t.*, Sul.

—**Of Drink.**—*Acon.*, Ant. cr., **Ant. t.**, Apomor, *Arn.*, ARS., Bry., Cham., *Chin.*, Cic., Cocc., *Con.*, *Crot. tig.*, Cup., **Dulc.**, Fer., **Ip.**, Nat. m., Nux v., Puls., Rhus, **Sec. c.**, Sil., Sul., *Sul. ac.*, *Verat. a.*

—**Fæcal.**—Bell., Bry., **Nux v.**, OP., Pb.

—**Of Food.**—Acon., **Am. carb.**, Anac., **Ant. cr.**, **Ant. t.**, *Arn.*, ARS., Bell., Bism., *Bor.*, Bov., BRY., **Calc. c.**, *Calc. ph.*, **Canth.**, Caps., Carb. v., *Cham.*, Chin., Cina, Cocc., Coff., *Colch.*, *Coloc.*, Con., **Crotal.**, *Crot. tig.*, *Cuar.*, *Cund.*, **Cup.**, *Dig.*, **Dros.**, EUP. PER., **FER.**, *Fer. ph.*, Graph., *Hyd. ac.*, Hyos., **Ign.**, *Iod.*, Ip., K. carb., *Kre.*, Lach., Laur., Led., **Lyc.**, *Mag. c.*, *Merc.*, Mos., Mur. ac., **Nat. m.**, *Nit. ac.*, NUX V., *Oleand.*, *Op.*, PHOS., *Pho. ac.*, PB., PULS., Rhus, *Ruta*, Sabi., Samb., **Sec. c.**, **Sep.**, SIL., **Stan.**, Sul., *Sul. ac.*, Thuj., *Ura.*, VERAT. A., *Zinc.*

—**Offensive Smelling.**—Ant. t., Arn., **Ars.**, *Bell.*, Bism., *Bry.*, *Calc. c.*, Cocc., Coff., *Crot. tig.*, Cup., Guai., Ip., *Led.*, *Merc.*, Nat. c., **Nux v.**, Op., **Phos.**, Pho. ac., Pb., Sec. c., SEP., **Stan.**, **Sul.**, Thuj., Valer., Verat. a.

—**Slimy.**—Acon., *Am. m.*, *Ant. cr.*, *Ant. t.*, ARG. N., **Ars.**, Bar. c., **Bell.**, *Bor.*, Bov., *Bry.*, Calc. c., Cannab. s., *Canth.*, Caps., **Cham.**, **Chin.**,

NAUSEA AND VOMITING—INTERNAL ABDOMEN. 77

Cina, Cocc., **Coc. c.**, Colch., **Con.**, *Coral.*, *Crot. tig.*, *Cup.*, **Dig.**, DROS, *Dulc.*, Fer., Graph., *Guai.*, *Hep.*, **Hyos.**, Ign., Iod., **Ip.**, *K. bi.*, *K. nit.*, *Kre.*, Lyc., Mag. c., **Merc.**, Merc. c., Mez., Mos., Nat. c., **Nit. ac.**, **NUX V.**, Oleand, *Phos.*, Phyt., *Pb.*, PULS., Samb., **Sec. c.**, Sil., Spig., *Stram.*, *Sul.*, Ter., Thuj., Valer., VERAT. A., Zinc.

—**Watery.**—*Acon.*, Am. carb., Ant. cr., *Ant. t.*, *Arg.*, **Arn.**, **Ars.**, *Asar.*, Bar. c., **Bell.**, Bov., BRY., **Cannab. s.**, CAUST., *Chin.*, Cina, Coc. c., Coloc., Con., Cup., Cyc., *Dros.*, Fer., Graph., Grat., *Guai.*, *Hep.*, Hyos., **Ip.**, Iris v., K. bi., K. carb., K. nit., *Kre.*, Laur., Mag. c., *Mag. m.*, Merc., Nat. c., **Nux v.**, *Oleand.*, *Ox. ac.*, Par., *Petrol.*, *Phos.*, *Pb.*, *Puls.*, ROB., Sars., Sec. c., Sep., *Sil.*, Spig., Stan., *Stram.*, Stro., **Sul.**, **Sul. ac.**, Tab., Thuj., VERAT. A., Verb., Zinc.

—**Of Worms.**—Acon., Anac., Ars., Cina, Coff., **Fer.**, *Hyos.*, Merc., Nat. m., Saba., Sec. c., *Sil.*, Spig., *Verat. a.*

Internal Abdomen.

Stomach.—*Ab. n.*, *Abrot.*, *Ac. ac.*, **Acon.**, *Acon. f.*, *Aesc.*, *Aeth.*, *Agar.*, Agn., *Aloe*, *Alumen.*, *Alum.*, *Ambr.*, Am. carb., Am. m., Anac., Ant. cr., Ant. t., Arg., ARG. N., *Arn.*, **ARS.**, **Asaf.**, Asar., Aur., **Bar. c.**, **Bell.**, **Bism.**, *Bor.*, Bov., BRY., *Cact.*, *Calad.*, CALC. C., Camph., *Cannab. s.*, **Canth.**, **Caps.**, *Carb. ac.*, *Carb. an.*, *Carb. v.*, *Carb. sul.*, **Caust.**, *Cham.*, **Chel.**, Chin., Cic., Cina, *Coca*, **Cocc.**, Coff., **Colch.**, Coloc., **Con.**, Croc., *Crotal.*, *Cup.*, Cyc., *Dig.*, Dros., Dulc., *Elaps.*, *Euphorb.*, Fer., **Glon.**, Graph., Grat., Guai., **Hell.**, Hep., *Hydras.*, Hyos., IGN., Iod., IP., *Iris v.*, K. BI., **K. carb.**, *K. chl.*, K. nit., Kalm., Kre., *Lach.*, Laur., Led., *Lith.*, **Lob. i.**, Lyc., Mag. c., Mag. m., Mang., *Mar.*, Meny., *Merc.*, Mez., Mos., Mur. ac., *Myr.*, **Nat. c.**, **Nat. m.**, *Nit. ac.*, Nux m., **NUX V.**, Oleand., Op., Par., Petrol., PHOS., *Pho. ac.*, Phyt., *Plat.*, Pb., Pod., PULS., Ran. b., **Ran. s.**, *Rat.*, Rheum, Rhodo., **Rhus**, *Rob.*, *Rumex*, *Ruta*, Saba., *Sabi.*, Samb., **Sang.**, Sars., Sec. c., Seneg., Sep., Sil., Spig., Spo., Squ., **Stan.**, *Staph.*, Stram., Stro., SUL., **Sul. ac.**, Tab., *Thea.*, Thuj., *Ura.*, *Valer.*, VERAT. A., *Verat. v.*, Verb., Zinc., Zing.

Diaphragm.—Apis, *Asc. t.*, Bism., Cact., *Cimic.*, Cup., *Ran. b.*

Hypochondria.—ACON., Alum., Am. m., Ant. cr., Ant. t., Arn., **Ars.**, **Asaf.**, Asar., Aur., Bell., Bism., Bov., Bry., **Calc. c.**, Camph., Cannab. s., *Canth.*, Caps., Carb. an., **Carb. v.**, Caust., Cham., CHIN., Cocc., Coc. c., Coff., Colch., Con., *Cup.*, Dig., Dios., Dros., Fer., Graph., Hell., Hep., Ign., *Ip.*, K. carb., K. nit., Lach., Laur., Led., *Lyc.*, Mag. c., Mag. m., Mang., *Mar.*, Meny., Merc., **Mos.**, Mur. ac., Nat. c., Nat. m., *Nit. ac.*, Nux v., Op., Phos., Pho. ac., Plat., Pb., Puls., RAN. B., Ran. s.

Rhodo., Rhus, *Ruta*, Saba., Sars., Sec. c., Sele., Seneg., **Sep.**, *Sil.*, Spig., Spo., Stan., **Staph.**, *Stro.*, **Sul.**, *Sul. ac.*, Tar., Thuj., Valer., *Verat. a.*, Verb., Zinc.

Liver (and Region.)—*Ab. c.*, *Abrot.*, **Abs.**, **ACON.**, **Aesc.**, **Agar.**, Agn., *All. c.*, **Aloe**, Alum., Ambr., Am. carb., **Am. m.**, Anac., **Ant. t.**, **Apoc. c.**, **Arg. n.**, Arn., **Ars.**, *Asaf.*, **Aur.**, Bap., Bar. c., *Bell.*, **BERB.**, Bov., **BRY.**, Calad., **CALC. C**, *Calc. f.*, *Calc. ph.*, *Camph.*, Cannab. s., Canth., **Carb. ac.**, **Carb. an.**, *Carb. v.*, **Card.**, *Caust.*, *Ced.*, **Cham.**, **CHEL.**, **Chin.**, *Cinnab.*, Clem., **Cocc.**, Colch., Coloc., Con., *Corn. c.*, Croc., **Crotal.**, **Cup.**, *Dig.*, Dros., Dulc., *Euo.*, Fer., *Fl. ac.*, *Gel.*, *Graph.*, *Grind.*, Hell., **Hydras.**, *Hydroc.*, Hvos., **Ign.**, *Iod.*, Ip., *Iris v.*, **K. CARB.**, K. nit., Kre., *Lach.*, *Laur.*, **LEPT.**, **Lyc.**, *Mag. c.*, **MAG. M.**, Mar., **MERC.**, *Merc. c.*, *Merc. d.*, Mos., *Mur. ac.*, *Myr.*, *Nat. c.*, **Nat. m.**, *Nat. s.*, *Nit. ac.*, Nux m., **Nux v.**, Op., Par., Petrol., **Phos.**, Pho. ac., Plat., **Pb.**, **POD.**, *Polyp.*, *Pru.*, *Pso.*, **Puls.**, *Ran. b.*, *Ran. s.*, Rhodo., *Rhus*, *Rob.*, **Ruta**, Saba., Sabi., *Sang.*, Sars., Sec. c., *Sele.*, Seneg., **SEP.**, *Sil.*, Spig., Spo., Stan., Staph., **SUL.**, *Sul. ac.*, *Tab.*, Tar., Thuj., *Trom.*, Valer., *Verat. a.*, Verb., *Vip.*, Zinc.

Spleen.—*Ab. c.*, *Abrot.*, Acon., Agar., Agn., *Alum.*, *Am. carb.*, *Am. m.*, Anac., Ant. t., *Aran.*, Arg., **Arn.**, **Ars.**, ASAF., Asar., Aur., Bar. c., Bell., Bism., **Bor.**, Bov., Bry., Calad., *Calc. ph.*, *Camph.*, **Cannab. s.**, Canth., Caps., Carb. an., Carb. v., Caust., **Cean.**, *Ced.*, *Cham.*, Chel., **CHIN.**, *Coc. c.*, Colch., Con., *Corn. c.*, *Crot. tig.*, **Dios.**, Dros., **Dulc.**, Fer., *Gel.*, Graph., *Grind.*, Guai., Hep., **IGN.**, *Iod.*, Ip., *K. nit.*, Kre., Laur., Lyc., *Mag. c.*, **Mag. m.**, Mang., *Mar.*, *Merc.*, *Mez.*, Mos., **Mur. ac.**, **Nat. c.**, *Nat. m.*, Nit. ac., Nux m., Nux v., Oleand., Petrol., *Phos.*, *Pho. ac.*, **Plat.**, **Pb.**, *Pso.*, Puls., **RAN. B.**, Ran. s., Rheum, *Rhodo.*, *Rhus*, **Ruta**, Saba., *Sars.*, Sec. c., *Sele.*, Seneg., Sep., *Sil.*, *Spig.*, Spo., **Stan.**, *Sul.*, **Sul. ac.**, Tar., Thuj., *Valer.*, Verat. a., *Verb.*, Vio. t., **Zinc.**

Abdomen in General.—*Abrot.*, *Ac. ac.*, Acon., Aesc., Aeth., Agar., Agn., *Alet.*, **Aloe**, *Alum.*, Ambr., Am. carb., **Am. m.**, Anac., Ant. cr., Ant. t., **Apoc. c.**, Arg., *Arg. n.*, Arn., **ARS.**, **Asaf.**, Asar., Aur. Bar. c., **Bell.**, Bism., Bor., *Bov.*, **Brach.**, *Brom.*, **BRY.**, *Calad.*, **Calc. c.**, *Calc. ph.*, Camph., *Cannab. s.*, **Canth.**, *Caps.*, **Carb. ac.**, Carb. an., Carb. v., *Carb. sul.*, Caust., *Cham.*, Chel., **CHIN.**, Cic., *Cina*, Clem., Coca, **Cocc.**, Coff., *Colch.*, **COLOC.**, Com., Con., Croc., **Crotal.**, *Crot. tig.*, **Cup.**, Cyc., Dig., **Dios.**, Dros., Dulc., *Elat.*, *Euphorb.*, Euphr., **Fer.**, *Fl. ac.*, *Gam.*, Graph., *Gent. l.*, *Gram.*, *Grat.*, Guai., **Hell.**, Hep., **Hydras.**, Hyd. ac., Hyos., **Ign.**, *Iod.*, Ip., *Jat.*, *Jug. r.*, **K. bi.**, **K. carb.**, K. nit., *Kre.*, *Lach.*, Laur., **Led.**, **Lyc.**, *Mag. c.*, *Mag. m.*, Mang., **Mar.**, **Meny.**, **Merc.**, **Merc. c.**, *Mez.*,

Mos., Mur. ac., Myr., **Nat**. c., *Nat. m.*, Nit. ac., *Nux m.*, NUX V., *Oleand.*, **Op.**, *Ox. ac.*, **Par.**, **Petrol.**, **Phos.**, *Pho. ac.*, **Plat.**, *PB.*, PO.)., **Pru.**, **PULS.**, *Ran. b.*, Ran. s., **Rheum**, *Rhodo.*, *Rob.*, **RHUS**, *Ruta*, *Saba.*, *Sabi.*, *Sul. ac.*, Samb., *Sang.*, *Sars.*, *Sec. c.*, Sele., *Seneg.*, **SEP.**, **Sil.**, *Spig.*, *Spo.*, *Squ.*, *Stan.*, **Staph.**, *Stram.*, *Stro.*, SUL., *Sul. ac.*, Tar., **Ter.**, *Thuj.*, *Valer.*, VERAT. A., *Verat. v.*, *Verb.*, Vio. t., *Xan.*, Zinc.

Epigastrium.—*Ab. c.*, Acon., **Aesc.**, **Agar.**, *Agn.*, *Aloe.*, *Ambr.*, *Am. carb.*, Am. m., *Anac.*, *Ant. cr.*, Ant. t., *Apoc. c.*, **Arn.**, *Ars.*, *Asaf.*, Asar., Aur., *Bar. c.*, *Bell.*, *Bor.*, Bov., BRY., Calad., **Calc.** c., *Calc. ph.*, Camph., Cannab. s., **Canth.**, **Caps.**, *Carb. ac.*, **Carb. v.**, CAUST., **CHAM.**, **Chel.**, CHIN., *Cic.*, **Cina**, COCC., *Colch.*, **Coloc.**, *Con.*, *Croc.*, *Crot. tig.*, **Cup.**, *Cyc.*, **Dig.**, *Dios.*, Dulc., Euphr., *Fer.*, **Gel.**, Guai., Hell., Hep., *Hyd. ac.*, Hyos., **Ign.**, **Iod.**, *Ip.*, *Iris v.*, *K. bi.*, *K. carb.*, K. nit., Lach., **Laur.**, **Lyc.**, Mag. m., *Mar.*, Meny., **Merc.**, MERC. C., *Merc. i. r.*, *Mez.*, *Mos.*, Mur. ac., *Nat. c.*, **Nat. m.**, *Nux m.*, NUX V., Oleand., *Op.*, *Ox. ac.*, *Par.*, *Petrol.*, **Phos.**, Pho. ac., *Phyt.*, Plat., *Pb.*, *Pod.*, PULS., *Ran. b.*, Ran. s., *Rhodo.*, *Rhus.* *Rumex*, *Ruta*, *Saba.*, Sabi., *Sal. ac.*, *Samb.*, *Sec. c.*, *Seneg.*, *Sep.*, Sil., Spig., *Spo.*, **Stan.**, **Staph.**, *Stram.*, *Stro.*, *Sul.*, Sul. ac., Tar., **Thea.**, Thuj., *Valer.*, Verat. a., *Verb.*, Vio. t., *Zinc.*

—**Umbilical Region.**—Acon., *Aesc.*, *Agar.*, *Alum.*, Ambr., Am. carb., **Am. m.**, **Anac.**, Ant. cr., Ant. t., *Apoc. c.*, **Arn.**, Ars., *Asaf.*, Bar. c., **Bell.**, **Bov.**, **BRY.**, *Calad.*, *Calc. c.*, **Calc. ph.**, Camph., Cannab. s., Canth., *Caps.*, *Carb. an.*, Carb. v., *Caust.*, *Cham.*, **Chel.**, **Chin.**, Cina, Cocc., *Colch.*, COLOC., *Con.*, **Crot. tig.**, *Dig.*, Dios., Dulc., *Gam.*, *Graph.*, Guai., *Hell.*, Hep., *Hyos.*, Ign., Iod., Ip., K. carb., *K. nit.*, KRE., Lach., *Laur.*, Mag. c., *Mag. m.*, *Mang.*, Mar., Meny., Merc., *Mez.*, **Mos.**, *Mur. ac.*, **Nat. c.**, **Nux m.**, Nux v., Oleand., *Op.*, Par., *Phos.*, PHO. AC., **Plat.**, PB., *Puls.*, *Ran. b.*, *Ran. s.*, **Rheum**, Rhodo., RHUS, Ruta, *Sabi.*, *Sars.*, Seneg., **Sep.**, *Sil.*, Spig., Spo., *Stan.*, Staph., Stram., **Stro.**, **Sul.**, **Sul. ac.**, Tar., Thuj., *Valer.*, VERAT. A., VERB., Vio. t., *Zinc.*

Sides.—*Agar.*, Agn., *Alum.*, Ambr., *Am. carb.*, Am. m., Anac., Ant. cr., Arn., Ars., ASAF., *Asar.*, Aur., *Bar. c.*, *Bell.*, Bism., Bor., Bov., **Bry.**, Calad., *Calc. c.*, Camph., *Cannab. s.*, **Canth.**, Caps., Carb. an., **CARB V.**, **Caust.**, *Cham.*, Chel., **CHIN.**, Cina, *Clem.*, **Cocc.**, *Coff.*, Colch., Coloc., Croc., Cyc., *Dig.*, *Dros.*, Dulc., *Euphorb.*, Fer., Graph., Guai., Hell., Hep., Hyos., **IGN.**, Iod., *Ip.*, K. carb., K. nit., *Kre.*, *Lach.*, Laur., **Led.**, **Lyc.**, Mag. c., **Mag. m.**, Mang., *Mur.*, *Meny.*, Merc., Mez., Mos., Mur. ac., **Nat. c.**, *Nat. m.*, **Nit. ac.**, Nux m., **Nux v.**, Oleand., Op., *Par.*, *Petrol.*, **Phos.**, **Plat.**, Pb., Puls., *Ran. b.*, *Ran. s.*, *Rheum*, *Rhodo.*, *Rhus*, *Ruta*, Saba., Sabi.

80 INTERNAL ABDOMEN.

Samb., *Sang.,* Sars., Sec. c., Seneg., *Sep.,* Sil., *Spig.,* Spo., *Stan.*, **Staph.**, Stro., Sul., TAR., Thuj., Valer., Vio. t., **Zinc**.

Loins.—*Acon., Agar., Agn., Ambr.,* Am. m., Anac., *Ant. cr.,* Arg., *Arn.* **Asaf., Aur.,** Bell., Berb., Bov., *Calc. c.,* Camph., Cannab. s., CANTH., *Carb. an.,* Carb. v., Caust., Cham., **Chel.,** *Chin.,* Cina, Clem., Cocc., *Colch.,* **Coloc.,** Dig., *Dros., Dulc.,* Euphorb., Hep., *Hyos.,* Ign., Iod., K. carb. **K. nit.,** Kre., Lach., Laur., Led., **Lyc.,** Mag. c., *Mar., Meny.,* Merc., **Mez.,** Nat. c., *Nit. ac.,* Nux v., Oleand., *Phyt.,* **Pb.,** *Puls.,* **Ran. b.,** *Ran. s.,* RHEUM., Rhus, *Ruta,* Saba., Sabi., **Samb.,** Sars., *Sec. c., Senec.,* **Sep.,** Spig., Spo., **Staph.,** Stro., Sul., **Tar.,** THUJ., Valer., Verat. a., Verb., *Vib. op.,* Vio. t., *Xan.,* ZINC.

Lower Abdomen.—*Acon., Aesc., Agar., Agn.,* ALOE, Alum., **Ambr.,** Am. carb., Am. m., *Anac.,* Ant. cr., **Ant. t.,** *Arg.,* **Arn., Ars.,** *Asaf., Asar.,* **Aur., Bar. c.,** BELL., Bism., Bor., Bov., BRY., Calad., **Calc. c.,** *Camph.,* Cannab. s., *Canth.,* **Caps.,** Carb. an., CARB. V., **Caust.,** Cham., *Chel.,* **Chin.,** Cic., Cina, *Clem.,* **Cocc.,** *Coc. c.,* Coff., *Colch., Coll.,* **Coloc.,** Con., *Conv., Croc.,* Cup., *Cyc.,* Dig., *Dros.,* Dulc., *Equi.,* Euphorb., Euphr., Fer., Graph., Guai., Hell., Hep., *Hyos.,* **Ign.,** Iod., **K. carb.,** K. nit., *Laur.,* Led., Lil. t., **LYC.,** Mag. c., *Mag. m.,* Mang., Mar., Meny., Merc., *Mez.,* Mos., *Nat. c.,* Nat. m., Nit. ac., Nux m., **Nux v.,** Oleand., Par., **Phos.,** *Pho. ac.,* Plat., Pb., **Puls.,** RAN. B., Rheum, Rhodo., *Rhus,* Ruta, Saba., *Sabi.,* Samb., Sars., *Sec. c.,* Seneg., SEP., **Sil.,** Spig., *Spo.,* SQU., Stan., Staph., *Stro.,* SUL., Sul. ac., **Tar.,** Thuj., *Valer.,* Verat. a., Verat. v., *Verb.,* Vib. op., Vio. t., Zinc.

Groins (Including Cœcum, Cœcal Region, Ilio-Cœcal Region, Iliac Region and Pourpart's Ligament).—*Agar., Amm. c.,* BAP., Berb., Bry., *Carb. sul.,* Chel., *Corn., Dios., Gins.,* Merc. c., *Osm.,* Phos., Pb., Sul., *Thuj.*

Inguinal Rings.—Agar., Agn., **Alum.,** *Am. carb.,* AM. M., Anac., *Ant. cr.,* Ant. t., *Arg.,* Ars., Asaf., Asar., AUR., Bar. c., *Bell.,* Berb., Bov., Calc. c., Camph., *Cannab. s., Canth., Caps.,* **Carb. an.,** Carb. v., Caust., Cham., Chel., *Chin.,* Cic., Clem., **Cocc.,** Coff., Coloc., Con., *Croc.,* Dig., Dros., Dulc., *Euphorb., Graph.,* Guai., Hell., **Ign.,** Iod., *K. carb.,* K. nit., Kre., Laur., **LYC.,** *Mag. c.,* Mag. m., **Mar.,** Meny., **Merc.,** *Mez.,* Mur. ac., Nat. c., Nat. m., *Nit. ac.,* NUX V., *Op., Osm.,* Par., Petrol., Phos., Pho. ac., *Plat.,* Pb., Ran. b., Ran. s., Rheum., **Rhodo., Rhus,** Saba., Sars., *Sep.,* **Sil., Spig.,** Spo., *Stan.,* Staph., Stram., **Stro., Sul.,** SUL AC., Tar., Thuj., *Valer.,* **Verat. a.,** Vio. t., *Zinc.*

Hernia.—**Alum.,** Am. carb., AM. M., Anac., Ant. cr., Arg., *Asar.,* AUR., *Bell., Calc. c.,* Camph., *Cannab. s., Caps.,* Carb. an., **Cham.,** Chin.,

EXTERNAL ABDOMEN—ABDOMEN.

Clem., **Cocc.**, Coff., *Coloc.*, Dig., Euphorb., *Graph.*, *Guai.*, Hell., *Ign.*, *K. carb.*, K. nit., LYC., *Mag. c.*, Mar., *Merc.*, Mez., Nat. m., **Nit. ac.**, NUX V., *Op.*, Petrol., Phos., Pho. ac., Plat., *Pb.*, Rheum, **Rhus**, Sep., **Sil.**, Spig., Spo., Stan., Staph., Stram., Stro., *Sul.*, SUL. AC., Thuj., VERAT. A., Zinc.

External Abdomen.

Pit of Stomach.—*Acon.*, **Aloe**, Alum., *Ant. cr.*, **Ant. t.**, **Arg. n.**, ARS., Asaf., Aur., *Bar. ac.*, Bar. c., **Bell.**, BRY., **Cact.**, **Calc. c.**, Caps., *Caust.*, *Cham.*, **Chel.**, Chin., **Cic.**, **Cocc.**, Coff., *Coloc.*, Con., *Corn. c.*, *Croc.*, *Dios.*, *Euphorb.*, Fer., **Hell.**, *Hep.*, *Ign.*, *K. bi.*, *K. carb.*, *Kalm.*, Lach., **Lyc.**, Mang., **Merc.**, Merc. c., Mez., Mos., Nat. c., NAT. M., *Nux v.*, *Oleand.*, Op., *Ox. ac.*, Petrol., *Phos.*, **Pho. ac.**, *Phyt.*, *Plat.*, *Pru.*, **Puls.**, *Ran. b.*, *Ran. s.*, *Ruta*, *Saba.*, Sabi., *Samb.*, Sec. c., *Sep.*, *Sil.*, *Spig.*, *Spo.*, Stan., *Sul.*, *Tab.*, *Verat. a.*, Zinc.

Abdomen Externally.—Acon., Alum., *Ambr.*, Am. m., Anac., Ant. cr., *Arg.*, Arn., *Ars.*, Asaf., Asar., Aur., Bar. c., **Bell.**, *Bov.*, BRY., *Calc. c*, Camph., Cannab. s., **Canth.**, Caps., Carb. v., Caust., Cham., Chel., *Chin.*, Cic., **Cocc.**, Colch., **Coloc.**, Con., Croc., Cup., Dig., *Dros.*, Euphorb., *Fer.*, Graph., Guai., **Hyos.**, Ign., Iod., Ip., K. carb., Lach., Led. *Lyc.*, Mag. c., *Mag. m.*, Mang., Meny., MERC., Mos., Mur ac., *Nat. c.*, *Nat. m.*, Nit. ac., NUX V., Oleand., Op., *Par.*, Petrol., Phos., Pho. ac., *Plat.*, Pb., PULS., Ran. b., *Ran. s.*, Rheum, Rhodo., Rhus, Ruta, Saba., *Sabi.*, *Samb.*, Sars., SELE., Seneg., **Sep.**, Sil., Spig., Spo., Squ., Stan., Staph., Stram., Stro., Sul., Sul. ac., Tar., *Thuj.*, *Valer.*, *Verat. a.*, *Vio. t.*, Zinc.

Rings Externally.—Alum., Ambr., Am. carb., *Am. m.*, ARS., *Aur.*, *Bov.*, Calc. c., Cannab. s., **Canth.**, Chin., Cic., Cocc., Dig., Euphorb., Graph., *Guai.*, K. carb., **Lyc.**, Mag. m., MERC., Mez., Mur. ac., Nat. c., Nit. ac., *Nux v.*, Pho. ac., **Puls.**, Sars., **Sele.**, Sep., **Sil.**, *Spig.*, Stro., *Sul.*, *Sul. ac.*, Thuj.

Mons Veneris.—Amm. c., Anac., Ant. t., Arg., Asaf., *Aur.*, Bell., *Calc. ph.*, Hell., Hyos., Meny., *Nat. c.*, Nat. m., *Nit. ac.*, *Nux v.*, Pb., RHUS, *Ruta*, Saba., *Sele.*, Staph., **Valer.**, *Vib. op.*, *Vio. t.*, Zinc.

Inguinal Glands.—*Ant. cr.*, Ars., *Asaf.*, Aur., *Bad.*, Bar. c., **Bell.**, CALC. C., *Cannab. s.*, *Cinnab.*, CLEM., *Con.*, **Dulc.**, *Graph.*, HEP., *Iod.*, Lyc., *Meny.*, MERC., Mez., *Nat. c.*, NIT. AC., Nux v., *Osm.*, Phos., Pho. ac., Puls., *Rheum*, *Rhus*, Sil., Spo., Stan., Staph., Stram., *Sul.*, THUJ.

Abdomen.

Left Side.—*Acon.*, Agar., Agn., ALUM., Ambr., **Am. carb.**, **Am. m.**, Anac., **Ant. cr.**, **Ant. t.**, **Apis.**, **Arg.**, Arn., Ars., ASAF., *Asar.*,

82 ABDOMEN—HYPOCHONDRIA.

Aur., Bar. c., **Bell.,** **Bov.,** *Brom.,* **Bry.,** **Calc. c.,** Camph., *Cannab.* s., Canth., *Caps.,* Carb. v., Caust., **Cham.,** Chel., *Chin.,* **Cina,** Cocc., Colch., Coloc., **Con.,** Croc., *Crot. tig.,* **Cup.,** Dig., DULC., *Euphorb.,* FL. AC., *Graph.,* *Grat.,* **Guai.,** HEP., *Ign.,* **Iod.,** *Jug. r.,* **K. carb.,** *Kre.,* Lach., Laur., *Led.,* Lyc., Mag. m., *Mang.,* Mar., Meny., Merc., Mez., **Millef.,** *Mur. ac., Nat. c.,* **Nat. m.,** *Nit. ac.,* Nux m., *Nux v.,* Oleand., **Op.,** **Par.,** Petrol., *Pho. ac.,* Plat., PB., *Pso.,* **Puls.,** **Ran. b.,** RHEUM, Rhodo., Rhus, *Ruta, Saba.,* Sabi., *Samb., Sars., Sele.,* Sep., Sil., **Spig.,** *Spo.,* Squ., Stan., *Staph.,* SUL., *Sul. ac.,* TAR., Thuj., **Valer.,** *Verb.,* Vio. t., Zinc.

Right Side.—Agar., *Agn.,* Ambr., Am. m., Anac., *Ant. cr.,* Apis., *Arg.,* *Arn.,* ARS., Asaf., **Aur.,** Bap., Bar. c., **Bell.,** *Bism.,* **Bry.,** *Calad.,* Calc. c., Camph., **Cannab. s., Canth.,** **Carb. an.,** Carb. v., **Caust.,** Chel., **Chin.,** *Cic., Clem.,* Cocc., *Colch.,* **Coloc.,** Con., *Croc.,* Cup., *Cyc.,* Dig., *Dros.,* Dulc., Fl. ac., Graph., **Guai., Ign.,** Iod., *Ip.,* **K. carb., K. nit.,** Kre., **Lach.,** Laur., **Lyc., Mag. m.,** *Mar.,* Meny., *Merc.,* Mez., Millef., *Mos.,* Nat. c., **Nat. m.,** Nit. ac., Nux m., *Nux v.,* Oleand., Petrol., *Phos.,* **Pho. ac.,** *Plat.,* Pb., **Pod.,** Pso., *Puls.,* Ran. b., *Ran. s.,* Rhodo., **Rhus,** Saba., *Sabi.,* Samb., *Sang.,* **Seneg., Sep.,** Sil., Spig., Spo., Squ., **Stan.,** *Stro.,* **Sul.,** Tar., **Thuj.,** Verb., *Vio. t.,* Zinc.

Hypochondria.

Left Side.—Acon., *Agar.,* **Agn.,** Alum., Am. carb., **Am. m.,** *Anac.,* Ant.cr., Apis, *Arg.,* Arn., Ars., **ASAF., Asar.,** *Aur.,* Bell., Bar., Brom., Bry., Calad., *Calc. c.,* **Cannab. s.,** Carb. an., **Carb. v., Caust., Cham.,** Chel., Chin., *Cocc., Coff., Con.,* Cup., Dig., *Dios.,* Dulc., Euphorb., **Fer.,** FL. AC., *Graph., Hep.,* IGN., *Iod., Ip.,* **K. carb., K. nit.,** Kre., Laur., Lyc., Mang., Mar., Merc., **Mez.,** Millef., Mos., **Mur. ac.,** *Nat. c., Nat. m.,* NIT. AC., *Nux v.,* Oleand., Par., Petrol., Phos., Pho. ac., *Plat.,* Pb., **Puls.,** Pso., **Ran. b.,** *Ran. s.,* Rheum, *Rhodo.,* Rhus, *Ruta,* Saba., *Sars., Sec. c., Seneg.,* Sep., *Sil.,* Spig., Squ., Stan., Staph., SUL., *Sul. ac.,* Valer., **Verb.,** *Vio. t.,* Zinc.

Right Side.—ACON., Aesc., *Agar.,* **Agn.,** Aloe, Alum., Ambr., AM. CARB., Am. m., Anac., *Ant. cr.,* Apis, *Arn., Ars., Asaf.,* Bap., BAR. C., BELL., Berb., Bor., BRY., Calad., **Calc. c., Canth.,** Carb. an., *Carb. v.,* Card., *Caust.,* **Chel.,** Chin., **Clem.,** COCC., Colch., Con., Dig., *Dios.,* Dulc., *Fer.,* Fl. ac., Graph., **Hep., Hydras.,** Hyos., Ign., Iod., Iris v., K. CARB., Kre., **Lach.,** Laur., *Led.,* LYC., Mag. m., Mang., Mar., **Merc.,** Millef., Mos., **Myr.,** *Nat. c.,* **Nat. m., Nat. s.,** Nit. ac., Nux m., NUX V., Par., Petrol., Phos., *Pho. ac.,* Plat., *Pb.,* **POD.,** *Pru., Pso.,* Puls., Ran. b., *Ran. s.,* Rhodo., *Rhus, Ruta,* **Saba.,** *Sabi., Sec. c.,*

Sele., Sep., Sil., *Spig.*, Stan., Staph., *Sul.*, *Sul. ac.*, *Tell.*, Valer., **Verat. a.**, Verb., Zinc.

Abdominal Rings.

Left Side.—*Agar.*, Agn., *Alum.*, *Ambr.*, **Am. carb.**, **Am. m.**, *Ant. cr.*, **Apis.**, *Arg.*, Arn., *Asar.*, Aur., Bell., *Berb.*, Calc. c., Camph., Cannab. s., Carb. an., *Chel.*, Cocc., *Dig.*, Dulc., **EUPHORB.**, Fl. ac., Graph., Ign., K. carb., Laur., Lyc., **MAG. C.**, *Mag. m.*, *Merc.*, **Nit. ac.**, Nux m., *Nux v.*, *Par.*, *Phos.*, Rhodo., Rhus, *Saba.*, Sabi., Sars., *Sep.*, Sil., *Spig.*, Spo., *Stan.*, *Staph.*, Sul., *Sul. ac.*, *Tar.*, *Verat. a.*, Vio. t., ZINC.

Right Side.—Agn., Alum., **Am. carb.**, **Am. m.**, *Apis.*, *Ars.*, Aur., *Bell.*, Bor., **CALC. C.**, Camph., Cannab. s., Canth., **Carb. an.**, **Carb. v.**, *Cic.*, *Clem.*, Cocc., Coloc., *Con.*, Dig., *Dros.*, Dulc., Fl. ac., Graph., *Hell.*, Iod., *Ip.*, **K. CARB.**, **LACH.**, Laur., **LYC.**, *Mang.*, *Mar.*, **Merc.**, Mez., **NUX V.**, *Oci.*, *Op.*, Petrol., *Pho. ac.*, *Pso.*, **PULS.**, *Ran. b.*, **RHODO.**, **RHUS**, *Ruta*, *Sabi.*, Sars., Seneg., *Sep.*, Sil., Spig., Spo., Stan., **Staph.**, Stro., Sul., **SUL. AC.**, **THUJ.**, *Valer.*, Verat. a., Zinc.

Flatulence.

Flatulence in General.—Acon., Agar., Agn., *Ail.*, *All. c.*, **ALOE**, Alum., *Ambr.*, Am. carb., Am. m., Anac., *Ant. cr.*, Ant. t., Apoc. c., Arg., **ARG. N.**, **ARN.**, Ars., Asaf., Asar., Aur., Bar. c., Bell., Bism., Bor., *Bov.*, Bry., Calad., *Calc. c.*, *Calc. i.*, *Calc. ph.*, Camph., Cannab. s., Canth., Caps., Carb. ac., Carb. an., **CARB. V.**, *Carb. sul.*, Caust., **CHAM.**, Chel., **CHIN.**, *Cic.*, *Cina*, *Clem.*, *Coca*, **COCC.**, *Coc. c.*, *Coff.*, *Colch.*, **COLOC.**, Con., Corn. c., Croc., Crotal., Crot. tig., *Cub.*, Cup., Cyc., *Dig.*, **DIOS.**, Dros., Dulc., *Euphorb.*, Euphr., Fer., *Fl. ac.*, Gam., *Gran.*, **GRAPH.**, Guai., Hell., Hep., *Hyos.*, IGN., Iod., Ip., K. bi., K. carb., *K. iod.*, K. nit., Kre., Lach., *Laur.*, Led., Lil. t., **LYC.**, Mag. c., *Mag. m*, Mang., **MAR.**, Meny., **MERC.**, *Merc. c.*, *Mez.*, Mur. ac., Nat. c., Nat. m., **NAT. S.**, Nit. ac., Nux m., **NUX V.**, *Oleand.*, **OP.**, *Osm.*, Par., Petrol., **PHOS.**, **PHO. AC.**, *Plat.*, **PB.**, **Pod.**, Pso., **PULS.**, Ran. b., Ran. s., **RAPH.**, *Rheum*, Rhodo., **Rhus**, Rob., *Rumex*, Ruta, *Saba.*, Sabi., *Sal. ac.*, Sang., Samb., *Sars.*, Sec. c., Sele., Seneg., Sep., **SIL.**, *Spig.*, Spo., Stan., Squ., **STAPH.**, Stram., *Stro.*, **SUL.**, *Sul. ac.*, Tar., Ter., Thuj., *Ura.*, Valer., **VERAT. A.**, Verb., Vio. t., Zinc., *Zing.*

Flatus Smelling of Bad Eggs.—*Ant. t.*, **Arn.**, *Coff.*, Kre., *Mar.*, Sep., Stan., **SUL.**, *Valer.*

—**Cold.**—Con.

—**Fetid.**—Acon., Agar., All. c., **ALOE**, Alum., Am. m., Ant. cr., *Ant. t.*, **Arn.**, **ARS.**, **ASAF.**, *Asar.*, Aur., Bar. c., Bell., **Bism.**, **Bor.**, *Bov.*,

FLATULENCE.

BRY., Calad., **Calc. c.**, **Calc. ph.**, Canth., *Carb. an.*, CARB. V., Caust., **Cham.**, Chin., *Cocc.*, Coff., **Coloc.**, Dios., Dros., Dulc., **Graph.**, *Guai.*, Hell., Hep., Ign., *Iod.*, *Ip.*, K. carb., K. nit., Kre., *Lach.*, Lyc., **Mag. c.**, **Mar.**, *Merc.*, Mur. ac., *Nat. c.*, Nat. m., **Nit. ac.**, Nux m., **Nux v.**, Oleand., *Op.*, *Pœo.*, Petrol., Phos., *Pho. ac.*, **Pb.**, PULS., Ran. b., Ran. s., Rheum, *Rhodo.*, Rhus, Ruta, Sabi., *Sars.*, Sec. c., *Sep.*, SIL., Spig., Squ., Staph., Stram., *Stro.*, SUL, *Sul. ac.*, Valer., Verat. a., Zinc.

—**Garlicky.**—Agar., *Mos.*, Phos.

—**Hot.**—*Acon.*, ALOE, Ant. t., *Cham.*, Cocc., Mag. m., **Mar.**, Nux v., Phos., Pb., Puls., *Staph.*, **Sul.**, Zinc.

—**Loud.**—Am. m., Canth., **Lach.**, Laur., *Mar.*, *Merc.*, Squ.

—**Moist.**—Carb. v.

—**Odorless.**—AGAR., *Ambr.*, Arn., **Bell.**, Cannab. s., Carb. v., Coff., Lyc., **Mar.**, Merc., Zinc.

—**Putrid.**—Acon., Alum., **Ant. t.**, *Arn.*, ARS., *Asar.*, *Aur.*, Bell., *Bov.*, *Bry.*, *Calad.*, **Calc. c.**, *Carb. ac.*, CARB. V., *Cham.*, *Chin.*, **Cocc.**, *Coff.*, Coloc., **Dulc.**, *Graph.*, *Hep.*, Ign., *Iod.*, *Ip.*, Kre., Lyc., *Mar.*, Merc., Nat. c., Nat. m., **Nit. ac.**, Nux m., **Nux v.**, Oleand., *Par.*, Puls., *Ruta,* Sabi., Sars., Sec. c., *Sep.*, Sil., Spig., *Staph.*, Stram., Sul., **Valer.**, Zinc.

—**Sour Smelling.**—*Arn.*, Bell., **Calc. c.**, *Cham.*, Coloc., Dulc., Graph., *Hep.*, *Mag. c.*, **Merc.**, Nat. c., Petrol., Phos., RHEUM, *Sep.*, Sul.

Borborygmi.—*Acon.*, Aesc., **Agar.**, Agn., **Aloe**, *Alum.*, *Ambr.*, *Am. carb.*, *Am. m.*, Anac., **Ant. cr.**, **Ant. t.**, Arg., Arn., Ars., *Asaf.*, Asar., *Aur.*, Bar. c., *Bell.*, *Bism.*, Bor., *Bov.*, Bry., **Calc. c.**, Canth., Caps., **Carb. ac.**, *Carb. an.*, **Carb. v.**, CAUST., **Cham.**, Chel., CHIN., *Cic.*, Cina, Clem., Cocc., **Coc. c.**, Coff., **Coloc.**, *Con.*, Croc., **Crot. tig.**, Cup., *Cyc.*, *Dig.*, DIOS., *Dulc.*, Euphorb., Euphr., Fer., **Gam.**, **Glon.**, *Graph.*, Guai., HELL., *Hep.*, Hyos., **Ign.**, Iod., Ip., **JAT.**, K. bi., K. carb., K. nit., *Laur.*, Led., LYC., Mag. c., *Mag. m.*, **Mar.**, Meny., **Merc.**, **Mez.**, Mos., *Mur. ac.*, Nat. c, **Nat. m.**, **Nit. ac.**, Nux m., NUX V., *Oleand.*, **Op.**, *Par.*, Petrol., PHOS., PHO. AC., **Plat.**, Pb., Pod., PULS., Ran. b., Ran. s., *Rheum*, *Rhodo.*, Rhus, Ruta, Saba., Sabi., Samb., **Sars.**, Sec. c., Sele., Seneg., **Sep.**, Sil., **Spig.**, Spo., **Squ.**, *Stan.*, Staph., *Stram.*, *Stro.*, SUL, *Sul. ac.*, *Tar.*, **Thuj.**, **Valer.**, **Verat. a.**, *Verb.*, Zinc.

Flatulent Pain.—Acon., Alum., *Ambr.*, Am. carb., Am. m., **Anac.**, Ant. cr., Ant. t., Arg., **Arn.**, **Asaf.**, *Asar.*, Aur., Bell., *Bism.*, Bry., Calc. c., Camph., Cannab. s., *Canth.*, *Caps.*, Carb. an., CARB. V., **Cham.**, Chel., CHIN., Cic., **Cocc.**, **Coc. c.**, Coff., Colch., Coloc., **Con.**, *Crot. tig.*, Cyc., **Dros.**, **Euphorb.**, **Fer.**, **Graph.**, *Guai.*, Hell., **Hep.**, **Hyos.**,

FLATULENCE—STOOL. 85

Ign., Iod., Ip., K. carb., Lach., *Laur.*, LYC., Mag. c., **Mar.**, **Menth.**,
Meny., *Mez.*, Nat. c., *Nat. m.*, *Nit. ac.*, Nux m., NUX V., Op., Par.,
Phos., *Plat.*, **Pb.**, **PULS.**, Ran. b., **Rheum**, **RHODO.**, *Rhus*, *Ruta*,
Sabi., Samb., *Sele.*, Seneg., Sep., *Sil.*, Spig., *Spo.*, Squ., STAPH., Sul.,
Sul. ac., Tar., *Thuj.*, Valer., VERAT. A., *Verb.*, Zinc.

Incarceration of Flatus.—Acon., Agar., *Ambr.*, Am. carb., Am. m.,
Ant. cr., **ANT. T.**, **Arn.**, **Asar.**, *Aur.*, *Bar. c.*, **Bell.**, *Bor.*, *Calc. c.*,
Camph., Cannab. s., **Canth.**, *Caps.*, *Carb. ac.*, *Carb. an.*, CARB. V., *Caust.*,
CHAM., **Chin.**, *Cic.*, COCC., *Coff.*, Colch., **Coloc.**, **Con.**, Euphorb.,
GRAPH., *Guai.*, Hell., *Hep.*, Hyos., IGN., *Iod.*, K. CARB., K. nit.,
Lach., LYC., *Mag. m.*, *Mar.*, *Meny.*, *Mez.*, *Mos.*, **Nat. c.**, **Nat. m.**, **Nat.
s.**, NIT. AC., **Nux m.**, NUX V., Op., Petrol., Phos., **Pho. ac.**, Plat.,
PB., **PULS.**, **RAPH.**, **Rheum**, *Rhodo.*, *Rhus*, Ruta, Saba., Sabi., Sele.,
Sep., Sil., Spig., *Spo.*, **Squ.**, Stan., STAPH., Stram., Stro., SUL., Sul. ac.,
Thuj., Valer., **Verat. a.**, Verb., Zinc.

Stool.

Diarrhœa.—Acon., *Aesc.*, **Aeth.**, **Agar.**, Agn., *Ail.*, *All. c.*, **Aloe.**,
Alst., *Alum.*, Ambr., Am. carb., **Am. m.**, Anac., **ANT. CR.**, **Ant. t.**,
Apis, APOC. C., Arg., ARG. N., ARN., ARS., ARS. IOD., Arum. t.,
Asaf., *Asar.*, *Aur.*, **Bap.**, *Bar. c* , *Bell.*, **Benz. ac.**, Bism., BAR., **Bov.**,
BRY., Calad., **Calc. c.**, **Calc. ph.**, Cannab. s., Canth., **CAPS.**, *Carb.
ac.*, Carb. an., *Carb. v.*, *Carb. sul.*, *Caust.*, CHAM., CHEL., CHIN.,
Chrom. ac., *Cic.*, **Cina**, *Cist.*, Clem., **Cocc.**, *Coff.*, Colch., COLOC.,
Con., **Corn. c.**, *Corn. f.*, Croc., *Crotal.*, CROT. TIG., Cup., Cyc., **Dig.**,
Dios., *Dirc.*, *Dros.*, DULC., ELAT., *Euphorb.*, **FER.**, *Fer. ph.*, *Fl. ac.*,
GAM., **Gel.**, *Gent. l.*, **Gran.**, *Graph.*, GRAT., Guai., *Hell.*, Hep., *Hydras.*,
Hyos., *Ign.*, Iod., Ip., IRIS V., JAL., JAT., K. BI., K. carb., *K. nit.*,
Lach., Laur., Led., LEPT., *Lyc.*, Mag. c., *Mag. m.*, Mang., Mar., MERC.,
Merc. c., **Merc. d.**, *Mez.*, *Mur. ac.*, *Nat. c.*, **Nat. m.**, **Nat. s.**, **Nit. ac.**,
Nux m., *Nux v.*, *Oenot.*, *Oleand.*, **Op.**, *Osm.*, *Ox. ac.*, *Par.*, **Petrol.**, PHOS.,
PHO. AC., **PHYT.**, *Plant.*, Plat., Pb., POD., **PSO.**, **PULS.**, Ran. b.,
Ran. s., **Raph.**, RHEUM, Rhodo., RHUS, RUMEX, Ruta, **Saba.**,
Sabi., **Sul. ac.**, **Sang.**, Sars., SEC. C., Seneg., **Sep.**, **Sil.**, *Spig.*, Spo., *Squ.*,
Stan., *Staph.*, **Stict.**, *Still.*, *Stram.*, Stro., SUL., SUL. AC., **Sum.**, *Tab.*,
Tar., **THUJ.**, *Trom.*, *Valer.*, VERAT. A., Verb., *Vio. t.*, Zinc.

—**Alternating with Constipation.**—Ant. cr., *Card.*, *Chel.*, Cimic.,
Pod., *Puls.*

—**Painful.**—*Agar.*, Alum., *Am. carb.*, *Am. m.*, Anac., Ant. t., ARS.,
Asaf., *Asar.*, Bar. c., Bell., Bor., *Bov.*, **Bry.**, Calad., Calc. c., Canth.,

86 STOOL.

Caps., Carb. an., *Carb. v.*, Caust., **Cham.**, *Chin., Colch., Coloc.,* Con., Croc., Cup., Dig., Dros., **Dulc.**, *Euphorb.*, Graph., Hell., Hep., *Ign.,* Ip., **JAL.**, K. carb., *K. nit.,* Laur., Lyc., Mag. c., Mag. m., Mang., Meny., **Merc.**, MERC. C., Mez., *Nat. c.,* Nat. m., **Nit. ac., Nux v.**, Op., Petrol., *Phos.*, Pb., Pod., *Puls.,* Raph., RHEUM, RHUS, Saba., Sars., Seneg., SENN., *Sep.,* Sil., *Spig.,* Spo., Stan., Staph., Stro., **Sul.,** Thuj., VERAT. A., Vio. t., Zinc.

—**Painless.**—Acon., *Ambr.,* Anac., Ant. t., *Apoc. c.,* Arn., ARS., Aur., *Bur. c.,* Bell., Berb., **Bism.**, *Bor., Bov.,* Bry., *Calc. c., Cannab. i., Canth., Carb. an.,* Carb. v., **Cham.**, **Chel.**, *Chin.,* Cic., *Clem., Cocc.,* Coloc., Con., Croc., **Crot. tig.,** Cup., Dig., *Dulc.,* **FER.**, *Form., Gel., Graph., Grat., Hell.,* **HYOS.**, *Ign.,* Ip., **Iris v.**, *K. nit., Laur.,* Led., **LYC.**, Mag. c., Mag. m., *Merc.,* Mur. ac., Nat. m., *Nit. ac.,* Nux m., Nux v., *Oleand.,* **Op.,** Petrol., **PHOS., PHO. AC., Plat., Pod.,** Puls., *Ran. b., Rhodo., Rhus,* Sabi., Sars., *Sec. c.,* Sep., Sil., *Spig.,* Spo., Staph., **STRAM.,** Stro., Sul., **Tab.,** Thuj., Valer., *Verat. a.,* Zinc.

Constipation.—*Ab. c., Ab. n.,* Acon., Agar., Agn., **Alum.,** *Ambr., Am. carb.,* **Am. m.,** Anac., *Ant. cr.,* Ant. t., Arg., Arn., *Ars., Asaf.,* Asar., Aur., Bar. c., **Bell.,** Bor., *Bov.,* **BRY.,** Calad., CALC. C., Camph., *Cannab. s.,* Canth., Caps., Carb. an., **Carb. v.,** *Carb. sul., Card.,* Caust., Cham., **Chel.,** *Chin.,* Cic., *Cina, Coca.,* COCC., COFF., *Colch.,* **Coll.,** *Coloc.,* **Con.,** Cup., Cyc., Dig., Dros., **Dulc.,** *Euon.,* Euphorb., Euphr., Fer., Gam., Graph., *Guai.,* Hell., *Hep., Hydras., Hyos.,* Ign., *Iod.,* **Iris v.,** K. carb., K. nit., Kre., *Lach.,* Laur., *Led.,* **Lil. t.,** LYC., *Mag. c., Mag. m., Mang.,* **Meny.,** **Merc.,** *Mez.,* **Mos.,** Nat. c., *Nat. m.,* NIT. AC., Nux m., **NUX V.,** *Oleand.,* **OP.,** Par., *Petrol.,* Phos., *Pho. ac., Phyt.,* **Plat.,** PB., **Pso.,** Puls., Ran. b., Rheum, *Rhodo., Rhus,* Ruta, **Saba.,** *Sabi.,* Sars., Sele., Seneg., Sep., **SIL.,** Spig., *Spo., Squ..* **Stan.,** STAPH., *Stram.,* Stro., **SUL.,** **Sul. ac.,** Thuj., **VERAT. A., Verb., Vib. op.,** Vio. o., Vio. t., Zinc.

—**On Account of Hard Fæces.**—Acon., **Aesc.,** *Agar.,* Agn., *Alum.,* **Am. carb.,** AM. M., *Ant. cr.,* Ant. t., Arg., Arn., *Ars., Asaf.,* Asar., Aur., *Bar. c., Bell.,* Bov., BRY., *Calc. c.,* Camph., *Cannab. s., Canth.,* Caps., **Carb. an.,** *Carb. v.,* **Caust.,** Cham., **Chel.,** Chin., *Cina, Coca, Cocc.,* Colch., Coloc., *Con.,* Cyc., Dulc., Euphr., Graph., *Guai.,* Hell., *Hep.,* Hyos., *Ign., Iod.,* K. carb., *K. nit.,* **Kre.,** Lach., *Laur.,* Led., *Lyc.,* **Mag. c.,** MAG. M., Mang., *Meny.,* **Merc.,** *Mez.,* Mur. ac., *Nat. c.,* NAT. M., **Nit. ac.,** Nux m., **Nux v.,** *Oleand.,* OP., Par., **Petrol.,** Phos., *Pho. ac.,* **Plat.,** PB., **Pru.,** Puls., *Ran. b.,* Rheum, *Rhodo.,* **Ruta,** Saba., *Sabi.,* Sars., Sele., Seneg., **Sep.,** SIL., *Spig.,* Spo., Squ., Stan., Staph., Stro., SUL., **Sul. ac.,** Thuj., **VERAT. A., VERB., Vib. op.,** Vio. t., ZINC.

STOOL. 87

—**On Account of Inactivity.**—Acon., Agn., **ALUM.**, Am. carb., **Am. m.**, Anac., Ant. cr., Ant. t., **Arn.**, Asaf., Aur., *Bar. c.*, Bov., **BRY.**, **Calc. c.**, **Camph.**, *Canth.*, Carb. an., **Carb. v.**, Caust., *Cham.*, **Chin.**, **Cocc.**, Coff., *Colch.*, Dulc., Euphr., Graph., **HEP.**, Hyos., **Ign.**, Iod., **K. CARB.**, K. nit., Kre., Lach., Lyc., Mag. c., **Mag. m.**, Mang., *Merc.*, Mez., Mos., Mur. ac., **Nat. c.**, **NAT. M.**, *Nit. ac.*, **NUX M.**, **NUX V.**, *Oleand.*, **Op.**, Par., Petrol., **PHOS.**, Pho. ac., *Plat.*, **Pb.**, **Puls.**, *Rheum*, *Rhodo.*, Rhus. **Ruta**, *Saba.*, *Sars.*, Sele., Seneg., **Sep.**, **Sil.**, *Spig.*, Squ., Stan., **Staph.**, Stram., Stro., **Sul.**, Sul. ac., *Tar.*, **Thuj.**, **Valer.**, **Verat. a.**, Verb., **Vib. op.**, Zinc.

Stool, Acrid.—*Acon.*, *Alum.*, Ant. cr., **ARS.**, *Bry.*, Calc. c., *Cannab. s.*, Canth., Caps., Caust., Cham., **CHIN.**, **Dulc.**, **Fer.**, Graph., Hell., **IGN.**, K. carb., Lach., **MERC.**, *Merc. d.*, Nat. c., *Nat. m.*, Nux m., **Nux v.**, Petrol., Phos., Pho. ac., Pod., **PULS.**, *Rheum*, *Sabi.*, Sars., **Sele.**, **Spo.**, Stan., Staph., Sul., Verat. a.

—**Like Beaten Eggs.**—*Nux m.*

—**Bilious.**—*Ars.*, Bism., **CHAM.**, Chin., **COLCH.**, *Coloc.*, *Crot. tig.*, Dulc., *Fl. ac.*, *Gel.*, **Ip.**, *Merc.*, **MERC. D.**, Nux v., *Oleand.*, Pso., **PULS.**, Sul., Verat. a.

—**Blackish (and Dark).**—*Aesc.*, **Ars.**, Asaf., Bap., Brom., Bry., Calc. c., Camph., *Carb. ac.*, *Chel.*, Chin., *Cic.*, Coca, Coloc., Corn. c., *Crotal.*, *Dros.*, Fer., Hep., Iod., *Jal.*, Lept., Merc. c., **Merc. i. f.**, **NUX V.**, Op., *Ox. ac.*, Petrol., **PHOS**, **PB.**, *Pso.*, Sec. c., *Squ.*, *Stram.*, Sul., **Sul. ac.**, *Verat. a.*

—**Bloody (and Dysentery).**—Acon., *Ail.*, Aloe, Alst., Alum., Ambr., Am. carb., Am. m., Anac., Ant. cr., Ant. t., **Apis**, Apoc. c., **ARG. N.**, Arn., Ars., Asar., Bap., Bar. c., **Bell.**, *Benz. ac.*, Bor., Bry., Calc. c., **CANTH.**, **CAPS.**, *Curb. ac.*, Carb. an., **Carb. v.**, *Carb. sul.*, Caust., Cham., Chin., Colch., **Coll.**, Coloc., *Con.*, Corn. c., **Croc.**, Crotal., Cup., Dros., Dulc., Fer., Graph., Hep., Hydras., Hyos., Ign., Iod., **IP.**, Jal., **K. bi.**, K. carb., K. chl., *K. iod.*, K. nit., Lach., **Led.**, Lyc., *Mag. m.*, **MERC.**, **MERC. C.**, **MERC. D.**, Mez., Mur. ac., **NAT. C.**, *Nat. m.*, *Nat. s.*, **Nit. ac.**, Nux m., **NUX V.**, *Osm.*, Ox. ac., Petrol., Phos., Pho. ac., **Phyt.**, Plat., Pb., Pod., **PULS.**, *Ran. b.*, *Raph.*, *Rat.*, Rhus, Ruta, *Saba.*, **Sabi.**, Sang., Sars., Sec. c., **Sele.**, **SEP.**, Sil., Squ., Stan., **Stram.**, **SUL.**, Sul. ac., *Sum.*, *Tan.*, Tar., Thuj., *T. om.*, Valer., Verat. a., *Zinc.*

—**Brownish.**—Aloe, Ant. t., Apis, Arg. n., **ARN.**, Arum. t., **Asaf.**, Bry., *Carb. ac.*, *Card.*, *Cic.*, Coloc., Crot. tig., *Cup.*, Graph., **K. BI.**, Merc., Merc. i. f., Mez., **OP.**, *Plant.*, **PSO.**, Raph., **Rheum**, **Rhus**, **RUMEX**, Saba., Sec. c., Sep., *Stram.*, *Trom.*

—**Burning.**—*Nit. ac.*, Pod.

—**As if Chopped.**—SUL. AC.

—**Like Chopped Eggs.**—*Puls., Rheum, Sul. ac.*

—**Like Chopped Spinach.**—Arg. n.

—**Curdy (Containing Cheesy Masses).**—PHOS., Still.

—**Flattened.**—*Puls.*

—**Forcible (Gushing).**—*Calc. ph.,* CROT. TIG., *Elat.,* **Gam.**, GRAT., **Jal.**, **JAT.**, **NAT. C.**, *Nat. s.,* **Phos.,** *Pod., Raph., Rheum.*

—**Frothy.**—*Ant. t., Apoc. c.,* **ARN.**, *Benz. ac., Bor., Carb. sul.,* Calc. c., *Canth.,* Chin., **Coloc.**, ELAT., GRAT., *Iod.,* **Ip.,** K. BI., **Mag. c.,** Merc., Op., *Plant., Rheum,* **Rhus,** *Ruta,* **Saba., Sul.,** *Sul. ac.*

—**Gray and Whitish.**—*Aesc.,* **Acon., Am. m.,** *Ant. t.,* **Apis, Arn., Ars.,** *Asar.,* **Aur., Bell.,** *Benz. ac.,* **Calc. c.,** *Carb. v., Caust., Cham., Chel., Chin., Cina,* **Cocc., Colch., Coll.,** *Crot. tig., Cub.,* **DIG.,** *Dios., Dol., Dros.,* **Dulc., Hell., Hep.,** *Hydras., Ign.,* **Iod.,** *K. bi.,* **Lach.,** *Lept.,* **Merc., Mez.,** *Naj., Nat. c.,* **Nux m., Nux v., Op., PHOS., PHO. AC., Pb., Puls.,** *Rheum, Rhus,* **Sep., Sil.,** *Spig., Spo.,* STILL., *Stro., Sul., Sul. ac., Thuj., Verat. a.*

—**Greasy.**—*Iod., Thuj.*

—**Green.**—**Acon., Am. m.,** *Ant. t.,* **Apis,** ARG. N., **Ars., Bell., Bor., Calc. ph.,** *Canth., Carb. an.,* CHAM., *Coloc.,* CROT. TIG., **Cup., Dulc.,** *Elat., Fer.,* GAM., GRAT., *Hep., Hydras.,* **IP.,** *Laur., Mag. c.,* **Merc., Merc. c., Merc. d.,** *Naj., Nit. ac.,* **Nux v.,** *Petrol.,* **PHOS., Pho. ac.,** POD., *Pso.,* PULS., *Raph., Rheum, Sal. ac., Sep.,* **Stan.,** SUL., *Sul. ac., Valer.,* **Verat. a.,** *Zinc.*

—**Insufficient.**—*Acon.,* **Agar., Alum.,** *Ambr., Am. m., Anac., Ant. cr., Arg.,* **ARN.,** *Asar., Bar. c.,* **Bell.,** *Bov., Bry., Calad., Calc. c., Camph., Canth.,* **Caps.,** *Carb. an., Carb. v.,* CHAM., **Chin., Cocc., Colch.,** *Euphr., Graph.,* **Hell.,** *Hep.,* **Hyos.,** Ign., **Ip.,** *K. carb.,* **Lach.,** *Laur.,* **Led., Lyc., Mag. c.,** MAG. M., *Mang.,* Merc., Mez., **NAT. C., Nat. m.,** *Nit. ac.,* **Nux m., NUX V.,** *Oleand.,* **Op.,** *Petrol.,* **Plat., Pb., Rhus,** *Ruta,* **Saba.,** *Sabi., Sars., Seneg.,* **Sep., SIL.,** *Spo., Squ.,* **Stan., Staph., SUL.,** *Thuj., Valer., Verb., Zinc.*

—**Involuntary.**—*Acon.,* **ALOE, Ant. t., Apis.,** *Apoc. c.,* **ARN., Ars., Bell.,** *Bry., Carb. ac., Carb. v., Carb. sul.,* **Chin.,** *Cina,* **Cocc.,** *Colch., Coloc., Cun., Crotal.,* **Cup.,** *Dig., Gel., Hell.,* HYOS., Ign., **K. bi.,** Lach. *Laur.,* Merc., **Mur. ac., Nat. m.,** *Nat. s.,* **Nux v.,** *Oleand.,* **Op.,** *Ox. ac.,* **Petrol., PHOS., PHO. AC., Puls.,** *Rhus,* **Sec. c., Sep., Spo., Squ.,** *Staph.,* **Sul., VERAT. A.,** *Zinc.*

—**Large.**—*Aesc., Aloe, Ant. cr.,* **Ant. t., Apis, Arg. n., Asaf.,** *Aur.* **BRY., Calc. c.,** *Chel.,* **Coloc.,** *Crot. tig.,* **Cup., Dulc.,** ELAT., **Gam.,**

STOOL.   89

Graph., *Grat.*, *Hydras.*, **Ign**., *K. bi.*, **K. CARB.**, *Jal.*, *Jat.*, **LEPT.**, **Merc.**, *Naj.*, *Nat. m.*, *Nux m.*, Nux v., **Petrol.**, **Phos.**, **Pod.**, Ran. b., **Raph.**, Ruta, Seneg., Stan., **SUL.**, *Sul. ac.*, *Thuj.*, **VERAT. A.**, **Vib. op.**, *Zinc.*

—**Offensive (and Putrid).**—Acon., Agar., **Alum.**, Am. m., Ant. cr. **Ant.t.**, **Apis**, **ARG. N.**, **Arn.**, **ARS.**, **ASAF.**, *Asar.*, **Aur.**, **Bap.**, Bar. c. **Bell.**, **Bism.**, **Benz. ac.**, **Bor.**, **Bov.**, **BRY.**, **Calad.**, *Calc. c.*, *Calc. ph.*, Canth., *Carb. ac.*, *Carb. an.*, **CARB. V.**, *Carb. sul.*, Caust., **Cham.**, Chin., *Cic.*, *Cocc.*, Coff., **Coloc.**, *Corn. c.*, *Crotal.*, **CROT. TIG.**, *Dig.*, Dros., Dulc., *Fl. ac.*, **Graph.**, *Guai.*, *Hell.*, Hep., Ign., *Iod.*, **Ip.**, *Jal.*, K. carb., K. nit., Kre., Lach., **LEPT.**, Lyc., Mag. c., **Mar.**, *Merc.*, **Merc. c.**, *Mur. ac.*, Nat. c., **Nat. m.**, **Nit. ac.**, *Nux m.*, **Nux v.**, Oleand., **Op.**, *Ox. ac.*, Oxyt., *Par.*, **Petrol.**, **Phos.**, *Pho. ac.*, **Pb.**, **POD.**, **PSO.**, **PULS.**, Ran. b., Ran. s., Rheum, *Rhodo.*, *Rhus*, Ruta, Sabi., *Sal. ac.*, *Sars.*, Sec. c., Sep., **SIL.**, Spig., Squ., **Staph.**, *Still.*, Stram., *Stro.*, **SUL.**, *Sul. ac.*, *Sum.*, *Valer.*, Verat. a., Zinc.

—**Purulent.**—*Apis*, Arn., Bell., Calc. c., Cannab. s., **Canth.**, Chin. Clem., *Cocc.*, Con., **Ign.**, Iod., *K. carb.*, Lyc., **MERC.**, **Nit. ac.**, Nux v. Petrol., **Puls.**, Sabi., *Sep.*, **SIL.**, **Sul**.

—**Putty-like.**—Merc. i. f.

—**Scanty. See Insufficient.**

—**Like Sheep Dung.**—*Agar.*, *Alum.*, Am. carb., **AM. M.**, Arn., Asar., Aur., **Bar. c.**, Bell., Bor., Bry., Carb. an., Card., Caust., Chel., Chin., Coca, **Coll.**, Graph., *Guai.*, **Iod.**, *K. carb.*, K. nit., Led., Mag. c., **MAG. M.**, *Mang.*, **MERC.**, **Nat. c.**, **NAT. M.**, **Nat. s.**, Nit. ac., Nux v., Oleand., **OP.**, Petrol., Phos., *Pho. ac.*, **Plat.**, **PB.**, Pru., Ruta, Sec. c., Sep., **SIL.**, Spig., *Stan.*, Staph., Stro., **SUL.**, **Sul. ac.**, Thuj., **VERB.**, Vio. o.

—**Slimy.**—Agar., **Aloe**, *Alum.*, Am. carb., Am. m., *Ant. cr.*, Ant. t., *Apis*, *Apoc. c.*, **ARG. N.**, Arn., Ars., **ASAR.**, Bap., Bar. c., *Bell.*, **BOR.**, *Bry.*, Calc. c., *Calc. ph.*, **CANTH.**, **CAPS.**, *Carb. ac.*, Carb. an., **Carb. v.**, *Caust.*, **CHAM.**, Chel., *Chin.*, Cic., Cina, *Coc. c.*, **COLCH.**, Col., Coloc., Con., *Crot. tig.*, Cup., Dig., Dros., *Dulc.*, *Fer.*, Gam., Graph., *Guai.*, **HELL.**, *Hep.*, *Hydras.*, **Hyos.**, Ign., *Iod.*, **IP.**, K. bi., K. carb., *K. iod.*, **K. nit.**, Lach., Laur., *Led.*, Lyc., Mag. c., **Mag. m.**, MERC., **MERC. C.**, **MERC. D.**, *Naj.*, *Nat. c.*, Nat. m., **Nit. ac.**, Nux m., **NUX V.**, *Ox. ac.*, Oxyt., Par., Petrol., **PHOS.**, *Pho. ac.*, **Phyt.**, POD., **PULS.**, *Raph.*, Rheum, Rhus, Ruta, *Saba.*, Sabi., Sec. c., Sele., Seneg., Sep., Sil., Spig., Squ., Stan., Staph., **SUL.**, **Sul. ac.**, Thuj., *Verat. a.*, Vio. t., Zinc.

—**Slipping Back Again.**—SIL.

—**Small (In Size).**—*Aesc.*, **AM. M.**, *Apis*, Apoc. c., **ARG. N.**, Asar.,

Bell., CAPS., Caust., Coloc., Crot. tig., *Fer.*, Graph., *Hyos.*, *K. chl.*, Merc., MERC. C., *Mur. ac.*, Nit. ac., Nux v., PHOS., PB., Puls., Sep., SIL., *Staph.*, Sul., Verat. a., ZINC.

—**Sour.**—*Arn.*, Bell., Calc. c., *Carb. sul.*, *Cham.*, Coloc., Dulc., Graph., Hep., *Jalap*, Mag. c., Merc., *Mez.*, Nat. c., Petrol., Phos., RHEUM, *Sep.*, SUL., *Sul. ac.*

—**Stringy.**—*Aesc.*, Ars., Asar., Calc. c., *Caps.*, *Carb. ac.*, Carb. v., Caust., *Chel.*, HELL., Hep., Ign., K. carb., MERC., Merc. c., Mez., Nat. c., Nux v., *Pb.*, Sars., SUL., SUL. AC., Verat. a.

—**Undigested.**—*Aesc.*, Aloe, *Alst.*, Ant. cr., *Apoc. c.*, Arg. n., *Arn.*, Ars., *Asar.*, *Bor.*, Bry., Calc. c., *Calc. ph.*, Cham., CHIN., *Coloc.*, *Con.*, FER., Graph., Hep., Meny., *Mez.*, *Nit. ac.*, Nux m., OLEAND., *Ox. ac.*, Phos., Pho. ac., POD., *Rheum*, Rhodo., Rhus, *Sang.*, *Sil.*, Squ., Sul., *Sul. ac.*, Valer.

—**Yellow.**—Aeth., Aloe, Apis, *Apoc. c.*, Arg. n., Asar., BOR., *Cannab. i.*, *Carb. sul.*, *Card.*, CHEL., China., Cocc., Colch., Coll., Coloc., Crot. tig., *Dig.*, Dios., DULC., GAM., Gel., *Gent. l.*, GRAT., Hep., *Hydras.*, Hyos., *Ip.*, Iris v., Lach., *Merc. c.*, Nat. s., PHOS., Pho. ac., POD., Raph., *Sang.*, SUL. AC.

Worms.—*Acon.*, Alum., *Ambr.*, *Anac.*, Ars., *Asar.*, Bar. c., Bell., Bor., CALC. C., Carb. an., Carb. v., Caust., Cham., Chin., *Cic.*, CINA., Coff., Colch., Coloc., Croc., *Cup.*, Dig., *Fer.*, Graph., Hyos., *Ign.*, Iod., *K. carb.*, Laur., Lyc., Mag. c., Mag. m., *Mar.*, Merc., Nat. c., *Nat. m.*, Nux m., Nux v., *Petrol.*, *Phos.*, **Plat.**, *Puls.*, Rhus, *Ruta*, Saba., *Sabi.*, Sec. c., Sep., SIL., Spig., *Spo.*, Squ., Stan., SUL., *Valer.*, Zinc.

Round Worms.—Acon., Anac., *Ars.*, Bar. c., Bell., Bor., Calc. c., Caust., Cham., *Chin.*, Cic., CINA, Coloc., Graph., Hyos., Iod., *K. carb.*, *Lyc.*, Mag. c., Mag. m., Merc., Nat. m., Nux m., Nux v., Petrol., Phos., Ruta, SABA., Sec. c., SIL., SPIG., SUL., Valer.

Tape Worm.—Alum., *Ambr.*, Anac., *Ars.*, CALC. C., Carb. an., Carb. v., Caust., *Chin.*, Cina., Coff., Colch., Croc., *Cucur.*, GRAPH., *Ign.*, *K. carb.*, Laur., Lyc., *Mag. m.*, *Mar.*, Merc., Nat. c., Nat. m., Nux v., Petrol., Phos., PLAT., PULS., Rhus, SABA., *Sabi.*, Sep., SIL., Spig., Spo., Stan., SUL., *Valer.*, Zinc.

Thread Worms.—Acon., Alum., *Ambr.*, Asar., CALC. C., CHIN., CINA, Colch., Croc., *Crot. tig.*, Dig., FER., Graph., Hyos., IGN., K. carb., Mag. c., MAR., *Merc.*, Nat. c., Nux m., Nux v., Petrol., *Phos.*, Plat., Rhus, Saba., Sabi., Sep., Sil., Spig., Spo., Squ., SUL., *Valer.*, Zinc.

Troubles Before Stool.—*Acon.*, Agar., *Agn.*, ALOE, Alum., Ambr., Am.

STOOL.

carb., *Am. m.,* Anac., **Ant.** t., Arn., *Ars.,* Asaf., *Asar.,* **Bar.** c., **Bell.,** Berb., *Bor.,* Bov., Bry., *Calad.,Calc. c.,* Camph., Cannab. s., *Canth.,* **Caps.,** *Carb. an.,* Carb. v., **Caust., Cham.,** Chel., Chin., Cina, *Cocc.,* Colch., **Coloc.,** Con., Croc., Cup., Cyc., *Dig.,* **Diosc.,** Dros., DULC., Euphorb., *Fer.,* Graph., Guai., Hell., Hep., *Hydras.,* Ign., *K. bi.,* **K.** Carb., K. nit., **Lach.,** Laur., *Lil. tig.,* Lyc., **Mag.** c., *Mang.,* Meny., MERC., **Mez.,** Mos., *Nat. c.,* Nat. m., Nit. ac., *Nux. v.,* Oleand., **Op.,** *Petrol.,* **Phos.,** Pho. ac., Plat., **Pod., Puls.,** Rheum, *Rhodo.,* Rhus, Ruta, Saba., Sars., Sec. c., Sele. Seneg., *Op.,* Sep., **Sil., Spig.,** Spo., **Stan.,** *Staph.,* Stram., *Sti* ., SUL., Sul. ac., *Thuj.,* Valer., VERAT. A., Vio. o., Vio. t., Zinc.

During Stool.—*Acon., Aesc.,* Agar., Agn., **Aloe,** *Alum.,* Ambr., *Am. carb.* **Am. m.,** *Anac.,* **Ant. cr., Ant.,** *Apis,* Arg., *Arg. n.,* Arn., ARS., Asaf. Asar., Aur., *Bar.* c., **Bell., Berb.,** *Bor.,* Bov., *Bry., Calad.,* **Calc.** c., Camph., Cannab. s., *Canth.,* **Caps.,** *Carb. an.,* Carb. v., *Caust.,* CHAM., Chel., Chin., Cocc., Colch., **Coloc.,** Con., **Crot. tig.,** Cup., Cyc., Dig., Dros., Dulc., *Euphorb.,* Fer., *Graph.,* Guai., *Hell.,* **Hep.,** Hyos., *Ign.,* Iod., **Ip.,** Iris. v., *K. bi., K. carb.,* K. nit., Kre., *Lach., Laur., Lyc.,* Mag. c., **Mag. m.,** Meny., MERC., **Merc.** c., Mez., Mos., *Murex., Mur. ac., Nat. c.,* **Nat. m.,** NIT. A C., *Nux. m.,* Nux. v., *Oleand.,* Op., Par., Petrol., **Phos.,** Pho. ac., Plat., Pb., **Pod.,** PULS., Ran. b., **Rheum,** *Rhodo.,* **Rhus,** Ruta, *Sabi.,* **Sars.,** *Sele.,* Seneg., SEP., SIL., SPIG., *Spo.,* Squ., Stan., **Staph.,** Stram., *Stro.,* SUL., **Sul ac.,** Tar., *Throm.,* Thuj., VERAT. A., Verb., Vio. t., *Zinc.*

After Stool.—Acon., *Aesc.,* Agar., Agn., **Aloe,** *Alum.,* Ambr., *Am. carb.,* **Am. m.,** Anac., Ant. t., Apoc. c., Arg., Arn., ARS., Asar., Bar. c., **Bell.,** Berb., *Bor.,* Bov., Bry., Calc. c., Camph., **Canth., Caps.,** *Carb. an.,* Carb. v., CAUST., Cham., Chin., *Cocc., Coloc.,* **Con.,** *Crot. tig., Cup.,* Dig., Dros., Dulc., Euphorb., Fer., Graph., *Hell., Hep.,* Hyos., *Ign.,* Iod., Ip., **Iris v.,** Jat., **K. br., K. carb.,** K. nit., **Lach.,** Laur., **Lept.,** *Lyc.,* Mag. c., **Mag. m.,** *Mar.,* MERC., **Merc.** c., **Mez.,** Mur ac., *Nat. c.,* **Nat. m.,** NIT. AC., *Nux m.,* NUX V., Oleand., Op., Petrol., PHOS., Pho. ac., *Plat.,* Pb., **POD., Puls.,** Rheum, Rhodo., *Rhus,* Ruta, Saba., Sabi., Sars., Sec. c. SELE., *Seneg.,* Sep., SIL., Spig, Spo., *Stan.,* **Staph.,** *Stro.,* SUL., Sul. ac., Tar., Thuj., Valer., **Verat.** a., *Zinc.*

—**Tenesmus.**—Acon., AESC., Agar., **ALOE,** *Alum.,* Ambr., Am. carb., **Anac.,** *Ant. cr.,* Ant. t., Apoc. c., *Arg.,* Arn., **Ars.,** *Asaf., Asar.,* Bar. c., **Bell.,** Bism., Bor., Bov., Bry., Calc. c., Camph., **Canth., CAPS.,** *Carb. an., Carb. v., Carb. sul., Caust.,* Chel., Chin., *Cic.,* Cocc., Coff., **COLCH., Col.,** Coloc., **Con., Corn.** c., Croc., CROT. TIG., **Cup.,** *Dig., Dulc.,* Euphorb., Fer., **Gam., Gran.,** Graph., *Hell.,* Hep., *Hydras.,*

Hyos., *Ign.*, Iris v., *K. carb.*, *K. chl.*, **K. nit.**, Lach., *Laur.*, **LIL. T.**, Lyc., Mag. c., **Mag. m.**, Mar., Meny., MERC., **MERC. C.**, **Merc. d.**, *Mez.*, Mos., Mur. ac., *Nat. c.*, *Nat. m.*, **Nit. ac.**, Nux m., **NUX V.**, Op., *Petrol.*, Phos., *Plat.*, Pb., Pod., Puls., *Ran. s.*, Rheum, Rhodo., *Rhus*, *Ruta*, *Saba.*, *Sars.*, Sec. c., Sele., Seneg., *Sep.*, *Sil.*, Spig., Squ., *Stan.*, Staph., Stram., Stro., SUL., Sul. ac., Tar., *Thuj.*, *Trom.*, *Verat. a.*, **Verb.**, Vib. op., Vio. o., *Vio. t.*, Zinc.

Ineffectual Tenesmus.—Acon., Aesc., Agar., Alum., Ambr., Am. carb., Am. m., *Anac.*, **Arn.**, *Ars.*, *Asaf.*, Bar. c., **Bell.**, *Bism.*, *Bov.*, **Calc. c.**, Canth., **CAPS.**, *Carb. an.*, *Carb. v.*, *Caust.*, Chin., **Cocc.**, **Colch.**, Coloc., Con., *Crot. tig.*, Cup., Dulc., Euphorb., **Gran.**, *Graph.*, **Hell.**, *Hep.*, Hyos., **Ign.**, Iod., *Ip.*, *K. carb.*, *K. nit.*, Kre., *Lach.*, *Laur.*, *Lil. t.*, Lyc., Mag. c., *Mag. m.*, Mang., MERC., Mez., Mos., **Nat. c.**, **Nat. m.**, *Nit. ac.*, Nux m., **NUX V.**, *Oleand.*, **Op.**, *Par.*, *Phos.*, Pho. ac., **Plat.** *Pb.*, Puls., **RHEUM**, Rhodo., **RHUS**, *Ruta*, *Saba.*, Sabi., *Sars.*, Sele., Seneg., Sep., **SIL.**, *Spig.*, *Spo.*, *Stan.*, **Staph.**, *Stram.*, Stro., **SUL.**, *Sul. ac.*, Tar., *Thuj.*, Valer., Verat. a., Vio. o., Zinc.

Anus.—*Acon.*, Aesc., *Agar.*, *Agn.*, *All. c.*, **ALOE**, Alum., *Ambr.*, *Am. curb.*, *Am. m.*, *Anac.*, **Ant. cr.**, Ant. t., **Apis**, Arn., **Ars.**, Asar., Aur., Bar. c., Bell., Berb., Bor., Bov., Bry., *Cact.*, **Calc. c.**, *Calc. ph.*, Camph., Cannab. i., Cannab. s., **Canth.**, Caps., Carb. an., **CARB. V.**, Caust.. Cham., *Chel.*, *Chin.*, Cic., Cina, *Cocc.*, **Colch.**, Coloc., *Con.*, *Croc.*, Crot. tig., Cup., Cyc., *Dios.*, *Dirc.*, Dulc., Euphorb., Euphr., *Fer.*, *Form.*, *Gam.*, *Gel.*, **GRAPH.**, *Ham.*, Hell., Hep., *Hydras.*, Hyos., **Ign.**, Iod., Ip., *Iris v.*, K. bi., K. CARB., K. nit., Kre., *Lach.*, *Laur.*, Led., *Lil. t.*, Lyc., Mag. c., Mag. m., Mang., *Mcr.*, Meny., **Merc.**, *Mez.*, Mos., **Mur. ac.**, *Nat. c.*, Nat. m., **NIT. AC.**, Nux m., **NUX V.**, Oleand., *Op.*, *Oxyt.*, **Pæo.**, *Petrol.*, **PHOS.**, *Pho. ac.*, *Phyt.*, *Plat.*, Pb., Pod., **Puls.**, Ran. b., Ran. s., **RAT.**, Rheum, Rhodo., *Rhus*, Ruta, *Saba.*, *Sabi.*, Sars., **Sec. c.**, Seneg., **SEP.**, **SIL.**, Spig., *Spo.*, Squ., *Stan.*, Staph., Stro., SUL., *Sul. ac.*, Thuj., Valer., Verat. a., Verb., **Vib. op.**, Zinc., Zing.

Hæmorrhoids.—Acon., Agar., **ALOE**, *Alum.*, Ambr., **Am. carb.**, Am. m., *Anac.*, **Ant. cr.**, Ant. t., **Apis**, *Apoc. c.*, Arn., Ars., Bar. c., **Bell.**, *Berb.*, Bor., Brom., **Cact.**, Calc. c., Canth., Caps., **Carb. an.**, Carb. v., Caust., Cham., Chin., *Cinnab.*, *Coll.*, Coloc., Cup., **Dios.**, *Euon.*, Euphr., **Fer.**, *Fer. ph.*, **GRAPH.**, *Hum.*, Hell., Hep., Hyos., **Ign.**, K. CARB., K. nit., *Lach.*, Led., Lyc., Mag. c., **Merc.**, *Millef.*, **MUR. AC.**, **Nat. m.**, **Nit. ac.**, **NUX V.**, *Pæo.*, *Petrol.*, Phos., *Pho. ac.*, **Pb.**, **Pod.**, **PULS.**, Ran. b., **Rat.**, Rhodo., *Rhus*, *Sabi.*, **SEP.**, **Sil.**, Spig., Stan., Staph., *Stram.*, Stro., SUL., **Sul. ac.**, *Thuj.*, Valer., Verat. a., **Verb.**, Zinc., Zing.

STOOL—URINARY ORGANS.

Rectum.—*Ab. c.*, *Acon.*, *ÆSC.*, *Agar.*, **Aloe**, **Alum.**, **Ambr.**, Am. carb., *Am. m.*, *Anac.*, Ant. cr., *Ant. t.*, Arn., **Ars.**, **Asar.**, *Aur.*, **Bell.**, *Berb.*, *Bor.*, Bov., *Bry.*, CALC. C., Camph., **Canth.**, Carb. an., *Carb. v.*, **Caust.**, Cham., *Chel.*, **Chin.**, *Cic.*, *Cina*, *Cinnab.*, *Cocc.*, *Colch.*, **Coll.**, **Coloc.**, *Con.*, *Conv.*, Cup., *Dulc.*, *Euphorb.*, Fer., *Gel.*, *Graph.*, *Hell.*, Hep., *Hydras.*, IGN., Iod., **K. carb.**, *Kre.*, *Lach.*, Laur., LIL. T., LYC., Mag. c., **Mag. m.**, Mang., *Mar.*, Meny., **Merc.**, MERC. C., *Mez.*, *Mur. ac.*, *Nat. c.*, NAT. M., NIT. AC., Nux m., NUX V., *Oleand.*, Op., *Petrol.*, PHOS., Pho. ac., *Phyt.*, Plat., Pb., *Pod.*, *Pru.*, **Puls.**, *Rhodo.*, *Rhus*, **Ruta**, **Saba.**, Sars., *Sele.*, SEP., **Sil.**, *Spig.*, Spo., Squ., *Stan.*, Staph., Stram., *Stro.*, SUL., Sul. ac., *Thuj.*, Valer., Verat. a., *Vib. op.*, Zinc.

Perineum.—AGN., ALUM., **Am. m.**, **Ant. cr.**, Ant. t., Ars., **Asaf.**, *Bell.*, Bov., Bry., Calc. c., Cannab. s., CARB. AN., CARB. V., *Caust.*, Chin., CYC., Graph., Hep., Ign., *Lil. t.*, **Lyc.**, Mag. m., Merc., *Mez.*, *Mur. ac.*, **Nux v.**, *Pæo.*, Petrol., Phos., **Pb.**, Rhodo., Rhus, Seneg., Sep., Spig., **SUL.**, **Tar.**, *Thuj.*

Urinary Organs.

Kidney.—Acon., *Alum.*, APIS, Arn., ARS., *Asc. c.*, BELL., BERB., *Bor. ac.*, *Bor.*, Camph., Cannab. i., **Cannab. s.**, CANTH., *Carb. ac.*, Ced., **Chel.**, *Chin.*, *Cinnab.*, Clem., Coccin., *Cocc.*, Coc. c., Colch., Crotal., **Dig.**, Dulc., *Eup. per.*, Fer., Fer. iod., *Hell.*, HELO., **Hep.**, *Hydras.*, Ip., K. CARB., K. chl., K. nit., *Merc.*, **Merc. c.**, *Nit. ac.*, Nux v., *Op.*, Oci., *Petrol.*, Phos., Pho. ac., Phyt., *Pic. ac.*, *Piper.*, Pb., *Puls.*, *Ran. s.*, *Rhus*, Samb., *Sec. c.*, *Senec.*, Squ., *Stro.*, **Sul.**, Ter., *Thlasp.*, *Thuj.*, *Trill.*, Zinc.

Bladder.—Acon., *All. c.*, Alum., Ambr., Am. carb., Am. m., Ant. cr., Ant. t., Apis, *Apoc. c.*, Arn., Ars., Asaf., Asar., Aspar., *Aur.*, Bell., BENZ. AC., *Bor. ac.*, **BRACH.**, Bry., **Calad.**, Calc. c., Calc. ph., Camph., *Cannab. s.*, CANTH., **Caps.**, Carb. an., **Carb. v.**, *Carb. sul.*, Caust., Cham., **Chel.**, CHIM., *Chin.*, *Cic.*, *Clem.*, *Coc. c.*, *Coff.*, *Colch.*, *Coloc.*, *Con.*, *Cub.*, *Dig.*, **Dulc.**, *Equi.*, *Eup. pur.*, Fer., *Fer. ph.*, *Gel.*, Guai., *Hell.*, Hep., *Hydras.*, HYOS., **Ign.**, Ip., *K. br.*, **K. carb.**, *Lach.*, Laur., **Led.**, *Lil. t.*, Lith., LYC., Mag. m., Mang., Meny., *Merc.*, Merc. c., Mez., *Mos.*, **Mur. ac.**, *Nat. m.*, Nit. ac., NUX V., *Op.*, **Parei.**, Petrol., *Petros.*, Phos., Pho. ac., **Pb.**, *Pop. t.*, Pru., PULS., Ran. b., *Rheum*, *Rhodo.*, *Rhus*, *Rhus a.*, RUTA, Saba., *Sabi.*, *Sant.*, Sars., Sec. c., *Senec.*, Seneg., **Sep.**, **Sil.**, Spig., **Squ.**, Stan., **Staph.**, *Sul.*, Sul. ac., Ter., Thuj., **URA.**, **Valer.**, Verat. a., *Zinc.*

Urethra.—Acon., *Agar.*, Agn., *Alum.*, *Ambr.*, Am. carb., Am. m., Anac., Ant. cr., *Ant. t.*, ARG. N., *Arn.*, *Ars.*, Asar., **Aspar.**, Aur., Bar.

c., Bell., Berb., Bor., *Bov.*, Bry., **Calc.** c., *Calc. ph.*, Camph., **Cannab. i.**, **CANNAB. S.**, **CANTH.**, **CAPS.**, Carb. an., *Carb. v.*, **Caust.**, *Ced.*, Cham., *Chel.*, Chin., Cic., **CLEM.**, Cocc., Coff., Colch., *Coloc.*, Con., Croc., *Crot. tig.*, **Cub.**, *Cup.*, Cyc., **Dig.**, Dulc., *Equi., Eryng., Eup. pur.*, Euphorb., *Fer., Fl. ac., Gel., Graph.*, Guai., Hell., *Hep., Hydras., Ign.*, Iod., Ip., **K. bi.**, *K. br., K. carb.*, K. nit., *Lach.*, Laur., Led., Lil. t., **LYC.**, **Mag. c.**, Mag. m., Mung., *Mar.*, **MERC.**, **Merc.** c., **Mez.**, Mur. ac., *Nat. c.*, **NAT. M.**, **Nit. ac.**, Nux m., Nux v., Op., *Ox. ac., Par., Parei.*, Petrol., **Petros.**, **PHOS.**, Pho. ac., Pb., *Pop. t., Pru.*, **Puls.**, R̄hodo., *Rhus*, Ruta, Saba., **Sabi.**, Samb., *Sars.*, Sec. c., **Sele.**, Seneg., **Sep.**, *Sil.*, Spig., Squ., Stan., *Staph., Still.*, Stram., **Sul.**, **TER.**, **THUJ.**, Verat. a., Vio. t., ZINC.

Prostate.—Acon., Aspar., Bar. c., *Caps., Chin., Clem., Cub., Dig., Nat. s.*, **Puls.**, *Rhus a., Senec., Thuj.*

Urine.

Acrid.—Ambr., Ant. t., **Arn.**, **Ars.**, Benz. ac., Bor., *Calc.* c., Camph., **Cannab. s.**, *Canth.*, **Caps.**, Carb. v., **Caust.**, Cham., Chin., **Clem.**, *Graph.*, Guai., **HEP.**, Ign., *Iod., K. carb.*, Laur., **Lith.**, **MERC.**, *Nat. m.*, **Nit. ac.**, **Par.**, Petrol., **Puls.**, Rhus, Sabi., *Sars., Seneg.*, **Sep.**, *Sul.*, **Thuj.**, *Verat. a.*

Albuminous.—*Abs.*, Acon., **Canth.**, *Carb. ac., Carb. sul., Ced., Colch., Dig., Euon., Glon., Helo.*, **K. chl.**, *Lach., Lith.*, **Merc.**, **MERC. C.**, *Nit. ac., Osm.*, Petrol., **Phos.**, *Pho. ac., Phyt.*, **PB**, *Sal. ac.*, Sec. c., *Sil., Sul. ac., Ter., Zinc.*

Ammoniacal Odor.—Ant. t., **ASAF.**, Benz. ac., *Bor.*, Calc. c., **Carb. ac.**, Carb. an., *Carb. v.*, Dig., *Equi.*, Graph., Iod., Kre., **Mos.**, **Nit. ac.**, *Parei.*, Petrol., Phos., Rhodo., *Stro.*, Vio. t.

Bloody.—Acon., Ambr., Ant. cr., **Ant. t.**, **ARG. N.**, **Arn.**, **Ars.**, *Bell., Benz. ac., Cact.*, **Calc. c.**, Camph., *Cannab. s.*, **CANTH.**, **Caps.**, *Carb. v., Carb. sul.*, Caust., Chel., *Chim., Chin., Coc. c.*, Colch., *Coloc.*, Con., Conv., *Crotal.*, *Cup.*, Dig., Dulc., Erig., Euphorb., *Ham., Hep.*, **Ip.**, **K. chl.**, Lach., Lyc., Merc., **Merc. c.**, **Mez.**, Millef., *Nat. m.*, Nit. ac., Nux v., Op., Petrol., **PHOS.**, *Pho. ac., Pic. ac.*, Pb., **PULS.**, *Rhus a*, **Saba.**, **Sars.**, Sec. c., Senec., **Sep.**, **Squ.**, **Sul.**, *Sul. ac.*, **TER.**, Thuj., *Uva.*, Zinc.

Cold.—Agar., *Nit. ac.*

Dark.—**ACON.**, *Aesc.*, Agn., Alum., Ambr., Am. carb., Am. m., **Ant. cr.**, **ANT. T.**, Apis, Arg. n., Arn., *Ars., Asaf., Aspar.*, Aur., Bar. c., **BELL.**, **BENZ. AC.**, Bov., **BRY.**, **Calc.** c., Camph., *Cannab. i., Cannab. s.*, **Canth.**, Carb. ac., Carb. v., Caust., *Ced.*, **CHEL.**, *Chin.*, Clem., Coff., **COLCH.**, **Coloc.**, Con., *Conv., Crotal., Crot. tig., Cup.*, **Dig.**, Dros., Dulc.,

URINE.

Elat., **EQUI.**, **Eup. per.**, *Eup. pur.*, *Fer. iod.*, *Glon.*, Graph., Hell., **Hep.**, Iod., **Ip.**, *K. bi.*, *K. carb.*, **K. chl.**, K. nit., Kre., *Lach.*, Led., Lith., *Lyc.*, **MERC.**, Mez., **Myr.**, Nat. c., **Nat. m.**, *Nit. ac.*, *Nux m.*, Nux v., Oleand., Op., *Osm.*, *Par.*, *Petrol.*, **Phos.**, Pho. ac., *Pic. ac.*, Plat., **PB.**, **Puls.**, Raph., *Rheum*, *Rhodo.*, Rhus, Sabi., *Sang.*, *Sant.*, Sars., **Sele.**, **Senec.**, **SEP.**, Sil., Squ., **Staph.**, Stro., Sul., *Sul. ac.*, Ter., Thuj., *Ura.*, Valer., **VERAT. A.**, **Vip.**

Flesh Colored.—*Coloc.*

Flocculent.—Ant. t., *Cannab. s.*, **CANTH.**, **Cham.**, *Eup. pur.*, K. carb., *K. nit.*, Merc., **MEZ.**, Par., Sars., Seneg., Squ., Zinc.

Frothy.—**Chel.**, *Crot. tig.*, Cub., Glon., *Lach.*, *Laur.*, Lyc., **Myr.**, Seneg., Spo., *Still.*

Glutinous.—Arg., Canth., **COLOC.**, *Cup.*, *Kre.*, *Pho. ac.*

Glycosuria.—Ars., *Helo.*, *Pho. ac.*, Sul., Ura.

Green.—Ars., Aur., Bov., **CAMPH.**, Chin., *Iod.*, *K. carb.*, Mag. c., **MERC.**, *Merc. c.*, Rheum., Rhodo., *Ruta*, *Sant.*, Sul., Verat. a.

Hot.—**ACON.**, Aesc., All. c., Aloe, *Alum.*, Am. m., Ant. t., **ARS.**, Bell., Bor., Bry., Calc. c., Camph., *Cannab. s.*, **CANTH.**, Caps., Carb. an., *Carb. sul.*, Caust., Cham., *Chim.*, Chin., **Clem.**, *Coc. c.*, Colch., Dig., Dulc., Fer., **HEP.**, Ign., Ip., K. bi., *K. carb.*, **Kalm.**, *Kre.*, Lyc., Merc., **Mez.**, Nat. c., Nat. m., **Nat. s.**, *Nit. ac.*, Nux v., Oleand., Par., *Phos.*, **Pho. ac.**, *Pop. t.*, Puls., Rhodo., Rhus, *Saba.*, Sabi., **Sars.**, *Senec.*, Seneg., Sep., Sil., Squ., *Staph.*, *Still.*, Stram., **Sul.**, Sul. ac., Ter., *Thuj.*, Verat. a., *Vesp.*, *Zinc.*

Milky.—Ant. t., **Aur.**, Cannab. s., Chin., **Chel.**, **Cina**, *Coloc.*, Con., Cyc., *Dulc.*, Hep., *Iod.*, Merc., *Mur. ac.*, *Phos.*, **PHO. AC.**, Rhus, Sul.

Offensive.—*Abs.*, Agar., Ambr., Ant. t., Ars., **BENZ. AC.**, Bor., *Caj.*, *Calad.*, Calc. c., Camph., *Carb. ac.*, *Carb. an.*, **Carb. v.**, *Chel.*, *Chim.*, *Coloc.*, *Conv.*, Cup., Dros., **DULC.**, *Guai.*, Kre., Lach., Merc., **Murex**, Nat. c., Nit. ac., Op., *Osm.*, Petrol., Phos., Pho. ac., Puls., Rhodo., *Sele.*, **SEP.**, *Sil.*, Stan., Sul., **Ter.**, Vio. t.

Pale.—Agar., Alum., Ambr., *Anac.*, Ant. cr., Ant. t., Arg. n., **Arn.**, Ars., Arum. t., Aur., Bell., Bism., Bry., Calc. c., **CANNAB. I.**, Cannab. s., Canth., Carb. v., Caust., *Ced.*, Cham., Chel., *Chin.*, Cocc., **Colch.**, Coloc., **CON.**, *Dig.*, Dros., *Dulc.*, Euphr., **Fl. ac.**, Gel., Hell., **Hep.**, Hyos., **IGN.**, *Iod.*, K. br., K. carb., **K. NIT.**, Kre., Lach., *Laur.*, Mag. c., Mag. m., *Mar.*, Meli., Merc., Mez., **Mos.**, *Mur. ac.*, Nat. c., **NAT. M.**, Nux v., Op., Par., Phos., **PHO. AC.**, Plant., *Plat.*, Pb., **Puls.**, *Rheum*, Rhodo., Rhus, *Samb.*, *Sant.*, Sars., Sec. c., SEP., Spig., Spo., **Squ.**, *Staph.*, Stram., Stro., Sul., Sul. ac., Thuj., Verat. a., **Verat. v.**, *Zinc.*

URINE.

Pellicle Fatty.—*All. c.*, *Calad.*, *Calc. c.*, *Canth.*, *Coca*, *Crot. tig.*, **Hep.**, *Iod.*, *Op.*, **PAR.**, **Petrol.**, **Phos.**, **Pso.**, **Puls.**, *Sars.*, **Sul.**

Profuse.—*Acon.*, **Agar.**, **Agn.**, *All. c.*, *Alum.*, **Ambr.**, **Am. m.**, **Ant. cr.**, **Ant. t.**, **Apoc. c.**, **ARG.**, *Arg. n.*, **Arn.**, **Ars'.**, **Arum. t.**, **Aesc.**, *Aspar.*, **Aur.**, **Bar. c.**, *Bell.*, **Bism.**, **Bov.**, **Bry.**, **Cact.**, **Calc. c**, *Calc. f.*, **Calc. Ph.**, **CANNAB. I.**, **Cannab. s.**, **Canth.**, *Carb. ac.*, *Carb. an.*, **Carb. v.**, **Caust.**, *Ced.*, **Cham.**, **Chel.**, **Chin.**, *Cic.*, **Cimic.**, **Cina**, **Clem.**, **Cocc.**, **Coff.**, *Colch.*, **Coloc.**, **Con.**, *Conv.*, *Crot. tig.*, **Cup.**, *Cyc.*, **Dig.**, **Dros.**, **Dulc.**, *Euphr.*, **GEL**, *Glon.*, **Graph.**, **Guai.**, **Hell.**, **Helo.**, **Hep.**, *Hyos.*, **Ign.**, **Iod.**, **K. br.**, **K. carb.**, **K. nit.**, *Kre.*, **Lach.**, *Led.*, **Lyc.**, **Mag. c.**, **Mang.**, **Mar.**, **Meli.**, **Merc.**, **Mos.**, *Murex*, **MUR. AC.**, *Nat. c.*, **Nat. m.**, **Nat. s.**, **Nit. ac.**, **Nux v.**, **Oleand.**, **Par.**, **Petrol.**, **Phos.**, **Pho. ac.**, **Plant.**, **Puls.**, **Rheum**, **Rhodo.**, **RHUS**, *Rhus a*, **Ruta**, *Saba.*, *Sabi.*, **Samb.**, *Sang.*, **Sars.**, **Sec. c.**, *Sele.*, **Seneg.**, **Sep.**, *Sil.*, **SPIG.**, **Spo.**, **SQU.**, **Stan.**, **Staph.**, *Still.*, *Stram.*, *Stro.*, **Sul.**, **Sul. ac.**, **Tab.**, **Tar.**, *Thuj.*, *Ura.*, *Valer.*, **Verat. a.**, **VERB.**, **Vib. op.**, **Vio. t.**, **Zinc.**

Purulent.—Acon., *Cannab. s.*, **CANTH.**, **Caps.**, **CLEM.**, *Con.*, **Ip.**, **K. carb.**, **Lyc.**, **Nat. m.**, *Nit. ac.*, **Nux v.**, **Petrol.**, *Pop. t.*, **Puls.**, **Sabi.**, **Sars.**, *Sep.*, *Sil.*, **Staph.**, **Sul.**

Red.—*Abs.*, **Acon.**, **Ant. t.**, **Bap.**, **Bell.**, **BERB.**, **BRY.**, *Calad.*, *Calc. ph.*, *Canth.*, *Carb. ac.*, *Carb. sul.*, **Card.**, *Ced.*, **Chel.**, *Crot. tig.*, *Cup.*, **Dig.**, *Form.*, **Grat.**, **Ip.**, **K. bi.**, *Laur.*, **Lith.**, **Merc.**, *Merc. c.*, **Op.**, *Phyt.*, **Rheum**, *Sal. ac.*, *Sant.*, *Sec. c.*, **Sele.**, *Senec.*, **Sul.**

Scanty.—Acon., **Aesc.**, **Agar.**, *Aloe*, **Ambr.**, **Am. carb.**, **Am. m.**, *Anac.*, *Ant. cr.*, **Ant. t.**, **Apis**, **Apoc. c.**, **Arg. n.**, **Arn.**, **ARS.**, *Aspar.*, **Aur.**, **Bar. c.**, **Bell.**, **Bism.**, **Bry.**, **Calc. c.**, **Camph.**, *Cannab. i.*, *Cannab. s.*, **CANTH.**, *Caps.*, **Carb. v.**, **Caust.**, *Ced.*, **Cham.**, **Chel.**, *Chim.*, **Chin.**, **Cic.**, **Clem.**, *Cocc.*, **Coff.**, **COLCH.**, **Coloc.**, **Con.**, *Conv.*, *Crotal.*, *Cup.*, **Cyc.**, **DIG.**, **Dros.**, **Dulc.**, **EQUI.**, *Eup. pur.*, *Euphorb.*, *Fer. iod.*, **GRAPH.**, **Grat.**, *Ham.*, **HELL.**, *Helo.*, **Hep.**, **Hyos.**, *Iod.*, **Ip.**, *K. bi.*, **K. carb.**, **K. chl.**, **K. nit.**, **Kalm.**, *Kre.*, **Lach.**, **Laur.**, *Led.*, **Lil. t.**, **Lith.**, *Lyc.*, **Mag. c.**, **Mag. m.**, **Mang.**, **Meny.**, **Merc.**, *Merc. c.*, *Mez.*, **Murex**, **Nat. c.**, **Nat. m.**, **Nat. s.**, **Nit. ac.**, *Nux m.*, **Nux v.**, **OP.**, *Ox. ac.*, **Par.**, **Petrol.**, **Phos.**, *Pho. ac.*, *Phyt.*, *Pic. ac.*, **PB.**, **Pru.**, **Puls.**, *Rat.*, **Rhus**, **RUTA**, *Saba.*, **Sabi.**, **Samb.**, **Sant.**, **Sars.**, *Sec. c.*, **Sele.**, **Senec.**, **Seneg.**, **Sep.**, *Sil.*, **Spo.**, **Squ.**, **Stan.**, **STAPH.**, *Stram.*, **Stro.**, **SUL.**, **Sul. ac.**, **TER.**, **Verat. a.**, **Vio. t.**, **Zinc.**

Slimy.—Ant. cr., **Arg. n.**, **Ars.**, *Aur.*, **Bry.**, **Calc. c.**, **Cannab. s.**, *Canth.*, **Caps.**, *Carb. v.*, **Caust.**, **Cham.**, *Chim.*, **Chin.**, **Cina**, *Coc. c.*, **Coloc.**, *Con.*, **Dulc.**, **Equi.**, *Eup. pur.*, **Hep.**, *Hydras.*, **Ip.**, **K. nit.**, **Merc.**, *Merc. c.*,

URINE.

Mez., *Nat. c.*, **NAT. M.**, *Nit. ac.*, **Nux v.**, *Parei.*, **Petrol.**, **Phos.**, **Pop. t.**, **PULS.**, Rheum, *Sars.*, *Sec. c.*, *Seneg.*, Sep., *Sul.*, Sul. ac., **Uva.**, **Valer.**

Sour Odor.—*Ambr.*, Calc. c., *Graph.*, **Merc.**, *Nat. c.*, Petrol.

Suppressed.—Apis, Apoc. c., *Asaf.*, *Bell.*, *Chim.*, *Colch.*, *Conv.*, *Crotal.*, **Cup.**, **Dig.**, *Dulc.*, *Hell.*, *Merc. c.*, **Phyt.**, Sec. c., **STRAM.**, Sul., Ter., *Verat. a.*, Zing.

Turbid.—Alum., **Ambr.**, Am. carb., *Anac.*, **Ant. t.**, *Ars.*, *Aspar*, *Aur.*, **Bell.**, BERB., Bov., *Bry.*, Calc. c., Camph., **Cannab. s.**, *Canth.*, Carb. an., Carb. v., *Carb. sul.*, **Card.**, Cham., **CHEL.**, *Chim.*, Chin., CINA, *Coca*, *Colch.*, **Coloc.**, CON., *Crot. tig.*, *Cup.*, *Cyc.*, *Dig.*, Dulc., Fer., *Hep.*, Hyos., **Ign.**, *Iod.*, *Ip.*, *K. carb.*, K. nit., Kre., Lach., Lyc., Mag. c., Mag. m., MERC., **Merc. c.**, Mez., *Mos.*, *Mur. ac.*, Nat. c., **Nat. m.**, Nit. ac., Nux v., *Op.*, Petrol., **Phos.**, *Pho. ac.*, *Pb.*, **Puls.**, Raph., Rhus, Ruta, SABA., Sars., Sec. c., Seneg., SEP., Sil., SUL., *Sul. ac.*, Valer., Verat. a., Vio. t., Zinc.

Becomes Turbid After Standing.—*Ambr.*, **Am. carb.**, Am. m., Arn., Aur., Bell., BRY., *Calc. c.*, Caust., CHAM., Chin., *Cina*, *Cocc.*, *Coloc.*, *Con.*, Dig., Dulc., *Graph.*, Hell., *Hep.*, Iod., *K. nit.*, *Laur.*, *Mang*, Merc., *Mez.*, Nat. c., *Par.*, *Petrol.*, Phos., PHO. AC., *Plat.*, Rhodo., Rhus, Sabi., *Sars.*, Seneg., *Sul.*, *Sul. ac.*, *Thuj.*, **Valer.**, Zinc.

Sediment in General.—*Acon.*, *Alum.*, AMBR., **Am. carb.**, Am. m., Anac., **Ant. cr.**, **Ant. t.**, *Arn.*, Ars., Aur., Bell., Bov., *Bry.*, Calc. c., *Cannab. s.*, CANTH., Caps., *Carb. ac.*, Carb. an., Carb. v., *Caust.*, *Ced.*, Cham., *Chim.*, Chin., Cina, Clem., *Coca*, Colch., COLOC., Con., *Crot. tig.*, Dig., Dulc., Euphorb., *Graph.*, Hep., Hyos., Ign., Iod., *Ip.*, *K. carb.*, *K. nit.*, Kre., *Lach.*, *Laur.*, Led., LYC., Mag. m., Mang., Meny., **Merc.**, Merc. c., **Mez.**, Nat. c., **Nat. m.**, **Nit. ac.**, *Nux m.*, Nux v., Oleand., Op., Par., Petrol., Phos., PHO. AC., Pic. ac., Plat., PULS., Rheum, Rhodo., *Rhus*, *Ruta*, *Sal. ac.*, *Samb.*, Sars., Sec. c., *Sele.*, Seneg., SEP., Sil., Spig., *Spo.*, Squ., *Still.*, SUL., *Sul. ac.*, Thuj., VALER., ZINC.

—**Bloody.**—Acon., Ant. t., Arn., *Calc. c.*, *Cannab. s.*, CANTH., Caps., Chin., *Coloc.*, Con., Dulc., Ip., Lyc., Merc., Mez., *Phos.* PHO. AC., PULS., Sec. c., SEP., *Sul.*, Sul. ac., Zinc.

—**Clayey.**—Am. m., *Anac.*, Canth., Ign., K. carb., Mang., Sars., Sep., Sul., Thuj., ZINC.

—**Flocculent.**—Ant. t., Benz. ac., Cannab. s., CANTH., *Cham.*, Coloc., K. carb., K. nit., *Merc.*, MEZ., Par., Phos., *Sars.*, *Seneg.*, Squ., Zinc.

—**Gray.**—Ant. t., Con., Hyos., Led., Mang., Spo.

—**Mealy.**—Ant. t., BERB., Calc. c., *Ced.*, Chin., *Graph.*, Hyos., Merc., *Nat. m.*, Pho. ac.

Sediment, Purulent.—Calc. c., Cannab. s., CANTH., CLEM., Con., K. carb., Lyc., Nit. ac., Petrol., Puls., Sabi., Sep., Sul.

—**Red.**—Acon., Alum., Ambr., Am. m., **Ant. cr., Ant. t., Arn., Bell.,** BERB., Bov., Cact., Calc. c., Cannab. s., CANTH., Carb. v., Chin., Coca, Coc. c., Coloc., Con., Dulc., Graph., Ip., K. carb., Kre., Lach., Laur. Lith., Lob. i., Lyc., Mang., Merc. c., **Mez.,** NAT. M., Nat. s., Nit. ac., Nux m., Op., Osm., Par., Petrol., Phos., Pho. ac., Plat., Pso., PULS., Rhodo., Ruta, Sars., Sec. c., Sele., Seneg., SEP., Sil., Squ., Still., Sul., Sul. ac., Thuj., VALER., Zinc.

—**Sandy.**—Acon., Alum., Ambr., Ant. cr., Ant. t., Arn., Cact., **Calc. c., Cannab. s.,** Canth., Chin., Cimic., Coc. c., Dios., Graph., Ip., K. br., K. carb., Lach., Led., LYC., Mang., Meny., **Merc., Nat. m.,** Nat. s., Nit. ac., Nux m., Nux v., Op., **Petrol.,** Phos., Pho. ac., Phyt., Piper, Puls., Rhodo., **Ruta, SARS.,** Sele., **Sep., Sil.,** Still., **Sul., Sul. ac.,** Thuj., Valer., Zinc.

—**Slimy (Gelatinous, Adherent).**—Ant. cr., Ars., Aur., Bry., Calad., Calc. c., Canth., Carb. v., Caust., Cham., Chin., Cina, Coca, Coloc., Con., Crot. tig., Dulc., Ip., K. nit., Merc., Nat. c., **Nat. m.,** Nit. ac., Nux v., Op., Petrol., Phos., Pho. ac., PULS., Rheum, Sars., Seneg., **Sep.,** Sul., Sul. ac., **Valer.**

—**Turbid.**—Alum., Ambr., Am. m., Bov., **Bry.,** Caust., Chin., Crot. tig., K. carb., K. nit., Laur., Mag. m., Merc., Par., Petrol., Phos., Pho. ac., Plat., Rhodo., Sars., Seneg., Thuj., Valer., Zinc.

—**White.**—Am. carb., Ant. t., **Bell.,** Benz. ac., Bry., Calc. c., Canth., Caps., Chin., Colch., Coloc., Con., Crot. tig., Dig., Dulc., Euphorb., Graph., Hep., Hydrang., Hyos., Ign., Kre., Led., **Nit. ac., Oleand.** Petrol., PHOS., Pho. ac., Phyt., RHUS, Seneg., Sep., Spig., Spo. Still., Sul., Valer., Zinc.

—**Yellow.**—Am. carb., Am. m., Anac., Bry., Canth., Cham., Chin., Cimic., Cup., Lach., Lyc., Mang., Phos., Pho. ac., Seneg., Sil., Spo., Sul. ac., Thuj., Zinc.

Micturition.

Tenesmus of Bladder.—Acon., Agar., Agn., Alum., Ambr., Am. carb., Am. m., Anac., Ant. cr., Ant. t., Apoc. c., Arg., Arn., Ars., Asar., Aspar., Aur., Bar. c., **Bell.,** Bism., Bor., Bov., Brach., BRY., Calc. c., Calc. ph., Camph., Cannab. i., Cannab. s., CANTH., Caps., Carb. an., Carb. v., Carb. sul., CAUST., Cham., **Chel.,** Chim., Chin., Cic., Cina, Clem., Cocc., Coc. c., Coff., Colch., COLOC., Con., Croc., Cup., Cyc., Dig., Dros., Dulc., EQUIS., Eup. pur., Euphorb., Fer., Graph., Guai., Hell., Hep., **Hyos.,** Ign., Iod., Ip., **K. carb.,** K. chl., K. nit., Kre., Lach.,

MICTURITION.

Laur., Led., LIL. T., *Lith.*, Lyc., Mag. c., Mag. m., Mang., Meny., MERC., MERC. C., Mos., Mur. ac., *Nat. c.*, *Nat. m.*, *Nit. ac.*, Nux m., NUX V., Oleand., **Oxyt.**, Par., *Parei.*, *Petrol.*, Phos., PHO. AC., Pb., *Pop. t.*, *Pru.*, PULS., Ran. b., Rhodo., **Rhus**, **Ruta**, Saba., SABI., **Samb.**, SARS., Sec. c., *Sele.*, *Senec.*, Seneg., SEP., *Sil.*, **Spig.**, Spo., SQU., *Stan.*, STAPH., Stram., Stro., SUL., **Tar.**, *Ter.*, Thuj., Valer., *Ve. at. a.*, **Verb.**, **Vio. t.**, Zinc.

Ineffectual.—Acon., *Agar.*, Alum., Am. carb., Anac., Ant. cr., *Apis*, Arn., *Ars.*, *Aur.*, Bar. c., *Bell.*, Bism., Bar., Bov., Bry., Calc. c., **Camph.**, **Cannab. i.**, Cannab. s., **CANTH.**, **Caps.**, Carb. an., Carb. v., **Caust.**, Ced., Chel., *Chin.*, *Cic.*, *Clem.*, Colch., **Coloc.**, *Con.*, Croc., Cup., DIG., *Dulc.*, Euphorb., **Graph.**, Guai., *Hell.*, *Hep.*, **Hyos.**, Iod., Ip., K. carb., K. nit., Lach., *Laur.*, Led., *Lyc.*, Mag. m., Mang., Merc., Merc. c., *Mur. ac.*, Nat. c., Nat. m., Nit. ac., Nux m., NUX V., **Op.**, Par., *Parei.*, *Petrol.*, **Petros.**, **Phos.**, Pho. ac., Pb., Pru., Puls., Rhus, *Ruta*, Saba., *Sabi.*, SARS., Sec. c., *Sep.*, *Sil.*, *Squ.*, Stan., Staph., Stram., Stro., **Sul.**, TER., Thuj., *Verat. a.*, Vio. t., Zinc.

By Drops.—Agar., Ant. cr., **Arn.**, Ars., BELL., Bov., Calc. c., Camph., CANNAB. I., Cannab. s., CANTH., *Caps.*, Carb. an., **Caust.**, Cham., *Chin.*, **Clem.**, Coff., *Colch.*, *Coloc.*, **Con.**, *Dig.*, Dros., Dulc., *Eryng.*, Euphorb., **Gel.**, *Graph.*, Guai., *Hell.*, K. carb., Kre., Led., Lyc., Mag. m., Merc., MERC. C., Nit. ac., Nux m., Nux v., Op., **Petrol.**, *Phos.*, *Pho. ac.*, PB., **Puls.**, Rheum, *Ruta*, Sabi., Samb., **Sant.**, Sec. c., **Sele.**, *Sil.*, Spig., Spo., **Staph.**, **Stram.**, SUL., **Thuj.**, **Verb.**, Zinc.

Dysuria.—Acon., *Ant. t.*, ARG. N., **Bell.**, **Canth.**, *Caps.*, Coc. c., Dig., *Equis.*, **Eup. pur.**, Lith., NUX V., Op., Phos., PB., *Pru.*, **Sant.**, Ter., Verat. a.

Too Frequent.—Acon., Aesc., *Agn.*, **All. c.**, Alum., Am. carb., **Am. m.**, *Anac.*, Ant. cr., Ant. t., ARG., *Arn.*, Ars., Aspar., BAR. C., *Bell.*, Bism., *Bor.*, Bry., **Cact.**, Calc. c., **Cannab. i.**, *Cannab. s.*, Canth., Caps., CAUST., *Ced.*, Cham., *Chel.*, Chin., Cic., Cina, *Clem.*, Cocc., Coff., *Colch..* Coloc., Con., *Crotal.*, Cup., Cyc., Dig., Dulc., *Eryng.*, *Eup. pur.*, Euphorb., Euphr., *Fl. ac.*, **GEL.**, Graph., *Guai.*, Hell., **Hyos.**, Ign., Iod., K. br., K. carb., K. NIT., **Kalm.**, Kre., Lach., Laur., *Led.*, LIL. T., *Lyc.*, Mag. c., Mag. m., **Meli.**, MERC., Mez., Mos., Mur. ac., Nat. c., **Nat. m.**, Nat. s., Nit. ac., *Oleand.*, *Ox. ac.*, Petrol., *Phos.*, Pho. ac., **Plant.**, Pb., Puls., *Rat.*, RHUS, Ruta, Sabi., Samb., **Sant. Sars.**, Sec. c., **Sele.**, Senec., *Seneg.*, Sep., *Sil.*, **Spig.**, Spo., SQU., Stan., STAPH., Stram., SUL., **Tar.**, Thuj., **Valer.**, Verat. a., **Verb.**, *Vesp.*, **Vio. t.**, Zinc.

Interrupted.—*Agar.*, Bov., Caps., *Cannab. i.*, Carb. an., *Caust.*,

CLEM., CON., Dulc., *Gel.*, K. carb., Led., *Op.*, *Pho. ac.*, Sabi., **Sul.**, Thuj., Zinc.

Involuntary.—Acon., *Am. carb.*, Ant. cr., *Ant. t.*, **Apis**, *Arn.*, **ARS.**, Bar. c., **Bell.**, Bor., *Bry.*, *Calc. c.*, Camph., *Cannab. i.*, Cannab. s., *Canth.*, Caps., *Carb. ac.*, Carb. an., *Carb. v.*, *Carb. sul.*, CAUST., Cham., *Chin.*, **Cic.**, *Cina*, Clem., *Cocc.*, Colch., Coloc., **Con.**, *Cup.*, Cyc., *Dig.*, Dulc., **Fer.**, *Gel.*, *Graph.*, Guai., *Hep.*, *Hyos.*, Ign., Iod., K. carb., **Kre.**, Lach., *Laur.*, Led., **Lyc.**, *Mag. c.*, Mag. m., Meny., **Merc.**, *Mur. ac.*, Nat. c., **NAT. M.**, *Nit. ac.*, Nux m., *Nux v.*, Op., *Ox. ac.*, Petrol., *Phos.*, *Pho. ac.*, Pb., **PULS.**, Rheum, **RHUS**, *Rhus a.*, Ruta, Sant., **Sec. c.**, *Seneg.*, Sep., Sil., **Spig.**, Spo., *Squ.*, Staph., *Stram.*, **Sul.**, Sul. ac., **Ter.**, Thuj., **Verat. a.**, *Zinc.*

Involuntary at Night.—*Acon.*, Am. carb., Ant. cr., Ant. t., *Arn.*, Ars., *Bar. c.*, **BELL.**, Benz. ac., Bor., **Bry.**, *Calc. c.*, Camph., *Cannab. s.*, Canth., Caps., Carb. an., Carb. v., **Caust.**, **Cham.**, *Chin.*, Cic., **Cina**, Clem., Cocc., Colch., Coloc., **Con.**, Cyc., Dig., **Dulc.**, *Equi.*, Fer., Graph., Guai., *Hep.*, *Hyos.*, *Ign.*, K. carb., **Kre.**, Lach., Laur., Led., *Lyc.*, Mag. c., Mag. m., Meny., **Merc.**, Mur. ac., Nat. c., *Nat. m.*, Nit. ac., *Nux v.*, **Op.**, Petrol., Phos., *Pho. ac.*, *Plant.*, Pb., *Pod.*, **PULS.**, *Rheum*, RHUS, *Ruta.*, Seneg., **Sep.**, SIL., **Spig.**, Spo., Squ., Staph., **Stram.**, SUL., Sul. ac., Thuj., Verat. a., *Vio. t.*, Zinc.

Retention of Urine.—Acon., Agar., **Apis**, ARN., **Ars.**, *Aur.*, **Bell.**, Bism., Calc. c., **Camph.**, Cannab. s., CANTH., *Caps.*, Carb. v., Caust., Chel., **Chin.**, Cic., Clem., *Colch.*, *Coloc.*, Con., *Cup.*, *Dig.*, Dulc., Euphorb., *Graph.*, Hell., **Hep.**, Hyos., Iod., Ip., Lach., **Laur.**, Led., LYC., Merc., Mez., Mur. ac., Nit. ac., **NUX V.**, OP., Pho. ac., Pb., Puls., Rhus, **Ruta**, Sabi., Sars., *Sec. c.*, Sep., Sil., Squ., Stan., Staph., STRAM., *Sul.*, Verat. a., Zinc.

Too Seldom.—Acon., *Agar.*, Alum., Am. carb., Am. m., **Arn.**, Ars., **Aur.**, *Bell.*, Bism., Bry., Calc. c., **Camph.**, Cannab. s., CANTH., Caps., *Carb. v.*, Caust., Chel., *Chin.*, *Cic.*, Clem., Colch., Coloc., Con., **Cup.**, Dig., Dulc., Euphorb., **Gam.**, Graph., Hell., **Hep.**, **Hyos.**, Iod., Ip., K. carb., Lach., **Laur.**, Led., Lyc., Merc., Mez., Mur. ac., Nat. s., Nit. ac., **Nux v.**, **Op.**, Par., Petrol., Phos., Pho. ac., Pb., Puls., Ruta, Sabi., Sars., Sec. c., Sep., Squ., Stan., Staph., Stram., Stro., Sul., *Sul. ac.*, *Verat. a.*, Zinc.

Troubles before Micturition.—*Aesc.*, Alum., Ant. t., **Apis**, **Arn.**, Asaf., **Aur.**, *Bell.*, BOR., Bry., Calc. c., *Cannab. s.*, CANTH., *Caps.*, Caust., Cham., Chel., *Chin.*, Cic., Cocc., *Coff.*, *Colch.*, COLOC., Con., Croc., Cup., Dig., *Dulc.*, Gel., *Graph.*, **Hep.**, **Hyos.**, **Kre.**, *Lith.*, **Meli.**, Merc., Mos., Nat. c., NUX V., *Op.*, **Pho. ac.**, Pb., PULS., *Rhodo.*, Rnus., Saba., Seneg., **Sep.**, **Sul.**, **Sul. ac.**, Tar., Thuj., **Zinc.**

MICTURITION—SEXUAL ORGANS.

Troubles at Beginning of Micturition.—Acon., *Canth.*, Caust., *Clem.*, Merc.

—During Micturition.—Acon., ALOE., *Alum.*, Ambr., Am. carb., *Anac.*, *Ant. cr.*, Ant. t., Apis, Arg. n., Arn., *Ars.*, Asaf., Asar., Bap., Bar. c., *Bell.*, Bor., Bov., *Bry.*, Calad., *Calc.* c., Camph., CANNAB. S, CANTH., *Caps.*, Carb. an., *Curb. v.*, *Carb. sul.*, *Caust.*, *Cham.*, Chel., *Chin.*, Clem., Colch., Coloc., Con., *Cub.*, *Cup.*, Cyc., Dig., Dulc., Euphorb., Fer., Fl. ac., *Graph.*, Guai., Hell., HEP., Hyos., *Ign.*, Ip., K. bi., *K. carb.*, K. nit., Kre., Lach., Laur., LIL. T., LYC., Mag. c., Mag. m., Mar., MERC., Merc. c., *Mez.*, *Mur. ac.*, *Nat. c.*, *Nat. m.*, Nit. ac., *Nux m.*, NUX V., *Op.*, Par., *Petrol.*, Phos., PHO. AC., Plat., Pb., PULS., Rheum, Rhodo., *Rhus.*, Ruta, Saba., Sabi., Sars., Sec. c., *Seneg.*, Sep., Sil., *Spig.*, Squ., Stan., *Staph.*, *Still.*, Stram., Stro., SUL., Sul. ac., THUJ., Verat. a., Vio. t., *Zinc.*

—At Close of Micturition.—Bry., Canth., Equi., Mez., Petrol., Phos., *Sars.*, *Sul.*

—After Micturition.—*Acon.*, Agn., Alum., Ambr., Anac., Ant. t., *Apis.*, Arg. n., Arn., Ars., *Asaf.*, *Asar.*, Bar. c., Bell., Bor., Bov., BRACH., Bry., Calc. c., Camph., CANNAB. I., Cannab. s., CANTH., Caps., Carb. v., *Chel.*, Chin., *Clem.*, Colch., COLOC., Con., *Cub.*, Dig., Fl. ac., Graph., *Guai.*, HEP., Ign., K. bi., *K. carb.*, Kre., *Lach.*, *Laur.* Led., *Lyc.*, Mag. c., Mar., MERC., Mez., *Mur. ac.*, Nat. c., NAT. M., Nit. ac., Nux v., Par., *Pare.*, Petrol., PETROS., Phos., *Pho. ac.*, Plat., Pb., Puls., *Rhodo.*, Rhus, Ruta, Saba., *Sars.*, Sele., *Seneg.*, Sep., Sil., Spig., Squ., *Stan.*, Staph., Sul., Sul. ac., THUJ., Verat. a., Vio. t., Zinc.

Sexual Organs.

Sexual Organs in General.—Acon., Agar., Agn., *Alum.*, *Ambr.*, Am. carb., Am. m., Anac., *Ant. cr.*, Ant. t., (Arg.), ARN., Ars., Asaf., (Asar.), *Aur.*, Bar. c., Bell., (Bism.), Bor., Bov., Bry., *Calad.*, Calc. c., Camph., Cannab. s., Canth., *Caps.*, Carb. an., *Carb. v.*, *Caust.*, Cham., Chel., Chin., (Cic.), (Cina), Clem., Cocc., *Coff.*, Colch., Coloc., *Con.*, Croc., Cup., (Cyc.), Dig., (Dros.), Dulc., Euphorb., Euphr., Fer., Graph., Guai., Hell., Hep., Hyos., Ign., *Iod.*, Ip., K. carb., K. nit., Kre., Lach., Laur., Led., Lyc., Mag. c., Mag. m., Mang., Mar., Meny., MERC., *Mez.*, (Mos.), Mur. ac., *Nat. c.*, Nat. m., NIT. AC., Nux m., NUX V., Op., (Par.), *Petrol.*, *Phos.*, Pho. ac., Plat., *Pb.*, PULS., Ran. s., (Rheum), Rhodo., Rhus, Ruta, Saba., Sabi., (Samb.), Sars., Sec. c., *Sele.*, Seneg., SEP., Sil., Spig., *Spo.*, Squ., Stan., Staph., (Stram.), SUL., Sul. ac., Tar., THUJ., Valer., Verat. a., Vio. t., *Zinc.*

SEXUAL ORGANS.

Male Organs in General.—Acon., Agar., Agn., *Alum., Ambr.,* **Am. carb.,** Am. m., Anac., *Ant. cr.,* Ant. t., Arg., *Arg. n.,* **ARN., Ars.,** Asaf., Asar., *Aur.,* Bar. c., **Bell.,** Bism., Bor., Bov., Bry., *Calad., Calc. c.,* Camph., **CANNAB. S., Canth.,** *Caps.,* Carb. an., *Carb. v., Caust.,* Cham., Chel., *Chin.,* Cic., Clem., Cocc., Coff., Colch., Coloc., *Con.,* Croc., Cup., (Cyc.), Dig., *Dios.,* Dros., Dulc., Euphorb., Euphr., Fer., **Graph.,** Guai., Hell., *Hep.,* Hyos., Ign., *Iod.,* Ip., **K. carb.,** K. nit., Kre., Lach., Laur., Led., Lyc., Mag. c., Mag. m., Mang., Mar., Meny., MERC., *Mez.,* (Mos.), Mur. ac., *Nat. c., Nat. m.,* NIT. AC., Nux m., **NUX V.,** Op., Par., *Petrol., Phos.,* **Pho. ac.,** Plat., *Pb.,* **PULS.,** Ran. s., **Rhodo.,** Rhus, Ruta, Saba., **Sabi.,** Samb., Sars., Sec. c., Sele., Seneg., **Sep.,** *Sil.,* Spig., *Spo.,* Squ., Stan., **Staph.,** Stram., SUL., Sul. ac., Tar., **THUJ.,** Valer., Verat. a., Vio. t., *Zinc.*

Penis.—Acon., Agar., *Agn., Alum., Ambr.,* Am. carb., Am. m., Anac., *Ant. cr., Ant. t.,* **ARN., Ars.,** Asaf., Asar., Aur., Bar. c., Bell., Bor., *Bov., Bry.,* **Calc. c.,** Camph., **Cannab. i., CANNAB. S., CANTH., Caps.,** Carb. an., *Carb. v.,* **Caust.,** Cham., *Chel., Chin.,* Cic., *Cinnab.,* **CLEM.,** Cocc., Coff., Colch., Coloc., **Con.,** Croc., *Crot. tig.,* Cup., Cyc., Dig., Dros., Dulc., Euphorb., Fer., **Graph.,** Guai., Hell., **Hep., Ign.,** *Iod.,* **Ip., K. carb.,** K. nit., Kre., *Lach.,* Laur., *Led.,* **Lyc.,** Mag. c., Mag. m., Mang., *Mar.,* MERC., *Merc. c., Mez.,* Mos., *Mur. ac., Nat. c.,* **Nat. m., Nit. ac.,** Nux m., **Nux v.,** Op., Par., *Petrol.,* **Phos., Pho. ac.,** *Pb.,* Puls., Ran. s., **Rhodo.,** *Rhus,* Ruta, *Saba.,* **Sabi.,** Samb., *Sars.,* Sec. c., Sele., Seneg., **Sep.,** Sil., *Spig.,* Spo., Squ., Stan., *Staph.,* Stram., SUL., THUJ., Verat. a., *Vio. t.,* **Zinc.**

Glans.—*Acon., Alum.,* Ambr., Ant. cr., Ant. t., Arn., *Ars.,* Asaf., Aur., Bell., Bor., Bry., *Calad.,* Calc. c., **Cannab. i., Cannab. s.,** *Canth.,* Caps., *Carb. v., Caust.,* Chin., *Cinnab.,* Coff., Colch., *Coloc.,* Con., *Coral., Crot. tig.,* Cup., Dig., Dros., Euphorb., Euphr., Graph., Hell., Hep., Ign., Iod., Ip., *K. carb.,* **Led., Lyc.,** Mag. m., Mang., MERC., **Mez.,** *Nat. c.,* **Nat. m., NIT. AC., Nux v., Osm.,** *Petrol.,* Phos., **Pho. ac.,** *Pso.,* Puls., Ran. s., *Rhodo.,* **Rhus, Sabi.,** Sars., Sele., Seneg., Sep., S.l., Spig., Spo., Squ., Stan., *Staph.,* **Sul., Sul. ac.,** *Tab.,* Tar., **THUJ.,** Valer., Vio. t., Zinc.

Foreskin.—*Acon.,* Agar., Alum., Arn., *Ars.,* **Bell.,** *Bry.,* **CALAD.,** *Calc. c.,* Camph., **Cannab. s.,** *Canth.,* Carb. v., *Caust.,* Cham., Chin., **Cinnab.,** Cocc., *Coloc.,* Con , *Coral.,* Croc., Euphorb., Euphr., *Form.,* **Graph., Hep., Ign.,** *Lach.,* Lyc., Mang., MERC., *Mez.,* Mur. ac., *Nat. c.,* **Nat. m.,** Nit. ac., *Nux v.,* **Osm.,** Phos., Pho. ac., Pb., *Puls.,* **Rhodo.,** Rhus, Sabi., *Sars.,* Sep., *Sil.,* **Sul.,** Tar., Thuj., Verat. a., *Vio. t.*

Testicles.—Acon., Agar., AGN., Alum., (Ambr.), *Am. carb.,* Ant. cr.,

SEXUAL ORGANS. 103

Ant. t., **Apis**, **Arg**., ARN., Ars., Asaf., AUR., Bar. c., Bell., **Berb.**,
Bism., *Bry.*, *Calc. c.*, (Camph.), Cannab. s., **Canth.**, *Caps.*, *Carb. v.*, *Caust.*,
Chel., Chin., *Cimic.*, *Cinnab.*, CLEM., *Cocc.*, Coff., *Coloc.*, **Con.**, *Cub.*,
Dig., *Dios.*, *Equi.*, Euphorb., Euphr., Graph., *Ham.*, Hep., Hyos., *Ign.*,
Iod., Ip., *Jab.*, *K. carb.*, K. nit., *Lyc.*, Mang., *Mar.*, Meny., **Merc.**,
Merc. c., **Mez.**, *Nat. c.*, Nat. m., **Nit. ac.**, **NUX V.**, *Osm.*, *Ox. ac.*, Petrol.,
Phos., **Pho. ac.**, Plat., *Pb.*, *Pso.*, PULS., RHODO., Rhus, Ruta, Saba.,
Sabi., Sele., **Sep.**, **Sil.**, *Spig.*, SPO., Squ., **Staph.**, *Still.*, **Sul.**, Sul. ac.,
Tar., **Thuj.**, Valer., Verat. a., **Zinc**.

Scrotum.—Acon., Agar., *Agn.*, Alum., *Ambr.*, Am. carb., Anac., *Ant. cr.*, Ant. t., **Apis**, **ARN.**, Ars., Aur., *Bar. c.*, Bell., Calc. c., Camph.,
Cannab. s., Canth., **Caps.**, *Carb. an.*, *Carb. v.*, Caust., Cham., *Chel.*, **Chin.**,
Clem., *Cocc.*, Coff., *Con.*, *Crot. tig.*, *Dig.*, Dulc., Euphorb., **Graph.**, Hell.,
Hep., *Hydras.*, *Ign.*, **Iod.**, *K. carb.*, Lach., *Lyc.*, Mag. m., **Mar.**, *Meny.*,
Merc., Mez., Mur. ac., *Nat. c.*, Nat. m., Nit. ac., **Nux v.**, PETROL.,
Pho. ac., **Plat.**, Pb., PULS., Ran. s., Rhodo., Rhus, Samb., *Sele.*, Sep.,
Sil., Spig., Spo., *Staph.*, **Sul.**, Thuj., *Vio. t.*, Zinc.

Spermatic Cord.—Agn., Alum., Ambr., Am. carb., *Am. m.*, *Ant. cr.*,
Arn., Bell., **Berb.**, Bry., Cannab. s., **Canth.**, Caps., *Chel.*, Chin., *Cimic.*,
CLEM., Colch., *Equi.*, Graph., *Ham.*, Iod., *K. carb.*, K. nit., *Mang.*,
Mar., Meny., Merc., Nat. c., *Nit. ac.*, Nux m., *Nux v.*, Osm., *Ox. ac.*,
Phos., **Pho. ac.**, Pb., PULS., *Rhodo.*, Saba., Sabi., *Sars.*, Sil., SPO., **Staph.**,
Sul., *Thuj.*, Verat. a., Zinc.

Female Organs in General.—Acon., Agar., Agn., *Alet.*, Alum.,
AMBR., Am. carb., *Ant. cr.*, Ant. t., *Arn.*, Ars., Asaf., Aur., Bell., *Bor.*,
Bov., *Bry.*, **Calc. c.**, *Calc. ph.*, *Camph.*, Cannab. s., **Canth.**, **Carb. an.**,
Carb. v., *Caust.*, Cham., Chel., Chin., Cina., Cocc., *Coff.*, Colch., Coloc.,
Con., Croc., Cup., Dig., Dros., Dulc., Fer., Graph., Hep., *Hyos.*, *Ign.*,
Iod., **Ip.**, **K. carb.**, K. nit., KRE., *Lach.*, Laur., Lil. t., **Lyc.**, Mag. c.,
Mag. m., Merc., Mez., Mos., Mur. ac., *Nat. c.*, *Nat. m.*, **Nit. ac.**, Nux m.,
NUX V., *Op.*, Petrol., *Phos.*, Pho. ac., Plat., Pb., *Pod.*, **PULS.**, Ran. b.,
Ran. s., **Rheum**, **Rhus**, Ruta, Saba., **Sabi.**, *Sars.*, SEC. C., **SEP.**, *Sil.*,
Stan., **Staph.**, SUL., Sul. ac., **THUJ.**, Verat. a., Zinc.

External Female Organs.—Acon., **Agar.**, Alum., **Ambr.**, Am. carb.,
Ant. t., **Ars.**, Ars. iod., Bell., Bor., *Bry.*, **Calad.**, Calc. c., **Canth.**,
Carb. ac., **Carb. v.**, Caust., Cham., *Chel.*, Chin., Cocc., *Coc. c.*, Coff., *Coll.*,
Coloc., Con., Croc., Dulc., **Fer.**, *Goss.*, *Graph.*, *Ham.*, Hep., Hyos.,
Hydras., *K. bi.*, K. carb., Kre., *Lil. t.*, *Lyc.*, **Merc.**, *Merc. c.*, Nat. c.,
Nat. m., **Nit. ac.**, *Nux v.*, Petrol., Plat., **Puls.**, Rhus, Sars., Sec. c., **SEP.**,
Sil., **Staph.**, **Sul.**, *Tare.*, **THUJ.**, Verat. a., Zinc.

SEXUAL ORGANS.

Vagina.—Ambr., *Arg. n.*, **Ars., Aur.**, **Aur. m. n.**, **Bell., BERB., Bor.**, Bry., CALC. C., *Calc. ph.*, **Canth.**, Carb. an., *Carb. v., Caul., Caust.,* Cham., *Chel.*, **Chin.**, Cinnab., *Cocc., Coff., Con.,* Croc., *Cub.*, Dulc., **Fer.**, *Graph.*, Hep., *Hydras.*, Hyos., Ign., Iod., **K CARB., Kre.**, *Lil. t.*, **Lyc.**, Mag. c., Mag. m., *Menth.*, **Merc., Mez.**, *Murex*, Nat. c., *Nat. m., Nit. ac.,* Nux m., **Nux v.**, *Petrol., Phos., Plat.*, **PB.**, *Pod.*, **Puls.**, Rheum, **Rhus**, *Sabi.*, Sars., *Sec. c.*, **SEP.**, *Sil.*, *Stan., Staph.*, **Sul.**, Sul. ac., *Tarent.,* Thuj., Zinc.

Uterus.—*Ab. c.*, Acon., *Alet.*, **ALOE, Ant. cr.**, Ant. t., **Arg., Arg. n.**, Arn., ARS., *Asaf.*, **Aur., Aur. m. n., BELL., Bor.**, Bov., *Bry.*, *Calad., Calc. c.*, **Calc. ph.**, *Calend.*, Camph., *Canth.*, *Carb. ac.*, **Carb. an.**, Carb. v., *Caul.*, Caust., **CHAM.**, *Chin.*, Cimic., Cina, *Cocc., Coff., Coll.*, **Con.**, *Conv.,* Croc., *Cub.*, Cup., Dros., **Fer.**, *Fer. iod.*, **Gel.**, *Graph.*, Ham., *Helo.*, *Hydras.*, Hyos., Ign., Iod., *Ip.*, **K. CARB.**, *K. iod.*, Kre., *Lach.*, *Lap.*, **LIL. T.**, Lyc., Mag. c., *Mag. m.*, Merc., **Merc. i. r.**, *Mez., Mos.*, Murex., Mur. ac., *Nat. c., Nat. m., Nit. ac.*, Nux m., **Nux v., Op.**, *Pall., Phos., Pho. ac.*, **PLAT.**, *Pod.*, **PULS.**, Rhus, Ruta, Saba., **SABI., SEC. C.,** *Senec.*, **SEP.**, *Stan.*, **Sul.**, Sul. ac., *Tarent., Ther., Thuj., Trill., Ust., Verat. a., Verat. v., Vib. op., Vib. pr., Visc.*, Zinc.

Ovaries.—*Abrot., Acon.*, Agar., Agn., *Ambr.*, **Am. b.**, *Ant. cr.*, **APIS, Arg., Arn., Ars., Asaf., Aur., Aur. m. n., Bell.**, Bry., *Cact.*, Calc. c., **CANTH., Carb. ac., Carb. an.**, *Carb. v., Carb. sul.*, Caust., *Chel.*, **Chin.**, Cimic., **COLOC.**, Dros., *Fer. ph.*, **Gel.**, *Graph., Guai., Ham.*, Hyos., *Ign., Iod., K. br.*, **K. carb., K. nit.**, Lach., Laur., **Lil. t.**, Lyc., *Meli.*, Merc., *Mez., Naj.*, Nat. c., *Nit. ac., Nux v.*, Pall., **Pb.**, *Pod.*, Puls., **Ran. b.**, *Ran. s., Rhus*, Ruta, *Saba.*, Sars., Sec. c., Sep., **STAPH.**, *Still., Sul., Tarent., Thea., Ther.*, **THUJ.**, *Ust.*, Vesp., *Vib. op., Xan.*, Zinc., *Ziz.*

Labor-like Pains.—*Acon.*, Ant. cr., Ant. t., **Apis**, Arn., Asaf., Aur., **BELL.**, *Bor.*, Bov., Bry., *Calc. c.*, Camph., *Canth.*, Carb. an., Carb. v., Caust., **CHAM.**, *Chin.*, **Cimic.**, Cina, *Cocc.*, Coff., Con., *Conv., Croc.*, Cup., Dros., **Fer., GEL.**, *Graph.*, Hyos., *Ign.*, Iod., *Ip.*, **K. CARB., Kre.**, *Lach.*, Lyc., Mag. c., *Mag. m.*, Merc., **Mos.**, Mur. ac., *Murex*, Nat. c., *Nat. m.*, Nux m., **Nux v., Op.**, Phos., *Pho. ac.*, **PLAT.**, *Pod.*, **PULS.**, Rhus, Ruta, Saba., Sabi., **SEC. C., SEP., Sil.**, *Stan.*, **Sul.**, Sul. ac., Thuj., *Ust.*, **Vip. op.**, *Xan.*, Zinc.

Labor Pains Cease.—*Arn.*, Asaf., **BELL.**, *Bor.*, Bry., Calc. c., *Camph.*, Carb. an., *Carb. v.*, **Caust., Cham.**, *Chin.*, Cocc., Coff., *Graph.*, Hyos., *Ign.*, **K. CARB.**, Kre., *Lyc.*, Mag. c., *Mag. m.*, Merc., Mos., *Nat. c.*, **Nat. m.**, *Nux m.*, Nux v., **OP.**, Phos., *Plat.*, **PULS.**, Rhus, Ruta, **SEC. C., Sep.**, Stan., *Sul.*, Sul. ac., **Thuj.**, Zinc.

SEXUAL ORGANS. 105

—**Too Severe.**—Acon., Ant. cr., Arn., *Aur.*, **Bell.**, CHAM., Chin., Cocc., Coff., *Con.*, Cup., Hyos., *Lyc.*, Mag. c., Nat. c., **Nux v.**, *Phos.*, Sec. c., SEP., Sul.

—**Spasmodic.**—Arn., Asaf., **Bell.**, Bry., Calc. c., Carb. an., Carb. v., *Caust.*, CHAM., **Cimic.**, **Cocc.**, *Cup.*, Fer., HYOS., *Ign.*, **Ip.**, *K. carb.*, Lyc., Mag. m., Mos., Nux m., **Nux v.**, *Op.*, Phos., PULS., **Sec. c.**, Sep., Stan., Stram., Zinc.

—**Weak (Inefficient, Flying in all Directions).**—*Arn.*,Asaf.,BELL., Bor., Bry., Calc. c., *Camph.*, Carb. an., *Carb. v.*, *Caul.*, **Caust.**, **Cham.**, Chin., Cimic., *Cocc.*, Coff., *Graph.*, Hyos., *Ign.*, K. CARB., Kre., *Lyc.*, Mag. c., *Mag. m.*, Merc., Mos., *Nat. c.*, **Nat. m.**, *Nux m.*, **Nux v.**, OP., Phos., *Plat.*, PULS., Rhus, **Ruta**, Saba., SEC. C., **Sep.**, Stan., *Sul.*, Sul. ac., *Thuj.*, Zinc.

After-Pains.—Acon., ARN., Asaf., *Aur.*, **Bell.**, Bor., Bry., *Calc. c.*, Carb. an., Carb. v., CHAM., *Chin.*, Cic., *Cina*, Cocc., **Coff.**, Con., Croc., **Cup.**, Fer., Graph., *Hyos.*, *Ign.*, Iod., Ip., **K. carb.**, Kre., Lach., Lyc., Nat. c., **Nat. m.**, Nux m., **Nux v.**, *Op.*, Plat., PULS., RHUS, **Ruta**, SABI., Sec. c., Sep., Sul., *Sul. ac.*, **Vib. op.**, Zinc.

Desire Too Weak.—Agar., **Agn.**, *Alum.*, Ambr., Am. carb., Anac., Ant. cr., Arn., **Bar. c.**, Bell., *Bor.*, **Calad.**, Calc. c., Cannab. s., Canth., Caps., Carb. an., Carb. v., *Carb. sul.*, CAUST., *Clem.*, Con., *Dig.*, Euphorb., Fer., *Graph.*, **Hep.**, Hyos., Ign., *K. carb.*, Laur., **Lil. t.**, *Lyc.*, **Mag. c.**, Mag. m., *Mar.*, **Meny.**, **Mur. ac.**, *Nat. m.*, *Nit. ac.*, Nux m., Oxyt., Petrol., **Phos.**, **Pho. ac.**, Plat., *Pso.*, **Rhodo.**, *Saba.*, Sabi., Sele., Seneg., Sep., Sil., Spig., Stan., Staph., *Sul.*, Sul. ac.

—**Too Strong.**—Acon., *Agar.*, Alum., Ambr., Anac., **Ant. cr.**, Arn., **Ars.**, Asaf., *Aur.*, **Bell.**, Bor., *Bov.*, *Cact.*, **Calc. c.**, CAMPH., *Cannab. s.*, CANTH., Caps., **Carb. v.**, Caust., Cham., CHIN., Clem., *Cocc.*, **Coff.**, *Coloc.*, CON., Croc., *Cub.*, *Dig.*, *Dulc.*, Fer., **Fl. ac.**, Graph., Hep., *Hyos.*, *Ign.*, **Iod.**, *K. br.*, K. carb., K. nit., Kre., **Lach.**, Laur., Led., *Lyc.*, Mag. m., Mang., *Meny.*, **Merc.**, Mez., **Mos.**, Mur. ac., **Murex**, Nat. c., **Nat m.**, Nit. ac., Nux m., NUX V., **Op.**, Par., Petrol., PHOS., *Pic. ac.*, PLAT., *Pb.*, PULS., *Raph.*, Rhodo., Rhus, *Ruta*, **Sabi.**, Sars., Seneg., Sep., **Sil.**, Spig., Stan., *Staph.*, **Stram.**, *Sul.*, Sul. ac., *Thuj.*, VERAT. A., Verb., Zinc.

Discharge of Prostatic Fluid.—Alum., AGN., *Am. carb.*, **Anac.**, Aur., Bell., Calc. c., Cannab. s., Carb. v., Caust., Dig., Euphorb., HEP., *Ign.*, Iod., K. carb., Lyc., NAT. C., Nat. m., *Nit. ac.*, Nux m., Petrol., Pho. ac., Plat., *Puls.*, SELE., SEP., **Sil.**, Spig., *Staph.*, **Sul.**, *Thuj.*, Zinc.

SEXUAL ORGANS.

Emissions.—Agar., **Agn.**, Alum., Ambr *Am. carb.*, *Anac.*, Ant. cr., **Arg.**, *Arn.*, *Ars.*, Aur., Bar. c., Bell., Bism., Bor., *Bov.*, **Calad.**, **Calc. c.**, Camph., Cannab. s., *Canth.*, *Caps.*, *Carb. an.*, *Carb. v.*, *Caust.*, Cham., CHIN., Cic., Clem., **Cob.**, Cocc., Coff., CON., Cyc., Dig., DROS., *Eryng.*, Fer., *Gel.*, Graph., Guai., Hep., Ign., **K. carb.**, Lach., Led., Lyc., Mag. c., Mag. m., **Merc.**, Mos., **Nat. c.**, Nat. m., *Nit. ac.*, Nux m., *Nux r.*, *Op.*, *Par.*, *Petrol.*, **Phos.**, PHO. AC., **Pic. ac.**, Plat., Puls., *Ran. b.*, Ran. s., Rhodo., Rhus, *Ruta*, Saba., *Sal. ac.*, Samb., **Sars.**, SELE., **Sep.**, **Sil.**, **Stan.**, Staph., Stram., Sul., *Tar.*, *Thuj.*, *Verb.*, Vio. o., **Vio. t.**, Zinc.

Erections.—*Agar.*, Agn., *Alum.*, Ambr., Am. carb., Am. m., *Anac.*, **Ant. cr.**, ARG. N., Arn., Ars., *Aur.*, Bar. c., *Calad.*, Calc. c., **Cannab. i.**, **Cannab. s.**, CANTH., *Caps.*, Carb. an., *Carb. v.*, Caust., Cham., **Chin.**, Clem., *Coloc.*, *Con.*, **Dig.**, Euphorb., Fer., Fl. ac., Graph., Hep., Hyos., Ign., **K. carb.**, *Lach.*, Led., *Lyc.*, **Mag. m.**, MERC., Mez., Mos., Mur. ac., NAT. C., **Nat. m.**, NIT. AC., NUX V., Op., *Par.*, *Petrol.*, **Petros.**, PHOS., Pho. ac., PIC. AC., **Plat.**, *Pb.*, PULS., Ran. b., Rhodo., **Rhus**, Saba., *Sabi.*, Sars., *Seneg.*, Sep., **Sil.**, *Spig.*, Stan., **Staph.**, Sul., *Sul. ac.*, *Tar.*, TER., THUJ., Valer., Verat. a., *Vio. t.*, *Zinc.*

Impotency.—*Agar.*, Alum., AGN., Am. carb., **Ant. cr.**, **Bar. c.**, CALAD., *Calc. c.*, **Camph.**, Cannab. s., Caps., Carb. an., Carb. v., *Carb. sul.*, *Caust.*, *Chin.*, **Cob.**, Coff., Coloc., CON., Dig., *Dios.*, Dulc., Euphorb., Fer., Graph., Hell., *Hep.*, Hyos., *Ign.*, Iod., *K. br.*, **K. carb.**, Kre., *Lach.*, LYC., *Mag. c.*, Mar., *Meny.*, Merc., Mos., *Mur. ac.*, Nat. c., **Nat. m.**, *Nit. ac.*, *Nux m.*, Nux v., Op., Petrol., **Phos.**, Pho. ac., *Pic. ac.*, Pb., **Pso.**, Rhodo., Ruta, Sabi., SELE., *Sep.*, Spo., Stan., *Stram.*, Sul., *Sul. ac.*, Thuj., Zinc.

Weak Sexual Power.—*Agar.*, AGN., Alum., Ambr., Am. carb., **Ant. cr.**, Arn., **Bar. c.**, Bor., CALAD., *Calc. c.*, **Camph.**, Cannab. s., Canth., Caps., Carb. an., Carb. v., *Caust.*, Chin., Coff., Coloc., CON., Dig., Dulc., Euphorb., Fer., GRAPH., Hell., *Hep.*, Hyos., Ign., Iod., K. carb., Kre., *Lach.*, LYC., *Mag. c.*, Mang., Mar., *Meny.*, Merc., Mos., *Mur. ac.*, Nat. c., *Nat. m.*, *Nit. ac.*, *Nux m.*, Nux v., Op., Petrol., *Phos.*, Pho. ac., Plat., Pb., Rhodo., Rhus, Ruta, Saba., Sabi., SELE., *Sep.*, Sil., Spo., Stan., SUL., Sul. ac., Thuj., *Zinc.*

Left Side.—*Abrot.*, *Agar.*, Alum., Ambr., **Am. b.**, *Am. m.*, Ant. cr., **Apis**, **Arg.**, *Aur.*, Bar. c., **Brom.**, *Bry.*, Calc. c., Cannab. s., *Chin.*, Clem., *Colch.*, *Con.*, *Euphr.*, *Fer. ph.*, **Fl. ac.**, Graph., **K. carb.**, *Lach.*, Lyc., **Mag. c.**, Mar., Meny., *Merc.*, Mez., *Naj.*, Nat. c., **Nit. ac.**, *Osm.*, Petrol., Pho. ac., *Pb.*, *Puls.*, Rhodo., *Rhus*, *Saba.*, Sele., *Sep.*, Sil., Spig., **Staph.**, **Tar.**, *Ther.*, THUJ., *Ust.*, *Vesp.*, *Xan.*, Zinc.

SEXUAL ORGANS—MENSTRUATION.

Right Side.—Acon., Alum., *Apis.*, *Arg.*, **Arn.**, *Ars.*, **Aur.**, *Bism.*, CALC. C., *Cannab. s.*, *Canth.*, CAUST., **Clem.**, *Coff.*, Coloc., Con., *Croc.*, Graph., HEP., Iod., Lach., *Lil. t.*, **Lyc.**, Mar., Meny., **Merc.**, Mez., *Murex*, *Mur. ac.*, Nit ac., NUX V., *Pall.*, Petrol., POD., PULS., *Rhodo.*, **Sabi.**, Sec. c., *Sele.*, Sil., Spig., SPO., **Staph.**, Sul., SUL. AC., Tar., *Valer.*, VERAT. A., Zinc.

Menstruation.

Abortion.—Acon., Ant. cr., **Apis**, *Arn.*, *Asar.*, BELL., **Bry.**, **Calc. c.**, *Cannab. s.*, **Canth.**, Caps., Carb. an., *Carb. v.*, *Carb. sul.*, CHAM., **Chin.**, **Cocc.**, Con., CROC., Cup., Cyc., **Fer.**, **Hyos.**, IP., K. carb., *Kre.*, *Lyc.*, Merc., Nat. c., *Nit. ac.*, Nux m., **Nux v.**, Op., *Phos.*, **Plat.**, **Pb.**, **Puls.**, **Rhus**, Ruta, SABI., SEC. C., SEP., *Sil.*, Stram., Sul., *Tan.*, *Trill.*, *Verat. a.*, Zinc.

Hæmorrhage, not at Menstrual Times.—*Ambr.*, *Arn.*, Asar., **Bell.**, Bov., Bry., CALC. C., *Canth.*, *Carb. v.*, CHAM., *Chin.*, **Cocc.**, *Coff.*, Croc., *Fer.*, **Hep.**, *Hyos.*, IP., *K. carb.*, *Lyc.*, Mag. m., Merc., *Murex*, *Nit. ac.*, *Nux v.*, Petrol., PHOS., Pb., *Puls.*, RHUS, SABI., Sec. c., *Sep.*, SIL., Stram., *Sul.*, Zinc.

Uterine Hæmorrhage.—Acon., Amyl., Ant. cr., **Apis**, **Apoc. c.**, **Arn.**, *Ars.*, BELL., Bor., Bov., Bry., CALC. C., *Canth.*, Caps., Carb. an., *Carb. v.*, Cham., CHIN., Cina, *Cinnam.*, Cocc., *Coff.*, Con., CROC., Cup., *Dig.*, *Erig.*, FER., HAM., Hyos., Ign., *Iod.*, IP., Kre., *Led.*, **Lyc.**, Merc., *Millef.*, *Nat. c.*, Nat. m., **Nit. ac.**, *Nux m.*, NUX V., *Op.*, **Phos.**, *Plat.*, Pb., **Puls.**, Rhus, Ruta, SABI., Samb., *Sang.*, SEC. C., Sep., *Sil.*, Stram., Sul., *Sul. ac.*, *Trill.*, *Ust.*, *Uva.*, *Visc.*, Zinc.

Menstruation Beginning. Delayed in Girls.—Acon., Agn., Am. carb., Aur., Bry., Calc. c., CAUST., *Chel.*, Cic., *Cocc.*, **Con.**, Croc., Cup., *Dig.*, Dros., *Dulc.*, Fer., GRAPH., Guai., Hyos., K. CARB., Lach., *Lyc.*, **Mag. c.**, Mag. m., Merc., **Nat. m.**, Petrol., Phos., **PULS.**, Saba., **Sabi.**, Sars., Sep., *Sil.*, Spig., Staph., Stram., Stro., SUL., *Valer.*, Verat. a., Zinc.

—**Too Early.**—Acon., *Aloe*, Alum., AMBR., Am. carb., **Am. m.**, **Arn.**, **Ars.**, **Asaf.**, **Asar.**, Bar. c., BELL., *Berb.*, Bor., BOV., Bry., Cact., CALC. C., *Calc. ph.*, Cannab. s., **Canth.**, *Carb. an.*, CARB. V., *Carb. sul.*, Caust., CHAM., *Chin.*, *Cimic.*, Cina, Cinnam., Clem., *Coc. c.*, COCC., Coff., Colch., Coloc., Con., Croc., *Crotal.*, Dig., Dulc., Fer., Form., Graph., Hell., *Hep.*, Hyos., Ign., *Iod.*, IP., *Jug. r.*, **K. carb.**, *K. nit.*, **Kre.**, Lach., Laur., Led., Lyc., Mag. c., *Mag. m.*, Mang., **Mez.**, *Mos.*, Mur. ac., Nat. c., Nat. m., Nit. ac., *Nux m.*, NUX V., Par., *Petrol.*,

PHOS., *Pho. ac.*, Plat., *Pb.*, Puls., Rhodo., RHUS, Ruta, SABI., **Sec c.**, *Senec.*, Sep., *Sil.*, Spig., *Spo.*, *Stan.*, Staph., Stram., Stro., Sul., **Sul ac.**, *Trill.*, Verat. a., Xan., Zinc.

—**Early and Scanty.**—Alum., Lep., **Nat. m.**

—**Gushing.**—Bell., *Coca*, *Cocc.*, Puls., *Sabi.*, *Trill.*

—**Late.**—*Acon.*, Agn., *Am. carb.*, Arn., Ars., *Aur.*, Bell., Bor., Bov., *Bry.*, Calc. c., Canth., Carb. an., CAUST., Cham., **Chel.**, Chin., *Cic.*, **Cocc.**, Colch., Coloc., CON., *Croc.*, CUP., *Dig.*, **Dros.**, DULC., Fer., *Goss.*, GRAPH., *Guai.*, Hell., Hep., *Hyos.*, Ign., Iod., K. CARB., *Lach.*, LYC., MAG. C., *Mag. m.*, **Merc.**, Nat. c., NAT. M., Nit. ac., Nux m., Nux v., Petrol., *Phos.*, Pho. ac., PULS., Rhodo., Rhus, Ruta, *Saba.*, **Sabi.**, *Sars.*, Sec. c., SEP., SIL., Spig., *Staph.*, *Stram.*, *Stro.*, SUL., Sul. ac., **Valer.**, *Verat. a.*, **Vib. op.**, Zinc.

—**Long.**—*Acon.*, Agar., *Am. carb.*, *Ars.*, *Asar.*, **Bar. c.**, **Bell.**, Bor., Bov., **Bry.**, Calc. c., **Canth.**, *Caust.*, *Chel.*, **Chin.**, Cina, **Cinnam.**, **Coff.**, Croc., Crotal., CUP., *Dulc.*, **Fer.**, Hyos., **Ign.**, *K. carb.*, K. nit., **Kre.**, *Laur.*, Led., LYC., Mag. c., **Merc.**, Nat. c., NAT. M., NUX V., **Phos.**, PLAT., Rhus, Saba., **Sabi.**, SEC. C., Sep., SIL., Stan., *Stram.*, *Sul.*, Sul. ac., Zinc.

—**Profuse.**—Acon., Agar., Aloe., Ambr., Am. carb., **Am. m.**, *Ant. cr.*, Arn., **Ars.**, Bar. c., **BELL.**, Bor., **BOV.**, Bry., *Cact.*, CALC. C., **Cannab. i.**, Cannab. s., **Canth.**, Caps., *Carb. ac.*, *Carb. an.*, **Carb. v.**, Caust., Cham., *Chel.*, Chin., *Cimic.*, *Cina*, **Cinnam.**, *Cit. ac.*, *Clem.*, *Coc. c.*, *Cocc.*, Coff., Coloc., Croc., *Crotal.*, Cup., *Cyc.*, *Dig.*, Dulc., FER., *Fer. ph.*, Gel., *Helo.*, Hep., Hyos., Ign., *Iod.*, IP., *K. nit.*, Kre., *Laur.*, Led., Lyc., Mag. c., Mag. m., Merc., Mez., *Mos.*, *Mur. ac.*, *Nat. c.*, **Nat. m.**, **Nit. ac.**, Nux m., NUX V., Op., Phos., *Pho. ac.*, PLAT., Pb., *Puls.*, Rhodo., Rhus, Ruta, Saba., SABI., *Samb.*, SEC. C., *Sele.*, Senec., **Sep.**, *Sil.*, Spig., Spo., *Stan.*, STRAM., Stro., *Sul.*, **Sul. ac.**, Tan., *Thlasp.*, *Trill.*, Ust., *Verat. a.*, *Vinc.*, Zinc.

—**Scanty.**—*Acon.*, *Agn.*, **Alum.**, AM. CARB., Arn., Asaf., Aur., *Bur. c.*, *Bor.*, Bov., Bry., Cact., Calc. c., Carb. an., Carb. v., **Caust.**, Chel., *Cic.*, **Cocc.**, Colch., CON., Croc., Cup., Dig., Dros., DULC., Euphr., Fer., Form., *Gnap.*, GRAPH., *Guai.*, Hep., Hyos., *Ign.*, Iod., Ip., K. CARB., Lach., Lyc., MAG. C., *Mag. m.*, *Mang.*, Merc., Mos., Nat. m., Nux v., Petrol., PHOS., Plat., PULS., Rhodo., Rhus, *Ruta*, Saba., Sabi., **Sars.**, Sep., Sil., Staph., Stram., Stro., SUL., Thuj., *Valer.*, Verat. a., **Vib. op.**, *Xan.*, Zinc.

—**Short.**—*Alum.*, AM. CARB., Bar. c., Bov., Carb. an., Colch., **Con.**, Dulc., Euphr., **Graph.**, Iod., Ip., *Lach.*, Lyc., *Mag. c.*, Mag. m., Mang.,

Merc., Mos., **Phos.**, Plat., PULS., Rhodo., *Ruta*, *Saba.*, Sars., Sil., SUL., Vib. op.

—**Suppressed.**—Acon., *Agn.*, *Alum.*, **Am. carb.**, **Ant. cr.**, Arn., Ars., Aur., **Bar. c.**, **Bell.**, *Bor.*, **Bry.**, **Calc. c.**, Carb. an., Carb. v., *Caul.*, **Caust.**, **Cham.**, Chel., Chin., *Cimic.*, **Cocc.**, Colch., *Coloc.*, CON., *Croc.*, **Cup.**, *Dig.*, Dros., DULC., Euphr., **Fer.**, *Fer. iod.*, *Gel.*, *Glon.*, *Goss.*, GRAPH., Guai., *Hell.*, *Hyos.*, *Ign.*, Iod., K. CARB., *Lach.*, LYC., *Mag. c.*, *Mag. m.*, Mang., *Merc.*, *Mos.*, **Nat. m.**, Nit. ac., *Nux m.*, *Op.*, *Ox. ac.*, Petrol., **Phos.**, Pho. ac., Plat., *Pod.*, PULS., *Rhodo.*, Rhus, *Ruta*, Saba., *Sabi.*, *Sars.*, Sec. c., *Senec.*, **Sep.**, SIL., **Staph.**, *Stram.*, Stro., SUL., Thuj., *Ust.*, **Valer.**, *Verat. a.*, *Verat. v.*, *Xan.*, **Zinc.**

Menses Acrid.—*Am. carb.*, Ars., Bar. c., *Bov.*, *Canth.*, Carb. v., Fer., Graph., Hep., K. CARB., **K. nit.**, **Rhus**, Sars., SIL., *Sul.*, Sul. ac., Zinc.

—**Bright.**—Am. carb., *Ant. t.*, **Arn.**, Ars., BELL., *Bar.*, Bov., Bry., *Calc. c.*, *Calc. ph.*, Canth., Carb. an., Carb. v., Chin., *Cinnam.*, Dig., Dros., DULC., Fer., *Form.*, Graph., **Ham.**, HYOS., **Ip.**, *K. nit.*, Kre., *Laur.*, Led., Mag. m., **Meli.**, Merc., *Millef.*, Nat. c., Nux m., **Phos.**, Puls., Rhus, *Saba.*, SABI., Sec. c., Sep., Sil., *Spig.*, **Stram.**, *Stro.*, Sul., *Trill.*, Ust., **Vip. op.**, *Zinc.*

—**Brown.**—BRY., *Calc. c.*, **Carb. v.**, Con., *Gnap.*, Puls., *Rhus.*

—**Clotted.**—*Aloe*, *Arn.*, **Bell.**, Bry., *Canth.*, Carb. an., *Caust.*, CHAM., **Chin.**, *Cimic.*, *Coc. c.*, *Coff.*, Con., *Croc.*, **Fer.**, *Hyos.*, Ign., Ip., Kre., *Mag. m.*, Merc., *Nit. ac.*, Nux m., Nux v., *Pho. ac.*, PLAT., Puls., RHUS, Sabi., Sec. c., Sep., *Spig.*, **Stram.**, *Stro.*, *Ust.*, *Xan.*, Zinc.

—**Dark.**—Acon. *Aloe,* **Am. carb.**, **Ant. cr.**, *Arn.*, *Asar.*, **Bell.**, Bism., Bov., Bry., *Cact.*, *Calc. ph.*, *Canth.*, Carb. ac., Carb. v., CHAM., *Chin.*, *Cimic.*, Cocc., *Coc. c.*, *Coff.*, Con., CROC., Cup., Dig., Dros., Fer., Graph., *Helo.*, *Ign.*, *Jug. r.*, K. nit., **Kre.**, **Lach.**, Led., *Lyc.*, **Mag. c.**, Mag. m., **Nit. ac.**, *Nux m.*, NUX V., Phos., *Pho. ac.*, *Plat.*, **Puls.**, Sec. c., *Sele.*, **Sep.**, *Spig.*, *Stram.*, *Sul.*, *Thlasp.*, *Ust.*, *Xan.*

—**Membranous.**—BOR., **Calc. ac.**, **Coll.**, Lach., Phos., Ust., **Vib. op.**

—**Offensive.**—Ars., **BELL.**, BRY., *Calc. ph.*, **Carb. an.**, Carb. v., Caust., Cham., Chin., **Croc.**, *Helo.*, *Ign.*, K. carb., Lach., Merc., Phos., Plat., *Rheum.*, **Sabi.**, Sec. c., *Sil.*, *Spig.*, Sul.

—**Tenacious.**—*Cact.*, CROC., **Cup.**, Mang., *Phos.*, *Sec. c.*

—**Watery.**—*Fer.*, *Goss.*, Ust.

Before Menstruation.—*Alum.*, **Am. carb.**, Am. m., *Asar.*, **Bar. c.**, Bell., Bor., BOV., Bry., CALC. C., *Calc. ph.*, Canth., Carb. an., **Carb. v.**, *Caust.*, Cham., Chin., Cina, Cocc., Coff., **Con.**, Croc., CUP., Dulc., *Fer.*

Gel., *Graph.*, Hep., **Hyos.**, Ign., *Iod.*, Ip., *K. carb.*, **K. nit.**, **Kre.**, *Lach.*, **LYC.**, *Mag. c.*, Mag. m., *Mang.*, **Merc.**, Mez., Mos., **Mur. ac.**, **Nat. c.**, **Nat. m.**, *Nux m.*, Nux v., Petrol., **Phos.**, **Pho. ac.**, **Plat.**, PULS., Rhus., Ruta, Saba., Sars., SEP., *Sil.*, Spig., Spo., *Stan.*, Staph., SUL., Sul. ac., Valer., VERAT. A., *Vib. op.*, ZINC.

At Beginning of Menstruation.—Acon., Asar., Bell., *Bry.*, *Cact.*, **Caust.**, **Cham.**, Cocc., *Coff.*, *Graph.*, HYOS., Ign., *Iod.*, *Ip.*, Lyc., *Mag. c.*, **Mag. m.**, Merc., Mos., *Nat. m.*, Nit. ac., **Phos.**, **Plat.**, **Puls.**, Ruta, Sars., **Sep.**, **Sil.**, **Staph.**

During Menstruation.—Acon., *Aloe*, Alum., Ambr., **AM. CARB.**, **Am. m.**, **Ant. cr.**, **Ars.**, **Asar.**, **Bar. c.**, *Bell.*, **Bor.**, BOV., Bry., Buf., **Calc. c.**, *Calc. ph.*, Cannab. s., *Canth.*, Caps., *Carb. an.*, *Carb. v.*, *Caust.*, **CHAM.**, Chel., *Chin.*, Cimic., **Cocc.**, **Coff.**, Con., Croc., *Crotal.*, Cup., Fer., *Fer. ph.*, *Gel.*, **GRAPH.**, Hep., **HYOS.**, **Ign.**, Iod., **K. CARB.**, **K. nit.**, **Kre.**, Lach., Laur., **Lyc.**, **Mag. c.**, **Mag. m.**, Merc., Mos., **Mur. ac.**, *Nat. c.*, **Nat. m.**, Nit. ac., Nux m., **NUX V.**, *Oenan.*, Op., Petrol., **Phos.**, **Pho. ac.**, Plat., **PULS.**, Rhodo., Rhus, *Sabi.*, Sars., Sec. c., Sele., **SEP.**, **Sil.**, Spo., Stan., *Stram.*, Stro., SUL., Sul. ac., *Thea.*, Verat. a., **Vib. op.**, ZINC.

After Menstruation.—*Alum.*, Am. carb., BOR., Bov., Bry., *Calc. c.*, Canth., *Carb. an.*, Carb. v., *Chel.*, Chin., **Con.**, Cup., Fer., GRAPH., **Iod.**, **K. carb.**, **KRE.**, Lach., **Lil. t.**, **Lyc.**, *Mag. c.*, *Merc.*, **Nat. m.**, **NUX V.**, **Nit. ac.**, **Phos.**, **Pho. ac.**, *Plat.*, Puls., Rhus, Ruta, *Sabi.*, **SEP.**, **Sil.**, **Stram.**, Sul., Sul. ac., Verat. a.

Leucorrhœa.

Leucorrhœa in General.—Acon. **Aesc.**, Agn., **ALUM.**, Ambr., **Am. carb.**, Am. m., Anac., Ant. cr., Ant. t., **Ars.**, Bar. c., **Bell.**, *Bor.*, **Bov.**, Bry., **CALC. C.**, *Calc. ph.*, Cannab. s., *Canth.*, *Carb. an.*, **Carb. v.**, *Caul.*, Caust., *Ced.*, *Cham.*, **Chel.**, **Chin.**, *Cinnab.*, **Cocc.**, Coff., **Con.**, *Cub.*, Dros., **Fer.**, Graph., Guai., Hep., *Hydras.*, Ign., *Iod.*, *K. carb.*, K. nit., **KRE.**, **Lyc.**, *Mag. c.*, Mag. m., Mang., **MERC.**, *Merc. i. r.*, *Mez.*, Mur. ac., *Nat. c.*, **Nat. m.**, *Nit. ac.*, Nux m., Nux v., Petrol., **Phos.**, **Pho. ac.**, Plat., Pb., **PULS.**, Ran. b., *Rhus*, Ruta, Sabi., Sars., Sec. c., Seneg., **SEP.**, **Sil.**, Squ., **Stan.**, Stro., **Sul.**, *Sul. ac.*, *Tarent.*, Thlasp., Thuj., Vio. t., Zinc.

—Acrid.—ALUM., *Am. carb.*, *Anac.*, Ant. cr., *Aral.*, **Arg.**, **Ars.**, **Bov.**, Calc. c., *Carb. ac.*, Cannab. s., Canth., Carb. an., **Carb. v.**, *Cham.*, Chin., *Clem.*, **Con.**, *Cub.*, **FER.**, Hep., *Ign.*, Iod., **K. carb.**, *K. iod.*, *Kre.*, **Lil. t.**, *Lyc.*, Mag. c., Mag. m., **MERC.**, *Merc. i. r.*, Mez., **Nat. m.**, *Nit. ac.*, **PHOS.**, Pho. ac., **PULS.**, *Ran. b.*, *Ruta*, *Sabi.*, **SEP.**, **Sil.**, **Sul.**, *Sul. ac.*, **Thuj.**

LEUCORRHŒA.

Leucorrhœa, Albuminous.—Am. m., BOR., Bov., Calc. ph., Mez., *Petrol., Stan.*

—**Bland.**—Calc. c., *Fer.*, Kre., Merc., Nat. m., Nux v., Puls., *Ruta,* Sep.

—**Bloody.**—Alum., Ant. t., *Ars.*, **Ars. iod.**, Canth., Carb. v., CHIN., *Chrom. ac.*, COCC., Con., *K. iod.*, Kre., *Lyc.*, Mag. m., *Murex,* **Nit. ac.**, Sep., *Sil., Sul. ac.*

—**Brown.**—*Am. m.,* LIL. T., Nit ac., Sec. c., *Thlasp.*

—**Burning.**—*Am. carb.*, **Ars.**, BOR., CALC. C., *Canth., Carb. an.,* Con., *K. carb.*, Kre., PULS., *Sul. ac.*

—**Green.**—Bov., Carb. v., MERC., *Merc. i. r., Murex,* Nat. m., **Nit. ac.**, Puls., Sec. c., Sep., *Thuj.*

—**Itching.**—Alum., Anac., Ars., CALC. C., Chin., Fer., K. carb., Kre., Merc., Pho. ac., *Sabi.,* Sep.

—**Milky.**—Am. carb., Bor., CALC. C., Calc. ph., *Carb. v., Chel.,* Con., Fer., Graph., Kre., Lyc., Nat. m., Phos., PULS., Sabi., Sep., Sil., *Sul.,* Sul. ac., Sum.

—**Offensive.**—*Aral.*, **Arg.**, **Ars.**, *Calc. ph., Calend., Carb. ac.,* Chin., *Cub., Helo.,* Kre., *Lach.,* Nat. c., **Nit. ac.**, Nux v., Sabi., Sec. c., Sep., *Thlasp.,* Ust.

—**Purulent.**—Calc. c., *Chin.*, **Cocc.**, Ign., *Kre.*, **Merc.**, Sabi., *Sec. c.,* Sep., *Sil.*

—**Slimy.**—Alum., Ambr., *Am. m.,* Ars., Bell., BOR., *Bov.,* Bry., Calc. c., Canth., Carb. an., Carb. v., *Chel.,* Cocc., Con., Fer., **Graph.**, Guai., *K. nit., Kre.,* MAG. C., Merc., **Mez.**, *Nat. m.*, **Nit. ac.**, *Nux v.,* Petrol., Phos., Pb., **Puls.**, *Sabi.,* Sars., Seneg., Sep., Stan., Sul., Sul. ac., Thuj., *Z n.*

—**Tenacious.**—Acon., Am. m., **Bor.**, **Bov.**, *Chel., Hydras., Mez.,* Nit. ac., Phos., Pho. ac., *Sabi.,* Stan., *Trill.*

—**Thick.**—Ambr., **Ars.**, **Bor.**, Bov., *Carb. v.*, Con., **Iod.**, Mag. m., *Nat. c., Nat. m.,* PULS., Sabi., Sep., Zinc.

—**Watery.**—*Am. carb.,* Ant. cr., **Ant. t.**, Arg., Ars., Carb. an., Carb. v., Cham., Chin., GRAPH., *K. iod.*, K. nit., Kre., Lil. t., Mag. c., Mag. m., Merc., Mez., PULS., **Sec. c.**, *Sep.,* Sil., *Stan.,* Sul.

—**Yellow.**—*Acon.,* Alum., **Ars.**, **Ars. iod.**, Bov., *Carb. an., Carb. v.,* Cham., Chel., Cub., Hydras., Iod., K. carb., **Kre.**, Lyc., *Murex,* Nat. c., Nit. ac., Nux v., **Pho. ac.**, Sabi., SEP., *Stan., Sul., Trill.,* Ust.

Accompanying Troubles of Leucorrhœa.—Alum., Ambr., Am. carb., Am. m., Anac., Ant. cr., *Ars.*, Bell., Bor., Bov., **Calc. c.**, Cannab. s., Canth., *Carb. an.,* Carb. v., Caust., Cham., Chin., Cocc., Con., Dros., F., Graph., Hep., *Ign.*, Iod., K. carb., K. nit., KRE., Lyc., *Mag. c.,*

Mag. m., MERC., Mez., *Nat. c.*, **NAT. M.**, Nit. ac., *Phos.*, Pho. ac., **Plat. Puls.**, Ran. b., Ruta, Sabi., Sec. c., **SEP., Sil.**, *Sul.*, *Sul. ac.*, Thuj., Zinc,

Respiration.

Anxious.—ACON., Am. carb., *Anac.*, **Ant. t.**, rn., **Ars., Bell., Bry., Camph.**, Cannab. s., **Cham.**, Chel., Cina, Coff., Colch., Croc., Fer., Hep., Ign., **IP.**, K. carb., Kre., *Lach., Laur.*, Lyc., *Nux v.*, Oleand., **Op., PHOS., Plat.,** *Pb.*, **PRU., PULS., Rhus.**, Ruta, Saba., **Samb., SEC. C.**, *Spig., Spo.*, SQU., STAN., Staph., **Stram., Ter.,** *Thuj.*, Valer., *Verat. a.*, *Vio. o.*, Vio. t.

Arrested.—Acon., *Alum.*, Am. carb, **Anac.**, *Ant. t.*, **Arn., Ars.,** Bar. c., *Bell.*, Bism., Bor., BRY., Calad., **Calc. c.**, Camph., Cannab. s., Canth., *Carb. ac.*, *Carb. an.*, Carb. v., *Carb. sul.*, Caust., Cham., CHLORUM, *Cic.*, Cina, Cocc., Coff., Croc., **Cup.**, *Cur., Dros., Euphorb.*, **Hell.,** Hep., Ign., *Ip*, *K. carb.*, K. nit., Kre., Laur., **Led.,** Lyc., *Mag. m.*, Merc., Mos., Mur. ac., *Naph., Nat. m*, Nit. ac., **Nux m**., *Op., Phos.*, Plat., Pb., **Pso., PULS.,** Ran. b., *Ran. s.*, Rhus, **Ruta**, Saba., Sabi., *Samb.*, Sele., **Sep.,** Sil., *Spig.*, Spo., *Squ.*, Stan., Staph., Stram., *Sul.*, Sul. ac., Tar., Valer., **Verat. a., Verb.**

Catching.—*Acon.*, Alum., *Apis*, Arn., **Arg. n.**, *Ars.*, *Bar. c.*, **Bell., BRY., CALAD.,** Camph., *Carb. ac.*, **Carb. an., Cham.,** *Cina, Cocc., Cup., Dig., Gel.,* Graph., *Hell.*, Ign., IP, K. carb., Kre., *Laur.*, Merc., Mos., *Mur. ac., Naj., Nit. ac*, *Nux v.*, Op., Phos., *Pb.*, *Puls.*, Sec. c., Sil., Spo., Squ., Stan., STRAM.

Cold, Hot and Offensive Breath. See under **Mouth.**

Deep.—*Acon.*, Agar., Am. carb., **Ant. cr.,** Arn., **Aur.,** Bell., BRY., Calc. c., Camph., Cannab. s., **CAPS.,** Cham., *Chin.,* Cic., *Cocc.*, Croc., **Cup.,** Dig., Dros., **Euphorb.,** Glon., *Hell.*, Hep., *Hyd. ac.*, *Ign*, IP., K. carb., Kre., LACH., Laur., Merc., MOS., Mur. ac., Nat. c., *Nux m.*, Nux v., *Oleand.*, OP., Par., Phos., *Plat.*, Pb., **Puls.,** Ran. b., Ran. s., Rhus, Sabi., Sars., *Sec. c.*, **SELE.,** Seneg., **SIL.,** Spo., **Squ.,** *Stan.*, **Stram.,** Thuj.

Irregular.—Acon., *Ant. t.*, Asar., BELL., Camph., *Canth.*, *Carb. ac.*, Cham., Chin., *Cic.*, CINA, *Cocc.*, Coff., *Crotal.*, CUP., DIG., *Dros.*, Ign., Iod., Ip., **Laur., Led.,** Mez., *Mos.*, OP., **Puls.,** Ruta, Sec. c., Sep., **Verat. a.,** Zinc.

Loud.—Acon., **Agar.,** *Alum.*, Ambr., Ant. cr., Ant. t., *Apis*, **Arn.,** Ars., Asar., Bell., Bry., Calad., **Calc. c.,** Camph., **Cannab. i.,** *Cannab. s.,* Caps., **Carb. ac.,** CHAM., CHIN., **Cimic.,** Cina, Cocc., Coloc., Dros., Dulc., Fer., *Gel.*, Glon., *Graph.*, Hep., **Hyd. ac., Hyos., Ign.,** Iod., **K.**

RESPIRATION.

carb., Laur., Lyc., Mag. m., *Mur. ac.*, **Nat. m.**, Nit. ac., **Nux v.**, **OP.**, Petrol., **Phos.**, Pb., **PULS.**, *Rheum, Rhus, Saba., Sabi.,* SAMB., *Sep., Sil., Sin.,* SPO., Squ., *Stan.,* **Stram.,** Sul., *Verat. a.*

Oppressed.—*Ab. c., Ab. n., Ac. ac.,* ACON., **Acon. f.,** *Aconin.,* **Agar.,** *All. c.,* Alum., Ambr., **Ammc.,** *Am. carb.,* Am. m., **Amyl.,** *Anac.,* **ANT. ARS.,** Ant. cr., **Ant. s., Ant. t.,** Aur., **Apis,** Arg., **Arg. n.,** Arn., **ARS.,** *Asaf.,* Asar., Aur., Bap., Bar. c., BELL., *Benz. ac.,* Bism., *Bor.,* Bov., **Brom., BRY., CACT.,** *Calad., Calc. ac.,* **Calc. c., Calc. ph.,** *Camph.,* **Cannab. i.,** *Cannab. s.,* Canth., **Caps.,** *Carb. an.,* **CARB. V.,** *Carb. sul., Caust., Cean.,* Cham., *Chel.,* **Chin.,** CHLORUM, **Cic.,** *Cina,* Coca, **Cocc., Cocc. c.,** *Coff.,* COLCH., Coloc., *Con.,* **Conv.,** Croc., **Crotal., CROT. TIG.,** *Cub.,* **CUP.,** *Cyc.,* **Dig.,** *Dirc.,* **Dros.,** Dulc., **Euphorb.,** Euphr., **FER.,** *Gel., Glon.,* Graph., *Grind.,* Guai., Hell., **Hep.,** *Hyd. ac., Hyos., Hyper.,* **IGN., IOD., IP., K. bi., K. br., K. carb., K. iod.,** *Kalm.,* **K. nit.,** Kre., Lach., *Laur.,* **Led., LOBI., Lyc., Mag. c., Mag. m.,** Mang., Mar., **Meli.,** Meny., *Meph., Merc.,* **Merc. c., Mez., Mos.,** Mur. ac., *Naph.,* **Nat. c., Nat. m.,** *Nat. s.,* Nit. ac., *Nux m.,* **NUX V.,** Oleand., **Op., Ox. ac.,** Par., Petrol., **PHOS., Pho. ac., Plat., Pb., Pru., PULS.,** Ran. b., Ran. s., Rheum, Rhodo., Rhus, *Ruta, Saba.,* Sabi., *Sal. ac.,* **Samb., Sang.,** Sars., **Sec. c.,** Sele., Seneg., **SEP.,** *Sil.,* **Spig.,** *Spo.,* **SQU., STAN.,** *Staph.,* **Stram.,** Stro., **SUL.,** Sul. ac., *Tub.,* Tar., Ter., Thuj., **Valer., VERAT. A., VERAT. V.,** Verb., *Vio. o.,* **Vio. t.,** Zinc., **Zing.,** *Ziz.*

Rapid.—ACON., **Acon. f.,** Agar., Alum., Ambr., *Am. carb.,* Anac., Ant. t., **Apoc. c.,** *Arn.,* ARS., *Asaf.,* Asar., *Aur.,* Bar. c., **BELL.,** Bor., Bov., **Brom., Bry.,** *Calc. c.,* **Calc. ph.,** *Camph.,* Cannab. s., *Canth.,* Carb. an., **CARB. V.,** Caust., *Ced., Cham.,* **Chel.,** *Chin.,* Cic., *Cina,* Cocc., *Coff.,* Coloc., Con., **Conv.,** *Crot. tig.,* **CUP.,** *Cyc.,* Dig., Dros., *Euphorb.,* Euphr., Fer., Glon., Guai., **Hep.,** *Hyos.,* Ign., **IP.,** *K. carb.,* **K. iod., K. nit.,** *Kre.,* Lach., Laur., Led., **Lob. i.,** LYC., Mag. c., **Mag. m., Merc.,** *Mez.,* **Mos., Nat. c., Nat. m.,** Nit. ac., Nux m., **Nux v., Op.,** Petrol., **PHOS., Pho. ac.,** *Plat.,* **Pb., Pru., Puls.,** Ran. b., *Rhodo.,* **Rhus,** *Ruta,* Saba., Sabi., *Samb.,* Sars., Sec. c., Seneg., **SEP., Sil.,** *Spig.,* **SPO.,** *Squ.,* **STAN.,** Staph., **Stram., SUL., Ter.,** Thuj., Verat. a., Vio. o., *Zinc.*

Rattling.—*Acon.,* Alum., **Am. carb.,** *Am. m.,* Anac., Ant. cr., **ANT. T.,** *Arn., Ars.,* **Bell., Bry.,** *Calc. c.,* Camph., Cannab. s., *Carb. an.,* Carb v., *Carb. sul., Caust.,* **Cham., Chel., Chin., Cina,** Cocc., Croc., **CUP.,** *Hyd. ac.,* Fer., **HEP., Hyos.,** Ign., **Ip., K. carb., Lach., Laur.,** *Led.,* **LYC.,** Merc., **Nat. c.,** *Nat. m.,* **Nit. ac.,** *Nux v.,* **Op.,** Par., *Petrol.,* **Phos., Puls.,** *Samb.,* **Sep.,** *Spo.,* Squ., **Stan., Stram.,** *Sul.*

RESPIRATION.

Sighing.—Acon., Agar., Am. carb., *Ant. cr.*, **Apis**, **Arg. n.**, *Bry.*, **Calc. ph.**, Camph., *Caps.*, Chin., CIMIC., **Cocc.**, Colch., *Crotal.*, DIG., *Euphorb.*, Gel., *Glon.*, Hell., *Ign.*, **Ip.**, *Lach.*, **Lob. i.**, *Naph.*, Nat. c., OP., PHOS., *Pho. ac.*, Pb., Puls., Ran. s., SEC. C., *Sele.*, Sil., SPO., **Stram.**

Slow.—Acon., Agar., Ant. cr., Arn., Asaf., *Aur.*, BELL., Bry., Calc. c., Camph., Cannab. i., Cannab. s., **Caps.**, *Carb. ac.*, Cham., *Chin.*, *Cic.*, Coff., *Croc.*, Cup., Dig., *Dros.*, Fer., *Gel.*, *Hell.*, **Hep.**, *Hydras.*, *Hyd. ac.*, *Hyos.*, Ign., Ip., K. carb., Kre., *Lach.*, *Laur.*, Lob. i., Merc., Mez., *Mos.*, Mur. ac., Nat. c., *Nux m.*, Nux v., Oleand., Op., Par., *Phos.*, *Plat.*, Pb., Puls., *Ran. b.*, Ran. s., Rhus, Ruta, Sars., Sec. c., Sele., Seneg., Sil., *Spo.*, *Squ.*, **Stan.**, Staph., Stram., Sul., Thuj., Zinc.

Sobbing.—Asaf., Calc. c., Led., Op., **Sec. c.**, Stram.

Suffocative Attacks.—*Ab. n.*, Acon., *Acon. f.*, *All. c.*, **Ambr.**, **Ammc.**, *Amyl.*, Anac., *Ant. cr.*, **Ant. t.**, Apis, **Aral.**, **Arg. n.**, Ars., Asar., Atrop., *Aur.*, Bad., **Bar. c.**, *Bell.*, **Benz. ac.**, Brom., Bry., Cact., Calad., *Calc. c.*, **Calc. ph.**, Camph., Cannab. i., *Cannab. s.*, Canth., **Caps.**, *Carb. an.*, **Carb. v.**, *Card. m.*, Caust., Cham., *Chen. a.*, Chin., Chlorum, Cic., *Cinnab.*, Cina, *Coca*, *Coc. c.*, Coc., Coff., Con., *Conv.*, *Coral.*, *Cub.*, **Cup.**, Cyc., Dig., Dros., Euphr., *Fer.*, *Gel.*, **Graph.**, *Grind.*, *Hell.*, HEP., **Hyd. ac.**, *Hyos.*, Ign., **Iod.**, IP., *K. bi.*, *K. iod.*, K. nit., Kre., LACH., *Lact.*, *Laur.*, Led., Lob. i., *Lyc.*, Mag. m., **Meli.**, *Meph.*, **Merc.**, MERC. C., *Mos.*, *Naj.*, Nat. m., Nit. ac., Nux m., Nux v., Op., **Ox. ac.**, Petrol., PHOS., **Phyt.**, *Plat.*, Pb., *Pru.*, **Puls.**, Ran. b., Rhus, *Rumex*, Saba., SAMB., Sec. c., Seneg., Sep., Sil., *Spig.*, SPO., *Stan.*, Staph., **Stram.**, **Sul.**, *Sum.*, *Tab.*, **Verat. a.**, Verat. v., Zing.

Superficial.—*Acon.*, Bell., **Cannab. i.**, *Canth.*, *Carb. ac.*, Chin., *Gel.*, Hep., Ign., Laur., *Lob. i.*, Mez., Nit. ac., Oleand., Op., PHOS., **Sil.**, Sul., Verat. a., Vio. o.

Accompanying Troubles of Respiration.—Acon., Alum., *Am. carb.*, Am. m., *Anac.*, Ant. cr., **Ant. t.**, *Arg.*, *Arn.*, ARS., *Asaf.*, Asar., Aur., Bar. c., *Bell.*, Bism., *Bor.*, Bov., **Bry.**, Calad., Calc. c., Camph., Cannab. s., Canth., Caps., *Carb. an.*, **Carb. v.**, *Caust.*, *Cham.*, Chel., **Chin.**, *Cic.*, *Cina*, Cocc., Coff., Colch., Coloc., *Con.*, Croc., CUP., Cyc., Dig., Dros., Dulc., Euphorb., Euphr., Fer., Graph., Guai., Hell., *Hep.*, Hyos., **Ign.**, Iod., IP., *K. carb.*, *K. nit.*, Kre., *Lach.*, Laur., Led., *Lyc.*, Mag. c., Mag. m., Mang., Mar., Meny., Merc., *Mez.*, Mos., Mur. ac., Nat. c., *Nat. m.*, Nit. ac., Nux m., Nux v., Oleand., *Op.*, Par., *Petrol.*, PHOS., *Pho. ac.*, *Plat.*, Pb., PULS., *Ran. b.*, Ran. s., Rheum, **Rhodo.**, Rhus, *Ruta*, Saba., **Sabi.**, *Samb.*, *Sars.*, Sec. c., Sele., Seneg., SEP., *Sil.*, Spig., *Spo.*, *Squ.*, *Stan.*, Staph., Stram., Stro., **Sul.**, Sul. ac., Tar., Thuj., Valer., **Verat. a.**, Verb., Vio. o., Vio t., Zinc.

Cough.

Cough in General.—ACON., Agar., Agn., Ail., Aloe, Alum., Ambr., Am. carb., Am. m., Ammc., Anac., Ant. cr., Ant., Arg., ARG. N., Arn., ARS., Asaf., Asar., Aur., Bar. c., Bell., Bism., Bor., Bov., Brom., BRY., Calad., CALC. C., Calc. i., Calc. ph., Camph., Cannab. i., Cannab. s., Canth., Caps., Carb. ac., Carb. an., Carb. v., Carb. sul., Caust., Cham., Chel., Chin., Cic., Cina, Cinnab., Clem., Coca, Cocc., COC. C., Cod., Coff., Colch., Coloc., Con., Croc., Crot. tig., Cub., Cup., Cyc., Dig., DROS., Dulc., Eup. per., Euphorb., Euphr., Fer., Graph., Guai., Hell., Hep., HYOS., Ign., IOD., Ip., K. bi., K. br., K. carb., K. nit., Kre., Lach., Lact., Laur., Led., Lob. i., Lyc., Mag. c., Mag. m., Mang., Mar., Meny., Merc., Merc. c., Mez., Mos., Mur. ac., Nat. c., Nat. m., Nit. ac., Nux m., Nux v., Oleand., Op., Osm., Ox. ac., Par., Petrol., PHOS., Pho. ac., Phyt., Plat., Pb., Pso., PULS., Ran. b., Ran. s., Rheum, Rhodo., RHUS, RUMEX, Ruta, Saba., Sabi., Sal. ac., Samb., SANG., Sang. n., Sars., Sec. c., Sele., Seneg., SEP., Sil., Sin., Spig., Spo., Squ., STAN., Staph., Stict., STRAM., Stro., SUL., Sul. ac., Tar., Ther., Thuj., Verat. a., Verb., Zinc.

—With Expectoration.—Acon., Aesc., Agar., Agn., Aloe, Alum., Ambr., Am. carb., Am. m., Anac., Ant. cr., Ant. t., Apis, Arg., Arn., ARS., Arum. t., Asaf., Asar., Aur., Bar. c., Bell., Bism., Bor., Bov., Bry., Calad., CALC. C., Cannab. s., Canth., Caps., Carb. an., Carb. v., Carb. sul., Caust., Cham., Chel., Chin., Cic., Cina, Cocc., Coc. c., Colch., Coloc., Con., Croc., Crot. tig., Cub., Cup., Dig., Dros., Dulc., Euphorb., EUPHR., Fer., Graph., Guai., Hep., Hyos., Ign., Iod., Ip., K. carb., K. nit., Kre., Lach., Laur., Led., LYC., Mag. c., Mag. m., Mang., Merc., Mez., Mur. ac., Nat. c., Nat. m., Nit. ac., Nux m., Nux v., Oleand., Op., Par., Petrol., PHOS., Pho. ac., Pb., PULS., Rheum, Rhodo., Rhus, Ruta, Saba., Sabi., Samb., Sec. c., Sele., Seneg., SEP., Sil., Spig., Spo., SQU., STAN., Staph., Stro., Sul., Sul. ac., Tar., Thuj., Verat. a., Zinc.

—Dry.—ACON., Aesc., Agar., ALL. C., Aloe, Alum., Ambr., Am. b., Am. carb., Am. m., Anac., Ant. cr., Ant. t., Apoc. c., Arg., Arn., Ars., Asaf., Asar., Asc. t., Aur., Bar. c., Bell., Bor., Bov., BROM., BRY., Calad., Calc. c., Calc. f., Calc. ph., Camph., Cannab. s., Canth., Caps., Carb. ac., Carb. an., Carb. v., Carb. sul., Caust., Cham., Chin., Cimic., CINA, Clem., Cod., Coc. c., Cocc., Coff., Colch., Coloc., CON., Croc., Cup., Cyc., Dig., Dios., Dros., Dulc., Eup. per., Euphorb., Euphr., Fer., Fer. ph., Graph., Guai., Hell., Hep., Hyos., Hyper., Ign., Iod., IP., K. br., K. carb., K. iod., K. nit., Kre., Lach., Laur., Led., Lyc., Mag. c., Mag. m., Mang., Mar., Merc., Mez., Mos., Mur. ac., Nat. c., NAT. M., Nit. ac., Nux m., Nux v., Oleand., Op., Osm., Ox. ac., Par.,

Petrol., **PHOS.**, PHO. AC., **Phyt.**, *Plat.*, **Pb., Pso., PULS.,** *Ran. s.,* Rheum, Rhodo., **Rhus, RUMEX,** Ruta, *Saba.,* **Sabi., Samb., SANG., Sang. n.,** Sars., Sele., **SENEG., SEP., Sil.,** *Spig.,* **SPO.,** Squ., **Stan., Staph.,** *Stict.,* **Still.,** Stram., *Stro.,* **Sul.,** *Sul. ac.,* Tar., **THUJ., Verat. a.,** Verb., Zinc., Ziz.

Convulsive.—**Agar., AMBR., Amb., Aral., Arn., Ars.,** *Bad.,* **Bell.,** *Calc. p.,* **Caps.,** *Carb ac., Carb. sul., Cereum.,* **Chel.,** *Cina,* **Coc. c., Con.,** *Coral., Croc., Crotal.,* **Cup., DROS.,** *Fer., Fer. ph., Iod.,* **Ip., K. br.,** *Lach., Lact.,* **LAUR.,** *Mos., Nat. a., Nit. ac., Op.,* **Osm.,** *Phyt.,* **Pso., Puls., Rhus, RUMEX,** *Samb.,* **SEP., Sil.,** *Spo., Squ.,* **STAN.,** *Stict., Still.,* Stram., *Thuj., Urt., Visc.,* Zinc.

Evening with, and Morning without, Expectoration.—Alum., Ant. cr., *Arg.,* **Arn., Ars., Aur.,** *Bar. c.,* **Bell., Bov., Bry.,** Calc. c., Cannab. s., Canth., *Caust., Chin.,* **Cina,** *Dig.,* **Graph.,** *Ign.,* **K. carb., K. nit.,** Kre., *Lyc.,* Mur. ac., Nat. c., *Nux v.,* Rhodo., Rhus, Ruta, Sep., Sil., Stan., Staph., Sul. ac., Thuj., Verat. a.

Morning with, and Evening without, Expectoration.—*Acon.,* Alum., **Ambr., Am. carb.,** *Am. m.,* **Ant. cr.,** *Ant. t.,* **Arn., Ars., Aur.,** Bar. c., *Bell.,* **BRY., Calc. c.,** *Caps.,* Carb. an., **CARB. V.,** *Caust.,* Cina, *Colch., Cup., Dig., Dros.,* Euphr., Fer., **HEP., Hyos.,** Ign., *Ip., K. carb.,* K. nit., Kre., Lach., Led., *Lyc.,* **Mag. c., Mag. m., Mang.,** *Mez.,* Mur. ac., Nat. c., **Nat. m., Nit. ac.,** *Nux v.,* **PAR., PHOS., Pho. ac., PULS.,** *Rheum,* Rhodo., **Rhus,** *Seneg.,* **SEP., Sil.,** *Spo.,* **SQU., Stan., Staph.,** Stro., Sul., **SUL. AC., Verat. a.,** Zinc.

Night with, Day without, Expectoration.—Alum., *Am. m.,* **Arn.,** Calc. c., *Caust.,* Euphr., Led., Phos., *Rhodo.,* SEP., **Staph.,** *Stict.,* Sul.

Day with, and Night without, Expectoration.—*Acon.,* Alum., *Am. c.,* Anac., Ant. t., *Arg., Arn.,* **ARS.,** Asaf., **Bell.,** Bry., **Calc. c., Caps.,** *Carb. an.,* **Caust., CHAM.,** *Chin.,* **Cocc.,** *Colch.,* **Con.,** Euphr., **Graph.,** Guai., **HEP., Hyos.,** *K. carb.,* Lach., **Mag. c.,** *Mag. m., Mang.,* **MERC., Nit. ac., Nux v., Op.,** Petrol., *Phos.,* **PULS.,** Rhus, **Saba., SIL.,** Squ., **Stan.,** Stro., *Sul.,* Verat. a., Zinc.

With Expectoration, which he is obliged to Swallow.—**Arn.,** Calad., *Cannab. s.,* **CAUST., Con.,** Dig., Dros., *K. carb., Lach.,* Nux v., Sep., Spo., *Staph.*

Expectoration Acrid.—Alum., Am. carb., *Am. m.,* Anac., **Ars.,** Asaf., *Aur.,* **Bell.,** Carb. v., **Caust.,** Cham., Con., Fer., *Fl. ac.,* Ign., Iod., Kre., Lach., *Laur., Lyc.,* Mag. m., **Merc.,** Mez., Nat. m., Nit. ac., *Nux v.,* **Phos., Puls.,** *Rhus,* **Sep., Sil.,** Spig., Squ., *Staph., Sul.,* Sul. ac., *Thuj., Verat. a.*

COUGH.

Expectoration, Albuminous.—*Agar.*, **Apis**, **ARG.**, Am. m., *Ant. t.*, **Arn.**, **Ars.**, Bar., Bov., Chin., COC. C., **Fer.**, **K. bi.**, **Laur.**, *Mez.*, *Nat. s.*, *Petrol.*, **PHOS.**, *Sang.*, Sele., *Seneg.*, *Sil.*, Stan.

—**Blackish.**—Chin., K. bi., *Lyc.*, *Nat. a.*, **Nux v.**, Rhus.

—**Bloody.**—Acal., **ACON.**, **Aloe**, Alum., Ambr., *Am. carb.*, Am. m., Anac., Ant. cr., *Apis*, **Aran.**, **Arn.**, **Ars.**, Asar., Aur., **Bell.**, *Bism.*, Bor., Bry., **Cact.**, **Calc. c.**, *Canth.*, Caps., *Carb. ac.*, Carb. an., Carb. v., Cham., Chin., Cina, *Cinnam.*, Con., *Coral.*, Croc., Crotal., *Crot. tig.*, *Cup.*, **Dig.**, Dros., *Dulc.*, **FER.**, *Fer. ph.*, Hep., Hyos., Iod., **IP.**, *K. carb.*, *K. nit.*, Kre., *Lach.*, Laur., Led., Lyc., **Mag. c.**, Mag. m., Mang., *Millef.*, **Merc.**, Mez., *Mur. ac.*, *Naj.*, Nat. c., **Nat. m.**, NIT. AC., *Nux m.*, *Nux v.*, *Op.*, PHOS., Pho. ac., Pb., **PULS.**, **Rhus**, *Saba.*, **Sabi.**, SEC. C., **Sele.**, **Sep.**, *Sil.*, Squ., **Stan.**, Staph., SUL., *Sul. ac.*, Tar., Thuj., Zinc.

— —**Acrid.**—*Am. carb.*, *Ars.*, *Canth.*, Carb. v., Hep., K. CARB., K. nit., Rhus, *Sars.*, SIL., Sul., Sul. ac., Zinc.

— —**Bright.**—ACON., Am. carb., **Arn.**, Ars., **BELL.**, Bor., Bry., *Dulc. c.*, Canth., Carb. an., *Carb. v.*, Chin., Cob., Dig., Dros., DULC., Fer., HYOS., *Ip.*, *K. nit.*, Kre., *Laur.*, **Led.**, Mag. m., Meli., *Merc.*, Nat. c., **Nux m.**, Phos., Puls., Rhus, *Saba.*, SABI., Sec. c., Sep., Sil., Sul., *Zinc.*

— —**Brownish.**—BRY., *Calc. c.*, **Carb. v.**, Con., Puls., *Rhus.*

— —**Clotted.**—*Arn.*, Bell., Bry., *Canth.*, Carb. an., *Caust.*, CHAM., Chin., Con., *Croc.*, Fer., Hyos., **Ip.**, Kre., *Mag. m.*, Merc., Nit. ac., **Nux v.**, *Pho. ac.*, Puls., RHUS, Sabi., Sec. c., Sep., *Spo.*, *Stram.*, *Stro.*, *Sul.*

— —**Dark.**—Acon., **Am. carb.**, **Ant. cr.**, *Arn.*, **Asar.**, *Bell.*, Bism., Bry., *Canth.*, Carb. v., CHAM., *Chin.*, Con., CROC., *Cup.*, Dig., Dros., *Caps.*, Fer., K. nit., **Kre.**, Led., *Lyc.*, **Mag. c.**, Mag. m., Nit. ac., *Nux v.*, NUX V., Phos., *Pho. ac.*, Puls., Sec. c., *Sele.*, Sep., Stan., *Sul.*

— —**Tenacious.**—CROC., **Cup.**, Mag. c., Sec. c.

—**Blood-streaked.**—Acon., Alum., *Am. carb.*, **Arn.**, Ars., Bad., *Bism.*, Bor., BRY., *Caust.*, CHIN., Cina, *Cinnab.*, Cocc., Con., **Crotal.**, *Cub.*, Dros., Dulc., Euphr., FER., *Fer. ph.*, Iod., **Ip.**, **K. carb.**, K. bi., Kre., Laur., Lyc., **Merc. c.**, *Nat. m.*, Nit. ac., Nux m., *Op.*, Phos., *Puls.*, *Sabi.*, *Sang. n.*, Sec. c., **Sele.**, Sep., Sil., Spo., Squ., **Stan.**, Sul. ac., *Ter.*, Zinc.

—**Cold.**—*Asaf.*, Bry., Cannab. s., *Caust.*, CORAL., *K. carb.*, Merc., Nit. ac., Nux v., **Phos.**, Rhus., Sul., *Verat. a.*

—**Frothy.**—*Ant. t.*, *Apis*, Arn., **Ars.**, *Canth.*, Cob., **Fer.**, Hep., *Ip.*, K. iod., Led., Merc., Nux v., Op., **Phos.**, Pb., **Puls.**, *Sil.*, Sul.

—**Gelatinous.**—*Aloe*, **ARG.**, *Arn.*, Bar. c., *Bry.*, Chin., Dig., **Fer.**, Laur.

COUGH.

Expectoration, Granular.—*Agar.*, **Bad.**, *Calc, ac.*, Chin., **Coc. c.**, **K. bi.**, Merc. i. r., *Nat. a.*, **Phos.**, *Pho. ac.*, *Sal. ac.*, **Sele.**, **Seneg.**, **Sep.**, **SIL.**, STAN.

—**Gray.**—AMBR., Anac., ARG., **Ars.**, *Calc. c.*, *Carb. an.*, *Chin.*, *Cinnab.*, *Coc. c.*, *Dig.*, *K. bi.*, K. carb., Kre., LYC., Mang., *Nat. ars.*, *Nux v.*, Phos., Rhus, **Seneg.**, *Sep.*, STAN., Thuj.

—**Green.**—*Ars.*, Asaf., Aur., Bor., Bov., Calc. c., *Calc. iod.*, Cannab. s., Carb. an., *Carb. v.*, Colch., Dros., *Dulc.*, *Fer.*, Hyos., Iod., *K. bi.*, K. carb., K. iod., *Kre.*, Led., Lyc., Mang., Merc., **Merc. i. r.**, **Nat. c.**, Nit. ac., Nux v., Par., *Phos.*, Pb., PSO., PULS., Rhus, Sang. n., Sep., Sil., STAN., Sul., Thuj.

—**Hardened.**—Agar., Am. m., Ant. cr., **Bry.**, Calad., **Coca**, *Coc. c.*, Con., Hep., Iod., K. bi., *K. carb.*, Kre., Lach., Mang., NAT. C., *Phos.*, *Puls.*, *Sal. ac.*, *Sang.*, Sang. n., Sep., Sil., Spo., Stan., Staph., Stro., *Sul.*, Thuj.

—**Milky.**—Am. carb., **Ars.**, *Aur.*, Carb. v., Fer., *Phos.*, *Puls.*, *Sep.*, *Sil.*, Sul.

—**Offensive Odor.**—Alum., **Ars.**, Asaf., *Aur.*, **Bell.**, BOR., CALC. C., Caps., *Carb. ac.*, Caust., Chin., *Cinnab.*, *Con.*, *Cub.*, *Graph.*, GUAI., Hep., *Iris v.*, *Kre.*, Led., Lyc., *Mag. m.*, Merc., NAT. C., *Nit. ac.*, *Nux v.*, Phel., **Pho. ac.**, *Pso.*, *Puls.*, Rhus, *Sabi.*, **Sep.**, **Sil.**, **Stan.**, **Sul.**, Thuj.

—**Orange-colored.**—K. carb., Phos., *Puls.*

—**Purulent.**—Acon., Am. carb., Anac., Arg., *Ars.*, Asaf., *Aur.*, Bell., Bry., CALC. C., *Calc. iod.*, *Carb. ac.*, Carb. an., Carb. v., Cham., CHIN., Cic., Cina, *Cinnab.*, *Cocc.*, **Cod.**, CON., *Coral.*, *Cup.*, Dros., Dulc., **Fer.**, *Grind.*, Graph., *Guai.*, *Hep.*, Hyos., Ign., Ip., K. CARB., **K. nit.**, Kre., Lach., *Led.*, LYC., Mag. c., Mag. m., Merc., **Nat. c.**, Nat. m., *Nit. ac.*, Nux m., Nux v., PHOS., Pho. ac., **Pb.**, *Puls.*, Rhus, Ruta, *Sabi.*, Samb., Sec. c., SEP., SIL., Stan., Staph., Stro., *Sul.*, Zinc.

—**Slimy.**—Acon., Agar., Agn., Ail., Alum., Ambr., *Am. b.*, Am. carb., *Am. m.*, Amnc., Ant. cr., Ant. t., **Arg.**, Arn., ARS., Asar., Aur., Bar. c., **Bell.**, *Bism.*, Bor., Bov., **Bry.**, CALC. C., Cannab. s., Canth., Caps., Carb. an., *Carb. v.*, *Caust.*, *Cham.*, CHIN., **Cina**, Cocc., **Coc. c.**, **Cod.**, Croc., *Crot. tig.*, Cup., *Dig.*, DROS., Dulc., EUPHR., *Fer.*, Graph., *Hep.*, Hyos., **Iod.**, Ip., *Iris v.*, *K. carb.*, K. nit., Kre., LACH., **Laur.**, LYC., *Mag. c.*, Mag. m., *Menth.*, Merc., **Merc. i. r.**, Mez., *Naj.*, **Nat. c.**, Nat. m., Nat. s., NIT. AC., Nux m., **Nux v.**, Oleand., *Op.*, *Osm.*, PAR., PHOS., *Pho. ac.*, *Pb.*, PSO., PULS., Rhodo., Rhus, **Rumex**, Ruta, Saba., Sabi., *Samb.*, Sang. n., Sec. c., **Sele.**, **Seneg.**, *Sep.*, *Sil.*, Spig., Spo., SQU., Stan., **Staph.**, *Sul.*, Sul. ac., Tar., Thuj., Verat. a., **Zinc**.

—**Tenacious.**—Acon., *Aesc.*, Agn., *Alum.*, **Am. b.**, Am. m., Amnc.,

COUGH.

Ant. cr., Ant. t., **ARG., Ars., Arum. t., Bad.,** Bar. c., *Bor.,* **BOV.,** *Bry.,* **Calc. c., Cannab. s.,** *Canth.,* Carb. v., *Caust.,* **Cham.,** Chin., **Coca,** Cocc., **COC. C.,** Colch., *Crot. tig., Dig.,* **Dros.,** *Dulc.,* Euphr., **Graph.,** *Hydras.,* *Iod.,* K. BI., *K. carb., Mag. m.,* **Mez.,** *Naj.,* Nat. c., Nux v., **Op.,** *Osm.,* **Par.,** Petrol., **PHOS.,** *Pho. ac., Phyt., Pb.,* **Puls.,** *Saba., Sabi.,* **Samb.,** SENEG., *Sep., Sil.,* Spig., *Spo.,* Squ., **STAN.,** Staph., *Verat. a.,* **Zinc.**

Expectoration, Watery.—Agar., Am. carb., Am. m., *Arg., Ars.,* Bov., Carb. an., *Carb. v.,* **Cham.,** Chin., *Dig.,* **Fer., Graph.,** Guai., *Lach., Laur.,* **Mag. c.,** *Mag. m., Merc.,* **Mez.,** Mur. ac., Nux v., Pb., Puls., *Seneg.,* Sep., *Sil.,* Squ., **Stan.,** *Sul.*

—**Whitish.**—*Acon.,* Ambr., **Am. b.,** *Am. m., Ant. t., Arg., Cina, Cob., Coc. c., Crot. tig.,* **K. bi.,** *Kre.,* Laur., **LYC.,** *Merc., Naj.,* Par., **Phos.,** Pho. ac., Rhus, *Seneg.,* **SEP.,** Sil., Spo., *Squ.,* Stro., *Sul.*

—**Yellow.**—Acon., *Aloe, Alum.,* Ambr., Am. carb., **Am. m.,** Anac., Ant. cr., Arg., **Ars.,** *Aur., Bar. c.,* Bell., *Bism.,* Bor., *Bov.,* **Bry.,** CALC, C., Carb. an., **Carb. v.,** Caust., Cham., Cic., **Coca,** *Coc. c.,* Con., *Crot. tig., Cub., Dig.,* **Dros.,** Graph., Hep., *Hydras.,* Ign., *Iod.,* Ip., **K. bi.,** *K. carb.,* **Kre.,** Lyc., *Mag. c.,* Mag. m., *Mang.,* **Merc.,** Mez., Mur. ac., **Nat. c.,** *Nat. m., Nit. ac.,* Nux v., Op., Par., **PHOS.,** *Pho. ac.,* Pb., PULS., Ruta, *Saba., Sabi., Sal. ac.,* **Sang. n.,** *Sele.,* Seneg., **Sep., Sil.,** Spig., **Spo.,** **STAN.,** Staph., *Sul., Sul. ac.,* Thuj., *Verat. a.,* Zinc.

Taste of the Expectoration like Old Catarrh.—*Bell., Ign.,* Mez., *Nux v., Phos.,* **PULS.,** Sabi., **Sul.,** Zinc.

—**Bitter.**—Acon., Arn., **Ars.,** *Bry.,* Calc. c., **CHAM.,** Chin., Con., Dros., Ign., K. carb., Lyc., *Merc.,* Nat. c., Nat. m., Nit. ac., *Nux v.,* **PULS.,** Saba., *Sep.,* Stan., Sul., *Verat. a.*

—**Burnt.**—*Bry., Cyc., Nux v.,* **Puls.,** *Ran. b., Saba.,* Squ., Sul.

—**Fatty.**—*Alum.,* **Asaf.,** CAUST., Cham., *Fl. ac., K. carb., Lyc.,* **Mag. m.,** *Mang., Merc. c.,* Mur. ac., Petrol., Phos., PULS., *Rhus, Suba., Sabi.,* Sil., Thuj.

—**Flat.**—Alum., *Am. m., Ant. cr., Arg.,* Arn., *Ars.,* Aur., *Bell.,* **Bry.,** Calc. c., *Caps.,* **Chin.,** Euphr., **Ign.,** Ip., K. carb., *Kre., Lyc.,* Nat. c., *Nat. m.,* **Par.,** Petrol., Phos., Pho. ac., *Puls.,* Rhus, Sabi., Stan., **Staph.,** Stro., *Sul.,* Thuj.

—**Foul.**—*Acon.,* **Arn., Ars., Bell.,** Bov., Bry., Calc. c., *Caps.,* Carb. an., **Carb. v.,** *Caust.,* **Cham.,** Cocc., *Con., Cup., Dig.,* Dros., Fer., *Iod.,* Ip., K. carb., *Lach.,* Lyc., *Merc., Nit. ac., Nux v.,* Phos., **Puls.,** *Rhus, Samb.,* Sep., **STAN.,** Staph., *Sul.,* Verat. a., Zinc.

—**Garlicky.**—Asaf.

—**Herby.**—Calad., **Nux v., Pho. ac., Puls.,** *Sars., Stan., Verat. a.*

Taste of Expectoration Metallic.—*Aga.*, *Alum.*, *Am. carb.*, *Bism.*, Calc. c., *Cocc.*, *Coloc.*, Cup., Fer., *Hep.*, Ip., Nat. c., *Nux v.*, *Ran. b.*, Rhus, *Sars.*, *Seneg.*, *Sul.*, Zinc.

—**Mouldy.**—BOR.

—**Nauseous.**—Ars., Asaf., *Bry.*, *Calc. c.*, Canth., Chin., Cina, Cocc., *Coc. c.*, *Dros.*, Iod., Ip., *K. carb.*, Led., Merc., *Nat. m.*, *Nux v.*, Phos., PULS., Saba., Samb., Sele., *Sep.*, Squ., Stan., Sul., *Zinc.*

—**Salty.**—Alum., *Ambr.*, Am. carb., *Ant. t.*, ARS., Bar. c., Bell., Bov., *Bry.*, *Calc. c.*, Cannab. s., *Carb. v.*, Chin., *Cocc.*, Con., Dros., Euphorb., *Graph.*, Hyos., *Iod.*, Lach., LYC., Mag. c., Mag. m., **Merc.**, **Nat. c.**, Nat. m., *Nat. s.*, Nit. ac., Nux m., Nux v., PHOS., Pho. ac., PULS., *Rhus*, SEP., Stan., *Sul.*, Sul. ac., Tar., *Verat. a.*

—**Sour.**—Ambr., Ant. t., Ars., **Bell.**, Bry., CALC. C., Carb. an., Carb. v., *Cham.*, Chin., *Coc. c.*, Con., *Crot. tig.*, Graph., *Hep.*, *Ign.*, Ip., **K. carb.**, *Lyc.*, Mag. m., Merc., Nat. c., *Nat. m.*, Nit. ac., NUX V., *Petrol.*, PHOS., *Pho. ac.*, Pb., **Puls.**, Rhus, Sabi., Sep., *Stan.*, Sul., **Tar.**

—**Sweetish.**—*Aesc.*, Acon., *All. c.*, *Alum.*, Am. carb., *Ant. t.*, *Ant. s. aur.*, *Ars.*, Asar., Aur., **Calc. c.**, Canth., Chin., *Cocc.*, *Coc. c.*, *Dig.*, *Dirc.*, Fer., Hep., Iod., Ip., *Iris v.*, *K. carb.*, Kre., Laur., *Lyc.*, Merc., *Nux v.*, PHOS., **Pb.**, Puls., *Rhus*, **Saba.**, *Samb.*, **Sang. n.**, Sele., *Sep.*, **Squ.**, STAN., Sul., Sul. ac., Zinc.

—**Of Tobacco Juice.**—Puls.

Troubles Associated with Cough.—Acon., Alum., *Ambr.*, *Am. carb.*, Am. m., *Anac.*, Ant. cr., *Ant. t.*, **Arg.**, Arn., Ars., Asaf., Asar., Aur., Bar. c., BELL., Bism., Bor., BRY., Calad., Calc. c., Camph., Cannab s., Canth., CAPS., *Carb. an.*, **Carb. v.**, *Caust.*, *Cham.*, **Chel.**, **Chin.**, Cina, Cocc., Coff., Colch., Coloc., *Con.*, Croc., *Cup.*, Dig., DROS., Dulc., Euphorb., Euphr., **Fer.**, Graph., Guai., Hell., **Hep.**, *Hyos.*, Ign., Iod., IP., **Iris v.**, *K. carb.*, **K. nit.**, *Kre.*, Lach., Laur., Led., *Lyc.*, Mag. m., **Mang.**, Mar., Meny., MERC., Mez., Mos., Mur. ac., *Nat. c.*, **Nat. m.**, **Nit. ac.**, Nux m., NUX V., Oleand., Op., *Osm.*, Par., Petrol., PHOS., *Pho. ac.*, Pb., PULS., Rhodo., RHUS, Ruta, *Saba.*, Sabi., *Samb.*, Sars., Sec. c., Sele., *Seneg.*, SEP., **Sil.**, Spig., SPO., **Squ.**, STAN., Staph., Stro., **Sul.**, Sul. ac., Thuj., Valer., **Verat. a.**, Verb., Zinc.

Before and After Coughing and After Expectoration. See under **Aggravations.**

Air-Passages.

Larynx.—Ac. ac., Acon., *Aesc.*, Agar., ALL. C., *Alum.*, *Alumen*, *Ambr.*, Am. carb., Am. m., Anac., *Ant. cr.*, *Ant. t.*, *Ant. s.*, *Aur.*, **Apis**, **Arg.**, Arg. n., Arn., Ars., Ars. iod., Arum. t., Asar., Bap., Bar. c., BELL.

AIR-PASSAGES. 121

Berb., Bor., Bov., BROM., *Bry.*, **Calad.**, *Calc. c.*, *Calc. f.*, Camph., Cannab. s., **Canth.**, Caps., Carb. an., Carb. v., *Carb. sul.*, **Caust.**, Cham., *Chel.*, *Chin.*, Chlorum., *Chrom. ac.*, Cic., **Cimic.**, Cina, *Cinnab.*, *Cit. ac.*, *Coca*, Cocc., *Coc. c.*, *Cod.*, **Coff.**, Colch., *Con.*, *Crotal.*, *Cub.*, **Cup.**, Dig., DROS., *Dub.*, Dulc., *Eup. per.*, *Euphr.*, Fer., *Fl. ac.*, Gel., *Glon.*, *Graph.*, Guai., Hell., **Hep.**, *Hydras.*, Hyos., *Ign.*, IOD., **Ip.**, **K. bi.**, *K. br.*, *K carb.*, **K. iod.**, *K. nit.*, Kre., **LACH.**, **Lact.**, Laur., *Lob. i.*, Lyc., Mag. c. *Mag. m.*, **Mang.**, *Meny.*, Merc., *Merc. c.*, *Merc. cy.*, **Mez.**, *Mos.*, Mur. ac., *Naj.*, *Nat. m.*, *Nit. ac.*, Nux m., **NUX V.**, Oleand., Op., **Osm.**, *Ox. ac.*, **Par.**, Petrol., **PHOS.**, *Pho. ac.*, *Phyt.*, Plat., Pb., *Pso.*, **PULS.**, Rhodo., *Rhus*, *Rumex*, Ruta, **Saba.**, *Sabi.*, *Samb.*, *Sang.*, *Sang. n.*, *Sele.*, **Seneg.**, *Sep.*, *Sil.*, Spig., **SPO.**, *Squ.*, **Stan.**, Staph., *Stram.*, Stro., **Sul.**, Sul. ac., Tar., Thuj., **Verat. a.**, Verb., *Wye.*, Zinc.

Trachea.—*Acon.*, Agar., Alum., Ambr., *Am. carb.*, Am. m., Anac., Ant. cr., *Arg.*, *Arn.*, Ars., Asar., Bar. c., **Bell.**, Bor., Bov., BROM., Bry., **Calad.**, Calc. c., Camph., **Cannab. s.**, *Canth.*, Caps., Carb. an., **Carb. v.**, *Caust.*, Cham., *Chin.*, Cic., Cina, Cocc., *Coc. c.*, Coff., Con., Cup., *Dig.*, Dros., *Eup. per.*, Euphorb., *Fer.*, Graph., **Hep.**, Hyos., Ign., **Iod.**, **Ip.**, *K. carb.*, *K. nit.*, *Kalm.*, Kre., *Lach.*, **Laur.**, *Led.*, Lyc., Mag. c., Mag. m., *Mang.*, **Mar.**, Merc., *Mez.*, Mos., Mur. ac., Nat. c., *Nat. m.*, **Nit. ac.**, NUX V., *Osm.*, **Par.**, Petrol., PHOS., *Pho. ac.*, Plat., Pb., **PULS.**, Rhodo., Rhus, **Rumex**, Saba., Sabi., Samb., *Sang.*, Sars., **Seneg.**, Sep., *Sil.*, SPO., Squ., **STAN.**, Staph., *Still.*, Stro., **Sul.**, Sul. ac., *Thuj.*, *Verat. a.*, Verb., *Zinc.*, Zing.

Secretion of Mucus.—Agn., Alum., *Ambr.*, Am. carb., Am. m., Ant. cr., **Ant. s. aur.**, *Ant. t.*, *Arg.*, ARG. N., Arn., Ars., Asar., *Aesc. c.*, Aur., Bar. c., Bell., Bism., Bor., Bov., **Bry.**, *Cact.*, **Calc. c.**, Camph., Cannab. s., Canth., *Caps.*, **Carb. ac.**, *Carb. an.*, Carb. v., Caust., *Cham.*, Chin., Chrom. ac., *Cina*, *Coca*, Cocc., **Coc. c.**, Coff., Colch., Con., *Cop.*, Croc., Cup., Dig., *Dros.*, Dulc., Euphorb., Graph., *Grind.*, Guai., Hep., **Hydras.**, Hyos., Ign., *Iod.*, IP., K. BI., **K. carb.**, K. nit., Kre., Lach., *Laur.*, **LYC.**, Mag. c., Mag. m., Mang., Mar., Merc., Mez., *Mos.*, Nat. c., Nat. m., **Nit. ac.**, *Nux m.*, *Nux v.*, Oleand., Op., **Osm.**, *Pœo.*, **Par.**, Petrol., **Phyt.**, PHOS., *Pho. ac.*, Plat., Pb., **Puls.**, Ran. b., Rhodo., Rhus, Ruta, Saba., Sabi., **Samb.**, Sars., Sele., *Senec.*, SENEG., *Sep.*, **Sil.**, Spig., Squ., **Stan.**, Staph., *Sul.*, Sul. ac., Tar., Thuj., Valer., *Verat. a.*, Verb., Zinc.

Voice not Clear.—Agar., *Am. carb.*, Anac., Ant. cr., Bar. c., Bell., Bry., *Calc. c.*, Camph., Carb. an., *Carb. v.*, **Caust.**, *Cham.*, Chin., Croc., Cup., Dros., Graph., *Hep.*, Hyos., **Mang.**, Menth., MERC., Nat. m. *Nux m.*, *Nux v.*, PHOS., Saba., Sars., **Sele.**, Spo., Stan., *Sul.*, Verb.

6*

AIR-PASSAGES.

Voice Croaking.—Acon., Ars., *Cinc*, Lach., Ruta, STRAM.

—**Deep.**—Arn., *Bar. c.*, Cham., **Chin.**, DROS., *Iod., Laur., Par.*

—**Hoarse.**—Acon., Agn., **ALL. C.**, *Aloe*, Alum., **Ambr.**, Am. carb., Am. m., Anac., *Ant. cr., Ant. t., Apis,* ARG. N., Arn., Ars., Asaf., ARUM. T., *Bar. c.*, BELL., *Bov.*, BROM., *Bry.*, *Calad.*, Calc. c., *Calc f.,* Calc. ph., Camph., Cannab. s., *Canth.*, **Caps.**, *Carb. an.*, CARB. V., *Carb. sul.,* Caust., Cham., Chel., Chin., *Cic.*, Cina, *Cinnab.*, *Coca,* Coc. c., Coff., Colch., Con., *Cop.*, Croc., *Cub.,* Cup., Dig., DROS., Dulc., *Eup. per.*, Fer., Graph., Hep., Hyos., Ign., IOD., K. BI., *K. carb.*, K. nit., Kre., Lach., *Laur.*, Led., Lyc., Mag. c., Mag. m., MANG., *Meny.*, Merc., Merc. i. r., Mez., *Mur. ac., Naj.*, Nat. c., Nat. m., Nit. ac., Nux m., Nux v., Oleand., Op., Osm., *Ox. ac.*, Par., Petrol., PHOS., Pho. ac., *Phyt.*, Plat., *Pb.*, Puls., Rhodo., Rhus, Ruta, *Saba.*, Samb., *Sang. n.*, Sec. c., Sele., Seneg., *Sep.*, Sil., Spig., SPO., STAN., Staph., *Stict.,* STRAM., Stro., Sul., Sul. ac., Tar., TELL., Thuj., **Verat. a., Verb.**, Zinc.

—**Hollow.**—Acon., *Ant. t.*, Ars., Bar. c., Bell., *Camph., Carb. v., Caust.,* Chin., Cina, Dig., Dros., Euphorb., *Hep., Ign.*, **Ip.**, Kre., Led., Nux m., *Op.*, Phos., Samb., *Sec. c.*, Sil., *Spig.*, SPO., **Stan.**, *Staph., Stram.*, VERAT. A., *Verb.*

—**Hissing.**—Bell., **Nux v.**, *Phos.*

—**Interrupted.**—Ars., Cic., Dros., Euphr., Mag. c., Spo.

—**Lost.**—*Ac. ac.*, Acon., *Ambr., Ant. cr., Ars.*, **Bar. c.**, Bell., *Bov.*, BROM., *Bry.*, *Calc. c.*, Camph., *Cannab. s., Canth., Carb. an.*, CARB. V., Caust., *Cham., Chen. a., Chin., Cod.*, Cup., Dig., **Dros.**, Gel., *Graph.,* Hep., Hyos., *Iod., K. br., K. carb.*, **K. iod.**, Lach., *Laur., Mang., Meny.*, Merc., Mur. ac., *Nat. c.*, Nat. m., Nit. ac., Nux m., Nux v., Oleand., Op., Petrol., PHOS., *Plat., Pb.*, Puls., Rhus, *Rumex*, Ruta, Saba., Samb., *Sang.*, Sele., Seneg., Sep., Sil., **Spo.**, Stan., Stram., *Sul.*, **Verat. a.**, Verb.

—**Murmuring.**—Hyos., Lach., Op., *Stram.*

—**Nasal.**—Bell., Bry., *Lach.*, Pho. ac., Staph.

—**Raised.**—*Cannab. i.*, Cup., Stan., STRAM.

—**Rough.**—*Aloe*, Alum., Ambr., Bor., Bry., *Calc. c.*, Carb. v., **Caust.**, *Cham.*, Chin., Coff., *Dros., Hep.*, **Hyos.**, *Iod.*, K. BI., *K. carb.*, K. nit., Kre., Lach., *Laur., Mang.*, Meny., Merc., Mez., *Nux m.*, **Nux v.**, PHOS., Pho. ac., *Pb.*, Puls., *Rhus*, Sars., Seneg., Spo., Stan., Staph., Stram., *Stro.*, Sul., *Sul. ac.*, Thuj., Verb., *Zinc.*

—**Shrieking (and Squeaking).**—Cup., *Laur.*, STRAM.

—**Soft (and Weak).**—Acon., **Ant. cr.**, *Ant. t.*, Bell., Camph., *Can-*

n&b. s., CANTH., *Caust.*, Cham., Chin., Fer., Gel., **HEP.**, Ign., Laur., Lyc., Mos., Nux v., Op., Par., Phos., Puls., Sec. c., Spo., *Stan.*, **Staph.**, Stram., VERAT. A.

Voice Toneless.—Agn., *Ambr.*, **Calad.**, Carb. an., *Chin.*, Cina, DROS., *Hep.*, Nat. c., Rhodo., Samb., *l o.*, STRAM.

—**Tremulous.**—*Acon.*, Ars., **Camph.**, Canth., *Cup.*, **Ign.**, **Merc.**, Nux m.

External Throat and Neck.

Throat, External.—*Acon.*, *Agar.*, Agn., *Alum.*, Am. carb., **Am. m.**, **Amyl.**, Anac., *Ant. cr.*, Ant. t., *Arg.*, **Arn.**, **Ars.**, Asaf., **Asar.**, Aur., *Bap.*, Bar. c., **BELL.**, *Berb.*, Bism., Bor., Bov., **Bry.**, **Calc. c.**, *Calc. ph.*, Camph., Cannab. s., *Canth.*, Caps., Carb. ac., Carb. an., *Carb. v.*, **Caust.**, Cham., **Chel.**, *Chin.*, **Cic.**, Cina, Clem., *Cocc.*, Coff., Colch., *Coloc.*, *Con.*, Croc., Cup., **Cyc.**, *Dig.*, Dulc., Euphorb., Fer., **Gel.**, **Graph.**, Guai., Hell., **Hep.**, Hyos., *Ign.*, **Iod.**, Ip., *K. carb.*, K. nit., *Kalm.*, Kre., **Lach.**, Laur., Led., **LYC.**, Mag. c., Mag. m., **Mang.**, Mar., Meny., **Merc.**, *Mez.*, Mos., Mur. ac., *Nat. c.*, Nat. m., *Nit. ac.*, Nux v., **Oleand.**, Op., *Par.* Petrol., **Phos.**, *Pho. ac.*, **Phyt.**, **Plat.**, Pb, **Puls.**, Ran. s., Rheum, *Rhodo.* Rhus, Ruta, *Sabi.*, Samb., *Sars.*, Sec. c., Sele., *Sep.*, *Sil.*, *Spig.*, **Spo.**, Squ., Stan., **Staph.**, Stro., *Sul.*, Sul. ac., **Tar.**, Thuj., *Verat. a.*, Verb. Vio. o., Zinc.

Nape.—Acon., Aesc., Agar., Agn., *Alum.*, Ambr., *Am. carb.*, **Am. m.**, Anac., *Ant. cr.*, Ant. t., Arg., **Arn.**, *Ars.*, Asaf., **Asar.**, Aur., **BAR. C.**, **Bell.**, Bar., Bov., **BRY.**, **CALC. C.**, Camph., Cannab. s., **Canth.**, Caps., Carb. an., **Carb. v.**, **Caust.**, Cham., Chin., *Cic.*, **CIMIC.**, Cina., Clem., *Coca*, Cocc., Colch., *Coloc.*, Con., Croc., Cup., *Cyc.*, Dig., Dros., *Dulc.*, Euphr., Fer., *Glon.*, **Graph.**, Guai., Hell., Hep., *Hyos.*, **Ign.**, Iod., Ip. K. carb., *K. nit.*, **Lach.**, *Laur.*, Led., **Lyc.**, *Mag. c.*, Mag. m., **Mang.**, Meny., **Merc.**, *Mez.*, Mos., **Nat. c.**, Nat. m., *Nit. ac.*, Nux m., **NUX V.**, Oleand., Op., *Par.*, *Petrol.*, *Phos.*, **Pho. ac.**, *Pic. ac.*, **Plat.**, Pb, **PULS.**, Ran. b., Rheum, Rhodo., **RHUS**, Ruta, Saba., *Sabi.*, Samb., *Sang.*, *Sars.*, Sec. c., **Sele.**, **Sep.**, **Sil.**, *Spig.*, **Spo.**, Squ., *Stan.*, **STAPH.**, Stro., **Sul.**, Tar., **Thuj.**, Valer., *Verat. a.*, Vio. o., Vio. t., Zinc.

Cervical and Submaxillary Glands.—Agn., *Alum.*, *Ambr.*, Am. carb., *Am. m.*, *Ant. cr.*, Ant. t., Arg., **Arn.**, *Ars.*, Asaf., Asar., **Aur.**, **ARUM. T.**, **BAR. C.**, **BELL.**, Bor., *Bov.*, *Bry.*, Calad., **Calc. c.**, *Calc. iod.*, *Calc. ph.*, Camph., *Canth.*, Caps., **Carb. an.**, Carb. v., Caust., **Cham.**, Chin., *Cic.*, Cina, **Clem.**, *Cocc.*, **Con.**, Coral., Crot. tig., Cup., Cyc., *Dulc.*, Euphorb., Fer., **Graph.**, Hell., Hep., Hyos., Ign., Iod., **K. carb.**, *K. chl.*, *K. iod.*, Kre., *Lach.*, Lyc., Mag. c., Mag. m., **MERC.**, Merc. c.,

Merc. i. r., Mez., Mur. ac., Nat. c., *Nat. m.*, **Nit. ac.**, *Nux v.*, Par., *Petrol.*, *Phos.*, *Pho. ac.*, Pb., **Pso.**, *Puls.*, *Ran. s.*, RHUS, Saba., Sars., Sele., Seneg., *Sep.*, Sil., Spig., **Spo.**, Squ., *Stan.*, STAPH., *Still.*, Stram, **Sul.**, *Sul. ac.*, Thuj., *Verat. a.*, Vio. t., Zinc.

Thyroid Gland.—Ambr., Am. carb., Bell., *Calc. c.*, **Calc. fl.**, *Carb. an.*, Caust., Con., Dig., *Fer.*, *Fl. ac.*, IOD., K. carb., *K. iod.*, Lyc., Mag. c., *Merc.*, **Nat. c.**, *Nat. m.*, Petrol., Phos., *Plat.*, *Sil.*, SPO., Sul.

Neck and Nape of Neck.

Left Side.—*Acon.*, Agn., Alum., *Am. m.*, *Anac.*, APIS, *Ant. cr.*, Arg., *Arn.*, Ars., ASAF., **Asar.**, Aur., *Bar. c.*, Bell., *Bor.*, *Bov.*, *Brom.*, *Bry.*, CALC. C., *Canth.*, *Carb. an.*, *Carb. v.*, Caust., *Cic.*, Cocc., Colch., *Coloc.*, *Croc.*, *Cyc.*, Fl. ac., *Guai.*, *Hyos.*, *Ign.*, K. carb., *Lach.*, Laur., Lyc., Mar., Merc., Mez., *Mos.*, *Nux v.*, Oleand., *Par.*, Pho. ac., *Pso.*, Rhodo., *Rhus*, Sabi., **Sele.**, *Sep.*, Sil., Spig., Spo., Squ., *Staph.*, **Stram.**, SUL., *Sul. ac.*, Tar., Thuj., *Verat. a.*, *Vio. t.*, Zinc.

Right Side.—Agn., *Alum.*, **Am. carb.**, Anac., Ant. cr., *Ant. t.*, Apis, *Arg.*, Asaf., Aur., **Bell.**, **Bism.**, Bry., *Calc. c.*, *Camph.*, Canth., *Caps.*, Carb. v., CAUST., *Chel.*, *Chin.*, *Cina*, Cocc., Colch., Coloc., **Con.**, *Cup.*, *Dulc.*, FL. AC., Guai., **Hep.**, **Iod.**, **K. carb.**, *K. nit.*, Lach., Laur., Led., Lyc., Mar., *Meny.*, MERC., Mez., *Nat. c.*, *Nat. m.*, NIT. AC., Nux v., Oleand., *Petrol.*, Pho. ac., *Plat.*, Pb., *Puls.*, Rhodo., Sabi., **Sars.**, Seneg., Sil., *Spig.*, Spo., Staph., *Sul.*, **Sul. ac.**, Thuj., Zinc.

Chest.

Internal.—*Abrot.*, *Ac. ac.*, Acon., **Aesc.**, *Agar.*, Agn., *Aloe*, *Alum.*, Ambr., **Amnc.**, *Am. carb.*, *Am. m.*, *Amyl.*, Anac., Ant. ars., Ant. cr., *Ant. s aur.*, ANT. T., **Apis**, *Apoc. c.*, Arg., **Arn.**, **Ars.**, Ars. iod., Arum. t., *Asaf.*, *Asar.*, Asc. t., Aur., *Bap.*, **Bar. c.**, Bell., Bism., *Bor.*, *Bov.*, *Brom.*, BRY., *Cact.*, *Caj.*, Calad., **Calc. ac.**, **Calc. c.**, **Calc. ph.**, Camph., *Cannab. s.*, *Canth.*, *Caps.*, **Carb. ac.**, **Carb. an.**, Carb. v., Carb. sul., Card. m., *Caust.*, Cham., **CHEL.**, **Chin.**, *Cic.*, *Cina*, *Cinnab.*, *Clem.*, **Cocc.**, *Coc. c.*, *Coff.*, Colch., *Coloc.*, *Com.*, Con., *Cop.*, *Croc.*, *Crotal.*, *Cub.*, Cup., Cyc., Dig., *Dios.*, *Dirc.*, **Dros.**, **Dulc.**, *Elaps.*, *Eup. per.*, *Euphorb.*, *Euphr.*, *Fer.*, Fer. iod., *Fer. ph.*, **Gel.**, *Gran.*, Graph., *Grind.*, Guai., *Hell.*, Hep., *Hydras.*, *Hyd. ac.*, Hyos., *Hyper.*, Ign., *Iod.*, **Iodof.**, IP., K. bi., K. carb., *K. iod.*, *K. nit.*, Kre., Lach., Laur., Led., *Lil. t.*, **Lob. i.**, Lyc., Mag. c., Mag. m., *Mang.*, Mar., *Meny.*, Merc., Mez., Mos., *Mur. ac.*, *Naj.*, *Naph.*, *Nat. a.*, *Nat. c.*, *Nat. m.*, *Nat. s.*, *Nit. ac.*, *Nux m.*, **Nux v.**, Op., **Osm.**, *Ox. ae.*, *Par.*, Petrol., PHOS., *Pho. ac.*, *Plat.*, Pb., *Pru.*, Pso., PULS., Ran. b., *Ran. s.*, Rheum, Rhodo., Rhus, *Rumex*, Ruta, Saba., *Sabi.*, Samb., SANG.

Sang. n., Sars., *Sec. c.*, *Sele.*, *Senec.*, SENEG., **Sep.**, *Sil.*, SPIG., *Spo.*, *Squ.*, STAN., **Staph.**, *Stict.*, Stram., Stro., SUL., Sul. ac., Tar., *Tarent.*, Ter., *Ther.*, *Thuj.*, Valer., Verat. a., *Verat. v.*, Verb., Vio. o., *Vio. t.*, Zinc., *Ziz.*

Upper Part.—Acon., Agn., **All. c.**, *Alum.*, Ambr., **Anac.**, *Ant. cr.*, Arg., Ars., Asaf., Aur., *Bar. c.*, **Bell.**, Bry., *Calc. c.*, Cannab. s., **Canth.**, Carb. v., Caust., Cham., Chel., Chin., Cic., *Cina*, Cocc., Colch., *Con.*, Cyc., *Dulc.*, Graph., Guai., Hyos., Iod., K. carb., Laur., *Lyc.*, MANG., Meny., *Merc.*, Mez., Nat. m., *Nit. ac.*, Oleand., Petrol., **Phos.**, *Pho. ac.*, **Plat.**, Pb., *Ran. b.*, Rhus., Ruta, Sars., *Seneg.*, **Sep.**, Sil., *Spig.*, STAN., Staph., Sul., *Sul. ac.*, Tar., Thuj., *Verat. a.*, Vio. t., Zinc.

Lower Part.—Acon., *Agar.*, Agn., Alum., Ambr., **Am. carb.**, Anac., Arg., **Arn.**, Ars., Asaf., *Asar.*, Aur., Bell., *Bism.*, Bov., *Bry.*, Calc. c., *Cannab. s.*, Canth., **Carb. v.**, Caust., Cham., CHIN., *Cic.*, Cocc., Colch., *Croc.*, *Dig.*, Dros., Dulc., Guai., Hell., Hep., Hyos., *Iod.*, K. CARB., K. nit., Kre., *Laur.*, Led., *Mag. c.*, Mang., *Mar.*, Merc., **Mez.**, **Mos.**, *Mur. ac.*, **Nat. c.**, *Nat. m.*, *Oleand.*, Op., Par., Petrol., *Phos.*, PHO. AC., Plat., Pb., **Puls.**, *Ran. b.*, Rheum, *Rhus*, Ruta, *Saba.*, SABI., *Samb.*, Sars., Seneg., Sep., *Sil.*, Spig., *Spo.*, SQU., Stan., Staph., *Stro.*, Tar., Thuj., Valer., Verat. a., Verb., *Vio. t.*, Zinc.

Sternum and Region.—Acon., Bry., **CACT.**, Chel., *Coc. c.*, *Cup.*, *Euphr.*, *Fer.*, *Hydras.*, *Nat. m.*, Nux v., Phos., *Pho. ac.*, *Ran. s.*, *Rumex*, Ruta, *Sabi.*, *Samb.*, **Sang.**, *Sang. n.*, *Sil.*, Spig., *Sul.*, Tell., *Verat. a.*

Heart and Region.—*Ab. n.*, ACON., *Aesc.*, *Agar.*, Alum., Ambr., Am. carb., **Amyl.**, **Anac.**, Ant. t., *Apis*, APOC. C., *Arg. n.*, **Arn.**, **ARS.**, *Ars. iod.*, Asaf., Asar., **Asc. c.**, *Aspar.*, **Aur.**, **Bar. c.**, BAR. M., *Bell.*, **Benz. ac.**, Bism., Bor., Bov., *Brom.*, **Bry.**, **CACT.**, **CALC. C.**, *Camph.*, Cannab. s., **Canth.**, *Carb. ac.*, Carb. an., *Crb. v.*, *Caust.*, *Cham.*, *Chin.*, Clem., Cimic., *Coca*, Cocc., *Coc. c.*, *Cod.*, **Colch.**, Coloc., Con., *Conv.*, Crotal., Croc., *Cup.*, Cyc., **DIG.**, Dulc., **Fer.**, **Gel.**, **Glon.**, *Graph.*, *Grind.*, Hell., Hep., *Hyd. ac.*, Hyos., Ign., Iod., Ip., *K. carb.*, K. nit., **KALM.**, Kre., **Lach.**, Laur., *Lil. t.*, *Lith.*, Lyc., *Lycps.*, Mag. c., Mag./m., Mang., *Magnol.*, Meny., **Merc.**, Mez., Mos., Mur. ac., *Naj.*, **Nat. c.**, NAT. M., *Nit. ac.*, Nux m., Nux v., Oleand., Op., *Ox. ac.*, *Par.*, Petrol., **Phos.**, Pho. ac., Phys., *Phyt.*, **Plat.**, Pb., *Pru.*, **PULS.**, *Ran. s.*, Rhodo., Rhus, Ruta, *Sabi.*, Sars., *Sec. c.*, Seneg., **Sep.**, Sil., SPIG., *Spo.*, Staph., Stro., Strop., SUL., *Sul. ac.*, *Tab.*, THEA., *Thuj.*, Valer., **Verat. a.**, *Verat. v.*, Verb., Vio. o., *Vio. t.*, Zinc.

Palpitation.—*Abs.*, ACON., *Aconin.*, AGAR., *Alum.*, Ambr., **Am. carb.**, AMYL., *Anac.*, Ant. t., **Arn.**, ARG. N., **ARS.**, Asaf., Asar.,

Aspar., Aur., Bar. c., **Bar. m., Bell.,** *Benz. ac.,* Bism., Bor., Bov., *Brom.,* Bry., **CACT., CALC. C., Camph., Cannab. i., Cannab. s.,** *Canth., Carb. ac., Carb. an.,* **Carb. v.,** Caust., *Ced., Cham., Chel.,* **CHIN., Chloral.,** *Cic.,* Cimic., Clem., *Coca,* Cocc., **Coc. c.,** *Coff.,* Colch., Coloc., **Con.,** *Conv.,* Croc., **Crotal., Cup.,** *Cyc.,* DIG., *Dulc.,* **Fer., Gel., Glon., Gran.,** *Graph., Grind.,* Hell., **Hep.,** *Hydras.,* Hyd. ac., Hyos., **Ign., IOD., Ip., K. carb., K. iod.,** *K. nit.,* **KALM.,** Kre., Lach., *Laur., Lil. t.,* **Lob. i.,** LYC., Mag. c., *Mag. m., Maynol.,* Mang., Meny., MERC., Mez., *Millef.,* Mos., *Mur. ac., Naj.,* **Nat. c.,** NAT. M., **Nit. ac.,** *Nux m.,* **Nux v.,** Oleand., Op., **Ox. ac.,** *Par.,* Petrol., **PHOS., Pho. ac., Phys.,** *Plat.,* **Pb., PULS.,** Ran. s., Rhodo., **Rhus.,** Ruta, Saba., *Sabi.,* **Sars.,** Sec. c., Sele., *Seneg.,* **SEP., Sil., SPIG.,** SPO., Staph., **Stram.,** *Stro.,* **SUL.,** *Sul. ac.,* **TAB.,** Thuj., Valer., **VERAT. A.,** Verb., **Vio. o.,** *Vio. t.,* Zinc.

Palpitation Anxious.—ACON., Alum., *Am. carb.,* Anac., *Ant. t.,* **Arn, Ars., Asaf., Aur.,** *Bell.,* Bor., *Bry.,* **CALC. C., Camph., Cannab. s.,** Carb. v., Caust., *Cham.,* **Chin.,** *Cocc.,* Colch., Coloc., Cup., *Dig.,* **Fer.,** Graph., Hyos., Ign., K. carb., Lach., Laur., LYC., *Mag. c.,* **Merc.,** Mos., *Nat. c.,* **Nat. m.,** *Nit. ac.,* Nux v., Oleand., Petrol., PHOS., **Plat.,** Pb., **PULS.,** *Rhus,* Ruta, **Sec. c.,** Seneg., **Sep.,** *Sil.,* **SPIG.,** *Spo.,* Staph., **SUL.,** Sul. ac., Thuj., Valer., *Verat. a., Vio. o.,* Vio. t., Zinc.

Heart's Action Intermittent.—Acon., *Agar.,* Alum., *Ars.,* Asaf., *Benz. ac.,* Bism., Bry., **Camph.,** Canth., *Caps., Carb. ac.,* Carb. v., CHIN., *Cic.,* **Con.,** DIG., Hep., *Hyos.,* **Iod.,** *K. br.,* **K. carb.,** Lach., Laur., **Lil. t.,** Mez., *Mur. ac.,* NAT. M., Nux v., Op., **PHO. AC.,** *Pb.,* **Rhus, Sabi., Samb., Sec. c., Sep., Stram., Sul.,** Thuj., *Verat. a.,* Zinc.

—**Tremulous.**—*Acon., Agar.,* Ambr., Ant. t., *Apoc. c.,* **Ars., Aur., Bell., CALC. C.,** *Camph.,* **Cic.,** Cina, *Cocc., Cod., Conv., Dig., Glon.,* Iod., *K. corb.,* **Kalm., Kre.,** Lach., **LIL. T., NAT. M.,** *Nux m.,* Phos., **Rhus,** Ruta, **Sabi., Sep., SPIG.,** Staph., Stram., *Thea.*

External Chest (Ribs and Muscles).—Acon., *Agar.,* Alum., *Ambr.,* Am. carb., *Am. m.,* Anac., Ant. cr., Ant. t., Arg., **ARN.,** *Ars.,* Asaf., Asar., Aur., Bar. c., *Bell.,* Bism., Bor., *Bov.,* Bry., Calad., **Calc. c.,** Camph., **Cannab. s., Canth.,** Caps., Carb. an., *Carb. v., Caust.,* Cham., *Chel.,* **Chin.,** *Cic.,* Cina, *Clem.,* Cocc., Colch., Coloc., *Con.,* Croc., **Cup.,** *Dig., Dros.,* **Dulc.,** Euphorb., Euphr., Fer., Graph., Guai., Hell., *Hep.,* Hyos., Ign., Iod., Ip., K. carb., *K. nit.,* Kre., *Lach.,* Laur., **Led., Lyc.,** Mag. c., Mag. m., *Mang.,* Mar., Meny., *Merc.,* **Mez.,** Mos., *Mur. ac., Nat. c.,* **Nat. m.,** Nit. ac., Nux m., Nux v., Oleand., Op., Par., Petrol., **PHOS.,** *Pho. ac., Plat.,* Pb., *Pso.,* **Puls.,** RAN. B., *Ran. s., Rheum,* Rhodo., **Rhus,** Ruta, Saba., *Sabi.,* Samb., *Sars.,* Sec. c., Sele., *Seneg.,* Sep., Sil., SPIG.,

Spo., *Squ.*, *Stan.*, **Staph.**, Stram., *Stro.*, SUL., Sul. ac., *Tar.*, Thuj., *Ust.*, Valer., **Verat. a.**, **Verb.**, *Vio. t.*, Zinc.

Mammary Glands.—Acon., Alum., Ambr., Am. carb., **Arn.**, Ars., Ars. iod., *Asaf.*, Bar. c., **BELL.**, **Bor.**, **BRY.**, *Buf.*, **Calc. c.**, *Calc. ph.*, Camph., *Cannab. s.*, *Canth.*, **CARB. AN.**, Carb. v., Caust., **CHAM.**, *Ced.*, *Cimic.*, **Clem.**, Cocc., *Coloc.*, CON., Croc., *Cund.*, Cup., Dig., Dulc., Fer., *Graph.*, Guai., **Hep.**, *Hydras.*, *Iod.*, K. carb., *K. iod.*, *Kre.*, *Laur.*, *Lyc.*, Mang., *Merc.*, Mez., Nat. c., Nat. m., *Nit. ac.*, Nux m., Nux v., Op., Petrol., **PHOS.**, Pho. ac., **PHYT.**, *Pb.*, **Puls.**, Ran. s., Rheum, *Rhus,* Ruta, *Sabi.*, Samb., *Sang.*, Sep., SIL., Sul., Thuj., *Ust.*, Verat. a., Zinc.

Nipples.—Acon., *Agar.*, **Arn.**, Bell., *Bism.*, *Bry.*, **Calc. c.**, Camph., Cannab. s., Carb. an., Caust., **Cham.**, Cic., Cocc., Con., *Crot. tig.*, GRAPH., **Hep.**, Ign., LYC., Mang., **Merc.**, *Merc. c.*, Mez., Mur. ac., Nit. ac., Nux v., *Par.*, Petrol., *Phos.*, *Phyt.*, Pb., **PULS.**, Ran. s., *Rheum*, Rhus, Saba., *Sabi.*, **Sars.**, Sep., *Sil.*, **SUL.**, Thuj., Zinc.

Milk Bad.—*Ac. ac.*, Bell., Bor., *Calc. ph.*, *Carb. an.*, CHAM., *Crotal.*, Ip., Lach., *Merc.*, Nux v., Op., Puls., **Rheum**, **Samb.**

—Diminished.—Agn., Bell., *Bry.*, **Calc. c.**, **Camph.**, *Cham.*, Chel., *Chin.*, DULC., Phos., **Pb.**, **Puls.**, Rhus, Samb., Sec. c., Sep., Sul., *Ust.*, Zinc.

—Increased.—Acon., *Asaf.*, **BELL.**, *Bor.*, **BRY.**, Calc. c., *Chin.*, Con., Iod., Nux v., *Phos.*, **PULS.**, Rhus, *Stram.*

Left Side.—Acon., *Agar.*, Agn., Alum., Ambr., *Am. carb.*, **AM. M.**, Anac., Ant. cr., **Ant. t.**, **Apis**, Arg., **Arn.**, Ars., *Asaf.*, Asar., *Asc. t.*, *Aur.*, Bar. c., *Bell.*, *Berb.*, *Bism.*, Bor., *Bov.*, Brom., *Bry.*, **Cact.**, *Calad.*, **CALC. C.**, *Camph.*, **Cannab. s.**, *Canth.*, **Caps.**, *Carb. an.*, **Carb. v.** Caust., **Cham.**, *Chel.*, Chin., Cic., **Cina**, Clem., **Cocc.**, *Coc. c.*, *Colch.*, Coloc., Con., Croc., Cup., Cyc., Dig., Dros., Dulc., EUPHORB., *Fer.* **FL. AC.**, Graph., Guai., *Hep.*, Hyos., **Ign.**, *Jat.*, **K. CARB.**, **K. iod.**, **K. nit.**, Kre., Lach., LAUR., Led., *Lil. t.*, LYC., *Mag. c.*, Mang., Mar., Meny., **Merc.**, Mez., Millef., *Mos.*, Mur. ac., *Nat. c.*, **Nat. m.**, *Nat. s.*, NIT. AC., Nux m., **NUX V.**, **Oleand.**, *Ox. ac.*, Par., Petrol,, **Phos.**, Pho. ac., *Plat.*, **Pb.**, Pso., *Puls.*, Ran. b., Ran. s., *Rheum*, **Rhodo.**, RHUS, Rumex, Ruta, Saba., Sabi., Sars., SENEG., **Sep.**, *Sil.*, **Spig.**, Spo., *Squ.*, STAN., **Staph.**, Stro., SUL., **Sul. ac.**, *Tur.*, **Thuj.**, *Ust.*, Valer., *Verat. a.*, **Verb.**, Vio. t., Zinc.

Right Side.—Acon., Aesc., Agar., *Agn.*, *Alum.*, Ambr., **Am. carb.**, **Am. m.**, Anac., Ant. cr., Ant. t., *Arg.*, **ARN.**, **Ars.**, **Asaf.**, Asar., **Aur.**. *Bap.*, Bar. c., **BELL.**, Bism., **Bor.**, Bov., **Brom.**, **BRY.**, Calad., *Calc. c.*, Camph., *Cannab. s.*, **Canth.**, Caps., **CARB. AN.**, *Carb. v.*, Caust., Cham.,

CHEL., Chin., Cic., Cina, Clem., *Cocc.*, **Colch.**, COLOC., Con., Croc., Cup., Cyc., **Dig.**, Dros., *Dulc.*, Euphorb., Fl. ac., *Graph.*, **Hep., Hyos.**, Ign., **Iodof.**, IOD., *Ip.*, K. carb., K. nit., Kre., **LACH.**, **Laur., Led.**, *Lob. i., Lyc.*, **Mag. m.**, Mang., *Mar.*, Meny., *Merc.*, Mez., Millef., **Mur. ac.**, *Murex*, Nat. c., *Nat. m., Nit. ac., Nux m., Nux v.*, Oleand., **Op.**, *Par.*, Petrol., **Phel., Phos.**, *Pho. ac.*, Plat., Pb., *Pso.*, **PULS., Ran. b.**, *Ran. s.*, Rheum, *Rhus*, Ruta., *Saba.*, Sabi., **Sang.**, Sars., Seneg., *Sep.*, SIL., *Spig.*, Spo., **Squ.**, Stan., Staph., Stro., **Sul.**, Sul. ac., **Tar.**, Thuj., Valer., **Verat. a.**, *Vio. t.*, Zinc.

Back.

Back in General.—Acon., AGAR., Agn., *Alum.*, Ambr., Am. carb., *Am. m.*, **Anac.**, *Ant. cr.*, Ant. t., **Apis**, Arg., ARN., ARS., *Asaf.*, Asar., Aur., *Bap., Bar. c.*, **BELL.**, **Berb.**, Bism., Bor., *Bov., Brom.*, **Bry., Cact.**, CALC. C., *Calc. ph.*, Camph., *Cannab. s., Canth., Caps., Carb. ac.*, Carb. an., **Carb. v.**, CAUST., *Cham.*, CHEL., **Chin.**, Cic., CIMIC., **Cina**, *Cub.*, COCC., *Coc. c., Coff., Colch.*, Coloc., *Con., Corn. f.*, Croc., Cup., Cyc., *Dig., Dios.*, Dros., *Dulc.*, EUP. PER., **Eup. pur.**, Euphorb., Euphr., Fer., **Graph.**, **Guai.**, Hell., *Helo., Hep., Hyos.*, **Hyper.**, *Ign.*, Iod., *Ip., Iris v.*, K. carb., K. nit., *Kalm., Kre., Lach.*, Laur., *Led.*, LYC., Mag. c., Mag. m., Mang., Mar., *Meny.*, **Merc.**, *Merc. c., Mez., Mos., Mur. ac.*, **Nat. c.**, **NAT. M.**, *Nit. ac.*, Nux m., NUX V., Oleand., Op., *Ox. ac., Par.*, **Petrol.**, PHOS., *Pho. ac., Phys.*, **Phyt.**, *Pic. ac., Plat.*, Pb., *Pso.*, PULS., *Ran. b.*, Ran. s., Rheum, *Rhodo.*, **Rhus, Ruta**, *Saba., Sabi., Samb., Sars., Sec. c.*, Sele., *Senec.*, Seneg., SEP., SIL., **Spig.**, Spo., Squ., Stan., *Staph., Stram.*, Stro., SUL., *Sul. ac., Tar.*, **Tarent.**, TELL., *Thuj., Trill.*, Valer., VERAT. A., Verb., *Vib. op.*, Vio. t., *Xan.*, **Zinc.**

Scapulæ.—*Ab. c.*, Acon., *Agar., Alum.*, Ambr., Am. carb., **Am. m.**, ғnac., Ant. cr., *Arg., Arn.*, **Ars., Asaf.**, Asar., Aur., **Bar. c., Bell.**, Bism., Bor., Bov., **Bry., Calc. c.**, *Calc. ph., Camph.*, Cannab. s., *Canth., Caps.*, Carb. an., Carb. v., **Caust.**, Cham., CHEL., CHIN., *Cic.*, Cina, *Cocc.*, Colch., *Coloc.*, Con., Croc., Cup., Cyc., Dig., Dros., **Dulc.**, *Fer.*, Graph., *Guai.*, Hell., **Hep.**, Hyos., Ign., Iod., Ip., **K. carb.**, K. nit., KRE., Lach., *Laur.*, Led., Lyc., Mag. c., *Mag. m.*, Mang., Mar., **Meny.**, MERC., *Mez.*, Mos., *Mur. ac.*, **Nat. c.**, *Nat. m.*, Nit. ac., **Nux v.**, Oleand., Op., Par., Petrol., **Phos.**, *Pho. ac.*, Plat., *Pb.*, **Puls.**, *Ran. b.*, Ran. s., *Rhodo.*, RHUS, *Ruta*, Saba., Sabi., *Samb..* Sars., Seneg., SEP., **Sil.**, *Spig.*, Spo., **Squ.**, Stan., *Staph.*, Stro., **Sul.**, Sul. ac., **Tar.**, Thuj., Valer., **Verat. a.**, Verb., **Vio. t.**, *Zinc.*

Between Scapulæ.—Acon., *Bell.*, *Con.*, *Meny.*, *Nat. c.*, *Petrol.*, *Phos.*, *Pho. ac.*, Rhus, *Sep.*, *Sil.*, *Tell.*

Dorsal Region.—Agar., *Bry.*, CHEL., *Chen. a.*, CHIN. S., CIMIC., *Cocc.*, *Dig.*, *Jug. c.*, *Ox. ac.*, Phos., *Pod.*, *Ruta*, *Stram.*, *Tell.*, Zinc.

Lumbar and Sacral Region (including Small of Back).*—*Ab. c.*, Acon., ÆSC., Agar., Aloe, *Alum.*, Ambr., *Am. carb.*, *Am. m.*, Anac., Ant. cr., Ant. t., *Arg*, **Arg. n.**, Arn., *Ars.*, Asaf., Asar., *Aur.*, Bap., *Bar. ac.*, Bar. c., Bell., Bor., Bov., Bry., Calad., **Calc. c.**, **Calc. ph.**, Cannab. s., CANTH., Caps., Carb. an., *Carb. v.*, CAUST., *Ced.*, Cham., Chel., Chim., Chin., CIMIC., **Cina**, *Clem.*, **Cocc.**, *Coc. c.*, Coff., *Colch.*, *Coloc.*, Con., *Conv.*, Croc., Cup., *Dig.*, *Dios.*, Dros., *Dulc.*, *Erig.*, **Equis.**, *Eup. per.*, Euphorb., *Fer.*, *Fer. iod.*, *Graph.*, Guai., Hell., *Helv.*, Hep., Hyos., Ign., Iod., Ip., *K. bi.*, **K. carb.**, *K. nit.*, **Kalm.**, Kre., Lach., Laur., Led., LIL. T., Lyc., *Mag. c.*, **Mag. m.**, Mang., Meny., **Merc.**, Mez., Mos., *Murex*, Mur. ac., **Nat. c.**, **Nat. m.**, *Nit. ac.*, Nux m., NUX V., *Onos.*, Op., *Ox. ac.*, *Oxyt.*, *Petrol.*, **Phos.**, *Pho. ac.*, **Phyt.**, *Pic. ac.*, Plat., Pb., *Pod.*, PULS., Ran. b., *Ran. s.*, **Rheum**, *Rhodo.*, RHUS, **Ruta**, Saba., **Sabi.**, Samb., Sars., Sec. c., *Sele.*, *Senec.*, Seneg., SEP., **Sil.**, Spig., Spo., Squ., *Stan.*, *Staph.*, *Stram.*, **Stro.**, SUL., *Sul. ac.*, *Tar.*, Tarent., Tell., Ter., Thuj., *Ust.*, Valer., **Verat. a.**, *Vib. op.*, Zinc.

Coccyx.—Agar., Agn., Alum., Am. carb., Am. m., Ant. cr., Arg., Arn., Asaf., *Bell.*, Bor., *Bov.*, Calc. c., Cannab. s., Canth., *Carb. an.*, Carb. v., Caust., Chin., *Cic.*, Colch., Croc., Dros., *Fl. ac.*, GRAPH. HEP., Ign., Iod., *K. bi.*, K. carb., *Lach.*, Laur., Led., Mag. c., **Merc.**, Mur. ac., Nux m., **Par.**, *Petrol.*, Phos., **Pho. ac.**, *Pic. ac.*, **Plat.**, Pb., RHUS, Ruta, *Sil.*, *Spig.*, Staph., **Sul.**, *Tarent.*, Thuj., *Valer.*, *Verat. a.*, Zinc.

---

* Boenninghausen makes four divisions of the back, namely: scapulæ, back in general., *kreuz* (which means the part of the back between the hips, corresponding to the region of the sacrum), and *steiss* (the region of the coccyx). He has no separate division, for what is known in common language as the small of the back, which we understand to be the lumbar region, extending from the hips to the ribs. There is no doubt that great confusion exists as to the location of sensations in the back, and the *kreuz* region is often translated small of back, but it is properly understood to mean the boundary line between the lumbar and sacral regions. The symptoms in the *Materia Medica* noted as "in the small of the back" are included under lumbar and sacral region, since the expression in use is so indefinite. Consult list under LOINS (in abdomen).

Left Side.—Acon., **Agar.**, Agn., **Alum.**, Ambr., *Am. carb.*, **Am. m.**, **Anac.**, Ant. cr., **Ant. t.**, **Apis**, **Arg.**, *Ars.*, *Asaf.*, Aur., **Bar. c.**, **Bell.**, *Berb.*, Bism., Bry., Calc. c., Cannab. s., Canth., Carb. an., *Carb. v.*, **Caust.**, Chel., **Chin.**, Cina, *Cocc.*, Colch., *Coloc.*, Con., *Croc.*, *Cup.*, *Dig.*, DROS., *Dulc.*, Euphorb., *Fer.*, *Fl. ac.*, **Graph.**, Guai., *Hell.*, **Hep.**, **Ign.**, Iod., **K. carb.**, *K. nit.*, *Kre.*, Laur., **Led.**, *Lyc.*, **Mang.**, **Mar.**, Meny., Merc., Mez., *Millef.*, *Mos.*, Mur. ac., *Nat. m.*, *Nat. s.* Nit. ac., Nux v., Oleand., *Ox. ac.*, Par., *Petrol.*, Phos., *Pho. ac.*, Plat., Pb., *Pso.*, **Puls.**, Ran. s., *Rhodo.*, **Rhus**, Ruta, Saba., Sabi., Sars., **Seneg.**, *Sep.*, **SIL.**, *Spig.*, Spo., **Squ.**, **Stan.**, *Staph.*, *Stro.*, **Sul.**, Sul. ac., Tar., *Thuj.*, **Valer.**, Verat. a., Verb., Vio. t., **Zinc**.

Right Side.—*Acon.*, Agar., Agn., Alum., Ambr., Am. carb., *Am. m.*, Anac., Ant. cr., *Ant. t.*, Apis, *Arg.*, **Arn.**, **Ars.**, Asaf., *Asar.*, *Aur.*, Bar. c., Bell., *Bor.*, *Brom.*, Bry., **CALC. C.**, Cannab. s., **Canth.**, **Carb. an.**, Carb. v., *Caust.*, **Chel.**, *Chen. a.*, **Chin.**, **CIC.**, Cina, Cocc., *Colch.*, **Coloc.**, Con., Cup., *Dig.*, *Dios.*, Dros., Dulc., *Erig.*, *Equis.*, **Euphorb.**, **FL. AC.**, **Guai.**, Hep., **Iod.**, *Jug. c.*, *K. carb.*, **Laur.**, **Lyc.**, **Mar.**, Meny., **Merc.**, Mez., Millef., Mur. ac., **Nat. m.**, Nit. ac,, **Nux v.**, **Oleand.**, Petrol., **Phos.**, *Phyt.*, Plat., **PB.**, *Pod.*, **Ran. b.**, Ran. s., Rhodo., Rhus, Ruta, *Saba.*, **Samb.**, *Sang.*, Sars., Sep., *Sil.*, Spig., Spo., Stan., Staph., **Sul.**, Sul. ac., **Tar.**, **Ter.**, Thuj., Verb., Vio. t., **ZINC**.

Upper Extremities.

Shoulder.—ACON., Agar., Agn., **Alum.**, **Ambr.**, Am. carb., **Am. m.**, Anac., Ant. cr., Ant. t., *Arg.*, *Arn.*, Ars., *Asaf.*, *Asar.*, Bar. c., **Bell.**, *Bor.*, Bov., **BRY.**, Calc. c., Camph., *Cannab. s.*, Canth., Carb. an., *Carb. v.*, *Caust.*, **Chel.**, Chin., *Cic.*, Cina, Coca., Cocc., Colch., Croc., Cup., *Dig.*, *Dios.*, Dros., Euphorb., **Fer.**, *Fer. ph.*, *Gran.*, Graph., Guai., *Hep.*, Hyos., Ign., *Iris. v.*, K. CARB., K. nit., *Kalm.*, *Kre.*, *Laur.*, **Led.**, **Lith.**, **Lyc.**, MAG. C., *Mag. m.*, Mang., Mar., Meny., **Merc.**, *Mex.*, Mos., Mur. ac., *Nat. c.*, Nat. m., *Nat. s.*, **Nux v.**, Oleand., Op., *Ox. ac.*, Par., Petrol., **Phos.**, Pho. ac., Plat., Pb., **PULS.**, *Ran. b.*, Ran. s., Rhodo., **RHUS**, *Ruta*, Saba., *Sabi.*, **Sal. ac.**, **Sang.**, Sars., Sep., *Sil.*, Spig., Spo., Squ., **Stan.**, *Staph.*, **Stram.**, **Stro.**, Sul., Sul. ac., Tar., Thuj., Valer., Verat. a., Verb., *Zinc*.

Axilla.—Agn., Am. carb., *Am. m.*, Anac., Arg., Arn., Ars., **Ars. iod.**, *Asar.*, *Aur.*, Bar. c., **Bell.**, Bor., Bov., Bry., Calc. c., Canth., **Caps.**, **CARB. AN.**, Carb. v., Caust., Chel., **Clem.**, Cocc., Coloc., **Con.**, *Crotal.*, Cup., Dig., Dulc., **HEP.**, Iod., **K. carb.**, Lach., *Laur.*, **Lyc.**, Mag. c., Mang., Mar., *Meny.*, Merc., Mez., *Nat. c.*, **Nat. m.**, **Nit. ac.**, Oleand.,

UPPER EXTREMITIES. 131

Petrol., PHOS., Pho. ac., *Phyt.*, Pb., Puls., Rhodo., Rhus, Ruta, Saba., Sele., Seneg., SEP., **Sil.**, *Spig.*, Spo., Squ., Stan., **Staph.**, SUL., **Sul. ac.**, Thuj., Valer., Verat. a., *Vio. t.*, Zinc.

Upper Arm.—*Abrot.*, Acon., Agar., *Agn.*, Alum., Ambr., **Am. carb.**, Am. m., Anac., **Ant. cr.**, Ant. t., *Arg.*, Arn., **Ars.**, **Asaf.**, *Asar.*, Aur., Bar. c., **Bell.**, Bism., *Bor.*, Bov., **Bry.**, Calc. c., Camph., *Canth.*, *Carb. ac.*, Carb. an., *Carb. v.*, Caust., *Chel.*, *Chin.*, Cina, Clem., COCC., Coff., Colch., Coloc., Con., *Croc.*, Cup., Cyc., Dig., Dros., *Dulc.*, *Eup. per.*, Euphorb., Euphr., FER., Graph., *Guai.*, Hell., Hep., **Ign.**, Iod., Ip., *K. carb.*, **K. nit.**, *Kalm.*, Kre., *Lach.*, *Laur.*, *Led.*, Lyc., Mag. c., Mag. m., Mang., Mar., Meny., Merc., **Mez.**, Mos., Mur. ac., Nat. c., Nat. m., Nit. ac., Nux m., Nux v., **Oleand.**, *Ox. ac.*, Par., Petrol., Phos., Pho. ac., *Phyt.*, Plat., Pb., *Puls.*, Ran. b., Ran. s., Rheum., Rhodo., *Rhus, Ruta,* Saba., *Sabi.*, Samb., *Sang.*, Sars., Sep., Sil., Spig., Spo., *Squ.*, **Stan.**, Staph., Stro., *Sul.*, Sul. ac., Tar., Thuj., **Valer.**, *Verat. a.*, Zinc.

Forearm.—Acon., Agar., Agn., *Alum.*, *Ambr.*, Am. carb., *Am. m.*, Anac., Ant. cr., Ant. t., Arg., Arn., Asaf., Aur., Bar. c., **Bell.**, **Bism.**, *Bor.*, **Bry.**, *Calad.*, **CALC. C.**, *Camph.*, Canth., *Caps.*, *Carb. ac.*, Carb. an., Carb. v., *Carb. sul.*, CAUST., Cham., Chel., Chin., *Cic.*, Cina, Clem., Cocc., Colch., Coloc., **Con.**, **Croc.**, *Cup.*, *Cur.*, *Cyc.*, Dig., Dros., *Dulc.*, *Eup. per.*, Euphorb., Euphr., *Graph.*, Guai., Hell., *Hep.*, *Hyos.*, Ign., K. carb., *Kre.*, Laur., Led., *Lyc.*, Mag. c., Mag. m., Mang., *Mar.*, Meny., MERC., Mez., *Mos.*, Mur. ac., **Nat. c.**, Nat. m., *Nit. ac.*, *Nux v.*, Oleand., *Op.*, *Ox. ac.*, Par., Petrol., Phos., **Pho. ac.**, *Plat.*, Pb., *Puls.*, Ran. b., Ran. s., Rheum, Rhodo., RHUS, Ruta, *Saba.*, Sabi., *Sal. ac.*, *Samb.*, **Sars.**, *Sec. c.*, **Sele.**, Seneg., Sep., *Sil.*, **Spig.**, *Spo.*, Stan., STAPH., *Still.*, *Stram.*, **Stro.**, *Sul.*, Sul. ac., Tar., Thuj., **Valer.**, Verat. a., Verb., Vio. t., *Zinc.*

Hand.—Acon., Act., *Agar.*, Agn., Alum., *Ambr.*, Am. carb., Am. m., **Anac.**, Ant. cr., **Ant. t.**, Arg., *Arn.*, **Ars.**, Asaf., Asar., Aur., *Bar. c.*, **Bell.**, *Bism.*, Bor., *Bov.*, Bry., **Cact.**, CALC. C., *Camph.*, **Cannab. i.**, Cannab. s., *Canth.*, Caps., *Carb. ac.*, Carb. an., *Carb. v.*, *Carb. sul.*, Caust., *Ced.*, *Cham.*, *Chel.*, **Chin.**, Cic., *Cina*, *Clem.*, *Cocc.*, *Coff.*, Colch., *Coloc.*, Con., Croc., **Cup.**, *Cur.*, Cyc., Dig., **Dros.**, *Dulc.*, Euphorb., Euphr., *Fer.*, *Ferph.*, **Fl. ac.**, *Graph.*, Guai., **Hell.**, *Hep.*, Hyos., Ign., Iod., Ip., *K. carb.*, *K. nit.*, **Kre.**, *Lach.*, *Laur.*, **Led.**, LYC., Mag. c., Mag. m., Mang., Mar., *Meli.*, MENY., **MERC.**, *Mez.*, Mos., *Mur. ac.*, **Nat. c.**, **Nat. m.**, *Nit. ac.*, Nux m., NUX V., Oleand., Op., *Ox. ac.*, Par., *Petrol.*, Phos., **Pho. ac.**, *Plat.*, Pb., *Pso.*, PULS., *Ran. b.*, Ran. s., Rheum, **Rhodo.**, Rhus, *Ruta*, Saba., Sabi., *Samb.*, *Sars.*, *Sec. c.*, **Sele.**, Seneg., SEP., Sil., Spig., Spo., Squ., **Stan.**, *Staph.*, **Stram.**, Stro., SUL., Sul. ac., **Sum.**, Tar., Thuj., Valer., **Verat. a.**, *Verb.*, Vio. o., Vio. t., **Zinc.**

UPPER EXTREMITIES.

Back of Hand.—Alum., Ars., *Bor., Bov., Bry.,* **Calc. c.,** *Camph.,* Caust., Cina, *Cyc., Dig., Euphorb.,* **Kre.,** *Lyc.,* Merc., *Mur. ac.,* NAT. C., *Nux v., Petrol.,* Pho. ac., *Puls.,* Rheum., RHUS, *Sal. ac.,* **Samb.,** SEP., *Sil.,* Spig., Stan., **Sul.,** *Thuj.*

Palm.—Acon., Agar., Alum., Ambr., *Am. m.,* ANAC., Asar., Bar. c., *Berb., Bism.,* **Bor.,** *Bry., Camph.,* Canth., Caps., Carb. v., Caust., *Cham., Chel.,* Chin., Coff., *Con.,* Dig., **Dulc.,** *Fer., Fer. ph.,* Hell., He*p.*, *Ign., Ip.,* K. carb., **Kre.,** Lach., *Laur.,* Led., Lyc., *Mag. c.,* Mang., **Merc.,** *Mez., Mur. ac.,* Nat. c., *Nat. m.,* **Nux v.,** *Petrol., Phos.,* Puls., RAN. B., Ran. s., *Rheum,* Rhus, Ruta, **Samb.,** SELE., *Sep., Sil.,* SPIG., Spo., Stan., Staph., SUL., *Verat. a.*

Fingers.—Acon., Agar., *Agn.,* Alum., **Ambr.,** Am. carb., AM. M., *Anac., Ant. s. aur.,* Ant. cr., *Ant. t.,* **Apis,** Arg., Arn., *Ars.,* Asaf., Asar., Aur., *Bar. c.,* **Bell.,** *Benz. ac., Bism., Bor., Bov., Brom.,* **Bry., Calc. c.,** *Calc. ph.,* Camph., Cannab. s., Canth., Carb. an., *Carb. v., Carb. sul.,* **Caul.,** Caust., *Ced.,* Cham., **Chel.,** Chin., Cic., **Cimic.,** *Cina,* Clem., *Cocc.,* Coff., **Colch.,** Coloc., Con., Croc., Crotal., Cup., Cyc., Dig., **Dios.,** Dros., Dulc., Euphorb., Euphr., Fer., *Fl. ac.,* Graph., *Guai., Hell., Hep., Hyos., Ign.,* Iod., **K. carb.,** K. nit., **Kre.,** *Lach.,* Laur., Led., *Lith.,* LYC., **Mag. c.,** Mag. m., *Mang.,* **Mar.,** Meny., Merc., *Mez., Mos., Mur. ac., Nat. c.,* **Nat. m., Nit. ac.,** *Nux v.,* Oleand., Op., *Or. ac.,* Par., *Petrol.,* **Phos., Pho. ac.,** *Plat., Pb.,* PULS., **Ran. b., Ran. s.,** Rheum, **Rhodo.,** RHUS, Ruta, **Saba.,** Sabi., *Sal. ac., Sars.,* **Sec. c.,** Sele., **Sep.,** SIL., **Spig.,** *Spo.,* **Stan.,** Staph., *Stro.,* SUL., Sul. ac., *Tar.,* THUJ., Valer., *Verat. a., Verb.,* Vio. t., *Zinc.*

—**Tips.**—Acon., Agar., *Ambr.,* AM. M., *Ant. cr.,* **Ant. t., Apis,** Ars., Asaf., Bar. c., **Bell.,** Bism., *Bor., Brom.,* **Bry.,** Calc. c., Cannab. s., Canth., Cham., **Chel.,** Chin., Coff., *Colch.,* Con., Croc., Cup., Dros., Fer., *Fl. ac.,* **Glon.,** Hell., Hep., **Kre.,** *Lach.,* Laur., MAR., Merc., Mez., Mur. ac., Oleand., *Petrol.,* **Phos.,** Pho. ac., **Puls.,** Ran. b., Ran. s., *Rhus, Saba.,* Sabi., Sars., **Sec. c.,** Sele., *Sep.,* **Sil., Spig.,** *Spo.,* Stan., **Staph.,** *Stro.,* Sul., Sul. ac., **Tar.,** THUJ., Valer., Verat. a., Verb., Zinc.

—**Between.**—Ambr., *Am. m.,* Ars., Aur., Camph., Caust., *Cyc.,* Fer., GRAPH., Hell., Kre., *Lach.,* **Laur., Nit. ac.,** *Pb.,* **Puls.,** Ran. s., **Rhodo.,** Rhus, SELE., *Sep., Sul.,* Sul. ac., Zinc.

—**Nails.**—Acon., Alum., Am. m., *Ant. cr.,* **Apis,** Ars., Bar. c., **Bell.,** *Bor., Bov., Calc. c.,* **Calc. ph.,** Caust., *Chel.,* Chin., Cocc., *Con.,* Dig., Dros., *Fl. ac., Form.,* Graph., Hell., *Hep.,* Iod., K. carb., Lach., Lyc., Mar., **Merc.,** Mur. ac., *Nat. m., Nat. s., Nit. ac., Par.,* Petrol., Pho. ac., **Plat.,** *Puls., Ran. b.,* Ruta, *Saba.,* **Sep.,** SIL., Squ., **Sul., Sul. ac., Thuj.**

UPPER EXTREMITIES. 133

Joints of Upper Extremities in General.—Acon., Agar., **Agn.**, *Alum.*, **Ambr., Am. carb.**, *Am. m.*, Anac., *Ant. cr.*, Ant. t., *Arg.*, *Arn.*, Ars., *Asaf.*, Asar., *Aur.*, *Bar.* c., **Bell., Benz. ac.**, Bism., Bor., **Bov., Bry.**, Calad., **CALC. C.**, Camph., Cannab. s., Canth., *Caps.*, *Carb. an.*, **Carb. v., CAUST.,** *Cham.*, Chel., *Chin.*, Cic., Cina, Clem., *Cocc.*, Coff., Colch., *Coloc.*, Con., *Croc.*, Cup., Cyc., *Dig.*, **Dros.**, Dulc., Euphorb., Euphr., *Fer.*, **Graph.**, Guai., **Hell.**, **Hep., Hyos.**, *Ip.*, **Ign.**, *Iod.*, **K. CARB., K. nit.**, *Kre.*, Lach., Laur., **LED., LYC.**, *Mag. c.*, Mag. m., **Mang.**, *Mar.*, *Meli.*, Meny., **MERC.**, *Mez.*, Mos., *Mur. ac.*, *Nat. c.*, **Nat. m.**, *Nit. ac.*, Nux m., *Nux v.*, Oleand., **Op.**, Par., **Petrol., Phos.**, *Pho. ac.*, **Phyt.**, Plat., Pb., **Puls.**, Ran. b., Ran. s., *Rheum*, **Rhodo.**, **RHUS, Ruta,** Saba., **Sabi.**, Samb., **Sars.**, Sec. c., Sele., Seneg., **SEP., Sil., Spig.**, *Spo.*, Squ., **Stan., Staph., Stro., SUL.**, **Sul. ac.**, Tar., Thuj., Valer., **Verat.** *a.*, **Verb.**, Vio. o., Vio. t., **Zinc.**

Shoulder Joint.—Acon., **Agn., Ambr.,** Am. carb., *Am. m.,* Ant. t., Arg., **Arn., Asaf.,** Asar., Bism., **Bov., Bry., CALC. C.,** Canth., *Caps.,* Carb. an., *Carb. v.,* **Caust.,** Cham., Chel., Chin., Cic., *Cocc.,* Colch., *Coloc.,* **Croc.,** Dig., *Dros.,* Euphorb., FER., **Graph.,** Hell., Hep., Hyos., IGN., *Iod.,* **K. CARB.,** Kre., Laur., **Led., Lith., Lith. lact.,** *Lyc.,* Mag. c., *Mag. m.,* **Mang., Mar., Merc.,** Mez., Mur. ac., Nat. c., **Nat. m.,** Nit. ac., Nux m., *Nux v.,* Oleand., Op., **Petrol.,** *Phos.,* Pho. ac., PULS., Ran. b., *Rhodo.,* RHUS, Ruta, Saba., **Sabi.,** Sars., SEP., Sil., Spig., Stan., STAPH., **Stro.,** SUL., *Sul. ac.,* Thuj., Valer., *Verat. a.,* Vio. t., Zinc.

Elbow.—Acon., Agar., *Agn., Alum.,* **Ambr.,** Am. carb., Am. m., *Anac.,* **Ant. cr.,** Ant. t., **Arg.,** Arn., Ars., Asaf., Aur. Bar. c., **Bell., Bov., Bry.,** Calad., *Calc. c.,* Camph., *Canth., Caps.,* Carb. an., *Carb. v.,* **CAUST.,** Cham., Chel., *Chin.,* Cic., Cina, Clem., *Cocc.,* Colch., *Coloc.,* Con., Croc., Cup., Dig., Dros., *Dulc.,* Euphr., *Graph.,* Hell., *Hep.,* Hyos., Ign., *Iod.,* **K. CARB., K. nit.,** Kre., *Laur.,* **Led.,** Lyc., Mag. c., Mag. m., *Mang.,* Mar., **Meny., Merc., Mez., Mur. ac.,** *Nat. c., Nat. m.,* Nux m., *Nux v.,* Oleand., Par., **Petrol.,** Phos., Pho. ac., Plat., *Pb.,* **Puls.,** Ran. b., Ran. s., Rheum, *Rhodo.,* **RHUS, Ruta,** Saba., *Sabi.,* Samb., **Sars.,** Sec. c., Seneg., SEP., *Spig., Spo.,* Stan., **Staph., Still., Stro.,** SUL., *Sul. ac.,* Tar., Thuj., *Valer., Verat. a.,* **Verb.,** Vio. o., Vio. t., **Zinc.**

—Bend.—Agn., Alum., *Am. m.,* **Anac.,** Ant. cr., **Arn.,** Bar. c., *Bell.,* Calc. c., *Canth.,* Carb. an., **Caust.,** Cic., Cina, *Clem.,* Colch., Coloc., Con., *Cup.,* Dros., Dulc., Graph., Hell., Hep., Hyos., Iod., **K. CARB., K. nit.,** Laur., *Lyc.,* Mar., *Meny.,* Mur. ac., **Petrol.,** Phos., Pho. ac., **Puls., Sep.,** *Spig.,* Staph., **Sul.,** Thuj., *Valer.,* Verat. a., *Zinc.*

—Tip.—*Agar., Alum.,* Arg., Asaf., Bar. c., **Bry.,** Carb. an., **Carb. v.,**

Caust., Dulc., Graph., HEP., Hyos., Kre., Lyc., *Merc.*, Mur. ac., **Nat. m.**, Oleand., *Pho. ac.*, Puls., Rhus, *Sabi.*, Sars., *Sep.*, Spig., *Spo.*, **Stan.**, Sul. ac., Valer.

Wrist.—Acon., Agn., *Alum.*, Ambr., **Am. carb.**, **Am. m.**, **Anac.**, Ant. cr., Ant. t., *Arg.*, Arn., **Ars.**, **Asaf.**, Asar., Aur., *Bar. c.*, Bell., **Benz. ac.**, *Bism.*, BOV., Bry., CALC. C., Canth., Caps., *Carb. an.*, **Carb. v.**, *Carb. sul.*, **Caul.**, **CAUST.**, Cham., Chel., Chin., Cic., Cina, Clem., Colch., Coloc., Con., Croc., *Cur.*, *Cyc.*, Dig., *Dros.*, Dulc., **Eup. per.**, Euphorb., Euphr., *Graph.*, Guai., *Hell.*, Hep., *Hyos.*, *Ign.*, *Iod.*, K. CARB., **K. nit.**, Kre., Lach., Laur., **Led.**, *Lyc.*, Mag. c., Mag. m., **Mang.**, Mar., *Meny.*, **Merc.**, Mez., Nat. c., Nat. m., *Nit. ac.*, Nux v., *Oxyt.*, Petrol., *Phos.*, Pho. ac., Pb., **Puls.**, Ran. b., Ran. s., Rheum, **Rhodo.**, **RHUS**, **RUTA**, Saba., SABI., *Sal. ac.*, Samb., *Sang.*, **Sars.**, Sec. c., Sele., Seneg., SEP., **Sil.**, Spig., Spo., Squ., **Stan.**, Staph., *Stict.*, **Stro.**, **SUL.**, *Sul. ac.*, Tar., *Thuj.*, Valer., *Verb.*, Vio. t., *Zinc.*

Finger Joints.—Acon., *Act.*, *Agn.*, Alum., Ambr., **Am. carb.**, Am. m., *Am. phos.*, *Anac.*, Ant. cr., Ant. t., Arg., Arn., Ars., Asar., *Aur.*, *Bar. c.*, **Bell.**, **Benz. ac.**, Berb., Bism., **Bor.**, *Bov.*, **Bry.**, CALC. C., Camph., Cannab. s., *Caps.*, Carb. an., *Carb. v.*, **Caul.**, **Caust.**, **Cham.**, *Chel.*, *Chin.*, *Cina*, *Clem.*, Cocc., Coff., **Colch.**, Coloc., Con., Croc., *Cup.*, *Cyc.*, Dig., *Dros.*, *Dulc.*, Euphr., Fer., *Gran.*, **Graph.**, **Hell.**, Hep., *Ign.*, Iod., *K. bi.*, **K. carb.**, **K. nit.**, *Kre.*, **Led.**, *Lith.*, LYC., Mag. c., *Mang.*, *Mar.*, Meny., Merc., *Mos.*, Nat. c., **Nat. m.**, *Nit. ac.*, Nux m., *Nux v.*, Oleand., Par., Petrol., Phos., Pho. ac., *Plat.*, Pb., **Puls.**, Ran. s., Rheum, *Rhodo.*, **Rhus**, *Ruta*, Saba., Sabi., *Sal. ac.*, Samb., *Sars.*, Sec. c., Seneg., SEP., **Sil.**, SPIG., *Spo.*, **Stan.**, Staph., *Stict.*, **Stro.**, SUL., *Sul. ac.*, Verat. a., Verb., Zinc.

Bones of Upper Extremities in General.—Acon., Agar., Alum., Am. carb., *Am. m.*, Anac., Ant. t., *Arg.*, Arn., ASAF., **Aur.**, *Bar. c.*, Bell., *Bism.*, Bov., **Bry.**, Calc. c., Canth., Carb. an., *Carb. v.*, Caust., **Cham.**, CHIN., COCC., Coloc., Con., *Croc.*, Cup., *Cyc.*, Dig., **Dros.**, *Dulc.*, Euphorb., Hell., Hep., **Ign.**, *Iod.*, Ip., *K. carb.*, Lach., Laur., *Led.*, **Lyc.**, Mag., c. Mang., *Mar.*, **Merc.**, **Mez.**, Nat. c., Nat. m., Nit. ac., Oleand., Par., Petrol., **Phos.**, Pho. ac., Plat., Pb., **Puls.**, **Rhodo.**, RHUS, **Ruta**, *Saba.*, Sabi., Samb., Sars., Sep., **Sil.**, *Spig.*, Spo., STAPH., Stro., **Sul.**, Sul. ac., Thuj., *Valer.*, *Verat. a.*, Verb., Zinc.

Left.—Acon., Agar., Agn., **Alum.**, Ambr., Am. carb., Am. m., ANAC., Ant. cr., *Ant. t.*, **Apis**, Arg., ARN., *Ars.*, ASAF., Asar., Aur., **Bar. c.**, *Bell.*, Bism., Bor., Bov., *Brom.*, Bry., *Calad.*, Calc. c., *Camph.*, Cannab. s., Canth., **Caps.**, Carb. an., *Carb. v.*, Caust., **Cham.**, Chel., *Chin.*, Cic., *Cina*, Clem., **Cocc.**, **Coff.**, Colch., Coloc., *Con.*, Croc., Cup., *Cyc.*, Dig., *Dios.*,

UPPER EXTREMITIES—LOWER EXTREMITIES. 135

Dros., Dulc., Euphorb., **Euphr.**, Fer., Fl. ac., *Glon.*, Graph., Guai., Hell., **Hep.**, *Hyos.*, *Ign.*, *Iod.*, Ip., K.CARB., *K. nit.*, **Kre.**, Lach., Laur., *Led.*, **Lyc.**, Mag. c., **Mag. m.**, Mang., **Már.**, *Meny.*, Merc., Mez., Millef., Mos., Mur. ac., Nat. c., *Nat. m.*, *Nat. s.*, *Nit. ac.*, Nux m., Nux v., **Oleand.**, *Op.*, *Par.*, **Petrol.**, Phos., **Pho. ac.**, Plat., Pb., *Pso.*, **Puls.**, Ran. b., *Ran. s.*, Rheum, Rhodo., RHUS, Ruta, Saba., SABI., Samb., Sars., Sec. c., *Sele.*, **Seneg.**, *Sep.*, *Sil.*, Spig., Spo., SQU., STAN., *Staph.*, *Stram.*, *Stro.*, SUL., Sul. ac., *Tab.*, **Tar.**, *Thuj.*, **Valer.**, *Verat. a.*, **Verb.**, Vio. o., **Vio. t.**, *Zinc.*

Right.—Acon., Agar., *Agn.*, Alum., **Ambr.**, Am. carb., *Am. m.*, Anac., *Ant. cr.*, Ant. t., *Apis*, Arg., Arn., **Ars.**, Asaf., Asar., **Aur.**, Bar. c., BELL., BISM., Bor., **Bov.**, Brom., BRY., Calad., CALC. C., Camph., **Cannab. s.**, **Canth.**, Caps., Carb. an., *Carb. v.*, CAUST., *Cham.*, **Chel.**, Chin., Cic., Cina, Clem., **Cocc.**, Coff., **Colch.**, COLOC., *Con.*, Croc., **Cup.**, Cyc., *Dig.*, Dros., *Dulc.*, Euphorb., Euphr., *Fer.*, Fl. ac., GRAPH., Guai., Hell., Hep., Hyos., **Ign.**, Iod., *Ip.*, *Iris v.*, K. carb., K. nit., Kre., **Lach.**, Laur., Led., **Lith.**, *Lyc.*, *Mag. c.*, Mag. m., **Mang.**, Mar., Meny., Merc., Mez., Millef., Mos., Mur. ac, **Nat. c.**, Nat. m., Nit. ac., Nux m., **Nux v.**, Oleand., Op., Par., *Petrol.*, PHOS., *Pho. ac.*, **Phyt.**, Plat., **Pb.**, Pso., PULS., *Ran. b.*, Ran. s., *Rheum*, RHODO., *Rhus*, Ruta, Saba., Sabi., Samb., **Sang.**, *Sars.*, Sec. c., Sele., Seneg., SEP., SIL., Spig., Spo., Squ., Stan., *Staph.*, Stram., Stro., *Sul.*, **Sul. ac.**, Tar., *Thuj.*, Valer., Verat. a., Verb., *Vio. o.*, Vio. t., *Zinc.*

Lower Extremities.

Loins (Region of Hips).—Acon., ÆSC., *Agar.*, Agn., **Alum.**, *Ambr.*, Am. carb., *Am. m.*, Anac., *Ant. cr.*, Ant. t., Arg., **Arn.**, *Ars.*, *Asaf.*, **Asar.**, Aur., Bar. c., **Bell.**, *Berb.*, Bov., *Bry.*, **Calc. c.**, Camph., *Cannab. s.*, **Canth.**, Carb. an., *Carb. v.*, CAUST., Cham., *Chel.*, *Chin.*, Cic., *Cina*, *Clem.*, **Cocc.**, Coff., **Colch.**, Coloc., *Con.*, Cyc., Dig., Dros., *Dulc.*, EUPHORB., Fer., *Graph.*, Hell., Hep., Hyos., Ign., **Iod.**, *Iris v.*, *K. bi.*, K. CARB., *K. nit*, Kre., **Lach.**, *Laur.*, Led., LYC., *Mag. c.*, Mag. m., Mang., *Mar.*, **Meny.**, Merc., **Mez.**, Mos., Mur. ac., *Nat. c.*, **Nat. m.**, *Nit. ac.*, Nux v., *Oleand.*, *Par.*, Petrol., Phos., Pho. ac., Plat., *Pb.*, **Puls.**, Ran. b., Ran. s., Rheum, Rhodo., Rhus, RUTA., Saba., **Sabi.**, Samb., Sars., Sec. c., Sele., Seneg., SEP., *Sil.*, Spig., Spo., *Stan.*, *Staph.*, Stram., *Stro.*, SUL., **Tar.**, *Thuj.*, *Trill.*, *Valer.*, Verat. a., Verb., Vio. o., Vio. t., **Zinc.**

Nates.—Alum., Ambr., *Am. m.*, **Ant. cr.**, Asaf., *Bar. c.*, Bell., *Berb.*, Bor., *Bry.*, Calc. c., Camph., Cannab. s., **Canth.**, Carb. v., **Caust.**, *Chin.*, Cina, Cocc., Coff., **Con.**, Croc., *Cyc.*, Dig., Dros., Dulc., GRAPH., Guai.,

LOWER EXTREMITIES.

Hep., *Hyos.*, Ign., Iod., **K. carb.**, *Lach.*, *Laur.*, **Lyc.**, Mag. c., *Mang.*
Meny., Merc., **Mez.**, Mur. ac., Nat. c., Nat. m., Nit. ac., Nux v., *Oleand.*,
Phos., Pho. ac., *Plat.*, **Puls.**, **Rhus**, Samb., *Sars.*, *Sele.*, **Sep.**, **Sil.**, Spig.,
Stan., STAPH., Stro., **Sul.**, Tar., *Ther.*, Thuj., Verat. a., Vio. t., **Zinc**.

Thigh.—*Acon.*, *Agar.*, Agn., Alum., Ambr., Am. carb., *Am. m.*, *Anac.*,
Ant. cr., Ant. t., **Apoc. c.**, Arg., **Arn.**, *Ars.*, *Asaf.* *Asar.*, *Aur.*, Bar. c.,
Bell., *Berb.*, Bism., Bor., *Bov.*, *Bry.*, Calad., *Calc. c.*, Calc. ph., Camph.,
Cannab. s., Canth., **Caps.**, *Curb. an.*, **Carb. v.**, *Caust.*, *Cham.*, Chel.,
CHIN., *Cic.*, Cina, *Clem.*, **Cocc.**, *Coc. c.*, Coff., Colch., **Coloc.**, Con.,
Croc., Cup., Cyc., *Dig.*, *Dios.*, Dros., Dulc., *Eup. pur.*, Euphorb., Euphr.,
Fer., Gnap., Graph., GUAI., *Hell.*, Hep., *Hyos.*, *Ign.*, Iod., Ip., **K. bi.**,
K. carb., K. nit., Kre., Lach., Laur., *Led.*, Lyc., Mag. c., **Mag. m.**, Mang.,
Mar., *Meny.*, MERC., **Mez.**, *Mos.*, *Mur. ac.*, *Nat. c.*, **Nat. m.**, *Nit. ac.*, Nux
m., **Nux v.**, *Oleand.*, *Ox. ac.*, Par., *Petrol.*, Phos., *Pho. ac.*, *Phyt.*, **Plat.**,
Pb., **Puls.**, *Ran. b.*, Ran. s., Rheum, *Rhodo.*, **Rhus**, *Ruta*, Saba., *Sabi.*,
Sal. ac., Samb., *Sars.*, Sele., Seneg., **Sep.**, *Sil.*, Spig., **Spo.**, *Squ.*, Stan.,
Staph., *Still.*, Stram., Stro., **Sul.**, Sul. ac., Tar., **Thuj.**, *Valer.*, Verat. a.,
Verb., Vio. t., *Visc.*, *Xan.*, Zinc.

—Anterior Part.—*Agar.*, Ambr., ANAC., Ant. cr., Arg., Asaf., *Aur.*,
Bar. c., Bell., *Berb.*, Bov., *Bry.*, Calc. c., *Cannab. s.*, *Chel.*, **Chin.**, Cina,
Coloc., Con., *Dig.*, Dros., *Dulc.*, Euphorb., *Euphr.*, **Gnaph.**, Hep., K. carb.,
Laur., Lyc., *Mag. c.*, Mang., *Meny.*, Merc., Mos., **Mur. ac.**, Nat. c., *Nat. m.*,
Nit. ac., Nux v., *Oleand.*, *Pho. ac.*, Plat., Pb., Puls., *Rhus*, Saba., **Sabi.**,
Samb., Sars., Sil., Spig., SPO., Stan., Staph., Tar., Thuj., *Valer.*, *Vib. op.*,
Vio. t., *Xan.*, Zinc.

—Posterior Part.—Agar., *Alum.*, Ambr., Am. carb., **Am. m.**, Anac.,
Ant. cr., *Ant. t.*, Asaf., *Aur.*, *Bar. c.*, Bell., **Berb.**, Bor., Calc. c., Camph.,
Cannab. s., **Canth.**, *Caps.*, *Carb. v.*, **Caust.**, Chin., Cina, Cocc., *Coff.*, **Con.**,
Croc., **Cyc.**, Dig., Dros., Dulc., Euphorb., Euphr., **Graph.**, Guai., Hep.,
Hyos., *Ign.*, Iod., **K. carb.**, Laur., *Led.*, **Lyc.**, Mag. c., Mag. m., *Mang.*,
Meny., **Merc.**, **Mez.**, *Mos.*, Mur. ac., Nat. c., Nat. m., Nit. ac., Nux v.,
Oleand., *Par.*, Phos., **Pho. ac.**, *Plat.*, Pb., Puls., Ran. b., Rheum, *Rhus*,
Samb., Sars., *Sele.*, Seneg., **Sep.**, *Sil.*, Spig., *Stan.*, **Staph.**, Stro., SUL.,
Sul. ac., Tar., Thuj., Valer., *Verat. a.*, Vio. t., ZINC.

—Outer Side.—Agar., Agn., *Alum.*, **Anac.**, Ant. cr., Arn., Asaf., *Aur.*,
Bar. c., *Bell.*, Bism., *Canth.*, Carb. an., Carb. v., **Caust.**, Chin., *Cocc.*,
Colch., *Euphorb.*, Laur., Mag. c., Mang., Meny., Merc., Mez., Mos., Mur.
ac., Nat. c., Nit. ac., Nux v., Oleand., PHO. AC., *Phyt.*, Rhus, Ruta,
Sars., *Spig.*, **Stan.**, Staph., **Sul.**, Tar., *Valer.*, **Zinc**.

—Inner Side.—Agn., Alum., Anac., Ant. cr., Arg., **Arn.**, Ars., *Asaf.*,

LOWER EXTREMITIES. 137

Bar. c., **Bell.**, *Berb.*, **Calc. c.**, *Camph.*, **Caps.**, *Carb. an.*, *Carb. v.*, **Caust.**, Chin., Cocc., Coff., Dig., **Graph.**, **Hep.**, Ign., Iod., **K. carb.**, *Kre.*, Laur., *Lyc.*, Mag. m., *Mang.*, Meny., **Merc.**, Mez., Mos., Mur. ac., Nat. c., Nat. m., *Nit. ac.*, Nux v., Oleand., Par., **PETROL.**, **Plat.**, *Pb.*, Ran. b., **RHODO.**, Rhus, Ruta, Saba., **Sabi.**, *Samb.*, Sars., **Sele.**, Sep., *Spo.*, **STAN.**, Staph., **SUL.**, Sul. ac., *Tar.*, Thuj., Verb., *Vio. t.*, Zinc.

Leg Below Knee.—*Abrot.*, **Acon.**, *Agar.*, *Agn.*, *Alum.*, *Ambr.*, *Am. cvrb.*, *Am. m.*, **Anac.**, *Ant. cr.*, Ant. t., Arg., *Arn.*, *Ars.*, **Asaf.**, Asar., **Atrop.**, Aur., *Bar. c.*, **Bell.**, *Berb.*, Bism., *Bor.*, *Bov.*, **Bry.**, Calad., **CALC. C.**, *Camph.*, Cannab. s., *Canth.*, Caps., Carb. an., Carb. v., *Carb. sul.*, **Caust.**, *Cham.*, *Chel.*, *Chin.*, Cic., *Cina*, Clem., Cocc., Coff., Colch., *Coloc.*, *Con.*, Croc., *Crotal.*, **Crot. tig.**, Cup., *Cyc.*, Dig., *Dios.*, Dros., Dulc., *Euphorb.*, Euphr., *Fer.*, *Fl. ac.*, *Gran.*, **Graph.**, *Grind.*, *Guai.*, *Ham.*, Hell., *Helo.*, Hep., Hyos., *Ign.*, Iod., *Ip.*, **K. carb.**, *K. nit.*, *Kre.*, *Kalm.*, Lach., Laur., *Led.*, **LYC.**, *Mag. c.*, Mag. m., Mang., *Mur.*, **Meny.**, **Merc.**, **Mez.**, Mos., Mur. ac., *Nat. c.* Nat. m., *Nit. ac.*, Nux m., **Nux v.**, *Oleand.*, Op., **Ox. ac.**, Par., *Petrol.*, **Phos.**, **Pho. ac.**, *Pic. ac.*, *Plat.*, **Pb.**, *Pso.*, **PULS.**, Ran. b., *Ran. s.*, Rheum, **Rhodo.**, **Rhus**, *Ruta.*, Saba., Sabi., Samb., Sars., *Sec. c.*, *Sele.*, Seneg., **SEP.**, **SIL.**, *Spig.*, Spo., Squ., *Stan.*, **STAPH.**, *Still.*, Stram., Stro., **Sul.**, Sul. ac., *Tar.*, *Tarent.*, Thuj., *Valer.*, Verat. a., Verb., Vio. t., Zinc.

Tibia.—**AGAR.**, *Agn.*, Alum., Ambr., Am. carb., **Anac.**, Ant. cr., Arn., Ars., **ASAF.**, Asar., Aur., Bar. c., **Bell.**, *Bism.*, Bry., **CALC. C.**, *Calc. ph.*, Cannab. s., Carb. an., *Caust.*, Cham., Chel., *Chin.*, Cina, Clem., Cocc., Coff., Colch., *Coloc.*, Con., Cyc., Dig., Dros., Dulc., Euphorb., Euphr., Guai., Hyos., *Ign.*, K. carb., Kre., Lach., Laur., *Lyc.*, Mag. c., Mag. m., **Mang.**, Meny., MERC., Mez., Mos., Mur. ac., Nat. c., Nit. ac., Nux v., Par., *Petrol.*, **PHOS.**, Pho. ac., **Plat.**, Pb., **PULS.**, **Rhodo.**, **RHUS**, *Saba.*, **Sabi.**, Samb., Sars., **Sep.**, Sil., *Spig.*, Spo., Stan., Staph., *Sul.*, Sul. ac., **Tar.**, *Thuj.*, Valer., Verat. a., Vio. t., Zinc.

Calf.—Acon., *Agar.*, Agn., **ALUM.**, Ambr., Am. carb., Am. m., **Anac.**, **Ant. cr.**, Ant. t., Arg., *Arn.*, **ARS.**, Asaf., Asar., Bar. c., Bell., *Benz. ac.*, Bism., Bor., *Bov.*, **Bry.**, **CALC. C.**, Calc. ph., Camph., Cannab. s., *Canth.*, **Caps.**, Carb. an., *Carb. v.*, *Caust.*, **Cham.**, **Chel.**, **Chin.**, Cina, *Coca*, *Cocc.*, Coff., Colch., **Coloc.**, Con., *Croc.*, **Cup.**, Cyc., Dig., Dulc., *Eup. per.*, Euphorb., **Euphr.**, **Fer.**, **GRAPH.**, *Guai.*, Hep., *Hyos.*, Ign., *Ip.*, *Jat.*, K. carb., K. nit., Kre., Lach., Laur., **Led.**, **Lyc.**, *Mag. c.*, Mag. m., **Mang.**, Mar., Meny., *Merc.*, *Mur. ac.*, **Nat. c.**, **Nat. m.**, **NIT. AC.**, **Nux v.**, *Oleand.*, Op., Par., *Petrol.*, Phos., Pho. ac., **Plat.**, *Pb.*, *Pod.*, **PULS.**, Rheum, **RHUS**, Ruta, *Saba.*, **Sabi.**, Samb., Sars., *Sec. c.*, Sele.,

7

SEP., Sil., Spig., STAN., STAPH., Stram., *Stro.*, SUL., **Tar.**, *Thuj.*, VALER., **Verat. a.**, *Vib. op., Vio. t.*, Zinc.

Tendo Achilles.—*Acon., Aesc., Alum.,* ANAC., *Ant. cr.*, Arg., Arn., *Bell.,* **Benz. ac.,** *Bism.,* Bry., Camph., Carb. an., *Caust.,* Chel., **Cimic.,** *Dios., Dulc.,* **Euphr.,** *Hep.,* K. carb., Kre., *Mar., Mez.,* MUR. AC., *Nat. c., Nat. m.,* Plat., *Puls.,* Ran. b., Rheum, Rhodo., *Rhus, Sabi.,* SEP., *Stan.,* **Staph., Sul.,** Sul. ac., Thuj., *Valer.,* ZINC.

Foot.—Acon., Agar., **Agn.,** *Alum., Ambr., Am. carb.,* **Am. m.,** *Anac.,* Ant. cr., **Ant. t., Apis,** Arg., ARN., **Ars.,** *Asaf.,* Asar., *Aur.,* **Bar. c., BELL.,** Bism., *Bor., Bov.,* **Brom.,** BRY., Calad., **Calc. c.,** *Camph., Cannab. s.,* Canth., *Caps.,* Carb. an., *Carb. v., Carb. sul.,* **Caust.,** *Ced., Cham.,* **Chel.,** *Chin.,* Cic., Cina, *Clem., Cocc., Coc. c., Coff.,* Colch., Coloc., *Con.,* Croc., **Crot. tig., Cup.,** Cyc., Dig., Dros., Dulc., **Elaps.,** Euphorb., **Fer.,** *Gel., Glon.,* **Graph.,** *Guai.,* **Hell.,** *Hep.,* Hyos., *Ign.,* Iod., Ip., **K. carb.,** K nit., **Kalm.,** *Kre.,* **Lach.,** *Laur., Led., Lith.,* LYC., Mag. c., *Mag. m.,* Mang., *Meli.,* **Meny.,** MERC., *Mez., Mur. ac.,* NAT. C., *Nat. m., Nit. ac.,* Nux m., **Nux v.,** *Oleand.,* Op., **Ox. ac., Par.,** *Petrol.,* **Phos.,** *Pho. ac.,* **Plat., Pb.,** PULS., Ran. b., Ran. s., Rheum, Rhodo., Rhus, Ruta, Saba., *Sabi.,* Samb., *Sars., Sec. c.,* **Sele.,** SEP., SIL., Spig., Spo., **Squ.,** Stan., Staph., **Stram.,** Stro., **Sul.,** *Sul. ac.,* Tar., *Thuj.,* Valer., **Verat. a.,** *Verb.,* Vio. t., Zinc.

Heel.—Agar., Agn., Alum., *Ambr., Am. carb.,* **Am. m.,** *Anac.,* **Ant. cr.,** Ant. t., *Arg.,* **Arn.,** Ars., Aur., Bar. c., Bell., Bism., *Bor.,* **Bry.,** **Calc. c.,** *Cannab. s.,* Canth., Caps., Carb. an., *Carb. sul.,* CAUST., Ced., Cham., *Chin.,* Cic., *Cina,* Clem., Cocc., *Colch.,* Cyc., Dros., *Euphorb.,* GRAPH., Hell., Hep., IGN., Iod., *K. carb.,* K. nit., Kre., Lach., Laur., LED., *Lyc., Mag. c.,* Mag. m., Meny., *Merc.,* Mez., *Mur. ac.,* NAT. C., Nit. ac., *Nux v.,* Oleand., **Par.,** Petrol., *Phos.,* Pho. ac., *Phyt.,* Plat., **Pb.,** PULS., *Ran. b.,* Ran. s., Rheum, Rhodo., Rhus, *Ruta,* SABI., Sars., **Sele.,** SEP., Sil., Spo., Stan., Staph., Stro., Sul., Sul. ac., Thuj., **Valer.,** *Verat. a., Vio. t.,* Zinc.

Back of Foot.—*Agar.,* **Anac.,** Ant. t., Arg., Ars., **Asaf.,** Aur., Bell., *Bism.,* **Bry.,** *Calc. c.,* CAMPH., Cannab. s., *Canth., Carb. an.,* CAUST., Chel., **Chin.,** Cocc., **Colch.,** *Coloc.,* Con., **Cup.,** *Cyc.,* Dig., Graph., Guai., **Hep.,** *Ign., K. carb.,* Lach., **Led., Lyc.,** *Mag. m.,* Mang., *Merc.,* Mez., Mos., **Mur. ac., Nat. c.,** Nat. m., Nit. ac., *Nux v.,* Oleand., *Par.,* Petrol., Phos., **Plat.,** Pb., **Puls.,** Ran. b., Ran. s., *Rheum,* **Rhus,** Ruta, Sabi., Sars., *Sep., Sil.,* SPIG., Spo., Stan., Staph., Stram., *Sul.,* TAR., **Thuj.,** Vio. t., **Zinc.**

Sole.—Acon., Agar., Agn., *Alum., Ambr., Am. carb.,* Am. m., *Anac.,*

LOWER EXTREMITIES. 139

Ant. cr., Ant t., *Arg., Arn., Ars.,* Asaf., Asar., Aur., *Bar. c.,* **Bell.,** *Berb.,* Bism., **Bor.,** Bov., **Bry.,** Calad., **Calc. c.,** **Cannab. i.,** **Canth.,** Carb. an., *Carb. v., Carb. sul.,* **Caust.,** *Ced., Cham., Chel.,* **Chin.,** Cic., Cina, Clem., Coff., *Colch.,* Coloc., Con., *Croc.,* CUP., Dig., Dros., Dulc., Euphorb., *Fer.,* **Graph.,** Hell., *Hep.,* Hyos., *Ign., K. carb.,* K. nit., **Kre.,** Lach., Laur., **Led.,** *Lith., Lyc.,* Mag. m., Mang., Meny., *Merc., Mez.,* MUR. AC., **Nat. c.,** Nat. m., Nit. ac., Nux m., *Nux v.,* Oleand., Par., **Petrol.,** **Phos.,** PHO. AC., *Phyt., Plat.,* **Pb.,** PULS., Ran. s., Rheum, Rhodo., *Rhus,* Ruta, *Saba., Sabi.,* Samb., *Sars.,* Sec. c., Sele., **Sep., Sil.,** *Spig.,* Squ., **Stan.,** *Staph., Stro.,* SUL., Sul. ac., TAR., **Thuj.,** Valer., Verat. a., Verb., *Vio. t.,* Zinc.

Toes.—Acon., Agar., Agn., *Alum.,* Ambr., **Am. carb.,** **Am. m.,** Anac., *Ant. cr.,* **Ant. t.,** Arg., ARN., *Ars., Asaf.,* Asar., **Aur.,** *Bar. c.,* **Bell.,** Bism., *Bor.,* Bov., Bry., Calad., *Calc. c.,* Camph., Cannab. s., Caps., **Carb. an., Carb. v.,** *Carb. sul.,* **Caul.,** CAUST., Cham., *Chel.,* **Chin.,** Cic., Cimic., Cina, *Clem.,* Cocc., *Colch.,* Con., *Cup.,* **Cyc.,** Dig., Dros., *Dulc.,* Euphr., *Fer.,* GRAPH., Guai., Hell., *Hep.,* Hyos., Ign., **K. carb.,** K. nit., **Kre.,** *Lach.,* Laur., **Led.,** *Lyc., Mag. c.,* Mag. m., Mar., **Merc., Mez.,** *Mos.,* Mur. ac., **Nat. c.,** *Nat. m., Nit. ac.,* Nux m., *Nux v.,* Oleand., *Par.,* *Petrol.,* **Phos., Pho. ac.,** PLAT., *Pb.,* Puls., *Ran. b.,* **RAN. S.,** Rheum, *Rhodo., Rhus, Ruta,* Saba., **SABI.,** *Sal. ac.,* Sars., **Sec. c., Sep., Sil.,** *Spig.,* Spo., Squ., **Staph.,** *Stro.,* SUL., Sul. ac., **Tar.,** THUJ., *Valer.,* Verat. a., Verb., Vio. t., Zinc.

—**Great.**—Agar., **All. c.,** *Alum.,* Ambr., **Am. carb.,** *Am. m., Anac.,* **Ant. cr.,** ARN., Ars., ASAF., ATROP., **Aur.,** Bar. c., *Benx. ac.,* Bism., *Bry., Calc. c., Cannab. s.,* Caps., Carb. an., CAUST., Chin., **Cimic.,** Clem., *Cocc., Colch., Con.,* Cup., **Cyc.,** *Dulc.,* Fer., *Graph., Hell., Hep.,* Iod., K. CARB., Laur., **Led.,** *Mag. c., Mar.,* Merc., **Mez.,** Mur. ac., **Nat. c.,** Nat. m., **Nit. ac.,** Nux v., *Oleand.,* Petrol., **Phos.,** Pho. ac., PLAT., *Pb.,* **Puls.,** Ran. b., *Ran. s.,* **Rhus,** Ruta, **Sabi.,** *Sars.,* Sep., SIL., **Staph.,** *Sul.,* Sul. ac., *Tar.,* **Thuj.,** Verat. a., Vio. t., ZINC.

—**Tips.**—*Acon.,* Alum., Ambr., *Am. carb.,* **Am. m.,** *Arn.,* Ars., **Asaf.,** *Bism.,* Calc. c., *Camph.,* Canth., *Caps.,* **Chin.,** Hep., K. CARB., Lach., Led., *Mos.,* **Mur. ac.,** Oleand., Phos., **Puls.,** *Ran. b.,* SEP., **Sil.,** Spig., **Thuj.,** Zinc.

—**Balls.**—Agar., **Ambr.,** Am. carb., *Am. m.,* **Ant. cr.,** Ant. t., *Ars., Asaf., Bar. c.,* BRY., CANNAB. S., Carb. an., Caust., Cina, Coff., **Colch.,** Con., *Cup.,* Dros., *Graph., Hell.,* **K. carb.,** Laur., **LED.,** Lyc., Mez., Mur. ac., **Nit. ac.,** PETROL., Pho. ac., Plat., Pb., **PULS.,** *Ran. s.,* **Rhus,** Saba., *Sabi.,* SPIG., Squ., *Tar.,* V10. t.

LOWER EXTREMITIES.

Nails.—*Alum.*, Ant. cr.. *Ars.*, Bor., *Bov.*, Calc. c., *Caust.*, Colch., *Con.*, *Dig.*, GRAPH., *Hell.*, Hep., *Mar.*, **Merc.**, Mos., Mur. ac., *Nat. c.*, Nat. m., Nit. ac., Nux v., Par., Pho. ac., Puls., Ran. b., SABA., **Sep.**, Sil., *Squ.*, *Sul.*, *Thuj.*

Corns. See Under **Skin.**

Joints of Lower Extremities in General.—Acon., Agar., Agn., Alum., Ambr., *Am. carb.*, Am. m., Anac., Ant. cr., Ant. t., **Arg.**, **Arn.**, Ars., Asaf., Asar., *Aur.*, Bar. c., *Bell.*, Benz. ac., Bism., Bor., Bov., **Bry.**, Calad., CALC. C., Camph., Cannab. s., Canth., *Caps.*, *Carb. an.*, Carb. v., CAUST., Cham., Chel., **Chin.**, Cic., Cina, Clem., *Cocc.*, *Coff.*, Colch., *Coloc.*, *Con.*, Croc., Cup., *Cyc.*, *Dig.*, Dros., Dulc., Euphorb., Euphr., **Fer.**, **Graph.**, Guai., *Hell.*, Hep., *Hyos.*, *Ign.*, Iod., *Ip.*, K. CARB., K. nit., Kre., Lach., Laur., LED., LYC., *Mag. c.*, Mag. m., Mang., *Mar.*, *Meli.*, **Meny.**, **Merc.**, *Mez.*, Mos., Mur. ac., Nat. c., NAT. M., *Nit. ac.*, Nux m., **Nux v.**, Oleand., **Par.**, **Petrol.**, **Phos.**, *Pho. ac.*, **Phyt.**, **Plat.**, Pb., *Puls.*, Ran. b., Ran. s., *Rheum*, Rhodo., RHUS, *Ruta*, Saba., *Sabi.*, Samb., Sars., Sec. c., Sele., Seneg., SEP., Sil., *Spig.*, Spo., Squ., **Stan.**, **Staph.**, STRO. SUL., Sul. ac., *Tur.*, Thuj., Valer., *Verat. a.*, Verb., Vio. t., **Zinc.**

Hip-Joint.—Acon., Agn., Alum., Am. carb., Am. m., **Ant. cr.**, Ant. t., Arg., **Arn.**, Asaf., Asar., *Aur.*, Bar. c., **Bell.**, BRY., CALC. C., Camph., *Caps.*, Carb. an., CAUST., Cham., Chel., *Chin.*, **Cocc.**, Colch., *Coloc.*, Con., Croc., Dros., *Dulc.*, *Euphorb.*, Euphr., **Fer.**, Graph., **Hell.**, Hep., Hyos., *Ign.*, Iod., **K. carb.**, K. nit., *Kre.*, LED., **Lyc.**, *Mag. c.*, Mag. m., *Meny.*, **Merc.**, *Merc. c.*, Mez., **Nat. m.**, *Nit. ac.*, Nux v., *Par.*, Petrol., Phos., *Pho. ac.*, Plat., Pb., *Puls.*, RHUS, Samb., Seneg., **Sep.**, Sil., *Stan.*, Staph., **Stro.**, Sul., Thuj., *Verat. a.*, Zinc.

Knee.—*Abrot.*, Acon., Aesc., Agar., Agn., Alum., Ambra., Am. carb., Am. m., **Anac.**, Ant. cr., Ant. t., **Apis**, **Arg.**, Arn., Ars., **Asaf.**, *Asar.*, ATROP., *Aur.*, Bar. c., *Bell.*, **Benz. ac.**, Bor., BRY., Calad., CALC. C., *Calc. f.*, *Calc. ph.*, *Calot.*, Camph., *Cannab. s.*, *Canth.*, *Caps.*, Carb. an., **Carb. v.**, **Caul.**, CAUST., Cham., Chel., CHIN., Cina, *Clem.*, *Cocc.*, Coff., Colch., *Coloc.*, *Con.*, *Croc.*, Cup., *Cyc.*, *Dig.*, *Dios.*, Dros., Dulc., Euphorb., Euphr., **Fer.**, *Fer. ph.*, **Graph.**, Guai., Hell., *Hep.*, Hyos., *Ign.*, *Iod.*, Ip., *K. carb.*, K. nit., Kre., *Lach.*, *Laur.*, LED., **Lyc.**, *Mag. c.*, Mag. m., Mang., Mar., *Meny.*, **Merc.**, Mez., Mos., *Mur. ac.*, *Nat. c.*, NAT. M., **Nit. ac.**, Nux m., NUX V., Oleand., *Oxyt.*, Par., PETROL., PHOS., *Pho. ac.*, *Phyt.*, *Plat.*, Pb., PULS., Ran. b., Ran. s., *Rheum*, *Rhodo.*, RHUS, *Ruta*, Saba., *Sabi.*, Samb., *Sars.*, Sele., Seneg., SEP., **Sil.**, **Spig.**, *Spo.*, **Stan.**, Staph., *Stict.*, Stro., SUL., *Sul. ac.*, *Tur.*, Thuj., *Valer.*, **Verat. a.**, *Verb.*, Vio. t., **Zinc.**

LOWER EXTREMITIES. 141

Knee, Hollow of.—Alum., *Ambr.*, Am. carb., Am. m., Ant. t., **Ars.,** Asaf., Asar., **BELL.,** Bor., Bry., Calc. c., Cannab. s., Carb. an., **Caust.,** Chel., *Chin.*, Cocc., Coloc., Con., Dig., *Dios.*, Dros., Euphorb., Euphr., Fer., Graph., Guai., Hell Hep., K. carb., *Kre.*, Lach., Laur., *Led.*, *Lyc.*, Mag. c., *Mang.*, Meny., **Merc.,** Mez., Mur. ac., **Nat. c., NAT. M., Nit. ac.,** **Nux v.,** Oleand., Par., **Petrol.,** Phos., Pho. ac., Plat., **Puls.,** Ran. b., **Ran. s.,** **Rheum, Rhus,** Ruta, Samb., *Sars.*, Sep., *Spo.*, Squ., **Stan.,** Staph., **Sul.,** Sul. ac., Tar., Thuj., *Valer.*, Verat. a., *Zinc.*

Patella.—*Acon.*, Alum., Am. carb., Anac., *Arg.*, Arn., **Asaf., BELL.,** Bry., Calc. c., **CAMPH., Cannab. s., Carb. ac.,** Carb. v., **Caust.,** *Chel., Chin.*, Cocc., *Con.*, Graph., Guai., Hell., *Kre.*, **Led.,** Lyc., Mar., Meny., Mez., Mur. ac., **Nit. ac.,** Nux v., *Ox. ac.*, Par., Phos., Pho. ac., Ran. b., *Rhus*, Samb., Sars., Sep., **Spig., Stan., Staph.,** Stro., *Sul.*, Tar., Thuj., Verb., *Vio. t.*, Zinc.

Ankle.—*Acon.*, Agar., *Agn.*, Alum., *Ambr.*, Am. carb., Am. m., Anac., Ant. cr., *Ant. s. aur.*, *Arg.*, Arn., *Ars.*, Asaf., Asar., Aur., **Bar. c.,** Bell., Bism., Bor., Bov., *Bry.*, **Calc. c.,** Camph., Caps., Carb. an., Carb. v., **Caul., CAUST.,** Chel., *Chin.*, Cic., *Clem.*, Cocc., *Colch.*, Coloc., Con., Croc., Cyc., Dig., **Dros.,** Dulc., Euphorb., Euphr., *Fer.*, *Fer. ph.*, Graph., Guai., *Hell.*, Hep., Hyos., *Ign.*, Iod., **K. carb.,** K. nit., *Kre.*, Lach., **Led.,** **LYC.,** Mag. m., *Mang.*, Mar., **Merc.,** Mez., Mos., Mur. ac., *Nat. c.*, **NAT. M.,** *Nit. ac.*, Nux v., Oleand., Par., **Petrol.,** Phos., *Pho. ac.*, Plat., Pb., **Puls.,** Ran. b., Ran. s., Rheum, Rhodo., **RHUS, Ruta,** Samb., Sars., Sec. c., Sele., Seneg., **SEP., Sil.,** *Spig.*, Spo., *Stan.*, Staph., **Stro., SUL.,** Sul. ac., Tar., Thuj., *Valer.*, Verat. a., Vio. t., **Zinc.**

Toe-Joints.—*Act.*, *Agn.*, Ambr., *Am. carb.*, Ant. cr., Ant. t., **Arg., Arn., AUR.,** Bell., **Benz. ac.,** *Bism.*, **BRY.,** *Calc. c.*, *Caps.*, *Carb. an.*, Carb. v., **CAUST., Cham.,** Chel., **Chin.,** Cina, Cocc., **Colch.,** Con., Cup., Cyc., Dros., **Fer.,** Graph., Hell., Hep., *Hyos.*, *K. bi.*, **K. CARB., LED., Lyc.,** Mag. c., MAR., *Meli.*, **Merc.,** Mez., Nat. c., *Nat. m.*, Nit. ac., **Nux v.,** *Petrol.*, **Phos.,** Pho. ac., Plat., Pb., *Puls.*, Ran. b., Ran. s., **Rhus, Ruta, SABI.,** Sec. c., **SEP.,** *Sil.*, Spig., Staph., *Stict.*, **Stro., SUL.,** *Tar.*, Verat. a., **ZINC.**

Bones of Lower Extremities in General.—Agar., Alum., Am. carb., Am. m., Anac., **Aran.,** Arg., Ars., *Asaf.*, **Aur.,** Bar. c., Bell., *Bism.*, Bor., **BRY., Calc. c.,** Cannab. s., Canth., Caps., Carb. an., Carb. v., Caust., **Chin.,** Cocc., Coloc., **Con.,** Cup., *Cyc.*, **Dros.,** Dulc., *Euphorb.*, Graph., *Guai.*, Hep., Iod., Ip., **K. carb.,** *K. nit.*, **Kre.,** Lach., Laur., *Led.*, **Lyc.,** Mag. c., Mag. m., Mar., MERC., *Mez.*, Mos., Mur. ac., Nat. c., **Nit. ac.,** Nux v., Oleand., Petrol., **PHOS., Pho. ac., PULS., Rhodo.,**

142   LOWER EXTREMITIES—SENSATIONS.

Rhus, RUTA, Saba., Sabi., Samb., Sars., Sep., SIL., Spig., STAPH.,
Stro., Sul., Thuj., Valer., Verat. a., Vio. t., Zinc.

Left.—Acon., Agar., Agn., Alum., AMBR., Am. carb., Am. m., Anac.,
Ant. cr., Ant. t., Apis, Arg., Arn., Ars., ASAF., Asar., Aur., Bar. c.,
Bell., Berb., Bism., Bor., Bov., Brom., Bry., Calad., CALC. C., Camph.,
Cannab. s., Canth., Caps., Carb. an., Carb. v., Caust., Cham., Chel., Chin.,
Cic., CINA., Clem., Cocc., Coff., Colch., Coloc., Con., Croc., Cup., Cyc.,
Dig., Dios., Dros., Dulc., Eup. pur., Euphorb., Euphr., FER., Fl. ac.,
Graph., Guai., Hell., HEP., Hyos., Ign., Iod., Ip., Iris v., K. carb., K.
nit., Kre., Jat., Lach., Laur., Led., LYC., Mag. c., Mag. m., Mang.,
Mar., Meny., Merc., Mez., Millef., Mos., Mur. ac., Nat. c., Nat. m.,
Nat. s., NIT. AC., Nux m., Nux v., Oleand., Op., Par., Petrol., Phos.,
Pho. ac., Plat., Pb., Pso., Puls., Ran. b., Ran. s., Rheum, Rhodo.,
RHUS, Ruta, Saba., Sabi., Samb., Sars., Sec. c., Sele., Seneg., Sep.,
SIL., Spig., Spo., Squ., Stan., Staph., Stram., Stro., SUL., Sul. ac., Tar.,
Thuj., Valer., Verat. a., Verb., Vio. o., Vio. t., Zinc.

Right.—Acon., Agar., Agn., Alum., Ambr., Am. carb., Am. m., Anac.,
Ant. cr., Ant. t., Apis, Arg., Arn., ARS., Asaf., Asar., Aur., Bar. c.,
BELL., Bism., Bor., Bov., Brom., BRY., Calad., Calc. c., Camph., Cannab. s., Canth., Caps., Carb. an., Carb. v., Caust., Cham., Chel., Chin.,
Cic., Cina., Clem., Cocc., Coff., Colch., COLOC., Con., Croc., Cup., Cyc.,
Dig., Dros., Dulc., Euphorb., Euphr., Fer., Fl. ac., GRAPH., Guai.,
Hell., Hep., Hyos., Ign., Iod., Ip., K, carb., K. nit., Kre., LACH., Laur.,
Led., Lyc., Mag. c., Mag m., Mang., Mar., Meny., Merc., Mez., Millef.,
Mos., Mur. ac., Nat. c., Nat. m., Nit. ac., Nux m., NUX V., Oleand.,
Op., Pall., Par., Petrol., Phos., Pho. ac., Plat., Pb., PSO., PULS., Ran.
b., Ran. s., Rheum, RHODO., Rhus, Ruta, Saba., Sabi., Samb., Sang.,
SARS., SEC. C., Sele., Seneg., SEP., Sil., Spig., Spo., Squ., Stan., Staph.,
Stram., Stro., Sul., Sul. ac., Tar., Ter., Thuj., Valer., Verat. a., Verb.,
Vio. o., Vio. t., Zinc.

Sensations.

Adhesion of Inner Parts, Sensation of.—Arn., Bry., Coloc., Dig.,
Euphorb., Hep., K. nit., Merc., Mez., Nux v., Par., Petrol., Phos., Pb.,
Puls., RHUS, Séneg., Sep., Sul., Thuj., Verb.

Air, Aversion t' Open.—Agar., Alum., Ambr., Am. carb., Am. m.,
Anac., Arn., Ars., Aur., Bell., Bry., CALC. C., Camph., Cannab. s., Canth.,
Caps., Carb. an., Carb. v., Caust., CHAM., Chel., Chin., Cic., Cina.,
COCC., COFF., Coloc., Con., Dig., Dros., Fer., Graph., Guai., Hep.,
IGN., Ip., K. CARB., K. nit., Kre., Lach., Laur., Led., Lyc., Mag. m.,

SENSATIONS. 143

Mang., *Mar.*, Meny., *Merc.*, **Mos.**, *Mur. ac.*, **NAT. C., Nat. m.,** *Nit. ac.*, **Nux m., NUX V.,** *Op.*, **PETROL.,** Phos., *Pho. ac.*, **Plat.,** *Pb.*, **Puls.,** Rhodo., **Rhus,** *Ruta,* Sabi., Sars., *Sele.,* Seneg., Sep., **SIL., Spig.,** *Staph.,* *Stram.,* Stro., **Sul., Sul. ac.,** *Thuj., Valer.,* Verat. a., Verb., **Vio. t.,** Zinc.

Air, Desire for Open.—Acon., **Agn.,** Alum., *Ambr.,* **Am. carb., Am. m.,** Anac., **Ant. cr.,** *Arg.,* **Arn.,** *Ars.,* Asaf., **Asar., AUR., Bar. c.,** Bell., **Bor.,** Bov., Bry., Calc. c., *Cannab. s., Caps.,* Carb. an., **Carb. v.,** *Caust.,* Cic., Cina, **CROC.,** Dig., *Gel.,* **Graph., Hell., Hep., Iod.,** K. carb., K. nit., Lach., *Laur.,* **Lyc., Mag. c.,** *Mag. m.,* Mang., Mar., *Meny.,* **Mez.,** Mos., Mur. ac., Nat. c., *Nat. m.,* Op., Phos., Pho. ac., **Plat.,** *Pb.,* **PULS.,** *Rhodo.,* Rhus, Ruta, *Sabi., Sars.,* Sele., Seneg., Sep., **Spig.,** *Spo., Stan.,* Staph., **Stram.,** *Stro.,* Sul., Sul. ac., **Tar.,** Thuj., Verat. a., Vio. t., Zinc.

Alive, Sensation of Something.—Anac., Asar., Bell., **Calc. ph.,** Cannab. s., Cocc., **CROC.,** Hyos., **Ign.,** Lach., Led., Mag. m., *Meny.,* Merc., Nat. m., Petrol., *Pb.,* **Puls.,** *Rhodo., Saba., Sec. c., Sil.,* Spo., *Sul.,* Tar., **THUJ.,** Vio. t.

Anxiety, General Physical.—*Acon., Agar.,* Am. m., **Amyl., Ant. t.,** **ARG. N., ARS.,** Bar. c., **Brom.,** Bry., **Calc. c., CAMPH.,** *Cannab. s.,* **Canth.,** Carb. v., **CHAM., Chel., Chin.,** *Cic.,* **Cocc.,** *Coff.,* **Colch.,** *Con.,* **Cup., DIG.,** Euphorb., *Fer.,* Guai., Ign., **Iod. IP.,** *Laur.,* **Lob. i., Lyc., Mar.,** Merc., Mez., *Mos.,* Mur. ac., Nat. m., **NUX V., PHOS., PHO. AC.,** Plat., *Pb.,* **PULS.,** Rhus, *Saba.,* Sabi., Sec. c., Seneg., **Sep., Stan.,** Staph., *Stram.,* **SUL.,** Sul. ac., Thuj., **Verat. a.,** Zinc.

Apoplexy.—**ACON.,** Anac., Ant. cr., Ant. t., Arn., Asar., **Aur.,** *Bov. c.,* **BELL.,** Bry., *Calc. c.,* Camph., Carb. v., **Chin., COCC., Coff.,** Con., Croc., Cup., *Dig.,* **Fer.,** Hep., **Hyos.,** *Ign.,* **Ip.,** *Kre.,* **LACH.,** *Laur.,* **Lyc.,** *Merc.,* Nat. m., Nit. ac., **Nux m., Nux v.,** Oleand., **OP.,** Phos., Pb., Puls., *Rhus,* Saba., *Samb.,* Sars., Sec. c., Sep., **Sil.,** *Stram.,* Sul., *Verat. a.,* Vio. o.

—**Hæmorrhagic.**—Acon., Aur., **Bell.,** Bry., *Calc. c.,* Camph., Chin., Cocc., *Coff., Fer.,* Ign., *Ip., Kre., Lach.,* **Lyc.,** Merc., Nux v., Oleand., *Rhus,* Saba., *Samb.,* Sep., Sul., Vio. o.

—**Nervous.**—Arn., Asar., *Bar. c.,* Bell., Bry., **Chin.,** *Coff.,* Cup., *Dig.,* Hyos., *Ign.,* Laur., Merc., *Nux v.,* Phos., *Puls.,* Rhus, *Sil., Stram.,* Vio. o.

Arthritic Nodes. See under **Bones.**

Ascending, Sensation of.—Am. m., **Asaf.,** Asar., Bor., *Hep.,* Laur., *Lyc.,* **Merc.,** Nat. c., *Nux v.,* **Phos., Plat.,** *Ran. b.,* Spig., *Sul. ac., Valer.,* **Verat. a.**

Asleep Feeling, in Single Parts.—Acon., *Agar., Alum., Ambr., Am. carb.,* Am. m., *Anac.,* Ant. cr., **Ant. t.,** Arg., Arn., Asaf., Asar.,

Aur., **Bar. c.**, Bell., Bor., *Bov.*, *Bry.*, **Calc. c.**, *Calc. ph.*, Camph., Cannab. s., Canth., *Caps.*, **CARB. AN.**, **Carb. v.**, *Caust.*, **Cham.**, Chel., **Chin.**, *Cic.*, Cina, COCC., Colch., **Coloc.**, Con., CROC., *Dig.*, Dros., Dulc., *Euphorb.*, *Euphr.*, Fer., GRAPH., Guai., Hep., *Hyos.*, **Ign.**, Iod., *Ip.*, **K. CARB.**, K. nit., Kre., Laur., *Led.*, **LYC.**, Mag. c., **Mag. m.**, Mang., *Mar.*, MERC., Mez., *Mos.*, Mur. ac., Nat. c., **Nat. m.**, *Nit. ac.*, **Nux v.**, *Oleand.*, **Op.**, **Par.**, Petrol., Phos., Pho. ac., Plat., *Pb*, **PULS.**, Rheum., **Rhodo.**, RHUS, Saba., Sabi., Samb., Sars., **Sec. c.**, **Sep.**, SIL., *Spig.*, Spo., Squ., Stan., Staph., **Stram.**, **Sul.**, *Sul. ac.*, *Thuj.*, Valer., **Verat. a.**, Zinc.

Ball Internally. (Compare with **Knotted Sensation.**)—*Acon.*, *Asaf.*, *Calc. c.*, **Cannab. i.**, *Caust.*, *Coloc.*, Con., *Crot. tig.*, *Graph.*, IGN., *K carb.*, **Lach.**, Mag. m., Nat. m., Par., **Phyt.**, Plat., Pb., Ruta., SEP., *Sil.*, Staph., *Stram.*, Sul., Valer.

Band, Sensation of a.—*Acon.*, Ambr., ANAC., Ant. cr., Ant. t., *Arg. n.*, Arn., Ars., Asaf., **Asar.**, Aur., **Bell.**, *Brom.*, *Bry.*, CACT., Calc. c., *Cannab. i.*, **CARB. AC.**, Carb. v., *Carb. sul.*, *Caust.*, CHEL., *Chin.*, *Cocc.*, *Coc. c.*, *Colch.*, Coloc., CON., *Croc.*, *Dig.*, *Gel.*, Graph., Hell., *Hyos.*, *Iod.*, Kre., Laur., *Lyc.*, **Merc.**, **Merc. i. r.**, Mos., **Nat. m.**, NIT. AC., *Nux m.*, **Nux v.**, Oleand., **Op.**, *Petrol.*, *Phos.*, **PLAT.**, PULS., *Saba.*, Sabi., *Sang.*, Sars., SIL., **Spig.**, Stan., SUL., *Sul. ac.*, Zinc.

Benumbing Pain.—*Acon.*, Agar., Agn., Am. carb., Anac., Ant. cr., Ant. t., Arg., Arn., *Asaf.*, *Asar.*, Aur., *Bell.*, Bov., Bry., **Calc. c.**, Cannab. s., Carb. an., *Chin.*, Cic., **Cina**, Cocc., Con., Croc., Cup., Cyc., Dros., Dulc., *Euphorb.*, Euphr., Hell., Hep., *Hyos.*, Ign., *K. nit.*, **Iris v.**, *Laur.*, Led., Mag. c., Mag. m., Mang., **Meny.**, **Mez.**, *Mos.*, Mur. ac., Nat. c., Nat. m., Nux m., OLEAND., Op., Par., *Phos.*, Pho. ac., *Plat.*, **Puls.**, **Rheum**, Rhus, *Ruta.*, SABA., Sabi., Samb., Seneg., Sep., *Stan.*, *Staph.*, Sul., Sul. ac., Tar., Valer., **Verat. a.**, VERB., Zinc.

Biting.—*Acon.*, Agar., Agn., Alum., **Ambr.**, Am. carb., Ant. cr., Ant. t., Arg., Arn., Ars., *Asar.*, Aur., *Bell.*, *Bry.*, Calad., *Calc. c.*, Camph., Cannab. s., **Canth.**, **Caps.**, Carb. an., **CARB. V.**, *Caust.*, Cham., **Chin.**, **Clem.**, Cocc., Colch., Coloc., *Con.*, Croc., **Dros.**, Dulc., **Euphorb.**, Euphr., *Graph.*, Hell., Hep., Hyos., Ign., Iod., Ip., **K. carb.**, K. nit., *Kre.*, Lach., Laur., Led., *Lyc.*, Mag. c., **Mar.**, Merc., Mez., Mos., *Mur. ac.*, Nat. c., *Nat. m.*, **Nit. ac.**, Nux m., **NUX V.**, Oleand., Op., *Pæo.*, Par., Petrol., **PETROS.**, Pho., Pho. ac., **Pru.**, **Puls.**, **Ran. b.**, **RAN. S.**, Rheum., *Rhodo.*, **Rhus**, Ruta., Saba., Sabi., Sars., *Sele*, **Seneg.**, **Sep.**, *Sil.*, *Spig.*, Squ., Stan., **Staph.**, Stram., Stro., SUL., Sul. ac., Thuj., *Valer.*, Verat. a., Vio. t., ZINC.

Blackness of External Parts.—Acon., *Agar.*, Alum., *Am. carb.*,

Ant. cr., Arn., Ars., *Asaf.,* Asar., *Aur.,* Bar. c., **Bell.,** *Bism., Bry.,* Calc. c., *Camph.,* Carb. v., Caust., Cham., **Chin.,** *Cic., Cina,* Cocc., **Con., CUP., Dig.,** Dros., *Hyos., Ign.,* Iod., Ip., Lach., *Lyc.,* MERC., Nat. m., Nit. ac., **Nux v.,** OP., *Phos.,* **Pho. ac.,** Pb., Puls., *Saba.,* **Samb.,** Sars., SEC. C, Sep., Sil., *Spig., Spo.,* Squ., Stan., *Stram.,* Thuj., VERAT. A.

Blow, Pain as After. (Compare **Bruised Pain.**)—*Acon.,* Alum., **Am. carb., Am. m.,** *Anac.,* ARN., Bar. c., *Bov.,* Bry., *Cannab. s.,* Caust., Cic., CINA, Cocc., Con., *Croc.,* Cup., Dros., Dulc., EUP. PER., **Fer.,** *Goss.,* Graph., *K. carb.,* Kre., *Lach., Laur., Led.,* Mag. c., Mag. m., *Mang., Mez.,* Mos., **Nat. c.,** *Nat. m.,* **Nux m., NUX V., Oleand., Phos.,** Pho. ac., PLAT., *Pb.,* PULS., Ran. b., RHODO., **Ruta,** Saba., *Sars., Sil.,* **Stan.,** Staph., Sul., *Sul. ac., Tar.,* Thuj., *Valer.,* Zinc.

Boring.—*Acon.,* Agar., *Aloe., Alum.,* Am. carb., Am. m., Anac., Ant. cr., Ant. t., *Apis,* Arg., ARG. N., *Arn.,* Ars., **Asaf., Aur.,** Bar. c., BELL., BISM., Bor., *Bov.,* **Calc. c.,** *Cannab. i., Canth.,* Caps., *Carb. an., Carb. v., Carb. sul.,* **Caust.,** Chin., *Cimic.,* **Cina,** *Clem.,* Cocc., *Coc. c., Colch., Coloc.,* Con., Cup., Cyc., *Dig., Dios.,* Dros., Dulc., Euphr., *Euphorb.,* Hell., **Hep.,** Ign., Ip., **K. carb.,** K. nit., Kre., Lach., *Laur.,* **Led.,** *Lyc., Mag. c., Mag. m.,* Mang., Meny., **Merc., Mez.,** *Mur. ac.,* **Nat. c., Nat. m.,** Nit. ac., Nux m., Nux v., Oleand., Par., Petrol., *Phos.,* **Pho. ac.,** Plat., Pb., PULS., Ran. b., RAN. S., Rhodo., *Rhus,* Ruta, *Saba., Sabi.,* Sele., Seneg., Sep., Sil., SPIG., Spo., *Stan.,* Staph., Stram., Stro., Sul., Tar., Thuj., Valer., Zinc.

—**Inward.**—Alum., *Bell.,* Calc. c., Cocc., **K. carb.,** Mang., Zinc.

—**Outward.**—Ant. cr., *Asaf., Bell.,* Bism., Bov., Calc. c., Dros., **Dulc.,** *Ip.,* Puls., Sep., Spig., Spo., **Staph.**

Bruised Pain (in general).—Acon., *Agar., Aloe,* Alum., Ant. cr., Ant. t., Arg., ARN., Asar., Bap., Bar. ac., *Berb.,* Bor. **Bry.,** Calc. c., Calend., *Canch.,* Canth., Carb. an., Carb. v., *Carb. sul.,* **Caust.,** Cham., Chel., CIC., CIMIC., Cina, *Clem.,* Con., *Crotal.,* Cup., Cyc., Dig., DROS., Dulc., Euphorb., Hep., Hyos., *Ign.,* Iod., Ip., *K. carb.,* K. nit., Lach., Led., *Mar.,* Nat. c., Nat. m., Nit. ac., **Nux m.,** *Nux v.,* **Oleand.,** *Par.,* Petrol., *Phos.,* **Plat.,** *Puls.,* Ran. b., Rhodo., RHUS, RUTA, Saba., Sabi., Sep., SIL., Spo., *Sul.,* **Sul. ac.,** Thuj., *Verat. a., Verb.,* Vio. o.

—**Externally.**—Acon., Agar., *Aloe,* Alum., *Am. carb., Am. m.,* Anac., Ant. t., **Apis,** Arg., ARN., *Ars.,* Asaf., Asar., *Aur.,* Bar. c., BELL., *Bov.,* Bry., Calad., **Calc. c.,** *Calend.,* Camph., *Cannab. s.,* **Canth.,** Caps., Carb. an., *Carb. v.,* Caust., *Ced.,* Cham., *Chel.,* CHIN., Cic., Cina, **Clem.,** COCC., Coff., Colch., Coloc., *Con.,* Croc., Cup., *Cyc.,* Dig., **Dros.,** Dulc., EUP. PER., Euphorb., **Fer.,** *Fl. ac.,* Form., **Gran.,** *Graph., Guai.,*

Hell., HEP., Hyos., **Ign.**, Ip., *K. carb.*, **Kalm.**, Kre., Lach., Laur., **Led.**, Lyc., Mag. c., *Mag. m.*, Mang., Meny., Merc., *Mez.*, Mur. ac., **Nat. c.**, NAT. M., *Nit. ac.*, Nux m., NUX V., **Ox. ac.**, Par., *Petrol.*, **Phos.**, Pho. ac., *Phyt.*, *Plat.*, Pb., Puls., RAN. B., Ran. s., Rheum, Rhodo., RHUS, RUTA, **Saba.**, SABI., Sars., Seneg., Sep., SIL., Spig., SPO., Squ., Stan., *Staph.*, Stram., *Stro.*, SUL., Sul. ac., Tar., Thuj., **Valer.**, VERAT. A., Vio. t., Zinc.

Bruised Pain, Internally.—*Acon.*, *Agar.*, *Alum.*, Ambr., *Am. m.*, Anac., **Apis**, *Arn.*, **Ars.**, Asaf., Aur., Bar. c., Bov., *Bry.*, CAMPH., *Cannab. i.*, Cannab.s., *Carb.ac.*, *Carb. an.*, *Carb. v.*, *Caust.*, Cham., CHIN, Cina, *Clem.*, Cocc., *Coff.*, Coloc., *Con.*, **Cup.**, Dros., Euphorb., Euphr., Fer., GEL., *Glon.*, Graph., **Hell.**, *Hep.*, *Ign.*, Iod., **Ip.**, K. carb., Kre., Lach., **Laur.**, Led., Lyc., Mag. c., Mag. m., Mang., Meny., *Merc.*, MERC. C., Mos., *Mur. ac.*, Nat. c., Nit. ac., **Nux v.**, Op., *Phos.*, Pho. ac., *Phyt.*, PULS., RAN. B., *Ran. s.*, Rhodo., Rhus, *Rumex*, Ruta, Sabi., Samb., Sars., *Sep.*, **Sil.**, Spig., *Spo.*, STAN., Staph., Stram., Stro., Sul., *Sul. ac.*, *Thuj.*, Valer., Verat. a., Vio. t., Zinc.

—**In Joints.**—Acon., *Agar.*,Anac., Ant. cr., **ARG.**, **ARN.**, Ars., **AUR.**, Bell., Bov., *Bry.*, *Calc. c.*, *Calend.*, *Camph.*, Carb. an., Carb. v., **Caust.**, Cham., CHIN., Cic., *Coff.*, Coloc., **Con.**, Croc., Cyc., **Dig.**, Dros., Dulc., Fer., *Graph.*, Hep., Hyos., *Ign.*, K. carb., **Led.**, Mag. c., **Mez.**, **Mur. ac.**, Nat. c., **Nat. m.**, Nit. ac., Nux v., *Par.*, *Phos.*, Pho. ac., Plat., **PULS.**, Rhus, **Ruta**, Saba., Sep., Spig., *Stan.*, Staph., **Sul.**, Sul. ac., *Thuj.*, *Valer.*, **Verat. a.**, *Vio. o.*, Zinc.

Bubbling.—*Ip.*, Puls., Rheum., *Squ.*

Burning, Externally.—Acon., Agar., *Aloe*, *Alum.*, Ambr., *Am. carb.*, Am. m., *Anac.*, Ant. cr., Ant. t., **Apis**, *Arg.*, **Arn.**, Ars., ARUM. T., Asaf., Asar., *Bar. c.*, *Bell.*, Berb., Bism., **Bor.**, Bov., **BRY.**, Calad., *Calc. c.*, Calc. ph., Camph., Cannab. s., **Canth.**, **Caps.**, *Carb. an.*, CARB. V., CAUST., Cham., **Chel.**, *Chin.*, Cic., Cimic., Cina, **Clem.**, *Cocc.*, *Coc. c.*, Coff., Colch., **Coloc.**, Con., **Corn. c.**, Croc., *Crotal.*, *Crot. tig.*, Cup., **Cyc.**, *Dig.*, Dros., Dulc., *Euphorb.*, EUPHR., **Fer.**, *Graph.*, Grat., Guai., Hell., *Helo.*, Hep., **Ign.**, Iod., Ip., **IRIS V.**, **K. bi.**, **K. carb.**, K. nit., *Kre.*, Lach., *Laur.*, Led., *Lob. i.*, **Lyc.**, Mag. c., *Mag. m.*, Mang., Mar., Meny., MERC., **Merc. c.**, *Mez.*, Mos., **Mur. ac.**, **Nat. c.**, NAT. M., Nit.'ac., Nux m., NUX V., **Oleand.**, **Op.**, *Pœo.*, Par., **Petrol.**, PHOS., PHO. AC., *Phyt.*, *Plat.*, Pb., Pru., **Pso.**, **Puls.**, Ran. s., **RAT.**, Rheum, Rhodo., **RHUS**, **Rumex**, *Ruta*, *Saba.*, Sabi., *Sal. ac.*, Samb., Sars., Sec. c., Sele., Seneg., **SEP.**, SIL., Spig., Spo., Squ., STAN., **Staph.**, Stram., *Stro.*, SUL., Sul. ac., Tar., Thuj., Valer., *Verat. a.*, Vio. t., **Zinc.**

SENSATIONS.

Burning, Internally.—*Ab. c.*, *Ac. ac.*, **ACON.**, *Acon. f.*, **Agar.**, *Alumen*, **Alum.**, **Ambr.**, **Am. br.**, *Am. carb.*, **Am. m.**, **Ant. cr.**, **Ant. t.**, **Apis**, **Arg.**, **Arg. n.**, **Arn.**, **ARS.**, **ARUM. T.**, **Asaf.**, **Asar.**, **Aur.**, **Bar. c.**, **BELL.**, **BERB.**, **Bism.**, **Bor.**, **Bov.**, **BRY.**, *Calad.*, **Calc. c.**, **Calc. ph.**, **Camph.**, **CANNAB. I.**, **Cannab. s.**, **CANTH.**, *Caps.*, *Carb. ac.*, *Carb. an.*, **Carb. v.**, *Carb. sul.*, **Caust.**, *Ced.*, *Cham.*, **Chel.**, **Chin.**, **Cic.**, **Cina**, **Clem.**, *Cocc.*, **Coff.**, **Colch.**, **Coloc.**, **Com.**, **Con.**, *Crot. tig.*, *Cund.*, **Cup.**, *Dig.*, **Dios.**, *Dol.*, **Dros.**, **Dulc.**, *Equis.*, *Eup. pur.*, **Euphorb.**, **Euphr.**, **Fl. ac.**, **Gam.**, **Graph.**, *Hell.*, *Hep.*, *Hydras.*, **Hyos.**, *Ign.*, **Iod.**, *Ip.*, **Iris v.**, **K. Bl.**, *K. carb.*, **K. iod.**, **K. nit.**, **Kre.**, **Lach.**, **Laur.**, **Led.**, **Lil. t.**, **Lith.**, **Lob. i.**, **Lyc.**, **Mag. c.**, *Mag. m.*, *Mang.*, **MERC.**, **MERC. C.**, **Merc. i. f.**, **MEZ.**, **Mos.**, *Mur. ac.*, *Nat. ars.*, **Nat. c.**, **Nat. m.**, **NIT. AC.**, *Nux m.*, **NUX V.**, **Op.**, **Osm.**, **Ox. ac.**, **Par.**, **Petrol.**, **PHOS.**, **Pho. ac.**, *Phyt.*, *Plat.*, *Pb.*, **PRU.**, **Pso.**, **PULS.**, **Ran. b.**, *Ran. s.*, *Rat.*, **Rhodo.**, **RHUS**, *Rob.*, **Rumex**, *Ruta*, **SABA.**, **Sabi.**, **SANG.**, **Sang. n.**, **Sars.**, **Sec. c.**, **Seneg.**, **SEP.**, **Sil.**, *Sin.*, **SPIG.**, **SPO.**, **Stan.**, *Staph.*, **Stram.**, **Stro.**, **SUL.**, *Sul. ac.*, **Tar.**, *Thea.*, **Thuj.**, **Tell.**, **Ter.**, *Ura.*, *Ust.*, *Uva.*, **Verat. a.**, *Verat. v.*, **Vio. o.**, **Vio. t.**, *Wye.*, **ZINC.**

—**Pain as From.**—**Agar.**, *Aloe.*, **Alum.**, **Ambr.**, **Apis**, **Arum. t.**, **Bap.**, **Bar. c.**, *Bell.*, **Berb.**, **Bry.**, **Cannab. s.**, *Caust.*, **Chin.**, **Coloc.**, **Fer.**, **Hyos.**, **Ign.**, **IRIS. V.**, **K. carb.**, **Lil. t.**, **Mag. m.**, **Merc.**, *Mez.*, *Mur. ac.*, **Nat. c.**, **Nux v.**, **Op.**, *Osm.*, **Par.**, **Phos.**, **Phyt.**, **Plat.**, **Puls.**, **Ran. s.**, **Saba.**, **Sang.**, **Sep.**, *Still.*, **Sul. ac.**, *Tarent.*, **Thuj.**, **Verat. a.**

Burns.—**Agar.**, **Alum.**, *Ant. cr.*, **ARS.**, **Calc. c.**, *Canth.*, **Carb. v.**, **Caust.**, *Cyc.*, **Euphorb.**, **Kre.**, *Lach.*, **Pb.**, **Ruta.**, **Sec. c.**, **Stram.**

Carphology.—*Arn.*, **Ars.**, **Arum. t.**, **Bell.**, *Chin.*, **Cocc.**, **Dub.**, **Dulc.**, **Colch.**, **HYOS.**, *Iod.*, **Mur. ac.**, **Op.**, **Phos.**, **Pho. ac.**, **Rhus**, **Stram.**, **Sul.**

Carried, Desired to be.—**Ant. t.**, **CHAM.**

Chewing Motions.—**Acon.**, *Bell.*, *Bry.*, **Calc. c.**, **Cham.**, *Hell.*, **Lach.**, **Mos.**, *Verat. a.*

Chlorosis (Anæmia).—**Ac. ac.**, *Ars.*, **Bar. c.**, **BELL.**, **CALC. C.**, **Carb. an.**, **Carb. v.**, **Caust.**, **Chin.**, **COCC.**, **Con.**, *Dig.*, **FER.**, *Graph.*, **Hell.**, **Ign.**, **K. carb.**, **LYC.**, *Merc.*, **Nat. m.**, **NIT. AC.**, **Nux v.**, **Oleand.**, **Phos.**, *Pho. ac.*, **PLAT.**, **Pb.**, **PULS.**, **Sabi.**, **Sep.**, **Spig.**, *Staph.*, **SUL.**, **Sul. ac.**, *Valer.*, **Zinc.**

Clamp, Sensation of an Iron.—**Cact.**, **Coloc.**

Clamp-like Pains Externally.—*Acon.*, **Alum.**, **Ambr.**, **Anac.**, **Arg. n.**, **Arg.**, **Arn.**, **Bar. c**, **Bell.**, **Bry.**, **Calad.**, **Calc. c.**, **Camph.**, **Cannab. s.**, **Carb. v.**, *Caust.*, **Cham.**, **Chel.**, **Cic.**, **Cina**, *Cocc.*, *Colch.*, **Coloc.**, **Croc.**, **Cyc.**, **Dig.**, **Dros.**, **Dulc.**, *Euphr.*, **Graph.**, **Hyos.**, *Iod.*, *K. carb.*, **K. nit.**,

148 SENSATIONS.

Kre., Led., *Lyc.*, Mang., Mar., Meny., Merc., *Mez.*, *Mos.*, Nat. c., **Nit. ac.**, Nux v., *Oleand.*, Petrol., Phos., *Pho. ac.*, PLAT., Puls., Ran. b., Rhodo., Rhus, Ruta, Saba., *Sep.*, *Sil.*, *Spig.*, Squ., Stro., Sul., Thuj., Valer., *Verat. a.*, Verb., Vio. t., *Zinc.*

Clamp-like Pains, Internally.—Acon., Agn., AMBR., Am. m., *Anac.*, Ant. t., *Arg.*, Arn., Ars. Asaf., Asar., Aur., Bar. c., *Bell.*, Bism., Bor., *Bry.*, Calc. c., Camph., Canth., Caps., Carb. an., **Carb. v.**, *Cham.*, Chel., Chin., *Cina*, **Cocc.**, Colch., Coloc., Con., Croc., Cyc., *Dig.*, Dros., Dulc., *Fer.*, Graph., Hyos., IGN., Iod., **K. carb.**, Lach., Led., Lyc., *Mag. c.*, **Mar.**, Meny., Merc., **Mez.**, *Mur. ac.*, Nat. m., **Nux v.**, Oleand., Petrol., *Phos.*, PHO. AC., PLAT., *Puls.*, Ran. s., *Rheum.*, *Rhodo.*, Rhus, Sabi., Sars., Sele., Seneg., Sep., Sil., Spo., Squ., *Stan.*, **Staph.**, Stram., Stro., Sul., Sul. ac., Thuj., Valer., *Verat. a.*, Zinc.

Clothing, Intolerance of.—Am. carb., *Apis*, ARG. N., Arn., Asaf., *Asar.*, *Bry.*, Calc. c., *Caps.*, *Carb. v.*, **Caust.**, Chin., *Coff.*, **Crotal.**, Hep., Ign., K. nit., *Kre.*, LACH., **Lyc.**, NUX V., Oleand., Op., Puls., **Ran. b.**, Sars., Sep., SPO., *Stan.*

Clucking (Gurgling).—Agar., Alum., **Ambr.**, *Am. carb.*, *Anac.*, **Ant. cr.**, Ant. t., *Arn.*, Ars., Asaf., Asar., Bar. c., **Bell.**, *Bov.*, *Bry.*, *Calc. c.*, Carb. an., Carb. v., *Cham.*, *Chel.*, Chin., *Cina*, Cocc., **Colch.**, Croc., Dig., *Graph.*, Hell., *K. carb.*, *Kre.*, **Lyc.**, Mag. c., Mag. m., Mang., *Mar.*, *Meny.*, Merc., Mag. m., **Nux v.**, *Oleand.*, *Par.*, Petrol., Phos., Pho. ac., Plat., *Pb.*, **Puls.**, RHEUM, Rhus, Ruta, Sabi., Sars., *Sep.*, *Sil.*, **Spig.**, Spo., SQU., Stan., Staph., Stro., *Sul.*, Sul. ac., **Tar.**, *Valer.*, Verb., *Vio. t.*, Zinc.

Clumsiness.—Asaf., *Calc. c.*, Camph., Chin., Euphr., Ign., *K. carb.*, *Mez.*, **Nat. c.**, Nat. m., *Pho. ac.*, Puls., Rheum, Ruta, *Saba.*, Sep., *Sil.*, Spo., Stan., Sul.

Coat of Skin Drawn Over Inner Parts, Sensation of.—Caust, *Cocc.*, Dros., Merc., Nux m., **Phos.**, Puls.

Cobweb, Sensation of.—Alum., Bar. c., Bor., *Brom.*, *Bry.*, *Calc. c.*, *Con.*, Graph., Mag. c., Pho. ac., Pb., *Ran. s.*, Sul. ac.

Cold, Tendency to Take.—ACON., Alum., Am. carb., Anac., Ant. cr., Arn., Ars., **Bar. c.**, **Bell.**, *Bor.*, BRY., Calc. c., *Camph.*, Carb. v., *Caust.*, CHAM., Chin., Cocc., *Coff.*, Coloc., **Con.**, Croc., Cup., Dig., Dros., DULC., Fer., Graph., *Hep.*, **Hyos.**, Ign., Iod., Ip., *K. carb.*, Led., *Lyc.*, Mag. m., **Merc.**, *Mez.*, **Nat. c.**, Nat. m., NIT. AC., Nux m., NUX V., Op., **Petrol.**, Phos., Pho. ac., Plat., Pso., **Puls.**, Rhus, Ruta, Sabi., Samb., Sars., Sele., **Sep.**, SIL., Spig., Stan., Staph., **Sul.**, Sul. ac., Valer., *Verat. a.*

SENSATIONS.

Coldness. See under **Fever.**

Comfortable Sensation.—Coff., Op., Pb., *Stram.*, Valer.

Constriction, Externally.—*Abrot.*, Acon., *Aconin.*, **Aesc.**, *Aeth.*, Agar., All. c., *Alum.*, **Ammc.**, Am. carb., *Am. m.*, **Amyl.**, Anac., Ant. cr., Ant. t., **Apis**, *Aral.*, Arg., *Arg. n.*, Arn., Ars., Arum. t., Asaf., Asar., Aur., Bar. c., Bell., *Berb.*, **Bism.**, Bor., Bov., Bry., **Cact.**, *Calc. ac.*, Calc. c., **Calc. ph.**, *Cannab. i.*, Cannab. s., *Canth.*, **Caps.**, *Carb. ac.*, Carb. an., *Carb. v.*, *Carb. sul.*, Caust., Cham., **Chel.**, Chin., CIMIC., Cina, COCC., Coff., Colch., **Coloc.**, *Cyn.*, Cup., *Dig.*, Dios., Dros., *Dulc.*, Euphr., **Fer.**, **Gel.**, **Glon.**, GRAPH., *Guai.*, **Hell.**, Hep., *Hyd. ox.*, HYOS., Iod., **Ip.**, *K. carb.*, K. nit., Kre., Lach., Laur., Led., *Lil. t.*, Lob. i., Lyc., Mag. c., Mag. m., Mang., Meny., MERC., Merc. c., Merc. i. r., Mez., *Mos.*, Mur. ac., *Naj.*, Nat. c., *Nat. m.*, NIT. AC., Nux m., NUX V., *Oleand.*, **Op.**, **Ox. ac.**, Par., Petrol., Phos., **Plat.**, PB., **Puls.**, Ran. b., Ran. s., Rheum, *Rhodo.*, RHUS, *Ruta*, *Saba.*, Sabi., Sars., Sec. c., **Sele.**, **Sep.**, *Sil.*, *Spig.*, **Spo.**, Squ., STAN., Staph., STRAM., Stro., Sul., Sul. ac., **Tab.**, Thuj., **Verat. a.**, Verb., Vio. t., *Zinc.*

—**Internally.**—Acon., **Aesc.**, *Agar.*, Agn., **Alum.**, Ambr., *Am. carb.*, *Amyl.*, *Anac.*, Ant. cr., Ant. t., **Arg.**, **Arn.**, **Ars.**, *Asaf.*, **Asar.**, *Aur.*, **Bap.**, *Bar. c.*, BELL., *Benz. ac.*, *Bism.*, *Bor.*, Bov., Brom., Bry., CACT., **Calad.**, **Calc. c.**, **Camph.**, *Cannab. i.*, Cannab. s., *Canth.*, **Caps.**, *Carb. an.*, *Carb. v.*, **Caust.**, Cham., **Chel.**, CHIN., Chlorum., *Cic.*, Cina, **Clem.**, **Cocc.**, Coff., Colch., COLOC., **Con.**, Croc., *Crotal.*, *Crot. tig.*, *Cub.*, **Cup.**, **Dig.**, *Dios.*, **Dros.**, Dulc., *Euphorb.*, Fer., *Glon.*, *Graph.*, Guai., *Hell.*, Hep., Hyos., IGN., Iod., **Ip.**, *K. carb.*, K. nit., Kre., Lach., Laur., Led., *Lyc.*, Mag. c., *Mag. m.*, *Mang.*, Mar., Meny., Merc., Merc. c., Mez., Mos., Mur. ac., **Naj.**, *Nat. ars.*, *Nat. c.*, NAT. M., NIT. AC., Nux m., NUX V., *Oleand.*, *Op.*, *Ox. ac.*, Par., Petrol., **Phos.**, **Pho. ac.**, PLAT., PB., PULS., *Ran. s.*, Rheum, *Rhodo.*, *Rhus*, Ruta, *Saba.*, Sabi., Samb., Sars., Sec. c., **Sele.**, *Seneg.*, **Sep.**, *Sil.*, **Spig.**, *Spo.*, **Squ.**, Stan., *Staph.*, **Still.**, STRAM., Stro., SUL., **Sul. ac.**, Sum., *Tar.*, **Thuj.**, *Valer.*, **Verat. a.**, **Verat. v.**, *Verb.*, Vio. t., *Zinc.*

—**In Joints.**—Acon., Am. m., ANAC., AUR., Calc. c., Carb. an., Chin., *Coloc.*, Fer., GRAPH., Kre., Lyc., Meny., NAT. M., NIT. AC., Nux m., *Nux v.*, **Petrol.**. *Ruta*, *Sil.*, Spig., Squ., ·Stan., Stro., Sul., *Zinc.*

—**Of Orifices.**—Acon., *Alum.*, *Ars.*, Bar. c., BELL., Brom., *Calc. c.*, Carb. v., **Chel.**, *Cic.*, Cocc., Colch., Con., *Crotal.*, Dig., Dulc., Fer., *Form.*, Graph., Hep., Hyos., *Ign.*, Iod., Ip., *Lach.*, Lyc., MERC., **Merc. c.**, *Mez.*, **Nat. m.**, NIT. AC., **Nux v.**, *Op.*, Phos., **Plat.**, Pb.,

Rat., *Rhodo.*, RHUS, *Saba.*, Sars., Sep., SIL., **Staph.**, **STRAM.**, Sul., Sum., Tar., Thuj., *Verat. a.*, Verat. v.

Consumption in General.—Acon., *Ambr.*, Am. carb., Am. m., Arg., Arn., **Ars.**, Aur., Bar. c., *Bell.*, Bor., Bry., Calad., **Calc. c.**, Canth., Carb. an., *Carb. v.*, Caust., Cham., Chin., Cocc., *Con.*, Cup., Dros., *Dulc.*, Fer., Graph., Guai., Hep., Hyos., Ign., IOD., Ip., K. CARB., K. nit., *Kre.*, Lach., *Laur.*, Led., LYC., Mang., Mar., *Merc.*, *Nat. m.*, *Nit. ac.*, Nux m., *Nux v.*, Op., Par., Petrol., PHOS., *Pho. ac.*, Pb., PULS., Ran. b., Rhus, Ruta, Saba., Samb., *Sars.*, Sec. c., Sele., *Seneg.*, **Sep.**, *Sil.*, Spig., Spo., Squ., STAN., Staph., Stram., Sul., Thuj., *Verat. a.*, Zinc.

Contractions (After Inflammation).—Acon., **Agar.**, *Alum.*, Ant. cr., Arg., *Arn.*, *Ars.*, Asaf., Bell., Bry., *Calc. c.*, Camph., Canth., Caust., *Chel.*, Chin., CIC., *Clem.*, **Cocc.**, Con., Dig., Dros., *Dulc.*, Euphorb., Hyos., Ign., Lach., Led., Mar., Meny., MERC., **Mez.**, *Nat. m.*, Nit. ac., NUX V., Op., *Petrol.*, Phos., Pb., **Puls.**, Ran. b., RHUS, Ruta, Saba., *Sep.*, Spo., Squ., Staph., *Stram.*, *Sul.*, Thuj., *Verat. a.*, Zinc.

—Of Extremities.—Acon., Alum., Ambr., Am. m., *Anac.*, Ant. cr., *Ant. t.*, Arg., Arn., Bell., Bism., CALC. C., *Cannab. i.*, *Carb. an.*, Carb v., **Caust.**, Cham., Chel., **Chin.**, *Cina*, Cocc., Coff., Colch., *Coloc.*, Con., **Cup.**, Cyc., Dig., *Dros.*, Euphorb., **Fer.**, GRAPH., Guai., Hep., **Hyos.**, *K. carb.*, K. nit., Laur., LYC., Mag. m., Meny., Merc., Nat. c., Nat. m., Nit. ac., *Nux v.*, *Ox. ac.*, Phos., *Plat.*, Pb., Rhus, Ruta, Saba, Sabi., Sars., SEC. C., Sep., Sil., Spig., Spo., Stan., *Stram.*, *Sul.*, Sul. ac., Verat. a.

Convulsions.—Acon., Agar., Ambr., Ant. t., Arn., *Ars.*, *Asaf.*, Aur., Bar. c., BELL., Bry., Buf., *Cact.*, Calc. c., Camph., *Cannab. i.*, Cannab. s., *Canth.*, *Carb. ac.*, Caust., Cham., *Cham. a.*, CIC., Cina., Clem., Cocc., *Coff.*, Colch., Coloc., Con., Croc., *Crotal.*, CUP., Dig., Dulc., Fer., *Gel.*, Glon., **Hell.**, *Hyd. ac.*, HYOS., Ign., *Iod.*, Ip., *K. br.*, Lach., *Laur.*, Lyc., Mag. c., Mag. m., *Meli.*, Merc., *Merc. c.*, **Mos.**, Nit. ac., **Mur. ac.**, Nux m., Nux v., *Oenan.*, *Oleand.*, OP., Petrol., Phos., **Phyt.**, Plat., PB., Puls., Ran. s., Rhus, *Ruta*, Saba., *Samb.*, *Sant.*, Sec. c., Sep., Sil., Spig., Squ., Stan., Staph., STRAM., Stro., Sul., **Tan.**, *Thea.*, Valer., **Verat. a.**, *Verat. v.*, *Zinc.*

—Clonic.—Acon., AGAR., *Alum.*, *Ambr.*, Am. carb., Am. m., Anac., Ant. t., Arg., Arn., **Ars.**, Asar., *Ast. r.*, Aur., Bar. c., BELL., Bor., **Bry.**, **Calc. c.**, *Camph.*, Cannab. s., *Canth.*, *Carb. v.*, Caust., CHAM., Chin., CIC., *Cimic.*, Cina, Clem., *Cocc.*, Coff., Coloc., **Con.**, Croc., CUP., Dig., *Dulc.*, **Graph.**, Guai., Hell., Hep., HYOS., Ign., *Iod.*, Ip., K. carb., Kre., Lach., *Laur.*, Lyc., *Mag. c.*, Mag. m., *Mang.*, Mar., Meny., Merc., **Mez.**, **Mos.**, Mur. ac., *Na' c.*, **Nat. m.**, Nit. ac., Nux m., *Nux v.*, Oleand.,

OP., *Petrol.*, *Phos.*, *Pho. ac.*, **Phys.**, **Plat.**, Pb., **Puls.**, Ran. b., Ran. s., Rheum, *Rhodo.*, *Rhus*, Ruta., Saba., Samb., Sars., **Sec. c.**, Sele., Seneg., SEP., Sil., Spig., Spo., *Squ.*, Stan., Staph., STRAM., Stro., Sul., Sul. ac., *Tan.*, *Tarent.*, Tar., *Thuj.*, *Verat. a.*, *Verat. v.*, *Visc.*, Zinc.

Convulsions With Consciousness. — *Ars.*, **Bell.**, Calc. c., *Camph.*, Canth., Caust., CINA, *Hell.*, Hyos., K. carb., Lyc., **Mag. c.**, Merc., Mur. ac., *Nat. m.*, *Nit. ac.*, Nux m., Nux v., *Phos.*, **Plat.**, Sep., Sil., STRAM., *Sul.*

— **Without Consciousness.** — Ant. t., *Ars.*, *Aur.*, **Bell.**, CALC. C., Camph., CANTH., *Cham.*, Chin., CIC., Cina, **Cocc.**, **Cup.**, Dig., Fer., HYOS., *Ip.*, *Lach.*, *Laur.*, Led., *Lyc.*, *Merc.*, Nat. m., Nit. ac., Nux v., Op., Phos., PB., **Sec. c.**, **Sep.**, Sil., Staph., *Stram.*, **Sul.**, *Verat. a.*

— **Epileptiform.** — Acon., *Agar.*, Alum., Am. carb., Ant. cr., Ant. t., Arg., **Arg. n.**, Arn., **Ars.**, Asaf., Aur., BELL., Bry., Buf., CALC. C., Camph., Canth., *Carb. sul.*, CAUST., Cham., Chin., CIC., CINA, **Cocc.**, Coloc., *Con.*, **CUP.**, Dig., Dros., Dulc., Fer., Hell., HYOS., *Ign.*, Iod., **Ip.**, *K. br.*, **K. carb.**, Lach., *Laur.*, Led., **Lyc.**, *Mag. c.*, Merc., *Mos.*, Mur. ac., **Nat. m.**, **Nit. ac.**, Nux m., **Nux v.**, *Oenan.*, Op., *Petrol.*, Phos., Pho. ac., *Plat.*, PB., Puls., Ran. b., Ran. s., *Rhus*, Ruta, **Sec. c.**, Sep., Sil., Stan., Staph., STRAM., SUL., Tar., Thuj., Valer., Verat. a., *Verat. v.*, Zinc.

— **With Falling.** — Agar., *Alum.*, Am. carb., Ars., BELL., Calc. c., *Canth.*, Caust., CHAM., *Cic.*, Cina, Cocc., **Con.**, **CUP.**, Dig., *Dulc.*, HYOS., Ign., **Iod.**, *Ip.*, Laur., *Lyc.*, Merc., Nit. ac., Op., Petrol., Phos., Pho. ac., *Pb.*, **Sec. c.**, Sep., *Sil.*, **Stan.**, Staph., **Stram.**, *Sul.*, Verat. a., Zinc.

— **Hysterical.** — Ars., **Asaf.**, *Aur.*, **Bell.**, **Bry.**, Calc. c., Cannab. s., **Caust.**, *Cham.*, *Cic.*, **Cocc.**, Coff., CON., Croc., Dig., *Hyos.*, **IGN.**, **Iod.**, **Ip.**, Lach., *Lyc.*, **Mag. m.**, Merc., **Mos.**, Nit. ac., Nux m., *Nux v.*, Op., Petrol., Phos., **Plat.**, *Pb.*, **Puls.**, Ruta, *Sep.*, *Stan.*, Staph., **Stram.**, *Sul.*, *Tarent.*, **Valer.**, *Verat. a.*, *Verat. v.*, Zinc.

— **Internal.** — Acon., Agar., Alum., Ambr., Am. carb., Anac., *Ant. cr.*, Ant. t., Arg., *Arn.*, Ars., **Asaf.**, Asar., Bar. c., **Bell.**, *Bism.*, Bor., Bov., Bry., Calad., Calc. c., *Camph.*, Canth., *Caps.*, Carb. an., **Carb. v.**, CAUST., Cham., *Chel.*, *Chin.*, Cina, COCC., *Coff.*, *Colch.*, Coloc., *Con.*, Cup., *Dig.*, Dulc., *Euphorb.*, Fer., *Graph.*, Hep., HYOS., IGN., *Iod.*, Ip., K. carb., *K. nit.*, Kre., Lach., *Laur.*, Led., **Lyc.**, *Mag. c.*, **Mag. m.**, Mar., Merc., Mos., Mur. ac., Nat. c., *Nat. m.*, *Nit. ac.*, *Nux m.*, NUX V., Op., *Petrol.*, Phos., *Pho. ac.*, Plat., *Pb.*, PULS., Rhodo., *Rhus*, Saba., *Sars.*, **Sec. c.**, Seneg., Sep., Sil., Spo., STAN., **Staph.**, *Stram.*, Stro., *Sul.*, Sul. ac., *Thuj.*, Valer., *Verat a.*, **Zinc.**

Convulsions With Opisthotonos.—Bell., *Bry., Canth.,* **Cham.,** CIC., Clem., *Cocc.,* Con., *Hyos.,* IGN., *Ip., Nux v., Op., Rhus,* Sec. c., **Stan.,** *Strc.m., Verat. v.*

—**With Stiffness.**—*Acon.,* Alum., *Am. carb., Ant. t., Arg.,* Ars., **Asaf.,** Bell., *Bry.,* **Campli.,** Canth., Caust., Cham., Chin., **Cic.,** *Cina,* Cocc., Coloc., Dros., Hell., Hyos., Ign., **IP.,** K. carb., Laur., *Led.,* Lyc., Merc., MOS., Nit. ac., Op., Petrol., Phos., PLAT., Pb., *Sec. c.,* Sep., Sil., *Stram.,* Sul., *Thuj.,* Verat. a., Zinc.

—**Tetanic, (Rigidity.)**—Acon., Alum., **Am. carb.,** Am. m., **Ant. t.,** Ars., *Asaf.,* Bell., *Bry.,* Calc. c., **Camph.,** *Cannab. i., Cannab. s., Canth.,* Cham., CIC., Con., **Cup.,** *Our., Dros.,* Hell., Hep., **Hyos.,** *Hyper.,* Ign., Ip., K. carb., Kre., *Laur., Led.,* **Lyc., Merc., Mos., Nux v., Op.,** PETROL., Phos., *Phys.,* **PLAT.,** Pb., Puls., Rhodo., Rhus, **Sec. c.,** Seneg., SEP., **Stram.,** *Sul., Verat. a., Verat. v.,* Zinc.

—**Tonic.**—Acon., *Alum., Am. carb.,* Am. m., Anac., Ant. t., **Arg.,** Arn., Ars., *Asaf.,* Asar., BELL., Bor., *Bry., Calc. c., Camph.,* Cannab. s., Canth., Caps., **Caust.,** Cham., Chin., CIC., Cina, Clem., **Cocc.,** Coloc., *Con.,* Cup., Cyc., Dig., *Dulc.,* Euphorb., Fer., *Graph.,* Guai., Hep., *Hyos.,* **Ign.,** Ip., *K. carb., Laur.,* Led., **Lyc.,** Mang., Meny., **Merc.,** Mez., **Mos.,** Nat. c., *Nat. m.,* Nit. ac., *Nux v.,* Oleand., *Op.,* PETROL., Phos., Pho. ac., PLAT., Puls., Rhodo., *Rhus,* Saba., Sars., Sec. c., Seneg., SEP., *Sil.,* Spig., Spo., *Stan.,* Stram., Sul., *Thuj.,* Verat. a., Zinc.

—**Uterine (Compare with Hysterical).**—Ars., *Bell.,* Bry., *Caust.,* COCC., *Coff.,* CON., Cup., Fer., **Ign.,** Ip., *Kre.,* Lyc., MAG. M., *Mos.,* Nat. m., Nux m., **Nux v.,** Phos., *Plat.,* Puls., Rhus, Sec. c., Sep., **Stan.,** Staph., Stram., Sul., Sul ac., Valer., Zinc.

Convulsive Movements.—*Acon.,* Agar., *Ant. t.,* **Arg. n.,** Arn., *Ars.,* Bar. c., BELL., Bry., Calc. c., **Camph.,** Cannab. s., **Canth.,** *Caust.,* CHAM., CIC., *Cina,* COCC., *Coff.,* Con., Croc., **CUP.,** Dig., *Dulc.,* **Hell.,** HYOS., IGN., **Iod., IP.,** *Lach., Laur., Lyc.,* Meny., Merc., *Mos.,* Nat. c., *Nux m.,* Nux v., Oleand., OP., Pb., Petrol., Phos., Pho. ac., Plat., Ran. s., Rheum, *Rhus,* Ruta, Saba., *Samb.,* SEC. C., *Spig.,* Spo., **Squ., Stan.,** Staph., STRAM., *Sul.,* Verat. a., Zinc.

Corroded Feeling (Compare with Sore Pain).—*Con.,* Mar., *Ruta.*

Cracking of Joints.—*Acon., Am. carb., Anac.,* Ant. cr., Ant. t., Bar. c., *Bry. Calad.,* Calc. c., **Camph., CAPS.,** Caust., *Cham.,* Chin., *Cic.,* **Cocc.,** Coloc., *Con.,* **Croc.,** Euphr., Hep., Ign., Ip., K. carb., Kit. nit., LED., *Lyc.,* Meny., **Merc.,** Mez., **Nat. c.,** *Nat. m.,* NIT. AC., **Nux v.,** PETROL., **Phos.,** *Puls.,* Ran. b., Rhus, Saba., Sabi., Sars., *Sele.,* Seneg., Spo., Stan., Sul., Thuj., Verat. a., Zinc.

Cracking Sensation Internally.—Bar. c., Calc. c., Caust., Cham.,

SENSATIONS. 153

Cocc., Coff., Graph., *K. carb., Meny.,* Nat. m., Nux v., Petrol., Saba., Sep., Spig.

Cramps, Internal.—*Acon.,* Agar., Ant. t., **Bell.,** *Bry.,* Calad., *Calc. c.,* Cina, Coloc., *Croc.,* CUP., Dios., Gel., Ign., *K. carb.,* MERC., **Mez.,** Mos., *Mur. ac., Naj.,* Nat. m., Petrol., Pho. ac., PLAT., **Pb.,** Pru., Puls., Ran. b., Ran. s., Samb., SANG., **Sec. c.,** Sil., Spo., *Staph.,* Sul., *Tarent.,* Thuj., Valer., Verat. a., *Verb.,* **Vib. op.,** Zinc.

—Of Joints.—*Acon.,* Am. m., **Anac.,** Arn., *Aur.,* Bar. c., **Bell.,** Bov., Bry., **CALC. C.,** *Camph.,* Cannab. s., *Canth., Caust.,* Cham., Chel., Chin., *Cic., Cocc.,* Colch., Con., Cup., Dulc., Euphorb., Hep., *Hyos., Ign.,* K. carb., K. nit., Kre., *Lach., Laur.,* Led., Lyc., Meny., *Merc.,* Mez., Nux v., Oleand., *Op.,* Par., Petrol., *Phos.,* **PLAT.,** *Pb., Rhus,* **Sec. c.,** Sele., Spig., Spo., Staph., *Stram.,* **Sul.,** *Verat. a.,* Verb.

—Of Muscles.—*Acon., Agar., Alum.,* **Ambr.,** Am. carb., Am. m., ANAC., *Arg.,* **Arn., Ars., Asaf.,** *Asar., Aur.,* Bar. c., **BELL.,** Bism., Bov., Bry., **CALC. C.,** Camph., **Cannab. s.,** Caps., *Carb. an., Carb. v.,* **Caust.,** *Cham.,* Chin., Cic., **CINA,** Clem., **Cocc.,** Colch., **Coloc.,** Con., Croc., Cup., *Dig., Dios., Dros.,* **Dulc.,** Euphorb., **Euphr.,** Fer., *Gel.,* **Glon.,** Graph., Hell., *Hep.,* Hyos., Ign., Iod., Ip., *Jab.,* **K. carb.,** *K. nit.,* Kre., Lach., **LYC.,** **Mag. c., Mag. m.,** *Mang.,* Meny., MERC., *Mez., Mos.,* **Mur. ac.,** Nat. c., Nat. m., **Nit. ac.,** Nux m., *Nux v., Oleand.,* Par., **Petrol.,** *Phos.,* Pho. ac., **PLAT., Pb.,** Ran. b., *Rhodo.,* **Rhus,** *Ruta,* Saba., Samb., **Sec. c., SEP., SIL.,** Spig., Spo., Squ., **Stan.,** Staph., Stram., *Stro.,* **SUL.,** Sul. ac., Thuj., **Valer.,** *Verat. a.,* **Verb.,** *Vib. op.,* Vio. o., Vio. t., Zinc.

Crawling (as of a Mouse).—Arn., Aur., BELL., CALC. C., *Nit. ac., Rhodo.,* Sep., Sil., SUL.

Creaking of Joints.—Agn., **Caps., Fer., Led.,** Nat. m., Petrol., Pb., Puls., *Rhus,* Sul.

Creeping, as of Little Animals.—Agn., **Alum.,** Arg., Bar. c., *Bor.,* Cannab. s., Caust., Chin., Dulc., *K. carb.,* Lach., **Laur.,** Nux v., Pb., Ran. b., Ran. s., *Rhodo., Rhus,* Saba., Sec. c., Staph., *Sul.,* Tar., Thuj.

Crepitation, Sensation of.—ACON., Alum., Ars., Aur., *Bar. c.,* Bry., CALC. C., Carb. v., Coff., Con., Lach., Mos., Nit. ac., Par., Phos., *Puls.,* RHEUM, Saba., Sabi., *Sep.,* **Spig.**

Crushing Sensation.—*Acon.,* Ant. cr., **Arg., ARN.,** *Caust.,* **Cic.,** Con., Dros., Iod., K. carb., Lach., *Led.,* Mar., *Nux m.,* **Oleand.,** *Par.,* Petrol., **Phos.,** *Plat.,* **Puls.,** *Rhodo., Rhus,* **RUTA,** Sep., **Stan.,** Sul., Sul. ac., Verat. a., *Verb.*

Cutting, Externally.—Acon., **Alum.,** Ambr., Anac., Ant. cr., *Arg.,*

Arn., Asaf., Asar., Aur., BELL., Bism., Bor., Brcm., Bry., CALC. C.,
Camph., Cannab. s., *Canth., Caust.,* Chin., Čina, *Clem.,* Colch., **Coloc.,**
Con., Conv., Dig., DROS., *Dulc.,* Euphorb., **Graph.,** Hell., Hep., *Hyos.,*
Ign., K. carb., Led., Lyc., Mag. m., Mang., *Mar., Meny.,* **Merc.,** *Mez.,*
Mos., **Mur. ac.,** NAT. C., Nat. m., Nit. ac., **Nux v.,** Oleand., *Osm., Oxyt.,*
Par., **PETROL.,** Phos., Pho. ac., Plat., *Puls.,* Ran. b., Rhodo., **Rhus,**
Ruta, *Saba.,* Samb., Sars., Seneg., **Sep.,** Sil., *Spig., Stan.,* **Staph.,** Stram.,
Sul., Sul. ac., *Thuj., Verat. a.,* **Vio. t.,** Zinc.

Cutting, Internally.—*Ab. n., Acon., Aesc., Aeth., Agar., Agn., All. c.,*
Alum., Ambr., Am. carb., Am. m., Anac., *Ant. cr., Ant. t., Arg., Arg. n.,*
Arn., *Ars., Asaf., Asar.,* Aur., Bar. c., BELL., **Berb.,** Bism., Bor., *Bov.,*
Bry., **Calad.,** CALC. C., *Calc. ph.,* Camph., *Cannab. i., Cannab. s.,*
CANTH., *Caps., Carb. an.,* Carb. v., *Caust.,* Cham., **Chel.,** Chin., Cic.,
Cina, Clem., Cocc., *Coc. c.,* Coff., *Colch.,* **Coll.,** COLOC., Con., *Conv., Croc.,*
Crotal., Crot. tig., Cub., Cup., Cyc., *Dig.,* DIOS., Dros., **Dulc.,** Fer., Elat.,
Equis., GAM., *Gel., Graph.,* Guai., Hell., Hep., *Hydras.,* HYOS., *Ign.,*
Iod., **Ip.,** *Iris v.,* K. CARB., *K. chl.,* **K. nit.,** *Lach., Laur.,* Led., LYC.,
Mag. c., *Mag. m., Mang.,* Mar., Meny., MERC., *Merc. c.,* Mez., Mos., **Mur. ac.,** *Nat. c.,* NAT. M., *Nit. ac., Nux m.,* NUX V., **Op.,** Par., Petrol.,
Phos., *Pho. ac.,* Plat., *Pb.,* PULS., Ran. b., Ran. s., Rheum, Rhodo.,
Rhus, Ruta, *Saba.,* Sabi., Samb., *Sars.,* Sele., Seneg., **Sep.,** SIL., Spig.,
Spo., Squ., **Stan., Staph.,** Stro., SUL., *Sul. ac., Thuj., Valer.,* VERAT. A., *Verb.,* **Vib. op.,** Vio. t., ZINC., *Zing.*

Cyanosis.—*Acon.,* Agar., Alum., *Am. carb., Ant. cr.,* **Ant. t.,** *Arn.,*
Ars., Asaf., Asar., *Aur.,* Bar. c., **Bell.,** *Bism.,* Bry., Calc. c., Camph.,
Carb. v., Caust., Cham., **Chel.,** Chin., Cic., Cina, *Cocc.,* **Con.,** CUP., DIG.,
Dros., Fer., Hep., Hyos., Ign., Ip., **K. chl.,** LACH., Led., Lyc., Mang.,
Merc., Mos., Mur. ac., *Nat. m.,* Nit. ac., Nux m., *Nux v.,* OP., **Phos.,** Pho. ac., Pb., *Puls.,* Ran. b., *Rhus,* Ruta, Saba., **Samb.,** Sars., **Sec. c.,** Seneg.,
Sil., Spo., Staph., Stram., Sul., Sul. ac., Thuj., VERAT. A.

Dead Feeling.—Acon., Ambr., *Am. m., Ant. cr., Ant. t.,* Asar., Bry.,
Calc. c., Cannab. s., Caust., **Chel.,** *Cic.,* Coff., *Con., Crotal.,* Cup., Cyc.,
Euphorb., Hep., Kre., *Lyc., Merc.,* Mur. ac., Nat. c., *Nat. m.,* Nit. ac.,
Nux v., Par., *Phos.,* Pho. ac., **Puls.,** *Rhus,* Samb., SEC. C., Sil., **Stan.,**
Sul., Thuj., Verat. a., *Zinc.*

Death, Apparent.—*Ant. t.,* Arn., **Carb. v.,** *Chin.,* **Coff.,** Laur., *Nit. ac.,* **Op.,** Phos., *Pho. ac.,* Stram.

Debility, Sensation of. (Compare with **Weakness** and **Weariness.**)
—Alum., Am. carb., **Ant. cr.,** Apis, *Apoc. c., Asaf., Bell.,* Bism., *Calc. c.,*
Cannab. s., *Caps.,* **Carb. v.,** Caust., Chel., CHIN., Cic., **Cocc.,** Coff.,

Colch., Coloc., *Con.*, Gel., Hydras., Hyos., Ign., Iod., K. carb., K. nit., Lach., Laur., Lo. i., Lyc., Mag. c., Mar., Meny., *Mos.*, Nat. m., Nux m., **Nux v.**, Op., Ox. ac., *Oxyt.*, *Petrol.*, Phos., PHO. AC., Pb., Ran. b., Rhodo., Rhus, RUTA, *Sele.*, Seneg., Sep., Spo., Stan., Stram., **Sul.**, SUL. AC., *Verat. a.*, **Valer.**, Vio. t.

Digging.—Acon., *Am. m.*, Ant. cr., *Arg. n.*, Bry., *Chel.*, **Coloc.**, *K. carb.*, Kre., Laur., Mag. c., *Mag. m.*, *Nux v.*, Rhus, Sul. ac.

Digging Up (Burrowing, Rooting Sensation.—Acon., Agar., Alum., Ambr., Am. carb., **Am. m.**, Anac., Ant. cr., *Ant.*, Arg., **Arn**, Ars., **Asaf.**, Asar., Aur., Bar. c., **Bell.**, *Bism.*, Bor., Bov., Bry., Calc. c., Cannab. s., Caps., Canth., Carb. an., Carb. v., Caust., Cham., Chel., *Chin.*, **Cina**, *Clem.*, *Cocc.*, Colch., **Coloc.**, Con., Croc., Dig., Dros., DULC., Euphorb., Fer., **Graph.**, Hell., Hep., *Ign.*, **K. bi.**, **K. carb.**, K. nit., Kre., Led., Lyc., Mag. c., *Mag. m.*, *Mang.*, Merc., Mez., Mur. ac., **Nat. c.**, *Nat. m.*, Nux m., *Nux v.*, Oleand., Petrol., **Phos.**, *Pho. ac.*, **Plat.**, *Puls.*, Rheum, **RHODO.**, *Rhus*, **Ruta**, *Saba.*, Sabi., Samb., *Seneg.*, **Sep.**, *Sil.*, SPIG., Spo., Squ., **Stan.**, *Staph.*, *Stro.*, *Sul.*, Thuj., *Valer.*, Zinc.

Dilated Sensation, Internally.—Acon., Agar., Anac., Ant. t., *Apis*, ARG. N., Arn., *Ars.*, **Asaf.**, Aur., **BELL.**, Berb., **Bism.**, Bov., Bry., *Caj.*, *Calad.*, *Cannab. i.*, **Caps.**, Carb v., *Cimic.*, Cina, *Cocc.*, **Coc. c.**, *Colch.*, COM., Con., Coral., *Crot. tig.*, Euphorb., **Gel.**, GLON., *Guai.*, *Hell.*, Hyos., **K. carb.**, Laur., *Meli.*, Merc., NAT M., Nux m., OLEAND., Op., **Par.**, Petrol., *Phos.*, *Plat.*, Pb., **Ran. b.**, *Ran. s.*, Rhodo., Sars., **Sep.**, **Spig.**, Stan., Sul., *Tar.*, Verat. a., Zinc.

Dislocations.—AGN., *Ambr.*, Am. carb., Am. m., **Arn.**, Bar. c., Bov., Bry., CALC. C., Cannab. s., **Carb. an.**, *Carb. v.*, *Caust.*, Con., Graph., Hep., Ign., K. nit., Kre., **LYC.**, Merc., Mez., Mos., NAT. C., NAT. M., Nit. ac., Nux v., PETROL., PHOS., **Puls.**, *Rhodo.*, RHUS, Ruta, Sabi., Sep., *Spig.*, Stan., Staph., Sul., Zinc.

Dislocation Easy.—Agn., *Am. carb.*, Bry., *Calc. c.*, Cannab. s., **Carb. an.**, *Carb. v.*, Con., Hep., K. nit., **Lyc.**, *Merc.*, NAT. C., **Nat. m.**, **Nit ac.**, Nux v., Petrol., Phos., RHUS, Ruta, Sul.

Distortion of Limbs.—*Acon.*, Arn., *Ars.*, Asaf., BELL., Bry., **Camph.**, **Canth.**, Cham., Chin., CIC., Cocc., **Cup.**, *Graph.*, Hell., **Hyos.**, *Laur.*, Merc., Nux v., Op., Petrol., PLAT., Pb., **Puls.**, Ran. b., Rheum, Ruta, Sec. c., Spig., *Stan.*, STRAM., *Sul.*, *Verat. a.*

Doubling Up of Body.—Ant. t., Cocc., **Coloc.**, *Sabi.*, Sec. c.

Drawing Downward Sensation.—Cannab. s., Chel., Coc. c., Lil. t., Merc., Mos., *Nux v.*, Zinc.

Drawing Inward of Soft Parts.—Acon., *Agar.*, Am. carb., Arn.,

Ars., Bar. c., Bell., **Calad.**, *Carb. v.*, Caust., Chel., Chin., *Coloc., Con., Crot. tig.*, **Cup., Dros.**, Dulc., Euphorb., *Euphr.*, Hell., K. carb., Lach., Laur., **Mos.**, Nat. c., *Nux v.*, PB., *Rhus*, Ruta, Sars., Sil., *Staph.*, Sul., Thuj., Valer., Zinc.

Drawing-Inward Sensation.—*Crot. tig.*, Dig., *Hep.*, Lil. t., Mur. ac., Nux v., *Pb.*, *Rhus*, Sul, *Verb.*

Dropsy, Externally.—*Ac. ac., Acon.*, ANT. CR., APIS, **Apoc. c.**, ARS., Asc. c., *Aur.*, **Bell., Bism.**, Bry., *Cact., Camph.*, **Canth.**, *Ced.*, Chel., CHIN., *Cinnab., Coca.*, COLCH., *Coloc.*, **Con.**, *Conv., Cop., Crotal.*, DIG., *Dub.*, Dulc., *Eup. pur.*, Euphorb., **Fer.**, Guai., HELL., Hyos., Iod., **K. carb.**, K. iod., *K. nit.*, Lach., **Led.**, *Lyc.*, Mar., **Merc.**, *Mez., Mur. ac.*, Nat. c., **Nit. ac., Nux m.**, OLEAND., OP., Phos., *Pic. ac.*, Plat., **Pb., Puls.**, Rhodo., *Rhus*, Ruta, **Sabi., Samb.**, Sars., *Sec. c.*, **Seneg., Sep.**, *Sil.*, Stram., SQU., Sul., **Verat. a., Verb.**, *Zinc.*

—**Internally.**—*Acon.*, Agn, *Ambr.*, Am. carb., Ant. cr., **Ant. t.**, *Apis*, Arg., *Arn.*, ARS., Aur., **BELL., Bry.**, Calc. c., Camph., Cannab. s., Canth., Caps., Carb. v., CHIN., Cina, COLCH., Coloc., Con., DIG., Dulc., Euphorb., *Fer.*, Guai., HELL., Hep., *Hyos.*, Ign., Iod., *Ip.*, *K. carb.*, *Lach.*, Laur., **Led.**, *Lyc.*, Mar., **Merc.**, Mez., Mur. ac., Nit. ac., *Nux v.*, Op., Phos., Pho. ac., Puls., **Rhus**, Saba., Samb., Sars., **Seneg.**, Sep., Sil., *Spig., Spo.*, **Squ.**, Stan., Stram., SUL., Verat. a., Vio. t.

Dryness of Internal Parts.—ACON., *Agar.*, Agn., *Aloe.*, *Alum.*, *Ambr.*, *Am. carb.*, Am. m., Anac., Ant. cr., **Ant. t.**, Apis, Arg. n., Arn., ARS., *Asaf., Asar.*, Aur., **Bap., Bar. c., BELL.**, Berb., Bor., Bov., BRY., CALAD., CALC. C., Camph., CANNAB. I., *Cannab. s.*, CANTH., Caps., *Carb. an., Curb. v., Carb. sul.*, Caust., *Ced.*, **Cham., Chel.**, *Chin.*, Cic., Cina, Clem., **Coca**, Cocc., *Coff.*, Colch., Con., *Crotal., Crot. tig.*, Croc., Cup., *Cyc.*, Dig., **Dios.**, Dros., *Dulc.*, Euphorb., Euphr., Fer., **Gel., Graph.**, Guai., Hell., Hep., Hyos., *Ign.*, Iod., *Ip.*, Jal., K. Bl., *K. br., K. carb.*, **K. iod.**, K. nit., Kre., Lach., *Laur.*, Led., **Lyc.**, *Mag. c., Mag. m.*, **Mang.**, Meny., Merc., **Merc. c.**, *Mez.*, Mos., Mur. ac., Nat. c., **NAT. M., Nit. ac.**, NUX M., Nux v., Oleand., Op., Par., *Petrol.*, PHOS., **Pho. ac.**, *Phyt.*, Plat., **Pb., Puls.**, Ran. b., Ran. s., Rheum, Rhodo., **RHUS**, Ruta, Saba., Sabi., Samb., *Sang., Sars., Sec. c.*, Sele., SENEG., **SEP., Sil.**, *Spig., Spo.*, Squ., Stan., **Staph., Stram., Stro.**, SUL., *Sul. ac.*, Tar., *Thuj.*, VERAT. A., VERAT. V., Zinc.

Dryness of Palms and Soles.—*Bism., Crotal.*, SUL.

Dry Sensation, Internally.—Acon., **Aesc.**, *Alumen.*, **ALUM., Am. m.**, Apis, Arg., Arg. n., *Arn.*, ARS., **Arum. t., Asaf., Asar.**, BAR. C., BELL., *Benz. ac.*, **Berb., Bry., Calad.**, Camph., CANNAB. I., *Cannab.*

SENSATIONS.

s., Canth., **Caps., Carb.** v., *Carb. sul.,* Caust., *Chin.,* Cic., *Cimic.,* Cina, Cinnab., *Cist.,* **Clem., Cocc.,** Coff., CON., *Cop.,* Croc., *Crot. tig., Dios.,* Dros., *Dub., Elaps.,* Euphorb., **Euphr.,** Fer., *Gam.,* Gel., *Hydras., Ign.,* Ip., K. Br., K. carb., K. chl., Lach., Laur., Mar., *Meli.,* Meny., Merc., **Mez.,** Mos., *Naj., Nat. ars.,* Nat. c., NAT. M., Nit. ac., NUX M., NUX V., Oleand., *Osm., Par., Petrol.,* PHOS., **Pho. ac.,** Phyt., Pb., Pod., Pso., PULS., Rheum, RHUS, Ruta, Saba., Sabi., SANG., **Sang. n.,** Sec. c., Seneg., Sep., Sil., *Sin.,* Spig., Squ., **Stan.,** Staph., *Stict.,* STRAM., SUL., Sul. ac., Tar., Thuj., Valer., VERAT. A., Vio. o., Vio. t., **Wye.,** ZINC.

Dry Sensation In Joints.—Canth., *Croc., Lyc.,* NUX V., *Pho.ac.,* PULS.

Dust, Internal Sensation of.—Am. carb., *Ars.,* **Bell.,** CALC. C., Chel., Cina, Dros., *Hep.,* Ign., Ip., *Mar., Pho. ac.,* Rheum, Sul.

Emaciation.—Ac. ac., *Alum.,* Ambr., Am. carb., **Am. m.,** *Anac., Ant. cr., Ant. t., Arg.,* Arn., **ARS., Ars. iod., Bar. c.,** *Bor.,* **Bry.,** Calc. c., *Calc. ph., Canth., Carb. sul.,* Cham., Chel., **CHIN.,** *Cina,* **Clem., Cocc.,** *Con., Crot. tig.,* Cup., Dig., Dros., *Dulc.,* Fer., **GRAPH.,** Guai., *Helo., Hep.,* Ign., IOD., **Ip.,** *K. carb.,* K. iod., Lach., **LYC.,** *Mag. c.,* Mag. m., Merc., *Mez., Nat c.,* NAT. M., NIT. AC., Nux m., NUX V., Op., Petrol., PHOS., **Pho. ac., PB.,** Puls., *Ruta, Samb.,* **Sars.,** Sec. c., *Sele., Sep.,* SIL., Spig., Spo., **STAN.,** Staph., *Stram.,* Stro., SUL., *Ura.,* Verat. a.

—**Of Affected Parts.**—*Ars.,* **Bry., Carb.** v., Dulc., Graph., Led., Mez., Nat. m., Nit. ac., Pho. ac., *Pb.,* Puls., *Sele., Sil.*

—**Of Certain Parts.**—*Bry.,* Calc. c., *Caps.,* Carb. v., *Con., Dulc,* Graph., Iod., Led., Mez., *Nat. m.,* Nit. ac., *Pho. ac.,* Sele., Sil.

Emptiness.—Acon., Agar., *Alum.,* Am. carb., **Am. m.,** *Ant. cr.,* Ant. t., Apoc. c., *Arg.,* Arn., Aur., **Bar. c., Bry.,** Calad., Calc. c., **Calc. ph.,** *Caps.,* **Carb. v.,** *Caust.,* Cham., Chin., *Cina,* **Coca,** COCC., Coff., *Colch.,* Coloc., Croc., **Crot. tig.,** Cup., **DIG.,** Dulc., Euphorb., *Fer., Gam.,* Gel., Glon., Graph., Guai., Hep., *Hydras.,* **IGN.,** Iod., *Ip.,* **K. carb.,** *K. nit.,* Lach., Laur., Lyc., *Mag. c.,* Mang., *Mar.,* Meny., **Merc.,** Mez., **Mur. ac.,** *Nat. c., Nat. m., Nux v.,* **Oleand.,** Op., Par., **Petrol.,** PHOS., Plat., Pb., POD., PULS., Rhus, Ruta, *Saba.,* **Sang.,** Sars., Seneg., SEP., *Spig.,* Squ., **STAN.,** Stram., *Sul.,* SUL. AC., **TAB.,** *Verat. a.,* Verb., *Vib. op., Zinc.*

Excitement, Nervous.—Acon., Agn., *Alum.,* **Ambr., Arg. n.,** BELL., *Calc. c.,* Canth., **Cham., Chin.,** Cic., **COFF.,** *Colch.,* Croc., *Dros.,* **Fer.,** Iod., Kre., Lach., *Laur.,* Mar., Meny., MOS., NUX V., Petrol., Phos., **Pho. ac.,** Plat., Puls., *Rhus,* Ruta, Saba., **Sep., Sil.,** Spo., Stram., *Sul.,* Valer., *Verat. a.,* Verb., Vio. o.

Excoriated Feeling, See Under **Skin.**
Extravasation. See under **Skin.**
—**Sensation of.**—Arn., Calc. c., *Chin., Fer.,* Nux v., *Par., Ruta, Sec.* c.; Sul. ac.

External Parts, Drugs Affecting.—Acon., Agar., Agn., *Alum.,* Am. m., *Anac.,* Ant. cr., *Arg.,* Arn., Ars., Asaf., Asar., *Aur.,* Bar. c., Bell., Bism., Bry., Calc. c., Cannab. s., Caps., Carb. an., Carb. v., **Caust.,** Cham., Chin., Cic., *Cina, Clem.,* Cocc., Colch., Coloc., Con., Croc., *Cyc.,* Dig., *Dros.,* Dulc., Euphorb., Euphr., Fer., *Graph.,* Hell., Hep., *Hyos.,* Ign., Ip., K. carb., K. nit., Kre., Lach., *Led.,* Mag. c., Mag. m., Mang., Mar., Meny., Merc., Mez., Mos. *Mur. ac.,* Nat. c., *Nat. m.,* Nit. ac., Nux m., Nux v., Oleand., Op., Par., Petrol., Phos., Pho. ac., *Phyt.,* **PLAT.,** Puls., Ran. b., *Ran. s., Rhodo.,* RHUS, *Ruta,* Saba., Sabi., *Samb.,* Sars., Sec. c., *Sele.,* Seneg., *Sep., Sil.,* Spig., *Spo.,* Squ., *Stan.,* Staph., Stram., Stro., Sul., *Sul. ac.,* Tar., *Thuj.,* Valer., Verat. a., Verb., Vio. o., *Vio. t.,* Zinc.

Faintness.—ACON., Aesc., *Agar., All. c.,* Ambr., *Am. m.,* **Ant. t.,** Arg. n., Arn., ARS., Bar. c., *Bell.,* Bor., Bov., BRY., Calad., *Calc. c.,* Camph., *Cannab. i.,* Cannab. s., Canth., *Carb. ac.,* Carb. v., *Carb. sul.,* Caust., CHAM, *Chel.,* CHIN., *Cic.,* Cimic., Cina, *Coca,* Cocc., *Coll.,* Coloc., Con., *Crotal., Crot. tig.,* DIG., *Dios.,* Dros., Dulc., Fer., *Gel., Gran.,* Graph., *Grind.,* Hell., Hep., *Hyd. ac.,* Hyos., *Ign.,* Ip., *K. carb.,* K. nit., Kre., Lach., *Laur., Led.,* Lil. t., Lyc., Mag. c., Mag. m., Merc., Mez., Mos., *Nat. m.,* Nit. ac., NUX M., NUX V., *Oleand.,* Op., Petrol., Phos., PB, POD., *Puls.,* Ran. b., *Ran. s., Rhus,* Ruta, *Saba.,* Sang., Sars., Sec. c., Seneg., SEP., Sil., Spig., Staph., STRAM., **Sul., Tab.,** *Thea., Valer.,* Verat. a., **Verat. v.,** Vib. op., Vio. o.

Falling Easily.—Anac., Asar., *Bell.,* Bov., *Camph.,* Caps., **Caust.,** *Cina,* Cocc., Colch., Cup., Dros., *Hell.,* Hyos., Ign., *Iod.,* Ip., **Mag. c.,** Mang., Merc., *Nat. c.,* Nat. m., *Nux m.,* Nux v., Phos., Pho. ac., *Plat.,* Pb, Puls., Saba., Sec. c., Spig., Spo., Stan., **Stram.,** Sul., VERAT. A.

Falling Forward Feeling, Internally.—*Dig.,* Nux v., Sul., Verat. a.

Falling Outward of Internal Parts, Sensation of.—Agn., Ant. cr., **BELL.,** Bov., *Bry.,* Chel., Cocc., *Con.,* Graph., K. carb., Kre., Laur., LIL. T., *Lyc.,* Merc., Mos., Nat. c., **Nux v., Plat.,** *Pb.,* Ran. b., **Sep.,** *Spig.,* Staph., Sul., Thuj., Zinc.

Festering, Pain as From. (Compare with **Ulcerative Pain, Externally.**—Agn., Am. carb., Anac., *Arn.,* Ars., *Asaf.,* Aur., Bar. c., **Bry.,** *Calc. c., Carb. v.,* Chin., Colch., *Con.,* Cyc., Dros., Euphorb., *Graph.,* Hep., Hyos., Iod., *K. carb.,* Kre., *Led., Nat. m.,* Nit. ac., Nux v., Par.,

Petrol., PHOS., PULS., RAN. B., *Rhodo.*, *Rhus*, Ruta, Sars., *Sec. c.*, SIL., *Stan.*, Staph., *Sul.*, *Tar.*, *Valer.*, Verat. a., Zinc.

Flabby Feeling.—Acon., Agar., *Ambr.*, Am. m., *Ant. t.*, Arg., Arn., ARS., Asar., **Bar. c.**, Bell., *Bov.*, Bry., *Calc. c.*, Canth., **Caps.**, *Carb. an.*, *Carb. v.*, CAUST., **Cham.**, Chel., *Chin.*, Cic., *Cina*, Coff., CROC., **Cyc.**, Dig., Euphorb., Euphr., Graph., Hep., IGN., Iod., **Ip.**, K. carb., K. nit., *Laur.*, LYC., Mag. c., *Mag. m.*, *Mar.*, Meny., Merc., **Mos.**, Mur. ac., NAT. C., *Nit. ac.*, Nux m., **Nux v.**, *Oleand.*, Par., *Petrol.*, PHOS., **Plat.**, *Puls.*, Rhodo., *Rhus*, **Saba.**, Sabi., Seneg., *Sil.*, *Spo.*, **Staph.**, Stro., SUL., Tar., *Thuj.*, VERAT. A., Zinc.

—**In Hard Parts.**—*Caust.*, Merc., Mez., Nit. ac., Nux m.

—**Internally.**—Calc. c., *Kre.*

Floating Sensation (on Waves).—Coff., Hyos., *Nux m.*, Par., Stict.

Forcings.—Alum., Ambr., Am. carb., Am. m., Anac., *Ant. cr.*, Arn., **Asaf.**, Aur., *Bell.*, Bism., Bor., Bry., *Calc. c.*, *Cannab. s.*, **Canth.**, Caps., Carb. an., Carb. v., *Caust.*, *Cham.*, Chel., Chin., Cina, Clem., COCC., Colch., Coloc., Con., *Croc.*, Dig., Dulc., *Graph.*, Hell., Hyos., Ign., Iod., *Ip.*, *K. carb.*, K. nit., Laur., Led., Lyc., Mag. c., Mag. m., *Mar.*, Merc., MOS., Nat. c., Nat. m., Nit. ac., NUX V., Phos., Plat., PULS., *Ran. b.*, *Rhodo.*, **Rhus**, **Sabi.**, Samb., Sars., Seneg., *Sep.*, Spig., Spo., Stan., Stram., Sul., Sul. ac., Thuj.

Formication, Externally.—ACON., Agar., Alum., *Ambr.*, *Am. carb.*, Am. m., Anac., Ant. cr., Ant. t., *Arg.*, ARN., *Ars.*, Asaf., Asar., Aur., Bar. c., *Bell.*, Bor., Bov., Bry., *Calc. c.*, Camph., Cannab. s., Caps., Carb. an., *Carb. v.*, Caust., Cham., **Chel.**, *Chin.*, Cic., Cina, Clem., **Cocc.**, COLCH., Coloc., *Con.*, **Croc.**, Dros., Dulc., Euphr., Fer., **Gran.**, *Graph.*, *Guai.*, Hep., Hyos., *Ign.*, Ip., **K. carb.**, K. nit., Kre., *Lach.*, *Laur.*, Led., Mag. c., Mag. m., Mang., *Mar.*, **Merc.**, Mez., Mos., *Mur. ac.*, **Nat. c.**, **Nat. m.**, Nit. ac., Nux m., NUX V., Oleand., Op., Par., Phos., **Pho. ac.**, **PLAT.**, **Pb.**, Puls., Ran. b., *Ran. s.*, Rheum, Rhodo., RHUS, **Saba.**, *Sabi.*, Samb., Sars., SEC. C., Sele., Seneg., SEP., Sil., SPIG., *Spo.*, Stan., Staph., Stram., Stro., **Sul.**, *Sul. ac.*, Tar., *Thuj.*, Valer., *Verat. a.*, Verb., Vio. t., Zinc.

—**Internally.**—Acon., *Acon. f.*, *Agar.*, Agn., *Alum.*, *Ambr.*, Am. carb., Am. m., *Ant. t.*, Arg., **Arn.**, *Ars.*, Asaf., Bar. c., Bell., **Bry.**, *Calc. c.*, **Canth.**, Carb. v., *Caust.*, *Chel.*, **Chin.**, Cic., *Cocc.*, COLCH., Coloc., *Cup.*, Dros., Dulc., Euphr., Graph., Guai., Hep., *Hyos.*, *Ign.*, Iod., *Laur.*, Led., Meny., Merc., *Mez.*, Nat. c., Nux m., Nux v., Phos., *Pho. ac.*, **PLAT.**, **Pb.**, **Puls.**, Rheum, *Rhodo.*, RHUS, **Saba.**, *Sabi.*, SANG., Sec. c., Sele., *Seneg.*, Sep., *Sil.*, *Spig.*, *Spo.*, *Stan.*, Staph., SUL., Tar., *Thuj.*, *Vio. o.*, Zinc.

Frozen Limbs.—AGAR., **Ars.**, Bell., **Bor.**, Bry., *Camph.*, **Carb. v.**, Colch., Hep., Mur. ac., NIT. AC., Nux v., Petrol., **Phos.**, Pho. ac., PULS., Sul., *Sul. ac.*

Full Feeling, Externally.—*Aconin.*, *Ars.*, *Caust.*, K. nit., Laur., Nux m., Par., **Phos.**, Verat. a.

—**Internally.**—ACON., *Aconin.*, *Aesc.*, *Agar.*, Alum., **Am. carb.**, *Am. m.*, *Amyl.*, *Anac.*, **Ant. cr.**, **Ant. t.**, **Apis**, **Arn.**, *Ars.*, **Asaf.**, *Asar.*, Aur., **Bar. c.**, **Bell.**, *Bor.*, Bov., Bry., *Cact.*, *Calc. c.*, *Calc. iod.*, Camph., *Cannab. i.*, Cannab. s., **Canth.**, **Caps.**, **Carb. an.**, **Carb. v.**, *Carb. sul.*, Caust., **Cham.**, Chel., CHIN., Cic., CIMIC., *Cocc.*, *Coff.*, **Colch.**, Coloc., *Com.*, Con., Croc., **Crot. tig.**, **Cyc.**, Dig., Fer., GLON., Graph., Guai., Ham., Hell., Hyos., *Ign.*, Iod., **Iris v.**, **K. carb.**, **K. nit.**, Kre., Lach., *Laur.*, Led., **Lyc.**, *Mag. c.*, Mag. m., Mang., MELI., Meny., *Merc.*, Mez., MOS., *Mur. ac.*, **Nat. ars.**, *Nat. c.*, Nat. m., **Nit. ac.**, **Nux m.**, Nux v., Oleand., Op., Par., *Petrol.*, PHOS., Pho. ac., **Phyt.**, **Plat.**, **Pb.**, **Pso.**, Puls., **Ran. s.**, *Rheum*, Rhodo., RHUS, *Ruta*, Saba., **Sabi.**, Sars., **Sep.**, *Sil.*, Spig., *Spo.*, Stan., Staph., *Stict.*, Stro., SUL., Sul. ac., Thuj., **Valer.**, Verat. a., *Verat. v.*, Verb., Zinc.

Full Habit (Compare with **Plethora** Under **Circulation**).—Acon., *Alum.*, Ambr., **Am. carb.**, Arn., Ars., *Aur.*, **Bar. c.**, BELL., Bov., BRY., CALC. C., Carb. an., *Carb. v.*, *Caust.*, Cham., Chin., Clem., Cocc., Con., **Croc.**, Dig., **Fer.**, Graph., Hep., *Hyos.*, Ign., Iod., **Ip.**, **K. carb.**, K. nit., Led., LYC., Mag. m., **Merc.**, Mos., Nat. c., NAT. M., Nit. ac., Nux v., Op., *Petrol.*, PHOS., **Pho. ac.**, Puls., Rhodo., **Rhus**, Sars., Sec. c., *Sele.*, *Seneg.*, SEP., SIL., Spig., Spo., Stan., Staph., Stram., **Stro.**, SUL., Thuj., *Valer.*, *Verat. a.*, Zinc.

Gnawing.—Ars., Caust., MERC., *Sil.*, Staph., *Sul.*

—**Externally.**—*Acon.*, *Agar.*, AGN., **Alum.**, Ambr., **Am. carb.**, *Arg.*, Arn., Aur., **Bar. c.**, **Bell.**, Bry., Calad., *Calc. c.*, **Canth.**, Caps., **Cham.**, *Cyc.*, *Dig.*, **Dros.**, Dulc., Euphorb., *Fer.*, **Glon.**, Graph., *Hell.*, *Hyos.*, Ign., **K. carb.**, Kre., *Laur.*, Led., **Lyc.**, *Mag. c.*, Mag. m., *Mang.*, **Meny.**, *Merc.*, *Mez.*, Mur. ac., *Nat. c.*, *Nux v.*, Oleand., Op., **Par.**, **Phos.**, Pho. ac., PLAT., **Pb.**, Puls., RAN. S., Rheum, *Rhodo.*, *Rhus*, **Ruta**, Samb., Sep., Sil., *Spig.*, SPO., Stan., STAPH., *Stro.*, *Sul.*, **Tar.**, Thuj., Verat. a., Zinc.

—**Internally.**—*Agar.*, Alum., *Am. m.*, Arg., **Ars.**, Bar. c., **Bell.**, Calad., Calc. c., Cannab. s., Canth., Carb. v., CAUST., *Chel.*, **Cocc.**, **Coloc.**, Con., **Cup.**, *Dig.*, Dros., Dulc., **Gam.**, Hep., *Iod.*, **K. bi.**, K. carb., **Kre.**, *Lach.*, Lyc., *Mar.*, Merc., *Mez.*, Nux v., *Oleand.*, Phos., *Pho. ac.*, **Plat.**, PULS., **Ran. s.**, Rhodo., RUTA., *Seneg.*, SEP., Sil., Stan., *Sul.*, Verat. a.

Gnawing In Joints.—Am. carb.,Canth., **Dros.**, Dulc.,Graph., *Mag. c., Mang.*, Phos., RAN. S., *Stro.*, Zinc.

Gout-like Pains (Arthritic).—Acon., Agar., AGN., *Alum.*, Ambr., *Am. carb.*, Am. m., *Anac., Ant. cr.*, Ant. t., ARG., **Arn.**, Ars., **Asaf.**, *Asar.*, Aur., **Bar. c.**, BELL., Bism., Bor., *Bov.*, BRY., **Calc. c.**, Camph., Cannab. s., Caps., *Canth., Carb. an., Carb. v.*, **Caust.**, *Cham.*, **Chel., Chin.**, Cic., Cina, Clem., **Cocc.**, COLCH., Coloc., Con., Cup., Cyc., Dig., *Dros., Dulc.*, Euphorb., Euphr., **Fer., Graph.**, Guai., *Hell.*, Hep., **Hyos., Ign.**, **Iod.**, K. CARB., *K. nit.*, Kalm., Kre., *Laur.*, LED., *Lyc.*, Mag. c., Mag. m., Mang., *Mar.*, **Meny.**, MERC., **Mez.**, Mos., Mur. ac., **Nat. c., Nat. m.**, Nit. ac., *Nux m., Nux v.*, Oleand., Par., *Petrol.*, **Phos.**, *Pho. ac.*, Plat. **Pb., Puls., Ran. b.**, Ran. s., *Rheum, Rhodo.*, RHUS, *Ruta, Saba.*, SABI, **Sal. ac.**, *Samb.*, **Sang.**, Sars., *Sec. c.*, **Sep.**, *Sil., Spig.*, SPO., Squ., **Stan., STAPH.**, Stram., **Stro.**, SUL., Sul. ac., *Tar.*, **Thuj.**, *Valer.*, Verat. a., Verb., Vio. o., *Vio. t.*, **Zinc.**

Grinding Pain.—*Agar., Cocc., Dios.*.

Griping (Clawing, Clutching).—Acon., *Aeth.*, AGAR., *Alum.*, **Am. carb.**, *Arn.*, **Asaf.**, Bar. c., **Bell., Bor., Bry.**, CALC. C., **Carb. an.**, *Carb. v., Caust.*, Cham., **CHEL.**, Chin., **COCC.**, *Coc. c.*, **Colch.**, COLOC., Con., *Crot. tig.*, **Cup.**, *Dig.*, DIOS., Dros., *Dulc.*, **Euphorb., Gran.**, *Graph.*, **Hep.**, Hyos., **IGN.**, Ip., **Iris. v., K. bi.**, K. carb., *K. nit., Kre.*, **Led.**, Lil. t., Lyc., Mag. c., *Mag. m.*, Meny., **Merc., Merc. d.**, Mos., *Nat. c.*, **Nat. m.**, *Nux m.*, Nux v., **OP.**, *Ox. ac.*, Petrol., **Phos., PULS., Rheum**, Samb., Sep., **SIL., STAN.**, Stro., **SUL.**, Sul. ac., Verat. a., **Zinc.**

Growing Pains.—*Bell.*, Guai., **Pho. ac.**

Hacking (As with a Hatchet).—*Aur.*, Pho. ac., **Ruta**, *Staph.*, Thuj.

Hæmorrhage (From Internal Parts).—Ac. ac., Acon., Agar.,*Aloe.*, Alum., *Ambr., Am. carb.*, Am. m., Anac., Ant. cr., Ant. t., Aran., Arg., Arg. n., **Arn.**, Ars., *Asar.*, **Bar. c., BELL.**, Bism., *Bor.*, Bov., **Bry.**, Cact., CALC. C., Cannab. s., **CANTH., Caps.**, *Carb. an.*, Carb. v., **Caust.**, Cham., **CHIN.**, Cina, **Cinnam.**, Clem., Cocc., **Coff.**, Colch., Coloc., Con., **Croc., Crotal.**, *Crot. tig., Cub.*, **Cup.**, Dig., **Dros.**, Dulc., *Erig.*, Euphr., FER., Graph., *Ham.*, Hep., **Hydras., Hyos.**, Ign., Iod., IP., K carb., *K. nit.*, Kre., **Lach., Led.**, Lyc., Mag. c., *Mag. m.*, **Meli.**,MERC., MERC. C., **Mez., MILLEF.**, Mos., *Mur. ac., Nat. c.*, NAT. M., NIT. AC., Nux m., NUX V., Op., *Petrol.*, **PHOS., Pho. ac.**, Plat., *Pb.*, **PULS.**, Rhodo., **Rhus**, Ruta, *Saba.*, SABI., *Sang.*, Sars., **Sec. c.**, Sele., SEP., **Sil.**, Squ., *Stan.*, Staph., **Stram.**, SUL., *Sul., ac., Tar., Ter., Thlasp., Thuj., Trill.*, Valer., Verat. a., **Zinc.**

8

Hair, Sensation of a.—Arg. n., Ars., *Carb. sul.*, *Coc. c.*, **K. bi.**, *Lyc.* *Nat. m.*, **Puls.**, Ran. b., SIL., Sul.

Hair, Sensation of Pulling. See Under **Skin.**

Hammering.—*Am. carb.*, Am. m., *Calc. c.*, Chin., Cic., Clem., Coff., *Dros.*, Fer., Hep., *Lach.*, *Mez.*, *Nat. m.*, **Phos.**, Sep., *Sil.*, SUL, *Tab.*, Thuj., Verb.

Hard Bed, Sensation of.—Acon., **Arn.**, Bry., Caust., *Con.*, *Dros.*, Graph., *K. carb.*, Mag. c., Mag. m., Nux m., *Nux v.*, *Phos.*, *Plat.*, Saba. SIL., Stan., Sul., Tar., Thuj., Verat. a.

Hardened (Muscles).—Alum., *Bar. c.*, Bry., **Carb. an.**, Carb. v., **Caust.**, *Con.*, Dulc., Hep., Hyos., *Iod.*, *K. carb.*, Lach., **Lyc.**, *Nat. c.*, *Nux v.*, Pho. ac., *Puls.*, Ran. b., *Rhodo.*, Rhus, Sars., Sep., Sil., Spo., *Sul.*, Thuj.

Heaviness, Externally.—*Acon.*, *Agar.*, *Agn.*, *Aloe*, **Alum.**, *Ambr.*, *Am. carb.*, *Anac.*, Ant. cr., *Ant. t.*, *Arn.*, Ars., **Ars. iod.**, Asaf., Asar., Aur., Bar. c., **BELL.**, Bor., Bov., **BRY.**, *Cact.*, *Calc. c.*, Camph., *Cannab. i.*, *Cannab. s.*, Canth., Caps., *Carb. ac.*, **Carb. v.**, *Carb. sul.*, Caust., Cham., Chel., **Chin.**, Cic., *Clem.*, *Cocc.*, Coff., Colch., Coloc., *Con.*, Croc., *Crotal.*, *Crot. tig.*, Cup., *Cur.*, Dig., *Dulc.*, Euphorb., Euphr., Fer., **Gel.**, Graph., Hell., Hep., *Ign.*, *Iod.*, Ip., *K. carb.*, **K. nit.**, **Kre.**, Laur., **Led.**, Lyc., Mag. c., Mag. m., *Mar.*, **Meli.**, *Meny.*, **Merc.**, **Mez.**, Mos., *Mur. ac.*, **Nat. c.**, **Nat. m.**, *Nit. ac.*, Nux m., **NUX V.**, Onos., Op., *Par.*, **Petrol.**, PHOS., *Pho. ac.*, *Pic. ac.*, Plat., *Pb.*, **Pso.**, **PULS.**, Ran. b., Rheum, Rhodo., **RHUS**, **Ruta**, Saba., *Sabi.*, Samb., Sars., Sec. c., **SEP.**, Sil., SPIG., Spo., Squ., STAN., Staph., Stram., Stro., SUL., Sul. ac., Thuj., *Valer.*, **Verat. a.**, Verb., Vio. o., **Zinc.**

—**Internally.**—ACON., **Agar.**, Agn., ALOE., *Alum.*, Ambr., **Am. carb.**, **Am. m.**, Anac., *Ant. t.*, *Arg. n.*, *Arn.*, *Ars.*, *Asaf.*, Asar., Aur., **Bar. c.**, **Bell.**, BISM., Bor., Bov., Bry., Calad., CALC. C., *Camph.*, **Cannab. i.**, Cannab. s., Canth., *Carb. ac.*, **Carb. an.**, **Carb. v.**, *Carb. sul.*, Caust., Cham., **CHEL.**, Chin., Cic., Clem., **Cocc.**, Coff., Colch., Coloc., **Con.**, Croc., **Cup.**, Dig., Dros., *Dulc.*, Euphr., Fer., GEL., Graph., Hell., Hep., Hyos., Ign., Iod., Ip., Iris. v., **K. carb.**, *K. nit.*, **Kre.**, Lach., **Laur.**, **Lob. i.**, Lyc., Mag. c., **Mag. m.**, *Mang.*, **Meny.**, Merc., *Mez.*, *Mos.*, **Mur. ac.**, *Nat. c.*, NAT. M., Nit. ac., **Nux m.**, NUX V., Oleand., Onos., Op., Par., PETROL., PHOS., *Pho. ac.*, Plat., Pb., Pru., PULS., Ran. b., Ran. s., Rheum, *Rhodo.*, RHUS, Ruta, **Saba.**, *Sabi.*, Samb., Sang., Sars., Sec. c., Sele., Senec., Seneg., SEP., SIL., Spig., *Spo.*, Squ., STAN., Staph., Stram., *Stro.*, SUL., Sul. ac., Tar., Thuj., **Valer.**, **Verat. a.**, Verb., Vio. o., Vio. t., *Zinc.*

SENSATIONS. 163

Hysteria (and Hypochondriasis).—*Acon.*, *Agn.*, Alum., Ambr., Am. carb., **Anac.**, Arn., **Ars.**, ASAF., Asar., AUR.. Bar. c., **Bell.**, Bov., Bry., *Calc. c.*, *Cannab. s.*, Canth., Caps., Carb. an., Carb. v., **Caust.**, *Cham.*, Chel., Chin., Cic., *Cocc.*, Coff., CON., *Croc.*, *Cyc.*, Dig., *Euphr.*, Fer., *Graph.*, *Hell.*, Hep., **Hyos.**, **Ign.**, **Iod.**, *Ip.*, K. carb., *Lach.*, **Lyc.**, Mag. c., **Mag. m.**, Meny., *Merc.*, *Mez.*, **Mos.**, NAT. C., **Nat. m.**, Nit. ac., Nux m., NUX V., *Op.*, **Phos.**, Pho. ac., PLAT., **Pb.**, **Puls.**, Raph., *Rheum,* Rhus, Ruta, **Sabi.**, Sars., *Sele.*, Seneg., **Sep.**, *Sil.*, Spig., Spo., **Stan.**, Staph., *Stram.*, Stro., **Sul.**, Sul. ac., *Ther.*, VALER., **Verat. a.**, *Verat. v.*, Vio. o., Vio. t., *Zinc.*

Immobility of Affected Parts.—Acon., Agar., Alum., Ambr., Am. carb., Am. m., Anac., Ant. cr., Arg., Arn., *Ars.*, Asar., Aur., *Bar. c.*, **Bell.**, Bov., *Bry.*, *Calc. c.*, Cannab. s., Canth., Caps., *Carb. v.*, **Caust.**, Cham., *Chel.*, Chin., Cic., COCC., *Colch.*, Coloc., *Con.*, Cup., Cyc., Dig., Dros., Dulc., Euphr., Fer., GEL., Graph., Guai., Hell., Hep., **Hyd. ac.**, Hyos., Ign., Iod., Ip., *K. carb.*, Lach., Laur., Led., *Lyc.*, Meny., Merc., Mez., Mur. ac., **Nat. m.**, Nit. ac., **Nux m.**, Nux v., *Oleand.*, *Op.*, Petrol., *Phos.*, Pho. ac., **Pb.**, Puls., Rhodo., RHUS, *Ruta,* Sabi., Sars., *Sec. c.* Sele., Seneg., *Sep.*, Sil., *Spig.*, Stan., Stram., *Stro.*, **Sul.**, Sul. ac., Tar., **Verat. a.**, Zinc.

Indurations (After Inflammation).—Agn., Alum., Ambr., **Arn.**, *Ars.*, Asaf., Aur., *Bar. c.*, BELL., **Bry.**, **Calc. c.**, Camph., Cannab. s., Caps., Carb. an., Carb. v., Caust., *Cham.*, Chel., CHIN., Cina, CLEM. Coloc., **Con.**, Cup., Cyc., Dulc., *Fer.*, **Graph.**, Hep., Hyos., Ign., Iod., K. carb., Led., **Lyc.**, Mag. c., MAG. M., *Merc.*, Mez., Nat. c., *Nux v.*, Op., *Phos.*, **Pb.**, **Puls.**, Ran. s., *Rhodo.*, Sec. c., Sele., *Sep.*, *Sil.*, Spig., Spo., *Staph.*, Stram., *Sul.*, Thuj., Valer., Verat. a.

Inflammation Externally.—Acon., Agar., Ambr., Am. carb., *Ant. cr.*, *Arn.*, ARS., *Asaf.*, Asar., Aur., *Bar. c.*, **Bell.**, *Bor.*, Bov., *Bry.*, **Calc. c.**, Camph., *Cannab. s.*, Canth., Caps., Carb. an., Carb. v., Caust., **Cham.**, Chel., Chin., Clem., Cocc., Coff., Coloc., Con., *Crotal.*, *Cup.*, *Dig.*, Dulc., Euphorb., Euphr., Fer., **Fl. ac.**, Graph., Hell., **Hep.**, *Hyos.*, *Ign.*, Iod., Ip., K. carb., K. nit., *Kre.*, Lach., *Led.*, **Lyc.**, Mag. c., Mag. m., Mang., Mar., **Merc.**, Mez., Mur. ac., *Nat. c.*, Nat. m., **Nit. ac.**, *Nux v.*, Op., Petrol., Phos., Pho. ac, *Pb.*, PULS., **Ran. b.**, **Rhus**, Saba., Sabi., Samb., *Sars.*, **Sep.**, SIL., Spig., Spo., Stan., STAPH., Stram., **Sul. ac.**, Tar., Thuj., Valer., *Verat. a.*, Zinc.

—**Internally.**—ACON., Agar., Alum., Ant. cr., Ant. t., **Apis**, Arg., Arn., **Ars.**, Arum. t., Asaf., Aur., Bar. c., BELL., **Berb.**, Bism., **Bor. ac.**, BRY., *Calad.*, *Calc. c.*, *Camph.*, **Cannab. s.**, CANTH., Caps., Carb. ac.,

Carb. v., **Cham.**, *Chin.*, Cic., Cina, Clem., *Cocc.*, *Coc. c.*, Coff., *Colch.*, Coloc., *Con.*, **Cub.**, Cup., *Dig.*, Dros., Dulc., *Equis.*, *Euphorb.*, Fer., Graph., *Guai.*, *Ham.*, Hell., *Hep.*, **Hyos.**, Ign., IOD, *Ip.*, **K. carb.**, K. chl., K. iod., K. nit., *Lach.*, Laur., *Lil. t.*, **Lyc.**, Mag. m., *Mang.*, MERC., *Mez*, Nat. c., *Nat. m.*, *Nit. ac.*, NUX V., Op., *Par.*, *Parei.*, Petrol., PHOS., *Pho. ac.*, *Phyt.*, **PB.**, *Pop. t.*, PULS., *Ran. b.*, Ran. s., Rheum, *Rhus*, Ruta, *Saba.*, Sabi., *Samb.*, *Sang.*, *Sang. n.*, SEC. C, *Senec.*, Seneg., *Sep.*, *Sil.*, Spig., *Spo.*, **Squ.**, Stan., *Stram.*, Stro., *Strop.*, **Sul.**, Sul. ac., TER., Thuj., *Uva.*, **Verat. a.**

Inflammation Of Mucous Membrane.—ACON., **Agar.**, **Agn.**, **All. c.**, Alum., Ambr., Am. carb, *Am. m.*, *Ammc.*, Anac., *Ant. cr.*, *Ant. t.*, **Arg.**, Arn., ARS., Asaf., Asar., Aur., *Bar. c.*, BELL., Bism., **Bor.**, Bov., **Bry.**, *Calad.*, **Calc. c.**, Camph., Cannab. s., **Canth.**, *Caps.*, Carb. an., Carb. v., Caust., **Cham.**, Chin., Cic., Cina, Clem., *Cocc.*, Coff., Colch., Coloc., *Con.*, Cup., Cyc., Dig., **Dros.**, Dulc., Euphorb., **Euphr.**, *Graph.*, Guai., Hell., **Hep.**, Hyos., Ign., *Iod.*, **Ip.**, K. BI., **K. carb.**, *K. iod.*, *K. nit.*, Kre., *Lach.*, Laur., **Lyc.**, Mag. c., Mag. m., *Mang.*, Mar., Meny., MERC., *Mez.*, Mos., Mur. ac., *Nat. c.*, **Nat. m.**, **Nit. ac.**, Nux m., NUX V., Op., **Osm.**, **Par.**, *Petrol.*, **Phos.**, *Pho. ac.*, Plat., Pb., PULS., *Ran. b.*, Ran. s., Rhodo., Rhus, Ruta, *Saba.*, Samb., Sars., Sec. c, *Sele.*, Seneg., **Sep.**, Sil., Spig., *Spo.*, **Squ.**, Stan., Staph., Stro., SUL., Sul. ac., Thuj., **Verat. a.**, *Zinc.*

Inflated Feeling.—*Berb.*, *Calc. ph.*, *Carb. ac.*, *Coloc.*, MEZ., Par., Puls., *Ran. b.*, Ter.

Internal Parts, Drugs Affecting.—Acon., Alum., *Ambr.*, Am. carb., Ant. cr., **Ant. t.**, *Ars.*, Asaf., Asar., Aur., *Bell.*, Bism., *Bor.*, Bov., Bry., *Calad.*, CALC. C., *Camph.*, Cannab. s., CANTH., Caps., *Carb. an.*, Carb. v., Caust., Cham., *Chel.*, **Chin.**, Cic., *Cocc.*, *Colch.*, Coloc., Con., Croc., Cup., *Dig.*, *Dulc.*, Euphorb., Fer., Graph., **Hell.**, Hep., Hyos., Ign., **Iod.**, *Ip.*, K. carb., *Kre.*, *Lach.*, Laur., Lyc., Mag. c., Mag. m., *Mang.*, Mar., Meny., Merc., Mez., Mos., Mur. ac., Nat. c., Nat. m., Nit. ac., *Nux m.*, NUX V., Oleand., *Par.*, Petrol., PHOS., *Pho. ac.*, Plat., *Pb.*, Puls., *Ran. b.*, Ran. s., *Rheum*, Rhodo., Rhus, Ruta, Saba., Sabi., Sars., Sec. c., **Seneg.**, Sep., Sil., Spig., Spo., *Squ.*, Stan., Staph., Stram., Stro., Sul., Sul. ac., Tar., Thuj., Valer., *Verat. a.*, Verb., *Vio. o.*, Zinc.

Irritability, Physical.—*Abs.*, Acon., *Agar.*, Ambr., Anac., Ant. cr., *Ant. t.*, ARN., Ars., *Asaf.*, Asar., Aur., *Bar. c.*, BELL., Bor., Bov., Bry., Calc. c., Camph., *Cannab. i.*, CANTH., Carb. v., *Carb. sul.*, Caust., **Cham.**, Chin., Cina, Cocc., COFF., *Con.*, Croc., Cup., Dig., **Fer.**, *Graph.*, Hell., Hep., Hyos., Ign., K. carb., *Kre.*, *Lach.*, Laur., *Lyc.* **Mag. c.**, Mag. m., Mang., **Mar.**, *Meny.*, MERC., Mez., *Mos.*, Nat. c.,

Nat. m., Nux m., **NUX V.**, Par., Petrol., **Phos.**, Pho. ac., *Plat.*, **Puls.**, *Rhus*, *Sabi.*, Sars., Sec. c., Sele., *Sep.*, SIL., Spig., *Spo.*, Squ., **Staph.**, Stram., Sul., *Tarent.*, *Valer.*, **Verat. a.**

Irritability, Physical, Lack Of.—Acon., *Agn.*, *Alum.*, Ambr., Am. carb., **Am. m.**, **Anac.**, Ant. cr., **Ant. t.**, Arn., **Ars.**, Asaf., Asar., Bar. c., *Bell.*, Bism., Bor., Brom., Bry., CALC. C., Camph., Cannab. s., Canth., Caps., **Carb. an.**, CARB. V., Caust., Cham., *Chel.*, *Chin.*, *Cic.*, *Clem.*, *Cocc.*, Colch., Coloc., CON., Croc., *Crot. tig.*, Cup., Dig., **Dulc.**, *Euphorb.*, Fer., GELS., *Graph.*, *Guai.*, Hell., Hep., *Hyos.*, *Ign.*, **Iod.**, **Ip.**, *K. carb.*, Lach., LAUR., Led., **Lyc.**, *Mag. c.*, Mag. m., Merc., **Mez.**, *Mos.*, *Mur. ac.*, Nat. c., Nat. m., **Nit. ac.**, *Nux m.*, Nux v., OLEAND., **OP.**, Petrol., *Phos.*, PHO. AC., Pb., Puls., **Rhodo.**, *Rhus*, Sec. c., Seneg., **Sep.**, Sil., Spo., Stan., Staph., **Stram.**, Stro., **Sul.**, Thuj., Valer., Verb., Zinc.

Itching (Including Tickling) Internally.—Acon., *Aesc.*, Agar., Alum., AMBR., Am. carb., Am. m., *Anac.*, Ant. t., Arn., Asar., Bar. c., Bell., Bor., Bov., Bry., Calc. c., *Caps.*, **Carb. ac.**, Carb. v., *Carb. sul.*, Caust., *Cham.*, Chin., *Cic.*, *Cina*, *Coca*, Cocc., **Coc. c.**, Colch., **Con.**, Croc., Cup., *Dig.*, **Dios.**, *Dros.*, **Dulc.**, Euphorb., **Fer.**, Gam., *Gran.*, Graph., Hep., Ign., IOD., **Ip.**, **K. bi.**, *K. carb.*, **Laur.**, Led., Mag. c., Mag. m., *Mar.*, *Meny.*, *Merc.*, Mos., Nat. c., *Nat. m.*, **Nit. ac.**, Nux m., **NUX V.**, Oleand., *Op.*, **Osm.**, Petrol., **PHOS.**, Pho. ac., Pb., **Puls.**, Rhodo., RHUS, RUMEX, Ruta, *Saba.*, *Sabi.*, SANG., Seneg., **Sep.**, Sil., *Sin.*, Spig., Spo., *Squ.*, Stan., Still., SUL., Tar., Thuj., Valer., *Verat. a.*, Zinc.

Jaundice. See Skin, Yellow.

Jerking Internally.—Acon., *Agar.*, *Ambr.*, Anac., *Arn.*, Ars., **Bell.**, Bov., *Bry.*, Calad., CALC. C., CANNAB. I., **Cannab. s.**, Caust., *Cic.*, Clem., *Coca*, Colch., *Con.*, *Croc.*, Dig., Dulc., GLON., Kre., **Lyc.**, *Maj. c.*, *Many.*, Mar., *Mez.*, *Mur. ac.*, *Nat. c.*, *Nat. m.*, Nux m., Nux v., *Petrol.*, *Phos.*, PLAT., PULS., Ran. s., *Rhodo.*, Rhus, Ruta, Samb., *Sep.*, **Sil.**, SPIG., **Spo.**, STAN., Stro., *Sul. ac.*, **Thal.**, *Thuj.*, **Valer.**

—**In Joints.**—Alum., *Bell.*, Bry., Graph., Nat. m., Puls., *Sil.*, Spig., Spo., Sul., **Sul. ac.**, **Verat. a.**

—**Muscles.**—Acon., **Agar.**, *Alum.*, **Anac.**, Ant. cr., **Ant. t.**, Arn., Ars., Asar., Bar. c., **Bell.**, Bry., *Cad. s.*, Calc. c., **Cannab. i.**, **Caps.**, *Carb. sul.*, **Cham.**, Chin., CIC., Cimic., Cocc., Colch., **Con.**, Cup., Dulc., *Euphorb.*, Euphr., Fer., Gel., Graph., Hyos., Ip., Lach., Mag. c., Meny., **Merc.**, Merc. c., **MEZ.**, Nat. m., Nit. ac., Nux m., **Nux v.**, Oleand., Op., Petrol., Phos., Pho. ac., Plat., Pb., Puls., Rhus, Ruta, *Saba.*, Sabi., SEP., *Sil.*, Spig., Stan., *Staph.*, STRAM., SUL., **SUL. AC.**, **Ter.**, Valer., Vio. t., ZINC.

Jerking As in Convulsions.—Acon., *Agar.*, Alum., AMBR., Ant. cr., Arg., *Arn.*, Ars., *Bell.*, *Bry.*, Calc. c., *Camph.*, *Cannab. s.*, *Caps.*, *Carb. v.*, CAUST., Cham., *Chin.*, Cic., Coloc., Cup., Dig., Dros., *Dulc.*, Hep., Hyos., Ign., *Ip.*, *K. carb.*, Lach., *Laur.*, *Lyc.*, *Mag. c.*, Meny., Merc., *Mez.*, Mur. ac., *Nat. c.*, NAT. M., Nit. ac., Nux v., *Op.*, Petrol., Phos., Plat., PB., Ran. b., *Rhodo.*, *Saba.*, Sec. c., *Sep.*, *Sil.*, *Squ.*, Staph., Stram., *Stro.*, Sul., Sul. ac., *Thuj.*, Verat. a., Vio. t., Zinc.

Jerking Pain, Externally.—*Acon.*, *Agar.*, Agn., Alum., *Ambr.*, Anac., Ant. cr., Ant. t., Arg., Arn., *Ars.*, ASAF., Asar., Aur., Bar. c., Bell., Bism., Bor., Bov., Bry., CALC. C., Camph., *Canth.*, Caps., *Carb. v.*, CAUST., *Cham.*, Chin., Cic., Cina, Clem., *Cocc.*, Coff., *Colch.*, Coloc., Con., Croc., Cyc., Dig., Dros., *Dulc.*, Graph., Hell., Hep., *Hyos.*, *Ign.*, Iod., *K. carb.*, Kre., Lach., *Laur.*, Led., Lyc., Mag. c., *Mang.*, Mar., MENY., Merc., Mez., Mos., *Mur. ac.*, Nat. c., NAT. M., Nit. ac., NUX V., *Oleand.*, Op., Par., Petrol., Phos., Pho. ac., Plat., Pb., PULS., Ran. b., *Ran. s.*, *Rheum*, *Rhodo.*, RHUS, Ruta, Saba., Sabi., Sec. c., Sep., Sil., *Spig.*, *Spo.*, Squ., Stan., *Staph.*, Stro., *Sul.*, Sul. ac., TAR., *Thuj.*, Valer., *Verat. a.*, Verb., Vio. t., Zinc.

Jerking Pain, Internally.—Acon., *Agar.*, *Aloe.*, *Ambr.*, Am. m., *Anac.*, *Arn.*, Ars., BELL., Bor., Bry., Calc. c., Cannab. s., Carb. v., *Caust.*, Cham., CHIN., *Clem.*, Cocc., Colch., *Con.*, Croc., Graph., IGN., K. CARB., *Lyc.*, *Mang.*, Mar., Meny., Merc., *Mez.*, Nat. m., NIT. AC., *Nux v.*, Petrol., *Pho. ac.*, Plat., *Pb.*, PULS., Ran. b., *Ran. s.*, *Rhus*, Sep., SIL., Spig., Stan., Stro., SUL., Sul. ac., THUJ., Valer.

Jumping, Internally.—Croc., Mos.

Knotted Sensation, Internally. (Compare with **Ball, Sensation of.**)—Ambr., *Ant. t.*, *Arn.*, Ars., Bry., Carb. an., Cham., Cic., *Con.*, Cup., *Gel.*, *Hyd. ac.*, Kre., LACH., Mag. m., Merc. i. r., Nux v., *Petrol.*, Phyt., *Puls.*, Rhus, Saba., *Sec. c.*, Sep., SPIG., Staph., *Stict.*, SUL.

Labor-Like Pains.—ACON., Ant. t., *Apis*, Arn., Asaf., Aur., BELL., Bor., Bry., Calc. c., Camph., *Canth.*, Carb. an., Carb. v., Caul., CHAM., Chin., Cimic., Cina, Cocc., Coff., Con., Conv., Croc., Cup., Dros., FER., GEL., Graph., Hyos., Ign., Iod., Ip., K. carb., Kre., Lach., Mos., *Murex.*, Nat. m., Nux m., Nux v., Op., Plat., Pod., PULS., Rhus, Ruta, Saba., SABI., Sec. c., Sep., Sil., Stan., Sul., Sul. ac., Ust., Vip. op., Xan.

Lie Down, Inclination To.—ACON., Alum., Ambr., Am. carb., Anac., Ant. cr., Ant. t., Arn., ARS., Asar., Bar. c., *Bell.*, Bism., Bor., Bry., CALAD., Calc. c., Canth., Caps., Carb. an., Carb. v., Caust., CHAM., Chel., *Chin.*, Cina, Cocc., Coff., Con., Croc., Cup., Cyc., Dig.,

SENSATIONS.

Dros., *Dulc.*, *Fer.*, Graph., **Guai.**, *Ign.*, *Ip.*, K. carb., *Lach.*, Led., **Lyc.**, Mag. c, Mag. m., Mar., *Merc.*, *Mez.*, Mur. ac., *Nat. c.*, *Nat. m.*, Nit. ac., NUX V., Op., Petrol., *Phos.*, Pho. ac., **Puls.**, *Ran. b.*, **Rhus**, Ruta, *Saba.*, *Sele.*, **Sep.**, SIL., **Spo.**, *Stan.*, Staph., **Stram.**, Stro., Sul., *Tar.*, *Thuj.*, *Verat. a.*, Zinc.

Lifted-Up Sensation.—Acon.

Light Sensation in Limbs.—*Agar.* **Asar.**, *Cannab. i.*, Chin., **Coff.**, *Dig.*, *Hyos.*, Nat. m., Nux v., Op., Rhus, Spig., **Stram.**, Thuj.

Looked At, Aversion To Being.—**Ant. cr.**, Cham., Cina.

Loose Feeling in Joints. Stram.

Loose, Sensation as if Skin were Hanging.—Ant. cr., Bell., *Kre.*, PHOS., Saba.

Malaise. (Compare **Sick Sensation.**)—Acon., Agar., *Alum.*, **Ambr.**, Ant. cr., *Ant. t.*, Arg., **Ars.**, *Asaf*, Asar., Bar. c., **Bap.**, **Bell.**, *Bor.*, Bov., Bry., *Cact.*, Calad., CALC. C., *Camph.*, Carb. v., *Carb. sul.*, **Caust.**, *Cham.*, Chel., Chin., **Cic.**, *Cina*, Coff., CON., Croc., CUP., *Eucal.*, *Euphr.*, Fer., *Fer. ph.*, Graph., **Hep.**, *Hyos.*, **Ign.**, *Ip.*, **K. carb.**, *Led.*, **Lyc.**, *Mag. c.*, Mag. m., **Mang.**, **Merc.**, Mez., *Mos.*, *Mur. ac.*, Nat. c., **Nat. m.**, *Nit. ac.*, **Nux v.**, Oleand., Op., *Petrol.*, Phos., *Plat.*, Pb., Puls., Rhus, Saba., Sabi., Sele., *Seneg.*, **Sep.**, SIL., Spig., **Spo.**, *Stan.*, Staph., **Stram.**, Stro., **Sul.**, Thuj., Valer., *Verat. a.*, Zinc.

Mobility, Increased.—Alum., Arn., **Bell.**, Camph., Caust., Cocc., *Coff.*, Con., *Cup.*, Hyos., Pho. ac., **Stram.**

Motion, Aversion To.—ACON., *Alum.*, Ambr., Am. carb., *Anac.*, Ant. cr., Ant. t., Arn., ARS., Asar., **Bar. c.**, *Bell.*, Bor., *Bry.*, CALAD., Calc. c., Canth., *Caps.*, Carb. an., Carb. v., Caust., Cham., **Chel.**, Chin., Cina, **Cocc.**, Coff., Con., Croc., Cup., **Cyc.**, **Dig.**, Dros., *Dulc.*, Fer., Graph., GUAI., Hyos., **Ign.**, Ip., **K. carb.**, *Lach.*, Led., **Lyc.**, Mag. c., Mag. m., Mar., *Merc.*, **Mez.**, Mur. ac., *Nat. c.*, **Nat. m.**, Nit. ac., NUX V., Op., Petrol., *Phos.*, Pho. ac., *Puls.*, Ruta, Sep., *Stan.*, Stro., Sul., *Tar.*, **Thuj.**, *Zinc.*

—**Desire For.**—*Acon.*, Agar., Alum., *Ambr.*, Am. carb., **Arn.**, **Ars.**, Asar., *Aur.*, Bell., Bor., *Bry.*, Calc. c., *Cannab. s.*, *Canth.*, *Caust.*, CHAM., CHIN., *Coff.*, *Coloc.*, Con., *Cup.*, Euphr., **FER.**, *Fl. ac.*, Hyos., Ign., **Iod.**, Ip., *Kre.*, Lyc., Mag. c., *Mag. m.*, Mang., *Mar.*, **Merc.**, Mos., Mur. ac., Nat. c. Nux m., Nux v., Op., *Pho. ac.*, Puls., *Ran. b.*, *Rhodo.*, RHUS, *Ruta*, Samb., Sec. c., Sep., *Sil.*, *Squ.*, Stan., Staph., Sul., Valer., *Verat. a.*,

—**Difficult.**—*Acon.*, Agar., Alum., Ambr., *Am. carb.*, *Am. m.*, *Anac.*, Ant. cr., Ant. t., Arg., *Arn.*, **Ars.**, Asar., Aur., Bar. c., BELL., Bor., Bov., Bry., **Calc. c.**, Camph., Cannab. s., Canth., *Caps.*, **Carb. an.**, Carb. v.,

CAUST., **Cham.**, Chel., *Chin.*, **Cic.**, Cina, **Cocc.**, Coff., Colch., **Coloc.**, *Con.*, *Croc.*, Cup., Cyc., *Dig.*, Dros., Dulc., Euphorb., Euphr., Fer., **Graph.**, *Guai.*, *Hell.*, Hep., *Hyos.*, Ign., Ip., K. carb., K. nit., Kre., Lach., Laur., *Led.*, LYC., Mag. c., Mag. m., *M(ng.*, Meny., **Merc.**, Mez., Mos., Mur. ac., *Nat. c.*, **Nat. m.**, Nit. ac., Nux m., **Nux v.**, *Oleand.*, Op., Par., PETROL., *Phos.*, Pho. ac., Plat., Pb., **Puls.**, Ran. b., Rheum, Rhodo., RHUS, Ruta, Saba., Sabi., *Sars.*, Sec. c., *Sele.*, Seneg., SEP., **Sil.**, **Spig.**, Spo., Squ., *Stan.*, **Staph.**, Stram., Stro., **Sul.**, Sul. ac., Tar., **Thuj.**, Valer., **Verat. a.**, Zinc.

Motion Involuntary.—Acon., *Alum.*, Aur., **Bell.**, Camph., *Canth.*, *Caust.*, Cham., Chin., **Cocc.**, Colch., *Con.*, Cup., *Gel.*, HYOS., Ign., K. carb., **Lach.**, Lyc., Meny., **Merc.**, *Mos.*, Nat. m., Nux m., **Op.**, Phos., Pb., Rhus., *Samb.*, Sep, *Spig.*, *Staph.*, STRAM., *Verat. a.*

—Sensation of.—Acon., Alum., Am. carb., Anac., Ant. t., Arn., Ars., Asar., Aur., BELL., *Bry.*, **Calc. c.**, Cannab. s., *Cham.*, Chin., *Cocc.*, CROC., Cyc., Dig., Dulc., Gran., Guai., Hyos., **Ign.**, Iod., *K. carb.*, Kre., Lach., *Laur.*, Led , Mag. m., *Meny.*, Merc., *Mos.*, Nat. *m.*, **Nux v.**, Petrol., Phos., Pho. ac., *Pb.*, Rheum, **Rhodo.**, **Rhus**, Saba., *Sec. c.*, **Sep.**, **Sil.**, Spig., Spo., Stro., SUL., *Tar.*, *Thuj.*, Verat. a., Vio. t., Zinc.

—Moving Up and Down.—*Fer.*, *Lach.*, Pb., **Spo.**

Mucous Secretions Increased.—*Ac. ac.*, Acon., *Agar.*, **Alum.**, Ambr., Am. carb., **Am. m.**, *Amnc.*, *Ant. cr.*, Ant. t., *Arg.*, *Arg. n.*, Arn., Ars., Asar., Aur., Bar. c., **Bell.**, Bism., **Bor.**, *Bov.*, *Bry.*, CALC. C., Camph., Cannab. s., *Canth.*, **Caps.**, *Carb. an.*, *Carb. v.*, *Caust.*, **Cham.**, Chel., **Chin.**, *Cina*, *Cocc.*, Coff., *Colch.*, Coloc., Con., Croc., Cup., *Dig.*, *Dros.*, DULC., Euphorb., **Euph.**, Fer., **Graph.**, Guai., Hell., *Hep.*, **Hyos.**, *Ign.*, *Iod.*, Ip., *K. carb.*, K. nit., Kre., Lach., *Laur.*, **Lyc.**, *Mag. c.*, Mag. m., Mar., MERC., *Mez.*, Nat. c., Nat. m., **Nit. ac.**, *Nux m.*, NUX V., Oleand., **Par.**, *Petrol.*, PHOS., Pho. ac., Plat., *Pb.*, *Pod.*, PULS., Ran. b., Rheum, Rhodo., *Rhus*, Ruta, Saba., Sabi., Samb., Sars., Sec. c., *Sele.*, **Seneg.**, Sep., *Sil.*, Spig., Spo., Squ., **Stan.**, Staph., SUL., *Sul. ac.*, TAB., Thuj., **Valer.**, Verat. a., *Zinc.*

Numbness Externally.—*Abrot.*, *Abs.*, **Acon.**, *Aconin.*, *Agar.*, Alum., Ambr., Am. carb., Am. m., *Anac.*, Ant. cr., **Ant. t.**, **Apis.**, Arn., Ars., Asaf., Asar., Aur., **Bap.**, Bar. c., **Bell.**, BERB., Bism., *Bov.*, Brom., Bry., Cact., Caj., Calc. c., Camph., Cannab. i., Cannab. s., Canth., Carb. an., Carb. v., Carb. ac., Carb. sul., Caust., Ced., *Cham.*, **Chel.**, Chin., Chloral., **Cic.**, *Cimic.*, Coca, COCC., Colch., *Coloc.*, **Con.**, Croc., Crotal., Cup., Cur., Dig., Dios., Dulc., Euphr., Fer., Gel., Glon., Gnap., *Graph.*, **Hell.**, Hep., Hyd. ac., HYOS., **Ign.**, Iod., *Ip.*, *Iris. v.*, *K. br.*, Kalm., Lach., Laur.,

SENSATIONS.

Led., LYC., Mag. m., Merc., Mez., **Mos.**, **Nux m.**, Nux v., OLEAND., Onos., OP, **Ox. ac.**, Oxyt., Par., Petrol., PHOS., PHO. AC., **Pic. ac.**, **Plat.**, PB., **Puls.**, Rhodo., Rhus, SEC. C., **Sep.**, **Sil.**, Spig., Spo., St ph., STRAM., Sul., Tab., Thea., **Urt.**, Valer., Verat. a., Verat. v., Verb., Zinc.

Numbness Internally.—Acon., Aconin., Ambr., Am. carb., **Ars.**, Asaf., Bar. c., **Bell.**, Bov., Calc. c., Carb. an., Carb. sul., Caust., Cham., Chin., Cina, Coff., Colch., Con., Crot. tig., Cup., Dig., Fer., GEL., Graph., **Hyos.**, Ign., **K. br.**, K. carb., Laur., Lyc., Mag. c., Mag. m., Merc., Mur. ac., Nat. m., Nit. ac., Nux m., Oleand., **Op.**, Petrol., Phos., PLAT., Pb., Puls., Ran. b., Rheum, Sars., Seneg., Sil., **Spig.**, Stan., Stram., Stro., Thuj., Valer., Verat. a.

—Of Suffering Parts.—Acon., Alum., Ambr., **Anac.**, Ant. t., Ars., Asaf., Aur., Bell., Bor., Bov., Bry., Calc. c., Cannab. s., Carb. an., Carb. v., Caust., Cham., Chel., Chin., Cic., Cina, **Cocc.**, Coff., Colch., Coloc., Con., Croc., Cup., Cyc., Dig., Dulc., Euphr., Fer., Graph., Hell., Hep., Hyos., Ign., Iod., K. carb., K. nit., Kre., **Lyc.**, Mag. m., Merc., Mez., Mur. ac., Nat. m., Nux m., Nux v., **Oleand.**, Petrol., Phos., Pho. ac., PLAT. **Puls.**, Rheum, Rhodo., **Rhus**, Ruta, Samb., Sec. c., Sep., Sil., Spo., Stan., Staph., Stram., Stro., Sul., Sul. ac., Thuj., Verat. a., Verb., Vio. o., Zinc.

Obesity.—Agar., Ambr., Am. m., Ant. cr., Ant. t., Arn., Asaf., Bar. c., **Bell.**, Bor., Bry., CALC. C., Camph., Canth., **CAPS.**, Cham., Chin., Cic., Clem., Cocc., Coloc., Con., Croc., **Cup.**, Dig., Euphorb., FER., Graph., Guai., Hell., **Hyos.**, Iod., Ip., K. bi., K. carb., Lach., Laur., **Lyc.**, Mag. c., Merc., Mur. ac., Nat. c., Nux m., Oleand., Op., Plat., Pb., **Puls.**, Rheum, Saba., Sars., Seneg., Sep., Sil., Spig., Spo., Stram., **Sul.**, Thuj., Verat. a., Vio. o.

Oppressive Pain (Pinching and Stricture).—Acon., Aconin., Agar., Am. m., **Amnc.**, Ant. cr., **Ant. t.**, APOC. C., Ars., Aspar., Aur., Bell., Bov., Bry., **Calad.**, Calc. c., CANNAB. I., **Cannab. s.**, Carb. ac., Caust., Cham., Chel., Chin., CHIN. S., Cic., Cina, **Cocc.**, Coc. c., Coff., Colch., Coloc., Con., Crot. tig., Dig., DROS., Euphr., FER., Fer. iod., Fer. phos., Glon., Gran., Hyos., Ign., Ip., K. bi., Kre., Lob. i., **Mag c.**, Mag. m, Mar., Meli., Millef., MOS., Naj., Nat. a., Nat. m., Nat. s. **Nit. ac.**, Nux m., Nux v., Op., Osm., Petrol., PHOS., Plat., Pb., **Pso.**, Pru., PULS., Rhus, Ruta, Saba., Samb., Sec. c., Seneg., SEP., Sil., SPIG., **Squ.**, STAN., Staph., Stict., SUL., Tab., **Verat. a.**, Vio. t., Zinc.

Pain, Blunt.—Carb. v., Cina, Hyos., Mur. ac., Nat. m., Rheum.

—Dull.—AGAR., Agn., All. c., Alum., Anac., Ant. cr., Ant. t., Asar., Bism., Bor., Bov., Bry., Calc. c., **Camph.**, Canth., Carb. v., Caust., Chel., Chin., Cic., Cina, Clem., Cocc., Coff., Coloc., Con., Cyc., Dros., **Dulc.**,

Euphorb., Fer., **Guai., Hell.,** *Helo.,* Hep., **HYOS., Ign.,** Kre., **Laur.,** Led., Lyc., Mang., Mar., Meny., Merc., Mez., Mos., *Nat. c., Nat. m.,* Nit. ac., NUX V., *Oleand.,* Phos., *Pho. ac., Plat.,* Pb., Puls., Ran. s., Rheum., Rhodo., Rhus, *Ruta,* Saba., Samb., Sars., Sec. c., Seneg., *Sep., Sil.,* Spig., *Spo.,* Squ., Stro., **Sul.,** Sul. ac., *Thuj., Verat. a.,* Verb., Vio. o., **Vio. t.,** Zinc.

Pain Jumping from Place to Place.—Acon., **Arn.,** *Ars., Asaf.,* **Belt.,** *Benz. ac., Bry.,* **Calc. ph.,** *Carb. sul.,* **Caul.,** *Ced., Chel.,* Chin., **Clem.,** Colch., Croc., Dios., Gel., Goss., Ign., *Iod.,* **K. BI., Kalm., LED., Mang., Nux m., Pb.,** *Phyt.,* **PULS.,** Rhodo., **Sabi., Sal. ac.,** *Sars.,* Sep., **Spig., Sul.,** Valer., *Zinc.*

Paralysis, Internally.—Acon., Ant. cr., **Ars.,** Bar. c., **BELL.,** Calc. c., Cannab. s., Canth., Caps., *Caust.,* Chin., Cic., **Cocc.,** Coloc,. Con., Cyc., Dig., **DULC.,** Euphr., **Gel.,** Graph., **HYOS.,** Ip., K. carb., Lach., **Laur.,** Lyc., Meny., Merc., *Mur. ac.,* Nat. m., **Nux m., Nux v., Op.,** Petrol., Phos., Pb., **Puls.,** Rheum., **Rhus,** Sec. c., Seneg., Sep., Sil., Spig., **STRAM.**

—Of Limbs.—**Acon.,** *Agar.,* **Alum.,** *Ambr.,* Am. m., *Anac.,* **Arg.,** *Arn., Ars.,* Asar., Aur., *Bar. c.,* **Bell.,** Bov., *Brom., Bry.,* **Calc. c.,** Cannab., s., *Carb. v., Carb. sul.,* **Caust.,** Cham., **Chel.,** *Chen. a., Chin.,* COCC., *Colch.,* Coloc., **Con.,** *Crotal.,* Cup., Cyc., Dig., **Dros., Dulc.,** *Fer.,* Graph., Guai., Hell., Hep., **Hyos.,** Ign., Iod., Ip., *K. carb.,* K. nit., *Kalm.,* Lach., Laur., Led., *Lyc.,* Merc., Mez., Mur. ac., Nat. c., **Nat. m., Nit. ac., Nux v.,** Oleand., *Op., Petrol.,* **Phos.,** Pho. ac., *Pic. ac.,* **Pb.,** Puls., Rhodo., **RHUS,** Ruta, Sabi., *Sars.,* **Sec. c.,** Sele., Seneg., Sep., **SIL.,** *Spig., Stan.,* Staph., Stram., *Stro.,* **SUL.,** Sul. ac., Tar., **Verat. a.,** Zinc.

—One-sided.—Acon., *Agar.,* **Alum.,** Am. m., **Anac.,** *Arg.,* Arn., Asar., *Bar. c., Bell.,* Bov., *Calc. c.,* Carb. v., *Carb. sul.,* Caust., Chel., *Chin.,* **Cocc.,** Colch., *Cyc.,* Dig., *Dulc.,* **Graph.,** *Guai.,* Hell., Hep., *Hyos.,* Ign., **K. carb.,** Lach., Laur., Led., Lyc., Merc., *Mez., Mur. ac.,* Nat. c., *Nat. m.,* Nit. ac., Nux v., *Oleand.,* Op., *Phos.,* **Pho. ac.,** Pb., Rhodo., *Rhus, Sabi.,* **Sars.,** Spig., Stan., *Staph., Stro.,* **Sul. ac.,** Tar., *Zinc.*

—Of Organs.—Acon., Agar., Agn., *Alum., Ambr.,* Am. carb., Am. m, **Anac.,** Ant. cr., Ant. t., *Arn., Ars.,* Asaf., *Asar., Aur.,* **Bar. c., BELL.,** Bism., *Bor.,* Bov., **Bry., Calc. c.,** Camph., *Cannab. s.,* Canth., **Caps.,** *Carb. ac.,* Carb. an., Carb. v., **Caust.,** Cham., *Chel., Chin.,* Cic., **Cocc.,** Colch., *Coloc.,* **Con.,** Croc., Cup., *Cyc.,* Dig., **Dros.,** DULC., Euphr., *Gel.,* **Graph.,** *Hell., Hep., Hyd. ac.,* HYOS., *Ign.,* Iod., Ip., *K. br.,* K. carb., Kre., Lach., **Laur.,** *Led.,* **Lyc.,** *Mag. c., Mag. m.,* Mang., Meny., *Merc., Mez., Mur., ac.. Nat. c., Nat. m.,* **Nit. ac.,** *Nux m.,* Nux v., Oleand., **OP.,**

SENSATIONS.

Par., *Petrol.*, **Phos.**, *Pho. ac.*, **Pb.**, PULS., Rheum, *Rhodo.*, **Rhus**, **Ruta**, Saba., Sabi., *Sul. ac.*, Sars., SEC. C., *Seneg.*, **Sep.**, **SIL.**, Spig., Spo., Squ., Stan., *Staph.*, **Stram.**, *Stro.*, **Sul.**, Sul. ac., Thuj., **Verat. a.**, *Verb.*, Zinc.

—**Painless.**—*Abs.*, *Acon.*, *Aeth.*, Alum., *Ambr.*, **Anac.**, **Arg. n.**, *Arn.*, Ars., Aur., **Bap.**, *Bar. ac.*, *Bar. c.*, Bell., Bov., Bry., **Cad. s.**, Calc. c., *Calc. m.*, Camph., CANNAB. I., Carb. v., *Carb. sul.*, Caust., *Cham.*, Chel., Chin., *Chloral.*, *Cic.*, COCC., *Colch.*, *Coloc.*, CON., *Crotal.*, Cup., *Cur.*, Fer., Gel., *Graph.*, Hell., *Hyd. ac.*, **Hyos.**, Ign., Ip., K. carb., *Kalm.*, *Laur.*, Led., LYC., **Merc.**, Nat. m., Nux m., *Nux v.*, OLEAND., Op., Phos., *Pho. ac.*, PB., **Puls.**, Rhodo., RHUS, **Sec. c.**, *Sil.*, Staph., *Stram.*, *Stro.*, Sul., **Verat. a.**, Zinc.

Paralytic Pain.—Acon., Agar., Agn., Alum., Ambr., Am. carb., *Am. m.*, Ant. cr., Arg., Ars., Asaf., *Asar.*, **Aur.**, Bar. c., BELL., **Bism.**, Bov., Bry., Calc. c., Cannab. s., Canth., *Carb. v.*, *Caust.*, **Cham.**, Chel., **Chin.**, CINA, COCC., Coff., COLCH., Coloc., *Con.*, Croc., *Crotal.*, CYC., *Dig.*, *Dros.*, Dulc., Euphorb., Euphr., Fer., Graph., Hell., Hep., Hyos., Ign., Iod., *K. carb.*, *K. nit.*, *Kre.*, Laur., Led., Lyc., Mag. c., *Mag. m.*, Mang., Mar., *Meny.*, Merc., **Mez.**, *Mos.*, *Mur. ac.*, Nat. c., **Nat. m.**, NUX V. Oleand., *Par.*, Petrol., *Phos.*, Pho. ac., *Plat.*, Pb., *Puls.*, Ran. s., Rhodo., Rhus, Ruta, Saba., SABI., *Sars.*, Sele., Seneg., *Sep.*, **Sil.**, Spig., *Stan.*, Staph., Stram., *Stro.*, Sul., Sul. ac., Thuj., Valer., **Verat. a.**, Verb, *Zinc*,

—**In Joints.**—*Acon.*, Agn., Ambr., Am. carb., Anac., *Arg.*, **Arn.**, Ars., Asar., AUR., *Bell.*, *Bism.*, Bov., CAPS., **Carb. v.**, Caust., *Cham.*, **Chin.**, Cina. *Cocc.*, *Colch.*, Coloc., *Con.*, **Croc.**, *Dig.*, **Dros.**, EUPHORB., Fer., *Gran.*, Graph., Hell., Ign., *K. carb.*, Led., *Lyc.*, Mag. m., Meny., Merc., Mez., Nat. c., *Nat. m.*, Nit. ac., *Nux v.*, Par., *Petrol.*, Phos., *Pho. ac.*, Pb.. Puls., *Rhus*, *Ruta*, *Saba.*, **Sabi.**, Samb., *Sars.*, Seneg., Sep., *Stan.*, STAPH., Stram., *Stro.*, Sul., VALER., *Verat a.*, *Verb.*, Rinc.

Paralytic Sensation, Internally.—*Acon.*, *Bry.*, *Caj.*, *Caust.*, Cina, Cocc., **Gran.**, *Ip.*, Lyc., Meny., **Nat. m.**, Phos., Puls Seneg., Sil., Sul.

Picking.—Ambr., Ars., Aur., Carb. an., CHIN., *Cocc.*, Dros., **Mez.**, Nux v., Rhus, *Ruta*, Stram., **Verb.**, Zinc.

Pierced by a Hot Iron, Sensation as if.—Alum., *Cannab. i.*

Pinching.—Agar., Alum., *Ambr.*, Anac., ARN., Ars., Asar., BELL., Bov., Bry., **Calc. c.**, Cannab. s., *Canth.*, **Caps.**, Carb. an., Carb. v., *Caust.*, Cham., Cina, *Clam.*, Cocc., Colch., Coloc., Con., *Croc.*, Dros., Dulc., Euphorb., *Guai.*, Hell., Hep., Ign., Iod., *K. carb.*, *K. nit.*, Kre., Laur., Lyc., Mag. m., *Mang.*, Mar., Meny., Merc., Mez., *Mur. ac.*, Nat. c., Nat. m., *Nit. ac.*, *Nux m.*, NUX V., Op., Par., Petrol., **Phos.**, **Plat.**, Puls., Ran. b., *Ran. s.*, **Rheum**, *Rhodo.*, Rhus, *Ruta*, Saba., Sabi.,

Sars., *Seneg. Sep.*, Sil., *Spig.*, **Spo.**, *Stan., Staph., Stro.*, **Sul.**, **Thuj.** *Valer., Verat. a., Verb., Zinc.*

Pinching, Externally.—Acon., Anac., *Ant. cr., Arg., Arn.*, **Bell.**, *Bry.*, **Calc. c.**, Cannab. s., **Caps.**, Carb. v., *Caust.*, Chel., *Chin., Cina*, **Clem.**, Cocc., Con., Crocc, Dig., Dros., *Dulc., Euphorb., Euphr.,* **Hyos.**, **Ip.**, **K. carb.**, Kre., Lcd., Mang., **MENY.**, **Mur. ac.**, Nat. c., Nit. ac., Nux v., Oleand., Osm., Par, Phos., Pho. ac., RHODO., Rhus, Ruta, SABA., Sabi., Samb., Sars., Sil., Spig., SPO., STAN., Staph., **Sul.**, *Sul. ac.*, Thuj., Verat. a., VERB., *Vio. t.*, **Zinc.**

—**Internally.**—Acon., **Agar.**, Agn., *Alum.*, **Am. carb.**, Am. m., Anac., *Ant. cr.*, Ant. t., Arg., Arn., Ars., *Asaf.*, Asar., *Aur.*, Bar. c., **Bell.**, Bism., *Bor.*, Bov., **Bry.**, CALC. C., Camph., **Cannab. s.**, Canth., Caps., *Carb. an.*, **Carb. v.**, *Caust., Cham.,* CHEL., **Chin.**, Cic., Cina, *Coc. c.*, COCC., Coff., **Colch.**, COLOC., Com., Croc., Cup., *Cyc., Dig.*, Dros., Dulc., Euphorb., Euphr., **Gam.**, GRAPH., *Guai.*, **Hell.**, Hep., Hyos., IGN., Iod., **Ip.**, **K. carb.**, Kre., LYC., Mag. c., Mag. m., Mang., **Mar.**, Meny., Merc., *Mez.*, Mos., Mur. ac., **Nat. c.**, **Nat. m.**, Nit. ac. *Nux m.*, Nux v., Oleand., Par., Petrol., Phos., *Pho. ac.*, Plat., Pb., **Puls.**, Ran. b., *Ran. s.*, Rheum, Rhodo., Rhus, **Ruta**, Saba., Sabi., Samb., Sars., Seneg., Sep., Sil., **Spig.**, Spo., *Squ.*, **Stan.**, Staph., *Stro.*, **Sul.**, Sul. ac., Tar., Thuj., Valer., **Verat. a.**, VERB,, *Vio. t.*, **Zinc.**

—**Together.**—Cocc., *Ran. s.*

Plucking, Sensation of.—Chin., *Cic.*

Plug, Sensation of, Externally. (Compare **Wedge**.)—*Agar., Arn.,* Hell., **Crot. tig.**, **K. bi.**, *Lach., Plat.*, Ruta.

—**Internally.**—*Acon.*, Agar., ALOE., Ambr., *Am. b.*, Am. carb., Anac., *Ant. cr.*, **Arg.**, Arn., Asaf., Aur., *Bar. c.*, **Bell.**, Bov., Calc. c., *Caust.*, Cham., *Chel.*, Cocc., *Coc. c., Coff.*, Con., *Croc.*, Dros., Fer., Graph., *Hell.*, Hep., IGN., *Iod.*, K. carb., Kre., *Lach.*, Led., Lyc., *Merc., Mez.*, Mur. ac., Nat. m., **Nux v.**, Oleand., Par., Plat., Pb., *Ran. s.*, Rhodo., **Ruta**, Saba., *Sabi., Sang.*, Sep., *Spig.*, **Spo.**, Staph., **Sul.**, THUJ.

Polypus.—Ambr., Ant. cr., *Aur.*, Bell., CALC. C., *Con.*, Graph., Hep., Lyc., **Mar.**, Merc., *Mez.*, Nat. m., Nit. ac., *Petrol.*, Phos., *Pho. ac.*, Puls., Sep., *Sil.*, STAPH., Sul., Sul. ac., *Thuj.*

Pressing (Simple Pain), Externally.—Abrot., Acon., Aesc., Agar., Agn., *Aloe*, Alum., Ambr., Am. m., **Anac.**, *Ant. cr.*, Ant. t., **Arg.**, *Arn.*, Ars., *Asaf.*, Asar., *Aur.*, Bap., Bar. c., **Bell.**, *Bism.*, Bor., Bov., **Bry.**, Calc. c., **Calc. ph.**, Camph., *Cannab. s., Canth.*, **Caps.**, Carb. an., **Carb. v.**, CAUST., *Ced.*, **Cham.**, *Chel.*, **Chin.**, Cic., Cimic., *Cinnab.*, Cina, *Clem.*, *Cob.*, **Cocc.**, Coff., *Colch.*, **Coloc.**, Con., Crot. tig., Cup., **Cvc.**, *Dig., Dios.,*

SENSATIONS. 173

Dros., *Dulc.*, *Elaps.*, **EUP. PER.**, *Euphorb.*, *Euphr.*, *Fer.*, **Gel.**, *Graph.*, **Guai.**, **Hell.**, **Hep.**, **Hyos.**, *Ign.*, **Iod.**, K. BI., *K. carb.*, *K. nit.*, **Kalm.**, **Kre.**, **Lach.**, *Laur.*, **Led.**, Lil. t., **Lyc.**, Mag. c., Mag. m., **Mang.**, *Mar.*, *Meny.*, **Merc.**, **Mez.**, *Mos.*, *Mur. ac.*, Nat. c., **Nat. m.**, **NIT. AC.**, Nux m., **Nux v.**, *Oleand.*, Ox. ac., *Par.*, *Parei.*, **Petrol.**, **Phos.**, **Pho. ac.**, *Phyt.*, *Plat.*, **Pb.**, **POD.**, *Pru.*, **PULS.**, *Ran. b.*, Ran. s., Rheum, **RHODO.**, **RHUS**, **RUTA**, *Saba.*, *Sabi.*, *Samb.*, **Sang.**, *Sars.*, *Seneg.*, **SEP.**, **SIL.**, **Spig.**, *Spo.*, **STAN.**, **STAPH.**, *Stro.*, **Sul.**, *Sul. ac.*, **Tar.**, *Thuj.*, *Ust.*, **Valer.**, **Verat. a.**, *Verb.*, *Vib. op.*, Vio. o., Vio. t., **Zinc.**

Pressing, Internally.—Acon., *Aesc.*, *Agar.*, **Agn.**, **Ail.**, **Aloe**, **Alum.**, **Ambr.**, *Am. carb.*, Am. m., **Anac.**, Ant. cr., *Ant. t.*, Arg, **ARG. N.**, **ARN.**, **ARS.**, **Arum. t.**, **ASAF.**, *Asar.*, **Aur.**, *Bar. c.*, **BELL.**, *Berb.*, **Bism.**, **Bor.**, **Bov.**, **BROM.**, **Bry.**, *Cact.*, **Calad.**, **CALC. C.**, **Camph.**, **Cannab. i.**, **Cannab. s.**, **CANTH.**, *Caps.*, **Carb. an.**, **CARB. V.**, *Carb. sul.*, **Caust.**, **Ced.**, *Cham.*, *Chel.*, *Chen. a.*, **CHIN.**, *Cic.*, **CIMIC.**, *Cina*, **Clem.**, **Cocc.**, Coc. c., **Cod.**, *Coff.*, **Colch.**, **COLOC.**, **Con.**, **Coral.**, **Croc.**, *Crot. tig.*, **CUP.**, **Cyc.**, **Dig.**, *Dios.*, *Dros.*, *Dulc.*, *Elaps.*, *Epiph.*, *Euphorb.*, *Euphr.*, **Fer.**, **Gam.**, **Gel.**, **Glon.**, *Goss.*, **Graph.**, **Guai.**, **HAM.**, **Hell.**, *Hep.*, *Hydras.*, **Hyd. ac.**, *Hyos.*, *Hyper.*, **Ign.**, *Iod.*, **Ip.**, *Iris v.*, *K. bi.*, **K. carb.**, **K. iod.**, *K. nit.*, **Kalm.**, **Kre.**, **LACH.**, **Laur.**, **Led.**, **Lept.**, **LIL. T.**, **Lith.**, **LYC.**, Mag. c., Mag. m., **Mang.**, *Mar.*, **MENY.**, **Merc.**, **Merc. c.**, *Merc. i. f.*, **Mez.**, **Mos.**, *Murex*, *Mur. ac.*, *Naj.*, *Nat. ars.*, *Nat. c.*, **NAT. M.**, **Nit. ac.**, *Nux m.*, **NUX V.**, *Oleand.*, *Onos.*, **OP.**, *Osm.*, **Ox. ac.**, *Par.*, **PETROL.**, **PHOS.**, **Pho. ac.**, Phys., **Phyt.**, Pic. ac., **Plat.**, **Pb.**, **Pod.**, **Pru.**, *Pso.*, **PULS.**, **RAN. B.**, *Ran. s.*, Rheum, Rhodo., **RHUS**, **Rumex**, **RUTA**, *Saba.*, **Sabi.**, *Samb.*, **SANG.**, **SANG. N.**, *Sars.*, **SEC. C.**, **SENEG.**, **SEP.**, **SIL.**, **SFIG.**, **SPO.**, **Squ.**, **STAN.**, *Staph.*, *Stict.*, **Stram.**, *Stro.*, **SUL.**, *Sul. ac.*, *Tab.*, **Tar.**, *Tarent.*, **Ter.**, **Thuj.**, **Usn.**, *Ust.*, **VALER.**, **VERAT. A.**, **Verat. v.**, Verb., *Vesp.*, *Vib. op.*, Vio o., Vio. t., *Vip.*, *Xan.*, **ZINC.**

—**Inward.**—Acon., *Agar.*, **Alum.**, **ANAC.**, Ant. cr., *Ant. t.*, **Asaf.**, *Asar.*, *Aur.*, Bar. c., *Bell.*, *Bism.*, *Bor.*, Bry., **Calc. c.**, Cannab. s., Carb. an., **Caust.**, **Chel.**, Chin., **Cocc.**, *Coff.*, Croc., *Cyc.*, **Dulc.**, Hell., Hep., *Ign.*, K. carb., **Kre.**, Laur., Mar., Mez., *Mos.*, Nit. ac., Nux m., **Nux v.**, Oleand., *Pho. ac.*, **PLAT.**, *Ran. s.*, Rheum, *Rhodo.*, Rhus, Ruta, Saba., Sabi., *Sars.*, Sep., Sil., **Spig.**, **STAN.**, **Staph.**, **Sul.**, Sul. ac., Tar., Thuj., Valer., Verb., Vio. t., **Zinc.**

—**Deep, Inward, with Instruments.**—Bov., *Verat. a.*

—**In Joints.**—Acon., **Aesc.**, **Agn.**, Alum., *Anac.*, *Arg.*, Asaf., Asar., *Bar. c.*, Bell., Calc. c., Camph., **Carb. an.**, Caust., Cham., Chel., *Chin.*

Clem., Colch., *Dios.*, Dulc., *Graph.*, Hep., Hyos., Ign., Iod., **K. carb.**, **Led.**, Meny., *Merc.*, Mez., *Mos.*, Nit. ac., Nux v., Petrol., Rhus, Saba., Sabi., *Sep.*, Sil., *Spo.*, Stan., *Staph.*, Stro., SUL., Tar., Thuj., *Vio. o.*, Vio. t., Zinc.

Pressing, As From a Load.—Ab. n., ACON., Aesc., Agar., *Aloe.*, **Alum.**, *Am. carb.*, **Am. m.**, **Ant. t.**, *Aran.*, Arg., **Arg. n.**, Arn., **Ars.**, Asaf, **Ambr.**, Asar., *Aur.*, **Bar. c.**, BELL., *Bism.*, Bor., Bov., BROM., BRY., **Cact.**, Calad., *Calc. c.*, Camph., Cannab. s., *Carb. an.*, Carb. v., Caust. *Cham.*, **Chel.**, Chin., Cina, *Cinnab.*, Cocc., Colch., Coloc., **Com.**, Con., Croc., *Corn. c.*, *Crot. tig.*, **Cup.**, *Dig.*, Fer., *Gel.*, Graph., Hell., Hep., Hyos., Ign., Iod., **IP.**, **K. carb.**, *K. chl.*, K. nit., **Kre.**, *Laur.*, *Led.*, LIL. T., Lyc., Mag. c., Mag. m., Mang., **Meli.**, MENY., Merc., Mos., **Nat. c.**, Nat. m., Nit. ac., *Nux m.*, NUX V., Oleand., **Op.**, PAR., Petrol., PHOS., **Pho. ac.**, Plat., Pb., **Pso.**, Puls., RAN. B., *Rheum*, Rhodo., RHUS, Saba., *Sabi.*, **Samb.**, Sars., **Sec. c.**, *Seneg.*, SEP., Sil., Spig., Spo., *Squ.*, Stan., *Staph.*, STICT., Stro., SUL., Sul. ac., Thuj., Valer., **Verb.**, Vio. o., *Zinc.*, *Zing.*

—**In Muscles.**—Agar., *Agn.*, Am. m., **Anac.**, Arg., Arn., **Asaf.**, **Asar.**, *Aur.*, *Bell.*, Bism., Bry., Calc. c., *Camph.*, Cannab. s., **Caps.**, **Carb. an.**, Caust., *Chel.*, Chin., Cina, Clem., *Cocc.*, Con., **Cup.**, CYC., Dig., *Dros.*, *Euphorb.*, Euphr., Graph., Hell., Hep., **Ign.**, K. nit., **Led.**, *Lyc.*, Mag. c., Mag. m., Mang., **Mar.**, *Meny.*, Merc., *Mez.*, **Mos.**, Mur. ac., Nat. c., *Nat. m.*, NUX M., *Nux v.*, Oleand., *Petrol.*, Phos., Pho. ac., **Plat.**, Pb., *Puls.*, *Ran. b.*, Ran. s., Rheum, Rhus, RUTA, Saba., *Sabi.*, *Samb.*, Sil., *Spig.*, *Spo.*, Stan., Staph., Stro., *Sul.*, Sul. ac., **Tar.**, *Thuj.*, **Valer.**, Verat. a., VERB., Vio. t., Zinc.

—**From Within Outward.**—Acon., **Aloe**, Alum., Am. carb., Am. m., Anac., Ant. cr., Arg., Arn., ASAF., Asar., *Aur.*, Bar. c., **Bell.**, *Berb.*, **Bism.**, *Bor.*, **BRY.**, Calc. c., Camph., *Cannab. s.*, *Canth.*, Caps., Carb. v., Caust., *Chel.*, Chin., CIMIC., *Cina,* Clem., Cocc., Coff., *Colch.*, *Coloc.*, Con., **Coral.**, Croc., Cup., Dig., **Dros.**, Dulc., Euphorb., **Fer.**, *Graph.*, Guai., Hell., Hep., **Ign.**, *Ip.*, K. carb., K. iod., K. nit., Kre., Lach., *Laur.*, Led., Lyc., Mag. m., Mang., **Mar.**, *Meli.*, *Meny.*, **Merc.**, Merc. c., **Mez.**, Mur. ac., Nat. c., **Nat. m.**, Nit. ac., Nux m., Nux v., Oleand., **Op.**, Par., Petrol., Phos., *Pho. ac.*, Plat., Pru., PULS., *Ran. b.*, Ran. s., Rheum, Rhodo., Rhus, Ruta, *Saba.*, Sabi., *Samb.*, Seneg., Sep., Sil., **Spig.**, Spo., Squ., Stan., Staph., Stro., SUL., Sul. ac., *Tar.*, **Thuj.**, VALER., Verb., *Vio. t.*, Zinc.

Pressing, Sticking, in Muscles.—Anac., *Asaf.*, Bell., Calc. c., Coloc., Cyc., *Dros.*, *Euphorb.*, Ign., Mur. ac., Oleand., *Plat.*, Sars., Sep., *Sul. ac.*, **Thuj.**

SENSATIONS.

Pressing, Tearing, in Joints.—Anac., *Arn.*, Asaf., Bell., Bism., Carb. v., Caust., Cham., Hyos., *Led.*, Lyc., Ruta, Spo., Stan.

Pressing, Tearing, in Muscles.—Agar., Anac., Arg., Arn., *Asaf.*, Asar., Aur., **Bell.**, *Bism.*, Calc. c., **Camph.**, Cannab. s., Carb. v., Chin., Colch., Cup., *Cyc.*, Hyos., *Led.*, *Meny.*, Petrol., Pho. ac., Ruta, *Sars.*, Sep., Spig., Spo., *Stan.*, Sul., Zinc.

Pressing Together.—*Acon.*, *Agar.*, ALUM., Ambr., Am. m., **Anac.**, Ant. cr., Ant. t., *Arg.*, **Arn.**, **Ars.**, *Asaf.*, ASAR., Aur., Bar. c., **Bell.**, **Bov.**, *Bry.*, *Calc. c.*, Camph., **Cannab. s.**, **Canth.**, *Caps.*, Carb. an., Carb. v., Caust., Cham., Chel., *Chin.*, Cic., Cina, COCC., Coff., Coloc., *Con.*, Cup., *Dig.*, **Dros.**, Dulc., *Euphorb.*, Fer., *Graph.*, *Guai.*, **Hell.**, *Hyos.*, *Ign.*, Iod., **Ip.**, *K. carb.*, *K. nit.*, Laur., Led., *Lyc.*, Mag. c., *Mag. m.*, Mar., *Meny.*, Merc., *Mez.*, **Nat. m.**, Nit. ac., *Nux m.*, NUX V., Oleand., Op., Petrol., Phos., *Pho. ac.*, PLAT., Pb., *Puls.*, *Ran. s.*, *Rhodo.*, *Rhus*, Ruta., Saba., Sabi., **Sars.**, *Seneg.*, Sep., *Sil.*, *Spig.*, Spo., Squ., **Stan.**, *Staph.*, Stram., Stro., SUL., **Sul. ac.**, *Tar.*, *Thuj.*, Valer., **Verat. a.**, Verb., Vio. o., *Zinc.*

Prickling Externally.—*Acon.*, *Aconin.*, Agar., **Ail.**, Alum., Ant. cr., *Ant. t.*, Bell., Calc. c., *Cannab. i.*, *Cannab. s.*, Caps., *Carb. sul.*, Caust., Coloc., *Con.*, Croc., **Dros.**, *Glon.*, Hep., *K. br.*, Laur., *Lyc.*, **Mez.**, *Mos.*, **Nux m.**, *Onos.*, PLAT., RAN. S., Ruta, *Saba.*, Sec. c., *Sep.*, Staph., Sul., Sul. ac., *Zinc.*

—**Internally.**—Abrot., *Acon.*, *Aconin.*, **Ail.**, Aur., Cannab. s., *Dios.*, *Lach.*, NIT. AC., Osm., Phos., Pho. ac., *Plat.*, **Ran. b.**, Saba., Sang., Sec. c., Seneg., Verb., *Vio. o.*

Puckering.—*Carb. sul.*, *Phyt.*, **Sep.**

Pullings.—Acon., Agar., Aloe, *Apis*, Arg. n., Bar. c., *Bell.*, Bry., Calc. ph., Cannab. i., Cannab. s., **Canth.**, Caps., *Carb. sul.*, *Card. m.*, **Caul.**, Caust., Chel., Cinnab., *Clem.*, **Cocc.**, *Coc. c.*, Coloc., *Com.*, *Con.*, *Crotal.*, Crot. tig., Cup., Dig., *Dios.*, Dulc., *Fer.*, Gran., Ip., K. bi., Lach., Lil. t., Merc., Mez., **Nux v.**, Petrol., Phos., Phyt., PULS., RHODO., RHUS, SABI., Sul. ac., Sec. c., Sep., Spig., Squ., Stan., Staph., Stram., SUL., Ter., Thuj., VALER., Verat. a., Zinc.

Rawness (and Roughness) **Internally.**—*Acon.*, **Aesc.**, *Agar.*, Aloe, Alum., Ambr., *Am. carb.*, *Am. m.*, Anac., Ant. cr., Arg., ARG. N., *Ars.*, Arum. t., Bar. c., **BELL.**, Bor., Bov., BROM., Bry., **Calc. c.**, *Cannab. s.*, Canth., Caps., Carb. an., CARB. V., *Carb. sul.*, Caust., Cham., Chel., *Chin.*, Cina, **Cocc.**, **Coc. c.**, Coff., Colch., Coloc., *Cop.*, Croc., *Cub.*, Cyc., **Dig.**, Dros., Dulc., Euphorb., Fer., **Gam.**, *Graph.*, Hell., Hep., **Hydras.**, **Hyos.**, **Ign.**, Iod., *Ip.*, *K. carb.*, **K. chl.**, K. nit., **Kre.**, **Lach.**, Laur., Led.,

Lyc., **Mag. c.**, *Mag. m.*, *Mang.*, Meny., Merc., **Mez., Mur. ac., Nat. c.**
Nat. m., **Nat. s.**, Nit. ac., *Nux m.*, NUX V., Oleand., **Osm., Par.,**
Petrol., PHOS., **Pho. ac.**, Phyt., Plat., **Pb.**, Puls., Ran. b., *Ran. s.*,
Rhodo., Rhus, *Saba.*, Sang., Sang. n., Sars., Seneg., Sep., Sil., Spig.,
Spo., Squ., **Stan.**, *Staph.*, Stram., *Stro.*, SUL., **Sul. ac.**, TAR., **Thuj.**,
Verat. a., Verb., **Zinc.**

Reeling.—Acon., Agar., Ant. cr., *Arg.*, Arn., **Ars., Asar.**, Aur.,
BELL., *Bov.*, **BRY.**, *Calc. c.*, **Camph., Cannab. s.**, Canth., **Caps.**, Carb.
an., Carb. v., *Carb. sul.*, Caust., *Cham.*, **Chel.**, *Chen. a.*, **Chin.**, Cic., **Cocc.,**
Coff., Colch., **Con.**, *Croc.*, **Cup.**, C: , Dros., Dulc., Euphorb., *Fer.*, **Gel.,**
Graph., **Hell.**, Hyos., Ign., **Ip.**, *K. br.*, *K. carb.*, **Laur.**, *Led.*, Mag. c.,
Mag. m., Mar., *Merc.*, **Mez.**, Mos., **Mur. ac.**, Nat. c., Nat. m., Nit. ac.,
Nux m., **NUX V.**, Oleand., *Onos.*, OP., *Oxyt.*, Par., Petrol., *Pho. ac.*,
Pb., *Puls.*, Rheum, *Rhodo.*, RHUS, *Ruta*, *Saba.*, Samb , Sars., **Sec. c.**,
Seneg., *Sep.*, Sil., *Spig.*, *Spo.*, STRAM., Stro., **Sul.**, *Tar.*, **Thuj.**, *Valer.*,
VERAT. A., Verb., Vio. o., Vio. t., Zinc.

Relaxation of Muscles.—Agar., Ambr., Ant. t., Arn., Asaf., *Bor.*,
Bry., CALC. C., Camph., Canth., **CAPS.**, **Cham.**, *Chin.*, Cic., **Clem.,**
COCC., **Con.**, Croc., *Cup.*, *Dig.*, **Dios.**, Euphorb., *Fer.*, **GEL.**, Graph.,
Hell., *Hydras.*, **Hyos.**, **Iod.**, **Ip.**, K. carb., *Lach.*, *Laur.*, **Lyc.**, *Mag. c.*,
Merc., **Mur. ac.**, *Nat. c.*, Nux m., Op., *Oxyt.*, Plat., Pb., *Puls.*, Rheum,
Saba., **Sec. c.**, **Seneg.**, *Sil.*, Spig., Spo., **Sul.**, Sul. ac., Thuj., *Verat. a.*,
Vio. o.

Restlessness.—Acon., *Aconin.*, *Agar.*, *All. c.*, Alum., Ambr., Am.
carb., ANAC., **Ant. t.**, *Apis*, **Arg. n.**, Arn., ARS., Asaf., *Asar.*, **Bap.,**
Bar. c., **BELL.**, Bry., Calc. c., **Camph., Cannab. s.**, *Canth.*, Carb. an.,
Carb. v., *Carb. sul.*, *Caust.*, *Cact.*, **Cham.**, **Chel.**, Chin., CIMIC., *Cina*,
Coca, *Cocc.*, Coff., Colch., *Coloc.*, *Con.*, Croc., *Crot. tig.*, **Cup.**, **Dig.**, *Dios.*,
Dub., *Dulc.*, Euphorb., Euphr., Fer., *Form.*, *Graph.*, **Hell.**, *Helo.*,
HYOS., Ign., **Iod.**, *Ip.*, *K. carb.*, **Kalm.**, Lach., **Led.**, *Lyc.*, Mag. c.,
Mag. m., Mang., Mar., Meny., MERC., **Mez., Mos.**, *Mur. ac.*, Nat. c.,
Nat. m., *Nit. ac.*, Nux m., **Nux v.**, Oleand., **Op.**, Par., Petrol., **Phos.**,
Pho. ac., Plat., **PB., PULS.**, Ran. b., **RHUS, Rumex, Ruta**, Saba.,
Sabi., Samb., SEC. C., **SEP.**, SIL., Spig., Spo., *Squ.*, **Stan., STAPH.,**
STRAM., SUL , *Tab.*, Tar., **Tarent., Tell.**, Thuj., *Valer.*, Verat. a., Vio.
t., ZINC.

Retraction of Soft Parts.—Acon., Ant. cr., Arn., Ars., **Bell.**, Bov.,
Calad., *Camph.*, Caps., *Carb. v.*, Chin., Cocc., Coloc., Dulc., Euphorb.,
Graph., Hep., *Hyos.*, Ign., *Laur.*, MERC., **Merc. c.**, Nat. c., *Nat. m.*,
Nux v., *Op.*, **Phos.**, Pho. ac., Rhus, Sep., Staph., *Stram.*, Squ., **Sul.,**
Thuj.

SENSATIONS.

Rigidity.—Acon., Am. carb., Am. m., Ant. t., Ars., Asaf., Bell., *Bry.*, Camph., *Cannab. i.*, Cannab. s., *Canth., Carb. ac., Carb. sul.*, CHEL., *Chen. a.*, Cic., Cimic., *Cina*, Cocaine, Colch., *Con., Dig.*, DROS., *Dulc., Guai.*, Hell., Hyos., *Ign., Ip.*, K. carb., KALM., Kre., LED., Lith., Lyc., Mos., Nux v., Oleand., *Oxyt., Petrol.*, Phyt., Plat., *Pb.*, Puls., RHUS, Sec. c., Sep., Stram., Sul., *Verat. a.*, Zinc.

—Of Joints of Extremities (Clumsiness).—*Abrot.*, Acon., *Aesc., Ambr., Am. m., Anac., Ars., Atrop., Aur.*, Bell., Bov., *Brom.*, BRY., Calc. c., *Cannab. i.*, Canth., Caps., Carb. an., Carb. v., *Carb. sul.*, Caul., Caust., Cham., *Chel., Chin.*, Cina, *Clem.*, Cocc., Colch., Coloc., Con., Dig., *Dros.*, Dulc., Euphorb., Euphr., *Fer.*, Graph., *Hell.*, Hep., Hyos., *Ign.*, K. carb., K. nit., *Kalm.*, Lach., Led., Lyc., Merc., Mez., *Nat. c., Nat. m.*, Nux m., Nux v., Ox. ac., PETROL., Phos., Pho. ac., Phyt., Pb., *Pru.*, Puls., Ran. b., Rheum, *Rhodo.*, RHUS, Ruta, *Sabi., Sars.*, Sec. c., SEP., SIL., *Stan., Staph.*, SUL., Sul. ac., Thuj., Verat. a., Zinc.

—Sensation of.—*Aesc.*, Agar., Alum., Am. m., Arg., ASAF., Bap., Berb., *Cannab. i.*, Calc. ph., *Caust., Cham.*, Chin., *Cina*, Cocc., *Dios.*, Dulc., Guai., Lach., Mang., *Meny.*, Mez., Mos., *Nit. ac.*, Petrol., Phos., Plat., Rhodo., *Saba.*, Sec. c., *Stict.*, SUL.

Roaring (Humming and Buzzing).—*Agn., Ambr., Ars.*, Aur., Bar. c., Bell., *Calc. c.*, Cannab. s., Carb. v., Caust., *Cic.*, Cocc., Coff., *Con., Croc., Fer., Graph.*, Hyos., Kre., Lach., Mar., Meny., *Mos.*, Mur. ac., NUX M., Nux v., OLEAND., Op., Phos., *Pho. ac., Plat.*, PULS., Rhus, *Saba., Sars.*, Sep., SPIG., Squ., Stan., *Staph.*, SUL., Thuj., Verat. a., *Vio. t.*, Zinc.

Rolling Sensation.—*Acon.*, Bell., *Graph.*, Ign., Plat., Pb., Rhus, Sep., Tar.

Sensitiveness Externally.—Acon., Aesc., *Agar., Aloe, Alum.*, Ambr., Am. carb., Am. m., Ant. cr., *Ant. t.*, Arg., ARN., *Ars., Asaf.*, Aur., Bap., Bar. c., BELL., Bor., Bov., Bry., *Calc. c., Calc. ph., Camph., Cannab. s.*, Canth., Caps., Carb. an., Carb. v., Caust., CHIN., Cimic., Cina, Clem., Coc., c.. Coff., Colch., Coloc., Con., Cup., Dig., Fer., Hell., Hep., Hyos., Ign., Ip., K. bi., *K. carb.*, K. nit., *Kre.*, LACH., Led., Lyc., Mag. c., *Mag. m.*, Mar., *Menth.*, Merc., Mez., Mos., Nat. c., Nat. m., *Nit. ac.*, Nux m., NUX V., Oleand., Op., *Par., Petrol.*, Phos., Pho. ac., Pb., *Pso.*, PULS., RAN. B., Ran. s., Rhus, *Saba.*, Sabi., *Sal. ac., Sars.*, Sec. c., Sele., Seneg., Sep., SIL., SPIG., *Spo.*, Squ., Stan., Staph., Stro., Sul., *Sul. ac.*, Thuj., *Verat. a.*, Zinc.

—Internally.—Acon., *Agar.*, Alum., Am. carb., Ant. cr., Ant. t., *Apis, Arn.*, Ars., Asaf., Aur., Bap., Bar. c., Bell., *Bism.*, Bor., Bov.

SENSATIONS.

Bry., *Calad.*, **Calc. c.**, Cannab. s., **CANTH.**, **Carb. an.**, *Carb. v.*, *Carb. sul.*, *Caust.*, **Cham.**, Chin., *Cic.*, **Clem.**, **Cocc.**, **Coc., c.**, *Coff.* Colch., **Coloc.**, **Con.**, Croc., *Crotal.*, *Cub.*, *Cup.*, Cyc. *Dulc.*, *Equis.*, *Fer.*, **Graph.**, Hell., *Helo.*, HEP., *Hyos.*, Iod., Ip., **K. bi.**, K. iod., LACH., Laur., Led., Lil. t., *Mag. c.*, **Mag. m.**, *Mang.*, Meny., **Merc.**, **Merc. c.**, **Mez.**, *Mos.*, **Nat. c.**, NAT. M., **Nit. ac.**, Nux v., Oleand., Osm., Par., PHOS., **Puls.**, Ran. b., Rhus, Ruta, *Sars.*, **Sec. c.**, Sele., *Seneg.*, Sep., SIL., *Spo.*, **Squ.**, **Stan.**, **Stram.**, *Stro.*, **Sul.**, Sul. ac., Tar., *Tarent.*, Thuj., Valer., Verat a., Zinc.

Sensitiveness To Pain.—Acon., **Agar.**, Ambr., *Am. carb.*, Anac., *Ant. cr.*, Ant. t., *Arn.*, **Ars.**, **Asar.**, AUR., **Bar. c.**, **Bell.**, *Bry.*, Calad., Calc. c., *Camph.*, Cannab. s., **Canth.**, **Caps.**, Carb. an., **Carb. v.**, **CHAM.**, Chin., *Cina*, **Cocc.**, COFF., Colch., **Con.**, **Cup.**, *Dig.*, *Fer.*, *Graph.*, Hell., Hep., **Hyos.**, *Ign.*, Iod., *Ip.*, *K. carb.*, Lach., Laur., Led., LYC., **Mag. c.**, Mag. m., Merc., Mur. ac., **Nat. c.**, Nit. ac., *Nux m.*, **Nux v.**, Oleand., Petrol., PHOS., *Pho. ac.*, **Pb.**, **Puls.**, Saba., Sabi., Sars., *Sele.*, Seneg., SEP., *Sil.*, **Spig.**, Squ., Staph., **Sul.**, Thuj., *Valer.*, Verat. a., *Vio. o.*, Zinc.

Scraped Feeling.—Acon., *Aesc.*, **Alumen**, **Arg. n.**, Arn. *Asaf.*, **Bell.**, BROM., *Bry.*, *Carb. sul.*, **Cham.**, **Chin.**, **Coc. c.**, **Coloc.**, **Con.**, *Crot. tig.*, **Dig.**, DROS., **K. bi.**, **K. chl.**, Lach., Led., Lyc., Mez., NUX V., Osm., Par., **Phos.**, *Pho. ac.*, *Phyt.*, PULS., Rhus, Rumex, Saba., *Sele.*, *Seneg.*, Spig., **Stan.**, SUL., *Tell.*, VERAT. A.

Screwing Together.—*Aeth.*, Alum., Ambr., **Atrop.**, Bov., *Canth.*, *Chel.*, *Clem.*, **Coloc.**, Nux m., Stro., **Sul.**, *Zinc.*

Scurvy.—Agn., *Alum.*, *Ambr.*, Ant. cr., Arg., **Ars.**, Aur., **Bell.**, Bor., Bov., Bry., Calc. c., Canth., *Caps.*, **Carb. an.**, CARB. V., *Caust.*, Chin., Cic., *Cit. ac.*, *Con.*, Dulc., Graph., *Hep.*, *Iod.*, K. carb., K. nit., *Kre.*, Lyc., Mag. m., MERC., MUR. AC., **Nat. m.**, *Nit. ac.*, Nux m., NUX V., Petrol., *Phos.*, Pho. ac., Rhus, *Ruta*, Sabi., *Sep.*, Sil., Stan., STAPH., *Sul.*, Sul. ac., Zinc.

Shattering (Broken to Pieces) **Pain.**—ARG., *Arn.*, **Bell.**, Bor., *Bov.*, Calc. c., **Canth.**, Caust., **Cham.**, **Chel.**, Cina, COCC., *Cup.*, **Dros.**, *Graph.*, *Hep.*, Hyos., IGN., Kre., *Lyc.*, *May. m.*, Merc., Mez., Mos., Nat. m., *Nux v.*, Par., *Phel.*, PHOS., *Pho. ac.*, Puls., *Rhodo.*, Rhus, RUTA., Samb., Sep., Staph., VERAT. A., Zinc.

—**In Joints.**—Bov., Calc. c., *Caps.*, Caust., Dros., *Hep.*, Merc., Mez., *Par.*, Sep.

Shortened Muscles.—Acon., *Ambr.*, *Am. carb.*, AM. M., Anac., *Arn.*, Ars., Aur., **Bar. c.**, Bov., *Bry.*, Calc. c., **Carb. an.**, Carb. v., CAUST., Cic., **Cimic.**, COLOC., Con., Croc., *Cup.*, Dig., Dros., *Euphorb.*, Euphr., **GRAPH.**, *Guai.*, **Hell.**, Hep., Hyos., *Ign.*, K. carb., Kre., *Lach.*, Led.,

Lyc., *Mag. c.*, **Merc.**, *Mez.*, Mos., *Nat. c.*, **NAT. M.**, **Nit. ac.**, **Nux v.**, *Ox. ac.*, Petrol., *Phos.*, *Pho. ac.*, Pb., **Puls.**, Ran. b., **Rheum**, **Rhus**, Sabi., Samb., **Sep.**, Sil., Spig., Stan., Sul., Sul. ac., Verat. a.

Shrivelling.—Am. m., **Arg. n.**, Arn., *Bism.*, Chin., Cup., **Merc.**, *Rhodo.*, Verat. a., Zinc.

Shuddering.—*Acon.*, Anac., **Am. m.**, **ARN.**, *Aur.*, **Bell.**, *Calc. c.*, Camph., Cannab. s., Caust., Chin., *Cic.*, Cina, **Cocc.**, Cup., *Hyos.*, Kre., Laur., **Led.**, Lyc., Mag. m., *Mang.*, Mez., **Nat. m.**, Nux m., **Nux v.**, Pho. ac., Puls., **Rhus**, Seneg., *Sep.*, **Sil.**, **Spig.**, Staph., **Valer.**, *Verat. a.*, Vio. t.

Shuddering Pain (as from Concussion).—**Am. carb.**, *Mang.*, Petrol.

Sick Sensation (Compare **Malaise**).—**ACON.**, Agar., **Alum.**, *Ambr.*, **Ant. cr.**, **Ant. t.**, Arg., **Ars.**, *Asaf.*, Asar., Bor. Bov., Bry., *Calc. c.*, *Camph.*, Canth., Caust., *Cham.*, **Chel.**, *Chin.*, *Cic.*, **Coff.**, **Con.**, **Croc.**, Euphr., Fer., Graph., Guai., *Hep.*, Ign., Ip., K. nit., *Led.*, *Lyc.*, Mag. m., *Mang.*, **Merc.**, **Mez.**, Mos., Mur. ac., *Nit. ac.*, **NUX V.**, Oleand., Op., Petrol., *Plat.*, Pb., **Puls.**, Rhus, *Ruta*, *Saba.*, **Sabi.**, Sec. c., Seneg., *Spig.*, Spo., *Stan.*, Staph., Stro., **Sul.**, Tar., *Thuj.*, *Verat. a.*, *Zinc.*

Side (Symptoms on One Side).—**Agar.**, *Agn.*, **ALUM.**, Ambr., Am., carb., *Am. m.*, **ANAC.**, **Ant. cr.**, *Ant. t.*, **Arg.**, *Arn.*, Ars., **ASAF.**, *Asar.*, Aur., **Bar. c.**, *Bell.*, Bism., Bor., *Bov.*, **BRY.**, **Calc. c.**, Camph., Cannab. s., **Canth.**, Caps., Carb. an., *Carb. v.*, *Caust.*, Cham., **Chel.**, *Chen. a.*, *Chin.*, Cic., **Cina**, Clem., *Cocc.*, Coff., Colch., Coloc., Con., Croc., Cup., **Cyc.**, *Dig.*, Dros., **Dulc.**, Euphorb., Euphr., Fer., *Graph.*, **Guai.**, *Hell.*, *Hep.*, Hyos., *Ign.*, Iod., *Iris v.*, K. **CARB.**, K. nit., *Kre.*, Lach., *Laur.*, **Led.**, Lyc., *Mag. c.*, *Mag. m.*, **Mang.**, *Mar.*, Meny., *Merc.*, **Mez.**, Mos., **Mur. ac.**, *Nat. c.*, Nat. m., *Nit. ac.*, *Nux m.*, *Nux v.*, **Oleand.**, **Par.**, Petrol., **Phos.**, **PHO. AC.**, **PLAT.**, *Pb.*, Puls., Ran. b., Ran. s., Rheum, *Rhodo.*, Rhus, Ruta, **Saba.**, *Sabi.*, Samb., **SARS.**, Sele., Seneg., *Sep.*, Sil., **Spig.**, Spo., *Squ.*, *Stan.*, **Staph.**, Stro., Sul., **SUL. AC.**, *Tar.*, *Thuj.*, **Valer.**, Verat. a., **VERB.**, Vio. o., Vio. t., **Zinc.**

—**Cross-wise, Left Upper and Right Lower.**—**Alum.**, **Anac.**, **Arn.**, Ars., *Bar. c.*, *Bell.*, *Brom.*, Camph., Caps., **Carb. an.**, Cham., *Chel.*, Chin., *Coff.*, Con., Cyc., Euphr., **Fl. ac.**, Hep., **K. carb.**, K. nit., *Lach.*, Laur., Led., Mag. m, *Mar.*, Meny., **Merc.**, Millef., Mur. ac., Nat. m., Nit. ca., *Nux m.*, Nux v., Oleand., Op., *Par.*, *Pho. ac.*, **Puls.**, Ran. s., Rhodo., Rhus, Saba., *Sabi.*, Samb., *Sars.*, Sec. c., *Seneg.*, Spo., **Squ.**, **Stan.**, *Staph.*, Stram., *Sul.*, **TAR.**, Thuj., Valer., **Verat. a.**, **Verb.**, Vio. t.

— —**Left Lower and Right Upper.**—*Acon.*, *Agar.*, Agn., **AMBR.**, **Am. carb.**, Am. m., Ant. cr. Ant. t., *Arg.*, Asar., *Bism.*, **Bor.**, **Bov.**, Bry.,

SENSATIONS.

Calad., Calc. c., Cannab. s., Carb. v., **Caust.**, Chel., Cic., *Cina.*, Colch., *Coloc.*, Croc., Cup., *Dig.*, Dulc., Euphorb., Euphr., **Fer.**, Graph., Hell., Hyos., *Ign.*, Iod., Ip., **Lyc.**, Mag. c., Mang., **Merc. i. f.**, Mez., *Mur. ac.*, Nat. c., *Nux v.*, PHOS., Plat., Pb., Ran. b., *Rheum, Rhus*, Ruta, Sele., Sil., Spig., SUL. AC., Vio. o.

Side, Left.—*Abrot., Acon., Agar.,* Agn., **All. c.,** *Aloe.,* Alum., Ambr., **Am. b.,** Am. carb., Am. m., **Anac., Ant. cr., Ant. t.,** Apis, Arg., **Arn.**, Ars., *Arum. t.,* ASAF., ASAR., Asc. t., *Aur., Aur. m. n., Bar. c.,* Bell., *Berb.,* Bism., Bor., *Bov.,* Brom., Bry., Calad., **Calc. c.,** *Camph., Cannab. s.,* Canth., CAPS., Carb. an., Carb. v., Caust., **Cham., Chel., Chin.,** *Cic.,* CINA, *Clem.,* Cocc., Coff., Colch., Coloc., *Con.,* CROC., **Crot. tig., Cup.**, *Cyc., Dig.,* Dros., **Dulc.,** EUPHORB., **Euphr., Fer.,** *Fer. ph.,* Fl. ac., *Gel.,* Graph., **Guai.,** Hell., Hep., Hyos., *Ign.,* Iod., Ip., *Iris v.,* K. carb., **K. chl.,** K. nit., **Kre.,** LACH., Laur., Led., Lith., Lyc., *Mag. c., Mag. m.,* Mang., Mar., Meny., **Merc., Merc. c., Merc. i. r.,** MEZ., *Millef.,* Mos., **Mur. ac.,** *Naj.,* Nat. c., *Nat. m., Nat. s.,* **Nit. ac.,** *Nux m., Nux v.,* Oleand., **Onos., Osm., Par.,** *Petrol.,* PHOS., Pho. ac., *Phys.,* Plat., Pb., Pso., Puls., Ran. b., **Ran. s.,** Rheum, **Rhodo.,** Rhus, Ruta, Saba., **Sabi.,** *Sal. ac., Samb.,* Sars., Sec. c., SELE., Seneg., SEP., *Sil.,* Spig., Spo., SQU., STAN., Staph., Stram., Stro., SUL., Sul., ac. *Tab.,* **Tar.,** *Ther.,* **Thuj.,** *Ust., Valer., Verat. a., Verb.,* Vesp., Vio. o., Vio. t., *Xan.,* Zinc.

Right.—*Ab. c., Abrot.,* Acon., **Agar., Agn., Alum.,** Ambr., Am. carb., **Am. m.,** Anac., Ant. cr., Ant. t., APIS, ARG., Arn., **Ars.,** Asaf., Asar., AUR., BAP., Bar. c., BELL., Bism., BOR., Bov., Brom., BRY., Calad., CALC. C., **Calc. ph.,** Camph., *Cannab. i., Cannab. s.,* CANTH., Caps., *Carb. an.,* Carb. v., **Caust.,** Ced., *Cham.,* **Chel.,** *Chen. a.,* Chin., Cic., Cina, Clem., **Cocc.,** *Coff.,* Colch., COLOC., **Con.,** Croc., Cup., Cyc., *Dig.,* **Dros.,** Dulc., Euphorb., *Euphr.,* **Fer.,** *Fl. ac., Form.,* Graph., *Guai.,* Hell., Hep., Hyos., **Ign., Iod., Ip.,** Iris, K. carb., *K. nit., Kalm.,* Kre., Lach., Laur., *Led., Lil. t.,* Lith., LYC., *Mag. c.,* **Mag. m., Mang., Mar.,** Meny., **Merc., Merc. i. f., Mez.,** Millef., **Mos.,** *Mur. ac.,* **Nat. c.,** Nat. m., **Nit. ac., Nux m.,** NUX V., Oleand., *Op.,* **Pall., Par., Petrol.,** *Phos.,* Pho. ac., *Phyt.,* Plat., Pb., Pod., Pru., *Pso.,* PULS., Ran. b., RAN. S., **Rheum, Rhodo.,** *Rhus,* Ruta, Saba., **Sabi.,** Samb., **Sang.,** SARS., SEC. C., Sele., *Seneg., Sep.,* Sil., Spig., Spo., *Squ.,* Stan., **Staph., Stram.,** Stro., **Sul.,** SUL. AC., Tar., *Tell.,* Thuj., *Valer., Verat. a.,* **Verb.,** Vio. o., Vio. t., Zinc.

Sit, Inclination To.—Acon., Agar., Alum., *Am. carb.,* **Am. m.,** Anac., Ant. cr., *Ant. t.,* Arg., *Arn.,* Ars., *Asar.,* Bar. c., **Bell.,** *Bor.,* Bry., **Calc. c.,** Camph., **Cannab. s.,** Canth., **Carb. v.,** Caust., **Chel., CHIN.,**

Cocc., Colch., CON., Croc., *Cup.*, *Cyc.*, Dulc., **Euphr.**, **GRAPH.**, GUAI., *Hell.*, *Hep.*, *Hyos.*, *Ign.*, **Iod.**, *Ip.*, K. carb., *Lach.*, *Laur.*, Lyc., Mag. c., Mag. m., **Mar.**, Merc., *Mez.*, Mur. ac., Nat. c., **Nat. m.**, **Nit. ac.**, NUX V., *Oleand.*, Op., Petrol., **PHOS.**, **Pho. ac.**, *Pb.*, **Puls.**, Ran. b., **Ran. s.**, *Rheum*, Rhodo., Rhus, Ruta., Sec. c., Sep., *Sil.*, Spo., SQU., *Stan.*, Stro., **Sul.**, **Tar.**, Verb., *Vio. t.*, Zinc.

Smaller Sensation.—*Agar.*, **Calc. c.**, Croc., **Euphr.**, **Glon.**, Kre.

Smarting. See **Sore Pain**.

Softness. See **Flabby Feeling**.

Sore Pain (Smarting), Externally.—*Abrot.*, **Aesc.**, *Agar.*, *All. c.*, **Aloe**, **Alum.**, *Ambr.*, Am. carb., **Am. m.**, *Anac.*, **Ant. cr.**, *Arg.*, **Arn.**, *Ars.*, Asaf., *Aur.*, *Bar. c.*, *Bell.*, **Berb.**, Bism., *Bor.*, **Bry.**, Calad., **Calc. c.**, **Calc. ph.**, *Calend.*, Camph., Cannab. s., *Canch.*, *Canth.*, **Carb. ac.**, Carb. an., *Carb. v.*, *Carb. sul.*, *Caul.*, **Caust.**, **Cham.**, *Chin.*, **Cic.**, Cimic., Cina, *Clem.*, Coff., *Colch.*, Coloc., *Con.*, Croc., *Crot. tig.*, Cup., *Cyc.*, Dig., *Dios.*, *Dros.*, *Equis.*, **EUP. PER.**, *Euphorb.*, **Euphr.**, Fer., **Fl. ac.**, *Form.*, *Gel.*, **GRAPH.**, **Grat.**, *Ham.*, **HEP.**, Hyos., Hyper., IGN., *Iod.*, Ip., **K. carb.**, Kre., *Lach.*, Led., *Lyc.*, Mag. c., *Mag. m.*, *Mang.*, **Mar.**, **Meny.**, **Merc.**, **MERC. C.**, Mez., Mos., **Mur. ac.**, *Nat. c.*, **Nat. m.**, *Nit. ac.*, NUX V., Oleand., *Oxyt.*, Par., Petrol., **Phos.**, *Pho. ac.*, **Phyt.**, **PLAT.**, Pb., **Puls.**, Ran. b., *Ran. s.*, *Rhodo.*, **Rhus**, *Ruta*, Saba., **Sabi.**, *Sal. ac.*, *Sang.*, Sars., Sec. c., *Seneg.*, **SEP.**, *Sil.*, Spig., Spo., **Squ.**, Stan., **Staph.**, Stro., **Sul.**, Sul. ac., Thuj., Valer., *Verat. a.*, ZINC.

—**Internally.**—*Ac. ac.*, Acon., **Aesc.**, *Agar.*, **Aloe**, **Alum.**, Ambr., Am. carb., **Am. m.**, *Anac.*, **Ant. cr.**, Ant. t., **Apis**, *Apoc. c.*, **Arg.**, **Arg. n.**, Arn., *Ars.*, **ARUM. T.**, *Asaf.*, Asar., Aur., **Bap.**, BAR. C., **BELL.**, **Berb.**, Bism., Bor., Bov., **BRACH.**, **BROM.**, Bry., **Calc. c.**, *Calc. ph.*, Camph., *Cannab. s.*, **CANTH.**, *Caps.*, Carb. ac., Carb. an., *Carb. v.*, **Caust.**, Cham., **Chel.**, **Chin.**, **Cic.**, **Cimic.**, Cina, *Cinnab.*, *Clem.*, Coca, Cocc., Coc. c., Coff., *Colch.*, **Coloc.**, Con., Croc., *Crotal.*, *Crot. tig.*, Dig., Dios., **Eup. per.**, Euphorb., Fer., *Fl. ac.*, **Gam.**, *Gel.*, *Graph.*, Hell., **Helo.**, Hep., **Hydras.**, IGN., *Iod.*, Ip., **K. bi.**, *K. carb.*, **K. iod.**, **K. nit.**, Kre., **LACH.**, Led., **Lil. t.**, *Lith.*, **Lyc.**, *Mag. c*, **Mag. m.**, **Mang.**, Mar., **MERC.**, **Mez.**, Mos., **Mur. ac.**, *Nat. c.*, **Nat. m.**, **Nat. s.**, **NIT. AC.**, *Nux m.*, **Nux v.**, Oleand., Onos., Osm., Petrol., **PHOS.**, **Pho. ac.**, Phyt., Plat., Pb., **Pod.**, **Puls.**, Ran. b., *Ran. s.*, Rhodo., **RHUS**, *Rumex*, Ruta., **Saba.**, **Sabi.**, Sang., **Sang. n.**, *Sars.*, *Seneg.*, **SEP.**, **Sil.**, *Sin.*, Spig., **SPO.**, **STAN.**, *Staph.*, *Stict.*, *Still.*, Stram., Stro., **Sul.**, **Sul. ac.**, *Tarent.*, Thuj., *Ust.*, **Valer.**, **Verat. v.**, Vio. o., **ZINC.**, **Zing**.

Splinters, Feeling of.—**Aesc.**, *Agar.*, **Alum.**, **Arg. n.**, **Carb. v.**, *Cic.*,

Colch., *Coll.*, Dol., Fl. ac., Hep., NIT. AC., *Petrol.*, Plat., *Ran. b.*, **Sil.**, *Sul.*

Splitting Pain (Bursting Asunder).—*Acon.*, Am. carb., Am. m., Anac., *Ant. cr.*, Ant. t., *Apis*, *Arg. n.*, Arn., Ars., Asaf., **Asar.**, *Bar. c.*, **BELL.**, *Bism.*, Bor., Bov., BRY., *Cact.*, CALC. C., Camph., Cannab. s., CAPS., *Carb. an.*, *Carb. v.*, CAUST., Cham., *Chel.*, *Chin.*, *Cimic.*, Cina, Cocc., Coff., Colch., **Coloc.**, **Con.**, Croc., Dig., Dulc., **Euphorb.**, Euphr., Fer., **Gel.**, Glon., *Graph.*, Guai., *Hell.*, Hep., *Hyos.*, *Hyper.*, IGN., Iod., Ip., **Iris v.**, **K. carb.**, *K. nit.*, Kre., Lach., Laur., Lyc., Mag. c., Mang., Merc., *Mez.*, Mos., Mur. ac., Nat. c., NAT. M., Nit. ac., Nux m., **Nux v.**, Oleand., Op., **Par.**, Petrol., *Phos.*, Pho. ac., Plat., Pb., *Pru.*, **Puls.**, RAN. B., Ran. s., Rhodo., Rhus, Saba., **Sabi.**, Samb., **Sang.**, Sars., *Seneg.*, SEP., SIL., SPIG., *Spo.*, Squ., *Stan.*, *Staph.*, Stram., **Stro.**, Sul., Sul. ac., Tar., *Thuj.*, *Usn.*, Valer., Verat. a., Verb., *Vip.*, Vio. t., *Zinc.*

Sprain From Lifting.—Alum., *Ambr.*, **Arn.**, *Bar. c.*, Bor., Bry., CALC. C., *Carb. an.*, *Carb. v.*, *Caust.*, *Chin.*, Cocc., Coloc., **Con.**, Croc., Dulc., Fer., **Graph.**, *Iod.*, *K. carb.*, Lach., **Lyc.**, Merc., *Mur. ac.*, **Nat. c.**, *Nat. m.*, Nit. ac., *Nux v.*, Oleand., *Phos.*, **Pho. ac.**, Plat., Rhodo., RHUS, Ruta, *Sep.*, **Sil.**, Spig., *Stan.*, Staph., *Sul.*, Sul. ac., Thuj., *Valer.*

Sprained Pain, Externally.—Acon., *Agar.*, *Agn.*, *Aloe*, Alum., Ambr., *Am. carb.*, Am. m., Anac., Ant. cr., Ant. t., ARN., Ars., **Asar.**, Aur., *Bar. c.*, *Bell.*, *Bov.*, **Bry.**, Calad., CALC. C., Camph., Canth., Caps., Carb. an., **Carb. v.**, Caust., Cham., *Chel.*, Chin., Cina, *Coca*, Cocc., Coloc., Con., Croc., Cup., *Cyc.*, Dig., Dros., Dulc., *Euphorb.*, *Graph.*, Hell., *Hep.*, Ign., Ip., *K. carb.*, *K. nit.*, *Kre.*, **Led.**, *Lyc.*, *Mag. c.*, Mag. m., Meny., **Merc.**, **Mez.**, *Mos.*, *Mur. ac.*, Nat. c., NAT. M., *Nit. ac.*, Nux m., *Nux v.*, Oleand., PETROL., **Phos.**, Pho. ac., Plat., Pb., **Puls.**, Ran. b., **Rhodo.**, RHUS, *Ruta*, *Sabi.*, *Sal. ac.*, Sars., Seneg., Sep., Sil., Spig., Spo., **Stan.**, Staph., SUL., Thuj., Valer., Verat. a., Verb., Zinc.

—**Internally.**—*Agar.*, *Aloe*, Alum., Ambr., Am. m., Caust., Dulc., *Euphorb.*, *K. carb.*, **Lyc.**, *Nux v.*, *Onos.*, Petrol., Plat., Rhodo., Spig., Staph., **Sul.**, Tar., Thuj.

—**In Joints.**—Acon., *Agar.*, *Agn.*, Alum., **Ambr.**, *Am. carb.*, Am. m., Anac., Ant. cr., Ant. t., **Arg. n.**, ARN., Ars., **Arum. t.**, Asar., Aur., *Bar. c.*, Bell., *Bov.*, Bry., Calad., **Calc. c.**, **Calc. ph.**, Camph., *Caps.*, Carb. an., Carb. v., **Caust.**, Cham., Chel., Chin., Cina, Cocc., Con., **Coral.**, Croc., Cyc., Dig., Dros., Dulc., Euphorb., *Fer.*, *Fl. ac.*, **Graph.**, Hell., Hep., IGN., Ip., K. carb., **K. nit.**, *Kre.*, LED., *Lyc.*, Mag. c., Mag. m., **Mang.**, Meny., **Merc.**, *Mez.*, *Mos.*, Mur. ac., Nat. c., Nat. m., Nit. ac., Nux m., *Nux v.*, Oleand., *Osm.*, **Petrol.**, PHOS., Pho. ac., Plat., Pb., *Pru.*, **PULS.**,

SENSATIONS.

Ran. b., **Rhodo.**, RHUS, *Ruta*, *Sabi.*, Sars., Seneg., *Sep.*, Sil., **Spig.**, Spo., *Stan.*, *Staph.*, SUL., Thuj., Valer., Verat. a., Verb., *Zinc.*

Startings.—Acon., Agn., Alum., Ambr., Am. carb., Am. m., Anac., Ant. cr., *Ant. t.*, **Apis**, **Arn.**, **ARS.**, **Atrop.**, Bar. c., BELL., Bism., *Bor.*, Brom., BRY., Calad., Calc. c., Canth., **Caps.**, *Carb. an.*, *Carb. v.*, **Caust.**, Cham., *Chel.*, **Chin.**, *Cimic.*, *Cina*., **Cocc.**, *Coff.*, Colch., *Con.*, Croc., *Dig.*, Dros., Dulc., *Euphorb.*, *Graph.*, Guai., **Hep.**, HYOS., **Ign.**, *Ip.*, **K. carb.**, *K. nit.*, Kre., Lach., Laur., *Led.*, *Lyc.*, *Mag. c.*, Mag. m., Mar., **Merc.**, Mez., *Nat. c.*, Nat. m., Nit. ac., Nux m., NUX V., Op., Petrol., *Phos.*, Pho. ac., Plat., *Pb.*, **Puls.**, Rhus, **Samb.**, *Sars.*, **Sele.**, Seneg., *Sep.*, **Sil.**, Spo., Stan., Staph., STRAM., STRO., **Sul.**, *Sul. ac.*, **Ther.**, Thuj., *Verat. a.*, Zinc.

Sticking, Extending Downward.—Ant. cr., Arn., **Asc. t.**, Bell., Bor., Canth., Caps., CARB. V., **Caust.**, *Chel.*, *Cimic.*, Cina, Coloc., *Dios.*, Dros., FER., *Gel.*, *Kre.*, *Lyc.*, Mang., *Mez.*, Nit. ac., Nux v., *Pall.*, Petrol., Pho. ac., **Phyt.**, Puls., Ran. s., RHUS, *Sabi.*, Sars., Sep., *Still.*, Squ Sul., Tar., *Ust.*, Valer., Zinc.

—**Externally.**—*Abrot.*, *Acon.*, *Aconin.*, AGAR., *Agn.*, ALOE ALUM., Ambr., Am. carb., AM. M., Anac., Ant. cr., Ant. t., *Apis*, *Arg.*, ARN., Ars., ASAF., Asar., Aur., BAR. AC., *Bar. c.*, BELL., Berb., Bism., Bor., *Bov.*, BRY., Calad., CALC. C., CALC. PH., Camph., CANNAB. I., Cannab. s., *Canth.*, CAPS., *Carb. ac.*, *Carb. an.*, Carb. v., *Carb. sul.*, CAUST., *Ced.*, Cham., *Chel.*, CHIN., CIC., Cimic., Cina, *Cinnab.*, CLEM., COCC., Coff., Colch., COLOC., CON., Croc., *Crotal.*, *Crot. tig.*, *Cup.*, *Cyc.*, Dig., *Dios.*, DROS., Dulc., Euphorb., *Euphr.*, FER., *Fer. ph.*, *Farm.*, *Gel.*, GRAPH., Guai., HELL., Hep., *Hydras.*, Hyos., IGN., Iod., Ip., K. bi., K. CARB., K. nit., *Kre.*, Lach., *Laur.*, Led., LITH., *Lyc.*, Mag. c., *Mag. m.*, *Mang.*, Mar., MENY., MERC., Mez., MOS., MUR. AC., *Naj.*, NAT. C., ˙NAT. M., NIT. AC., Nux m., NUX V., *Oleand.*, OX. AC., PAR., Petrol., PHOS., *Pho. ac.*, PHYT., *Plat.*, PB., PULS., RAN. B., RAN. S., Rheum, Rhodo., RHUS, Ruta, SABA., SABI., Samb., SANG., Sars., Sele., Seneg., SEP., SIL., SPIG., Spo., Squ., STAN., STAPH., *Still.*, Stram., *Stro.*, SUL., *Sul. ac.*, TAR., THUJ., VALER., Verat. a., *Verb.*, *Vio. o.*, VIO T., ZINC.

—**Internally.**—*Abrot.*, Acon., Aesc., Agar., Agn., *All. c.*, *Aloe*, Alum., Ambr., *Ammc.*, Am. carb., *Am. m*, *Anac.*, Ant. cr., Ant. t., *Apis*, Arg., Arg. n., Arn., **Ars.**, ASAF., **Asar.**, Aspar., Aur., *Bar. c.*, Bell., BERB., Bism., BOR., Bov., BRY., Cact., *Calad.*, *Calc. ac.*, **Calc. c.**, *Calc. ph.*, Camph., CANNAB. I., CANTH., Caps., Carb. an., *Carb. v.*, *Carb. sul.*, *Card.*, **Caust.**, Cham., CHEL., CHIN., Cic., *Cimic.*, **Cina**, *Clem.*, *Cocc.*, **Coc. c.**, Coff., Colch., *Coll.*, **Coloc.**, Con., Croc., *Crot. t. j.*,

Cup., Cyc., *Dig., Dios.,* **Dol.,** Dros., **Dulc.,** Euphorb., **Euphr., Fer., Gam.,** *Gel.,* **Glon.,** Graph., Guai., Hell., Hep., *Hydras.,* Hyos., **IGN.,** Iod., **Ip., K. bi., K. carb., K. iod.,** *K. nit.,* **Kalm., Kre.,** LACH., **Laur.,** *Led.,* Lyc., **Mag. c., Mag. m.,** Mang., Mar., *Meny.,* MERC., MERC. C., *Merc. i. r., Merc. n., Mez.,* Mos., *Mur. ac.,* **Naj., Nat. c., Nat. m., Nat. s.,** NIT. AC., Nux m., **Nux v.,** *Oleand, Op., Ox. ac.,* **Par.,** Petrol, *Phel.,* PHOS., Pho. ac., *Phyt., Plant.,* Plat., PB., *Pru.,* **PULS.,** RAN. B., Ran. s., Rheum., Rhodo., **Rhus,** Rumex, *Ruta,* **Saba.,** Sabi., *Samb., Sang.,* Sars., Sec. c., Sele., Seneg., SEP., SIL., SPIG., *Spo.,* SQU., **Stan., Staph.,** Stram., *Stro.,* **Sul.,** *Sul. ac., Tab.,* Tar., Thal., **Ther., Thuj.,** *Valer.,* Verat. a., *Verb.,* **Vio. t., Zinc.,** Ziz.

Sticking Inward.—Acon., *Alum.,* Am. m., Arg., **ARN., Asaf.,** Bar. c., *Bell., Bov.,* **Bry., Calc. c.,** *Cannab. s.,* **CANTH., Caps.,** *Carb. v., Caust., Cina,* Clem., Cocc., Coloc., Croc., Dros., Guai., *Hyos.,* **Ign.,** *Ip.,* Laur., Mang., *Meny., Mez.,* Nux v., Oleand., Par., *Petrol.,* Phos., Pho. ac., **Phyt., Pb.,** RAN. B., *Rhus,* **Sabi.,** Samb., Sel., *Squ., Staph., Sul. ac.,* Tar., Thuj., *Verb.*

—**In Joints.**—Acon., Agar., **Agn.,** *Alum.,* Am. carb., *Am. m.,* Anac., *Ant. cr.,* Ant. t., *Apis, Arg.,* **Arn., Ars., Asaf.,** *Asar.,* Bar. c., **Bell., Bov., BRY., CALC. C.,** Camph., Canth., Caps., *Carb. an., Carb. v., Carb. sul.,* **Caust.,** *Chel.,* Chin., Cina , Clem., **Cocc.,** *Coloc.,* **Con.,** Dros., *Dulc.,* Euphorb., *Euphr.,* **Fer.,** Graph., *Guai.,* HELL., Hep., Hyos., **Ign.,** *Iod.,* **K. CARB., K. nit., Kre.,** *Laur., Led.,* Lyc., *Mag. c.,* **Mag. m.,** MANG., **Meny., MERC., Merc. c.,** Mez., Mos., *Mur. ac., Nat. c.,* **Nat. m.,** *Nit. ac.,* Nux m., *Nux v.,* Oleand., Par., *Petrol.,* Phos., *Pho. ac.,* Plat., Pb., **Puls.,** Ran. s., Rheum., **Rhodo.,** RHUS, Ruta, Saba., **Sabi.,** Samb., Sars., Sep., SIL., SPIG., *Spo.,* Squ., **Stan., Staph.,** Stro., SUL., **Sul. ac., TAR., THUJ.,** *Valer., Verat. a.,* Verb., *Vio. t.,* **Zinc.**

—**In Muscles.**—*Acon.,* Agar.,*Agn.,* **Alum.,** Ambr., Am. carb., **Am. m.,** Anac., *Ant. cr.,* Ant. t., *Arg.,* **Arn.,** Ars., ASAF., Asar., Aur., *Bar. c.,* **BELL.,** Bism., Bor., *Bov.,* BRY., Calad., **CALC. C.,** Camph., Cannab. s., **Canth.,** Caps., *Carb. an.,* Carb. v., **Caust.,** Cham., *Chel.,* **Chin.,** Cic., Cina, Clem., **Cocc.,** Colch., Coloc., **Con.,** Croc., Cup., *Cyc.,* Dig., **Dros.,** *Dulc.,* Euphorb., *Euphr.,* Fer., **Graph.,** *Guai.,* **Hell.,** Hep., Hyos., **Ign.,** Iod., **K. carb.,** K. nit., *Kre.,* Lach., **Laur.,** Led., *Lyc.,* Mag. c., *Mag. m.,* Mang., Mar., **Meny.,** MERC., *Mez.,* Mos., **Mur. ac., Nat. c., Nat. m., Nit. ac.,** Nux m., *Nux v., Oleand.,* **Par.,** Petrol., **Phos.,** *Pho. ac.,* Plat., Pb., **PULS.,** *Ran. b.,* **Ran. s.,** Rheum., Rhodo., RHUS, Ruta, **Saba., Sabi.,** Samb., **Sars.,** Sep., Sil.,SPIG., Spo., Squ., **Stan.,** STAPH., *Stro.,* **SUL.,** *Sul. ac.,* **TAR., THUJ.,** Valer., Verat. a., *Verb.,* **Vio. t., Zinc.**

SENSATIONS.

Sticking Outward.—Alum., *Am. m.*, Ant. cr., ARG., *Arn.*, ASAF., Asar., **Bell.**, *Bry.*, **Calc. c.**, Cannab. s., *Canth.*, *Carb. v.*, Caust., Cham., CHEL., CHIN., Clem., *Cocc.*, Coff., *Colch.*, CON., *Dros.*, **Dulc.**, Hell., *Hyos.*, *K. carb.*, **Lach.**, **Laur.**, **Lith.**, **Lyc.**, *Mang.*, Meny., MERC., **Mez.**, *Mur. ac.*, **Nat. c.**, Nat. m., *Nit. ac.*, Oleand., PHEL., Phos., *Pho. ac.*, *Phyt.*, PRU., Puls., *Rhodo.*, Rhus, **Saba.**, Sabi., **Sil.**, SPIG., SPO., STAN., **Staph.**, Stro., SUL., **Tar.**, *Ther.*, Thuj., VALER., Verat. a., Verb., Vio. o., *Vio. t.*

—**Transversely.**—Acon., Ambr., Anac., Arg., **Atrop.**, **Asc. c.**, BELL., Bov., *Bry.*, *Calc. c.*, Canth., *Caust.*, Cham., Chin., *Cimic.*, Cocc., *Cup.*, *Dig.*, **K. bi.**, *K. carb.*, Laur., Lyc., Merc., *Mur. ac.*, Phos., **Pb.**, **Ran. b.**, *Rhodo.*, Rhus, Seneg., **Sep.**, Spig., **Stict.**, *Stro.*, **Sul.**, Sul. ac., Tar.

—**Upward.**—Acon., Alum., Arn., *Ars.*, Bar. c., BELL., *Bry.*, Calc. c., *Canth.*, Carb. v., Caust., **Cham.**, *Chin.*, *Cimic.*, Cina, Coloc., *Dios.*, **Dros.**, Euphr., *Gel.*, Glon., Guai., K. carb., **Lach.**, **Lith.**, *Mang.*, **Meny.**, Merc., Nat. s., Petrol., PHYT., *Puls.*, Rhus, *Rumex*, Ruta, SEP., **Spo.**, Stan., Sul., Tar., Thuj.

—**Burning in Joints.**—Mez., Plat., Pb., Sul. ac., *Thuj.*

— —**In Muscles.**—Alum., Am. m., *Anac.*, **Arg.**, Arn., ASAF., Aur., Bar. c., *Bry.*, *Calc. c.*, Caust., Cic., *Cina*, COCC., Colch., **Dig.**, Ign., Laur., Lyc., Mag. c., *Mang.*, Merc., MEZ., Mur. ac., NUX V., **Oleand.**, *Plat.*, *Pb.*, Rhodo., RHUS, **Saba.**, Sabi., Samb., Sep., Spig., *Stan.*, STAPH., SUL. AC., *Tar.*, THUJ., Vio. t.

—**Crawling.**—Am. m., Anac., Arg., ARN., Bar. c., Caust., Chin., K. carb., Meny., Mez., Plat., Saba., **Sep.**, Sil., Spig., Staph., Thuj., *Zinc.*

—**Drawing.** See **Tearing.**

—**Jerking.**—Arn., Bry., **Calc. c.**, *Carb. sul.*, Caust., CINA, Cocc., Coff., **Coloc.**, Euphorb., *Guai.*, **Lyc.**, *Mang.*, **Meny.**, *Mez.*, Mur. ac., NUX V., Pho. ac., Pb., *Sep.*, Sil., Spo., SQU., Stan., Zinc.

—**Pressing in Joints.**—Pho. ac., *Sars.*, *Staph.*, Zinc.

— —**In Muscles.**—Am. m., *Anac.*, Arg., *Arn.*, **Asaf.**, Bar. c., Bell., *Calc. c.*, Chin., Colch., Dros., *Euphorb.*, *Ign.*, K. carb., *Mez.*, **Mur. ac.**, Phos., Rhus, Ruta, Saba., SARS., Spo., Stan., *Staph.*, Tar., **Thuj.**, Verb., Vio. t., Zinc.

—**Tearing in Joints.**—Acon., Ars., Asaf., **Asar.**, *Carb. v.*, Caust., *Clem.*, *Dulc.*, Fer., *Merc.*, Mur. ac., Puls., Sabi., Stan., STAPH., Sul. *Sul. ac.*, Tar., Thuj., Verb., *Zinc.*

— —**In Muscles.**—*Acon.*, *Agn.*, Alum., Ambr., Am. carb., Am. m., ANAC., *Arg.*, **Ars.**, Asaf., *Asar.*, Aur., Bell., Bism., Bor., CALC. C.,

Camph., *Cannab. s.*, Canth., Caps., *Caust.*, **Chin.**, *Cina*, *Clem.*, *Coloc.*, Con., *Cyc.*, *Dig.*, Dros., GUAI., *Hell.*, K. carb., Kre., Led., MANG., Merc., *Mez.*, *Mur. ac.*, *Nat. m.*, Nux v., Oleand., Phos., *Pho. ac.*, PULS., Rheum, **Rhus**, Ruta, Sabi., Samb., **Sars.**, *Sep.*, Sil., Spig., *Spo.*, Squ., Staph., *Sul. ac.*, Tar., THUJ., *Verb.*, Zinc.

Sticking, Tensive.—Asaf., **Calc. c.**, *Cina*, *Clem.*, Cocc., Dig., K. carb., Mang., *Nat. m.*, *Oleand.*, Pho. ac., Ruta, SPIG., **Staph.**, *Stan.*, Sul., **Tar.**, Vio. t.

Stiffness. See **Rigidity.**

Stopped Feeling, Internally.—Bism., Bry., Cham., Chel., *Chin.*, *Guai.*, *Meny.*, Nat. c., *Nux m.*, OP., Phos., Puls., Rhus, Sep., *Spig.*, *Spo.*, *Verb.*

Strangling Pain (Constriction).—Acon., Agar., Ambr., **Am. carb.**, *Asar.*, Bell., Bry., *Cact.*, Cannab. s., Canth., Carb. an., *Chel.*, Cocc., Coff., Cup., Dig., Dros., Graph., Hep., Ign., Kre., Mag. c., Nat. c., **Nux v.**, **Phos.**, Pb., PULS., Ran. s., Sabi., Spo., Stram., Sul., Sul. ac., **Sum.**, *Verat a.*, Zinc.

Strength, Sensation of.—*Agar.*, **Coff.**, OP., Stram.

Surging (in Body).—*Acon.*, *Alum.*, *Ars.*, *Cannab. i.*, Carb. v., Caust., Cina, Cocc., Dig., Dulc., Fer., GLON., **Graph.**, Hyos., *Laur.*, *Mag. m.*, Mang., **Meli.**, Merc., **Nux v.**, Pb., Rhodo., Sars., *Seneg.*, **Sep.**, *Spo.*, Thuj.

Swellings in General.—Acon., Agar., Agn., *Alum.*, Ambr., **Am. carb.**, Am. m., Anac., *Ant. cr.*, APIS, *Arg.*, **Arn.**, ARS., Asaf., *Aur.*, **Bar. c.**, BELL., Bism., *Bor.*, Bov., BRY., Calad., **Calc. c.**, Camph., *Cannab. s.*, **Canth.**, *Caps.*, Carb. an., *Carb. v.*, *Caust.*, **Cham.**, *Chel.*, **Chin.**, *Cic.*, Clem., Cocc., Coff., Colch., Coloc., *Com.*, Con., *Cop.*, Croc., *Crotal.*, Cup., Cyc., *Dig.*, Dros., *Dulc.*, *Euphorb.*, Euphr., Fer., *Graph.*, Guai., **Hell.**, **Hep.**, *Hyos.*, *Ign.*, *Iod.*, **K. carb.**, *K. nit.*, *Kre.*, *Lach.*, Laur., **Led.**, **Lyc.**, *Mag. c.*, Mag. m., Mang., Mar., MERC., *Mez.*, Mos., Mur. ac., *Naj.*, **Nat. c.**, *Nat. m.*, **Nit. ac.**, *Nux m.*, NUX V., Oleand., *Op.*, Par., **Petrol.**, **Phos.**, **Pho. ac.**, **Pb.**, PULS., Ran. b, *Rhodo.*, RHUS, *Ruta*, Saba., Sabi., Samb., Sars., *Sec. c.*, *Seneg.*, Sep., **Sil.**, **Spig.**, *Spo.*, Squ., *Stan.*, Staph., **Stram.**, Stro., Sul., Sul. ac., Thuj., Valer., *Verat. a.*, **Vip.**, Zinc.

—Of Affected Parts.—ACON., ACT., *Agn.*, Alum., Ant. cr., *Ant. s.*, *aur.*, **Apis**, *Arn.*, **Ars.**, **Ars. iod.**, Asaf., *Aur.*, Bar. c., BELL., Bov., BRY., **Calc. c.**, *Cannab. s.*, **Canth.**, Carb. an., Carb. v., **Caust.**, *Ced.*, Cham., Chin., *Cic.*, Clem., *Cocc.*, Coc. c., *Colch.*, **Coll.**, Con., CROTAL., *Crot. tig.*, *Cub.*, Cup., *Dig.*, Dulc., *Euphorb.*, EUPHR., **Fer.**, *Fer. ph.*, **Fl. ac.**, GEL., Graph., **Guai.**, Hell., **Hep.**, Hydras., Ign., **Iod.**, K. CARB.,

SENSATIONS.

K. iod., Lach., Led., Lyc., *Mag. c.*, Mang., MERC., MERC. C., **Mur. ac.**, **Nat. c.**, **Nat. m.**, **Nit. ac.**, **Nux v.**, *Ox. ac.*, Petrol., Phos., *Pho. ac.*, Pb., **Pso.**, PULS., Ran. b., RHODO., RHUS, Ruta, *Sabi.*, **Samb.**, Sang., Sars., Sec. c., SEP., SIL., Spig., SPO., **Stan.**, **Stram.**, SUL., Thuj., **Valer.**, Zinc.

Swellings, Inflammatory.—ACON., *Agn.*, Alum., Am. carb., *Ant. cr.*, Apis, *Arn.*, Ars., Asaf., Bar. c., **Bell.**, Bry., CALC. C., *Cannab. s.*, CANTH., Carb. an., Carb. v., **Caust.**, Chin., Cocc., Colch., Con., Cup., *Euphorb.*, Graph., Guai., *Hep.*, Iod., K. CARB., Led., **Lyc.**, *Mag. c.*, MERC., *Nat. c.*, **Nat. m.**, **Nit. ac.**, Nux v., *Petrol.*, **Phos.**, **Pb.**, **Puls.**, RHUS, Sabi., Samb., Sars., Sec. c., SEP., **Sil.**, *Spo.*, Stan., SUL., Thuj., Zinc.

—**Puffy.**—Acon., *Am. carb.*, Am. m., ANT. CR., *Arn.*, **Ars.**, **Asaf.**, Aur., *Bar. c.*, **Bell.**, Bry., CALC. C., CAPS., *Ced.*, Cham., Chin., Cina, Cocc., Colch., *Coloc.*, Con., CUP., Dig., Dros., *Dulc.*, FER., *Graph.*, *Guai.*, Hell., *Hyos.*, Ip., *K. carb.*, Kre., Lach., Laur., *Led.*, *Lyc.*, Mag. c., Mar., Merc., Mez., *Mos.*, Nat. c., Nit. ac., Nux m., Nux v., **Oleand.**, Op., Phos., *Phyt.*, **Pb.**, **Puls.**, Rheum, Rhus, Samb., Sars., Seneg., Sep., *Sil.*, **Spig.**, *Spo.*, Staph., *Stram.*, *Sul.*

Swollen Sensation.—Acon., *Aconin.*, *Agar.*, *Aloe.*, Alum., Ambr., Am. m., Anac., Ant. cr., Ant. t., *Apis*, **Aran.**, Arg., *Arn.*, *Ars.*, Asaf., Asar., **Aur.**, **Bap.**, Bar. c., **Bell.**, Bism., *Bov.*, **Bry.**, *Caj.*, *Calad.*, Calc. c., Calc. ph., *Cannab. i.*, Canth., **Caps.**, *Carb. ac.*, *Carb. sul.*, *Carb. v.*, Caust , **Ced.**, Cham., *Chin.*, *Cimic.*, Cina, **Cocc.**, Coc. c., *Colch.*, **Coloc.**, Com., *Con.*, **Coral.**, *Crotal.*, *Crot. tig.*, Cup., Cyc., Dig., *Dulc.*, Euphorb., Euphr., Glon., GUAI., *Hell.*, Hep., *Hyos.*, **Ign.**, Ip., K. carb., **K. nit.**, Kre., LACH., **Laur.**, Led., Lyc., Mag. c., Mang., MERC., MERC. I. F., *Mez.*, Mos., Nit. ac., *Nux m.*, **Nux v.**, *Oleand.*, Op., **PÆO.**, **PAR.**, Petrol., Phos., Pho. ac., Plat., **Pb.**, **PULS.**, Ran. b., *Ran. s.*, Rhodo., RHUS, Saba., *Sabi.*, Samb., **Sang.**, Sars., Seneg., *Sep.*, Sil., SPIG., Spo., *Stan.*, Staph., Stram., **Sul.**, *Sul. ac.*, Tar., Thuj., Valer., Verat. a., *Zinc.*

Tearing Away Sensation.—*Act.*, Coloc., *Dig.*, Hep., K. BI., Led., Mos., Nux v., *Pœo.*, Petrol., Phos., Pb., RHUS, Sep., Sul., *Thuj.*

—**Asunder.**—Agar., *Alum.*, Am. m., Anac., Arn., *Ars.*, Asar., Calc. c., *Carb. an.*, Carb. v., **Caust.**, COFF., Colch., *Con.*, Dig., Fer., Graph., *Ign.*, Mar., **Mez.**, *Mur. ac.*, Nat. m., NIT. AC., NUX V., Op., Puls., Rhus, Sabi., *Sep.*, Spig., Staph., *Sul.*, Sul. ac., Thuj., Zinc.

—**Downward.**—Acon., Agar., Agn., *Alum.*, Anac., Ant. cr., **Ant. t.**, Ars., Asaf., Aur., **Bar. c.**, BELL., Bism., **Bry.**, Calc. c., **Canth.**, CAPS., **Carb. v.**, Caust., **Chel.**, **Chin.**, *Cina*, Colch., **Coloc.**, Con., Croc., Dulc.,

Euphr., Fer., Graph., Ign., **K. carb.**, K. nit., Laur., **LYC.**, **Mag. c.,** **Meny.**, **Merc.**, Mez., *Mur. ac.*, **Nat. c.**, *Nat. m.*, Nit. ac., **Nux v.**, Phos., *Pho. ac.*, **Puls.**, Rhodo., **RHUS**, Sabi., *Sars.*, *Seneg.*, **Sep.**, *Sil.*, **Spig.**, Squ.. Stan., Staph., SUL., Thuj., Valer., **Verat. a.**, *Verb.*, Zinc.

Tearing, Externally.—ACON., *Aesc.*, **Agar.**, *Agn.*, **Alum.**, **Ambr.**, **Am. carb.**, **Am. m.**, **Anac.**, *Ant. cr.*, *Ant. t.*, Arg., **ARN.**, **Ars.**, **Asaf.**, Asar.,Aur., *Bar. c.*, BELL., Berb., **Bism.**, *Bor.*, Bov., *Brom.*, BRY., *Cact.,* Calad., **Calc. c.**, *Calc. ph.*, Camph., Cannab. s., *Canth.*, **Caps.**, **Carb. an.**, **Carb. v.**, Caust., Ced., **Cham.**, *Chel.*, CHIN., Cic., *Cina*, Clem., *Cocc.*, Coff., *Colch.*, **Coloc.**, *Con.*, Croc., Cup., Cyc., Dig., Dros., **Dulc.**, *Euphorb.*, Euphr., **Fer.**, **Gam.**, *Graph.*, Guai., Hell., Hep., Hyos., **Ign.**, Iod., Ip., K. bi., K. CARB., **K. iod.**, K. nit., Kre., Lach., Laur., *Led.*, **LYC.**, *Mag. c.*, **Mag. m.**, *Mang.*, *Mar.*, Meny., **Merc.**, **Mez.**, Mos., *Mur. ac.*, **Nat. c.**, NAT. M., NIT. AC., Nux m., **Nux v.**, Oleand., Op., Par., Petrol., Phos., Pho. ac., *Phyt.*, Plat., *Pb.*, PULS., **Ran. b.**, Ran. s., Rheum, **Rhodo.**, Rhus, Ruta, Saba., *Sabi.*, Samb., *Sars.*, Sec., c., **Sele.**, Seneg., **Sep.**, SIL., **Spig.**, *Spo.*, Squ., Stan., *Staph.*, *Stram.*, **Stro.**, SUL., Sul. ac., *Tar.*, *Thuj.*, **Valer.**, *Verat. a.*, Verb., Vio. o., Vio. t., ZINC.

—Internally.—*Acon.*, Aesc., **Agar.**, *Agn.*, *Aloe*, **Alum.**, **Ambr.**, Am. carb, Am. m., *Anac.*, Ant. cr., **Ant. t.**, *Apis*, **Arg.**, *Arn.*, *Ars.*, Asaf., Asar., **Aur.**, *Bar. c.*, BELL., Berb., *Bism.*, *Bor.*, Bov., BRY., Calad., *Calc. c*, Camph., Cannab. s., Canth., **Caps.**, Carb. an., Carb. v., *Carb. sul.*, Caust., **Cham.**, **Chel.**, *Chin.*, Cic., Cina, Clem., *Cocc.*, *Coff.*, Colch., **Coloc.**, CON., Croc., *Crotal.*, *Cup.*, *Cyc.*, *Dig.*, *Dios.*, Dros., Dulc., Euphorb., Euphr., Fer., **Gran.**, Graph., Guai., Hell., Hep., Hyos., **Ign.**, Iod., *Ip.*, *K. carb.*, K. nit., **Kalm.**, Kre., **Lach.**, Laur., Led., **LYC.**, *Mag. c.*, Mag. m., *Mang.*, Mar., **Meny.**, MERC., Mez., *Mos.*, Mur. ac., *Nat. c.*, **Nat. m.**, Nit. ac., Nux m., NUX V., Oleand., Op., Par., Petrol., **Phos.**, Pho. ac., Plat., *Pb.*, PULS., Ran. b., Ran. s., **Rhodo.**, Rhus, *Ruta*, Saba., Sabi., Samb., *Sang.*, Sars., Sec. c., *Sele.*, Seneg., SEP., SIL., SPIG., Spo., Squ., **Stan.**, *Staph.*,*Stram.*, Stro., SUL., Sul. ac., **Tar.**, Thuj., *Uva.*, Valer., Verat. a., **Verat. v.**, Verb., Vio. o., Vio. t., **Zinc.**

—In Joints.—Acon., *Agar.*, **Agn.**, *Alum.*, **Ambr.**, *Am. carb.*, *Am. m.*, *Anac.*, Ant. t., ARG., *Arn.*, **Ars.**, *Asaf.*, Asar., Aur., Bar. c., BELL., Bism., **Bov.**, Bry., *Cact.*, **Calc. c.**, Camph., *Canth.*, Carb. an., *Carb. v.*, CAUST., *Cham.*, Chel., Chin., Cic., Cina, *Clem.*, *Cocc.*, *Colch.*, **Coloc.**, Con., Cup., Cyc., Dig., **Dros.**, Dulc., Euphr., **Fer.**, Graph., Guai., Hell., *Hep.*, *Hyos.*, **Ign.**, Iod., K. CARB., **K. nit.**, Kre., Laur., **Led.**, LYC., Mag. c., *Mag. m.*, Mang., **Mar.**, Meny., MERC., Mez., Mos., *Mur. ac.*, *Nat. c.*, Nat. m. Nit. ac., Nux m., **Nux v.**, Oleand., *Par.*, Petrol., **Phos.**, Pho. ac., Pb.,

SENSATIONS.

PULS., *Ran. b.*, Rheum., *Rhodo.*, RHUS, *Ruta*, Saba., *Sabi.*, *Samb.*, **Sars.**, Sec. c., **Sep.**, *Sil.*, *Spig.*, *Spo.*, *Stan.*, **Staph.**, STRO., SUL., Tar., Thuj., Valer., Verat. a., Verb., Vio. o., ZINC.

Tearing In Muscles.—*Acon.*, *Agar.*, Agn., *Alum.*, **Ambr.**, Am. carb., Am. m., Anac., Ant. cr., Ant. t., Arg. *Arn.*, **Ars.**, **Asaf.**, Asar., **Aur.**, *Bar. c.*, **Bell.**, **Bism.**, Bor., Bov., **Bry.**, CALC. C., Camph., **Canth.**, Caps., **Carb. an.**, CARB. V., CAUST., Cham., **Chel.**, **Chin.**, Cic., **Cina**, Clem., Cocc., **Colch.**, Coloc. *Con.*, Croc., Cup., *Cyc.*, Dig., *Dros.*, **Dulc.**, *Euphorb.*, *Fer.*, **Graph.**, *Guai.*, Hell., **Hep.**, Hyos., *Ign.*, *Iod.*, Ip., K. CARB., K. nit., Kre., Lach., Laur., Led., LYC., **Mag. c.**, **Mag. m.**, **Mang.**, Mar., Meny., MERC., *Mez.*, Mos., **Mur. ac.**, **Nat. c.**, **Nat. m.**, NIT. AC., *Nux v.*, *Oleand.*, Par., Petrol., **Phos.**, *Pho. ac.*, Plat., *Pb.*, **Puls.**, Ran. b., Rheum, RHODO., *Rhus*, **Ruta**, Saba., *Sabi.*, *Samb.*, *Sars.*, Sec. c., *Sele.*, *Seneg.*, SEP., SIL., *Spig.*, Spo., Squ., **Stan.**, STAPH., STRO., SUL., Sul. ac., Tar., *Thuj.*, Valer., Verat. a. *Verb.*, Vio. o., Vio. t., ZINC.

—**Outward.**—*All. c.*, *Amm. c.*, **Bell.**, Bov., **Bry.**, **Calc. c.**, Cannab s., *Caust.*, **Cocc.**, Cyc., *Elaps.*, Euphorb., *Ip.*, Mang., Mez., Mur. ac., Nat. c., *Par.*, Pho. ac., PRU., **Puls.**, **Rhus**, Sil., Spig., Spo., Stram.

—**Upward.**—*Acon.*, *Alum.*, **Anac.**, Ant. cr., *Arn.*, **Ars.**, *Asaf.*, *Aur.*, BELL., Bism., Bor., *Calc. c.*, Carb. v., *Caust.*, Chin., Clem., *Colch.*, **Con.**, Dulc., Euphr., *Mag. c.*, Meny., Merc., **Nat. c.**, *Nat. m.*, **Nit. ac.**, **Nux v.**, Phos., Pho. ac., *Puls.*, Rhodo., *Rhus*, *Samb.*, Sars., SEP., SIL., SPIG., *Spo.*, Stro., Sul., Thuj., *Valer.*

—**Burning, in Joints.**—Carb. v., Nat. c., *Nit. ac.*

— —**In Muscles.**—Bell., **Carb. v.**, Caust., *K. carb.*, Led., Lyc., **Nit. ac.**, Ruta, Sabi., Tar., Zinc.

—**Cramp-like, in Joints.**—*Anac.*, Ars., *Aur.*, Bov., K. carb., OLEAND., Phos., **Plat.**

— —**In Muscles.**—ANAC., Ant. cr., Arg., Asaf., *Aur.*, Bism., **Calc. c.**, *Caust.*, Chel., **Chin.**, *Dulc.*, Euphorb., Graph., Iod., K. carb., *Mang.*, Meny., Mos., **Mur. ac.**, NAT. C., Nat. m., Nux v., **Petrol.**, Phos., Pho. ac., **PLAT.**, Ran. b., *Ruta*, Samb., *Sil.*, **Stan.**, Stro., Thuj., *Valer.*

—**Jerking, in Joints.**—Acon., *Caust.*, CHIN., Cup., Laur., Mang., Oleand., RHUS., **Sul.**

— —**In Muscles.**—*Acon.*, Agar., Agn., Alum., *Bell.*, *Calc. c.*, Camph., CHIN., *Cina*, **Cup.**, Dig., Dulc., Guai., *Lyc.*, Mang., Merc., Nat. c., Phos., *Pho. ac.*, Plat., PULS., Rhus, Spig., **Staph.**, Stro., Sul., Sul. ac.

—**Paralytic, in Joints.**—BELL., Carb. v., Chel., *Chin.*, *Cocc.*, Con., *Dig.*, K. carb., Meny., Nat. m., Nit. ac., Phos., *Sars.*, *Stan.*, STAPH.

— —**In Muscles.**—Agn., Ant. cr., Asaf., Carb. v., **Chin.**, Cic., **Cina**,

Cocc., Con., Dig., *Graph.*, **Hell.**, K. **CARB.**, *Mez.*, *Mos.*, Nat. m., Nit. **ac.**, Phos., **Sabi.**, **Sars.**, Seneg., Sil., *Stan.*, Verb.

Tearing, Pressing, in Joints.—Agn., Anac., *Arg.*, Bism., CARB.V., *Chin.*, Coloc., *Graph.*, Guai., K. *carb.*, *Lyc.*, Mez., Pho. ac., Ruta, Saba., Sars., Sep., *Stan.*, Staph., Zinc.

—— **In Muscles.**— Acon., Ambr., Anac., Ant. cr., *Arg.*, Arn., Asar., *Bism.*, *Camph.*, Cannab. s., CARB. V., Caust., *Chin.*, Colch., Cup., Cyc., Dig., Euphorb., Guai., **K. carb.**, K. nit., Laur., Led., *Lyc.*, *Mar.*, Pho. ac., Ran. b., Ruta, Sabi., Sars., Sep., Spig., STAN., **Staph.**, Stro., Sul. Vio. t., Zinc.

—**Sticking, in Joints.**—Agn., Bar. c., Chin., *Colch.*, Dulc., Graph., *Hyos.*, LED., Mag. c., Merc., Mur. ac., Nat. c., Nat. m., Puls., *Sabi.*, Sep., Staph., Zinc.

—— **In Muscles.**—Acon., Agn., Ambr., Ant. t., Arg., Arn., Bar. c., Bell., Bry., *Camph.*, Cannab. s., Canth., Caps., *Chin.*, *Cic.*, **Colch.**, Coloc., Con., Dros., Dulc., **Euphorb.**, Guai., Hyos., Ign., *Iod.*, *K. carb.*, **Lyc.**, Mag. c., Mang., Mar., *Merc.*, Mur. ac., Nat. m., Phos., *Pho. ac.*, Rheum, Sars., Spo., *Staph.*, Sul., *Thuj.*, ZINC.

Tension, Externally.—*Acon.*, *Agar.*, Agn., *Aloe*, **Alum.**, Ambr., *Am. carb.*, **Am. m.**, *Anac.*, Ant. cr., Ant. t., *Arg.*, **Arn.**, Ars., **Asaf.**, Asar., **Aur.**, BAR. C., **Bell.**, Bism., *Bor.*, Bov., **BRY.**, *Calc. c.*, Camph., Cannab. s., **Canth.**, Caps., **Carb. an.**, Carb. v., CAUST., *Cham.*, **Chel.**, *Chin.*, Cic., Clem., Cocc., *Colch.*, COLOC., CON., Croc., *Crotal.*, **Cup.**, *Dig.*, Dros., Dulc., *Euphorb.*, Euphr., Fer., *Glon.*, Graph., Guai., Hell., Hep., Hyos., Ign., Iod., Ip., **K. carb.**, K. nit., *Kre.*, Lach., Laur., **Led.**, *Lyc.*, Mag. c., *Mag. m.*, Mang., Mar., *Meny.*, **Merc.**, **Mez.**, *Mos.*, *Mur. ac.*, *Nat. c.*, Nat. m., *Nit. ac.*, *Nux m.*, **Nux v.**, Oleand., Op., *Par.*, Petrol., PHOS., *Pho. ac.*, **PLAT.**, Pb, **PULS.**, Ran. b., **Rheum**, *Rhodo.*, RHUS, Ruta, *Saba.*, **Sabi.**, Samb., *Sars.*, Sec. c., Seneg., **Sep.**, *Sil.*, Spig., Spo., Squ., *Stan.*, **Staph.**, Stram., STRO., SUL., Sul. ac., Tar., Thuj., Valer., *Verat. a.*, VERB., **Vio. o.**, Vio. t., **Zinc.**

—**Internally.**—*Acon.*, *Aconin.*, *Aesc.*, *Agar.*, Agn., *Alum.*, Ambr., Am. m., Anac., Ant. cr., **Ant. t.**, Arg., Arn., **Ars.**, ASAF., Asar., **Aur.**, *Bar. c.*, **BELL**, Berb., Bov., *Bry.*, **Calc. c.**, Camph., **Cannab. s.**, **Caps.**, **Carb. ac.**, Carb. an., *Carb. v.*, **Caust.**, *Cham.*, **Chel.**, *Chin.*, Cic., **Clem.**, Cocc., *Coc. c.*, *Coff.*, *Colch.*, **Coloc.**, *Com.*, *Con.*, Croc., *Crot. tig.*, **Cup.**, Cyc., *Dig.*, Dros., **Dulc.**, Euphorb., Euphr., *Fer.*, **Gel.**, Glon., **Graph.**, Hell., Hep., *Hyd. ac.*, **Hyper.**, Hyos., *Ign.*, Iod., Ip., *K. carb.*, **K. nit.**, Kre., Lach., Laur., Led., *Lob. i.*, LYC., Mag. c., *Mag. m.*, Mang., Mar., *Meny.*, **Merc.**, *Mez.*, *Mos.*, *Mur. ac.*, *Naj.*, *Nat. c.*, *Nat. m.*, **Nit. ac.**, *Nux m.*,

NUX V., Oleand., *Op.*, *Osm.*, PAR., Petrol., PHOS., Pho. ac., *Plat.*, Pb., PULS., RAN. B., Ran. s., Rheum, *Rhodo.*, Rhus, Ruta, Saba., Sabi., Samb., Sec. c., Seneg., SEP., *Sil.*, Spig., *Spo.*, Squ., Stan., Staph., Stram., STRO., SUL., Sul. ac., *Tab.*, Tar., Thuj., Valer., Verat. a., Verb., Zinc.

Tension In Joints.—*Acon.*, Anac., Ant. t., **Arg.**, *Arn.*, *Ars.*, Asaf., Bell., Bov., BRY., Calc. c., **Caps.**, *Carb. an.*, *Carb. v.*, CAUST., Cham., Colch., *Coloc.*, Con., **Croc.**, Dig., *Dros.*, *Euphorb.*, Euphr., *Graph.*, Hell., Hep., Iod., **K. carb.**, K. nit., Kre., Lach., *Laur.*, **Led.**, LYC., Mag. c., Mang., Mar., Merc., Mez., *Mur. ac.*, NAT. M., Nit. ac., *Nux v.*, Par., *Petrol.*, *Phos.*, Plat., PULS., *Rheum*, **Rhodo.**, RHUS, Ruta, Samb., Seneg., SEP., Sil., Spig., *Spo.*, **Stan.**, SUL., *Sul. ac.*, Verat. a., Verb., Zinc.

—Muscles.—ACON., Am. m., *Anac.*, Ant. cr., **Arn.** *Ars.*, Bell., *Cannab. i.*, Cannab. s., *Canth.*, *Carb. v.*, *Caust.*, Chin., *Dulc.*, Graph., **Guai.**, *K. carb.*, Lach., **Led.**, **Mos.**, Nat. c., **Nat. m.**, NIT. AC., NUX V., Oleand., PHOS., *Pho. ac.*, **Plat.**, Pb., Puls., Rhus, SEP., Sil., **Stan.**, Staph., Sul., Verb., Zinc.

Threads.—Bry., *Ign.*, Lach., Osm., Par., Plat., VALER.

Throbbing (Including "Klopfen" and "Pulsiren," of Bœnninghausen, Externally.—Acon., Agar., Alum., Ambr., Am. carb., Am. m., *Anac.*, Ant. t., **Arg.**, *Arn.*, Ars., Asaf., Bar. c., *Bell.*, *Berb.*, *Bov.*, *Brom.*, *Bry.*, CALC. C., *Calc. ph.*, *Cannab. s.*, Canth., Carb. v., *Carb. sul.*, Caust., *Cham.*, Chel., *Chin.*, Cina, *Clem.*, *Cocc.*, Coc. c., *Coff.*, **Coloc.**, Con., Croc., Dig., Dros., Dulc., Euphr., Fl. ac., *Gel.*, GLON., Graph., Guai., *Hell.*, Hep., *Hyos.*, Ign., K. bi., K. CARB., K. nit., Kre., LACH., Laur., Lyc., *Mag. c.*, *Mag. m.*, Mang., *Mar.*, Merc., Mez., Mur. ac., **Nat. c.**, **Nat. m.**, Nit. ac., Nux m., Nux v., OLEAND., *Op.*, Par., *Petrol.*, Phos., *Pho. ac.*, *Phys.*, Plat., Pb., *Puls.*, Ran. b., Rheum, Rhodo., *Rhus*, Ruta, SABA., Sabi., Samb., *Sars.*, Sec. c., Seneg., **Sep.**, **Sil.**, *Spig.*, *Spo.*, Squ., Stan., Staph., Still., Stram., Stro., SUL., Sul. ac., Tar., Thuj., Verat. a., Zinc.

—Internally.—ACON, *Aconin.*, *Aeth.*, *Agar.*, *Aloe*, ALUM., Ambr., Am. carb., Am. m., Amyl, *Anac.*, Ant. cr., ANT. T., Arg. n., *Arn.*, Ars., **Asaf.**, *Asar.*, Aur., Bar. c., Bell., Bor., *Bov.*, BRY., Cact., *Calad.*, CALC. C., *Calc. ph.*, Camph., CANNAB. I., Cannab. s., *Canth.*, **Caps.**, Carb. an., *Carb. v.*, Carb. sul., *Caust.*, Ced., Cham., Chel., *Chin.*, Cic., COCC., Coff., Colch., Coloc., Con., Croc., Crotal., Crot. tig., Cyc., **Dig.**, Dros., *Dulc.*, FER., *Gel.*, GLON., *Graph.*, *Hell.*, Hep., *Hyos.*, Ign., Iod., Ip., K. carb., K. nit., Kre., Lach., **Laur.**, Led., *Lyc.*, Mag. c., *Mag. m.*, Mang., MELI., Merc., Merc. c., Mez., Mos., *Murex*, Nat. c., **Nat. m.**,

Nit. ac., Nux m., **Nux v.**, Oleand., *Op., Par., Petrol.*, **PHOS., Pho. ac.,** *Phys., Pic. ac.,* **Plant.**, Plat., Pb., **Pso.**, **PULS.**, *Ran. b.,* Rheum, *Rhodo.,* **Rhus**, Ruta, **Saba.**, Sabi., **Sang.**, Sars., Sec. c., Sele., *Seneg.*, **SEP.**, **SIL.**, **Spig.**, Spo., Stan., **Stram.**, Sul., Sul. ac., **Thuj.**, *Verat. a., Verat v.,* Verb., Zinc.

Throbbing In Joints.—*Am. m.*, *Arg.*, Brom., Dros., **Merc.**, Mez., Oleand., Pho. ac., *Rhodo., Rhus,* **Ruta**, *Saba.,* Spig., *Thuj.*

Thrusts (Pushing Pain).—Acon., **Agar.**, Alum., *Am. carb.,* Am. m., **Anac.**, *Ant. t.,* **ARN.**, *Asaf., Asar.,* Aur., *Bar. c.,* **Bell.**, *Bov., Bry.,* *Calc. c., Camph.,* **Cannab. s.,** *Caust.,* Cham., *Chin.,* Cic., **CINA**, *Clem.,* Cocc., Colch., **Con.**, **Croc.**, *Cyc.,* Dig., Dros., **Dulc.**, *Euphorb.,* Fer., Graph., **Hell.**, *Hep.,* Hyos., **Ign.**, Iod., *Ip.,* K. carb., K. nit., Lach., Mang., Mar., Merc., **Mez.**, **Mur. ac.**, Nat. c., **Nat. m.**, Nux m., *Nux v.,* Oleand., Par., Petrol., **PLAT.**, Puls., Rhodo., Rhus, **RUTA**, Samb., Sars., Spig., Squ., Stan., Sul., **SUL. AC.**, Tar., *Verat. a.,* Vio. o., Vio. t.

Tickling Internally.—See Itching Internally.

Touch, Illusions Of.—Acon., **Alum.**, Anac., *Arn., Ars.,* **Asaf.**, Asar., *Bar. c.,* **Bell.**, Bism., *Bor.,* Bov., *Bry.,* **Calc. c.,** Cannab. s., Canth., Caps., *Caust.,* Chel., *Cocc., Coc. c.,* Coloc., **Con.**, **Croc.**, Dros., Dulc., *Graph.,* Guai., **Hell.**, *Hep.,* Hyos., **Ign.**, Iod., K. carb., *K. nit.,* **Kre.**, Lach., Laur., *Lyc.,* Mag. c., Mag. m., Meny., Merc., *Mos.,* Nat. c., Nat. m., Nux m., *Nux v.,* Oleand., **Op.**, **Par.**, Phos., Pho. ac., Plat., Pb., **Puls.**, *Ran. b., Ran. s.,* Rheum, *Rhodo.,* **RHUS**, Ruta, *Saba.,* Samb., Seneg., *Sep.,* Sil., **Spig.**, *Spo.,* Squ., Staph., **Stram.**, **Sul.**, *Sul. ac.,* Tar., Thuj., *Valer.,* Verat. a., Verb.

Trembling, Externally.—*Abrot., Abs., Ac. ac.,* **Acon.**, *Acon. f.,* Agar., *Agn.,* Alum., *Ambr.,* Am. carb., Am. m., *Amyl,* **Anac.**, Ant. cr., **Ant. t.**, Apis, **ARG. N.**, **Arn.**, **Ars.**, *Asaf.,* Aur., Bar. c., **Bell.**, Bism., **Bor.**, Bov., **Bry.**, *Buf., Cud., Calad.,* **Calc. c.,** Camph., **Cannab. s.,** Canth., **Caps.**, Carb. ac., Carb. v., *Carb. sul.,* **Caust.**, Cham., Chel., *Chin.,* **CIC.**, **CIMIC.**, **Cina**, *Clem.,* Cocc., *Cod., Coff.,* Colch., Coloc., **CON.**, Croc., **Crotal.**, **Crot. tig.**, Cup., *Cur.,* Dig., *Dios.,* Dros., **Dulc.**, Euphr., *Fer.,* **GEL.**, *Glon.,* Graph., **Hep.**, **Hyos.**, *Ign.,* Iod., *K. br.,* *K. carb.,* *Kalm.,* Kre., Lach., Laur., Led., *Lyc.,* Mag. c., Mag. m., Mang., Mar., Meny., **MERC.**, **Merc. c.**, **Mez.**, Mos., Nat. c., **Nat. m.**, Nit. ac., Nux m., **Nux v.**, Oleand., *Onos.,* **OP.**, Par., Petrol., **Phos.**, Pho. ac., **PLAT.**, Pb., **Pso.**, **PULS.**, Ran. b., Ran. s., Rheum, Rhodo., **RHUS**, *Ruta,* Saba., Sabi., Samb., *Sars.,* Sec. c., Seneg., Sep., Sil., Spig., Spo., *Stan.,* Staph., **STRAM.**, *Stro.,* **SUL.**, *Sul. ac., Turent., Thea.,* **Thuj.**, Valer., **Verat. a.**, Verb., Vio. o., **Zinc.**

SENSATIONS.

Trembling, Internally.—Ambr., **Ant. t.**, **Arg. n.**, Asaf., **Bell.**, **Brach.**, *Bry.*, Calad., CALC. C., *Camph.*, *Caps.*, *Carb. v.*, *Carb. sul.*, **Caust.**, Cina, Cocc., Colch., Con., Crotal., Cyc. Eup. per., Graph., IOD., K. carb., *K. nit.*, Kre., *Lil. t.*, **Lyc.**, **Mar.**, Merc., *Mos.*, **Nat. m.**, Nit. ac., *Nux m.*, **Nux v.**, *Par.*, Petrol., **Phos.**, *Plat.*, **Puls.**, RHUS, Ruta, Saba., *Sabi.*, Samb., **Sep.**, *Sil.*, **Spig.**, Stan., STAPH., Stro., Sul., Sul. ac., Valer.

Trickling Sensation, Like Drops.—Ambr., Arn., Bell., CANNAB. S., Sep., Spig., *Thuj.*, Verat. a.

Twingings.—*Aloe*, *Alum.*, AM. M., Ant. cr., *Apis*, *Aur.*, Bell., *Berb.*, Bov., *Canth.*, *Carb. an.*, *Caust.*, Chel., *Cocc.*, *Coloc.*, Crot. tig., Dros., Iod., K. carb., LAUR., Lyc., Mag. c., *Mag. m.*, Merc., MOS., Mur. ac., *Phos.*, Pho. ac., *Plant.*, PB., *Pru.*, *Rhus*, Sabi., Sars., Seneg., Sil., Staph., *Stro.*, Sul. ac., **Valer.**

Twistings.—Agar., Alum., Am. m., Anac., Ant. cr., Ant. t., Arg. n., Ars., *Asaf.*, *Bar. c.*, **Bell.**, *Berb.*, **Bry.**, Calad., Calc. c., **Caps.**, *Canth.*, *Cham.*, Cina, Con., Dig., **Dios.**, Dros., Dulc., **Ign.**, Ip., *K. nit.*, Led., **Merc.**, *Mez*, Nat. c., *Nat. m.*, *Nux m.*, Nux v., Oleand., Ox. ac., Phos., Pho. ac., **Plat.**, Pb., *Pod.*, Ran. b., Ran. s., Rhus, Ruta, Saba., Sabi., Sars., Seneg., Sep., SIL., *Staph.*, Sul., *Sul. ac.*, *Valer.*, VERAT. A.

Twitchings, Externally.—Acon., Agar., Agn., *Alum.*, Ambr., *Am. carb.*, *Am. m.*, Ant. cr., Ars., ASAF., *Atrop.*, *Bar. c.*, Bell., Bov., Brom., Bry., *Buf.*, **Calc. c.**, *Camph.*, *Cannab. i.*, Canth., *Caps.*, *Carb. ac.*, Carb. v., *Caust.*, Chel., Chen. a., Chin., Cic., *Cina*, Cimic., *Clem.*, Cod., Colch., Coloc., Con., Croc., Crotal., Cup., Dros., Graph., *Guai.*, Hell., *Hyos.*, *Ign.*, Ip., *K. br.*, K. CARB., Kre., Lyc., *Mag. m.*, Meny., Merc., MEZ., Mur. ac., NAT. C., Nat. m., Nux v., *Op.*, *Ox. ac.*, *Par.*, Petrol., *Phos.*, Plat., Pb., Puls., *Rhodo.*, Rhus, Ruta, Sabi., Sele., Seneg., Sep., Sil., **Spig.**, Stan., STRAM., Stro., *Sul.*, Tan., Tar., Thuj., *Valer.*, Vio. t., ZINC.

—**Internally.**—*Atrop.*, Bov., **Cannab. s.**, Seneg.

—**Of Muscles.**—*Acon.*, *Ambr.*, Ant. cr., **Ant. t.**, **Arg.**, Arn, *Ars.*, Asaf., Asar., Bar. c., **Bell.**, Bism., Bov., *Bry.*, Calc. c., Cannab. s., Carb. v., *Carb. sul.*, *Caust.*, Cham., Chin., Cic., **Clem.**, *Cocc.*, Cod., Coloc., Con., Croc., Cup., Dig., Graph., Hell., *Hyos.*, *Ign.*, IOD., Ip., *K. br.*, K. CARB., Lach., Laur., Mang., *Mar.*, Meny., Merc., MEZ., Nat. c., *Nat. m.*, Nit. ac., Nux v., Oleand., Op., Par., Phos., *Plat.*, Pb., Puls., *Ran. s.*, *Raph.*, Rheum, Rhus, Sec. c., Sep., Sil., *Spig.*, Spo., Stan., Sul., *Sul. ac.*, *Tar.*, Vio. t.

Ulcerative Pain, Externally. (Compare **Festering, Pains as From.**)—Acon., Agar., Alum., *Ambr.*, *Am. carb.*, AM. M., Anac., Ant. cr., Arg., Arn., Ars., Aur., Bar. c., *Bell.*, Bov., BRY., Camph., Cannab.

194 SENSATIONS.

?., **Canth.,** *Caps.,* Carb. an., Carb. v., **Caust.,** *Ced.. Cham., Chin.,* **Cic.,** *Cocc.,* Colch., Cyc., *Dros.,* Dulc., Fer., **Graph.,** *Hep.,* **Ign., K. carb.,** *K. nit.,* Kre., Lach., Laur., *Mag. c., Mag. m.,* **Mang.,** Mar., **Merc., Mur. ac.,** *Nat. c.,* **Nat. m.,** Nit. ac., **Nux v.,** *Petrol., Phos.,* Pho. ac., *Plut.,* PULS., RHUS, *Ruta, Sars.,* **Sep.,** SIL., *Spig., Spo., Staph.,* Sul., *Sul. ac.,* Thuj., Verat. a., Zinc.

Ulcerative Pain, Internally.—Acon., **Am. carb., Arg. n., Ars., Bell.,** *Bor., Bov.,* **Bry., Cannab. s.,** *Canth.,* **Caps.,** *Carb. an.,* Carb. v., *Carb. sul.,* **Caust.,** *Cham.,* Chel., *Cocc.,* **Coloc.,** *Cup.,* Dig., **Gam.,** *Hell., Hep.,* K. carb., *Kre.,* LACH., *Laur., Mag. c., Mag. m., Mang.,* **Merc.,** *Mur. ac.,* Nit. ac., **Nux v.,** Phos., Pho. ac., **Pso.,** PULS., *Ran. b.,* **Rhus,** *Ruta,* Saba., Sep., *Sil., Spig., Stan., Staph.,* Stro., **Sul.,** Valer., *Verat. a.*

Undulating Pains.—Acon., *Anac.,* Ant. t., Arn., *Asaf.,* Chin., *Cocc.,* Dulc., Mar., Mez., Oleand., Plat., Rhodo., Sep., Spig., Vio. t.

Unsteadiness (Staggering).—*Acon.,* Agar., Agn., Alum., Ant. t., **Arn., Ars., Asar.,** Aur., **Bell.,** Bism., Bry., Camph., *Carb. sul., Caust.,* Cham., Chel., *Chin.,* **Cic.,** *Cina,* COCC., Coff., Colch., Cup., Cyc., *Dig.,* Dulc., Euphorb., Fer., Hep., *Hyos., Ign.,* Ip., **K. carb.,** K. nit., Lach., *Lyc.,* Meny., Merc., Nat. c., **Nat. m.,** Nit. ac., Nux m., **Nux v.,** Oleand., Op., *Ox. ac., Par.,* Petrol., *Phos.,* Pho. ac., Plat., Pb., Ran. s., Rhodo., Rhus, Ruta, Saba., *Sabi., Sele.,* Sep., Sil., Spig., *Spo., Stan.,* **Staph.,** Stram., *Sul.,* **Tar.,** VERAT. A., *Vio. o.,* Vio. t., Zinc.

Valve in the Throat, Sensation of.—*Iod.,* **Spo.**

Veins. See under **Circulation.**

Vibrations.—Am. carb., BELL., Bism., *Caps., Caust., Clem.,* Con., *Dig.,* Hep., Hyos., Ign., *Iod.,* K. carb., K. nit., *Lyc., Mag. o.,* Mos., **Nit. ac.,** *Nux v.,* Petrol., Sars., **Sep.,** *Sil.,* Stan., *Stro.,* SUL., Verb.

Warm Feeling.—Agar., Agn., Alum., Am. carb., Ant. t., Ars., Asaf., Asar., Bov., *Bry.,* Calc. c., Camph., CANNAB. S., *Canth.,* Caps., *Caust.,* Chel., *Chin.,* Cina, *Cocc.,* COFF., Colch., *Croc.,* Cyc., *Euphorb.,* Graph., *Hell.,* Ign., **Iod.,** Ip., *K. carb.,* K. nit., Kre., **Laur.,** Mag. c., *Mag. m.,* **Mang.,** Mar., Merc., *Nat. c.,* Nat. m., Nux m., **Nux v.,** *Phos.,* Pho. ac., Plat., **Puls.,** Ran. b., Rheum, Rhodo., *Rhus,* **Saba.,** Sabi., *Sumb.,* Sars., *Sec. c.,* Seneg., Staph., Sul., SUL. AC., *Thuj.,* Valer., **Verat. a.,** Zinc.

Washing, Dread Of.—AM. CARB., *Am. m.,* ANT. CR., Bar. c., **Bell.,** Bor., Bov., Bry., Calc. c., **Canth.,** Carb. v., **Cham.,** CLEM., Con., *Dulc., K. carb.,* K. nit., Laur., Lyc., Mag. c., Merc., **Mez.,** Mur. ac., Nat. c., *Nit. ac., Nux m.,* Nux v., Phos., **Puls.,** RHUS, **Sars.,** SEP., Sil., SPIG., Stan., **Staph.,** Stro., SUL., *Sul. ac.,* Zinc.

SENSATIONS.

Water Dashing Against Inner Parts, Sensation of.—*Bell.*, Cina, CROT. TIG., *Dig.*, Fer., Hell., *Laur.*, *Pho. ac.*, Rhodo., Spig.

Water, Dread Of.—Ars., BELL., Coloc., Canth., *Cup.*, HYOS., Iod., Lach., Merc., Phos., Ruta, *Saba.*, STRAM.

Weakness. (Consult **Weariness and Debility.**)—*Ab. c.*, *Abrot.*, *Ac. ac.*, **Acon.**, *Acon. f.*, **Aconin.**, **Aesc.**, **Agar.**, *Agn.*, **Ail.**, *All. c.*, **Aloe**, *Alum.*, **Ambr.**, *Am. carb.*, *Am. m.*, **Anac.**, Ant. cr., ANT. T., **Apis**, **Arg.**, Arg. n., ARN., ARS., *Ars. iod.*, Asaf., Asar., Bap., Bar. ac., *Bar. c.*, **Bell.**, Bism., Bor., *Bov.*, *Brom.*, **Bry.**, *Buf.*, *Cact.*, *Caj.*, *Calad.*, CALC. C., **Calc. ph.**, Camph., *Cannab. i.*, **Cannab. s.**, Canth., Caps., *Carb. ac.*, Carb. an., *Carb. v.*, *Carb. sul.*, Caust., *Ced.*, **Cham.**, Chel., CHIN., **Cic.**, Cina, Clem., *Coca*, Cocc., *Coff.*, Colch., Coloc., Com., **CON.**, Corn. c., Croc., CROTAL., Crot. tig., Cup., *Cur.*, Cyc., **Dig.**, Dros., **Dulc.**, *Equis.*, *Eucal.*, *Eup. per.*, Euphorb., Euphr., FER., GEL., *Glon.*, **Gran.**, Graph., Guai., Hell., *Helo.*, Hep., **Hyd. ac.**, Hyos., Ign., IOD., **Ip.**, *K. bi.*, K. CARB., *K. chl.*, *K. nit.*, K. iod., *Kalm.*, Kre., Lach., *Laur.*, **Led.**, LYC., Mag. c., Mag. m., Mang., Mar., Meny., MERC., MERC. C., MERC. CY., Mez., *Mos.*, MUR. AC., *Nat. c.*, NAT. M., NIT. AC., **Nux m.**, NUX V., Oleand., Op., Par., Petrol., PHOS., PHO. AC., **Phyt. Pic. ac.**, **Plat.**, PB., *Pso.*, **Puls.**, RAN. B., *Ran. s.*, **Rheum**, **Rhodo.**, RHUS, Rumex, Ruta, Saba., Sabi., Samb., Sang., Sars., SEC. C., Sele., Seneg., SEP., SIL., *Spig.*, SPO., SQU., STAN., Staph., Stram., *Stro.*, Strop., SUL., SUL. AC., TAB., Tar., TELL., TER., *Thea*, Thuj., Valer., VERAT. A., **Verat. v.**, Verb., Vio. t., **Zinc.**

—**Of Joints.**—ACON., Agar., Agn., Alum., *Am. carb.*, Anac., Ant. t., ARN., Asar., Aur., Bar. c., *Bell.*, *Bor.*, *Bov.*, Bry., CALC. C., Cannab. s., Canth., Carb. an., Carb. v., **Caust.**, Chin., Clem., *Cocc.*, Colch., Con., Cup., Cyc., *Dig.*, Dros., Dulc., Euphorb., **Fer.**, Hep., Hyos., Ign., K. CARB., K. nit., Kre., Lach., **Led.**, LYC., Mang., MERC., *Mez.*, *Mos.*, **Nat. m.**, Nit. ac., Nux m., **Nux v.**, Oleand., *Oxyt.*, Par., Petrol., **Phos.**, Pho. ac., *Plat.*, Pb., PSO., *Puls.*, Ran. b., Rheum, *Rhodo.*, RHUS, *Ruta*, Saba., Sars., SEP., Sil., Spo., *Stan.*, **Staph.**, *Stro.*, SUL., Sul. ac., Tar., Thuj., *Valer.*, **Verat. a.**, Vio. o., *Zinc.*

—**Nervous.**—*Acon.*, Agn., **Alum.**, Ambr., Am. carb., Arn., *Ars.*, **Asar.**, Aur., Bar. c., Bell., Bry., **Calc. c.**, Camph., Carb. an., Carb. v., *Carb. sul.*, *Cham.*, CHIN., Cic., Cocc., Coff., Colch., Con., Croc., Cup., *Cur.*, Dig., Graph., Hell., *Hep.*, Hyos., Ign., Iod., K. nit., Lach., *Laur.*, Led., **Lyc.**, Mar., Merc., Mos., Mur. ac., **Nat. c.**, *Nat. m.*, Nit. ac., Nux m., NUX V., Op., Petrol., PHOS., *Pho. ac.*, **Plat.**, **Pb.**, PULS., *Rhus*, Sabi.,

Sars., Sec. c., *Sele.*, *Sep.*, SIL., Spig., Spo., **Stan.**, Staph., *Stram.*, **Sul.**, Sul. ac., **Valer.**, Verat. a., Vio. o., Zinc.

Weakness, Paralytic.—Alum., *Am. m.*, Ars., *Bell.*, **Bism.**, *Bry.*, Calc. c., Camph., *Canth.*, Carb. v., **Caust.**, Cham., *Chel.*, Chin., Cina, COCC., **Colch.**, *Con.*, *Dig.*, *Dros.*, Euphorb., *Fer.*, *Hell.*, K. nit., Laur., Merc., Mez., Mos., Nat. c., *Nux v.*, Oleand., Pho. ac., Pb., **Puls.**, **Rhodo.**, Rhus, *Saba.*, *Sil.*, Stan., Stro., Valer., *Verat. a.*

Weariness. (Compare with **Weakness.**)—Alum., Acon., Agar., Ambr., *Am. carb.*, *Anac.*, Ant. cr., **Ant. t.**, *Arg.*, Arn., Ars., Ars. iod., Asaf., *Asar.*, Aur., Bar. c., *Bell.*, *Bism.*, Bov., **Bry.**, **Calc. c.**, **Calc. ph.**, Camph., CANNAB. S., Canth., Caps., **Carb. ac.**, Carb. an., Caust., Cham., Chel., *Chin.*, Cic., *Cimic.*, *Cina*, *Clem.*, *Cocc.*, **Coc. c.**, *Coff.*, Colch., Coloc., **Con.**, CROC., Cyc., Dig., Dros., *Dulc.*, Euphorb., Euphr., Fer., *Fer. ph.*, GEL., *Graph.*, **Ham.**, Hell., *Helo.*, **Hep.**, **Hyos.**, *Ign.*, Ip., *K. carb.*, K. nit., *Kre.*, Lach., Laur., *Led.*, *Lyc.*, **Mag. c.**, Mang., Mar., Meny., **Merc.**, *Mez.*, Mos., Mur. ac., *Nat. c.*, Nat. m., Nit. ac., *Nux m.*, Nux v., Oleand., Op., **Par.**, Petrol., *Phos.*, Pho. ac., PIC. AC., **Plat.** Pb., PULS., Ran. b., Rheum, Rhodo., **Rhus**, RUTA, *Saba.*, Sabi., S. nb., Sars., Sec. c., *Seneg.*, SEP., Sil., Spig., *Spo.*, Squ., *Stan.*, *Staph.*, Stram., Stro., **Sul.**, Sul. ac., *Thuj.*, Valer., **Verat. a.**, Verb., Vio. o., ZINC.

Wedge, Sensation of. (Compare **Plug.**)—Ant. cr., *Apoc. c.*, Bov., Caust., Dros., Par., *Spo.*, *Thuj.*

Whirling.—Ant. t., *Arg.*, Croc., *Nux v.*, Petrol., Ran. b., *Saba.*, Sep., Sil., Sul., Tar.

Whiteness (of Parts Usually Red).—Ambr., Anac., *Ars.*, BOR., *Calc. c.*, Canth., Caust., Coloc., *Fer.*, HELL., *K. carb.*, Lyc., MERC., **Merc. c.**, Nat. c., **Nit. ac.**, Nux v., *Oleand.*, Op., *Petrol.*, *Phos.*, **Pb.**, Puls., Sabi., Sec. c., Sep., **Staph.**, *Sul.*, **Sul. ac.**, *Valer.*, *Verat. a.*, Vio. t., Zinc.

Wind, Sensation of.—Canth., Chel., **Coral**, Graph., Nux v., *Oleand.*, Puls., Rhus, Sabi., Spig., Squ., Stram.

—**Cold.**—*Camph.*, *Croc.*, **Laur.**, Mos., *Rhus*, Samb.

Wooden Sensation.—K. nit.

Wringing Pain.—Alum., Anac., Ars., Bor., Calc. c., **Dig.**, *Dio.*, K. carb., Merc., *Thuj.*

Glands.

Air Passing Through, Sensation of.—Spo.

Atrophy.—Ars., Cham., *Chin.*, CON. IOD., **K. carb.**, **Nit. ac.**, *Nux m.*, Pho. ac., Sec. c., *Sil.*, Verat. a.

Boring.—Bell., Puls., *Saba.*

GLANDS.

Bruised Pain.—*Arg.*, Arn., *Ars.*, **Carb. an.**, Caust., **Cic.**, CON., *Cup.*, Iod., K. carb., Phos., *Plat.*, **Pso.**, Puls., Rhodo., *Rhus*, Ruta, **Sep.**, Staph., Sul., *Sul. ac.*

Burning.—ARS., **Bell.**, **Cannab. s.**, Carb. v., *Cocc.*, **Hep.**, Laur., Merc., **Phos.**, *Phyt.*, Rheum, *Sil.*

Burrowing.—Acon., Am. m., *Arn.*, Asaf., **Bell.**, Bov., Bry., *Calc. c.*, Dulc., K. carb., Nat. c., *Phos.*, Plat., **Rhodo.**, *Rhus*, Ruta, Sep., *Spig.*, Stan.

Constricting Pain.—Am. carb., *Chin.*, Ign., Nux v., **Puls.**, *Spo.*

Contractions.—Acon., Alum., Arn., *Bell.*, Bor., *Chin.*, Cocc., Con., Ign., Iod., Lyc., *Mang.*, *Nit. ac.*, **Nux v.**, Phos., *Pb.*, *Puls.*, *Rhus*, Sep, *Sul.*, Sul. ac.

Crawling.—*Acon.*, **Arn.**, Cannab. s., *Canth.*, CON., *Merc.*, Nat. c., *Pho. ac.*, **Plat.**, Puls., *Rhodo.*, **Rhus**, *Sabi.*, Sep., Spo., Sul., Zinc.

Creeping.—Bell., Calc. c., *Laur.*, Sep., **Spo.**, Sul.

Cutting.—*Arg.*, **Bell.**, *Calc. c.*, *Con.*, Graph., Ign., **Lyc.**, *Nat. c.*, Pho. ac., **Sep.**, *Sil.*, Staph., Sul.

Gnawing.—Bar. c., Cham., *Mez.*, Pho. ac., **Plat.**, *Ran. s.*, Spo., *Staph.*

Heaviness.—**Bell.**, Chin., *Cup.*, Merc., Nux v., **Phos.**, Puls., *Rhus*, Sil., Stan., Staph., *Sul.*

Indurations.—*Agn.*, *Ambr.*, *Am. carb.*, Ant. cr., *Arn.*, Ars., Aur., **Bar. c.**, BELL., Bov., **Bry.**, *Calc. c.*, *Calc. f.*, Camph., Cannab. s., Canth., Caps., **Carb. an.**, Carb. v., Caust., *Cham.*, Chin., CLEM., Cocc., Coloc., CON., Cup., Cyc., *Dig.*, *Dulc.*, *Fer.*, Graph., Hep., Hyos., Ign., Iod., *K. carb.*, **Lyc.**, **Mag. m.**, Mang., Merc., *Nat. c.*, *Nit. ac.*, Nux v., Petrol., *Phos.*, *Pb.*, Puls., Rhodo., *Rhus*, Sep., *Sil.*, *Spig.*, Spo., *Squ.*, Staph., *Sul.*, Thuj., Verat. a.

Inflammation.—Acon., Arn., *Ars*, Aur., **Bar. c.**, BELL., *Bry.*, Calc. c., Camph., *Canth.*, **Carb. an.**, Carb. v., *Cham.*, *Clem.*, Con., Dulc., *Hep.*, K. carb., Lach., Laur., *Lyc.*, MERC., *Nit. ac.*, **Nux v.**, Petrol., PHOS., Pho. ac., **Pb.**, Puls., *Rhus*, Samb., Sars., **Sil.**, Spig., Squ., *Staph.*, **Sul.**, Sul. ac., Thuj., Verat. a., Zinc.

Injuries.—Arn., Cic., CON., **Dulc.**, *Hep.*, **Iod.**, Merc., **Phos.**, **Puls.**, *Rhus*, Sil., Sul.

Itching.—*Am. carb.*, Anac., Ant. cr., Canth., Carb. an., **Carb. v.**, Caust., Cocc., CON., *K. carb.*, Mag. c., *Merc.*, **Phos.**, Ran. s., Rheum, Rhus, *Sabi.*, Sep., **Sil.**, Spo.

Jerking Pain.—Arn., *Asaf.*, Aur., **Bell.**, Bry., **Calc. c.**, *Caps.*, *Caust.*, Chin., Clem., Graph., Lyc., *Meny.*, Merc., Nat. c., **Nat. m.**, Nit. ac., *Nux v.*, Petrol., **Puls.**, *Rhus*, Sep., Sil., *Sul.*

GLANDS.

Living, Feeling of Something.—Ign., Merc., Rhodo., **Spo.**, Sul.

Numb Feeling.—Anac., Asaf., Bell., Cocc., *Con.*, *Lyc.*, **Plat.**, Puls., Rhus, *Sep.*, Sil., Spo.

Painfulness in General.—Acon., Alum., Ambr., **Am. carb.**, *Ant. cr.*, Ant. t., ARN., *Ars.*, **Aur.**, Bar. c., BELL., *Bry.*, **Calc. c.**, **Cannab. s.**, Canth., **Carb. an.**, *Carb. v.*, **Caust.**, Cham., *Chin.*, *Cic.*, *Clem.*, Coloc., Con., Dulc., *Graph.*, Hell., Hep., Ign., **Iod.**, *K. carb.*, LYC., Mag. c., MERC., *Nat. m.*, **Nit. ac.**, *Nux v.*, *Petrol.*, PHOS., Pho. ac., **Puls.**, Rheum, *Rhus*, Sele., Sep., *Sil.*, **Spig.**, *Spo.*, Squ., Stan., **Staph.**, Stram., Sul., *Sul. ac.*, Thuj., *Verat. a.*

—**Blunt.**—*Asar.*, Carb. v., *Hyos.*, Mur. ac.

Pinching.—*Bry.*, Calc. c., *Meny.*, Mur. ac., **Rhodo.**, Rhus, *Saba.*, Stan., Sul., *Verat. a.*

Pressings.—*Arg.*, *Ars.*, *Aur.*, **Bell.**, Calc. c., Carb. v., *Caust.*, Chin., Cina, Cocc., Cyc., *Ign.*, K. carb., Lyc., Mang., Mar., Meny., **Merc.**, *Osm.*, Par., *Pho. ac.*, Puls., Rheum, Rhus, Sabi., **Spo.**, *Stan.*, **Staph.**, **Stram.**, Sul., Verat. a., *Zinc.*

—**Inward.**—Aur., Calc. c., *Cocc.*, Cyc., Rheum, **Staph.**, Zinc.

—**Outward.**—Arg., Cina, *Ign.*, Lyc., Mang., *Mar.*, Meny., **Merc.**, *Par.*, Puls., *Rhus*, **Spo.**, Sul.

Pulsation.—Am. m., Arn., *Asaf.*, Bell., Bov., Bry., **Calc. c.**, *Caust.*, *Cham.*, Clem., K. carb., *Lyc.*, MERC., Nat. c., *Nit. ac.*, Phos., Rhodo., Saba., *Sep.*, Sil., Sul., Thuj.

Quivering.—Bell., *Calc. c.*, K. carb., *Mez.*, Nat. c., *Sil.*

Sensitiveness.—Arn., **Aur.**, BAR. C., Bell., **Cham.**, Chin., *Clem.*, Cocc., CON., *Crotal.*, Cup., *Graph.*, Hep., Ign., K. carb., Laur., **Lyc.**, Mag. c., *Nat. c.*, Nit. ac., Nux v., *Petrol.*, PHOS., Pho. ac., Puls., **Sep.**, Sil., *Spig.*, Squ., *Sul. ac.*, Zinc.

Smarting.—Alum., Ant. cr., Arn., Bry., Calc. c., Caust., Cic., Clem., Con., *Graph.*, *Hep.*, Ign., K. carb., *Mar.*, Merc., Mez, Nat m., *Nux v.*, Phos., **Plat.**, Puls., Rhus, **Sep.**, Staph., Sul., Sul. ac., Zinc.

Squeezing.—Anac., *Bell.*, **Calc. c.**, *Carb. v.*, Caust., *Chin.*, Iod., K. carb., Lyc., Nat. c., Pho. ac., **Plat.**, *Saba.*, Sep., Sil.

Sticking.—Acon., Agn., *Alum.*, **Am. m.**, Arg., **Arn.**, **Asaf.**, Bar. c., BELL., Bor., Bry., **Calc. c.**, *Carb. an.*, Caust., *Chin.*, Cocc., **Con.**, Cup., Cyc., Euphorb, *Graph.*, Hell., Hep., Ign., Iod., *K. carb.*, Kre., Lach., Lyc., MERC., Mez., *Mur. ac.*, *Nat. c.*, **Nat. m.**, *Nit. ac.*, *Nux v.*, **Phos.**, Pho. ac., Pb., PULS., Ran. s., Rheum, Rhus, Saba., Sep., *Sil.*, Spig., **Spo.**, Stan., *Staph.*, **Sul.**, Sul. ac., *Thuj.*, Verat. a., Zinc.

Swelling.—*Acon.*, Agn., Alum., *Ambr.*, *Am. carb.*, Am. m., Ant. cr.,

GLANDS.

Ant. t., Arg., *Arn.*, **Ars.**, Ars. iod., **Arum. t.**, Asaf., Aur., BAR. C., Bar. m., **BELL.**, Bor., Bov., **Bry.**, Calad., **Calc. c.**, *Calc. ph.*, Camph., Cannab. s., **Canth.**, Caps., **Carb. an.**, *Carb. v.*, **Caust.**, Cham., *Chin.*, Cic., *Cist.*, **Clem.**, Cocc., Coloc., **CON.**, Croc., Cup., **Cyc.**, *Dig.*, Dulc., Euphorb., *Fer.*, Graph., Hell., Hep., Hyos., Ign., *Iod.*, K. carb., K. chl., K. iod., *Lach.*, Led., **LYC.**, Mag. c., **Mag. m.**, Mang., Mar., MERC., *Merc. d*, Merc. i. r., Mez., Mur. ac., **Nat. c.**, **Nat. m.**, NIT. AC., Nux v., Petrol., **PHOS.**, *Pho. ac.*, **Phyt.**, *Pb.*, *Pso.*, **Puls.**, Ran. b., Ran. s., Rhodo., RHUS, Ruta, Saba., Sabi., Samb., Sars., *Sep.*, **Sil.**, *Spig.*, Spo., *Squ.*, Stan., *Staph.*, *Stram.*, Stro., SUL., Sul. ac., **Thuj.**, Verat. a., Vio. o., Zinc.

Swelling, Bluish.—Arn., Ars., *Aur.*, **Carb. an.**, Carb. v., Con., *Hep.*, **Lach.**, Mang., Merc., **Puls.**, Sil., Sul. ac.

—**Cold.**—Ars., Asaf., *Bell.*, **Cocc.**, CON., *Cyc.*, Dulc., Lach., *Rhodo.*, Spig.

—**Hard.**—Agn., Ant. cr., *Arn.*, Ars., *Asaf.*, Bry., *Caust.*, Chin., CON., *Dig.*, Graph., Lach., *Led.*, *Merc.*, Mez., Nux v., **Phos.**, **Puls.**, RHUS, Sabi., *Samb.*, Spo., Stro., Sul.

—**Hot.**—Acon., Am. carb., *Ant. cr., Arn., Asaf.*, BELL., BRY., Calc. c., Canth., **Carb. an.**, Carb. v., *Chin.*, **Clem.**, *Cocc.*, Euphorb., Hep., K. carb., *Led.*, MERC., Nux v., Petrol., PHOS., *Puls.*, *Rhus*, Sars., Sil., Sul.

—**Inflammatory.**—Acon., Agn., Am. carb., *Ant. cr.*, Arn., *Ars.*, Asaf., Bad., Bell., Bor., Bry., *Calc. c.*, **Carb. an.**, *Carb. v.*, Caust., *Cinnab.*, Cocc., Con., Hep., Hyos., Lyc., **Mang.**, MERC., Mez., Mur. ac., Nat. c., *Petrol.*, Phos., *Puls.*, Rhus, Sars., *Sil., Sul.*, Thuj.

—**Like Knotted Cords.**—Calc. c., Dulc., *Hep.*, Iod., Lyc., *Rhus.*

—**Painful.**—*Acon.*, Ant. cr., **Arn.**, *Aur.*, Bell., Calc. c., Canth., **Carb. an.**, *Chin.*, Clem., *Coral.*, Iod., Nit. ac., *Nux v.*, Phyt., Puls., *Rhus*, Sil., *Spig.*, Stan., Staph.

—**Painless.**—Calc. c., Con., *Dulc.*, Ign., *Nit. ac.*, Pho. ac., *Pb.*, Sep., Sil., Staph., *Sul.*

Swollen Feeling.—Ant. cr., *Aur.*, **Bell.**, *Bry.*, Carb. v., Chin., *Clem.*, Con., Dulc., *Hep., Ign.*, K. nit., Lach., *Merc.*, Nit. ac., Nux m., Nux v., PULS., Rhus, *Sabi.*, Spig., Spo., *Staph.*, Zinc.

Suppuration.—Bell., *Calc. c.*, Canth., Coloc., Dulc., HEP., Hyos., Ign., *Kre.*, Lach., Lyc., Merc., Nit. ac., *Petrol.*, Phos., Sars., *Sep.*, SIL., Squ., Sul.

Tearing.—Agn., *Ambr.*, Am. carb., Arn., Bar. c., Bell., Bov., Bry., *Calc. c.*, Cannab. s., **Caps.**, *Carb. an.*, Carb. v., *Caust.*, Cham., CHIN.,

Cocc., Con., Cyc., *Dulc.*, *Fer.*, *Graph.*, *Ign.*, **K. carb.**, Kre., *Lyc.*, *Merc.*, Mez., *Nat. c.*, Nit. ac., *Nux v.*, Phos., *Puls.*, Rhodo., *Rhus*, Sele., *Seneg.*, *Sep.*, Sil., *Sul.*, Thuj., *Zinc.*

Tension.—Alum., Ambr., Arg., *Arn.*, Aur., **Bar. c.**, *Bell.*, *Bov.*, **Bry.**, Calc. c., *Carb. an.*, **Caust.**, *Clem.*, Coloc., Con., Dulc., *Graph.*, *K. carb.*, Lyc., Merc., Mur. ac., Nux v., **PHOS.**, **Puls.**, Rhus, Saba., Sabi., *Sep.*, Sil., **Spo.**, Staph., *Stro.*, **Sul.**, Thuj.

Tickling.—**K. carb.**, Plat.

Ulcerative Pain.—Am. carb., **Am. m.**, Aur., Bell., *Bry.*, Calc. c., Canth., *Caust.*, Cham., Chin., *Cic.*, Cocc., *Graph.*, Hep., *Ign.*, *K. carb.*, Mar., *Merc.*, Mur. ac., Nat. c., *Nat. m.*, Nit. ac., Petrol., PHOS., Puls., Rhus, Ruta, Sil., Staph., Sul. ac., *Zinc.*

Ulcers.—Ambr., Ant. cr., Arn., ARS., Asaf., *Aur.*, **Bell.**, *Calc. c.*, **Canth.**, *Carb. an.*, Carb. v., Caust., Clem., *Coloc.*, Con., Cup., *Dulc.*, Hep., Hyos., Ign., K. carb., *Kre.*, **Lach.**, Lyc., *Merc.*, Nit. ac., PHOS., *Pho. ac.*, Rhus, Sars., Sep., SIL., Spo., Squ., **Sul.**, *Sul. ac.*, *Thuj.*, Zinc.

—**Cancerous.**—Arn., ARS., *Aur.*, **Bell.**, Calc. c., Carb. an., Carb. v., Caust., Clem., CON., **Cup.**, *Dulc.*, **Hep.**, K. carb., **Kre.**, Lyc., Merc., Nit. ac., Phos., Pho. ac., Rhus, **Sep.**, **Sil.**, *Squ.*, SUL., Sul. ac., Zinc.

—**Spongy.**—CARB. AN., *Clem.*, Kre., **Lach.**, **Merc.**, *Nit. ac.*, Rhus, *Sep.*, SIL., **Sul.**, Thuj.

Bones.

Absence of Marrow, Sensation of.—Lyc.

Band, Sensation of.—*Aur.*, Chin., Con., *Graph.*, Kre., *Lyc.*, *Merc.*, *Nat. m.*, NIT. AC., Petrol., *Phos.*, PULS., Saba., *Sil.*, SUL.

Boring.—*Agar.*, *Asaf.*, *Aran.*, *Aur.*, **Bar. c.**, Bell., *Brom.*, Calc. c., *Clem.*, *Dulc.*, *Hell.*, Hep., Lach., *Lyc.*, Mang., **Merc.**, **Mez.**, *Nat. c.*, *Nat. m.*, Phos., Pho. ac., **Puls.**, *Rhodo.*, Rhus, Saba., Sabi., **Sep.**, **Sil.**, Spig., Staph., *Sul.*, Thuj.

Broken, Pain as if.—Aur., Bry., *Cup.*, Hep., **Nat. m.**, Puls., Ruta, *Sep.*, *Ther.*, Verat. a., Vib. op.

Bruised Sensation.—Acon., *Agar.*, **Am. m.**, Asaf., Aur., Bar. c., Bov., Calc. c., Cannab. s., Chin., COCC., **Coral.**, Cup., Graph., HEP., Ign., **Ip.**, Led., Mag. c., Mez., Nat. m., *Nux v.*, Par., Petrol., *Phos.*, **Puls.**, RUTA, Saba., Sep., Sil., Spig., Valer., **Verat. a.**, Zinc.

Burning.—Ars., Asaf., Aur., Bry., *Carb. v.*, Caust., *Euphorb.*, **Form.**, Lach., *Lyc.*, *Merc.*, MEZ., Nat. c., Nit. ac., Par., *Phos.*, **Pho. ac.**, **Puls.**, Rhus, Ruta, Sabi., **Sep.**, Sil., Staph., **Sul.**, Thuj., ZINC.

Burrowing.—*Aran.*, *Asaf.*, Calc. c., **Carb. an.**, **Cocc.**, Dulc., **Mang.**, Rhodo., *Ruta*, Sep., Spig., *Thuj.*

BONES.

Caries.—Ars., ASAF., *Aur.*, Bell., Bry., Calc. c., *Calc. ph.*, Caps., *Chin.*, Clem., *Con.*, Cup., Dulc., *Euphorb.*, Fer., *Fl. ac.*, *Graph.*, *Guai.*, Hep., Iod., *Kre.*, Lach., LYC., MERC., Mez., Nat. m., Nit. ac., Op., Petrol., Phos., Pho. ac., *Puls.*, Rhodo., Rhus, *Ruta*, Sabi., *Sec. c.*, Sep., SIL., Spo., Staph., Sul., *Ther.*, Thuj.

—**Of Periosteum.**—*Ant. cr.*, ASAF., *Aur.*, Bell., Chin., Cyc., Hell., Merc., Mez., PHO. AC., *Puls.*, Rhodo., Rhus, *Ruta*, Sabi., Sil., *Staph.*

Cold Feeling.—Aran., Ars., Calc. c., *Lyc.*, Sep., Sul., Zinc.

Constriction.—Am. m., Anac., *Aur.*, *Chin.*, Cocc., Coloc., Con., Graph., Kre., *Lyc.*, *Merc.*, *Nat. m.*, NIT. AC., *Nux v.*, Petrol., *Phos.*, PULS., Rhodo., Rhus, Ruta, Saba., Sep., *Sil.*, Stro., SUL., Zinc.

Crawling.—Acon., Arn., *Cham.*, Colch., Merc., Nat. c., Nat. m., Nux v., Pho. ac., Plat., Pb., Puls., Rhodo., Rhus, Saba., *Sec. c.*, Sep., Spig., *Sul.*, Zinc.

Curvature. (See **Softening.**)

Cutting in Long Bones.—*Calc. ac.*, *Osm.*, *Saba.*

Drawing as from a Thread Through Shafts.—Bry.

Gnawing.—Am. m., *Arg.*, BELL., *Brom.*, Canth., Dros., Graph., *K. iod.*, Lyc., Mang., *Phos.*, Puls., Ruta, *Samb.*, Staph., Stro.

Gouty Nodes.—*Agn.*, Acon., Ant. cr., Arn., Aur., Bry., CALC. C., *Carb. an.*, Caust., Cic., Cocc., *Colch.*, Dig., Graph., *Hep.*, *Lach.*, Led., LYC., *Meny.*, Merc., Nit. ac., *Puls.*, Rhodo., Rhus, *Sabi.*, Staph., *Sul.*

Healing of Broken Bones Slow.—*Asaf.*, Calc. c., Fer., *Lyc.*, Merc., Mez., *Nit. ac.*, Phos., Pho. ac., Puls., *Ruta*, Sep., Sil., Staph., *Sul.*

Inflammation.—Acon., *Ars.*, Asaf., Aur., Bell., *Bry.*, Calc. c., Chin., *Clem.*, Coloc., *Con.*, Cup., Dig., Euphorb., *Guai.*, Hep., Iod., Kre., Lach., Lyc., Mag. m., *Mang.*, MERC., *Mez.*, Nat. c., Nit. ac., Phos., Pho. ac., Pb., PULS., *Rhus*, Sep., SIL., Spig., STAPH., Sul., Thuj., Verat. a.

—**Of Periosteum.**—Ant. cr., Asaf., Aur., *Bell.*, *Chin.*, Led., Merc., Mez., Pho. ac., *Puls.*, Rhus, *Ruta*, Sil., *Staph.*

Injuries.—Arn., Calc. c., Con., Hep., Iod., Phos., Pho. ac., Puls., Rhus, RUTA, Sil., *Staph.*

Itching.—Cyc., K. nit., *Phos.*, Verat. a.

Jerks.—Phos., Rhodo.

Jerking Pain.—ASAF., Aur., Bell., Calc. c., *Caust.*, Chin., Clem., *Colch.*, Lyc., Merc., Nat. m., Nux v. Petrol., Phos., Puls., Rhodo., Rhus, Sep., Sil., SUL., Valer.

Loosened From Flesh, Feeling as if.—Bry., *Canth*, Dros., Ign., Kre., Led., Mos., Nat. m., *Nit. ac.*, *Nux v.*, RHUS, Staph., Sul., Thuj.

Necrosis.—ARS., *Asaf.*, Bell., Con., Euphorb., Kre., **Merc.**, **Phos.**, Pho. ac., *Pb.*, Sabi., *Sec. c.*, *Sil.*, Sul., *Ther.*, *Thuj.*

Painfulness in General.—Acon., Agar., Agn., Am. carb., *Am. m.*, Anac., **Arg.**, Arn., *Ars.*, **ASAF.**, **Aur.**, Bar. c., *Bell.*, Bism., *Bry.*, Calc. c., Calc. ph., Cannab. s., *Canth.*, **Caps.**, Carb. an., *Carb. v.*, Caust., Cham., Chel., **Chin.**, *Chin. s.*, Cic., **Cinnab.**, Clem., **Cocc.**, *Colch.*, *Coloc.*, Con., Cup., *Cyc.*, Dig., *Dios.*, *Dros.*, Dulc., EUP. PER., *Euphorb.*, Fer., Fl. ac., *Glon.*, *Graph.*, *Guai.*, *Hell.*, *Hep.*, Ign., Iod., Ip., *K. carb.*, Kre., *Lach.*, Led., **Lyc.**, Mag. c., Mag. m., *Mang.*, Mar., MERC., *Merc. i. f.*, **Mez.**, Nat. c., *Nat. m.*, NIT. AC., Oleand., Op., Petrol., Phos., PHO. AC., *Pb.*, **PULS.**, Ran. s., **Rhodo.**, Rhus, RUTA, *Saba.*, **Sabi.**, Samb., *Sars.*, Sec. c., Sep., Sil., *Spig.*, Spo., **Staph.**, *Still.*, *Stro.*, **Sul.**, Thuj., *Valer.*, *Verat. a.*, *Vio. t.*, Zinc.

—**Of Periosteum.**—*Ant. cr.*, ASAF., *Aur.*, Bell., Bry., Camph., **Chin.**, Colch., Coloc., **Cyc.**, Hell., *Ign.*, *Led.*, *Mang.*, **Merc.**, **Mez.**, PHO. AC., *Phyt.*, *Puls.*, Rhodo., *Rhus*, Ruta, Saba., *Sabi.*, Sil., Spig., Staph.

—**Paralytic.**—Aur., Bell., Chin., **Cocc.**, *Cyc.*, *Dig.*, Led., *Mez.*, Nat. m., *Nux v.*, Petrol., *Puls.*, Rhus, *Sabi.*, Sil., *Staph.*, Verat. a., Zinc.

Pinching.—Bell., Calc. c., *Cina*, *Ign.*, Mez., *Osm.*, *Petrol.*, **Pho. ac.**, *Plat.*, VERB.

Pressure.—*Anac.*, **Arg.**, Ars., Asaf., *Aur.*, Bell., Bism., *Bry.*, *Cannab. i.*, Canth., *Carb. sul.*, Cham., Cocc., *Colch.*, Coloc., Con., Cup., Cyc., Dros., Graph., *Guai.*, Hell., *Hep.*, *Ign.*, **K. carb.**, K. nit., *Merc.*, *Mez.*, *Nux m.*, **Oleand.**, Phos., *Plat.*, *Puls.*, Rhodo., Rhus, Ruta, **Sabi.**, Sil., Spo., Stan., **Staph.**, Thuj., *Valer.*, *Verat. a.*, Vio. t., Zinc.

—**Sticking.**—Mez., Staph.

—**Tearing.**—Arg., Bell., Cham., Coloc., Thuj.

Pulsation.—Asaf., **Calc. c.**, Carb. v., *Lyc.*, **Merc.**, Nit. ac., Phos., Rhodo., Ruta, *Saba.*, Sep., *Sil.*, Sul., Thuj.

Scraping in Periosteum.—Asaf., CHIN., Coloc., PHO. AC., *Puls.*, RHUS, Saba., Spig.

—**Long Bones.**—*Bry.*, Saba.

Sensitiveness.—*Asaf.*, **Aur.**, *Bell.*, *Bry.*, *Calc. c.*, Carb. an., *Chel.*, *Chin.*, **Chin. s.**, *Cup.*, EUP. PER., *Guai.*, *Hyper.*, Lach., *Lyc.*, Merc., **Merc. c.**, *Mez.*, Nat. c., PHOS., Puls., Rhus, Sil., Stram., *Sul.*, TELL., Zinc.

—**Of Periosteum.**—Ant. cr., Aur., *Bell*, Bry., Chin., Ign., LED., **Merc.**, **Mez.**, **Pho. ac.**, Puls., Rhus, *Ruta*, *Sil.*, Spig., Staph.

Smarting.—*Hep.*, Ign., Merc., **Pho. ac.**, Sep.

Softening.—Am. carb., ASAF., **Bell.**, CALC. C., *Calc. f.*, *Calc. ph.*,

BONES.

Cic., *Fer.,* **Hep.,** Iod., **Ip., Lyc., MERC.,** *Mez.,* **Nit. ac.,** Petrol., **Phos., Pho. ac.,** Pb., **Puls.,** Rhodo., *Ruta,* **Sep., SIL., Staph., Sul.,** *Ther.*

Sticking.—Acon., Agar., *Agn.,* **Am. carb.,** Anac., **Ant. cr., Arg.,** *Ars.,* **Asaf., Aur., BELL., BRY., CALC. C.,** Canth., **Carb. v., CAUST.,** *Ced.,* Chel., **Chin.,** Cocc., *Coff.,* Colch., **CON., Dros.,** *Dulc.,* Euphorb., *Graph.,* **HELL.,** Iod., **K. carb., Kalm.,** Lach., *Lyc.,* **Mag. c.,** *Mang.,* **MERC.,** Mez., *Nit. ac.,* Nux v., Par., *Petrol.,* **Phos.,** *Pho. ac.,* **PULS., Ran. s., Ruta,** *Sabi.,* Samb., **SARS., SEP.,** *Sil.,* Spig., *Staph.,* **Stro., SUL., Thuj.,** *Valer.,* Verb., Vio. t., Zinc.

—**Burning.**—Arg., Euphorb., *Par., Phyt.,* Zinc.

—**Pressing.**—Anac., Ruta.

—**Tearing.**—Acon., Ars., Chel., Merc., Phos., Thuj.

Swelling.—Am. carb., **ASAF., Aur.,** Bell., *Bry.,* **CALC. C., Calc. ph.,** Carb. an., *Clem., Coloc.,* Con., Dig., *Dulc.,* Euphorb., Fer., *Fl. ac., Guai., Hep.,* Iod., *Kre.,* Lach., **Lyc.,** Mang., **Merc., Mez.,** Nat. c., Nat. m., **Nit. ac.,** Petrol., **Phos., PHO. AC.,** Pb., **PULS.,** Rhodo., *Rhus,* Ruta, *Sabi.,* Sep., **SIL.,** Spig., **STAPH., SUL.,** Thuj., Verat. a.

—**Of Periosteum.**—*Ant. cr.,* **ASAF., Aur.,** Bell., Bry., *Chin.,* Mang., Merc., *Mez.,* **PHO. AC.,** *Puls.,* Rhodo., Rhus, Ruta, Sabi., Sil., *Staph.*

Swollen Feeling.—*Ant. cr.,* **Bell.,** Chel., Guai., **Puls.,** *Rhus, Spig.*

Tearing.—Acon., **Agar.,** Alum., **Am. m.,** Anac., **Arg.,** *Arn.,* Ars., Asaf., **AUR., Bar. c., Bell.,** Berb., *Bism.,* Bor., Bov., *Bry., Calc. ph.,* **Cannab. s.,** *Canth.,* **Caps., Carb. v., Caust.,** *Cham.,* **Chel., CHIN., Cina, Cocc.,** Coloc., *Con. Crot. tig.,* **Cup., Cyc.,** Dig., **Dros.,** Dulc., Fer., Graph., Hell., *Hep.,* Ign., Iod., **K. CARB., K. nit., LACH., Laur., Lyc.,** Mag. c., Mag. m., *Mang.,* Mar., **MERC.,** Merc. c., **Mez.,** *Nat. c.,* Nat. m., *Nit. ac.,* Nux v., Phos., Pho. ac., *Pb.,* **Puls., RHODO.,** Rhus, Ruta, Sabi., Samb., Sars., *Sep.,* **SPIG.,** *Spo.,* Stan., **Staph.,** Stro., Sul., Sul. ac., **Tab.,** *Thuj.,* Valer., *Verat. a.,* Verb., Zinc.

—**In Periosteum.**—Bry., **Mez.,** *Pho. ac.,* Rhodo.

—**Burning.**—Sabi.

—**Cramplike.**—*Aur.,* Oleand., **Valer.**

—**Jerking.**—Agn., Bry., **CHIN.,** *Cup.,* Mang.

—**Paralytic.**—Bell., Bism., Chel., *Chin.,* Cocc., Dig.

—**Pressive.**—**ARG.,** Arn.,*Asaf., Bism., Bry.,* Coloc., **CYC., Mar., Staph.**

—**Sticking.**—Bell., *Cina,* Mur. ac., Sabi.

Tension.—*Agar.,* **Asaf., BELL.,** *Bry., Cimic., Cocc.,* **Con.,** *Crotal., Dig., Dulc.,* K. bi., *Merc., Nit. ac., Rhodo.,* **Ruta, Sul., Valer.,** Zinc.

Ulcerative Pain.—Am. carb., **Am. m., Bry.,** Caust., Cic., Graph., Ign., Mang., Nat. m., **Puls.,** *Rhus.*

Skin.

Adherent.—Arn., Par.

—**To Ulcers on the Bone.**—Arn., Asaf., Aur., Chin., Hell., Merc. Pho. ac., Puls., Ruta, Sabi., Sil., Staph.

Biting.—Agn., Alum., Am. carb., **Am. m.**, Ant. cr., Arn., Bell., Bor., Bov., Bry., **Calc. c.**, Camph., Canth., Caps., Carb. an., **Carb. v.**, Caust., Cham., Chel., Chin., Cocc., Coc. c., **Colch.**, Coloc., Con., Dros., EUPHORB., Hell., **Ip.**, Kre., **Lach.**, **LED.**, **Lyc.**, Mag. c., Mang., Merc., **Mez.**, Mur. ac., Nat. c., Nat. m., Nux v., Oleand., Op., Petrol., Phos., Pho. ac., **Plat.**, PULS., Ran. b., Ran. s., Rhodo., Rhus, Ruta, Sele., Sep., Sil., Spig., **Spo.**, Stro., **Sul.**, Thuj., Verat. a., Vio. t., Zinc.

Blood Sweating.—Arn., Calc. c., Cham., Chin., Clem., Coca., Crotal., Lach., Lyc., Nux m., **Nux v.**, Petrol.

Bruised Pain.—Arg., Arn., Cic., Dros., Dulc., Oleand., Plat., Rhus, Sul. ac.

Burning.—ACON., Agar., Alum., Ambr., Am. carb., Am. m., Anac., Ant. cr., Arg., **Arn.**, ARS., Asaf., Asar., Aur., Bar. c., BELL., Bism., Bov., BRY., Calad., **Calc. c.**, Camph., Cannab. s., Canth., **Caps.**, Carb. an., Carb. v., Caust., Cham., Chel., Chin., Cic., Clem., Cocc., Coff., Colch., Coloc., Con., Cup., Cyc., Dig., Dros., Dulc., Euphorb., Fer., Graph., Guai., Hell., **Hep.**, Hyos., Ign., Iod., K. carb., K. nit., Kre., LACH., Laur., Led., LYC., Mag. c., Mag. m., Mang., Mar., Meny., **Merc.**, **Mez.**, Mos., Mur. ac., Nat. c., Nat. m., Nit. ac., Nux v., Oleand., Op., Par., Petrol., PHOS., Pho. ac., Plat., Pb., Puls., Ran. b., Rhodo., Rhus, Ruta, Saba., Sabi., Samb., Sars., Sec. c., Sele., Seneg., Sep., SIL., Spig., Spo., Squ., Stan., Staph., Stram., Stro., Sul., Sul. ac., Thuj., Valer., Verat. a., Vio. o., Vio. t., Zinc.

—**As from Flames.**—Vio. o.

—**As from Sparks.**—Sec. c., Sele.

Chilblains.—AGAR., Ant. cr., Arn., Ars., Asar., Aur., Bell., Bry., Carb. an., Carb. v., Cham., Chin., Cocc., Colch., Croc., Crotal., Cyc., Hep., Hyos., Ign., K. carb., Lyc., Mag. c., **Nit. ac.**, Nux m., Nux v., Op., PETROL., Phos., Pho. ac., PULS., Rheum, Rhus, Ruta, Sep., Stan., Staph., Sul., Sul. ac., Thuj., Zinc.

—**Blue.**—Arn., Bell., K. carb., PULS.

—**Crawling In.**—Arn., Colch., Nux v., Rhus, Sep.

—**Inflamed.**—Ars., Bell., Cham., Hep., Lyc., Nit. ac., Phos., **PULS.**, Rhus, Staph., Sul.

—**Painful.**—Arn., Bell., Chin., Hep., Lyc., Mag. c., **Nit. ac.**, Nux v., Petrol., Phos., Pho. ac., Puls., Sep.

Chilblains, Vesicular.—Ant. cr., Bell., *Carb. an.*, Chin., Cyc., *Mag. c.* Nit ac., *Phos.*, RHUS, Sep., Sul.

Clamminess. See Fever, Sweat Clammy.

Coldness.—Acon., Agar., *Agn.*, Alum., *Ambr.*, Am. carb., Am. m., Anac., Ant. cr., **Ant. t.**, *Apis*, Arn., *Ars.*, Asaf., Asar., Aur., Bar. c., **Bell.**, Bism., Bov., *Bry.*, *Calad.*, Calc. c., **Camph.**, Cannab. s., *Canth.*, **Caps.**, *Carb. ac.*, *Carb. an.*, **Carb. v.**, Caust., *Cham.*, **Chel.**, Chin., *Cic.*, Cina, Cocc., Coff., Colch., Coloc., *Con.*, Croc., **Crotal.**, *Cup.*, Cyc., DIG., **Dios.**, Dros., *Dulc.*, Euphorb., Euphr., Fer., *Graph.*, *Hell.*, Hep., **Hyd. ac.**, *Hyos.*, *Ign.*, Iod., IP., *K. bi*, *K. carb.*, *K. nit.*, Kre., Laur., *Led.*, Lyc., Mag. c., Mag. m., Mang., Mar., *Meny.*, Merc., Merc. c., **Mez.**, **Mos.**, Mur. ac., *Nat. c.*, *Nat. m.*, Nit. ac., **Nux m.**, **Nux v.**, Oleand., Op., *Par.*, Petrol., **Phos.**, *Pho. ac.*, *Plat.*, *Pb.*, Puls., *Ran. b.*, *Rhodo.*, RHUS, Ruta, Saba., Sabi., **Samb.**, *Sang.*, *Sars.*, SEC. C., Sele., Seneg., SEP., Sil., Spig., Spo., *Squ.*, *Stan.*, Staph., *Stram.*, Stro., SUL., Sul. ac., Tab., Tar., *Thuj.*, Valer., VERAT. A., Verb., Zinc.

Color, Blackish.—Acon., Ant. cr., Asaf., *Chel.*, Crotal., *Nit. ac.*, Sec. c., Spig.

—**Blue.**—Acon., *Am. carb.*, *Arn.*, **Ars.**, Aur., **Bap.**, **Bell.**, Bism., Bry., Calc. c., *Camph.*, Carb. v., Coca, Cocc., Con., *Cop.*, Crotal., **Cup.**, DIG., *Gel.*, LACH., Merc., *Naj.*, *Nat. m.*, NUX V., OP., **Ox. ac.**, Phos., *Pho. ac.*, *Pb.*, Puls., Rhus, *Samb.*, **Sec. c.**, Sil., Spo., **Stram.**, Thuj., VERAT. A., *Vip.*

—**Dirty.**—Bry., Fer., Iod., *Merc.*, Phos., *Pso.*, Sec. c.

—**Pale.**—Ars., Bar. c., BELL., CALC. C., Carb. an., Carb. v., Caust., Chin., COCC., **Con.**, *Dig.*, FER., *Graph.*, Hell., Ign., *K. carb.*, LYC., *Merc.*, Nat. m., NIT. AC., Nux v., Oleand., Phos., *Pho. ac.*, PLAT., Pb., PULS., Sabi., SEC. C., **Sep.**, Spig., *Staph.*, SUL., Sul. ac., *Valer.*, VERAT. A., Zinc.

—**Red.**—Acon., Agar., *Agn.*, *Am. carb.*, *Ant. cr.*, **Apis**, **Arn.**, BELL., Bov., Bry., Calc. c., *Camph.*, *Canth.*, Carb. v., *Chin.*, Cocc., *Coc. c.*, *Coll.*, **Com.**, Con., *Cop.*, *Crotal.*, Cyc., **Dulc.**, Euphorb., Fer. ph., GRAPH., Hyos., Ign., *Kre.*, Lach., Led , Lyc., Mar., MERC., Nat. m., *Nit. ac.*, **Nux v.**, *Oleand.*, Op., *Pæo.*, *Petrol.*, Phos., Pho. ac., *Phyt.*, Pb., Puls., RHUS, *Ruta*, Saba., *Sec. c.*, Sep., Sil., *Spo.*, Squ., Stan., STRAM., Sul., Sul. ac., Tar., TELL., Zinc.

—**Yellow.**—Acon., Agar., Aloe, Ambr., Am. m., *Ant. cr.*, *Ant. t.*, Arn., Ars., Asaf., Aur., Bell., Bry., *Calc. c.*, Cannab. s., **Canth.**, Carb. v., *Card. m.*, *Caust.*, *Ced.*, Cham., Chel., *Chen. a.*, Chin., Cina, Coca, Cocc., CON., *Corn. c.*, *Corn. f.*, Croc., CROTAL., Cup., *Dig.*, *Dol.*, Dulc., Euphorb.,

Fer., *Gel.*, Graph., Hell., *Hep.*, *Hydras.*, Ign., Iod., *Iris v.*, *K. bi.*, K. carb., *Lach.*, *Laur.*, *Lept.*, **Lyc.**, *Mag. m.*, Merc., *Merc. c.*, *Myr.*, Nat. c., *Nat. m.*, *Nat. s.*, **Nit. ac.**, NUX V., **Op.**, Petrol., **Phos.**, Pho. ac., PB., *Pod.*, *Puls.*, Ran. b., Rheum, *Rhus*, Saba., Sec. c., SEP., Sil., **Spig.**, **Sul.**, Sul. ac., *Tar.*, *Verat. a.*, *Vip.*

Comedones.—Dig. Dros., *Graph.*, **Nat. c.**, *Nit. ac.*, Saba., Sabi., *Sul.*

Contractions.—Alum., Am. m., *Anac.*, *Asar.*, Bell., *Bism.*, Bry., Carb. v., **Chin.**, *Cocc.*, *Cup.*, **Fer.**, Graph., K. carb., Kre., *Lyc.*, Merc., *Nat. m.*, *Nit. ac.*, **Nux v.**, Oleand., Par., Petrol., Phos., **Plat.**, Pb., Puls., Ran. s., Rhodo., RHUS, Ruta, Saba., *Sec. c.*, **Sele.**, *Sep.*, Sil., Spig., *Stan.*, *Stro.*, Sul., Sul. ac., Zinc.

Corns.—*Agar.*, *Ambr.*, **Am. carb.**, Anac., ANT. CR., Arg., Arn., *Bar. c.*, *Bor.*, Bov., **Bry.**, **Calc. c.**, Camph., Carb. an., Carb. v., *Caust.*, *Cocc.*, Con., Graph., *Hep.*, Ign., Iod., *K. carb.*, K. nit., LYC., Nat c., *Nat. m.*, Nit. ac., *Nux v.*, Petrol., *Phos.*, *Pho. ac.*, Puls., *Ran. b.*, **Ran. s.**, Rhodo., Rhus, Ruta, SEP., SIL., Spig., Staph., **Sul.**, Sul. ac., Thuj., Verat. a.

—**With Boring.**—Bor., *Calc. c.*, Caust., Hep., K. carb., Nat. m., Phos., Puls., **Ran. s.**, Rhodo., **Sep.**, **Sil.**, *Spig.*, Thuj.

—**With Burning.**—Am. carb., Arg., Bar. c., Bor., **Bry.**, *Calc. c.*, *Carb. v.*, *Caust.*, Graph., Hep., *Ign.*, K. carb., **Lyc.**, Nat. c., *Nux v.*, Petrol., *Phos.*, *Pho. ac.*, Puls., *Ran. s.*, Rhus, Sep., *Sil.*, Spig., Staph., **Sul.**, Thuj.

—**Horny.**—Ant. cr., *Ran. b.*, Sul.

—**Inflamed.**—Bor., *Calc. c.*, Hep., **Lyc.**, Nit. ac., Phos., Puls., *Rhus*, Sep., SIL., *Staph.*, *Sul.*

—**With Jerking.**—Anac., Cocc., *Nux v.*, *Phos.*, Puls., *Rhus*, SEP., Sul., *Sul. ac.*

—**With Pressing.**—Agar., *Anac.*, **Ant. cr.**, Arg., Bov., **Bry.**, *Calc. c.*, Carb. v., **Caust.**, Graph,, *Ign.*, Iod., LYC., Phos., *Pho. ac.*, Ruta, Sep., Sil., **Staph.**, SUL., Verat. a.

—**Sensitive.**—*Agar.*, **Am. carb.**, **Arn.**, Bar. c., Bov., Bry., **Calc. c.**, Camph., Carb. an., Carb. v., **Hep.**, Ign., *K. carb.*, *Lith.*, LYC., *Nat. c.*, Nat. m., Nit. ac., **Nux v.**, *Petrol.*, *Phos.*, Puls., Ran. b., **Ran. s.**, Rhus, Sep., SIL., Spig., Staph., Sul., Sul. ac., Thuj., Verat. a.

—**Smarting.**—Agar., Ambr., **Ant. cr.**, Arn., *Bry.*, *Calc. c.*, Camph., *Caust.*, *Graph.*, **Hep.**, IGN., K. carb., *Lyc.*, *Nat. m.*, Nux v., *Phos.*, Pho. ac., Puls., *Rhus*, SEP., *Sil.*, Staph., *Sul.*, Sul. ac., Verat. a.

—**With Stitches.**—Agar., Am. carb., **Ant. cr.**, Arg., Arn., *Bar. c.*, Bor., Bov., **BRY.**, CALC. C., Carb. an., *Caust.*, Cocc., Graph., Hep., *Ign.*, *K. carb.*, K. nit., **Lyc.**, Nat. c., *Nat. m.*, Nit. ac., Petrol., *Phos.*, **Pho. ac.**,

Puls., **Ran. s.**, Rhodo., RHUS, **Sep.**, Sil., *Spig.*, *Staph.*, SUL., Sul. ac., *Thuj.*, Verat. a.

Corns, With Tearing.—*Am. carb.*, *Arn.*, Bry., *Calc. c.*, Caust., Cocc., *Ign.*, *K. carb.*, LYC., Nat. c., Nux v., *Rhus.*, Sep., SIL., Sul., Sul. ac.

—**With Throbbing.**—*Calc. c.*, K. carb., Lyc., *Sep.*, *Sil.*, Sul.

Cracks.—Alum., Ant. cr., Arn., Aur., Bar. c., Bry., CALC. C., Carb. an., Carb. v., Cham., Cyc., GRAPH., Hep., *K. carb.*, Kre., Lach., Lyc., *Mag. c.*, Mang., Mar., Merc., *Nat. c.*, Nat. m., Nit. ac., *Osm.*, Petrol., Phos., PULS., Rhus, Ruta, Sars., SEP, *Sil.*, SUL., *Vio. t.*, Zinc.

—**After Washing.**—Ant. cr., *Bry.*, CALC. C., *Cham.*, K. carb., Lyc., Nit. ac., Puls., *Rhus*, *Sars.*, SEP., SUL., Zinc.

—**Deep, Bloody.**—Merc., *Petrol.*, Puls., **Sars.**, *Sul.*

Cutting.—BELL., **Calc. c.**, *Dros.*, Graph., Ign., *Lyc.*, Mur. ac., **Nat. c.**, Pho. ac., Rhus, Sep., *Sil.*, Sul. ac., **Vio. t.**

Desquamation.—Acon., *Agar.*, AM. CARB., Am. m., Ant. t., **Ars.**, Aur., Bar. c., BELL., Bov., Calc. c., *Canth.*, Caps., Carb. an., *Caust.*, Cham., *Clem.*, **Coloc.**, *Con.*, *Dig.*, Dulc., Euphorb., *Fer.*, Graph., **Hell.**, *Iod.*, K. carb., Laur., **Mag. c.**, *Merc.*, MEZ., Mos., Nat. c., Nat. m., OLEAND., *Op.*, Par., **Phos.**, Pho. ac., Plat., Pb., Puls., Ran. s., **Rhus**, *Saba.*, Sec. c., Sele., **Sep.**, *Sil.*, Spig., Staph., *Sul.*, Sul. ac., Tar., **Verat. a.**

Hard.—Am. carb., Ant. cr., Bar., *Graph.*, Ran. b., Sep., *Sil.*, Sul.

—**Sensation of.**—Agar., Alum., *Am. carb.*, Apis, *Arum. t.*, **Bar. c.**, Calc. c., K. bi., Lach., *Merc.*, Phos., Pho. ac., Phyt., Rhus, *Sep.*, SUL.

Dryness.—Acon., *Acon. f.*, Alum., *Ambr.*, Am. carb., Ant. cr., Ant. t., Arg., Arn., Ars., Asaf., *Bar. c*, BELL., Bism., Bor., BRY., CALC. C., *Camph.*, **Cannab. s.**, *Canth.*, Carb. an., Carb. v., *Caust.*, CHAM., CHIN., Clem., *Cocc.*, Coff., COLCH., *Coloc.*, Con., *Crotal.*, DULC., EUP. PER., *Fer.*, Graph., Hell., Hep., Hyos., Hyd. ac., Ign., Iod., Ip., K. CARB., K. nit., Kre., Lach., Laur., LED., *Lith.*, LYC., Mag. c., Mang., MAR., Merc., *Mez.*, Mur. ac., Nat. c., *Nat. m.*, Nit. ac., NUX M., *Nux v.*, OLEAND., OP., Par., PHOS., Pho. ac., *Phyt.*, Plat., PB., Puls., Ran. b., Ran. s., Rhodo., **Rhus**, *Ruta*, Saba., *Samb.*, SEC. C., SENEG., Sep., SIL., Spig., **Spo.**, Squ., Stapn., Stram., Stro., SUL., Sul. ac., Valer., *Verat. a.* VERB., Vio. o., *Vio. t.*

—**Burning.**—ACON., Alum., Ambr., Am. m., *Anac.*, Ant. cr., Ant. t., Arg., Arn., ARS., *Bar. c.*, BELL., *Bism.*, BRY., Calc. c., *Camph.*, **Cannab. s.**, Canth., Caps., *Carb. v.*, *Caust.*, *Cham.*, **Chel.**, *Chin.*, Clem.,

Cocc., Coff., *Colch.*, Coloc., Con., Croc'., *Cup.*, Cyc., **Dulc.**, **Fer.**, *Graph.*, **Hell.**, *Hep.*, Hyos., *Ign.*, *Ip.*, **K. carb.**, K. nit., *Kre.*, LACH., Laur., **Led.**, LYC., Mang., **Merc.**, Mos., Mur. ac., *Nat. c*, Nat. m., **Nit. ac.**, *Nux m.*, NUX V., OP., Par., PHOS., Pho. ac., PULS., Ran. b., Rheum, *Rhodo.*, Rhus, *Ruta*, *Saba.*, Sabi, **Samb. Sec. c.**, Sele., **Sep.**, **Sil.**, *Spig.*, *Spo.*, **Squ.**, **Stan.**, Staph., STRAM., *Stro.*, **Sul.**, Sul. ac., Tar., *Thuj.*, VALER., Verat. a., Vio. t., *Zinc.*

Eruptions in General.—Acon., *Agar.*, Agn., Alum., Ambr., **Am. carb.**, *Am. m.*, Anac., **Ant. cr.**, Ant. t., Arg., *Arn.*, ARS., Asaf., Asar., Aur., **Bar. c.**, *Bell.*, Bism., *Bor.*, Bov., Bry., Calad., CALC. C., Camph., Cannab. s., *Canth.*, Caps., **Carb. an.**, Carb. v., CAUST., *Cham.*, Chel., Chin., **Cic.**, Cina., Clem., *Cocc.*, *Coff.*, *Colch.*, Coloc., **Con.**, Croc., *Cup.*, Cyc., Dig., Dros., **Dulc.**, *Elaps*, *Euphorb.*, Euphr., Fer., **Graph.**, Guai., **Hell.**, *Hep.*, Hyos., *Ign.*, Iod., **Ip.**, **K. carb.**, K. nit., *Kre.*, *Lach.*, Laur., **Led.**, LYC., *Mag. c.*, Mag. m., Mang., Mar., **Meny.**, **Merc.**, *Mez.*, Mos., Mur. ac., *Nat. c.*, NAT. M., **Nit. ac.**, Nux m., *Nux v.*, **Oleand.**, Op., Par., **Petrol.**, Phos., Pho. ac., Plat., *Pb.*, **Puls.**, Ran. b., Ran. s., Rheum., *Rhodo.*, RHUS, Ruta, Saba., Sabi., Samb., **Sars.**, *Sec. c*, Sele., Seneg., SEP., SIL., *Spig.*, Spo., Squ., Stan., **Staph.**, Stram., *Stro.*, SUL., *Sul. ac.*, Tar., Thuj., Valer., *Verat. a.*, Verb., **Vio. t.**, *Zinc.*

—**On Covered Parts.**—Led., *Thuj.*

—**On Hairy Parts.**—K. carb., Lyc., Merc., **Nat. m.**, *Nit. ac.*, Pb ac., RHUS.

—**Abscesses.**—*Ant. cr.*, Ant. t., *Ars.*, **Ars. iod.**, *Asaf.*, *Bry*, Calc. c., Caps., Cic., *Cocc.*, Con., **Croc.**, *Crotal.*, *Dulc.*, **Hep.**, *K. carb.*, Mag. c., *Merc.*, *Mez.*, *Nat. c.*, Nat. m., *Pæo.*, Petrol., **Puls.**, Sec. c., *Sep.*, SIL., Staph., *Sul.*

—**Biting.**—*Agn.*, Alum., *Am. carb.*, **Am. m.**, Ant. cr., *Arn.*, Ars., **Bell.**, Bor., Bov., **Bry.**, **Calc. c.**, Camph., Canth., Caps., *Carb. an*, Carb. v., **Caust.**, Cham., Chel., *Chin.*, Cocc., **Colch.**, Coloc., Con., Dros., EUPHORB., Hell., **Ip.**, Lach., **LED.**, **Lyc.**, Mag. c., *Mang.*, Merc., **Mez.**, Mur. ac., *Nat c.*, **Nat. m.**, *Nux v.*, **Oleand.**, Op., *Petrol.*, Phos., *Pho. ac.*, *Plat.*, **PULS.**, *Ran. b.*, *Ran. s.*, Rhodo., *Rhus*, Sele., *Sil.*, Spig., **Spo.**, *S.ill.*, Stro., **Sul.**, Thuj., Verat. a., Vio. t.

—**Blackish.**—Ant. cr., ARS., Asaf., **Bell.**, **Bry.**, *Hyos.*, **Lach.**, Mur. ac., Nit. ac., *Ran. b.*, **Rhus**, Sec. c., *Sep.*, Sil., Spig., *Still.*

—**Blood-Boils.**—Arn., Bry., Sec. c.

—**Burning.**—*Agar.*, Alum., **Ambr.**, **Am. carb.**, *Am. m.*, Anac., Ant. cr., Ant. t., *Arg.*, ARS., Aur., Bar. c., **Bell.**, *Bov.*, Bry., *Calad.*, Calc. c., **Cannab. s.**, *Canth.*, *Caps.*, CARB. AC., **Carb. an.**, Carb. v., CAUST.,

SKIN.

Chin., CIC., *Clem.*, Cocc., Coff., Colch., *Com.*, **Con.**, *Crot. tig.*, Dig., Dulc., Euphorb., Guai., Hell., **Hep.**, *Ign.*, *K. carb.*, *K. nit.*, *Kre.*, **Lach.**, Laur., *Led.*, **Lyc.**, Maug., Mar., MERC., **Mez.**, *Nat. c.*, *Nat. m.*, *Nit. ac.*, **Nux v.**, *Oleand.*, *Par.*, Petrol., Phos. *Pho. ac.*, Plat., *Pb.*, **Puls.**, **Ran. b.**, RHUS, *Saba.*, Sars., Seneg., *Sep.*, **Sil.**, *Spig.*, Spo., *Squ.*, *Stan.*, **Staph.**, Stram., *Stro.*, **Sul.**, *Thuj.*, *Urt.*, Verat. a., Vio. o., Vio. t., Zinc.

Eruptions, Carbuncles.—Ant. t., ARS., BELL., Caps., *Crotal.*, **Hyos.**, Lach., *Mur. ac.*, *Phyt.*, *Pic. ac.*, *Rhus*, *Sec. c.*, **Sil.**

—**Chapping.**—*Alum.*, Ant. cr., *Arn.*, *Aur.*, Bry., Calc. c., *Cham.*, **Cyc.**, Graph., Hep., K. carb., *Kre.*, **Lach.**, *Lyc.*, Mag. c., *Mang.*, Merc., Nat. c., *Nat. m.*, *Nit. ac.*, *Petrol.*, **PULS.**, **Rhus**, Ruta, *Sars.*, SEP., Sil., SUL., *Vio. t.*, Zinc.

—**Chicken-pox.**—*Acon.*, ANT. CR., Ant. t., *Ars.*, Asaf., Bell., Carb. v., Caust., Cyc., *Ip.*, **Led.**, Nat. c., Nat. m., PULS., Rhus, Sep., Thuj.

—**Clustered.**—**Agar.**, Calc. c., Ran. b , *Rhus*, **Staph.**, Verat. a.

—**Confluent.**—Agar., Ant. t., Chloral., Cic., *Hyos.*, Pho. ac., *Valer.*

—**Coppery.**—Alum., **Ars.**, *Calc. c.*, *Cannab. s.*, CARB. AN., *Carb. v.*, **Kre.**, *Led.*, **Mez.**, Rhus, Ruta, **Verat. a.**

—**Corroding** (Phagadenic).—Alum., *Am. carb.*, Bar. c., Bor., Calc. c., Carb. v., *Caust.*, CHAM., *Chel.*, **Clem.**, **Con.**, Croc., GRAPH., Hell., **Hep.**, *K. carb.*, **Lach.**, Lyc., *Mag. c.*, Mang., Merc., *Mur. ac.*, **Nat. c.**, *Nat. m.*, Nit. ac., Nux v., *Oleand.*, *Par.*, PETROL., Phos., Pho. ac., Pb., **Rhus**, *Sars.*, Sep., SIL., Squ., Staph., *Sul.*, Tar., Vio. t.

—**Desquamating.**—Acon., AM. CARB., Am. m., *Ars.*, Aur., BELL., **Clem.**, *Cup.*, Dulc., *Hell.*, Lach., **Led.**, Mag. c., Mar., *Merc.*, **Mez.**, Oleand., **Phos.**, *Pho. ac.*, Puls., Ran. b., *Sec. c.*, SEP., Sil., **Staph.**, Sul., *Verat. a.*

—**Dry.**—Alum., *Ars.*, BAR. C., **Bov.**, Bry., Cact., CALC. C., **Carb. v.**, *Caust.*, **Clem.**, Cocc., Cup., Dulc., *Graph.*, Hydr. ac., Hyos., *Kre.*, LED., *Lyc.*, **Mag. c.**, *Mar.*, **Merc.**, Nat. c., Nat. m., Par., Petrol., Phos., Pho. ac., *Rhus*, Sars., SEP., SIL., Stan., **Staph.**, *Sul.*, Valer., VERAT. A., Vio. t., Zinc.

—**Erysipelas.**—ACON., **Am. carb.**, **Am. m.**, *Ant. cr.*, APIS, **Arn.**, **Ars.**, *Bar. c.*, BELL., **Bor.**, **Bry.**, Calc. c., *Calend.*, **Camph.**, **Canth.**, **Carb. an.**, *Carb. v.*, Caust., Chin., **Clem.**, *Crotal.*, *Crot. tig.*, Dulc., EUPHORB., GRAPH., **Hep.**, *Hyos.*, Iod., Ip., *Jug. c.*, K. carb., *K. iod.*, **Lach.**, **Lyc.**, *Mag. c.*, Mang., MERC., Mur. ac., *Nat. c.*, Nat. m., Nit. ac., Petrol., **Phos.**, Pho. ac., *Pb.*, **Puls.**, *Ran. b.*, Rhodo., RHUS, Ruta, Saba., *Samb.*, Sars., Sep., *Sil.*, Spo., Stan., Staph., *Stram.*, **Sul.**, Thuj., **Verat v.**, Zinc.

SKIN.

Eruptions, Erysipelas, Gangrenous.—Acon., ARS., Bell., Camph., Chin., *Hyos.*, *Lach.*, Mur. ac., Rhus, Sabi., Sec. c., Sil.

— —**With Swelling.**—Acon., *Am. carb.*, Apis, *Arn.*, *Ars.*, BELL., *Bry.*, *Calc. c.*, Canth., Carb. v., Caust., Chin., Euphorb., *Hep.*, *K. carb.*, *Lyc.*, Mag. c., MERC., Nat. c., Nat. m., *Nit. ac.*, Petrol., Phos., Pho. ac., *Puls.*, RHUS, Ruta, *Samb.*, Sars., *Sep.*, Sil., Sul., Thuj., Verat. v.

— —**Vesicular.**—Am. carb., Ars., *Bar. c.*, Bell., Bry., *Canth.*, Carb. an., Chin., *Euphorb.*, Graph., *Hep.*, Lach., Petrol., *Phos.*, Ran. b., RHUS, Saba., Sep., Staph., *Sul.*

—**Fine (Miliary.** Compare **Granular).**—*Agar.*, Alum., Ars., Bell., Bry., *Carb. v.*, Clem., Cocc., *Con.*, *Cop.*, Dulc., Graph., Hep., Iod., Ip., Kre., *Led.*, Merc., Mez., *Nat. m.*, Nux v., *Par.*, Phos., *Pho.*, *ac.*, *Puls.*, *Rhus*, Sars., SUL., Valer., Zinc.

—**Flat.**—Am. carb., *Ant. cr.*, Ant. t., Ars., Asaf., BELL., *Carb. an.*, *Euphorb.*, LACH., Lyc., Merc., Nat. c., *Nit. ac.*, *Petrol.*, Phos., Pho. ac., *Puls.*, *Ran. b.*, Sele., Sep., Sil., Staph., *Sul.*, Thuj.

—**Furuncles.**—*Agar.*, Alum., Am. carb., *Am. m.*, Anac, Ant. cr., Ant. t., Apis, ARN., *Ars.*, *Aur.*, BELL., Brom., *Bry.*, Calc. c., *Calc. ph.*, *Carb. an.*, Carb. v., *Chin.*, Cocc., *Coc. c.*, *Crotal.*, Euphorb., Graph., Hep., Hyos., Ign., *K. nit.*, Kre., LACH., Laur., Led., LYC., Mag. c., *Mag. m.*, Merc., Mez., Mur. ac., Nat. c., Nat. m., Nit. ac., *Nux m.*, Nux v., Petrol., Phos., Pho. ac., *Phyt.*, *Pic. ac.*, Puls., *Rhus*, Sec. c., Sep., *Sil.*, *Spo.*, *Stan.*, Staph., Stram., Sul., *Sul. ac.*, Thuj., *Zinc.*

— —**Large.**—Ant. t., Hep., *Hyos.*, Lyc., Nat. c., Nit. ac., Phos.

— —**Small.**—ARN., *Mag. c.*, Sul., Zinc.

—**Gooseflesh (In the House).**—Calc. c.

— —**In Open Air.**—Sars.

—**Granular (Compare Fine).**—Agar., Am. carb., Ars., Cocc., Kre., *Led.*, Nux v., *Par.*, Valer.

—**Gritty.**—Am. carb., *Graph.*, Hep., *Nat. m.*, Phos., Zinc.

—**Hard.**—Ant. cr., Ran. b., Rhus, Spig., Valer.

—**Itch** (Scabies).—*Ambr.*, Ant. cr., *Ant. t.*, Ars., Bry., Calc. c., *Canth.*, *Carb. an.*, CARB. V., CAUST., *Clem.*, Coloc., *Con.*, Cup., Dulc., *Graph.*, *Guai.*, Kre., Lach., *Led.*, *Lyc.*, Mang., *Merc.*, *Mez.* Nat. c., Petrol., Pho. ac., Pso., Puls., Saba., SELE., SEP., *Sil.*, *Squ.*, Staph., SUL., *Sul. ac.*, Tar., *Valer.*, Verat. a., Zinc.

— —**Bleeding.**—Calc. c., *Dulc.*, Merc., *Sul.*

— —**Dry.**—Ars., Calc. c., *Caust.*, Clem., *Cup.*, *Dulc.*, Graph., Kre., Led., Lyc., *Merc.*, Nat. c., *Petrol.*, Pho. ac., SEP., SIL., Staph., Sul., Valer., Verat. a., Zinc.

SKIN. 211

Eruptions, Itch, Fatty.—Ant. cr., Caust., Clem., Cup., Kre., MERC., Sele., Sep., *Squ.*, *Sul.*

— — **Moist.**—Calc. c., **Carb. v.,** *Caust., Clem.,* Con., Dulc., **Graph.,** *Kre.,* Lyc., Merc., Petrol., *Sep.,* Sil., Squ., *Staph., Sul.*

— — **Suppressed.**—Alum., *Ambr.,* Ant. cr., Ant. t., *Ars., Carb v.,* **Caust.,** Dulc., **Graph.,** Kre., Lach., Nat. c., *Nat. m.,* Pho. ac., **Sele., Sep.,** Sil., Sul., Verat. a., *Zinc.*

— — **Suppressed with Mercury and Sulphur.**—Agn., *Ars.,* Bell. Calc. c., *Carb. v.,* CAUST., **Chin.,** *Dulc.,* Hep., Iod., *Nit. ac.,* Puls., Rhus Sars., Sele., SEP., *Sil.,* Staph., Thuj., *Valer.*

—**Itching.**—Acon., **Agar.,** Agn., Alum., Ambr., **Am. carb.,** *Am. m.,* Anac., Ant. cr., Ant. t., *Arg., Arn.,* ARS., **Ars. iod.,** Asaf., *Bar. c,* Bell., *Bov.,* Bry., Calad., Calc. c., **Canth.,** Caps., Carb. an., *Carb. v.,* CAUST., Cham., Chel., Cic., Cina, Clem., Cocc., *Con., Crot. tig.,* Cup., Dig., Dulc., Graph., Hep., Ign., *Ip.,* Jug. c., *K. br.,* **K. carb.,** *K. nit.,* Kre., Lach., *Laur.,* Led., *Lyc.,* Mag. c., Mag. m., Mang., Mar., **Merc., Mez.,** Nat. c., *Nat. m.,* NIT. AC., **Nux v.,** Oleand., **Par.,** *Petrol.,* Phos., Pho. ac., Pb., *Puls.,* Ran. b., Ran. s., RHUS, *Saba.,* Sabi., *Sars.,* Sele., SEP., **Sil.,** *Spig., Spo.,* Squ., Stan., STAPH., Stram., *Stro.,* SUL., Tar., *Thuj.,* Valer., *Verat. a.,* Vio. t., *Zinc.*

—**With Jerking Pain.**—Asaf., *Calc. c.,* **Caust.,** *Cham.,* Chin., *Cup.,* Lyc., Puls., Rhus, Sep., *Sil.,* Staph.

—**With Maggots.**—Aur., *Bry., Calc. c.,* Graph., Nat. c., *Nat. m.,* Nit. ac., Pb., *Sabi.,* SELE., *Sul.*

—**Measles.**—ACON., Ars., **Bell.,** Bry., *Carb. v.,* Cham., Chin., Chloral., *Coff., Cop., Crotal., Dros., Euphr., Gel.,* Hyos., Ign., **Ip.,** Mag. c., Nux v., *Phos.,* PULS., Rhus, Stram., *Sul.*

—**Milk-Crust.**—Ambr., Ant. cr., Ars, **Bar. c.,** *Bell*, *Bry.,* CALC. C., *Carb. an.,* Carb v., Cham., **Cic.,** Dulc., Graph., *Hep.,* Led., *Lyc.,* **Merc., Mez.,** *Nat. m.,* Oleand., Phos., RHUS, SARS., **Sep.,** *Sil.,* Staph., *Sul.,* **Vio. t.**

—**Moist.**—*Alum.,* Anac., Ant. cr., *Ars.,* **Ars. iod.,** Bar. c., **Bell.,** Bov., Bry., *Calc. c., Canth.,* Carb. an., CARB. V., *Caust., Cic.,* Clem., *Con., Dulc.,* GRAPH., *Hell.,* Hep., *Hydras.,* **Jug. c.,** *K. carb.,* Kre., Lach., Led., LYC., Merc., MEZ., Nat. c., *Nat. m., Nit. ac.,* Oleand., Petrol., Phos., Pho. ac., RHUS, *Ruta,* Sabi., *Sars.,* Sele., Sep., *Sil., Squ.,* Staph., *Still.,* Sul., Sul. ac., Tar., *Tell.,* Thuj., *Vinc., Vio. t.,* Zinc.

—**Nettle-rash.**—Acon., Am. carb., *Am. m.,* Ant. cr., Ant. t., APIS., Ars., Bar. c., **Bell.,** Bov., **Bry.,** CALC. C., Carb. an., *Carb. v.,* CAUST., Chin., *Chloral.,* Cic., Coca, Cocc., Con., Cup., *Cub.,* DULC., **Graph.,**

SKIN.

HEP., *Ign.*, *Ip.*, K. carb., Kre., Lach., Led., **Lyc.**, **Mag. c.**, *Merc.*, **Mez.**, *Nat. c.*, **Nat. m.**, *Nit. ac.*, *Nux v.*, **Petrol.**, Phos., Pho. ac., **Puls.**, RHUS, *Ruta*, Sec. c., Sele., **Sep.**, *Sil.*, Staph., Stram., **Sul.**, *Ter.*, Thuj., *Urt.*, Valer., **Verat. a.**, Zinc.

Eruptions, Nodular (Wheals and Hives).—Agar., Alum., Am. carb., *Am. m.*, Anac., **Ant. cr.**, *Ant. t.*, APIS, Ars., *Aur.*, *Bar. c.*, Bell., **Bry.**, CALC. C., Cannab. s., Canth., Caps., *Carb. an.*, *Carb. v.*, CAUST., Chel., Chin., Chloral., *Cic.*, Cocc., *Con.*, **Cop.**, Dig., Dros., DULC., *Graph.*, *Hell.*, Hep., Ign., Iod., Ip., K. carb., *K. nit.*, Kre., LACH., **Led.**, Lyc., **Mag. c.**, *Mag. m.*, **Mang.**, *Merc.*, MEZ., *Mur. ac.*, *Nat. c.*, **Nat. m.**, Nit. ac., *Nux v.*, *Oleand.*, Op., Petrol., Phos., Pho. ac., Puls., RHUS, Ruta, Sabi., Sec. c., *Sele.*, Sep., Sil., *Spig.*, Spo., Squ., Stan., **Staph.**, Stram., *Sul.*, Sul. ac, *Tar.*, Thuj., *Valer.*, **Verat. a.**, Verb., Vio. t., *Zinc.*

——**Rosy Red (Erythema).**—Antip., Bell., Bry., Chloral., *Coca*, *Cop.*, *Crot. tig.*, *Gel.*, *Jug. c.*, *K. br.*, *K. iod.*, *Merc.*, **Nat. c.**, *Petrol.*, Phos., *Phyt.*, RHUS, *Sil.*, STRAM., *Ter.*

—**Painful.**—*Agar.*, Ambr., **Ant. cr.**, *Arg.*, ARN., Ars., Asaf., *Aur.*, Bar. c., BELL., Cannab. s., Canth., *Caps.*, **Chin.**, **Clem.**, **Con.**, Cup., Dulc., Guai., **Hep.**, K. carb., Lach., *Led.*, Lyc., **Mag. c.**, Mag. m., *Merc.*, Nat. c., NUX V., Par., Petrol., *Phos.*, PHO. AC., **Puls.**, Ran. b *Ran. s.*, *Rhus*, Ruta, *Sele.*, *Seneg.*, **Sep.**, SIL., Spig., Spo., *Squ.*, SUL., Thuj., *Valer.*, **Verat. a.**, *Verb.*

—**Painless.**—Ambr., Anac., Ant. cr., *Ant. t.*, Bell., Cham., **Cocc.**, Con., *Cyc.*, Dros., **Hell.**, Hyos., Lach., *Laur.*, LYC., Oleand., Phos., Pho. ac., Puls., *Rhus*, Samb., **Sec. c.**, Spig., *Staph.*, **Stram.**, Sul.

—**Pimples.**—Acon., Agar., *Aloe*, *Alum.*, Ambr., Am. carb., *Am. m.*, Anac., ANT. CR., Ant. t., *Arg.*, Arn., ARS., Aur., Bar. c., **Bell.**, Bov., **Bry.**, Calc. c., *Calc. ph.*, **Canth.**, *Caps.*, Carb. an., *Carb. v.*, CAUST., **Cham.**, *Chel.*, Chin., *Cina.*, *Clem.*, **Cocc.**, Coc. c., **Con.**, *Crotal.*, *Crot. tig.*, Cup., Cyc., Dros., **Dulc.**, Euphr., *Gel.*, **Gam.**, *Graph.*, *Hell.*, *Hep.*, Iod., *K. br.*, *K. carb.*, K. nit., **Led.**, Lyc., *Mag. c.*, Mag. m., Mang., **Merc.**, Mez., Mos., *Mur. ac.*, *Nat. c.*, **Nat. m.**, NIT. AC., Nux v., Par., *Petrol.*, Phos., Pho. ac., **Pb.**, Puls., Rhus, Saba., *Sars.*, *Sele.*, Seneg., SEP., *Sil.*, *Spig.*, Spo., Squ., *Stan.*, **Staph.**, *Stro.*, SUL., *Sul. ac.*, Tar., **Thuj.**, Valer., *Verat. a.* Vio. t., ZINC.

—**Purulent.**—*Ant. cr.*, *Ant. t.*, Ars., Bell., *Cic.*, *Clem.*, Cocc., Con., Cyc., Dulc., Euphr., *Hep.*, *Jug. c.*, Led., **Lyc.**, Mag. c., MERC., NAT. C., *Nat. m.*, *Petrol.*, Pb., Puls., RHUS, Samb., *Sars.*, Sec. c., SEP., *Sil.*, *Spig.*, **Staph.**, *Sul.*, Tar., Thuj., Verat. a., Vio. o., Vio. t., Zinc.

—**Pustules.**—*Agar.*, *Am. m.*, **Ant. cr.**, ANT. T., Ant. s. aur., *Arn.*,

SKIN. 213

Ars., Bell., *Bry., Calc. ph., Carb. sul.,* Cham., *Chel., Cic., Clem.,* Cocc., *Crotal., Crot. tig., Cyc., Euphorb.,* Gnap., Hyos., K. bi., K. br., *K. iod., Lach.,* Merc., *Mez.,* Nit. ac., *Nux v.,* Op., *Pho. ac.,* Puls., RHUS, *Sec. c., Sil., Squ.,* Staph., SUL., Thuj., *Vio. t.*

Eruptions, Rash.—ACON., Alum., *Am. carb., Am. m.,* Ant. cr., Ant. t., *Arn.,* Ars., Asaf., Bell., *Bov.,* BRY., Calad., *Calc. c., Canth.,* Carb. v., Caust., Cham., Chin., *Clem., Coff.,* Cup., Dig., *Dulc.,* Euphr., *Graph., Hell., Hyos.,* IP., Jug. c., Lach., Led., Mar., MERC., Mez., Nat. m., *Nux v.,* Op., *Phos.,* Pho. ac., Puls., Rheum, Rhus, Ruta, *Sars.,* Sec. c., Sele., Sep., *Sil., Spo.,* Staph., STRAM., Sul., *Valer.,* Verat. a., *Vio. t., Zinc.*

— —Purple.—ACON., *Bell.,* Coff.

— —Scarlet.—ACON., *Am. carb.,* Ars., *Bell.,* BRY., Carb. v., Caust., *Coff., Dulc.,* Hyos., Ip., Lach., Merc., Phos., Pho. ac., Rhus, *Sul.*

— —White.—*Agar.,* ARS., *Bov.,* Bry., *Ip., Phos., Sul.,* Valer.

—Roseola.—ACON., Bell., BRY., Carb. v., Coff., Ip., *Merc.,* Phos., PULS., *Rhus, Sars.,* Sul.

—Scabby.—Alum., Ambr., *Am. carb., Am. m.,* Ant. cr., *Ant. s. aur., Ant. t., Ars.,* Bar. c., Bell., *Bov.,* Bry., CALC. C., *Caps.,* Carb. an., *Carb. v.,* Cham., Cic., Clem., CON., Dulc., GRAPH., Hell., Hep., *K. carb., Kre.,* Led., LYC., Mag. c., Merc., MEZ., Mur. ac., *Nat. m.,* NIT. AC., Nux v., Oleand., *Pœo., Par.,* Petrol., Phos., Pb., Puls., Ran. b., RHUS, Saba., *Sabi.,* Sars., Sep., Sil., Spo., Squ., Staph., Sul., *Thuj., Verat. a.,* Vio. t., Zinc.

—Scaly.—*Agar.,* Am. m., Ant. cr., ARS., Aur., Bell., *Bor., Cact., Cic.,* CLEM., *Cup., Dulc.,* Hep., Hydroc., Hyos., K. bi., *K. carb.,* Led., Mag. c., *Mar.,* Merc., *Mez.,* Oleand., *Petrol.,* PHOS., Pb., Rhus, SEP., Staph., Sul.

—Scarlatina.—*Acon.,* AM. CARB., *Am. m., Arn.,* Ars., Bar. c., BELL., Bry., *Carb. v., Caust.,* Cham., *Coff.,* Croc., *Crotal.,* Dulc., Euphorb., *Hep.,* Hyos., Iod., *Ip., Jug. c., Lach.,* MERC., *Phos.,* Pho. ac., Rhus, *Stram.,* Sul.

— —Smooth.—Am. carb., BELL., Euphorb., Hyos., *Merc.*

—Small-pox.—*Am. m.,* Ant. cr., ANT. T., *Arn., Ars.,* Bell., Bry., Canth., Cham., *Clem., Cocc., Hyos.,* MERC., Nit. ac., Puls., RHUS, *Sil.,* Stram., Sul., *Thuj.*

— —Black.—Ant. cr., ARS., Bell., *Bry.,* Hyos., Lach., *Mur. ac.,* RHUS, Sec. c., Sep., *Sil.,* Spig.

—Smarting.—Acon., Agar., Alum., *Ambr.,* Ant. cr., ARG., Ars., Aur., Bar. c., Bry., Calc. c., Cannab. s., *Canth.,* Caps., Carb. an., Chel., Chin., Cic., Coff., Colch., Dol., Dros., *Fer.,* GRAPH., Hell., HEP.,

Ign., *K. carb.*, *Lyc.*, *Mag. c.*, **Mang.**, Mar., *Merc.*, *Mez.*, *Nat. c.*, **Nat. m.**, Nit. ac., *Nux v.*, *Oleand.*, **Par.**, *Petrol.*, Phos., **Pho. ac.**, **Puls.**, Ran. b., Rhus, *Ruta*, *Sabi.*, *Sars.*, Sele., SEP., *Sil.*, Spig., Spo., **Squ.**, *Staph.*, Sul., *Valer.*, Verat. a., Zinc.

Eruptions, Stinging.—*Acon.*, Alum., Am. m., *Ant. cr.*, *Arn.*, **Ars.**, *Asaf.* Bar. c., **Bell.**, Bov., Bry., *Calc. c.*, Camph., *Canth.*, Caps., *Carb. v.*, Caust., *Cham.*, Chin., **Clem.**, Cocc., *Con.*, **Cyc.**, Dig., Dros., Graph., Guai., Hell., Hep., *Ign*, K. carb., Kre., **Led.**, *Lyc.*, *Mag. c.*, **Merc.**, *Mez.*, Mur. ac., Nat. c., *Nat. m.*, NIT. AC., Nux v., *Petrol.*, Phos., **Plat.**, PULS., Ran. b., Ran. s., Rhus, *Saba.*, **Sabi.**, *Sele.*, **Sep.**, SIL., Spo., *Squ.*, Staph., Stro., SUL., *Thuj.*, Verb., **Vio. t.**, Zinc.

—With Swelling.—Acon., Am. carb., *Arn.*, Ars., **Bell.**, *Bry.*, Calc. c., *Canth.*, Carb. v., *Caust.*, Chin., Cic., Con., Euphorb., *Hep.*, **K. carb.**, Lyc., Mag. c., MERC., Nat. c., *Nat. m.*, *Nit. ac.*, Petrol., *Phos.*, Pho. ac., **Puls.**, RHUS, Ruta, Samb., *Sars.*, Sep., *Sil.*, Sul., Thuj.

—With Tearing Pain.—Acon., *Arn.*, Ars., *Bell.*, **Bry.**, Calc. c., *Canth.*, Carb. v., *Caust.*, Clem., Cocc., Dulc., *Graph.*, K. carb., LYC., Merc., *Mez.*, Nat. c., Nit. ac., *Nux v.*, Phos., Puls., Rhus, Sep., Sil., Staph., Sul., Zinc.

—Tense.—Alum., Ant. t., Arn., Bar. c., Bell., Bry., *Canth.*, Carb. an, CAUST., *Cocc.*, *Con.*, Hep., K. carb., Mez., Oleand., **Phos.**, *Puls.*, RHUS, Sabi., Sep., Spo., *Staph.*, **Stro.**, *Sul.*, Thuj.

—Transparent.—Cina, Merc., RAN. B.

—With Ulcerating Pain.—*Am. carb.*, **Am. m.**, Ant. cr., Ars., Bar. c., Caps., *Caust.*, Con., *Graph.*, K. carb., Laur., **Mang.**, Merc., **Phos.**, Puls., Rhus, Sep., SIL., Staph., *Sul.*, Tar., *Zinc.*

—Unhealthy (Suppurating).—Alum., *Am. carb.*, Bar. c., Bor., Calc. c., Carb. v., *Caust.*, CHAM., *Chel.*, *Cic.*, **Clem.**, **Con.**, Croc., GRAPH., Hell., **Hep.**, *K. carb.*, *Lach.*, Lyc., *Mag. c.*, Mang., *Merc.*, *Mur. ac.*, Nat. c., NIT. AC., Nux v., *Oleand.*, *Par.*, PETROL., Phos., Pho. ac., Pb., *Pso.*, Rhus, Sep., SIL., Squ., Staph., *Sul.*, Tar., Vio. t.

—Vesicular.—*Agar.*, Alum., *Am. carb.*, **Am. m.**, **Ant. cr.**, **Ant. t.**, *Arg.*, ARS., Aur., *Bar. c.*, **Bell.**, Bov., **Bry.**, *Buf.*, Calad., Calc. c., *Cannab. s.*, **Canth.**, *Caps.*, *Carb. ac.*, **Carb. an.**, *Carb. v.*, **Caust.**, *Cham.*, Chin., Cic., Clem., Cocc., Con., *Cop.*, *Corn. c.*, *Crotal.*, CROT. TIG., *Cyc.*, Dig., Dulc., EUPHORB., *Fl. ac.*, Graph., Hell., Hep., *Hyos.*, K. carb., K. iod., K. nit., Kre., LACH., Laur., Mag. c., Mang., Merc., Mez., Nat. c., *Nat. m.*, NIT. AC., Oleand., Op., *Osm.*, Petrol., PHOS., *Pho. ac.*, Plat., **Pb.**, **Pso.**, Puls., RAN. B., **Ran. s.**, Rheum, RHUS, Ruta, Saba.,

Sabi., Sars., *Sal. ac.*, **Sec. c.**, *Sele.*, Seneg., **Sep.**, *Sil.*, Spig., *Spo., Squ.,* Staph., *Stram.*, SUL., *Sul. ac.*, Tar., Tell., *Thuj.*, Verat. a., Zinc.

Eruptions, Vesicular, Blue.—Ars., Bell., Con., Lach., RAN. B., *Rhus.*

— —**Bloody.**—Ars., *Aur.*, Bry., Canth., *Carb. ac., Nat. m.,* **Sec. c.,** *Sul.*

— —**Gangrenous.**—Acon., **Ars.,** *Bell.,* Camph., *Carb. v.,* Lach., Mur. ac., Ran. b., **Sabi., Sec. c.**

—**Whitish.**—*Agar.,* ARS., Bor., *Bov.,* Bry., *Ip.,* Phos., *Sul.,* Thuj., **Valer.,** Zinc.

—**With White Tips.**—Ant. cr., Ant. t., *Puls.*

—**Yellow.**—Agar., Ars., *Cic.,* Cocc., *Cup.,* **Euphorb.,** Hell., Led., Lyc., *Kre.,* Merc., Nat. c., Nit. ac., Par., *Sep.,* Spo., Valer.

—**Zoster (Zona).**—Ars., Bry., *Ced.,* Cham., *Crotal., Dol.,* Graph., MERC., Nat. c., *Puls.,* Ran. b., RHUS, *Sele.,* Sil., *Sul.*

Excrescences, Bunions.—Am. carb., *Pb.,* Phos., Pho. ac., SIL., *Zinc.*

—**Condylomata.**—*Calc. c., Cinnab., Euphr.,* Lyc., **Nit. ac.,** Phos., Pho. ac., Sabi., *Staph.,* THUJ.

—**Cysts, Sebaceous.**—*Agar.,* Ant. cr., BAR. C., CALC. C., *Coloc.,* Graph., Hep., *K. carb.,* Nit. ac., Sabi., *Sil., Spo.,* Sul.

—**Fleshy.**—*Ars.,* Staph., Thuj.

—**Fungus** (Cauliflower).—ANT. CR., Ars., *Clem.,* Con., *Iod.,* **Kre.,** LACH., *Petrol.* Phos., Rhus, Sabi., SIL., Staph., *Sul.*

— —**Hæmatodes.**—*Ant. t.,* ARS., *Bell., Calc. c.,* CARB. AN., **Carb. v.,** *Clem.,* Kre., Lach., **Lyc.,** Merc., Nit. ac., Nux v., PHOS., Rhus, Sep., SIL., Staph., Sul., *Thuj.*

— —**Medullary.**—*Bell.,* Carb. an., Phos., Sil., Sul., Thuj.

—**Horny.**—Ant. cr., *Mez.,* Ran. b., Sul.

—**Moles.**—Calc. c., *Carb. v.,* Graph., Nit. ac., *Petrol., Pho. ac., Sil.,* **Sul.,** *Sul. ac.*

—**Polypi.**—Ambr., *Aur., Bell.,* CALC. C., CON., *Graph.,* Hep., Lyc., **Mar.,** Merc., Mez., *Nat. m., Nit. ac.,* Petrol., PHOS., *Pho. ac.,* Puls., **Sang.,** Sil., STAPH., *Sul., Sul. ac.,* Thuj.

—**Swellings, Inflamed** (Puffy Bunches).—*Ars.,* Carb. an., Hep., Nat. c., Phos., Sil., Sul.

Extravasations.—ARN., Bry., *Cham.,* Chin., *Chloral., Coca,* **Con.,** *Crotal., Dulc.,* Euphr., Fer., Hep., Lach., Laur., *Led.,* Nux v., Par., Phos., Pb., Puls., *Rhus,* Ruta, Sec. c., Sul., SUL. AC.

Flabbiness.—*Agar.,* Ant. t., *Bor.,* CALC. C., **Caps.,** *Cham.,* **Chin.,** *Clem.,* Cocc., *Con.,* Croc., Cup., Dig., Euphorb., Fer., Graph., Hell.,

SKIN.

Hyos., **Iod.**, Ip., Lach., **Lyc.**, Mag. c., *Merc.*, Nat. c., Puls., Rheum, **Saba.**, Sec. c., *Seneg.*, Sil., *Spo.*, *Sul.*, Sul. ac., **Verat. a.**

Fatty.—*Agar.*, Aur., **Bar. c.**, **Bry.**, *Calc. c.*, Chin., *Mag. c.*, **Merc.**, **Nat. m.**, Pb., *Pso.*, *Sele.*, Stram.

Formication.—Acon., *Acon. f.*, *Aconin.*, *Agar.*, Agn., Alum., Am. carb., *Apis*, **Aran.**, Arg., **Ars.**, *Aur.*, **Bar. ac.**, **Bar. c.**, *Bor.*, Bov., Calc. c., *Cannab. s.*, **Canth.**, *Caps.*, *Carb. v.*, *Carb. sul.*, Caust., **Fer.**, **Hyper.**, *Laur.*, Led., **Lyc.**, Mag. c., *Mag. m.*, Mang., *Mur. ac.*, **Nat. c.**, Nit. ac., Nux v., Oleand., *Onos.*, **Phos.**, **Pho. ac.**, **Plat.**, Ran. b., Ran. s., RHODO., *Rhus*, **Saba.**, SEC. C., *Sil.*, Spig., *Spo.*, **Staph.**, SUL., **Urt.**, **Vio. t.**, Zinc.

Gangrene (From Burns or Gangrenous Sores).—Agar., Alum., *Ant. cr.*, ARS., *Calc. c.*, **Carb. v.**, CAUST., *Cyc.*, Euphorb., **Kre.**, *Lach.*, *Mag. c.*, *Rhus*, Ruta, *Sec. c.*, Stram.

—**Cold.**—Ant. t., ARS., Asaf., *Bell.*, **Canth.**, *Caps.*, Carb. v., Con., *Crotal.*, Euphorb., Lach., Merc., PB., Ran. b., SEC. C., **Sil.**, **Squ.**, *Sul.*, *Sul. ac.*

—**Hot.**—Acon., *Ars.*, *Bell.*, Mur. ac., **Sabi.**, **Sec. c.**

—**Moist.**—CHIN., Hell.

Gnawing (Compare **Itching, Corroding**).—*Agar.*, AGN., *Alum.*, Ambr., Anac., *Ant. cr.*, Arg., Ars., **Bar. c.**, Bell., *Bism.*, Bry., *Canth.*, *Caps.*, *Cham.*, Clem., Cocc., Con., **Cyc.**, **Dig.**, **Dros.**, Euphorb., Graph., Guai., Hell., Hyos., *K. carb.*, Led., LYC., **Meny.**, Merc., Mez., Nat. c., Nux v., OLEAND., *Par.*, **Phos.**, **Pho. ac.**, PLAT., *Puls.*, Ran. s., Rhodo., *Rhus*, Ruta, Sep., Spig., *Spo.*, Squ., Stan., STAPH., Sul., *Tar.*, Thuj., Verat. a.

Hair of Head Falls Out.—Ambr., *Am. carb.*, Am. m., *Ant. cr.*, **Ars.**, Aur., Bar. c., Bell., *Bov.*, Calc. c., *Canth.*, Carb. an., **Carb. v.**, Caust., Chel., Colch., *Con.*, *Cyc.*, *Dulc.*, Fer., *Fl. ac.*, GRAPH., *Hell.*, Hep., *Ign.*, Iod., K. CARB., Kre., *Lach.*, Lyc., Mag. c., Merc., Nat. c., NAT. M., NIT. AC., Op., *Par.*, Petrol., PHOS., *Pho. ac.*, *Pb.*, *Rhus*, Sabi., **Sars.**, Sec. c., Sele., SEP., *Sil.*, Staph., SUL., Sul. ac., *Zinc.*

—**On Forehead.**—Ars., *Bell.*, *Hep.*, Merc., Nat. m., Phos., Sil.

—**Occiput.**—Calc. c., Carb. v., Hep., **Petrol.**, Sep., *Sil.*, Staph., **Sul.**

—**Sides.**—*Bov.*, Graph., *K. carb.*, Pho. ac., Staph., *Zinc.*

—**Temples.**—*Calc. c.*, K. carb., Lyc., *Merc.*, NAT. M., *Par.*, Sabi.

—**Vertex.**—BAR. C., *Calc. c.*, Carb an., **Graph.**, Hep., Lyc., *Nit. ac.*, Pb., *Sele.*, **Sep.**, *Sil.*, Zinc.

—**In Bunches.**—*Calc. ph.*, **Phos.**

—**Beard.**—Agar., *Ambr.*, **Calc. c.**, **Graph.**, Nat. c., **Nat. m.**, Nit. ac., Pb., Sil.

SKIN.

Hair Falls Out, Eyebrows.—Agar., **Bell.**, *Caust.*, Hell., K. CARB., *Par. Pho. ac.*, Pb., *Sele.*

—**Moustache.**—Bar. c., **K. carb.**, *Pb.*

—**Mons Veneris.**—*Bell.*, Hell., *Nat. c.*, **Nat. m.**, Nit. ac., Rhus, *Sele.*

—**Nostrils.**—Calc. c., *Caust.*, **Graph.**, Sil.

—**Whole Body.**—Ars., **Calc. c.**, *Carb. v.*, **Graph.**, *Hell.*, K. carb., Nat. m., Op., Phos., *Sabi.*, *Sec. c.*, Sul.

Hair Feels Pulled.—Acon., *Alum.*, Aur., *Bar. c.*, *Bry.*, *Canth.*, *Caust.*, *Chin.*, K. carb., K. nit., Kre., **Laur.**, *Lyc.*, **Mag. m.**, Mur. ac., **Phos.**, Pho. ac., Rhus, *Sele.*

Hard, Like Callosities.—Am. Carb., **Ant. cr.**, *Bor.*, GRAPH., *Lach.*, Ran. b., *Rhus*, SEP., Sil., Sul.

—**Like Parchment.**—*Acon.*, ARS., **Chin.**, *Dig.*, Dulc., *K. carb.*, Led., Lyc., Phos., Sil., *Squ.*

—**With Thickening.**—Am. carb., *Ant. cr.*, Ars., Bor., *Cic.*, Clem., Dulc., *Graph.*, *Hydr. ac.*, Lach., Par., **Ran. b.**, RHUS, SEP., *Sil.*, Sul., *Thuj.*, Verat. a.

Inactivity.—Alum., *Ambr.*, ANAC., **Ant. cr.**, Ant. t., **Ars.**, Bell., Bry., *Calc. c.*, Camph., *Carb. an.*, *Carb. v.*, Caust., Cham., Chin., *Cocc.* CON., Cyc., Dig., Dulc., *Graph.*, Hell., *Hep.*, *Iod.*, **Ip.**, K. CARB., Lach. Laur., Led., LYC., Merc., Mur. ac., *Nat. c.*, *Nat. m.*, **Nit. ac.**, Nux v. Oleand., *Op.*, Petrol., Phos., PHO. AC., Plat., *Pb.*, Puls., *Rhodo.*, Rhus Ruta, Sabi., *Sars.*, **Sec. c.**, *Sep.*, Sil., Spo., *Squ.*, Staph., Stram., **Sul** Thuj., *Verat. a.*, Zinc.

Indurations.—Am. carb., **Ant. cr.**, *Ars.*, **Ars. iod.**, Bar. c., Bov. *Buf.*, **Chel.**, *Chin.*, Cic., Clem., *Con.*, Dulc., Graph., K. carb., *Lach.*, Led., *Lyc.*, Par., Phos., **Ran. b.**, RHUS, SEP., Sil., Squ., SUL., *Thuj.*, Verat. a.

Inelasticity.—Ant. cr., *Ars.*, **Bov.**, **Cup.**, *Dulc.*, *Lach.*, Ran. b., **Rhus**, Sep., **Verat. a.**

Inflammation.—Acon., Agn., Alum., Ant. cr., Apis, Arn., **Ars.**, Asaf., *Bar. c.*, **Bell.**, *Bor.*, Bry., *Calc. c.*, Camph., Cannab. s., *Canth.*, Caust., CHAM., Cina, Cocc., Colch., *Com.*, Con., Croc., *Crotal.*, Euphorb., Graph., HEP., Hyos., Kre., Lach., Lyc., Mang., MERC., *Mez.*, Nat. c., Nat. m., **Nit. ac.**, *Petrol.*, Phos., Pb., PULS., Ran. b., **Rhus**, *Ruta*, Sep., SIL., Staph., Sul., Verat. a., Zinc.

—**Inclination to.**—Alum., Ars., **Asaf.**, **Bar. c.**, *Bell.*, **Bor.**, *Calc. c.*, *Camph.*, Canth., CHAM., *Chel.*, Con., Croc., *Euphorb.*, *Graph.*, **Hep.**, Hyos., *Lach.*, Mang., **Merc.**, *Nat. c.*, Nat. m., **Nit. ac.**, Petrol., *Pb.*, **Puls.**, Ran. b., SIL., *Staph.*, **Sul.**

SKIN.

Itching in General.—Acon., AGAR., **Agn.**, *Aloe.*, **Alum.**, **Ambr.**, *Am. carb.*, *Am. m.*, *Anac.*, *Ant. cr.*, Ant. t., *Apis*, **Arg.**, *Arn.*, *Ars.*, Asaf., Asar., Aur., **Bar. c.**, **Bell.**, Bism., Bor., *Bov.*, Bry., Calad., *Calc. c.*, Camph., Cannab. s., *Canth.*, *Caps.*, Carb. an., *Carb. v.*, **Carb. sul.**, Caust., Cham., **Chel.**, *Chin.*, Cic., Cina, **Clem.**, **Cocc.**, *Coc. c.*, *Coff.*, *Colch.*, *Coll.*, Coloc., *Con.*, Croc., Cup., *Cyc.*, *Dig.*, *Dios.*, *Dol.*, *Dros.*, Dulc., *Euphorb.*, Euphr., *Fl. ac.*, *Gam.*, **Graph.**, Guai., Hell., *Hep.*, Hyos., *Ign.*, Iod., Ip., *K. br.*, **K. carb.**, K. nit., Kre., **Lach.**, Laur., **Led.**, LYC., Mag. c., Mag. m., Mang., Mar., **Menth.**, Meny., MERC., **Mez.**, Mos., *Mur. ac.*, Nat. c., NAT. M., **Nit. ac.**, **Nux v.**, Oleand., Op., *Par.*, **Petrol.**, **Phos.**, *Pho. ac.*, **Plat.**, Pb., **PULS.**, *Ran. b.*, Ran. s., Rheum, *Rhodo.*, **RHUS**, *Rumex*, Ruta, **Saba.**, *Sabi.*, *Sal. ac.*, Samb., **Sars.**, Sec. c., *Sele.*, Seneg., SEP., SIL., Spig., SPO., Squ., Stan., STAPH., Stram., Stro., SUL., *Sul. ac.*, Tab., Tar., *Tarent.*, Thuj., **Urt.**, Valer., *Verat. a.*, Vio. o., **Vio. t.**, *Zinc.*,

—**Biting.**—Alum., **Agn.**, *Am. carb.*, *Am. m.*, *Ant. cr.*, Arn., Bell., Bor., Bov., **Bry.**, *Calc. c.*, Camph., *Canth.*, Caps., Carb. an., *Carb. v.*, **Caust.**, Cham., Chel., *Chin.*, Cocc., *Colch.*, Coloc., Con., *Dros. Dulc.*, **Euphorb.**, Hell., *Ip.*, **Lach.**, LED., **Lyc.**, Mag. c., Mang., **Merc.**, Mez., Mur. ac., Nat. c., Nat. m., *Nux v.*, OLEAND., Op., **Paeo.**, Petrol., Phos., *Pho. ac.*, **Plat.**, PULS., *Ran. b.*, *Ran. s.*, Rhodo., *Rhus*, *Sele.*, **Sep.**, Sil., *Spig.*, Spo., Stro., **Sul.**, *Thuj.*, Verat. a., Vio. t., *Zinc.*

—**Burning.**—Acon., **Agar.**, Alum., *Ambr.*, Am. carb., *Anac.*, *Ant. cr.*, *Arg.*, *Arn.*, ARS., Asaf., Asar., Aur., **Bar. c.**, **Bell.**, Bism., Bov., BRY., *Calad.*, *Calc. c.*, Camph., Cannab. s., Canth., *Caps.*, Carb. an., *Carb. v.*, Caust., Cham., Chin., Cic., Clem., *Cocc.*, *Coff.*, *Colch.*, Coloc., **Com.**, Con., Cup., Dig., Dros., Dulc., *Euphorb.*, Graph., Guai., Hell., **Hep.**, *Hyos.*, *Ign.*, Iod., **Jug. c.**, **K. carb.**, K. nit., Kre., LACH., Laur., *Led.*, **LYC.**, Mag. c., Mang., Mar., Meny., **Merc.**, **Mez.**, Mur. ac., Nat. c., Nat. m., Nit. ac., *Nux v.*, *Oleand*, Op., Petrol., **Phos.**, *Pho. ac.*, *Plat.*, Pb., **PULS.**, *Ran. b.* Rhodo., Rhus, Ruta., *Saba.*, Samb., Sars., Sec. c., *Sele.*, Seneg., **Sep.**, SIL., Spig., *Spo.*, Squ., Stan., *Staph.*, Stram., Stro., **SUL.**, Sul. ac., *Thuj.*, Valer., Verat. a., Vio. o., *Vio. t.*, Zinc.

—**Corroding** (Compare **Gnawing**).—*Agar.*, AGN., *Alum.*, Ambr., Anac., *Ant. cr.*, *Arg.*, Ars., **Bar. c.** Bell., Bism., *Bry.*, *Canth.*, **Caps.**, Cham., **Clem.**, *Cocc.*, Con., *Cyc.*, *Dig.*, *Dros.*, Euphorb., *Graph.*, Guai., Hell., Hyos., *K. carb.*, Led., LYC., *Meny.*, *Merc.*, *Mez.*, Nat. c., Nux v., OLEAND., *Par.*, Phos., *Pho. ac.*, PLAT., *Puls.*, *Ran. s.*, Rhodo., *Rhus*, Ruta, Sep., *Spig.*, **Spo.**, *Squ.*, Stan., STAPH., *Sul.*, Tar., *Thuj.*, *Verat. a.*

—**Crawling.**—Acon., *Alum.*, *Ambr.*, *Am. carb.*, Ant. cr., *Arg.*, **Arn.**, *Ars.*, Asaf., **Bar. c.**, *Bell.*, *Bry.*, *Calc. c.*, Camph., **Canth.**, Caps., *Carb. v.*,

Caust., *Chel.*, *Chin.*, Cina, COLCH., *Con.*, *Croc.*, Euphr., *Graph.*, Guai., Hep., *Ign.*, K. carb., *Lach.*, *Led.*, **Lyc.**, Mar., **Merc.**, *Mur. ac.*, *Nat. c.*, *Nat. m.*, Nux. v., *Par.*, *Pho. ac.*, PLAT., Pb., PULS., **Ran. b.**, Ran. s., *Rhodo.*, **RHUS.**, Saba., Sabi., **Sec. c.**, Sele., SEP., *Sil.*, SPIG., *Spo.*, *Squ.*, Staph., SUL., Sul. ac., *Thuj.*, Verat. a., *Vio. t.*, Zinc.

Itching, Creeping.—*Agn.*, Alum., Am. carb., *Arg.*, Aur., **Bar. c.**, Bor., Bov., Calc. c., Cannab. s., Caps., *Carb. v.*, *Caust.*, Laur., Led., LYC., Mag. c., Mag. m., Mang., *Mur. ac.*, Nat. c., Nit. ac., Nux v., Oleand., Phos., *Pho. ac.*, Plat., *Ran. b.*, Ran. s., Rhodo., Rhus, Saba., Sec. c., Sil., *Spig.*, *Spo.*, STAPH., SUL., Zinc.

—**Jerking.**—*Calc. c.*, Caust., **Lyc.**, Nat. m., *Puls.*, Rhus.

—**Smarting.**—Alum., Ambr., **Arg.**, Aur., *Bry.*, *Calc. c.*, Cannab. s., Cic., Colch., Dros., **Graph.**, *Hep.*, *K. carb.*, Led., *Lyc.*, Mag. c., Mang., Merc., Mez., Nat. c., Nat. m., Nit. ac., *Nux v.*, Oleand., Par., Petrol., PLAT., **Puls.**, Rhus, Ruta, Sabi., Sars., **Sep.**, *Sil.*, *Squ.*, *Staph.*, **Sul.**, Valer., Verat. a., Zinc.

—**Sticking.**—Acon., *Agn.*, Alum., *Am. m.*, Anac., Ant. cr., *Apis*, Arg., **Arn.**, Ars., *Asaf.*, Asar., Aur., **Bar. c.**, *Bell.*, Bov., BRY., Calad., *Calc. c.*, Camph., Cannab. s., *Canth.*, Caps., Carb. an., Carb. v., **Caust.**, Cham., Chel., *Chin.*, Clem., **Cocc.**, Colch., **Con.**, **Cop.**, Cyc., Dig., **Dros.**, Dulc., Euphorb., *Euphr.*, GRAPH., Guai., *Hell.*, Hep., Hyos., *Ign.*, Iod., K. carb., K. nit., Kre., *Lach.*, *Laur.*, Led., *Lyc.*, Mag. c., Mag. m., Mang., Mar., *Meny.*, **Merc.**, *Mez.*, Mos., **Mur. ac.**, Nat. c., **Nat. m.**, *Nit. ac.*, Nux v., Oleand., Op., *Par.*, Petrol., Phos., Pho. ac., *Plat.*, Pb., PULS., Ran. b., *Ran. s.*, Rheum, Rhodo., RHUS, Ruta, Saba., *Sabi.*, Samb., *Sars.*, Sele., Sep., Sil., Spig., SPO., *Squ.*, Stan., Staph., Stram., Stro., **Sul.**, Sul. ac., *Tar.*, Thuj., Verat. a., VIO. T., Zinc.

—**Tearing** (Including Drawing).—**Bell.**, *Bry.*, **Lyc.**, *Sil.*, Staph., *Sul.*, Zinc.

—**Tickling.**—Acon., *Agar.*, Alum., **Ambr.**, Am. m., **Arg.**, *Bry.*, Calc. c., anth., *Caps.*, Chel., *Chin.*, Cocc., Dig., Dros., Euphorb., Euphr., Ign., Mang., **Mar.**, **Merc.**, Mur. ac., Phos., **Plat.**, *Pru.*, *Puls*, Ruta, SABA., Sep., SIL., Spig., *Spo.*, *Squ.*, *Staph.*, Sul., Tar.

—**Voluptuous.**—*Ambr.*, *Anac.*, Arg., Meny., **Merc.**, *Mur. ac.*, Plat., Puls., *Saba.*, Sep., Sil., Spig., Spo., SUL.

—**Aggravated and Ameliorated by Scratching.** See **Agg.** and **Amel., Scratching.**

—**Changing Place on Scratching.**—*Anac.*, Calc. c., Carb. an., Chel., Cyc., Ign., Mag. c., Mag. m., Mez., Spo., Staph., Sul. ac., Zinc.

—**Unchanged by Scratching.**—*Acon.*, Agar., Agn., Alum., *Ambr.*,

SKIN.

Am. carb., Am. m., Ant. cr., Ant. t., **Arg.**, *Arn.*, Asaf., *Aur.*, Bar. c., **Bell.**, *Bism.*, Bor., **Bov.**, *Calad.*, Camph., Carb. an., Carb. v., Caust., *Cham.*, *Chel.*, Cina, *Clem.*, Cocc., Coff., *Colch.*, Coloc., Croc., Cup., Dig., *Euphorb.*, Euphr., *Hell.*, Hyos., *Iod.*, **Ip.**, Laur., **Mag. m.**, *Mar.*, Mur. ac., Nat. c., Nux v., Op., Plat., *Pru.*, **PULS.**, **Ran. s.**, *Rheum*, Rhus, Ruta, Samb., Sec. c., Seneg., *Sil.*, **Spig.**, SPO., Stan., *Stram.*, Sul. ac., *Tar.*, Valer.

Itching, After Scratching Biting.—*Am. carb.*, **Am. m.**, Bry., *Calc. c*, Canth., Carb. an., *Carb. v.*, **Caust.**, Chin., Con., Dros., Euphorb., Hell., Ip., *Kre.*, **LACH**, **Led.**, Lyc., Mang., *Merc.*, **Mez.**, Nat. c., Nat. m., *Nux v.*, OLEAND., *Petrol.*, Pho. ac., **Puls.**, Ran. b., Ruta, Sele., Sep., Sil., **Spo.**, Sul., Zinc.

— —**Blisters.**—**Am. carb.**, **Am. m.**, *Ant. cr.*, *Ars.*, Bar. c., Bell., Bry., *Caust.*, Chin., **Cyc.**, *Dulc.*, Graph., **Hep.**, K. carb., *Kre.*, **LACH.**, Laur., Mang., Merc., *Nat. c.*, Nat. m., **Phos.**, Ran. b., RHUS, Sabi., *Sars.*, Sele., Sep., *Spo.*, *Sul.*

— —**Oozing of Blood.**—*Calc. c.*, Chin., **Lach.**, Lyc., *Nux v.*, SUL.

— —**Bloody.**—Alum., *Calc. c.*, *Chin.*, Cocc., *Cyc.*, **Dulc.**, Euphorb., *Hep.*, Hyos., K. carb., K. nit., *Lach.*, *Lyc.*, MERC., *Nit. ac.*, **Par.**, Petrol., SUL.

— —**Burning.**—Agar., Ambr., **Am. carb.**, *Am. m.*, *Anac.*, *Arn.*, **Ars.**, **Bell.**, Bov., Bry., Calad., *Calc. c.*, Cannab. s., Canth., *Caps.*, Carb. an., Carb. v., CAUST., Chel., Cic., *Cocc.*, Con., *Cyc.*, Dros., **Dulc.**, *Euphorb.*, Graph., **Hep.**, *K. carb.*, Kre., LACH., Laur., Led., **Lyc.**, Mag. c., Mag. m., Mang., MERC., *Mez.*, *Mos.*, *Nux v.*, **Oleand.**, Par., **Phos.**, Pho. ac., *Puls.*, *Ran. b.*, Rhodo., RHUS, *Saba.*, Sabi., Samb., Sars., Sele., Seneg., **Sep.**, SIL., *Spig.*, Spo., Squ., *Staph.*, *Stro.*, SUL., *Thuj.*, Verat. a., Vio. t., Zinc.

— —**Eruption.**—Agar., Alum., AM. CARB., *Am. m.*, *Ant. cr.*, Arn., **Ars.**, Bar. c., Bell., *Bov.*, Bry., **Calc. c.**, Canth., *Carb. an.*, **Carb. v.**, CAUST., Chin., *Cic.*, Con., **Cyc.**, *Dulc.*, Euphorb., *Graph.*, Hell., **Hep.**, Ip., **K. carb.**, Kre., *Lach.*, Laur., LYC., Mag. c., **Merc.**, *Mez.*, Nat. c., *Nat. m.*, *Nit. ac.*, Nux v., Oleand., Petrol., Phos., Pho. ac., Pb., **Puls.**, Rhodo., RHUS, *Sabi.*, Sars., Sep., Sil., *Spo.*, Squ., Staph., *Stro.*, SUL., Sul. ac., *Thuj.*, Verat. a., *Vio. t.*, Zinc.

— —**Erysipelas.**—**Am. carb.**, Ant. cr., *Arn.*, **Ars.**, **Bell.**, Bor., *Bry.*, *Calc. c.*, Canth., *Carb. an.*, Carb. v., **Graph.**, **Hep.**, Hyos., **Lach.**, **Lyc.**, Mag. c., MERC., Nat. c., *Nit. ac.*, *Petrol.*, **Phos.**, Puls., Ran. b., RHUS, Samb., Sil., Spo., **Sul.**, *Thuj.*

— —**Excoriation.**—Agar., *Am. carb.*, Ant. cr., *Arn.*, Bar. c., Calc. c.,

Caust., Chin., Dros., GRAPH., Hep., K. carb., Kre., Lach., Lyc., Mang. Merc., Oleand., PETROL., Phos., Pb., Puls., Rhus, Ruta, Sabi., Sep., Sil., Squ., Sul., Sul. ac.

Itching, after Scratching Gnawing.—Agar., Alum., Ant. cr., Bar. c., Canth., Caps., Cyc., Dros., K. carb., Led., Lyc., OLEAND., Par., Phos., Pho. ac., Puls., Rhus, Ruta, Spo., Staph., Tar., Verat. a.

— —**Hives.**—Agar., Alum., Am. carb., Am. m., Ant. cr., Ars., Bar. c., Bry., Calc. c., Carb. an., Carb. v., Caust., Cic., Cocc., Con., DULC., Graph., Hell., Hep., Ip., LACH., Led., Lyc., Mag. c., Mag. m., Mang., Merc., MEZ., Nat. c., Nat. m., Nit. ac., Nux v., Oleand., Petrol., Puls., RHUS, Ruta, Sele., Sep., Sil., Spig., Staph., Sul., Thuj., Verat. a., Zinc.

— —**Moisture.**—Alum., Ars., Bar. c., Bell., Bov., Bry., Calc. c., Carb. an., Carb. v., Caust., Cic., Con., Dulc., GRAPH., Hell., Hep., K. carb., Kre., LACH., Led., LYC., Merc., Mez., Nat. c., Nat. m., Nit. ac., Oleand., Petrol., RHUS, Ruta, Sabi., Sele., Sep., Sil., Squ., Staph., Sul., Sul. ac., Tar., Thuj., Vio. t.

— —**Numbness.**—Ambr., Anac., Con., Cyc., Lach., Lyc., OLEAND., Phos., Pho. ac., Pb., Sep., Sul.

— —**Pain.**—Agar., Alum., Ars., BAR. C., Bell., Calc. c., Cups., Chin., Cocc., Con., Euphr., Kre., Led., Nat. m., Nux v., Par., Petrol., Pho. ac., Pb., Puls., Rhus, Sele., Sep., SIL., Squ., Staph., SUL., Thuj., Verat. a.

— —**Pimples.**—Am. carb., Am. m., Ant. cr., Bry., Caust., Chin., Cocc., Con., Cyc., Dros., Dulc., Graph., Hep., K. carb., Laur., Merc., Nat. c., Nat. m., Nit. ac., Petrol., Phos., Pho. ac., Puls., Rhus, Saba., Sabi., Sars., Sele., SEP., Sil., Spo., Squ., Staph., Stro., Sul., Verat. a., Zinc.

— —**White Pimples.**—Agar., Ars., Bov., Bry., Ip., Sul.

— —**Pustules.**—Am. m., Ant. cr., Ars., Bell., Bry., Cyc., Hyos., Merc., Puls., RHUS, Sil., Staph., Sul.

— —**Rash.**—Am. carb., Am. m., Ant. cr., Bov., Bry., Calc. c., Caust., Dulc., Graph., Ip., Lach., Led., Merc., Mez., Phos., Pho. ac., Puls., Rhus, Sars., Sele., Sil., Spo., Staph., Sul., Verat. a., Vio. t., Zinc.

— —**Redness.**—Agar., Am. carb., Ant. cr., Arn., Bell., Bov., Canth., Chin., Dulc., Graph., Kre., Lyc., Mar., Merc., Nat. m., Nux v., Oleand. Op., Petrol., Pho. ac., Puls., RHUS, Ruta, Spo., Tar.

— —**Red Streaks.**—Carb. v., Euphorb., Par., Pho. ac., Saba.

— —**Scales.**—Alum., Am. carb., Am. m., Ant. cr., Ars., Bar. c., Bell., Bov., Bry., Calc. c., Caps., Carb. an., Carb. v., Cic., Con., Dulc., Graph., Hep., K. carb., Kre., Led., LYC., Merc., Mez., Nat. m., Petrol., Phos.,

Puls., *Ran. b.*, RHUS, Saba., Sabi., *Sars.*, *Sep.*, *Sil.*, **Staph.**, SUL., Thuj., Verat. a., *Vio. t.* Zinc.

Itching, after Scratching Smarting Pain.—Agar., *Alum.*, Ambr., Ant. cr., *Arg.*, *Bar. c.*, *Bry.*, *Calc. c.*, Cannab. s., *Canth.*, **Caps.**, *Cic.*, Dros., Graph., **Hep.**, K. carb., Led., *Lyc.*, Mag. c., *Mang.*, Merc., **Mez.**, Nat. c., *Nat. m.*, *Nit. ac.*, Nux v., OLEAND., *Par.*, **Petrol.**, Phos., Pho. ac., *Puls.*, **Rhus**, *Sabi.*, Sars., Sele., SEP., *Sil.*, Squ., **Staph.**, SUL., Verat. a., Zinc.

— —**Spots.**—Am. carb., *Ant. cr.*, *Bell.*, Calc. c., *Cocc.*, *Cyc.*, Graph., Mag. c., *Mang.*, Merc., Nit. ac., **Phos.**, Pho. ac., **Rhus**, Saba., Sep., Sil., **Sul.**, Sul. ac., Verat. a.

— —**Stitches.**—Alum., Am. m., *Arn.*, Ars., *Asaf.*, BAR. C., Bell., **Bry.**, *Calc. c.*, Cannab. s., *Canth.*, **Caust.**, Chel., *Chin.*, *Cocc.*, Con., **Cyc.**, Dros., *Dulc.*, Graph., Hell., K. carb., *Lach.*, Lyc., Mar., Merc., Mez., *Nit. ac.*, Par., *Pho. ac.*, Puls., Ran. b., RHUS, Ruta, Saba., Sars., Sele., *Sep.*, *Sil.*, Spo., Squ., Staph., Stro., SUL., *Tar.*, *Thuj.*, Vio. t., Zinc.

— —**Suppurative Pain.**—Arn., *Asaf.*, Bar. c., *Bry.*, *Calc. c.*, Carb. v., *Con.*, Cyc., Graph., *Hep.*, K. carb., Led., Nat. m., *Petrol.*, **Phos.**, **Puls.**, *Ran. b.*, Rhus, SIL., Staph., **Sul.**, Zinc.

— —**Swelling.**—*Ant. cr.*, Arn., *Ars.*, Bell., *Bry.*, Calc. c., *Canth.*, **Caust.**, Chin., Con., *Dulc.*, Hep., K. carb., *Kre.*, LACH., *Led.*, Lyc., *Mang.*, **Merc.**, *Mez.*, Nat. m., Nit. ac., Phos., **Puls.**, **Rhus**, *Sabi.*, Samb., Sep., Sil., Sul., *Sul. ac.*

— —**Tearing.**—*Ars.*, Bell., Bry., *Calc. c.*, *Cyc.*, **Lyc.**, Puls., Rhus, Sep., *Sil.*, Staph., SUL.

— —**Tension.**—*Caust.*, Lach., *Pho. ac.*, Ruta, Spig., **Stro.**

— —**Skin Becomes Thick.**—Ant. cr., Ars., *Cic.*, **Dulc.**, Graph., Lach., *Ran. b.*, RHUS, Sep., Thuj., Verat. a.

— —**Tickling.**—Agar., *Ambr.*, Caps., *Chin.*, Cocc., *Mar.*, Merc., SABA., Sil., Spig.

— —**Ulcerative Pain.**—*Am. carb.*, AM. M., Bell., *Bry.*, *Caust.*, *Chin.*, Cic., Graph., *Hep.*, *K. carb.*, Mag. m., Mang., *Merc.*, Nat. m., *Phos.*, **Puls.**, RHUS, *Sep.*, Sil., Spig., *Staph.*, Sul. ac., *Thuj.*, Verat. a.

— —**Ulcers.**—Ant. cr., Ars., *Asaf.*, Bar. c., Bell., *Bry.*, Calc. c., Carb. an., Carb. v., **Caust.**, Chin., *Con.*, Graph., Hep., *Kre.*, LACH., **Lyc.**, Mang., **Merc.**, **Mez.**, Nat. c., **Nit. ac.**, Petrol., Phos., Pho. ac., *Puls.*, Ran. b., Rhus, *Sabi.*, Sep., Sil., *Staph.*, SUL., Thuj.

Lousiness.—*Ars.*, Lach., Merc., *Oleand.*, **Pso.**, Saba., *Staph.*, Sul.

Moisture.—*Alum.*, Ars., Bar. c., *Bell.*, **Bov.**, Bry., Calc. c., Carb. an., CARB. V., *Caust.*, *Cic.*, **Clem.**, Con., *Dulc.*, GRAPH., *Hell.*, Hep., K. **carb.**, Kre., **Lach.**, Led., LYC., *Merc.*, *Mez.*, Nat. c., *Nat. m.*, *Nit. ac.*,

SKIN.

Oleand., **Petrol.**, **Phos.**, **Pho. ac.**, **RHUS**, *Ruta*, Sabi., **Sele.**, **Sep.**, *Sil.*, *Squ.*, Staph., Sul., Sul. ac., Tar., Thuj., *Vio. t.*

Nails Generally Affected.—Alum., Am. m., *Ant. cr.*, **Ars.**, Aur., Bar. c., Bell., *Bor.*, Bov., *Calc. c.*, *Caust.*, Chel., Chin., Cocc., Colch., *Con.*, Dig., Dros., **GRAPH.**, *Hell.*, *Hep.*, Iod., K. carb., Lach., Lyc., *Mar.*, **Merc.**, Mos., Mur. ac., **Nat. m.**, **Nit. ac.**, *Nux v.*, *Par.*, Petrol., Pho. ac., Plat., **Puls.**, *Ran. b.*, Rhus, Ruta, **Saba.**, Sec. c., *Sep.*, **SIL.**, **Squ.**, **SUL.**, Sul. ac., Thuj.

—**Brittle.**—*Alum.*, Calc. c., *Dios.*, *Fl. ac.*, **Graph.**, *Merc.*, **Saba.**, Sep., **Sil.**, Sul.

—**Blue.**—*Aesc.*, **Aur.**, Chel., Chin., **Cic.**, *Cocc.*, **Dig.**, **Dros.**, Gel., **Nat. m.**, **NUX V.**, Petrol., **Sil.**, **VERAT. A.**

—**Deformed.**—*Alum.*, Calc. c., **GRAPH.**, Merc., **Saba.**, Sep., *Sil.* Sul.

—**Discolored.**—*Ant. cr.*, **Ars.**, **Graph.**, Mur. ac., **Nit. ac.**, Ox. ac., **Sil.**, Sul.

—**Falling Off.**—Ant. cr., *Ars.*, *Form.*, *Hell.*, Merc., Sec. c., **Squ.**, Thuj.

—**Furrowed.**—*Ars.*, *Fl. ac.*, **Saba.**, **SIL.**

—**Growing Inward.**—Colch., *Graph.*, *Mar.*, *Sil.*, Sul.

—**Growing Very Slowly.**—Ant. cr.

—**Jerking Pain.**—Alum., *Calc. c.*, *Caust.*, **Graph.**, Mos., **Nat. m.**, Nit. ac., *Nux v.*, **Puls.**, *Rhus*, Sep., *Sil.*, Sul.

—**Painful.**—Am. m., *Ant. cr.*, Bell., **Caust.**, **Graph.**, *Hep.*, K. carb., *Mar.*, **Merc.**, Nat. m., *Nit. ac.*, *Nux v.*, Par., **Petrol.**, *Puls.*, Ran. b., Rhus, **Saba.**, Sep., **Sil.**, *Squ.*, Sul.

—**Scaling Off.**—Merc.

—**Sensitive.**—Calc. c., Con., Hep., Merc., Nat. m., **Nux v.**, Petrol., Pho. ac., Sep., **Sil.**, *Squ.*, *Sul.*, Thuj.

—**Smarting.**—*Alum.*, Ant. cr., Calc. c., Caust., **GRAPH.**, *Hep.*, Merc., Nat. m., *Nux v.*, Puls., **Sep.**, *Sul.*

—**Splitting.**—Ant. cr., Sil., Squ.

—**Sensation of Splinters Under.**—Colch., Fl. ac., *Hep.*, Nit. ac., Petrol., Plat., Ran. b., Sil., Sul.

—**Spotted.**—*Alum.*, Ars., Nit. ac., Sep., Sil., *Sul.*

—**Thick.**—*Alum.*, **Ant. cr.**, Calc. c., **GRAPH.**, Merc., **Saba.**, Sep., *Sil.*, Sul.

—**Ulcerated.**—*Alum.*, Am. m., *Ant. cr.*, **Ars.**, Aur., Bar. c., Bell., Bor., Bov., **Calc. c.**, Caust., Chin., *Con.*, *Crotal.*, *Fl. ac.*, **Graph.**, Hep., **Lach.**, **Lyc.**, Mar., **Merc.**, **Mur. ac.**, Nat. m., **Nit. ac.**, Petrol., Pho. ac.,

Plat., **Puls.**, *Ran. b.*, **Rhus**, **Ruta**, Saba., **Sang.**, Sec. c., *Sep.*, SIL., *Squ.*, SUL., Sul. ac., Thuj.

Nails, Ulcerative Pain.—**Am. m.**, **Bell.**, **Calc. ph.**, *Caust.*, *Chin.*, GRAPH., *Hep.*, *K. carb.*, **Merc.**, Mos., Mur. ac., **Nat. m.**, *Nux v.*, PULS., Ran. b., **Rhus**, **Ruta**, Sep., **Sil.**, *Sul.*, Sul. ac., *Thuj.*

—**Yellow.**—*Ambr.*, Ant. cr., Ars., *Aur.*, **Bell.**, *Bry.*, Calc. c., *Canth.*, *Carb. v.*, Caust., *Cham.*, Chel., *Chin.*, CON., *Fer.*, Hep., *Ign.*, *Lyc.*, **Merc.**, Nit. ac., **Nux v.**, *Op.*, *Pb.*, Puls., SEP., SIL., *Spig.*, Sul.

Numbness (and Fuzziness).—*Acon.*, **Ambr.**, ANAC., Ant. t., *Cham.*, *Con.*, Cyc., **Hyper.**, Lach., **Lyc.**, Nux v., **Oleand.**, *Phos.*, **Pho. ac.**, *Plat.*, Pb., SEC. C., Sep., Stram., *Sul.*

Pressure, Deep Inward, From Instruments.—BOV., *Verat. a.*

Prickling.—Acon., *Aconin.*, Agar., Ant. t., **Apis**, Bell., Cannab. s., Croc., *Dros.*, Lyc., *Mez.*, Mos., **PLAT.**, **Ran. s.**, *Saba.*, Sep., **SUL.**, Zinc.

Rawness.—Bell., CALC. C., *Graph.*, Iod., K. carb., *Laur.*, Merc., NIT. AC., *Oleand.*, **Petrol.**, Phos., Pho. ac., **Rhus**, Ruta, *Sars.*, SEP., Sul.

Sensitiveness in General.—Acon., Agar., Alum., Am. m., Ant. cr., Ant. t.; Apis, *Arn.*, Ars., Aur., Bar. c., **BELL.**, Bov., **Bry.**, **Calc. c.**, *Camph.*, Cannab. s., *Canth.*, **Caps.**, Carb. an., Carb. v., Cham., CHIN., **Coff.**, Colch., **Con.**, **Fer.**, *Gel.*, *Hep.*, Ign., **Ip.**, K. carb., **Kre.**, *Lach.*, Led., *Lyc.*, **Mag. c.**, MERC., *Mez.*, **Mos.**, *Nat. c.*, **Nat. m.**, *Nux m.*, **Nux v.**, Oleand., Ox. ac., Par., PETROL., *Phos.*, PHO. AC., PB., *Puls.*, Ran. b., Ran. s., **Rhus**, **Sang.**, Sars., Sec. c., Sele., Sep., SIL., Spig., *Spo.*, Stan., Staph., Squ., SUL., Sul. ac., **Thuj.**, **Verat. a.**, Zinc.

Sore, Becomes (Decubitus).—Agar., Ambr., *Am. carb.*, Am. m., *Ant. cr.*, ARN., Ars., *Bap.*, Bar. c., Bell., Bov., **Calc. c.**, *Calc. ph.*, *Canth.*, Carb. an., Carb. v., *Caust.*, *Cham.*, CHIN., Coff., Colch., Dros., Euphr., *Fl. ac.*, GRAPH., **Hep.**, *Hydras.*, Ign., *K. carb.*, **Kre.**, LACH., **Lyc.**, Mag. m., *Mang.*, **Merc.**, Mez., **Nat. c.**, *Nat. m.*, Nit. ac., Nux v., *Oleand.*, Op., PETROL., *Phos.*, Pho. ac., *Pb.*, Puls., Rhus, *Ruta*, Sele., SEP., SIL., Spig., *Squ.*, Sul., *Sul. ac.*, Ter., Zinc.

—**In a Child.**—Ant. cr., Bar. c., Bell., **Calc. c.**, CHAM., **Chin.**, *Ign.*, Kre., **Lyc.**, *Merc.*, Puls., *Ruta*, **Sep.**, *Sil.*, Squ., SUL.

Sore Feeling in General.—Acon., Agar., **Alum.**, Ambr., *Ant. cr.*, *Arg.*, **Arn.**, **Ars.**, *Aur.*, Bar. c., *Bor.*, **Bry.**, Calc. c., Cannab. s., Canth., Caps., Carb. an., Carb. v., *Caust.*, Chel., Chin., **Cic.**, CIMIC., Coff., *Colch.*, *Crotal.*, **Dros.**, EUP. PER., *Fer.*, **Glon.**, **Graph.**, Hell., HEP., Ign.,

SKIN.

K. carb., Led., Lyc., Mag. c., *Mang.*, Mar., **Merc.**, *Mez.*, Mos., *Nat. c.*, **Nat. m., Nit. ac.,** Nux v., Oleand., *Par.,* **Petrol.,** *Phos.*, Pho. ac., **Plat., Puls.,** Ran. b., **Rhus,** Ruta, Sabi., Sars., Sele., SEP., *Sil.*, Spig., Spo., *Squ., Staph.,* **Still.,** Sul., *Sul. ac.,* Valer., Verat. a., ZINC.

Spots, Black.—Ars., Lach., *Rhus,* Sec. c.

—**Blue.**—Ant. cr., ARN., *Ars.,* Bar. c., Bry., *Con.,* Fer., *Lach.,* **Led.,** Mos., Nit. ac., Nux m., *Nux v.,* Op., *Rhus,* Ruta, Sec. c., Sil., Sul. **Sul. ac.**

—**Burning.**—Am. carb., Am. m., **Ars.,** Bell., *Canth.,* Chel., Croc., Fer., Iod., **K. carb.,** *Lyc.,* Mag. c., *Merc.,* **Mez.,** PHO. AC., *Rhus, Sul.,* Sul. ac.

—**As if Burnt.**—Ant. cr., **Ars.,** *Carb. v.,* Caust., **Cyc.,** Euphorb., *Hyos.,* Kre., Rhus, Sec. c., Stram.

—**Confluent.**—Bell., Cic., *Hyos.,* Pho. ac., *Valer.*

—**Death Spots in Old People.**—*Ars.,* Bar. c., **Con.,** Lach., Op.

—**Like Flea-bites.**—Acon. (Stram.)

—**Freckles.**—**Am. carb.,** Ant. cr., Ant. t., *Bry.,* **Calc. c.,** Carb. v., *Con., Dros.,* Dulc., **Graph.,** Hyos., Iod., *K. carb.,* Lach., Laur., **LYC.,** *Merc., Mez.,* **Nat. c., Nit. ac.,** *Nux m., Petrol.,* PHOS., Pb., **Puls.,** Sec. c., Sep., *Sil.,* Stan., SUL., Thuj.

—**Gangrenous.**—*Cyc.,* **Hyos.,** *Sec. c.*

—**Green.**—Arn., Ars., CON., *Nit. ac.,* Sep., Sul. ac.

—**Itching.**—Agn., Am. m., *Arn.,* **Con.,** Dros., *Euphorb.,* **Graph.,** *Iod.,* K. carb., Led., *Lyc.,* Merc., *Mez., Nat. m.,* Op., Par., *Sep., Sil., Spo.,* Sul. ac.

—**Liver.**—*Am. carb,* Ant. cr., Ant. t., *Arn.,* Ars., **Aur.,** *Bry., Calc. c.,* Canth., **Carb. v.,** Caust., **Con.,** *Cop.,* Dros., **Dulc.,** *Fer.,* **Graph.,** *Hyos.,* Iod., *K. bi.,* K. carb., LACH., Laur., LYC., MERC., **Mez.,** Nat. c., NIT. AC., Nux v., *Petrol,* Phos., *Pb.,* Puls., Ruta, Saba., SEP., Sil., Stan., SUL., Thuj.

—**Of Petechiæ.**—**Apoc. c.,** *Arn.,* ARS., *Bell.,* BRY., *Crotal., Cup.,* Hyos., *Lach.,* **Led.,** *Nat. m., Nux v.,* **Phos.,** RHUS, Ruta, Sec. c., *Sil.,* Squ., Stram., *Sul. ac., Ter.*

— —**Red.**—*Acon., Agn.,* Alum., Ambr., AM. CARB., Am. m., Ant. t. *Apis,* **Arn.,** *Ars.,* Aur., *Bar. c.,* **BELL.,** Brom., **Bry.,** Calad., **Calc. c.,** Canth., Caps., Carb. an., *Carb. v.,* Caust., Cham., *Chel., Chin.,* Clem., *Coc. c.,* COCC., Coff., **Con.,** *Croc.,* Cup., **Cyc.,** Dros., *Dulc.,* **Graph.,** Hep., *Hyos., Iod.,* Ip., K. carb., *K. nit., Lach.,* **Led.,** *Lyc.,* **Mag. c.,** Mag. m., Mar., **Merc.,** Mez., *Nat. c.,* Nat. m., **Nit. ac.,** Nux v., Op., Par., PHOS., Pho. ac., *Pb.,* Puls., Rhodo., Rhus, SABA., Sec. c., SEP., **Sil.,** *Spo., Squ., Stan.,* **Stram., Sul., Sul. ac.,** *Verat. a.,* **Zinc.**

Spots of Petechiæ, Bluish.—Bell., Phos.

— —**Brownish.**—Cannab. s., NIT. AC., **Phos.**

— —**Coppery.**—Alum., **Ars.**, *Calc. c., Cannab. s.,* CARB. AN., *Carb. v.,* Kre., LACH., *Led.,* **Mez.,** *Phyt.,* Rhus, Ruta, **Verat. a.**

— —**Fiery.**—Acon., Bell., *Stram.*

— —**Pale.**—Mar., *Nat. c.,* Phos., Sil.

— —**Becoming Pale in the Cold.**—Saba.

— —**Violet.**—*Phos.,* Verat. a.

— —**Like Red Wine.**—Cocc., *Sep.*

—**Scarlet.**—*Acon.,* AM. CARB., *Am. m.,* Arn., **Ars.,** *Bar. c.,* BELL., Bry., *Carb. v., Caust.,* Cham., *Coff.,* **Croc.,** Dulc., Euphorb., *Hep.,* **Hyos.,** Iod., *Ip., Lach.,* MERC., *Phos.,* Pho. ac., Rhus, **Stram.,** Sul.

—**Smarting.**—Bry., **Fer.,** *Hep.,* **Led.,** Nat. m., *Pho. ac.,* Sil., *Verat. a.*

—**Stinging.**—*Canth.,* Chel., *Nit. ac.,* Puls., SIL.

—**White.**—Alum., Am. carb., ARS., **Aur.,** Carb. an., *Coca,* **Phos.,** Sep., SIL., Sul.

—**Yellow.**—Ambr., **Ant. t.,** ARN., Ars., *Canth.,* **Con., Fer.,** Iod., K. carb., *Lach.,* **Lyc.,** Nat. c., *Petrol.,* **Phos.,** Ruta, *Saba.,* Sep., Stan., SUL.

Sticking.—Acon., Agar., *Agn.,* Alum., *Am. m.,* Anac., Ant. cr., *Apis,* **Arn.,** *Ars.,* **Asaf.,** BAR. C., *Bell.,* BRY., **Calc. c.,** *Cannab. s.,* **Canth.,** Caps., Carb. v., *Carb. sul., Caust., Chel.,* Chin., Clem., Cocc., Colch., **Con.,** Cyc., *Dig., Dios., Dros.,* Dulc., Euphr., GRAPH., *Guai., Hell.,* Hep., Hyos., *Ign.,* Iod., *K. carb., K. nit.,* Kre., Lach., *Lyc.,* Mag. c., *Mar. Meny.,* **Merc.,** *Mez.,* Mur. ac., Nat. c., Nat. m., **Nit. ac.,** *Nux v.,* Oleand., *Par.,* Phos., Pho. ac., *Plat.,* Pb., **PULS.,** *Ran. b., Ran. s.,* Rhodo., RHUS, *Ruta,* **Saba.,** Sabi., *Sars., Sele.,* **Sep.,** Sil., Spig., SPO., Squ., Stan., Staph., Stro., **Sul.,** Sul. ac., **Tar.,** Thuj., Verat. a., VIO. T., *Zinc.*

—**Burning.**—Acon., Alum., Anac., Apis, Arg., Arn., *Ars.,* ASAF., Bar. c., *Bell.,* **Bry.,** Calc. c., *Cannab. s., Caps.,* Carb. v., *Caust.,* Cina, **Cocc.,** Colch., *Dig., Dros.,* Dulc., *Hell., Hep., Hyos., Ign.,* Iod., K. carb., *Lach.,* **Lyc.,** Mag. c., *Meny.,* **Merc., Mez.,** Nux v., *Oleand.,* **Phos.,** Pho. ac., *Plat.,* **Puls.,** Ran. b., *Ran. s.,* Rhus, *Saba.,* Samb., *Sele.,* Sep., **Sil.,** Spig., *Spo., Squ., Stan.,* STAPH., Sul., Sul. ac., THUJ., *Vio. t.*

Stings of Insects.—*Acon., Ant. cr.,* **Apis, Arn.,** Ars., Bell., **Calad.,** Caust., *Coloc., Lach., Led., Merc.,* Seneg., Sep., Sil., Sul.

Swelling, General, External.—*Acon.,* Agn., *Aloe.,* Am. carb., **Ant. cr.,** APIS, **Arn.,** ARS., **Ars. iod.,** Asaf., *Aur.,* **Bar. c., Bell.,** Bor.,

SKIN.

BRY., *Calc. c.*, *Canth.*, Carb. an., Carb. v., *Caust.*, Chel., **Chin.**, CIC., Cina, Clem., *Cocc.*, *Colch.*, Coloc., *Con.*, **Cop.**, Cyc., *Dig.*, **Dulc.**, EUPHORB., Fer., *Fl. ac.*, Graph., *Hell.*, *Hep.*, **Hydroc.**, *Hyos.*, *Iod.*, *K. bi.*, *K. br.*, *K. carb.*, K. nit., Kre., Lach., **Led.**, **Lyc.**, Mag. c., Mang., MERC., Mez., Mur. ac., Nat. c., *Nat. m.*, *Nit. ac.*, NUX V., Oleand., Op., Petrol., **Phos.**, Pho. ac., *Pb.*, PULS., *Rhodo.*, RHUS, Ruta, **Sabi.**, **Samb.**, Sars., Sec. c., Seneg., Sep., *Sil.*, Spig., Spo., Squ., Stram., Stro., SUL., Sul. ac., **Thuj.**, Verat. a.

Swelling of Affected Parts.—*Acon.*, Agn., Ant. cr., *Arn.*, *Ars.*, Asaf., Aur., BELL., **Bry.**, **Calc. c.**, **Canth.**, Carb. an., Carb. v., **Caust.**, Chin., Clem., *Cocc.*, *Con.*, Dig., *Dulc.*, *Euphorb.*, Fer., Graph., Hell., **Hep.**, Iod., K. CARB., *Lach.*, Led., **Lyc.**, *Mag. c.*, Mang., MERC., Mur. ac., *Nat. c.*, **Nit. ac.**, *Nux v.*, *Petrol.*, **Phos.**, *Pho. ac.*, Pb., PULS., *Rhodo.*, RHUS, Ruta, *Sabi.*, **Samb.**, Sars., Sec. c., SEP., Sil., Spig., **Spo.**, *Stram.*, SUL., Thuj.

—**Bluish-black.**—Acon., Am. carb., Arn., ARS., *Aur.*, **Bell.**, *Carb. v.*, Con., **Dig.**, *Hep.*, LACH., Mang., **Merc.**, Nux v., Op., *Phos.*, Pho. ac., Pb., PULS., *Samb.*, Sec. c., Seneg., *Sil.*, *Sul. ac.*, **Verat. a.**

—**Burning.**—Acon., *Ant. cr.*, Arn., ARS., **Bell.**, BRY., *Calc. c.*, Carb. an., Carb. v., *Caust.*, *Chin.*, *Cocc.*, Colch., Coloc., *Crotal.*, *Dulc.*, *Euphorb.*, Hell., *Hep.*, *Hyos.*, Iod., *K. carb.*, **Lach.**, Led., LYC., Mang., **Merc.**, *Mez.*, Nat. c., *Nux v.*, Op., PHOS., Pho. ac., Puls., Rhus, *Samb.*, Sec. c., *Sep.*, **Sil.**, *Spig.*, Spo., Squ., Stan., SUL.

—**Cold.**—Ars., *Asaf.*, Bell., *Cocc.*, **Con.**, *Cyc.*, Dulc., Lach., *Rhodo.*, Sec. c., *Spig.*

—**Crawling.**—*Acon.*, Arn., Caust., Chel., *Colch.*, *Con.*, Lach., **Merc.**, Nat. c., *Nux v.*, Pho. ac., Puls., RHUS, Sec. c., **Sep.**, *Spig.*, Sul.

—**Dropsical.**—Acon., ANT. CR., ARS., Aur., **Bell.**, BRY., *Canth.*, Chel., CHIN., *Colch.*, Coloc., *Con.*, **Dig.**, **Dulc.**, Euphorb., *Fer.*, Gnai., HELL., Hyos., *Iod.*, *K. carb.*, K. nit., Lach., **Led.**, **Lyc.**, **Merc.**, Mez., Mur. ac., Nat. c., *Nit. ac.*, Oleand., Op., *Phos.*, Pb., PULS., Rhodo., **Rhus**, *Ruta.*, Sabi., **Samb.**, Sars., Sec. c., *Seneg.*, Sep., Sil., SQU., Stram., SUL., TELL., *Verat. a.*

—**Hard.**—Acon., Agn., *Ant. cr.*, Arn., Ars., *Asaf.*, Bell., BRY., Calc. c., **Caust.**, *Chin.*, Cina, Con., Dig., *Dulc.*, Graph., Hell., Hep., Lach., Led., **Lyc.**, **Merc.**, Mez., Nux v., PHOS., Pho. ac., Pb., PULS., RHUS, Sabi., **Samb.**, Sep., *Sil.*, Spo., Squ., Stro., Sul., Ther.

—**Inflamed.**—Acon., Agn., Am. carb., *Ant. cr.*, Arn., **Ars.**, *Asaf.*, Bell., Bor., BRY., Calc. c., Canth., *Carb. v.*, Caust., Cocc., *Colch.*, Con., *Crotal.*, **Hep.**, Hyos., Lach., *Lyc.*, **Mang.**, MERC., Mez., Mur. ac., Nat.

c., *Nit. ac.*, Petrol., *Phos.*, PULS., **Rhus**, Sars., Sep., **Sil.**, Sul., *Thuj.*, Verat. a.

Swelling, Pale.—Arn., Ars., Bell., BRY., *Calc. c.*, Chin., Cocc., Con., Dig., Fer., Graph., Hell., **Iod.**, K. carb., *Lach.*, **LYC.**, **Merc.**, **Nit. ac.**, Nux v., Phos., Pb., *Puls.*, Rhus, Sep., Spig., Sul.

—**Puffy.**—Acon., *Am. carb.*, **Am. m.**, ANT. CR., *Arn.*, **Ars.**, **Asaf.**, Aur., *Bar. c.*, Bell., Bry., CALC. C., CAPS., Cham., Chin., Cina, *Cocc.*, Colch., *Coloc.*, Con., CUP., Dig., Dros., *Dulc.*, FER., Graph., *Guai.*, Hell., *Hyos.*, Ip., *K. carb.*, Kre., Lach., Laur., *Led.*, *Lyc.*, Mag. c., Mar., *Merc.*, Mez., *Mos.*, Nat. c., Nit. ac., Nux m., Nux v., **Oleand.**, Op., Phos., Pb., **Puls.**, Rheum, Rhus, Samb., Sars., **Seneg.**, Sep., *Sil.*, **Spig.**, *Spo.*, Staph., *Stram.*, *Sul.*

—**Shining.**—Arn., *Ars.*, BRY., *Merc.*, **Rhus**, *Sabi.*, Sul.

—**Spongy.**—Ant. cr., ARS., *Bell.*, Calc. c., **Carb. an.**, Carb. v., Caust., *Clem.*, *Con.*, Graph., Iod., *Kre.*, LACH., *Lyc.*, *Merc.*, Nit. ac., Nux v., Petrol., **Phos.**, Pho. ac., *Rhus*, *Sabi.*, Sep., SIL., **Sul.**, *Thuj.*

—**Stinging.**—Acon., Agn., Ant. cr., *Arn.*, Ars., BRY., *Canth.*, CAUST., Chel., *Chin.*, **Cocc.**, *Con.*, *Cyc.*, Dig., Fer., *Graph.*, K. nit., Lach., *Led.*, Mag. c., Mang., Mez., **Nit. ac.**, Nux v., PULS., **Rhus**, Ruta., *Saba.*, Sep., *Sil.*, Spo., **Sul.**, Thuj.

—**White.**—Ant. cr., APIS, **Ars.**, *Bell.*, BRY., *Calc. c.*, *Chin.*, Dig., Euphorb., Graph., Hep., *Iod.*, Kre., LYC., *Merc.*, **Nux v.**, **Puls.**, Rhodo. Rhus, Sabi., *Sep.*, *Sil.*, Sul.

Swollen Sensation.—*Alum.*, **Am. m.**, Ant. cr., Arn., **Ars.**, Aur., BELL. Bry., *Canth.*, **Caps.**, Carb. v., **Chin.**, Cocc., *Con.*, Dig., *Dulc.*, *Guai.*, Hep., Hyos., Ign., **K. nit.**, Kre., *Lach.*, **Laur.**, *Merc.*, *Nit. ac.*, Nux m., Nux v., **Par.**, Plat., PULS., RHUS, Sabi., Sars., Seneg., Sep., Sil., **Spig.**, *Spo.*, Stan., Staph., Sul., *Sul. ac.*, *Verat. a.*, Zinc.

Tension.—*Agn.*, *Alum.*, Am. carb., Am. m., Anac., Arg., **Arn.**, *Asaf.*, *Asar.*, Aur., **Bap.**, **Bar. c.**, *Bell.*, Bor., *Bry.*, Calc. c., Canth., **Carb. an.**, CAUST., Cham., Chin., Colch., **Coloc.**, **Con.**, Dig., Euphorb., Hell., Hep., Iod., *K. carb.*, Kre., *Lach.*, Laur., Led., Lyc., Mag. m., Mang., Meny., Merc., *Mez.*, Mos., Mur. ac., Nat. c., Nat. m., Nit. ac., Nux v., *Oleand.*, *Par.*, Petrol., **Phos.**, *Pho. ac.*, **Plat.**, **Puls.**, Rhodo., Rhus, *Ruta*, *Saba.*, *Sabi.*, Sars., Sep., Sil., Spig., *Spo.*, Stan., Staph., STRO., **Sul.**, Tar., *Thuj.*, Verat. a., *Verb.*, **Vio. o.**, Vio. t., *Zinc.*

Tetter in General (Herpetic).—Agar., *Alum.*, *Ambr.*, Am. carb., Anac., ARS., Aur., *Bar. c.*, Bell., BOV., Bry., Calad., CALC. C., Caps., Carb. an., Carb. v., **Caust.**, Chel., Cic., CLEM., Cocc., CON., *Cup.*, Cyc., DULC, GRAPH., Hell., *Hep.*, Hyos., K. carb., **K. nit.**, **Kre.**, *Lach.*, **Led.**, LYC.,

SKIN.

Mag. c., Mag. m., Mang., **Mar.**, MERC., Mez., Mos , *Mur. ac.*, **Nat. c.**, *Nat. m.*, *Nit. ac.*, Nux v., *Oleand.*, Par., **Petrol.**, Phos., *Pho. ac.*, Pb., Puls., *Ran. b.*, Ran. s., RHUS, Ruta, Saba., *Sars.*, SEP., SIL., Spig., Spo., Squ., Stan., **Staph.**, SUL., Sul. ac., Tar., Thuj., Valer., Verat. a., *Vio. t.*, Zinc.

Tetter, Burning.—Agar., **Alum.**, *Ambr.*, **Am. carb.**, Anac., ARS., Aur., Bar. c., *Bell.*, *Bov.*, Bry., Calad., **Calc. c.**, Caps., *Carb. an.*, *Carb. v.*, CAUST., Cic., *Clem.*, Cocc., **Con.**, *Dulc.*, Hell., *Hep.*, K. carb., K. nit., Kre., Lach., Led., **Lyc.**, Mang., Mar., MERC., *Mez.*, Nat. c., Nat. m., *Nux v.*, Oleand., Par., Petrol., Phos., *Pho. ac.*, Pb., *Puls.*, *Ran. b.*, RHUS, Saba., Sars., *Sep.*, **Sil.**, Spig., Spo., Squ., Stan., *Staph.*, **Sul.**, Thuj., Verat. a., *Vio. t.*, Zinc.

—**Chapping.**—Alum., Aur., Bry., **Calc. c.**, *Cyc.*, *Graph.*, *Hep.*, K. carb., Kre., *Lach.*, *Lyc.*, Mag. c., Mang., *Merc.*, Nat. c., Nat. m., Nit. ac., Petrol., **Puls.**, **Rhus**, Ruta, Sars., SEP., *Sil.*, SUL., Vio. t., Zinc.

—**Corrosive.**—Alum., Am. carb., Bar. c., **Calc. c.**, Carb. v., Caust., Chel., **Clem.**, **Con.**, GRAPH., Hell., *Hep.*, K. carb., Lach., *Lyc.*, Mag. c., Mang., *Merc.*, Mur. ac., *Nat. c.*, *Nit. ac.*, Nux v., Oleand., Par., **Petrol.**, Phos., *Pho. ac.*, Pb., **Rhus.**, **Sep.**, SIL., *Squ.*, *Staph.*, *Sul.*, Tar., *Vio. t*

—**Dry.**—Alum., *Ars.*, Bar. c., Bov., Bry., **Calc. c.**, Carb. v., Caust. *Clem.*, Cocc., Cup., **Dulc.**, *Graph.*, Hyos., Kre., **Led.**, *Lyc.*, *Mag. c.*, *Mar.*, **Merc.**, Nat. c., Nat. m., Par., *Petrol.*, *Phos.*, Pho. ac., *Rhus*, *Sars.*, SEP., SIL., Stan., *Staph.*, *Sul.*, Valer., **Verat. a.**, *Vio. t.*, Zinc.

—**Gray.**—Ars.

—**Itching.**—*Agar.*, Alum., Ambr., *Am. carb.*, Anac., **Ant. t.**, *Ars.*, Bar. c., Bell., Bov., *Bry.*, *Calad.*, *Calc. c.*, Caps., Carb. an., Carb. v., **Caust.**, Chel., Cic., CLEM., Cocc., **Con.**, Cup., *Dulc.*, **Graph.**, Hep., *Jug. c.*, *K. carb.*, *Kre.*, Lach., Led., *Lyc.*, Mag. c., Mag. m., Mang., **Merc.**, *Mez.*, Nat. c., Nat. m., **Nit. ac.**, Nux v., *Oleand.*, *Par.*, Petrol., Phos., Pho. ac., Pb., Puls., *Ran. b.*, Ran. s., RHUS, Saba., Sars., SEP., **Sil.**, Spig., Spo., *Squ.*, Stan., **Staph.**, **Sul.**, Tar., Thuj., Valer., Verat. a., *Vio. t.*, Zinc.

—**Jerking.**—Calc. c., *Caust.*, Cup., Lyc., *Puls.*, RHUS, Sep., Sil., Staph.

—**Mealy.**—ARS., *Aur.*, Bry., CALC. C., **Dulc.**, *Graph.*, *Kre.*, Lyc., *Phos.*, Sep., SIL., *Sul.*

—**Moist.**—Alum., *Ars.*, Bar. c., Bell., **Bov.**, Bry., *Cact.*, *Calc. c.*, Carb. an., **Carb. v.**, Caust., Cic., *Cist.*, **Clem.**, Con., *Dulc.*, GRAPH., Hell., Hep., *K. carb.*, *Kre.*, Lach., Led., LYC., *Merc.*, Mez., Nat c., Nat. m.,

230 SKIN.

Nit. ac., Oleand., *Petrol.*, Phos., Pho. ac., *Ran. b.*, RHUS, Ruta, SEP., *Sil.*, Squ., *Staph.*, *Sul.*, Sul. ac., Tar., **Tell.**, Thuj., Vio. t.

Tetter, Red.—*Am. carb.*, *Bry.*, *Cic.*, **Clem.**, **Dulc.**, *Led.*, **Lyc.**, **Mag. c.**, **Merc.**, Petrol., Pho. ac., Staph.

—**Ring-worms.**—Clem., Mag. c., **Nat. c.**, *Nat. m.*, SEP., **Tell.**

—**Scabby.**—*Alum.*, Ambr., Am. carb., *Ars.*, *Bar. c.*, *Bell.*, *Bov.*, *Bry.*, CALC. C., Caps., *Carb. an.*, Carb. v., *Cic.*, *Clem.*, CON., **Dulc.**, GRAPH., Hell., *Hep.*, K. carb., Kre., *Led.*, LYC., Mag. c., **Merc.**, Mez., *Mur. ac.*, Nat. m., Nit. ac., Nux v., Oleand., Par., Petrol., Phos., Pb., *Puls.*, *Ran. b.*, RHUS, *Sars.*, **Sep.**, Sil., Squ., *Staph.*, SUL., Thuj., Verat. a., *Vio. t.*, Zinc.

—**Scaly.**—Agar., *Ars.*, *Aur.*, Bell., Cic., CLEM., Cup., *Dulc.*, Hep., Hyos., K. carb., *Led.*, *Mag. c.*, Mar., **Merc.**, *Oleand.*, **Phos.**, Pb., *Rhus*, *Sep.*, Staph., **Sul.**

—**Stinging.**—Alum., **Ars.**, *Bar. c.*, *Bell.*, Bov., *Bry.*, Calc. c., Caps., Carb. v., Caust., CLEM., Cocc., *Con.*, *Cyc.*, *Graph.*, Hell., *Hep.*, K. carb., Kre., *Led.*, *Lyc.*, Mag. c., **Merc.**, Mez., Mur. ac., Nat. c., Nat. m., **Nit. ac.**, Nux v., Petrol., Phos., **Puls.**, *Ran. b.*, Ran. s., **Rhus**, Saba., SEP., Sil., Spo., Squ., *Staph.*, **Sul.**, Thuj., *Vio. t.*, Zinc.

—**Suppurating.**—*Ars.*, Bell., Cic., *Clem.*, Cocc., *Con.*, Cyc., *Dulc.*, Hep., *Jug. c.*, Led., **Lyc.**, Mag. c., MERC., **Nat. c.**, Nat. m., Petrol., Pb., Puls., RHUS, Sars., SEP., *Sil.*, Spig., *Staph.*, *Sul.*, Tar., Thuj., Verat. a., *Vio. t.*, Zinc.

—**Tearing.**—*Ars.*, Bell., *Bry.*, **Calc. c.**, Carb. v., Caust., *Clem.*, Cocc., *Dulc.*, *Graph.*, K. carb., LYC., *Merc.*, Mez., Nat. c., Nit. ac., Nux v., Phos., Puls., *Rhus*, **Sep.**, Sil., *Staph.*, **Sul.**, Zinc.

—**With Whitish Crusts.**—*Ars.*, **Graph.**, **Lyc.**, Zinc.

—**Yellowish.**—Agar., *Ars.*, Cic., Cocc., Cup., Hell., Kre., Led., *Lyc.*, **Merc.**, *Nat. c.*, Nit. ac., Par., *Sep.*

—**Yellowish-brown.** —**Lyc.**, **Nat. c.**

Tightness.—**Acon.**, Anac., Ant. cr., *Arn.*, Ars., *Bar. c.*, Bell., **Carb. v.**, **Caust.**, *Con.*, Dulc., *Guai.*, K. carb., Led., *Mos.*, Nat. m., NIT. AC., Nux v., Oleand., Petrol., PHOS., Pho. ac., **Plat.**, Pb., *Puls.*, *Rhus*, Ruta, Sabi., **Sep.**, Stan., Staph., **Stro.**, *Sul.*, Vio. t., Zinc.

Ulcerative Pain.—Alum., Ambr., *Am. carb.*, AM. M., Anac., Ars., *Bell.*, Bov., **Bry.**, Canth., Caps., *Caust.*, Cham., **Chin.**, **Cic.**, Cocc., Dros., Fer., GRAPH., *Hep.*, *Ign.*, **K. carb.**, **K. iod.**, K. nit., Kre., Lach., Laur., Mag. c., *Mag. m.*, **Mang.**, Merc., *Mur. ac.*, Nat. c., **Nat. m.**, Nit. ac., *Nux v.*, Petrol., Phos., Pho. ac., PULS., RHUS, *Ruta*, Sars., **Sep.**, *Sil.*, Spig., Spo., Stan., *Staph.*, Sul., **Sul. ac.**, Tar., **Thuj.**, *Verat. a.*, *Zinc.*

SKIN.

Ulcers in General.—Acon., Agar., Alum., Ambr., Am. carb., Anac., Ant. cr., Ant. t., Arg., Arn., ARS., ASAF., Aur., Bar. c., **Bell.**, Bor., Bov., **Brom., Bry., Calc. c.**, Calc. ph., Camph., Canth., Carb. ac., Carb. an., **Carb. v.**, Caust., Cham., Chel., Chin., Cic., Cina, Clem., Cocc., Coff., Colch., Con., Croc., Cup., Cyc., Dig., Dros., Dulc., Euphorb., Graph., Guai., HEP., Hydras., Hyos., Ign., Iod., Ip., K. bi., K. carb., K. CHL., Kre., LACH., Led., LYC., Mang., MERC., Mez., Mur. ac., Nat. c., Nat. m., **Nit. ac.**, Nux m., Nux v., Pœo., Par., Petrol., **Phos., Pho. ac.**, Pb., Pso., PULS., Ran. b., Ran. s., **Rhus**, Ruta, Sabi., Samb., Sars., Sec. c., Sele., Seneg., **Sep.**, SIL., Spo., Squ., **Staph.**, Stram., Stro., SUL., Sul. ac., Tar., Thuj., Verat. a., Zinc.

—**Biting.**—Ars., Bell., Bry., Calc. c., Carb. an., Caust., Cham., Chin., Colch., Dig., **Euphorb.**, Graph., **Lach., Led., Lyc.**, Mang., Merc., Mez., Nat. c., Petrol., Pho. ac., PULS., Ran. b., Rhus, Ruta, Sele., Sil., Staph., Sul., Sul. ac., Thuj.

—**Black.**—Ant. t., ARS., **Asaf.**, Bell., Carb. v., Con., Euphorb., Grind., Ip., Lach., **Pb.**, Rhus, SEC. C., **Sil.**, Squ., Sul., Sul. ac.

— —**At Base.**—ARS., Ip., Pb., Sil., Sul.

— —**At Margins.**—**Ars.**, Lach., Sil., Sul.

—**Bleeding.**—Ant. t., Arg., Arn., ARS., **Asaf.**, Bell., **Carb. v.**, Caust., Con., Croc., Dros., **Hep.**, Hydras., Hyos., Iod., **K. carb.**, Kre., Lach., LYC., MERC., Mez., Nat. m., **Nit. ac.**, PHOS., Pho. ac., Puls., Rhus, Ruta, Sabi., Sec. c., Sep., Sil., **Sul.**, Sul. ac., Thuj., Zinc.

— —**At Edges.**—ARS., Asaf., Caust., Hep., Lach., **Lyc.**, Merc., Phos., Pho. ac., Puls., Sep., **Sil.**, Sul., Thuj.

—**Bluish.**—Arn., Ars., Asaf., Aur., Bell., Bry., Calc. c., Carb. v., Con., Hep., LACH., Mang., Merc., Pho. ac., Sec. c., Seneg., Sil., Staph., Verat. a.

—**With Boring.**—Arg., Aur., Bell., Calc. c., Caust., Chin., Hep., K. carb., Nat. c., Nat. m., Puls., Ran. s., Sep., **Sil., Sul.**, Thuj.

—**With Bruised Pain.**—Arn., Cham., Chin., Cocc., **Con.**, HEP., Hyos., Nat. m., Nux v., Rhus, Ruta, **Sul.**

—**Burning.**—Ambr., ARS., Asaf., Aur., Bar. c., **Bell.**, Bov., Bry., Calc. c., Carb. an., **Carb. v.**, CAUST., Cham., Chin., Clem., **Con.**, Dros., Graph., **Hep.**, Ign., K. carb., Kre., Lach., LYC., Mang., MERC., **Mez.**, Mur. ac., Nat. c., Nat. m., Nit. ac., Nux v., Petrol., Phos., Pho. ac., Pb., **Puls.**, Ran. b., RHUS, Sars., Sec. c., Sele., Sep., SIL., Squ., **Staph.**, Stro., Sul., Thuj., Zinc.

— —**In Circumference.**—Ars., **Asaf.**, Bell., Caust., Cham., Hep., Lach., Lyc., Merc., Mez., Mur. ac., Nat. c., Nux v., Petrol., Phos., PULS., **Rhus**, Sep., **Sil., Staph.**

Ulcers, Burning In Margins.—ARS., *Asaf*, *Carb. an*, **Caust.**, Clem., **Hep.**, *Lach.*, LYC, MERC., *Mur. ac.*, Petrol., Phos., Pho. ac., *Puls.*, Ran. b., *Sep.*, SIL., Staph., *Sul.*, Thuj.

—**As if Burnt.**—Alum., Ant. cr., ARS., *Bar. c*, Bell., Bry., Calc. c, **Carb. v.**, *Caust.*, **Cyc.**, Hyos., *Ign.*, **Lach.**, *Kre.*, *Nux v.*, *Puls.*, *Saba.*, *Sec. c.*, *Sep.*, Stram.

—**Burrowing.**—Asaf., Bell., Bry., Calc. c, *Chin.*, Nat. c., Phos., Ruta, *Sep.*, Stro., Sul.

—**Cancerous.**—*Ambr.*, Ant. cr., ARS., *Aur.*, *Bell.*, Calc. c, *Carb. an.*, *Carb. v.*, Caust., Chel., Clem., *Con.*, Dulc., *Hep.*, *Kre.*, **Lach.**, **Merc.**, *Nit. ac.*, Phos., *Rhus*, Sars., **Sep.**, SIL., Spo., Squ., *Staph.*, SUL., *Thuj.*

—**With Cold Feeling.**—Ars., BRY., *Merc.*, Petrol., Pb., *Rhus*, Sil., Thuj.

—**With Crawling.**—*Acon.*, Ant. t., ARN., *Bell.*, Caust., *Cham.*, **Clem.**, *Colch.*, Con., Croc., Graph., *Hep.*, K. carb., *Lach.*, *Merc.*, Nat. c., Nat. m., *Nux v.*, *Pho. ac.*, Pb., *Puls.*, Ran. b., RHUS, Sabi., *Sec. c.*, SEP., Spo., *Staph.*, *Sul.*, Sul. ac., Thuj.

—**Crusty.**—*Ars.*, Bar. c., **Bell.**, Bov., Bry., CALC. C, Carb. an., Cic., Clem., CON., Graph., *Hep.*, Led., LYC., **Merc.**, Mur. ac., *Puls.*, Ran. b., Rhus, Sars., **Sep.**, SIL., Staph., SUL., Vio. t.

—**With Cutting.**—BELL., **Calc. c.**, *Dros.*, Graph., Ign., *Lyc.*, Mur. ac., **Nat. c.**, Pho. ac., Rhus, Sep., *Sil.*, Sul. ac.

—**Deep.**—*Ant. cr.*, Ars., *Asaf.*, *Aur.*, **Bell.**, CALC. C, *Carb. v.*, Caust., Chel., Clem., **Con.**, *Hep.*, *K. bi.*, Kre., *Lach.*, Led., **Lyc.**, *Merc.*, *Mur. ac.*, Nat. c., Nat. m., **Nit. ac.**, *Petrol.*, Phos., *Pho. ac.*, PULS., *Rhus*, *Ruta*, Sabi., Sele., *Sep.*, SIL., Staph., Stram., Sul., *Thuj.*

—**With Elevated, Indurated Margins.**—ARS., *Asaf.*, *Bry.*, Carb. an., *Caust.*, Cic., Cina., Clem., Hep., Lach., **Lyc.**, **Merc.**, Mur. ac., *Petrol.*, Phos., Pho. ac., **Puls.**, Ran. b., *Sep.*, SIL., Staph., *Sul.*, Thuj.

—**Eruptions Around.**—*Lach.*, Rhus.

—**Fistulous.**—*Ant. cr.*, Ars., **Asaf.**, *Aur.*, Bell., BRY., CALC. C, *Calc. ph.*, **Carb. v.**, *Caust.*, Chel., Clem., **Con.**, *Hep.*, Kre., *Lach.*, Led., LYC., Merc., Nat. c., Nat. m., **Nit. ac.**, *Petrol.*, Phos., Pho. ac., PULS., Rhus, *Ruta*, Sabi., Sele., *Sep.*, SIL., Staph., Stram., **Sul.**, *Thuj*

—**Foul.**—Am. carb., *Ars.*, *Asaf.*, Aur., Bell., Bor., *Bry.*, **Calc. c.**, Carb. v., Caust., Chel., **Chin.**, Cic., Con., Cyc, *Graph.*, HEP., *Kre.*, *Lyc.*, Mang., *Merc.*, Mez., MUR. AC., Nat. c., *Nit. ac.*, Nux m., Nux v., Phos., **Pho. ac.**, Pb., *Puls.*, Rhus, Ruta, Sabi., Sec. c., *Sep.*, SIL., Staph., **Sul.**, Sul. ac., Thuj.

—**With Gnawing Pain.**—Agn., *Bar. c.*, Bell., Calc. c., *Cham.*, Cyc.,

Dros., Hyos., *K. carb.*, Led., *Lyc.*, Mang., *Merc.*, Mez., Nat. c., *Phos.*, *Pho. ac.*, Plat., Puls., **Ran. s.**, Rhus, *Ruta,* STAPH., *Sul.*, Thuj.

Ulcers, Indolent.—Agn., Anac., ARS., **Calc. c.**, *Camph.*, *Carb. an.*, Carb. v., CON., Dulc., *Euphorb.*, Graph., *Iod.*, Ip., K. carb., *Lach.*, Laur., LYC., Mur. ac., *Nit. ac.*, *Oleand.*, **Op.**, Phos., **Pho. ac.**, *Pb.*, Rhus, Sec. c., **Sep.**, Sil., Stram., **Sul.**, Zinc.

—**Indurated.**—*Agn.*, *Arn.*, **Ars.**, **Asaf.**, Aur., Bar. c., **BELL.**, **Bry.**, Calc. c., Carb. an., *Carb. v.*, Caust., Cham., Chel., **Chin.**, Cic., Cina, Clem., Con., Cup., Cyc., Dulc., *Graph.*, **Hep.**, Hyos., Iod., **Lach.**, Led., LYC., **Merc.**, Mez., Nat. c., Nux v., *Phos.*, *Pb.*, PULS., Ran. b., Ran. s., Sele., *Sep.*, **Sil.**, *Staph.*, **Sul.**, Thuj., Verat. a.

— —**Areola.**—Arn., **Ars.**, ASAF., Bell., Caust., Cham., Cina, *Hep.*, LACH., **Lyc.**, *Merc.*, Mez., Nat. c., Nux v., Petrol., Phos., PULS., Sep., *Sil.*, Staph., Sul.

— —**Margins.**—ARS., **Asaf.**, *Bry.*, Carb. an., Caust., Cic., Cina, *Clem.*, **Hep.**, **Lach.**, LYC., MERC., Petrol., Phos., Pho. ac., **Puls.**, Ran. b., Sep., SIL., Staph., *Sul.*, Thuj.

—**Inflamed.**—ACON., Agn., Ant. cr., *Arn.*, ARS., *Asaf.*, Bar. c., **Bell.**, Bor., Bov., **Bry.**, *Calc. c.*, Caust., *Cham.*, Cina, Cocc., *Colch.*, Con. Croc., Cup., Dig., HEP., Hyos., Ign., Kre., Led., **Lyc.**, Mang., MERC., *Mez.*, Nat. c., *Nit. ac.*, Nux v., *Phos.*, Pb., **Puls.**, Ran. b., **Rhus**, *Ruta*, Sars., Sep., SIL., **Staph.**, *Sul.*, Thuj., Verat. a., Zinc.

—**Itching.**—*Alum.*, Ambr., Am. carb., Anac., *Ant. cr.*, *Ant. t.*, Arn., **Ars.**, Bar. c., *Bell.*, Bov., Bry., *Calc. c.*, *Canth.*, Carb. v., **Caust.**, *Cham.*, Chel., **Chin.**, *Clem.*, Con., Dros., **Graph.**, HEP., Ip., K. nit., Kre., *Lach.*, Led., LYC., *Merc.*, Mez., Nat. c., Nat. m., *Nit. ac.*, Nux v., Petrol., *Phos.*, **Pho. ac.**, Puls., **Ran. b.**, Rhus, Ruta., Saba., Sars., Sele., **Sep.**, SIL., Squ., **Staph.**, Sul., *Thuj.*, Verat. a., Vio. t., Zinc.

— —**Around Them.**—*Agn.*, Ant. t., *Ars.*, **Bell.**, *Caust.*, Clem., HEP., **Lach.**, **Lyc.**, Merc., Mez., Nat. c., Nux v., Petrol., Phos., Pho. ac., PULS., *Rhus*, Sabi., Sep., SIL., *Staph.*, Sul.

—**With Jagged Margins.**—*Hep.*, Lach., MERC., **Pho. ac.**, Sil., *Staph.*, Sul., Thuj.

—**With Jerking Pain.**—Arn., **Asaf.**, Aur., *Bell.*, Bry., Calc. c., CAUST., *Cham.*, *Chin.*, Clem., *Cup.*, Graph., *Lyc.*, *Merc.*, Nat. c., **Nat. m.**, *Nit. ac.*, *Nux v.*, Petrol., PULS., **Rhus.**, Sep., SIL., *Staph.*, Sul.

—**Lardaceous.**—*Ant. cr.*, **Ars.**, Cup., Hep., *Kre.*, MERC., **Nit. ac.**, *Sabi.*, Sul., Thuj.

— —**At Base.**—Ars., *Hep.*, **Merc.**, *Nit. ac.*

—**Painless.**—Ambr., Anac., Ant. t., Arn., **Ars.**, Aur., Bar. c., **Bell.**,

Bov., *Bry.*, Camph., Carb. an., Cham., *Chel.*, Chin., Cic., **Cocc.**, **Con.**, Croc., Graph., **Hell.**, **Hyos.**, *Ign.*, Ip., *Laur.*, Led., **LYC.**, *Merc.*, Nux m., Nux v., **Oleand.**, Op., Phos., **PHO. AC**, **Plat.**, **Puls.**, *Rhus*, *Sec. c.*, Staph., **Stram.**, *Sul.*, Verat. a., Zinc.

Ulcers Surrounded by Pimples.—Acon., **Ars.**, Bell., **Caust.**, Cham., Hep., **Lach.**, *Lyc.*, Merc., Mez., Mur. ac., Nat. c., Petrol., Phos., Puls., *Rhus*, **Sep.**, *Sil.*, Staph., Sul.

—**Pressing.**—Camph., *Carb. v.*, Chin., **Graph.**, *Mez.*, PÆO., **Par.**, SIL.

—**With Proud Flesh.**—Alum., Ant. cr., ARS., Bell., *Carb. an.*, Carb. v., Caust., **Cham.**, *Clem.*, *Graph.*, Kre., **Lach.**, Merc., **Petrol.**, Phos., Sabi., SEP., SIL., *Staph.*, **Sul.**, *Thuj.*

—**Pus Blackish.**—*Bry.*, *Chin.*, Lyc., **Sul.**

— —**Bloody.**—Ant. t., Arg., Arn., ARS., ASAF., *Bell.*, **Carb. v.**, **Caust.**, Con., Croc., Dros., HEP., Hyos., Iod., *K. carb.*, Kre., *Lach.*, Lyc., MERC., Mez., Nat. m., **Nit. ac.**, *Phos.*, Pho. ac., **Puls.**, *Rhus*, Ruta, Sabi., Sec. c., *Sep.*, **Sil.**, *Sul.*, Sul ac., Thuj., Zinc.

— —**Brownish.**—Anac., *Ars.*, **Bry.**, Calc. c., *Carb. v.*, Con., Puls., Rhus, **Sil.**

— —**Cheesy.**—*Merc.*

— —**Copious.**—Acon., *Arg.*, **Ars.**, **Asaf.**, Bry., **Calc. c.**, *Canth.*, Chin., Cic., Graph., Iod., K. carb., Kre., *Lyc.*, Mang., **Merc.**, Mez., Nat. c., Phos., *Pho. ac.*, **PULS.**, Rhus, Ruta, Sabi., **SEP.**, **Sil.**, *Squ.*, Staph., Sul., Thuj.

— —**Corrosive.**—Am. carb., Anac., ARS., Bell., Calc. c., **Carb. v.**, CAUST., Cham., Chel., *Clem.*, Con., Cup., *Graph.*, **Hep.**, Ign., Iod., *Kre.*, Lach., **Lyc.**, MERC., Mez., *Nat. c.*, Nat. m., **Nit. ac.**, *Nux v.*, Phos., Pb., *Puls.*, Ran. b., **Ran. s.**, RHUS, Ruta, *Sep.*, SIL., Spig., **Squ.**, *Staph.*, Sul., *Sul. ac.*, Zinc.

— —**Gelatinous.**—*Arg.*, Arn., Bar. c., Cham., Fer., *Merc.*, *Sep.*, Sil.

— —**Gray.**—*Ambr.*, Ars., Carb. an., CAUST., Chin., **K. chl.**, *Lyc.*, Merc., Sep., **Sil.**, Thuj.

— —**Green.**—Ars., **Asaf.**, **Aur.**, Carb. v., **Caust.**, *Clem.*, Kre., *Merc.*, Nat. c., *Nux v.*, Phos., **Puls.**, *Rhus*, Sep., **Sil.**, Staph.

— —**Ichorous.**—Am. carb., Ant. t., ARS., **Asaf.**, Aur., Bov., *Calc. c.*, CARB. V., **Caust.**, **Chin.**, Cic., Clem., *Con.*, Dros., *Graph.*, **Hep.**, K. carb., Kre., *Lyc.*, Mang., MERC., **Mez.**, Mur. ac., NIT. AC., Nux v., Phos., *Pho. ac.*, Pb., *Ran. b.*, **Ran. s.**, RHUS, Sec. c., *Sep.*, SIL., **Squ.**, **Staph.**, *Sul.*

— —**With Maggots.**—*Ars.*, Calc. c., **Merc.**, **Saba.**, Sil., *Sul.*

Ulcers, Pus Offensive.—Am. carb., **Ars.**, **Asaf.**, *Aur.*, Bell., Bov., Bry., **Calc. c.**, *Calc. ph.*, *Carb. v.*, Caust., Chel., **Chin.**, Cic., Con., Cyc., **Graph.**, *Grind.*, HEP., *Hydras.*, *Kre.*, **Lyc.**, Mang., **Merc.**, **Mez.**, *Mur. ac.*, *Nat. e.*, NIT. AC., Nux m., Nux v., PÆO., *Petrol.*, Phos., PHO. AC., Pb., Puls., *Rhus*, Ruta, Sabi., *Sec. c.*, **Sep.**, **Sil.**, *Staph.*, SUL, Sul. ac., Thuj., *Vinc.*

— — —**Like Old Cheese.**—Hep., *Sul.*

— — —**Like Herring-brine.**—*Graph.*, **Tell.**

— —**Scanty.**—Acon., Ars., *Bar. c.*, **Bell.**, *Bov.*, Bry., CALC. C, *Carb. v.*, Caust., Chin., Cina, *Clem.*, Coff., **Cup.**, Dros., **Dulc.**, *Graph.*, **Hep.**, Hyos., Ign., Ip., Kre., LACH., *Led.*, Lyc., *Mag. c.*, MERC., Nux v., *Petrol.*, *Phos.*, **Plat.**, Pb., Puls., Rhus, *Sars.*, **Sep.**, SIL., *Spo.*, *Staph.*, Sul., Verat. a.

— —**Smelling Sour.**—*Calc. c.*, Graph., HEP., **Merc.**, **Nat. c.**, *Sep.*, Sul.

— —**Like Tallow.**—*Merc.*

— —**Tenacious.**—*Ars.*, *Asaf.*, Bov., Cham., **Con.**, *Merc.*, Mez., *Phos.*, Pho. ac., *Sep.*, Sil., Staph., *Vio. t.*

— —**Thin.**—Ant. t., ASAF, Carb. v., CAUST., Dros., Iod., K. carb., Lyc., MERC., *Nit. ac.*, Pb., Puls., *Ran. b.*, *Ran. s.*, *Rhus*, *Ruta*, **Sil.**, Staph., Sul., Thuj.

— —**Watery.**—Ant. t., **Ars.**, Asaf., Calc. c., *Carb. v.*, CAUST., *Clem.*, Con., Dros., *Graph.*, Iod., K. carb., *Lyc.*, MERC., *Nit. ac.*, Nux v., Pb., Puls., **Ran. b.**, Ran. s., Rhus, *Ruta*, **Sil.**, *Squ.*, *Staph.*, *Sul.*, Thuj.

— —**Whitish.**—*Am. carb.*, *Ars.*, **Calc. c.**, Carb. v., **Hell.**, **Lyc.**, MEZ., Puls., *Sep.*, *Sil.*, *Sul.*

— —**Yellow.**—*Acon.*, Ambr., Am. carb., Anac., Arg., *Ars.*, *Aur.*, Bov., *Bry.*, **Calc. c.**, Caps., **Carb. v.**, **Caust.**, *Cic.*, **Clem.**, Con., Croc., *Dulc.*, Graph., Hep., Iod., *K. nit.*, *Kre.*, *Lyc.*, Mang., **Merc.**, MEZ., *Nat. c.*, **Nat. m.**, **Nit. ac.**, Nux v., **Phos.**, PULS., *Rhus*, Ruta, Sec. c., Sele., **Sep.**, **Sil.**, Spig., **Staph.**, Sul., Sul. ac., *Thuj.*, Vio. t.

—**Red Areola.**—Acon., Ant. cr., Arn., ARS., Asaf., Bar. c., *Bell.*, Bor., Bry., *Calc. c.*, Cham., Cocc., Cup., HEP., Hyos., Ign., Kre., **Lach.**, **Led.**, **Lyc.**, **Merc.**, Mez., Nat. c., *Nit. ac.*, Nux v., *Petrol.*, *Phos.*, Pho. ac., Pb., PULS., Ran. b., **Rhus**, Sars., *Sep.*, SIL., **Staph.**, *Sul.*, **Thuj.**, Verat. a., Zinc.

—**Reopening of Old.**—*Lach.*, Sil.

—**Salt-rheum.**—Ambr., ARS., *Calc. c.*, Chin., **Graph.**, LYC., Merc., Nat. c., *Petrol.*, *Phos.*, **Puls.**, SEP., *Sil.*, **Staph.**, Sul., Zinc.

—**Sensitive.**—Alum., Am. carb., Anac., **ARN.**, **Ars.**, **ASAF.**, Aur.,

Bell., Carb. an., **Caust.**, *Cham.*, *Chin.*, Cic., **Clem.**, *Cocc.*, Coff., **Con.**, Croc., *Cup.*, Dig., *Dulc.*, **Graph.**, HEP., Hyos., Iod., *Kre.*, **Lach.**, Led., Lyc., **Merc.**, Mez., *Mur. ac.*, Nat. c., Nat. m., Nit. ac., *Nux v.*, Petrol., *Phos.*, **Pho. ac.**, Puls., Ran. b., Ran. s., Rhus, Sabi., Sele., **Sep.**, **Sil.**, Squ., Sul., Thuj., *Verat. a.*

Ulcers, Sensitive at Margins.—ARS., ASAF., *Caust.*, *Clem.*, HEP., Lach., Lyc., MERC., Mur. ac., Petrol., Phos., *Pho. ac.*, *Puls.*, Ran. b, *Sep.*, SIL., Sul., Thuj.

— —**In Their Vicinity.**—Ars., ASAF., *Bell.*, *Caust.*, Cocc., **Hep.**, LACH., *Lyc.*, *Merc.*, Mez., Mur. ac., Nat. c., Nux v., Petrol., Phos., PULS., Rhus, *Sep.*, *Sil.*

—**Smarting.**—Alum., Ambr., Ant. cr., Arn., *Ars.*, Bell., *Bry.*, *Calc. c.*, Caust., Cic., **Graph.**, HEP., Hyos., *Ign.*, K. carb., *Lyc.*, **Merc.**, Mez., Nat. m., *Nux v.*, Phos., **Pho. ac.**, PULS., *Rhus*, **Sep.**, *Sil.*, Staph., **Sul.**, Sul. ac., Thuj., *Zinc.*

—**Spongy.**—Alum., *Ant. cr.*, Ant. t., ARS., *Bell.*, Calc. c., CARB. AN., *Carb. v.*, Caust., *Cham.*, **Clem.**, Con., Graph., Iod., *Kre.*, LACH., Lyc., *Merc.*, Nit. ac., Nux v., *Petrol.*, **Phos.**, Pho. ac., Rhus, Sabi., **Sep.**, SIL., Staph., Sul., Thuj.

— —**At Margins.**—ARS., **Carb. an.**, Caust.,*Clem.*, **Lach.**, Lyc., Merc., Petrol., *Phos.*, Pho. ac., *Sep.*, SIL., *Staph.*, *Sul.*, *Thuj.*

—**Spotted.**—*Arn.*, Ars., CON., Ip., **Lach.**, Sul. ac.

—**Stinging.**—Acon., Alum., Ant. cr., Arn., ARS., **Asaf.**, *Bar. c.*, Bell., Bov., Bry., *Calc. c.*, Camph., Canth., *Carb. v.*, Cham., *Chin.*, Clem., Cocc., *Con.*, *Cyc.*, Graph., **Hep.**, K. nit., *Led.*, Lyc., Mag. c., Mang., MERC., *Mez.*, Mur. ac., *Nat c.*, Nat. m., NIT. AC., *Nux v.*, Petrol., *Phos.*, PULS., *Ran. b.*, Rhus, Saba., *Sabi.*, Sars., Sele., **Sep.**, SIL., Spo., Squ., Staph., SUL., Thuj.

— —**In Areola.**—Acon., **Ars.**, ASAF., *Bell.*, Cham., Cocc., **Hep.**, *Lyc.*, **Merc.**, Mez., Mur. ac., Nat. c., Nux v., *Petrol.*, Phos., PULS., *Rhus*, Sabi., *Sep.*, **Sil.**, *Staph.*, **Sul.**

— —**At Margins.**—ARS., **Asaf.**, *Bry.*, Clem., **Hep.**, Lyc., MERC., Mur. ac., *Petrol.*, Phos., **Puls.**, Ran. b., *Sep.*, SIL., *Staph.*, Sul., Thuj.

—**Superficial.**—*Am. carb.*, *Ant. cr.*, Ant. t., Ars., Asaf., *Bell.*, Carb. an., Carb. v., *Chin.*, LACH., Lyc., **Merc.**, Nat. c., *Nit. ac.*, *Petrol.*, Phos., **Pho. ac.**, *Puls.*, *Ran. b.*, **Sele.**, **Sep.**, **Sil.**, Staph., *Sul.*, Thuj.

—**Suppurating.**—*Acon.*, Ambr., *Am. carb.*, Anac., Ant. cr., Ant. t., Arg., Arn., **Ars.**, ASAF., *Aur.*, Bar. c., **Bell.**, Bov., Bry., *Calc. c.*, **Canth.**, Caps., Carb. an., **Carb. v.**, CAUST., Cham., C^hel., *Chin.*, Cic.,*Clem.*, Cocc., **Con.**, Croc., Dros., *Dulc.*, *Graph.*, Hell., HEP., Hyos., Ign., Iod., Ip., K.

carb., K. nit., *Kre.*, *Lach.*, Led., **Lyc.**, Mang., MERC., *Mez.*, *Mur. ac.*, Nat. c., Nat. m., **Nit. ac.**, *Nux v.*, Petrol., *Phos.*, Pho. ac., Pb., PULS., *Ran. b.*, *Ran. s.*, RHUS, *Ruta*, Saba., *Sabi.*, Sars., Sec. c., Sele., Sep., SIL., Spig., Spo., *Squ.*, **Staph.**, **Sul.**, Sul. ac., Thuj., Vio. t., Zinc.

Ulcers, With Suppurative Pain.—Am. carb., *Anac.*, *Arn.*, Ars., **Asaf.**, Aur., *Bar. c.*, Bry., **Calc. c.**, **Carb. v.**, Chin., Colch., **Con.**, *Cyc.*, Dros., Euphorb., Graph., **Hep.**, Hyos., Iod., *K. carb.*, Kre., *Led.*, Nat. m., Nit. ac., Nux v., Par., *Petrol.*, PHOS., **PULS.**, Ran. b., Rhus, Ruta, Sars., Sec. c., SIL., Staph., Sul., *Valer.*, Verat. a., Zinc.

—Swollen.—Acon., Agn., Arn., *Ars.*, Aur., *Bar. c.*, **BELL.**, **Bry.**, *Calc. c.*, Carb. an., *Carb. v.*, *Caust.*, Cham., Cic., Cocc., *Con.*, Dulc., Graph., **Hep.**, Iod., **K. carb.**, Led., *Lyc.*, Mang., MERC., Nat. c., *Nat. m.*, *Nit. ac.*, Nux v., Petrol., *Phos.*, Pho. ac., Pb., **PULS.**, **Rhus**, Sabi., Samb., SEP., **Sil.**, Staph., SUL.

— —Areola.—Acon., *Ars.*, **Bell.**, Caust., Cham., **Hep.**, *Lyc.*, **Merc.**, Nat. c., Nux v., Petrol., Phos., PULS., *Rhus*, **Sep.**, *Sil.*, Staph.

— —Margins.—Ars., *Bry.*, Carb. an., Caust., Cic., **Hep.**, *Lyc.*, MERC., Petrol., Phos., Pho. ac., **Puls.**, **Sep.**, SIL., **Sul.**

—With Tearing.—**Ars.**, Bell., *Bry.*, **Calc. c.**, *Canth.*, Carb. v., Caust., *Clem.*, Cocc., **Cyc.**, *Graph.*, K. carb., LYC., **Merc.**, Mez., Nat. c., Nit. ac., Nux v., Phos., **Puls.**, *Rhus*, Sep., **Sil.**, Staph., SUL., Zinc.

—Tense.—*Arn.*, Asaf., Aur., Bar. c., *Bell.*, *Bry.*, *Calc. c.*, *Carb. an.*, Carb. v., **Caust.**, Cham., Chin., *Clem.*, *Cocc.*, CON., *Hep.*, Iod., *K. carb.*, Kre., Lach., *Lyc.*, **Merc.**, *Mez.*, Mur. ac., Nat. c., Nit. ac., *Nux v.*, Petrol., **Phos.**, Pho. ac., PULS., Rhus, *Sabi.*, *Sep.*, *Sil.*, Spo., Staph., STRO., SUL., Thuj., Zinc.

— —Areola.—Asaf., Bell., *Caust.*, Cham., Cocc., Hep., **Lach.**, Lyc., Merc., Mez., Mur. ac., Nat. c., Nux v., Petrol., *Phos.*, Pho. ac., PULS., *Rhus*, Sabi., Sep., Sil., Staph., **Stro.**, Sul.

—Throbbing.—*Acon.*, Arn., *Ars.*, **Asaf.**, Bar. c., Bell., Bov., Bry., **Calc. c.**, *Caust.*, Cham., Chin., *Clem.*, Con., *Hep.*, Hyos., Ign., **K. carb.**, **Lyc.**, MERC., Mez., *Mur. ac.*, *Nat. c.*, Nat. m., *Nit. ac.*, Petrol., *Phos.*, Pho. ac., *Puls.*, Rhus, *Ruta.*, Saba., Sars., Sep., Sil., Staph., **SUL.**, *Thuj.*

—With Thrusts in Them.—Arn., Cic., **Clem.**, Mez., *Mur. ac.*, Plat., **Ruta**, *Sul. ac.*

—Unhealthy.—Alum., Am. carb., *Bar. c.*, **Calc. c.**, *Carb. v.*, Caust., Cham., Chel., *Clem.*, **Con.**, Croc., **Graph.**, Hell., HEP., K. carb., **Lach.**, Lyc., Mag. c., Mang., **Merc.**, Mur. ac., *Nat. c.*, **NIT. AC.**, Nux v., Petrol., *Phos.*, *Pho. ac.*, Pb., Rhus, Sep., SIL., *Squ.*, **Staph.**, **Sul.**

238 SKIN.

Ulcers, Varicose.—Ant. t., **Ars.,** *Crotal.,* *Grind.,* *Hydras.,* **Kre., Lach., LYC.,** *Merc., Mez.,* **Puls., Sil.,** *Sul., Thuj.,* **Zinc.**

—**Surrounded by Vesicles.**—**Ars.,** Bell., *Caust., Hep.,* **LACH.,** Merc., **MEZ.,** Nat. c., Petrol., Phos., Rhus, *Sep.*

—**With White Spots.**—Ars., *Con.,* **LACH.,** Phos., *Sep*, Sil., Sul.

Unhealthy.—Alum., Am. carb., **Apis,** *Bar c.,* **Bor., Calc. c.,** *Calend.,* **Caps.,** Carb. v., Caust., **CHAM.,** *Chel.,* Clem., *Con.,* Croc., Fl. ac., **Graph.,** Hell., **HEP.,** K. carb., **LACH., Lyc.,** Mag. c., *Mang., Merc.,* Mur. ac., **Nat. c.,** *Nit. ac.,* Nux v., **PETROL.,** Phos., Pho. ac., Pb., *Rhus, Sep.,* **SIL.,** Squ., **Staph.,** Sul.

Veins, see **Circulation, Blood-vessels.**

Warts in General.—Ambr., *Am. carb.,* Anac., Ant. cr., **Ars., Bar. c., BELL.,** Bor., Bov., **CALC. C.,** Carb. an., Carb. v., **CAUST.,** Chel., Cup., **DULC.,** Euphorb., Euphr., *Fl. ac.,* **Hep.,** K. carb., Lach., *Lyc.,* **Nat. c.,** *Nat. m., Nat. s.,* **NIT. AC.,** *Petrol.,* Phos., **Pho. ac.,** Ran. b., Rhus, *Ruta,* Sabi., Sars., **Sep.,** *Sil.,* Spig., *Staph.,* **SUL.,** Sul. ac., **THUJ.**

—**Bleeding.**—*Cinnab.,* **Nit. ac.**

—**Burning.**—*Ars.,* Lyc., **Petrol.,** Phos., **Rhus,** *Sep.,* Sul.

—**Hard.**—Ant. cr., *Dulc., Ran. b.,* Sil., Sul.

—**Horny.**—Ant. cr., *Ran. b.,* Sul.

—**Indented.**—Calc. c., Euphr., *Lyc., Nit. ac.,* **Pho. ac.,** Sabi., *Staph.,* Thuj.

—**Inflamed.**—*Am. carb.,* Bov., **Calc. c.,** *Caust.,* Hep., *Lyc., Nit. ac.,* Rhus, *Sep.,* Sil., Staph., *Sul.*

—**Large.**—*Caust.,* Dulc., Nat. c., **Nit. ac.**

—**Pedunculated.**—*Dulc., Lyc.,* Pho. ac., Staph., **Thuj.**

—**Small.**—Bar. c., **Calc. c.,** *Dulc.,* Hep., Rhus, Sars., Sep., Sul.

—**Smooth.**—Dulc.

—**Stinging.**—*Ant. cr.,* Bar. c., **Calc. c.,** Caust., *Hep., Lyc.,* **Nit. ac.,** Rhus, Sep., Sil., Staph., *Sul.*

—**Suppurating.**—*Ars.,* Bov., *Calc. c.,* **Caust., Hep.,** Sil., *Thuj.*

—**Throbbing.**—Calc. c., K. carb., *Lyc.,* **Petrol.,** Sep., Sil., Sul.

—**Surrounded by a Circle of Ulcers.**—*Ars.,* **Nat. c.,** Phos.

—**Withered.**—**Ars.,** *Calc. c., Camph.,* Caps., Cham., **CHIN.,** Clem., Cocc., Croc., **Fer.,** Hyos., **Iod.,** *K. carb., Lyc.,* Merc., *Phos.,* **Pho. ac.,** Rheum, *Rhodo.,* **Sars.,** SEC. C., Seneg., *Sil.,* Spo., *Sul.,* **Verat. a.**

Wounds in General.—Arn., Bor., *Calend.,* Carb. v., Cic., Con., Croc. Euphr., **Hep.,** Iod., Kre., **Lach.,** *Merc.,* Mez., *Nat. c.,* Nat. m., **Nit. ac., Phos.,** *Pho. ac.,* Pb., **Puls.,** *Rhus,* Ruta, Seneg., Sil., **Staph.,** *Sul.,* **Sul. ac.,** Zinc.

Wounds Bleeding Freely.—Arn., Carb. v., Croc., *Hep.*, Kre. LACH., *Merc.*, Nat. m., PHOS., *Pho. ac.*, *Puls.*, Rhus, **Sul.**, *Sul. ac.*, *Zinc.*

—**With Injuries of Bones.**—Con., **Pho. ac.**, *Puls.*, Sil., RUTA.

—**Bruises.**—ARN., Cic., **Con.**, *Euphr.*, Hep., Iod., *Puls.*, **Ruta**, Sul., Sul. ac.

—**Cuts.**—Arn., Merc., *Nat. c.*, Pho. ac., Sil., STAPH., *Sul.*, Sul. ac.

—**With Injuries of Glands.**—Arn., Cic., CON., Hep., Merc., *Phos.*, Puls., **Sil.**, Sul.

—**Old Wounds Break Out.**—Carb. v., Con., *Croc.*, Lach., Nat. c., **Nat. m.**, PHOS., **Sil.**, Sul.

—**Penetrating.**—Carb. v., *Cic.*, Hep., **Hyper.**, Led., NIT. AC., *Pb.*, Sil., *Sul.*

—**With Sprained Muscles.**—*Arn.*, Nat. c., Nat. m., Phos., RHUS.

Wrinkled.—*Ambr.*, Am. carb., **Ant. cr.**, *Bry.*, Camph., *Canch.*, Cham., **Cup.**, Graph., *Hell.*, **Lyc.**, Merc., *Mur. ac*, Nux v., *Pho. ac.*, Pb., *Rheum*, Rhodo., *Rhus*, Saba., *Sars.*, SEC. C., **Sep.**, *Spig.*, *Stram.*, Sul., **Verat. a.**, Vio. o.

Sleep.

Yawning.—*Acon.*, **Aesc.**, *Agar.*, *Alum.*, Ambr., Am. carb., Am. m., Anac., Ant. cr., **Ant. t.**, Arg., **Arn.**, **Ars.**, Asaf., Asar., Aur., *Bar. c.*, **Bell.**, Bor., Bov., *Bry.*, Calad., *Calc. c.*, Camph., Cannab. s., *Canth.*, Caps., Carb. an., *Carb. v.*, CAUST., *Cham.*, CHEL., *Chin.*, Cic., CINA, Clem., Cocc., Coff., Colch., Con., CROC., **Cup.**, Cyc., *Dig.*, Dros., Dulc., Euphorb., *Euphr.*, Fer., Graph., Guai., Hell., *Hep.*, IGN., *Ip.*, *K. carb.*, **K. nit.**, Lach., **KRE.**, **Laur.**, Led., **Lyc.**, Mag. c., *Mag. m.*, Mang., Mar., **Meny.**, *Merc.*, Mez., *Mos.*, **Mur. ac.**, *Nat. c.*, **Nat. m.**, Nit. ac., NUX V., Oleand., Op., Par., Petrol., **Phos.**, *Pho. ac.*, *Plat.*, Pb., **Puls.**, Ran. b., Rheum, Rhodo., RHUS, Ruta, **Saba.**, Sabi., **Sars.**, Sec. c., Seneg., **Sep.**, Sil., Spig., *Spo.*, **Squ.**, Stan., Staph., Stram., Stro., *Sul.*, Sul. ac., Tar., Thuj., Valer., *Verat. a.*, Verb., *Vio. o.*, *Zinc.*

—**Without Sleepiness.**—Acon., Alum., Am. m., Ant. t., Arn., *Bry.*, Canth., Caust., Cham., Chin., Cup., Cyc., *Hep.*, Ign., *Lach.*, Laur., Mag. c., *Mos.*, Nat. m., Phos., PLAT., RHUS, Sep., Spig., *Squ.*, Staph., Sul., Vio. o.

—**With Stretching.**—Acon., Agar., Alum., Ambr., Am. carb., *Ant. c.*, Arn., ARS., Bar. c., **Bell.**, *Bor.*, Bov., Brom., *Bry.*, Calc. c., Cannab. s., *Canth.*, Caps., **Carb. v.**, Caust., CHAM., *Chin.*, Cocc., *Dios.*, Dros., Fer., Graph., *Guai.*, Hell., *Hep.*, Ign., **Ip.**, Kre., Laur., Led., Mag. c., Merc., Mez., *Mur. ac.*, Nit. ac., NUX V., *Oleand.*, Petrol., Phos., *Pho.*

SLEEP.

ac., *Plat.,* Pb., PULS., Ran. b., RHUS, *Ruta,* **Saba.,** Sec. c., Seneg., **Sep.,** Sil., **Spo.,** Squ., Stan., **Staph., Sul.,** *Valer.,* Verat. a., *Verb.,* Zinc.

Yawning, Ineffectual.—Acon., *Cham.,* Croc., Ign., **Lyc.,** Phos., *Ruta,* Stan.

—**Spasmodic.**—Ant. t., Arn , *Bry.,* Croc., Cup., **Hep.,** Ign., Laur., Mos., Nat. m., **PLAT.,** RHUS, **Sep.,** Staph., Squ., Sul.

—**Associated Troubles, see Agg., Yawning.**

Falling Asleep Late.—Acon., Agar., *Agn., Alum.,* Ambr., Am. carb., *Am. m.,* Anac., *Ant. cr., Ant. t.,* Arn., ARS., *Asar.,* Aur., *Bar. c.,* **Bell.,** Bism., **Bor., BRY., Calad.,** CALC. C., Camph., Cannab. s., Canth., Caps., **Carb. an.,** CARB. V., *Caust.,* Cham., *Chel.,* Chin., Clem., Cocc., Coff., Coloc., **Con.,** *Cyc.,* Dig., Dulc., *Euphorb.,* Euphr., Fer., **Graph.,** *Guai.,* **Hep.,** Hyos., **Ign.,** Ip., **K. carb.,** K. nit., *Kre.,* Lach., *Laur.,* Led., **Lyc.,** *Mag. c., Mag. m.,* Mang., **Mar.,** MERC., Mez., *Mos.,* **Mur. ac.,** *Nat. c., Nat. m., Nit. ac.,* Nux m., **Nux v.,** Par. Petrol., PHOS., *Pho. ac,* Plat., Pb., **PULS,** Ran. b., Ran. s., Rheum, Rhodo., RHUS, *Saba.,* Sabi., Samb., *Sars.,* **Sele.,** Seneg., **SEP., Sil., Spig.,** *Spo., Stan.,* Staph., *Stro.,* **Sul.,** Sul. ac., Tar., *Thuj.,* **Valer.,** *Verat. a.,* Verb., *Vio. t.,* Zinc.

—**Impossible After Waking Once.**—Am. carb., *Ars.,* **Aur.,** Bar. c., **Bell.,** Bor., *Calc. c.,* Carb. v., Caust., Clem., *Cocc.,* Con , Cyc., **Dulc., Fer.,** Graph., K. carb., Laur., Led., Lyc., *Mag. c.,* Mag. m , Mang.,**Merc.,** Mez., Mur. ac., **NAT. M.,** Nux v., **Phos.,** Pho. ac·, *Puls.,* **Ran. b.,** Ran. s., Rhus, Ruta, *Sabi.,* Sars., Sele., Sep., SIL., Spo., **Sul.,** Sul. ac., Zinc.

—**Prevented by Various Symptoms.**—Acon., Agar., *Agn.,* Alum., Ambr., Am. carb., *Am. m.,* Anac., Ant. cr., *Arn.,* ARS., Asar., *Aur.,* Bar. c., **Bell.,** Bism., Bor., **BRY., Calad.,** CALC. C, Camph., Canth., *Caps.,* **Carb. an.,** CARB. V., *Caust.,* Cham., Chel., **Chin.,** Clem., *Cocc.,* Coff., Coloc., Con., Cyc., Dig., *Dulc.,* Euphorb., Euphr., **Graph.,** *Grind., Guai.,* **Hep., Ign.,** *Ip.,* **K. carb.,** K. nit., **Kre.,** *Lach., Laur.,* Led., **Lyc.,** *Mag. c., Mag. m.,* Mang., Mar., MERC., Mez., Mos., Mur. ac., *Nat. c., Nat. m.,* Nit. ac., Nux m., *Nux v.,* Par., Petrol., PHOS., *Pho. ac.,* Plat., Pb., PULS., *Ran. b.,* Rheum., Rhodo., RHUS, Saba., *Sabi.,* Samb., **Sars.,** *Sele.,* Seneg., **SEP., Sil.,** Spig., *Spo.,* Stan., Staph., *Stro.,* SUL., Sul. ac., Tar., *Thuj.,* Verat. a., **Verb.,** *Vio. t.,* Zinc.

Waking In Distress.—*Cina,* **Dig.,** Euphr., *Hyos.,* **LACH., Nat. m.,** Puls., Sep., *Tan.*

—**Early.**—Acon., Alum., Ambr., Am. carb., Am. m., Ant. cr., Ant. t., Arn., **Ars.,** *Asaf.,* **Aur.,** Bar. c., *Bor.,* Bry., Calad., *Calc. c.,* Cannab. s., Canth., **Caps.,** Carb. v., *Caust.,* Cham., Chin., Cocc., **Coff.,** *Con.,* Croc., Cyc., Dros., **Dulc.,** Euphr., Fer., *Graph.,* Guai., Hell., *Hep.,* Ign., Iod.,

K. CARB., *K. nit.*, *Kre.*, *Lach.*, *Lyc.*, **Mag. c.**, *Mang.*, *Merc.*, *Mez.*, **Mur. ac.**, NAT. C., *Nat. m.*, *Nit. ac.*, NUX V., Oleand., Phos., *Pho. ac.*, *Plat.*, Pb., Puls., RAN. B., *Ran. s.*, *Rhodo.*, Rhus, Saba., Sabi., Samb., *Sars.*, *Sele.*, **Sep.**, **Sil.**, Spo., Squ., *Staph.*, SUL., **Sul. ac.**, Thuj., Verat. a., *Verb.*, Vio. t.

Waking Frequently At Night.—Acon., Agar., Agn., *Alum.*, **Ambr.**, *Am. carb.*, *Am. m.*, Anac., *Ant. cr.*, Ant. t., *Arn.*, **Ars.**, Aur., *Bar. c.*, *Bell.*, **Benz. ac.**, *Bism.*, Bor., *Bov.*, Bry., Calad., CALC. C., Cannab. s., **Canth.**, Caps., **Carb. an.**, *Carb. v.*, **Caust.**, Cham., Chel., **Chin.**, Cic., Cina, *Clem.*, Cocc., *Coff.*, Colch., **Con.**, Croc., Cyc., **Dig.**, Dros., Dulc., Euphorb., **Euphr.**, Fer., Graph., Guai., HEP., *Hyos.*, Ign., **Ip.**, **K. carb.**, K. nit., Kre., *Lach.*, Laur., Led., **Lyc.**, *Mag. c.*, *Mag. m.*, Mang., Mar., Meny., **Merc.**, Mez., Mos., *Mur. ac.*, *Nat. c.*, **Nat. m.**, **Nit. ac.**, Nux m., **Nux v.**, Oleand., Op., Par., *Petrol.*, PHOS., *Pho. ac.*, *Plat.*, PULS., Ran. b., Ran. s., Rheum, Rhodo., **Rhus**, *Ruta*, *Saba.*, *Sabi.*, *Samb.*, *Sars.*, *Sele.*, Seneg., SEP., **Sil.**, Spig., Spo., Stan., Squ., **Staph.**, Stram., *Stro.*, SUL., *Sul. ac.*, Tar., Thuj., Valer., Verat. a., Vio. o., *Vio. t.*, **Zinc**.

—**Late.**—Agar., *Alum.*, Ambr., *Anac.*, Ant. cr., Ant. t., *Arn.*, *Asaf.*, Bell., Bism., Bor., *Bry.*, CALC. C., Canth., *Carb. v.*, **Caust.**, Clem., *Cocc.*, Con., Croc., Dig., Dulc., **Euphr.**, GRAPH., Hep., *Hyos.*, Ign., *K. carb.*, K. nit., Kre., *Laur.*, Led., Lyc., Mag. c., **Mag. m.**, Merc., Nat. c., *Nat. m.*, *Nit. ac.*, NUX V., Petrol., **Phos.**, Pho. ac., Plat., *Puls.*, Ran. b., Rhodo., *Rhus*, SEP., **Sil.**, *Spig.*, Stram., **Sul.**, *Sul. ac.*, *Verat. a.*, *Verb.*, Zinc.

—**Associated Symptoms.** See Aggravations, Waking.

Position in Sleep.

Lies on Abdomen.—Bell., *Calc. c.*, *Cocc.*, **Coloc.**, Ign., Puls., Stram.

Arms and Hands Over Head.—*Calc. c.*, Chin., *Coloc.*, Nux v., *Plat.*, PULS., Rheum, Ruta, Thuj., Verat. a.

—**Under Head.**—Acon., Ambr., Ant. t., *Ars.*, Bell., *Cocc.*, Coloc., Ign., Meny., **Nux v.**, *Plat.*, Puls., Rhus, Saba., Spig., Vio. o.

—**On Abdomen.**—Cocc., Puls.

—**On Back.**—Acon., Ambr., Ant. cr., *Ant. t.*, Arn., Ars., *Aur.*, Bism., BRY., Calc. c., *Chin.*, **Cic.**, Coca, *Coloc.*, Dig., Dros., **Fer.**, **Ign.**, Kre., Lyc., Nux v., Par., *Phos.*, Plat., PULS., Rhodo., **RHUS**, Ruta, Saba., Spig., Stan., Stram., Sul., Verat. a., *Vio. o.*

Head Inclined Forward.—Acon., Cic., Cup., Staph., Vio. o.

—**Backward.**—Bell., Chin., *Cic.*, **Cina**, Cup., Hep., *Hyos.*, Ign., Nux v., *Sep.*, **Spo.**, Stan., Vio. t.

Head Inclined To One Side.—*Cina*, Spo., Tar.

—Hanging Low Down.—*Arn.*, *Hep.*, Nux v., **Spo.**

Knees Bent.—Ambr., *Vio. o.*

—Spread Apart.—**Cham.**, *Plat.*, **Puls.**, Vio. o.

Legs Crossed.—Rhodo.

—Drawn Up.—Anac., *Carb. v.*, **Cham.**, **Chin.**, **Mang.**, **Meny.**, **Plat.**, **Puls.**, Rhodo., *Stram.*

—Stretched Out.—Agar., *Bell.*, **Cham.**, **Chin.**, **Dulc.**, *Plat.*, **Puls.**, *Rhus.*

—One Stretched Out, The Other Drawn Up.—Stan.

On Side.—Acon., **Alum.**, **Bar. c.**, Bor., *Caust.*, **Colch.**, Fer., K. nit., Merc., Mos., Nat. c., *Nux v.*, **Phos.**, Ran. b., Saba., *Sabi.*, Spig., *Sul.*

Sitting.—A**r**s., **Bar.**, *Cannab. s.*, Caps., Carb. v., *Chin.*, Cic., **Cina**, Dig., *Hep.*, K. nit., **Lyc.**, *Phos.*, *Puls* Rhus, *Sabi.*, *Spig.*, **Sul.**

Sleepiness During the Day.—Acon., *Agar.*, *Agn.*, **Aloe.**, **Alum.**, Ambr., *Am. carb.*, Am. m., **Anac.**, **ANT. CR.**, **ANT. T.**, **APIS**, Arg., *Arn.*, **Ars.**, **Asaf.**, Asar., Aur., *Bar. c.*, **Bell.**, Bism., Bor., Bov., **Brom.**, **Bry.**, Calad., **Calc. c.**, **Calc. ph.**, **Camph.**, **CANNAB. I.**, *Cannab. s.*, *Canth.*, **Caps.**, **Carb. an.**, **Carb. v.**, *Carb. sul.*, **Caust.**, **Cham.**, **Chel.**, **Chin.**, *Cic.*, **Cina**, **Clem.**, **Cocc.**, **Coff.**, **Colch.**, **Coloc.**, **Con.**, *Cop.*, *Corn. c.*, *Corn. f.*, **CROC.**, *Crotal.*, *Cup.*, **Cyc.**, *Dig.*, Dros., Dulc., **Eup. pur.**, Euphorb., Euphr., Fer., *Form.*, **Fl. ac.**, *Graph.*, Guai., *Hell.*, Hep., Hyos., Ign., Ip., *K. br.*, **K. carb.**, K. nit., Kre., *Lach.*, **Laur.**, Led., *Lyc.*, Mag. c., *Mag. m.*, Mang., Mar., *Merc.*, **MERC. C.**, Mez., **Mos.**, Mur. ac, **Nat. c.**, **Nat. m.**, *Nit ac.*, **NUX M.**, **NUX V.**, Oleand., **OP.**, *Ox. ac.*, Par., *Petrol.*, **PHOS.**, **PHO. AC.**, **POD.**, Plat., *Pb.*, **PULS.**, *Ran. b.*, Rheum., *Rhodo.*, **Rhus**, *Ruta*, Saba., Sabi., **Samb.**, *Sars.*, *Sec. c.*, *Sele.*, Seneg., **Sep.**, **Sil.**, **Spig.**, Spo., Squ., Stan., **Staph.**, **Stram.**, Stro., **SUL.**, **Sul. ac.**, Tar., **THUJ.**, Valer., **Verat. a.**, **Verb.**, Vio. o., *Vio. t.*, *Zinc.*

—Morning.—Agar., *Alum.*, Ambr., *Anac.*, Ant. cr., Ant. t., *Arn.*, *Asaf.*, Bell., Bism., Bor., Bry., **CALC. C.**, Canth., *Carb. v.*, **Caust.**, Clem , *Cocc.*, **Con.**, Croc., Dig., Dulc., Euphr., **GRAPH.**, *Hep.*, Hyos , Ign. *K. tarb.*, K. nit., Kre., *Laur.*, Lea., *Lyc.*, Mag. c., **Mag. m.**, **Merc.**, Nat. c., *Nat. m.*, *Nit. ac.*, NUX V., Petrol., **Phos.**, **Pho. ac.**, Plat., **Puls.**, Ran. b., Rhodo., *Rhus*, SEP., **Sil.**, *Spig.*, Stram., **Sul.**, *Sul. ac.*, *Verat. a.*, Verb., Zinc.

—Forenoon.—*Agar.*, Alum., *Am. carb.*, **ANT. CR.**, *Ant. t.*, Bar. c., Bism., Calc. c., **Cannab. s.**, *Carb. an.*, **Carb. v.**, Con., *Cyc.*, *Dros.*, Dulc., Graph., Hell., K. carb., Lyc., Mag. m., **Mos.**, **Nat. c.**, **Nux v.**, Puls., Rhus, SABA., *Sars.*, **Sele.**, **Sep.**, Sil., Spig., Staph., **Sul. ac.**, Zinc.

SLEEP

Sleepiness in Afternoon.—Acon., **Agar.**, Alum., *Am. carb.*, **Anac.**, Ant. cr., Ant. t., Ars., Asaf., *Aur., Bar. c.*, Bell., *Bov.*, Bry., Calc. c., *Canth.*, Caps., *Carb. an.*, **Carb. v.**, *Caust.*, Chel., CHIN., *Cic.*, Cina, *Clem.*, Coff., Con., **Croc.**, *Cyc.*, Dulc., Euphorb., Fer., *Graph.*, Guai., Hyos., Ign., K. carb., **Lach.**, *Laur.*, **Merc.**, Mez., Mur. ac., *Nat. c.*, *Nat. m.*, Nux m., NUX V, *Par.*, Petrol., **Phos.**, *Pho. ac.*, Plat., PULS., *Ran. b.*, Rheum. Rhodo., **RHUS**, **Ruta**, Saba., Sep., *Sil.*, Spig., *Spo.*, Squ., **Staph.**, Stro., **SUL.**, Sul. ac., Thuj., **Verb.**, *Vio. t.*, Zinc.

—**Evening.**—Agar., Alum., Am. carb., *Am. m.*, Anac., *Ant. cr.*, **Ant. t.**, Arn., ARS., *Asaf.*, Bar. c., *Bell.*, Bor., **Bov.**, Calad., CALC. C., Carb. v., *Caust.*, Chin., *Cina*, Cocc., Con., Croc., Cic., *Dros.*, Dulc., Graph., *Hep.*, Ign., K. CARB., *Lach.*, Laur., Lyc., Mag. m., *Mang.*, Mos., *Nat. m.*, NUX V., Par., *Petrol.*, Phos., **Pho. ac.**, *Plat.*, Pb., PULS., Ran. b., Rhodo., *Rhus*, Ruta, Sars., Sele., Seneg., Sep., **Sil.**, Spig., Squ., Sul., Thuj., Valer.

—**Associated Symptoms.**—*Acon.*, Agar., Ambr., ANT. T., *Arg.*, **Ars.**, Asaf., Bell., **Bor.**, *Calad.*, Caps., **Cham.**, Chel., *Chin.*, Cic., *Cina*, Cocc., **Con.**, *Croc.*, Cyc., *Dig.*, *Euphr.*, Fer., Hell., *Hep.*, **Ign.**, **K. carb.**, Kre., Lach., **Laur.**, Led., Mag. c., *Merc.*, **Mez.**, **Nat. m.**, **Nit. ac.**, NUX M., Nux v., **Op.**, Petrol., *Phos.*, **Pho. ac.**, **Plat.**, Pb., PULS., Ran. b., **Rhodo.**, *Rhus*, **Saba.**, *Sabi.*, Sep., Stan., **Staph.**, *Stram.*, Stro., Sul. ac., Tar., *Thuj.*, *Verat. a.*, Verb., *Vio. o.*, Vio. t.

Sleepiness, Caused by Various Things.—*Acon*, Agar., *Am. carb.*, Anac., Ant. cr., ANT. T., Arn., Ars., Asaf., Asar., *Aur.*, Bar. c., Bism., Bov., Bry., *Calc. c.*, Caps., *Carb. v.*, Caust., Cham., Chel., **Chin.**, Cic., Cina, Clem., Cocc., Coff., Con., *Croc.*, Cyc., Dros., Euphr., Fer., Graph., Hyos., Ign., K. carb., Lach., Laur., Lyc., Mag. c., *Merc.*, Mos., Mur. ac., *Nat. c.*, **Nat. m.**, Nit. ac., NUX M., Nux v., Op., Par., *Petrol.*, Phos., *Pho. ac.*, *Plat.*, Pb., *Puls.*, Ran. b, Rheum, RHUS, *Ruta*, **Saba.**, Sabi., Sele., Sep., **Sil.**, Spig., *Stan.*, Staph., **Sul.**, **Tar.**, Thuj., Verb., Zinc.

Sleep, Anxious.—Acon., ARS., Bell., Cham., **Cocc.**, Dulc., *Fer.*, Hep., Ip., **K. carb.**, Merc., *Op.*, *Petrol.*, *Rhus*, Samb., *Verat. a.*

—**Comatose.**—*Acon.*, *Agn.*, Anac., Ant. cr., ANT. T., Arn., Ars., *Asaf.*, Bar. c., **Bell.**, Bry., Calc. c., **Camph.**, Carb. v., Caust., Cham., Cic., Clem., *Cocc.*, Coloc., **Con.**, CROC., **Cup.**, Cyc., Dig., Euphorb., *Hell.*, Hyos., Ign., K. carb., Lach., *Laur.*, Led., Lyc., Merc., *Mos.*, Nit. ac., NUX M., Nux v., Oleand., **OP.**, Petrol., Phos, Pho. ac., **Pb.**, **Puls.**, Rhus, Ruta, *Sec. c.*, Sep., Stan., *Stram.*, Sul., VERAT. A., Zinc.

—**Intoxicated with.**—*Agn.*, **Ant. t.**, *Bell.*, **Bry.**, Calc. c., **Camph.**,

Carb. v., Caust., Clem., Coff., **Con.**, CROC., K. carb., Lach., Lyc., **Mez.**, NUX M., **Op.**, *Phos., Pho. ac.,* PULS., Stan., Zinc.

Sleep Restless.—*Abrot.,* ACON., Agar., Agn., Alum., *Ambr.,* Am. carb., Am. m., *Anac.,* Ant. cr., Ant. t., Arn., ARS., **Ars. iod., Asaf.,** Asar., **Aur.,** BAR. C., BELL., *Bor.,* Bov., **Bry.,** Calad., Calc. c., Camph., *Cannab. s.,* Canth., Caps, Carb. an., Carb. v., Caust., **Cham.,** *Chel.,* CHIN., Cic., **Cimic.,** Cina, *Clem., Coca,* Cocc., Coff., Colch., Coloc., *Con.,* Croc., Cup., Cyc., **Dig.,** Dros., *Dulc.,* Euphorb., **Fer., Gel.,** *Graph.,* Guai., Hell., Hep., Hyos., Ign., Iod., *Ip.,* **K. carb.,** K. nit., Kre., Lach., Laur., *Led.,* **Lyc.,** *Mag. c.,* Mag. m., Mang., **Mar.,** Meny., Merc., Mez., *Mos.,* **Mur. ac.,** Nat. c., *Nat. m.,* **Nit. ac.,** Nux m., **Nux v.,** *Oleand.,* Op., **Par., Petrol., Phos.,** *Pho. ac.,* **Pic. ac., Pb., Plat.,** PULS., *Ran. b.,* Ran. s., **Raph.,** *Rheum.,* Rhodo., RHUS, **Rumex,** *Ruta,* Saba., Sabi., Samb., Sars., Sec. c., Sele., **Seneg.,** Sep., SIL., Spig., *Spo.,* **Squ.,** Stan., *Staph.,* **Stram.,** Stro., SUL., Sul. ac., **Tar., Thuj.,** *Valer., Verat. a.,* Verb., Vio. t., Zinc.

—**Somnambulistic.**—ACON., **Agar.,** Alum., **Anac.,** *Ant. cr.,* Bell., **Bry.,** Croc., *Cyc.,* **Ign.,** *Lach.,* Lyc., Mar., Nat. m., OP., Petrol., **Phos., Plat.,** Rheum., Sep., *Sil.,* Spig., *Spo.,* Stan., *Stram.,* **Sul.,** Zinc.

—**Sound.**—*Acon.,* Agn., Alum., *Anac., Ant. cr.,* ANT. T., Ars., *Bar. c.,* **Bell.,** Bor., Bry., Calc. c., *Camph.,* CANNAB. I., *Caust.,* Cham., Chin., Cic., Cocc., *Con.,* **Croc.,** Cup., Cyc., *Dig.,* Hell., Hyos., Ign., Kre., **Laur., Led.,** Merc., Mos., NUX M., OP., *Petrol., Phos.,* Pho. ac., Pb., **Puls.,** Rhodo., Rhus, *Ruta,* Saba., Sec. c., Sele., **Seneg.,** Sep., *Spig.,* Stan., Stram., Sul., **Verat. a.,** *Zinc.*

—**Stupid.**—Agn., *Anac.,* Ant. t., BELL., **Bry.,** *Calad.,* Calc. c., **Camph.,** Carb. v., *Carb. sul., Caust.,* Cham., Chin., **Cic.,** Clem., *Cocc., Coloc.,* **CON., Croc.,** Dig., *Dios.,* Euphorb., *Euphr.,* Fer., GRAPH., Hep., **Hyos., Ign.,** K. carb., K. nit., Lach., LED., **Lyc.,** *Nat. m.,* NUX M., NUX V., OP., **Phos.,** *Pho. ac., Pb.,* **Puls.,** Ran. b., Sec. c., **Seneg.,** Spig., Stan., **Stram., Valer.,** *Verat. a.,* Zinc.

—**Unrefreshing.**—Acon., Agar., *Alum.,* **Ambr.,** Am. carb., *Am. m., Anac.,* Ant. cr., *Ant. t., Arn.,* Ars., Asaf., Aur., Bar. c., *Bell.,* Bism., Bor., Bov., BRY., **Calc. c.,** *Camph.,* Cannab. s., Caps., Carb. an., Carb. v., *Carb. sul.,* **Caust.,** Cham., *Chel.,* **Chin.,** Cic., Cina, *Clem.,* Cob., Cocc., Coff., CON., *Corn. c.,* Croc., **Dig.,** Dros., Euphorb., Euphr., *Fer.,* Graph., *Guai.,* HEP., Ign., *Ip., K. carb.,* K. nit., Kre., Lach., Laur., Led., **Lyc.,** *Mag. c., Mag. m.,* Mar., Meny., *Merc.,* Mez., Mos., Mur. ac., Nat. c., **Nat. m., Nit. ac.,** Nux m., Nux v., Oleand., OP., **Petrol.,** Phos., *Pho. ac.,* **Puls.,** *Ran. b.,* Rheum., Rhodo., *Rhus,* Ruta, *Saba.,* Samb., Sec. c., **Sele.,**

Sep., **Sil.**, *Spig.*, Spo., Squ., *Stan.*, **Staph.**, *Stram.*, Stro., SUL., Tar., Thuj., Valer., *Verat. a.*, Vio. t., *Zinc.*

Sleep, Associated Symptoms, see Aggravations, Sleep.

Sleeplessness in General.—Acon., Agar., Alum., *Ambr., Am. carb., Am. m.,* Anac., Ant. cr., Ant. t., ARG. N., Arn., ARS., Asaf., Asar., Aur., Bap., *Bar. c.,* **Bell.,** Bism., **Bor.,** BRY., *Calad.,* CALC. C., *Camph.,* *Cannab. s.,* **Canth.,** Caps., Carb. an., *Carb. v.,* **Caust.,** CHAM., Chel., CHIN., *Cic., Cimic.,* Cina, Clem., Coca, **Cocc.,** COFF., Colch., **Con.,** Cup., Cyc., Dig., Dros., *Dulc.,* Euphr., Fer., **Graph.,** Guai., Hell., HEP., HYOS., **Ign.,** Iod., *Ip., K. br.,* K. CARB., **K. iod.,** K. nit., **Kre.,** Lach., *Laur.,* **Led.,** *Lyc., Mag. c.,* Mag. m., Mang., Mar., MERC., Mez., *Mos.,* Mur. ac., **Nat. c., Nat. m., Nit. ac.,** Nux m., **Nux v.,** Oleand., **Op.,** Petrol., PHOS., *Pho. ac., Plat.,* PB., PULS., **Ran. b.,** *Ran. s., Raph.,* Rheum, **Rhodo.,** RHUS, Ruta, Saba., *Sabi., Samb.,* Sars., *Sec. c,* **Sele.,** *Senec.,* SEP., SIL., Spig., Spo., Squ., Stan., *S'aph.,* Stram., Stro., SUL., *Sul. ac.,* Tar., **Tarent.,** *Thea.,* **Thuj.,** Valer., *Verat. a.,* Verb., Vio. o., Vio. t., Zinc.

—**Before Midnight.**—Acon., Agar., *Alum.,* Ambr., **Am. carb.,** *Am. m.,* Anac., Ant. cr., *Ant. t.,* Arn., **Ars.,** *Asar.,* Aur., *Bar. c.,* **Bell.,** Bism., **Bor.,** BRY., Calad., CALC. C., Camph., Cannab. s., Canth., Caps., Carb. an., CARB. V., *Caust.,* Cham., *Chel.,* **Chin.,** Clem., Cocc., COFF., Coloc., **Con.,** Cyc., Dig., Dulc., *Euphorb.,* Euphr., Fer., **Graph.,** *Guai.,* **Hep.,** Hyos, **Ign.,** Ip., K. carb., K. nit., **Kre.,** Lach., *Laur.,* **Led.,** Lyc., *Mag. c., Mag. m.,* Mang., **Mar.,** MERC., Mez., *Mos.,* **Mur. ac.,** *Nat. c., Nat. m., Nit. ac.,* Nux m., **Nux v.,** Par., Petrol., PHOS., *Pho. ac.,* Plat., Pb., **PULS., Ran. b.,** Ran. s., Rheum, Rhodo., RHUS, *Saba.,* Sabi., Samb., *Sars.,* Sele., Seneg., SEP., **Sil.,** Spig., *Spo., Stan,* Staph., Stro., **SUL.,** Sul. ac., Tar., Thuj., **Valer.,** *Verat. a.,* Verb., Vio. t., Zinc.

—**After Midnight.**—*Acon.,* Alum., Ambr., *Am. carb.,* Am. m., *Ant. cr.,* Ant. t., Arn., ARS., **Asaf.,** Aur., Bar. c, *Bor., Bry.,* Calad., *Calc. c.,* Cannab. s., *Canth.,* CAPS., Carb. v., *Caust.,* Cham., Chin., Cocc., COFF., *Con.,* Croc., Cyc., Dros., **Dulc.,** *Euphr.,* Fer., *Graph,* Guai., Hell., **Hep.,** Ign., *Iod.,* K. CARB., *K. nit.,* Kre., *Lach.,* Lyc., **Mag. c.,** *Mang.,* Merc., Mez., Mur. ac., **Nat. c.,** Nat. m., *Nit. ac.,* NUX V., Oleand., Phos., *Pho. ac., Plat.,* Pb., Puls., Ran. b., **Ran. s.,** Rhodo., *Rhus,* Saba., *Sabi., Samb.,* Sars., *Sele.,* **Sep.,** SIL., Spo., Squ., *Staph.,* Sul., **Sul. ac.,** Thuj., Verat. a., *Verb.,* Vio. t.

—**Though Sleepy.**—Acon., Am. carb., Am. m., *Arn.,* **Ars.,** *Bar. c.,* **BELL.,** *Bor.,* Bry., Calad., **Calc. c.,** Camph., Canth., *Carb. v.,* **Caust., CHAM.,** Chel., *Chin., Cic.,* Cina, Clem., *Cocc.,* Coff., **Con.,** Euphr., Fer.,

Graph., Hep., *Hyos.*, **K. carb.**, *Lach., Laur.,* Lyc., *Mag. m.,* **Merc.**, *Mos.*, **Nat. c.**, **Nat. m.**, *Nit. ac.,* Nux v., OP., PHOS., Pho. ac., Pb., **PULS**, *Ran. b.*, Rhodo., **Rhus**, Saba., Sabi., Samb., *Sele.*, **SEP**, **Sil.**, Spig., Staph., **Sul.**, Sul. ac., *Verat. a.*, Vio. o., Zinc.

Symptoms Causing Sleeplessness.—*Acon.*, Agar., Alum., *Ambr., Am. carb., Am. m.,* Anac., Ant. cr., Ant. t., *Arn.*, **ARS.**, Asaf., *Aur., Bar. c.,* **Bell.**, Bism., *Bor.,* BRY., Calad., **CALC. C.**, **Calc. ph.**, *Camph.*, Cannab. s., Canth., *Caps., Carb. an.,* **Carb. v.**, *Caust.,* CHAM., Chel., **Chim.**, CHIN., Cic., Cina, Clem., *Cocc.,* COFF., Colch., **Con.**, Cup., *Cur.,* Cyc., Dig., Dros., *Dulc., Euphr.,* Fer., Graph., *Guai.,* Hell., Hep., HYOS., Ign., Iod., *Ip.,* **K. carb.**, K. nit., Kre., Lach., Laur., *Led.,* Lil. t., Lyc., **Mag. c.**, **Mag. m.**, Mang., *Mar.,* MERC., Mez., *Mos.,* Mur. ac., *Nat. c.,* **Nat. m.**, *Nit. ac.,* Nux m., *Nux v.,* Oleand., *Op.,* Petrol., PHOS., *Pho. ac., Plat.,* Pb., **PULS.**, *Ran. b.*, Ran. s., Rheum, **Rhodo.**, **RHUS**, Ruta, *Saba.*, **Sabi.**, Samb., **Sars.**, **Sele.**, SEP, **Sil.**, Spig., *Spo., Squ.,* Staph., Stan., Stram., *Stro.,* SUL., Sul. ac., *Tar.,* Thuj., Valer., *Verat. a.*, Vio. t., Zinc.

Dreams.

Dreams in General.—Acon., Agar., Agn., Alum., *Ambr., Am. carb.,* Am. m., *Anac., Ant. cr., Ant. t., Arg.,* **ARG. N.**, **Arn.**, **Ars.**, Asaf., Asar., *Aur., Bar. c., Bell.,* Bism., *Bor., Bov.,* BRY., Calad., **Calc. c.**, *Calc. f., Calc. ph.,* Camph., **Cannab. i.**, *Cannab. s., Canth.,* **Caps.**, Carb. an., *Carb. v., Caust., Cham.,* Chel., CHIN., **Cic.**, Cina, *Clem.,* Cocc., Coff., *Coloc.,* **Con.**, *Croc.,* Cyc., **Dig.**, *Dios.,* Dros., Dulc., Euphorb., Euphr., Fer., **Gran.**, **Graph.**, Guai., Hell., *Hep., Hyos.,* Ign., Iod., Ip., *K. carb.,* K. nit., Kre., Lach., Laur., *Led., Lyc.,* MAG. C., *Mag. m., Mang., Mar.,* Meny., **Merc.**, Mez., *Mos.,* Mur. ac., **Nat. c.**, **Nat. m.**, *Nat. s., Nit. ac.,* Nux m., NUX V., *Oleand., Op., Par., Petrol.,* PHOS., **Pho. ac.**, *Plat., Pb.,* **PULS.**, Ran. b., Ran. s., Rheum, Rhodo., RHUS, Ruta, **Saba.**, **Sabi.**, Samb., *Sars.,* Sec. c., Sele., Seneg., **Sep.**, SIL., Spig., Spo., Squ., **Stan.**, Staph., *Stram., Stro.,* SUL., Sul. ac., *Tar.,* Thuj., *Valer.,* Verat. a., Verb., *Vio. t.,* Zinc.

—**Anxious.**—*Abrot.,* ACON., *Agar.,* Agn., *Alum.,* Ambr., *Am. carb.,* Am. m., **Anac.**, Ant. cr., *Ant. t.,* Arg., **Arg. n.**, **ARN.**, **Ars.**, Asar., Aur., Bap., *Bur. c.,* **Bell.**, Bism., Bor., *Bov.,* **Bry.**, *Calc. c., Calc. ph.,* **Cannab. i.**, Cannab. s., *Canth.,* Caps., *Carb. ac., Carb. an.,* **Carb. v.**, *Caust., Cham.,* **Chin.**, Cina, Clem., *Coca, Cocc.,* Coff., Coloc., Con., **Croc.**, Dig., *Dios.,* Dros., Euphorb., Euphr., Fer., **GRAPH.**, *Guai.,* Hell., **Hep.**, Hyos., Ign., *Iod.,* Ip., *K. br.,* **K. carb.**, *K. nit.,* **Kre.**, Lach., *Laur.,* **Led.**, Lyc., MAG. C., **Mag. m.**, *Mang.,* Mar., Merc., Merc. i. r., *Mez., Mur.*

ac., *Nat. c.*, **Nat. m.**, *Nit. ac.*, **NUX V.**, *Op.*, Par., **Petrol.**, **PHOS.**, *Pho. ac.*, *Plat.*, *Pb.*, **PULS.**, *Ran. b.*, **Ran. s.**, Raph., *Rheum*, Rhodo., **RHUS**, **Saba.**, Sabi., **Sars.**, *Sele.*, **Sep.**, **SIL.**, *Spig.*, Spo., Squ., *Stan.*, *Staph.*, **Stram.**, Stro., **SUL**, **Sul. ac.**, *Tar.*, **THUJ.**, Valer., **Verat. a.**, *Verb.* Zinc.

Anxious, of Animals.—*Am. carb.*, **Am. m.**, ARN., *Bell.*, Bov., *Hyos.*, *Merc.*, Nux v., Phos., Ran. s., *Sil.*, *Sul. ac.*

—**Of Battle.**—*Bry.*, Fer., Plat., Thuj., Verb.

—**Of the Dead.**—Alum., Am. carb., **Anac.**, **Arn.**, **ARS.**, *Aur.*, Bar. c., *Brom.*, Bry., *Calc. c.*, Cocc., Con., **Graph.**, Iod., **K. Carb.**, Laur., Lyc., MAG. C., *Mag. m.*, Mur. ac., Nit. ac., **Phos.**, *Pho. ac.*, *Plat.*, Ran. b., Ran. s., Rheum, *Sars.*, Spo., *Sul. ac.*, **THUJ.**, *Verb.*, Zinc.

—**Of Difficulties.**—AM. M., *Anac.*, Ant. t., ARS., Cannab. s., Caps., Croc., **Graph.**, Mag. c., *Mag. m.*, Mur. ac., **Phos.**, Plat., Rhus.

—**Of Falling.**—**Am. m.**, *Aur.*, *Bell.*, Caps., Chin., **Dig.**, Fer., Guai., Hep., Ign., K. nit., *Kre.*, *Mag. m.*, Merc., Mez., Pb., Sabi., *Sars.*, Sul., THUJ.

—**Of Fire.**—*Alum.*, Am. carb., **Anac.**, Ant. t., *Ars.*, Bar. c., *Bell.*, Calc. c., Clem., Croc., Euphr., HEP., *Kre.*, *Laur.*, MAG. C., MAG. M., Nat. m., **Phos.**, Plat., Rhodo., **Rhus**, *Spig.*, Stan., Stro., *Sul.*, *Sul. ac.*

—**Of Ghosts.**—*Alum.*, Bov., **Carb. v.**, *Ign.*, *K. carb.*, *Sars.*, *Sil.*, Spig.

—**Of Bad Luck.**—*Alum.*, **Am. m.**, *Anac.*, Ant. cr., **Arn.**, *Ars.*, Bar. c., **Bell.**, Cannab. s., Carb. an., **Cham.**, **Chin.**, *Cocc.*, Croc., **GRAPH.**, Guai., *Ign.*, **K. carb.**, K. nit., Laur., *Led.*, **LYC.**, Mang., *Merc.*, Mur. ac., **NUX V.**, Op., Petrol., **Phos.**, Pho. ac., **PULS.**, *Ran. b.*, Rhus, **Sars.**, Sele., Spo., Stan., *Staph.*, **Sul.**, **Sul. ac.**, THUJ., Verat. a., *Verb.*, Zinc.

—**Of Quarrels.**—*Alum.*, Am. carb., Ant. cr., **Arn.**, *Aur.*, *Bap.*, *Brom.*, Bry., *Calc. c.*, Canth., *Caust.*, Cham., Con., Guai., *Hep.*, **Mag. c.**, Nat. c., NUX V., Op., Phos., Pho. ac., Plat., *Puls.*, Sabi., *Sele.*, Spig., **Stan.**, Staph., Tar., Verat. a.

—**Of Shooting.**—**Am. m.**, Hep., *Merc.*

—**Of Sickness.**—*Am. m.*, Anac., Asar., *Bor.*, **Calc. c.**, Cocc., Dros., Hep., K. carb., Kre., NUX V., *Phos.*, *Sil.*, Squ., Zinc.

—**Of Thieves.**—*Alum.*, *Aur.*, *K. carb.*, MAG. C., *Mag. m.*, **Merc.**, Nat. c., **Nat. m.**, Pb., Sil., Verat. a.

—**Of Thunder.**—Arn., Ars., Euphr., Nat. c.

—**Of Water.**—*Alum.*, AM. M., Bov., *Dig.*, Fer., **Graph.**, Ign., Iod., K. carb., K. nit., **Mag. c.**, *Nag. m.*, *Merc.*, Nat. c., *Ran. b.*, *Sil*, Valer., **Verat. a.**

Confused.—*Acon.*, *Alum.*, Bar. c., **Bry.**, *Cannab. s.*, Canth., Caust.,

Chin., Cic., Cina, *Clem.*, Croc., Dulc., Euphorb., **Hell.**, Laur., **Led.**, Lyc., *Mag. c.*, Mang., **Nat. c.**, Petrol., *Phos.*, Plat., **Pb.**, **Puls.**, Ruta, Saba., Sabi., **Sep.**, *Sil.*, Spig., Stan., Sul., Thuj., *Valer.*

Confused, Continued.—Acon., Anac., Ant. t., *Arn.*, Asaf., **Bry.**, **Calc. c.**, Chin., Coff., Euphorb., *Graph.*, IGN., *Lach*, Merc., **Nat. c.**, *Nat. m.*, **Puls.**, Sep., *Sil.*, Spig., Staph., Zinc.

— —**After Waking.**—*Acon.*, Anac., Arn., *Bry.*, **Calc. c.**, Chin., Euphorb., Graph., Ign., Merc., **Nat. c.**, *Nat. m.*, **Puls.**, Sep., Sil., Zinc.

—**Continuation of Former Ideas.**—Ant. t., Asaf., Ign., *Puls.*, **Rhus.**

Historical.—Caust., *Cham.*, Croc., Hell., **Mag. c.**, Merc., **Phos.**, Sele., *Sil.*, Stram.

With Indifference.—Alum., *Anac.*, Arg., Ars., *Bell.*, **Bry.**, Canth., Cham., Chel., **Chin.**, *Cic.*, Cina, Clem., *Cocc.*, Coff., *Con.*, Euphorb., Hep., *Ign.*, K. carb., *Lach.*, Lyc., **Mag. c.**, Merc., *Nat. m.*, **Nux v.**, *Phos.*, Pho. ac., Plat., **Puls.**, Rhodo., **Rhus**, Sabi., Sars., Sele., **Sep.**, *Sil.*, Stan., Staph., Stro., **Sul.**, *Vio. t.*

—**Indifferent to the Day's Business.**—Arg., *Bell.*, BRY., Canth., Chel., *Cic.*, Cina, Euphorb., *Hep.*, K. carb., **Led.**, *Lyc.*, **Mag. c.**, *Merc.*, **Nux v.**, Phos., Pho. ac., Plat., **Puls.**, **Rhus**, Sabi., Sars., Sele., *Sil.*, Stan., Staph., *Sul.*

Of Mental Effort.—Acon., Ambr., *Anac.*, Arn., **Bry.**, Camph., Carb. an., **Chin.**, Cic., Clem., Dulc., *Graph.*, IGN., Iod., K. nit., **Lach.**, Laur., Led., Mar., *Mos.*, Mur. ac., **Nat. m.**, NUX V., Oleand., Op., Par., **Phos.**, Pho. ac., Pb., Puls., *Rhus*, Saba., Sabi., Sars., Sec. c., Spo., Staph., Sul., Thuj., *Vio. t.*, Zinc.

—**Of Excelling in Mental Work.**—Acon., *Anac.*, Arn., *Bry.*, Camph., Carb. an., Graph., **Ign.**, *Lach.*, Nux v., Puls., Rhus, *Saba., Sabi., Thuj.*

Pleasant.—Acon., Agn., Alum., Ambr., Am. carb., *Am. m.*, Ant. cr., Ant. t., Arn., *Ars.*, Asaf., **Aur.**, *Bar. c.*, Bell., *Bism.*, Bor., Bov., *Bry.*, CALC. C, *Cannab. s.*, Canth., **Carb. an.**, *Carb. v.*, Caust., Cham., Chel., Chin., Cic., Clem., *Cocc.*, Coff., Coloc., Con., Croc., *Cyc.*, Dig., Dros., Euphorb., **Graph.**, Hell., *Hyos.*, Ign., **K. carb.**, K. nit., Kre., **Lach.**, Laur., **Led.**, Lyc., **Mag. c.**, *Mag. m.*, Mang., Mar., Meny., *Merc.*, Mez., Mur. ac., NAT. C., **Nat. m.**, *Nit. ac.*, Nux m., Nux v., *Oleand.*, OP., Par., Petrol., **Phos.**, Pho. ac., Plat., *Pb.*, PULS., Ran. b., *Rhodo.*, **Saba.**, *Samb.*, Sars., SEP., Sil., *Spig.*, Spo., Squ., *Stan.*, STAPH., *Stram.*, Stro., Sul., Tar., *Thuj.*, Valer., *Verat. a.*, VIO. T., *Zinc.*

—**Of Dancing.**—*Mag. c.*, Mag. m.

—**Fantastic.**—Ambr., Ant. t., Ars., *Bar. c.*, CALC. C., **Carb. an.**, *Carb. v.*, Cham., Con., *Fer. iod.*, **Graph.**, Hell., **K. carb.**, K. nit., *Lach.*,

DREAMS.

Lyc., Merc., **Nat. c.**, NAT. M., Nit. ac., *Nux v.*, OP., **Sep.**, *Sil.*, Spo., Sul., Zinc.

Pleasant, Of Festivities.—*Ant. cr.*

—**Of Gold.**—*Cyc.*, Puls.

—**Intellectual.**—*Ign.*

—**Full of Imagination.**—Ars., **Calc. c.**, Cham., Hell., *K. carb.*, **Lach**. Merc., Nit. ac., *Spo.*

—**Journeys.**—Am. carb., *Am. m.*, **Mag. c.**, Mag. m., **Nat. c.**, **Op.**

—**Joyful.**—Asaf., Caust., *Coff.*, **Croc.**, Dig., **Lach.**, Laur., *Mag. c.*, Mez., OP., *Phos.*, Squ., *Sul.*

—**Of Love.**—Acon., Agn., *Alum.*, Am. m., **Ant. cr.**, Arn., Ars., Aur., *Bism.*, Bor., Bov., *Calc. c.*, **Cannab. i.**, **Canth.**, Carb. an., Caust., Chel., *Chin.*, Clem., **Cob.**, Cocc., Coloc., **Con.**, **Cop.**, Euphorb., **Graph.**, *Hyos.*, Ign., *K. carb.*, Kre., **Lach.**, Led., Lyc., *Mag. c.*, Mag. m., Meny., Merc., Mez., Mur. ac., NAT. C., *Nat. m.*, Nit. ac., Nux m., NUX V., **Oleand.**, OP., *Ox. ac.*, Par., **Phos.**, PHO. AC., **Plat.**, **Puls.**, Ran. b., *Rhodo.*, **Saba.**, *Samb.*, Sars., **Sele.**, **Sep.**, **Sil.**, *Spig.*, **Stan.**, STAPH, *Stram.*, **Sul.**, Tar., *Thuj.*, Valer., *Verat. a.*, VIO. T., Zinc.

Unremembered.—Agn., *Arn.*, *Aur.*, **Bell.**, Bov., *Bry.*, Canth., Carb. an., Carb. v., **Cic.**, Cocc., **Con.**, Croc., **Hell.**, Ign., Iod., Ip., *Lach.*, *Laur.*, Lyc., Mag. c., Mag., m., *Meny.*, *Merc.* Mur. ac., *Nat. m.*, Phos., Pho. ac., Plat., *Rhus*, **Saba.**, Samb., Sars., **Sele.**, Seneg., **Spig.**, Stan., Staph., *Stram.*, **Sul.**, Sul. ac., **Tar.**, *Verat. a.*

Vexatious.—Acon., Agar., **Alum.**, *Ambr.*, *Am. carb.*, Am. m., *Anac.*, Ant. cr., Arn., *Ars.*, ASAR., Bor., Bov., **Bry.**, *Calc. c.*, **Cannab. i.**, Cannab. s., Caust., Cham., Chel., *Chin.*, *Cina*, Cocc., **Con.**, *Dig.*, Dros., **Gel.**, Hep., **Ign.**, Kre., Lach., Led., *Lyc.*, *Mag. m.*, **Mos.**, Mur. ac., *Nat. c.*, Nat. m., *Nat. s.*, Nit. ac., **Nux v.**, *Op.*, Petrol., *Phos.*, Pho. ac., Plat., Puls., *Rheum*, Rhus, Ruta, Sabi., Sars., Sep., *Sil.*, Spo., Staph., Stro., **Sul.**, Zinc.

—**Disgusting.**—Am. carb., Anac., Chel., Kre., *Mag. m.*, Mur. ac., *Nat. m.*, Nux v., Phos., **Puls.**, *Sul.*, Zinc.

—**With Humiliation.**—*Alum.*, Am. carb., Arn., **Asar.**, Con., Led., Mag. m., **Mos.**, Mur. ac., *Staph.*

—**Of Illusions of Hope.**—*Ign.*

—**Of Sick People.**—Ign., *Mos.*, Rheum, Staph.

—**With Strivings.**—Cina, Nux v., *Rhus*, Sabi.

—**Of Vermin.**—Chel., *Mur. ac.*, **Nux v.**, Phos.

Vivid.—Acon., *Ambr.*, Anac., Arg., Ant. t., **Arn.**, *Ars.*, Aur., Bar. c., **Bell.**, Bism., **Bry.**, Calad., **Calc. c.**, *Calc. f.*, *Calc. ph.*, Cannab. s.,

Canth., Caps., *Carb. a*., Carb. an., *Carb. v.*, *Cham.*, Chin., Cic., *Clem.*, Cocc., Coff., Coloc., Con., *Croc.*, *Dros.*, Euphorb., Fer., **Fer. iod.**, *Graph.*, Guai., **Ign.**, Iod., Ip., K. carb., *Lach.*, Laur., *Led.*, Lyc., **Mag. c.**, **Mar.**, *Meny.*, **Merc.**, Mez., *Mos.*, *Mur. ac.*, **Nat. c.**, *Nat. m.*, Nit. ac., Nux m., **Nux v.**, *Op.*, Petrol., PHOS., Pho. ac., Plat., Puls., Ran. b., *Rheum*, RHUS, Ruta, Saba., Samb., **Sep.**, SIL., *Spig.*, Stan., *Staph.*, *Stram.*, SUL., Tar., Thuj., *Valer.*, Verat. a., *Vio. t.*, Zinc.

Dreams, Waking.—Acon., Am. carb., Anac., **Arn.**, *Ars.*, Bell., Bry., Calc. c., Camph., **Cham.**, *Graph.*, Hell., **Hep.**, *Hyos.*, *Lach.*, **Merc.**, Nux m., **Nux v.**, *Oleand.*, *Op.*, *Phos.*, **Pho. ac.**, Puls., Ran. s., Rheum, Samb., Sele., *Sil.*, *Stram*, *Thuj.*, Verat. a.

Circulation.

Blood, Anæmia.—Ac. ac., Acon., Alum., **Arn.**, Arg., ARS., **Bell.**, Bov., Bry., **Calc. c.**, *Carb. v.*, *Ced.*, *Cham.*, CHIN., Cina, Coff., *Coloc.*, Con., *Cup.*, Cyc., *Dig.*, **Fer.**, Ign., Iod., K. carb., Lyc., Mag. c., Mag. m., **Merc.**, Mez., *Nat. c.*, *Nat. m.*, Nit. ac., Nux m., *Nux v.*, *Phos.*, **Pho. ac.**, PB., *Pso*, PULS., *Rhodo.*, Rhus, *Ruta*, *Sabi.*, **Sep.**, *Sil.*, Spig., SQU., **Stan.**, STAPH., Sul., *Valer.*, Verat. a., *Zinc.*

—**Congestion.**—ACON., Aloe., Alum., Ambr., **Am. carb.**, Am. m., Ant. cr., **Apis**, **Arn.**, *Asaf.*, **Aur.**, *Bar. c.*, BELL., Bor., Bov., **Bry.**, CACT., **Calc. c.**, Camph., Cannab. s., Canth., *Carb. an.*, **Carb. v.**, Caust., Cham., Chel., CHIN., Clem., Cocc., *Coff.*, *Colch.*, Coloc., Con., *Conv.*, *Croc.*, *Cup.*, *Cyc.*, Dig., Dulc., FER., Glon., Graph., *Guai.*, Hell., **Hep.**, *Hyos.*, Ign., Iod., *K carb.*, K. nit., Lach., *Laur.*, Led., Lyc., Mag. c., Mag. m., Mang., MELI., *Merc.*, Mez., *Mos.*, *Nat. c.*, **Nat. m.**, Nit. ac., Nux m., NUX V., Op., Petrol., **Phos.**, Pho. ac., Plat., *Pb.*, PULS., Ran. b., Rhodo., Rhus, Sabi., Samb., Sec. c., **Seneg.**, **Sep.**, Sil., Spig., **Spo.**, Squ., Staph., **Stram.**, SUL., Sul ac., Tar., Thuj., *Valer.*, Verat. a., Verat. v., VIO. O.

— —**Internally.**—Aloe, Apis, Ars, CACT., Camph., Canth., Colch., *Conv.*, *Cup.*, Glon., Hell., MELI., *Sep.*, Verat. a., *Verat. v.*

—**Orgasm.**—ACON., *Aloe*, Alum., Ambr., **Am. carb.**, *Am. m.*, Amyl., *Ant. t.*, Arg., ARG. N., **Arn.**, *Ars.*, AUR, *Bar. c.*, BELL., **Bov.**, **Bry.**, CALC. C., Cannab. i., Cannab. s., *Carb. an.*, **Carb. v.**, Caust., Chom., Chin., Con., **Croc.**, Cup., Dig., Dulc., FER., GLON., *Guai.*, **Hep.**, Ign., Iod., K. carb., KRE., Lach., LYC., *Mag. m.*, Merc., *Mos.*, **Nat. m.**, Nit. ac., Nux m., *Nux v.*, Op., Petrol., Phos., Pho. ac., Polyp., **Puls.**, Rhus, *Saba.*, **Sabi.**, Samb., *Sang.*, Sars., Seneg., **Sep.**, **Sil.**, SPO., Stan., *Staph.*, STRAM., SUL., Thuj., **Verat. a.**

CIRCULATION.

Blood, Plethora (Compare with **Full-blooded**).—Acon., Alum., Am. carb., *Arn.*, Ars., Aur., *Bar. c*., **BELL.**, Bry., **Calc. c.**, Canth., *Chel.*, Chin., Coloc., Croc., Cup., **Dig.**, Dulc., FER., *Graph.*, Guai., Hep., HYOS., Ign., **K. carb.**, K. nit., Lach., **Lyc.**, Merc., Mos., Nat. c., **Nat. m.**, Nit. ac., **Nux v.**, Op., Phos., Pho. ac., **PULS.**, **Rhus**, Sabi., *Sele.*, Sep., *Sil.*, Stram., Sul., *Thuj.*, Verat. a.

—**Sensation as if Blood Stagnated.**—*Acon.*, Bell., Bry., Caust., Croc., Dig., *Gel.*, Hep., Ign., **Lyc.**, *Nux v.*, *Oleand.*, Puls., *Rhodo.*, **Saba.**, Seneg., *Sep.*, Sul., Zinc.

Blood Vessels, Burning.—Ars., Bry., Hyos., Op., Rhus, Verat. a.

—**Cold Feeling.**—Acon., *Ant. t.*

—**Distention.**—Acon., *Alum.*, Am. carb., **Arn.**, *Ars.*, **Bar. c.**, **Bar. m.**, **BELL.**, Bry., *Calc. c.*, *Calc. f.*, Camph., *Chel.*, **CHIN.**, *Cic.*, *Coloc.*, *Con.*, **Croc.**, *Cyc.*, FER., Graph., *Ham.*, HYOS., *Lach.*, *Lyc.*, *Meny.*, Mos., *Nat. m.*, *Nux v.*, Oleand., Op., **Phos.**, *Pho. ac.*, **Pb.**, PULS., Rhodo., Rhus, *Sars.*, Sep., Sil., *Spig.*, *Spo.*, Staph., Stro., Sul., THUJ., *Vip.*, Zinc.

—**Inflammation.**—Acon., Ant. t., *Ars. iod.*, BAR. C., **Cup.**, *Ham.*, Lach., Spig.

—**Like a Net-work.**—*Carb. v.*, **Caust.**, *Clem.*, *Lyc.*, **Plat.**, THUJ.

—**Pulsation.**—Acon., Anac., Ant. t., *Ars.*, Asar., BELL., *Bov.*, Bry., Calad., *Calc. c.*, Canth., Caps., **Carb. an.**, *Carb. v.*, *Clem.*, Coloc., *Con.*, *Cup.*, Graph., Hell., Hep., Ign., Iod., K. carb., K. nit., Kre., MELI., Merc., Nat. c., *Nat. m.*, Nit. ac., Nux v., Phos., Pho. ac., *Pb.*, **Puls.**, Rhus, *Saba.*, Sabi., Sars., Sele., Sep., Sil., Staph., **Stram.**, Stro., SUL., Thuj., Zinc.

—**Stitches.**—*Merc.*

—**Varicose.**—Ambr., Ant. t., ARN., Ars., *Calc. c.*, *Calc. f.*, *Calc. ph.*, **Carb. v.**, Caust., *Clem.*, Coloc., Fer., *Fl. ac.*, Graph., *Ham.*, Kre., Lach., Lyc., Mag. c., *Millef.*, Nat. m., Nux v., Pb., PULS., *Sil.*, Spig., **Sul.**, *Sul. ac.*, Thuj., Vip., Zinc.

Pulse, Abnormal in General.—ACON., *Agar.*, Agn., *Ambr.*, Am. carb., Am. m., Ant. cr., Ant. t., Arg., Arn., ARS., Asaf., Asar., *Aur.*, *Bar. c.*, BELL., *Bism.*, Bor., *Bov.*, Bry., Calad., *Calc. c.*, Camph., *Cannab. s.*, Canth., Caps., **Carb. an.**, **Carb. v.**, Caust., *Cham.*, *Chel.*, **Chin.**, *Cic.*, Cina, Cocc., *Colch.*, Coloc., Con., Croc., CUP., **Dig.**, Dulc., Fer., *Gel.*, Graph., Guai., Hell., **Hep.**, HYOS., *Ign.*, IOD., *Ip.*, **K. carb.**, *K. nit.*, KRE., *Lach.*, **Laur.**, Led., *Lyc.*, Mang., *Meny.*, **Merc.**, Mez., *Mos.*, *Mur. ac.*, *Nat. m.*, Nit. ac., Nux m., *Nux v.*, Oleand., OP., Par., *Petrol.*, **PHOS.**, **PHO. AC.**, *Plat.*, *Pb.*, *Puls.*, Ran. b., Ran. s., Rheum, Rhod., **RHUS**,

Saba., *Sabi.*, *Samb.*, **Sec.** c., Seneg., **Sep.**, SIL., *Spig.*, Spo., Squ., ***Stan.***, Staph., STRAM., *Stro.*, **Sul.**, *Sul. ac.*, *Thuj.*, *Valer.*, VERAT. A., Vio. o., Vio. t., *Zinc.*

Pulse, Full.—ACON., *Ant. t.*, **Arn.**, Asaf., Asar., *Bar. c.*, BELL., Bism., Bry., Camph., *Canth.*, **Chel.**, *Chin.*, Colch., Coloc., Con., **Cup.**, DIG., Dulc., *Fer.*, **Glon.**, Hell., Hep., HYOS., *Ign.*, *Iod.*, K. NIT., *Lach.*, *Led.* Merc., Mez., **Mos.**, *Mur. ac.*, Nat. m., *Nux v.*, Oleand., **Op.**, Par., *Petrol.*, Phos., *Pho. ac.*, Pb., *Ran. b.*, *Ran. s.*, **Sabi.**, Samb., **Sep.**, *Sil.*, **Spig.**, Spo., STRAM., *Sul.*, **Tab.**, *Verat. a.*, **Verat. v.**, Vio. o.

—**Hard.**—ACON., *Ant. t.*, **Arn.**, *Ars.*, Asaf., Asar., *Bar. c.*, BELL., Bism., BRY., *Cact.*, Calad., Camph., **Canth.**, *Cham.*, CHEL., **Chin.**, *Cina*, Cocc., *Colch.*, *Coloc.*, **Cup.**, Dig., Dulc., **Fer.**, Hell., Hep., HYOS., **Ign.**, *Iod.*, Lach., **K.** nit., **Led.**, Merc., Mez., **Mos.**, Mur. ac., Nat. m., Nit. ac., *Nux v.*, Oleand., *Op.*, Par., Petrol., Phos., *Pho. ac.*, Pb., *Ran. b.*, Ran. s., *Sabi.*, Samb., Sec. c., Seneg., **Sep.**, **Sil.**, *Spig.*, Spo., Squ., STRAM., *Strop.*, *Sul.*, Valer., *Verat. a.*, **Verat. v.**, Vio. o., Zinc.

—**Imperceptible.**—ACON., Agn., Ant. t., **Ars.**, Bell., *Cact.*, Cannab. s., *Carb. ac.*, CARB. V., Cic., **Cocc.**, CUP., Dulc., Fer., Guai., Hell., Hyos., *Iod.*, **Ip.**, Kre., *Laur.*, **Merc.**, Nux v., **Op.**, Phos., *Pho. ac.*, **Plat.**, Puls., Rhus, Sec. c., SIL., *Stan.*, Stram., Sul., Sul. ac., VERAT. A., Zinc.

—**Intermittent.**—Acon., **Agar.**, Alum., *Ars.*, Asaf., Bism., **Bry.**, Camph., Canth., *Caps.*, *Carb. ac.*, Carb. v., CHIN., **Colch.**, *Conv.*, *Crotal.*, DIG., *Gel.*, **Glon.**, **Hep.**, *Hyos*, K. **carb.**, *K. chl.*, *Lach.*, *Laur.*, MERC., *Merc. cy.*, Mez., *Mur. ac.*, *Naj.*, *Nat. ars.*, NAT. M., *Nit. ac.*, Nux v., **Op.**, *Phyt.*, PHO. AC., *Pb.*, **Rhus**, Sabi., **Samb.**, SEC. C., **Sep.**, Stram., Sul., *Thea.*, Thuj., *Verat. a.*, Zinc.

—**Irregular.**—Acon., **Agar.**, Alum., *Amyl.*, *Ant. cr.*, *Apoc. c.*, ARS., Ars. iod., Asaf., Aur., Bell., Bism., **Bry.**, *Cact.*, *Canth.*, **Caps.**, *Carb. ac.*, Carb. v., *Cham.*, CHIN., **Cimic.**, Colch., Con., DIG., *Gel.*, **Glon.**, Hep., Hyos., *K. carb.*, **Kalm.**, Lach., *Laur.*, **Lob. i.**, Mang., Merc., Merc. c., *Merc. cy.*, Mez., *Mur. ac.*, NAT. M., Nux v., *Oleand.*, **Op.**, PHO. AC., *Phyt.*, **Pb.**, Rhus, Sabi., **Samb.**, **Sang.**, Sec. c., Seneg., Sep., **Sil.**, **Spig.**, **Still.**, STRAM., **Sul.**, *Tab.*, *Thea.*, Thuj., *Valer.*, Verat. a., *Verat. v.*, Zinc.

—**Rapid.**—*Ac. ac.*, ACON., Ambr., *Amyl.*, Ant. cr., *Ant. t.*, *Apis*, Arg., Arn., ARS., **Ars. iod.**, Asaf., Asar., Aur., Bar. c., BELL., Bism., Bor., BRY., Calc. c., Camph., *Canth.*, *Carb. v.*, Ced., Cham., *Chin.*, Cina, Cocc., **Colch.**, *Coloc.*, Con., Croc., **Crotal.**, Cup., DIG., *Gel.*, **Glon.**, Guai., **Hep.**, **Hyos.**, *Ign.*, IOD., *Ip.*, K. carb., *K. chl.*, K. nit., Kre., *Lach.*,

FEVER. 253

Led., *Lob. i.*, Lyc., Meny., MERC., *Merc. cy.*, Mez., Mos., **Mur. ac.**,
Nat. m., Nit. ac., Nux v., Oleand., Op., Par., Petrol., Pb., PHOS.,
PHO. AC., Puls., R...b., *Ran. s.*, Rheum, **Rhus**, Sabi., *Samb.*, SEC.
C., *Seneg.*, Sep., SIL., **Spo.**, STAN., Staph., STRAM., SUL., Sul. ac.,
Tab., Ter., Valer., Verat. a., *Verat. v.*, Zinc.

Pulse More Rapid than the Beat of the Heart.—Acon., Arn.,
Rhus, Spig.

—**Slow.**—Acon., *Acon. f.*, **Agar.**, Agn., Ant. cr., **Ant. t.**, Arn.,
Ars., **Bell.**, Camph., **CANNAB. I.**, *Cannab. s.*, **Canth.**, Chin., Cic.,
Colch., Coloc., **Con.**, **Cup.**, DIG., Dulc., **Gel.**, *Glon.*, **Hell.**, Hep., *Hyd. ac.*, Hyos., Ign., *K. br.*, K. carb., *K. chl.*, *K. nit.*, **Kalm.**, Laur., *Lob. i.*,
Meny., Merc., *Merc. cy.*, Mos., Mur. ac., **Nux m.**, OP., Par., Petrol.,
Phos., Puls., Rhodo., Rhus, *Samb.*, **Sang.**, *Sec. c.*, *Sil.*, Spig., Squ.,
STRAM., *Strop.*, Tab., Thuj., **Verat. a.**, **Verat. v.**

—**Slower than the Beat of the Heart.**—Agar., Cannab. s., **Dig.**,
Dulc., *Hell.*, K. nit., *Laur.*, Sec. c., *Verat. a.*

—**Small.**—ACON., Agar., Ant. cr., **Ant. t.**, *Arn.*, ARS., *Asaf.*, *Aur.*,
Bar. c., **Bell.**, *Bism.*, Bry., **Camph.**, *Cannab. s.*, Canth., *Carb. ac.*, CARB.
V., **Cham.**, Chin., *Cic.*, *Cina*, **Cocc.**, Colch., Con., **CUP.**, DIG., *Dulc.*,
Fer., **GUAI.**, Hell., **Hyos.**, Ign., **Iod.**, **Ip.**, K. carb., *K. chl.*, K. nit.,
Kre., *Lach.*, **LAUR.**, Lob. i., Mang., Meny., **Merc.**, *Merc. cy.*, Mur. ac.,
Nat. m., **Nux m.**, *Nux v.*, Op., Phos., Pho. ac., **Plat.**, *Pb.*, Puls., Ran.
b., Ran. s., Rhodo., *Rhus*, Saba., **Samb.**, SEC. C., Seneg., SIL., Spig.,
Squ., **Stan.**, Staph., STRAM., *Sul.*, **Sul. ac.**, **Tab.**, **Ter.**, Thuj., Valer.,
VERAT. A., Vio. o., *Zinc.*

—**Soft.**—*Ac. ac.*, Acon., *Aconin.*, Agar., Agn., Ant. cr., ANT. T., *Apis*,
Apoc. c., Arn., *Ars.*, *Bar. c.*, **Bell.**, Bism., **Camph.**, *Cannab. i.*, *Cannab. s.*,
Canth., **Carb. ac.**, CARB. V., *Cham.*, *Chin.*, Cic., **Cocc.**, Colch., Con.,
Conv., *Crotal.*, **CUP.**, DIG., Dulc., Fer., **Gel.**, Guai., *Hell.*, Hep., *Hyd. ac.*, Hyos., **Iod.**, **Ip.**, **Jal.**, *K. bi.*, *K. br.*, *K. carb.*, *K. chl.*, K. nit., Kalm.,
Kre., Lach., *Laur.*, **Lob. i.**, Mang., **Merc.**, MUR. AC., *Naj.*, *Nat. ars.*,
Nat. m., Nux v., *Oleand.*, **OP.**, **Ox. ac.**, Phos., *Pho. ac.*, **Phyt.**, Plat.,
Pb., *Puls.*, Ran. s., Rhodo., *Rhus*, **Sang.**, *Sec. c*, Seneg., *Sil.*, Spig.,
STRAM., *Sul. ac.*, **Tab.**, **TER.**, Thuj., Valer., VERAT. A., **Verat. v.**

—**Tremulous.**—Ambr., ANT. T., **Ars.**, *Aur.*, **Bell.**, CALC. C.,
Camph., *Carb. ac.*, **Cic.**, *Cina*, **Cocc.**, *Dig.*, *Gel.*, **Hell.**, Iod., K. carb., **Kre.**,
Lach., *Nat. m.*, Nux m., Phos., **Rhus**, Ruta, Sabi., Sep., SPIG., Staph.,
Stram.

—**Unchanged** (with Various Symptoms).—*Agar.*, Agn., **Alum.**, Am.
carb., *Am. m.*, **Anac.**, Ant. cr., **Arg.**, **Asaf.**, *Asar.*, Bism., **Bor.**, **Calad.**,

FEVER.

Camph., Cannab. s., Canth., **Caps.**, *Caust.*, Chel., Cic., **Cina**, **Clem.**, Cocc., *Coff.*, Colch., Coloc., **Cyc.**, DROS., *Dulc.*, **Euphorb.**, EUPHR., *Graph.*, Hell., Ip., K. nit., Lach., Laur., *Led.*, Lyc., MAG. C., *Mag. m.*, Mang., **Mar.**, Meny., *Mez.*, Mur. ac., NAT. C., Nit. ac., Nux m., **Oleand.**, **Par.**, *Plat.*, *Ran. b.*, **Ran. s.**, **Rheum**, *Rhodo.*, **Ruta**, **Sec. c.**, *Sele.*, Sep., Spig., Spo., Squ., *Stro.*, *Sul. ac.*, **Tar.**, Valer., **Verb.**, *Vio. o.*, *Vio. t.*, Zinc.

Chilliness in General.
—ACON., *Agar.*, Agn., **Alum.**, *Ambr.*, **Am. carb.**, **Am. m.**, *Anac.*, *Apis*, Ant. cr., **Ant. t.**, ARAN, *Arg.*, **Arg. n.**, **Arn.**, ARS., *Asar.*, Aur., Bar. c., *Bell.*, **Berb.**, Bism., Bor., **Bov.**, BRY., *Cact.*, **Calad.**, **Calc. c.**, *Calc. ph.*, Camph., Cannab. s., **Canth.**, **Caps.**, *Carb. ac.*, **Carb. an.**, *Carb. v.*, *Carb. sul.*, *Caust.*, *Ced.*, **Cham.**, *Chel.*, **Chin.**, Cic., *Cimic.*, *Cina*, Clem., **Cocc.**, **Coff.**, **Colch.**, *Coloc.*, *Con.*, *Conv.*, *Croc.*, **Cup.**, **Cyc.**, Dig., *Dios.*, **Dros.**, Dulc., *Elat.*, **Eup. per.**, **Euphorb.**, Euphr., **Fer.**, **Gel.**, **Gran.**, **Graph.**, *Guai.*, *Hell.*, **Hep.**, Hyos., **Ign.**, Iod., Ip., *K. bi.*, **K. carb.**, *K. nit.*, **Kre.**, Lach., *Laur.*, **Led.**, **Lept.**, **Lob. i.**, LYC., *Mag. c.*, Mag. m., *Mang.*, *Mar.*, MENY., **MERC.**, **Mez.**, *Millef.*, Mos., *Mur. ac.*, Nat. c., NAT. M., *Nit. ac.*, **Nux m.**, NUX V., Oleand., Op., *Oxyt.*, Par., *Petrol.*, PHOS, **Pho. ac.**, *Plat.*, *Pb.*, **Poly.**, PULS., **Ran. b.**, Ran. s., Rheum, *Rhodo.*, RHUS, Ruta, *Saba.*, *Sabi.*, Samb., **Sang.**, Sars., **Sec. c.**, Sele., **Seneg.**, **Sep.**, SIL., SPIG., *Spo.*, *Squ.*, **Stan.**, **Staph.**, Stram., Stro., SUL., Sul. ac., *Tar.*, *Ther.*, *Thuj.*, Valer., VERAT. A., Verb., Vio. t., *Zinc.*

—In Certain Parts.
—*Acon.*, Agar., *Agn.*, *Alum.*, *Ambr.*, **Am. m.**, Anac., **Arg.**, **Arn.**, **Ars.**, *Asar.*, Aur., *Bar. c.*, **Bell.**, **Berb.**, Bor., **Bov.**, Brom., Bry., *Calc. c.*, Camph., **Caps.**, *Carb. ac.*, Carb. v., Caust., *Chel.*, **Chin.**, Coc. c., *Coff.*, **Colch.**, *Conv.*, Croc., **Cup.**, *Dig.*, Dros., *Dulc.*, Eucal., **Euphr.**, **Fer.**, **Gam.**, **Gel.**, *Glon.*, *Guai.*, *Hell.*, **Hep.**, Hyos., IGN., Ip., **K. carb.**, K. iod., *Kalm.*, Kre., LACH., **Lept.**, **Lyc.**, Mag. c., *Meny.*, *Merc.*, *Mez.*, Mur. ac., *Nat c.*, *Nat. m.*, *Nux m.*, NUX V., Op., Par., *Petrol.*, **Phos.**, Pho. ac., Plat., *Pb.*, **Poly.**, PULS., **Ran. b.**, **Raph.**, **Rhus**, *Saba.*, *Samb.*, Sars., SEP., SIL., SPIG., **Spo.**, Squ., **Stan.**, **Staph.**, Stro., SUL., Thuj., Trom., VERAT. A., *Verb.*, Zinc.

—Internally.
—*Acon.*, *Agar.*, *Agn.*, *Alum.*, Ambr., ANAC., Ant. cr., **Ant. t.**, Arn., **Ars.**, Asaf., Bar. c., **Bell.**, **Bov.**, Bry., CALC. C., Camph., **Canth.**, **Caps.**, **Carb. an.**, *Carb. v.*, *Caust.*, **Cham.**, Chel., Chin., **Coff.**, Colch., Con., Croc., *Dig.*, Dros., Euphr., **Gam.**, **Graph.**, **Hell.**, Hep., **Ign.**, Ip., **K. carb.**, K. nit., *Kre.*, **Lach.**, Laur., **Lyc.**, Mag. c., Mang., *Meny.*, **Merc.**, **Mez.**, Mos., Nat. c., *Nat. m.*, Nit. ac., NUX V., Oleand., **Paeo.**, Par., **Phos.**, Pho. ac. Plat., *Pb.*, Puls., *Ran. b.*, Rhus, Ruta,

Saba., Sars., Sec. c., Sep., *Sil.*, **Spig.**, Spo., **Squ.**, Stro., **SUL**, Sul. ac., Thuj., Valer., Verat. a., Zinc.

Chilliness, One-sided.—Alum., *Ambr.*, Anac., **Ant. t.**, **Bar. c.**, **Bell.**, **Bry.**, **Caust.**, *Cham.*, **Chin.**, **Cocc.**, **Croc.**, Dig., *Ign.*, *K. carb.*, **Lyc.**, Nat. c., **Nux v.**, *Par.*, *Phos.*, Pho. ac., Plat., **PULS.**, **Rhus**, Ruta, *Saba.*, **Sars.**, *Spig.*, Stan., Stram., *Sul.*, Sul. ac., Thuj., **Verb.**

—**Becomes Chilled Easily.**—Acon., *Agar.*, **Agn.**, Alum., *Ambr.*, *Am. carb.*, Am. m., *Anac.*, Ant. cr., *Ant. t.*, Arn., ARS., **Asar.**, Bar. c., Bell., Bism., Bor., **Bov.**, *Brom.*, BRY., *Calad.*, **Calc. c.**, *Camph.*, Cannab. s., Canth., Caps., *Carb. an.*, **Carb. sul.**, *Carb. v.*, **Caust.**, Cham., Chel., CHIN., Cic., *Cimic.*, Cina, *Cist.*, **Clem.**, **Cocc.**, **Coff.**, Croc., Cup., *Dig.*, Dros., Dulc., Euphorb., *Euphr.*, Graph., *Guai.*, **Hell.**, **Hep.**, Hyos., *Ign.*, Ip., K. carb., K nit., Kre., *Laur.*, Led., **Lyc.**, *Mar.*, **Menth.**, Meny., **Merc.**, **Mez.**, Mos., Mur. ac., Nat. c., **NAT. M.**, Nit. ac., Nux m., **NUX V.**, Oleand., Op., *Par.*, Petrol., PHOS., Pho. ac., *Plat.*, Pb., **PULS.**, Ran. b., Ran. s., Rhodo., **Rhus**, **Rumex**, Ruta, **Saba.**, Sabi., Samb., Sars., Sec. c., Seneg., Sep., SIL., SPIG., Spo., *Squ.*, Stan., *Staph.*, Stram., Stro., **Sul.**, Tar., Thuj., Valer., *Verat. a.*, Vio. t., Zinc.

Chilliness with Gooseflesh.—Ant. t., Asar., *Bar. c.*, Bell., Bor., Bry., Camph., Cannab. s., Canth., Chel., *Chin.*, **Croc.**, *Hell.*, *Ign.*, Laur., Mang., Mur. ac., *Nat. m.*, Nux v., *Par.*, Phos., Ran. b., Rhodo., Saba., Sabi., Sars., Spig., Stan., Staph., Sul. ac., *Thuj.*, **Verat. a.**

—**With Shivering.**—Acon., *Agar.*, Am. carb., Anac., **ARN.**, Ars., **Bell.**, **BRY.**, Calc. c., Camph., *Cannab. s.*, Canth., **Caps.**, Carb. v., *Cham.*, Chel., **CHIN.**, Cic., *Cina*, Cocc., Fer., *Hell.*, Ign., Iod., Ip., Kre., *Laur.*, Led., Lyc., *Mang.*, Mur. ac., *Nat. m.*, Nux m., **Nux v.**, *Petrol.*, Pho. ac., **Rhus**, Ruta, Saba., Sabi., Samb., Sec. c., Spig., Spo., Stram., Valer., *Verat. a.*

—**With Thirst.**—ACON., Am. m., Anac., **Ant. cr.**, Arn., *Ars.*, Bar. c., Bell., *Bor.*, Bov., BRY., Calad., **Calc. c.**, Camph., *Cannab. s.*, **Caps.**, Carb. v., **CHAM.**, *Chin.*, CINA, Croc., Dros., Dulc., EUP. PER., **Hep.**, Ign., *Ip.*, K. carb., *K. nit.*, Kre., Lach., Laur., Led., Mag. m., *Merc.*, Mez., *Mur. ac.*, *Nat. c.*, **NAT. M.**, **NUX V.**, Op., Pb., Phos., Puls., Ran. b., **Rhus**, *Ruta*, Saba., *Sec. c.*, Sep., Sil., *Spo.*, Squ., Stan., Staph., **Sul.**, Thuj., Valer., VERAT. A.

—**Without Thirst.**—*Agar.*, Agn., Alum., Am. carb., **Am. m.**, *Ant. cr.*, Ant. t., ARS., *Asar.*, *Aur.*, Bell., Bor., Bov., *Bry.*, Calad., Calc. c., Camph., Canth., *Caps.*, Carb. v., *Caust.*, Chin., *Cina*, Cocc., *Coff.*, Coloc., Con., **Cyc.**, Dros., Dulc., Euphorb., Guai., **HELL.**, Hep., Hyos., Ip., K. carb., *K. nit.*, Kre., Lach., Led., Mang., Meny., Mur. ac., *Nat. c.*, Nat.

m., Nit. ac., NUX M., **Nux v.**, Oleand., Op., *Petrol.*, PHOS., *Pho. ac.*, PULS., Rhodo., **Rhus**, SABA., Sabi., *Samb.*, Sars. Sep., SPIG., **Spo.**, Squ., *Staph.*, Stram., **Sul.**, Tar., *Thuj.*, Verat. a., Zinc.

Chilliness, With Trembling.—Acon., *Agn.*, Anac., ANT. T., Arn., Bell., **Bry.**, *Calc. c.*, *Cannab. s.*, Canth., *Carb. sul.*, *Chin.*, Cic., *Cina*, Cocc., Con., Croc., Led., Mar., *Merc.*, *Nux v.*, Oleand., Op., *Par.*, Phos., *Plat.*, **Puls.**, Rhus, *Saba.*, **Sil.**, *Stram.*, **Sul.**

—Symptoms During Chill.—Acon., Agar., Agn., *Alum.*, Ambr., Am. carb., Am. m., *Anac.*, Ant. cr., *Ant. t.*, *Arn.*, ARS., Asar., Aur., Bar. c., *Bell.* **Bor.**, *Bov.*, BRY., *Calad.*, **Calc. c.**, *Camph.*, *Cannab. s.*, Canth., **Caps.**, Carb. an., *Carb. v.*, Caust., **Cham.**, Chel., **Chin.**, Cic., *Cina*, *Cocc.*, Coff., Coloc., *Con.*, Croc., Cup., Cyc., Dig., **Dros.**, Dulc., Euphorb., Fer., **Graph.**, **Hell.**, **Hep.**, Hyos., **Ign.**, Iod., Ip., *K. carb.*, K. nit., **Kre.**, *Lach.*, Laur., Led., **Lyc.**, Mag. m., Mang., Mar., Meny., *Merc.*, *Mez.*, Mur. ac., *Nat. c.*, **Nat. m.**, Nit. ac., *Nux m.*, NUX V., Oleand., Op., Par., Pb., *Petrol.*, Pho. ac., *Phos.*, Plat., PULS., *Ran. b.*, Rhodo., RHUS, *Ruta*, Saba., Sabi., Samb., Sars., Sec. c., Sele., *Seneg.*, *Sep.*, Sil., *Spig.*, Spo., Squ., Stan., Staph., Stram., Stro., *Sul.*, Sul. ac., Tar., *Thuj.*, Valer., **Verat. a.**, Vio. t, Zinc.

Heat.—*Ac. ac.*, ACON., *Aconin.*, *Agar.*, Agn., *All. c.*, *Aloe*, Alum., Ambr., Am. b., Am. carb., Am. m., **Amyl**, *Anac.*, Ant. cr., Ant. t., Arg., **Arn.**, Ars., Asaf., Asar., **Bar. c.**, BELL., Bism., **Bor.**, Bov., BRY., Cact., Calad., **Calc. c.**, *Calc. iod.*, Camph., Cannab. s., *Canth.*, **Caps.**, Carb. an., *Carb. v.*, *Caust.*, Ced., **Cham.**, Chel., *Chin.*, Cic., Cina, Clem., Cocc., *Coff.*, Colch., Coloc., **Con.**, *Corn. f.*, Croc., *Cub.*, Cup., Cyc., Dig., Dros., *Dulc.*, Euphorb., Fer., *Graph.*, Guai., Hell., **Hep.**, Hyos., **Ign.**, Iod., *Ip.*, *K. carb.*, K. nit., Kre., LACH., Laur., Led., *Lyc.*, *Mag. c.*, *Mag. m.*, Mang., Mar., Meny., MERC., *Merc. c.*, Mez., Mos., Mur. ac., Nat. c., Nat. m., **Nit. ac.**, Nux m., NUX V., Oleand., *Op.*, Par., **Petrol.**, PHOS., **Pho. ac.**, *Phyt.*, Plat., Pb., **PULS.**, Ran. b., *Ran. s.*, Rheum, *Rhodo.*, RHUS, Ruta, *Saba.*, Sabi., *Samb.*, **Sang.**, Sars., SEC. C, *Sele.*, Seneg., **Sep.**, **Sil.**, *Spig.*, Spo., Squ., Stan., *Staph.*, *Stram.*, Stro., **Sul.**, Sul. ac., Tar., *Thuj.*, VALER., Verat. a., *Vio. t.*, **Zinc.**

—Externally.—ACON., *Agar.*, Alum., *Ambr.*, Am. carb., Am. m., *Anac.*, Ant. cr., Ant. t., *Arg.*, **Arn.**, ARS., *Asaf.*, Asar., *Bar. c.*, BELL., Bism., Bor., Bov., BRY., *Calad.*, **Calc. c.**, *Camph.*, Cannab. s., Canth., **Caps.**, *Carb. an.*, **Carb. v.**, *Caust.*, **Cham.**, Chel., Chin., Cic., Cina, **Cocc.**, Coff., *Colch.*, Coloc., Con., Coral., Croc., Cup., Cyc., Dig., Dros., Dulc., Euphorb., Fer., Graph., Guai., *Hell.*, **Hep.**, **Hyos.**, IGN., *Iod.*, Ip., **K. carb.**, *K. nit.*, Kre., **Lach.**, *Laur.*, Led., **Lyc.**, Mag. c., Mag. m., *Mang*,

FEVER. 257

Mar., Meny., **Merc.**, *Mez.*, Mos., *Mur. ac.*, *Nat. c.*, Nat. m., Nit. ac., Nux m., Nux v., Oleand., **Op.**, Par., *Pb.*, Petrol., **Phos.**, *Pho. ac.*, Plat., **Puls., Ran. b.**, Ran. s., Rheum., Rhodo., RHUS, Ruta, Saba., Sabi., *Sal. ac., Samb.*, Sars., *Sec. c., Sele.*, Seneg., **Sep.**, SIL., Spig., *Spo.*, Squ., *Stan., Staph.*, STRAM., Stro., **Sul.**, Sul. ac., *Tar.*, Thuj., Valer., Verat. a., Vio. t., *Zinc.*

Heat, Internally.—ACON., Alum., Ambr., Am. carb., Am. m., *Anac.*, Ant. cr., Ant. t., *Apis*, Arg., **Arn.**, ARS., Asaf., Asar., Bar. c., BELL., **Benz. ac.**, Bism., Bor., Bov., BRY., *Calad.*, **Calc.** c., *Camph.*, Cannab. s., **Canth.**, Caps., Carb. an., *Carb. v., Caust.*, **Cham.**, Chel., *Chin., Cic.*, Cina, Cocc., *Coff.*, Colch., Coloc., **Con.**, Croc., *Cup.*, Dig., Dros., *Dulc.*, *Euphorb., Glon., Graph.*, Guai., **Hell.**, Hep., Hyos., Ign., Iod., *Ip.*, *K. carb.*, K. nit., Kre., Lach., Laur., Led., *Lyc., Mag. c., Mag. m., Mang.*, Mar., Meny., **Merc.**, *Mez., Mos., Mur. ac., Nat. c.*, Nat. m., *Nit. ac.*, Nux m., NUX V., Oleand., Op., **Ox. ac.**, Par., Petrol., **Phos.**, PHO. AC., Plat., Pb., **Puls.**, *Ran. b.*, Ran. s., Rhodo., RHUS, Ruta, SABA., *Sabi., Samb., Sars.*, **Sec. c.**, Seneg., **Sep.**, *Sil.*, **Spig.**, *Spo., Squ.*, **Stan.**, Staph., Stram., Stro., *Sul.*, Sul. ac., Tar., Thuj., Valer., **Verat. a.**, Vio. t., Zinc.

—**In Special Parts.**—Acon., Agar., Agn., *Alum., Ambr., Am. carb., Am. m.*, **Amyl.**, Anac., Ant. cr., Ant. t., Arg., **Arn.**, ARS., *Asaf., Asar.*, **Aur., Bap.**, *Bar. c.*, **BELL.**, Berb., Bism., BOR., *Bov., Brom.*, BRY., Calad., **Calc. c.**, *Camph.*, Cannab. s., **Canth.**, Caps., *Carb. ac., Carb. an.*, **Carb. v.**, *Caust., Ced.*, **Cham., Chel.**, *Chin., Cic., Cimic.*, **Cina, Clem., Cocc.**, *Coc. c.*, **Coff., Colch.**, Coloc., *Con.*, **Corn. c.**, *Corn. f.*, Croc., *Cup.*, Cyc., *Dig.*, **Dros.**, Dulc., *Euphorb.*, Euphr., FER., *Fer. ph., Fl. ac., Glon.*, **Graph.**, Guai., **Hell.**, *Hep.*, **Hyos.**, *Ign.*, Iod., Ip., *K. bi., K. carb., K. iod.*, K. nit., *Kre.*, Lach., Laur., Led., **Lil. t.**, Lyc., Mag. c., *Maj. m., Mang.*, Mar., Meny., MERC., **Mez.**, Mos., *Mur. ac., Nat. c.*, **Nat. m.**, **Nit. ac.**, Nux m., NUX V., Oleand., OP., *Par.*, Petrol., PHOS., PHO. AC., *Phyt., Plat.*, Pb., PULS., *Ran. b.*, Ran. s., Rheum, Rhodo., **Rhus**, RUTA, Saba., Sabi., Samb., SANG., *Sars.*, Sec. c., Sele., *Seneg.*, **Sep.**, SIL., *Sin., Spig.*, SPO., *Squ.*, **Stan.**, *Staph.*, STRAM., *Stro.*, SUL., Sul. ac., **Tar.**, Thuj., Valer., **Verat. a.**, Verb., Vio. o., Vio. t., *Zinc.*

——**Externally.**—ACON., Agar., Agn., *Alum., Ambr., Am. carb., Am. m.*, Anac., Ant. cr., Ant. t., **Apis**, Arg., **Arn.**, ARS., *Asaf. Asar.*, Aur., **Bar. c.**, BELL., Bism., BOR., *Bov.*, BRY., Calad., **Calc. c** *Calc. ph.*, Camph., *Cannab. s., Canth.*, **Caps.**, *Carb. an.*, **Carb. v.**, Caust. *Ced.*, Cham., Chel., Chin., Cic., *Cina*, Clem., Cocc., Coff., Colch., *Coloc.*, **Con.**, Croc., CUP., Cyc., *Dig.*, **Dros., Dulc.**, Euphorb., Euphr., **Fer.**, Fl. **ac.**, *Gel.*, **Glon.**, Graph., Guai., Hell., *Hep.*, Hyos., *Ign.*, Ip., **K. carb.**, *K.*

12

FEVER.

iod., K. nit., Kre., Lach., Laur., Led., **Lyc.**, Mag. c., Mag. m., M*a*ng., **Mar.**, **Meli.**, *Meny.*, MERC., MERC. I. R., *Mez.*, Mos., *Mur. ac*, *Nat. c.*, **Nat. m.**, **Nit. ac.**, Nux m., **Nux v.**, *Oleand.*, Op., *Par.*, *Petrol.*, PHOS., PHO. AC., *Plat.*, Pb., **Puls.**, Ran. b., Ran. s., Rheum, *Rhodo.*, *Rhus*, Ruta, **Saba.**, Sabi., *Samb.*, Sars., Sec. c., *Sele.*, Seneg., **Sep.**, Sil., **Spig.**, Spo., Squ., **Stan.**, **Staph.**, Stram., *Stro.*, SUL., Sul. ac., *Tar.*, **Thuj.**, Valer., *Verat. a.*, *Verb.*, Vio. o., Vio. t., Zinc.

Heat, Special Internally.—ACON., **Aloe.**, Alum., Ambr., *Am. carb.*, *Am. m.*, Ant. cr., *Ant. t.*, Arg., **Arn.**, *Ars.*, *Asaf.*, Asar., Aur., Bar. c., **BELL.**, *Bism.*, *Bor.*, *Bov.*, BRY., *Calad.*, **Calc. c.**, **Camph.**, Cannab. s., **CANTH.**, Caps., *Carb. an.*, **Carb. v.**, *Caust.*, **Cham.**, *Chel.*, Chin., **Cic.**, *Cimic.*, Cina, *Cocc.*, Coc. c., Coff., Colch., *Coloc.*, Con., Croc., *Crot. tig.*, *Cup.*, Dig., Dros., *Dulc.*, **Euphorb.**, Euphr., Fer., *Fl. ac.*, *Graph.*, Guai., Hell., Hep., Hyos., *Ign.*, *Iod.*, Ip., *K. carb.*, K. nit., Kre., Lach., LAUR., Led., **Lyc.**, Mag. c., *Mag. m.*, *Mang.*, Meny., **MERC.**, **Mez.**, Mos., Mur. ac., *Nat. c.*, **Nat. m.**, **Nit. ac.**, *Nux m.*, **Nux v.**, Oleand., Op., *Par.*, Petrol., PHOS., **Pho. ac.**, *Plat.*, *Pb.*, POD., **Puls.**, *Ran. b.*, Ran. s., Rhodo., *Rhus*, Ruta, **Saba.**, Sabi., **Sang. n.**, *Sars.*, **Sec. c.**, Seneg., **Sep.**, **Sil.**, *Spig.*, Spo., Squ., **Stan.**, Staph., Stram., Stro., SUL., Sul. ac., Tar., Thuj., *Verat. a.*, Vio. o., Vio. t., *Zinc.*

— —**One-sided.**—Alum., Ambr., Anac., Ant. t., *Arn.*, *Bar. c.*, **Bell.**, BRY., *Caust.*, *Cham.*, Chin., Cocc., Croc., Dig., Ign., K. carb., **Lyc.**, Nat. c., **Nux v.**, Par., **Phos.**, **Pho. ac.**, Plat., PULS., *Rhus*, Ruta, Saba., Sars., Spig., *Stan.*, Stram., **Sul.**, Sul. ac., Thuj., *Verb.*

—**Anxious.**—ACON., Ambr., Am. carb., *Anac.*, Arg., **Arn.**, ARS., Asaf., **Bell.**, *Bov.*, Bry., **Calc. c.**, **Carb. v.**, Caust., *Cham.*, Chin., *Coff.*, Colch., Con., *Cyc.*, Dros., Euphorb., Fer., *Graph.*, Hep., Hyos., **Ign.**, *Ip.*, Laur., *Lyc.*, Mag. c., **MERC.**, Nat. m., **Nit. ac.**, NUX V., *Op.*, Par., Petrol., PHOS., **Pho. ac.**, *Plat.*, Pb., **PULS.**, Rhodo., **Rhus**, Ruta, Sep., Sil., *Spig.*, Spo., **Stan.**, Stram., SUL., Thuj., Verat. a., Vio. t., Zinc.

—**Dry.** See **Skin, Dryness, Burning.**

—**In Flushes.**—*Ac. ac.*, Acon., *Agn.*, Alum., **Ambr.**, Am. carb., Am. m., Ant. t., **Arn.**, *Ars.*, Asaf., *Bap.*, Bar. c., **Bell.**, *Bism.*, Bor., Bov., Brom., Bry., Calc. c., Cannab. s., Canth., *Carb. an.*, **Carb. v.**, Caust., *Ced.*, Cham., *Chin.*, Cocc., Coff., Coloc., **Corn. c.**, Croc., Cup., *Dig.*, Dros., FER., GRAPH., Hep., *Ign.*, *Iod.*, *Jab.*, **K. carb.**, Kre., *Lach.*, Laur., LYC., *Mag. c.*, Mag. m., **Mar.**, Meny., *Merc.*, **Nat. c.**, Nat. m., **Nit. ac.**, **Nux v.**, Oleand., Op., **Ox. ac.**, Petrol., PHOS., Pho. ac., *Plat.*, Pb.,

FEVER.

Puls., Ran. b., *Rhus*, *Ruta*, Saba., *Sabi.*, Samb., SANG., Seneg., SEP., SIL., *Spig.*, Spo., Stan., *Staph.*, SUL., THUJ., **Valer.**, Vio. t., *Zinc.*

Heat With Thirst.—ACON., Agar., *Am. m.*, *Anac.*, *Ant. cr.*, Ant. t., *Arn.*, ARS., *Asar.*, Bar. c., **Bell.**, Bism., *Bor.*, *Bov.*, **Bry.**, *Calad.*, CALC. C., Canth., Caps., Carb. an., Carb. v., Caust., **Cham.**, *Chin.*, Cic., Cina, Cocc., Coff., **Colch.**, Coloc., Con., *Croc.*, *Cup.*, Dig., Dros., Dulc., EUP. PER., Guai., HEP., **Hyos.**, Ign., Iod., Ip., *K. carb.*, *Laur.*, *Lyc.*, **Mag. m.**, MERC., Mez., Mos., *Nat. c.*, **Nat. m.**, *Nit. ac.*, Nux m., Nux v., Op., *Petrol.*, Phos., Pho. ac., *Plat.*, Pb., **Puls.**, **Ran. s.**, Rhodo., RHUS, Ruta, Saba., SEC. C., *Sep.*, SIL., Spig., *Spo.*, *Stan.*, Staph., *Stram.*, Stro.; SUL., *Sul. ac.*, Thuj., *Valer.*, *Verat. a.*, Verb., Zinc.

—Without Thirst.—Acon., **Agn.**, Ambr., Am. m., Anac., Ant. t., APIS, *Arg.*, Arn., **Ars.**, **Asaf.**, Bell., Bor., Bry., Calad., Calc. c., **Camph.** Canth., **Caps.**, Carb. v., Cham., *Chel.*, Chin., Cina, Cocc., *Coff.*, Coloc., *Con.*, **Cyc.**, Dig., **Dros.**, Dulc., *Euphorb.*, GELS., Guai., HELL., Hep., *Ign.*, *Ip.*, K. carb., K. nit., Lach., Laur., *Led.*, Mag. c., **Mang.**, MENY., Merc., Mos., **Mur. ac.**, Nat. c., Nat. m., Nit. ac., NUX M., Nux v., Oleand., *Op.*, PHOS., **Pho. ac.**, Pb., PULS., *Rheum*, Rhodo, Rhus, *Ruta*, Saba., *Sabi.*, Samb., Sars., **Sep.**, SPIG., Spo., **Squ.**, Staph., Stram., Sul., Tar., Thuj., Valer., Verat. a., Vio. t.

—With Inclination To Uncover.—ACON., Ars., *Asar.*, Aur., *Bor.*, Bry. Calc. c., Carb. v., *Cham.*, *Chin.*, Coff., **Fer.**, *Ign.*, **Iod.**, Lach, *Led.*, Lyc., Merc., Mos, **Mur. ac.**, Nit. ac., Nux v, **Op.**, *Phos.*, *Plat.*, PULS., Rhus, *Sec. c.*, *Seneg.*, Sep., **Spig.**, **Staph.**, *Sul.*, *Thuj.*, **Verat. a.**

—With Dread of Uncovering.—Acon., *Agar.*, *Ant. cr*, *Arg.*, Arn., **Ars.**, Asar., Aur., *Bell.*, Bor., Bry., *Camph.*, **Canth.**, Caps., Carb. an., *Cham*, *Chin.*, *Cic.*, **Clem.**, *Cocc.*, Coff., **Colch.**, **Con.**, *Graph.*, Hell., **Hep.**, Ign., *Kre.*, *Lach.*, Led., **Mag. c.**, *Mag. m.*, Meny., *Merc.*, **Mur. ac.**, *Nat. c.*, *Nat. m.*, Nux m., NUX V., Phos., Pho. ac., PULS., Rheum, *Rhodo*, Rhus, *Saba.*, SAMB., Sep., **Sil.**, SQU., Staph., *Stram.*, STRO., Thuj.

—Associated Symptoms.—ACON., Agar., Agn., Alum., Am. carb., Am. m., Anac., Ant. t., Arg., *Arn.*, ARS., Asaf., Asar., BELL., *Bor.*, Bov., **Bry.**, Calad., Calc. c., *Camph.*, Canth., **Caps.**, **Carb. v.**, Cham., Chel., *Chin.*, Cic., *Cina*, Cocc., *Coff.*, Colch., Coloc., Con., Croc., Cup., Cyc., Dig., Dros., Dulc., Euphorb., Fer., Graph., Hell., Hep., *Hyos.*, Ign., Iod., Ip., *K. carb.*, Kre., *Lach.*, Laur., Led., Lyc., Mag. c., Mag. m., Mang., Mar., Meny., *Merc.*, *Mos.*, Mur. ac., *Nat. c.*, NAT. M., *Nit. ac.*, NUX V., Oleand., OP., Par., *Petrol.*, PHOS., Pho. ac., Plat., Pb., **PULS.**, Ran. b., Ran. s., Rheum, Rhodo., **Rhus**, *Ruta*, *Saba.*, **Sabi.**,

260 FEVER.

Samb., Sars., **Sep.**, *Sil.*, Spig., Spo., Squ., Staph., *Stram.*, **Sul.**, **Tar.**, Thuj., *Valer.*, **Verat. a.**, *Vio. t.*, Zinc.

Coldness in General.—Acon., *Acon. f.*, Aconin., **Agar.**, *Agn.*, *Aloe*, Alum., *Ambr.*, Am. carb., Am. m., Anac., Ant. cr., **Ant. t.**, **Apis**, ARAN., *Arg. n.*, *Arn.*, **ARS.**, Asaf., Asar., *Aur.*, *Bar. c.*, *Bell.*, Bism., Bor., Bov., Bry., *Calad.*, Calc. c., *Calc. ph.*, CAMPH., **Cannab. i.**, *Cannab. s.*, *Canth.*, **Caps.**, *Carb. an*, **Carb. v.**, **Caust.**, *Cham.*, **Chel.**, **Chin.**, Cic., Cina, *Cocc.*, Coff., Colch., Coloc., **Con.**, *Conv.*, Croc., *Crotal.*, **Cup.**, Cyc., **Dig.**, Dros., *Dulc.*, Euphorb., Euphr., *Fer.*, *Graph.*, **Hell.**, Hep., *Hyd. ac.*, *Hyos.*, Ign., Iod., **Ip.**, Jat., *K. carb.*, K. nit., Kalm., Kre., Lach., *Laur.*, Led., *Lyc.*, Mag. c., Mag. m., *Mang.*, Mar., Meny., *Merc.*, *Merc. cy.*, *Mez.*, *Mos.*, Mur. ac., *Nat. c.*, *Nat. m.*, **Nit. ac.**, Nux m., **Nux v.**, Oleand., **Op.**, *Ox.* Par., *Petrol.*, **Phos.**, *Pho. ac.*, *Plat.*, **Pb.**, Pod., PULS., RAN. B., HUS, Ruta, **Saba.**, Sabi., Samb., *Sars.*, SEC. C., Sele., Seneg., **Sep.**, **Sil.**, Spig., Spo., Stan., *Squ.*, Staph., Stram., Stro., **Sul.**, *Sul. ac.*, Tar., Thuj., *Trom.*, Valer., VERAT. A., Verb., Zinc.

—Of Special Parts.—Acon., **Agar.**, **Agn.**, **Alum.**, **Ambr.**, *Am. carb.*, Am. m., Anac., Ant. cr., **Ant. t.**, *Apis*, **Arn.**, **ARS.**, Asaf., Asar., *Aur.*, *Bar. c.*, **Bell.**, *Berb.*, Bism., Bor., *Bov.*, **BROM.**, *Bry.*, **CALAD.**, **Cact.**, **Calc. c.**, Camph., **Cannab. i.**, *Cannab. s.*, **Canth.**, **Caps.**, *Carb. ac.*, *Carb. an*, *Carb. v.*, *Carb. sul.*, CAUST., *Ced.*, **Cham.**, **Chel.**, **Chin.**, *Cic.*, **Cina**, *Co. c.*, Coc. c., *Coff.*, *Colch.*, Coloc., **Con.**, Croc., *Crotal.*, **Crot. tig.**, **Cup.**, Cyc., DIG., **Dros.**, *Dulc.*, Elaps., *Eup. pur.*, Euphr., **Fer.**, **Gel.**, Glon., **Graph.**, *Grat.*, **Hell.**, Hep., **Hyd. ac.**, *Hyos.*, Ign., IP., **Jab.**, K. bi., **K. carb.**, **K. chl.**, **K. nit.**, *Kalm.*, Kre., **Lach.**, *Laur.*, **Led.**, **Lyc.**, Mag. c., Mag. m., *Mang.*, Mar., **Meli.**, MENY., MERC., *Merc. c.*, Merc. cy., **Mez.**, Mos., Mur. ac., NAT. C., **Nat. m.**, **Nit. ac.**, *Nux m.*, **Nux v.**, Oleand., **Op.**, **Ox. ac.**, *Par.*, Petrol., PHOS., *Pho. ac.*, *Plat.*, Pb., Polyp., PULS., *Ran. b.*, **Ran. s.**, *Rhodo.*, **RHUS**, Ruta, Saba., *Sabi.*, **Samb.**, *Sang.*, *Sars.*, SEC. C., *Sele.*, Seneg., SEP., SIL., Spig., Spo., **Squ.**, *Stan.*, Staph., STRAM., Stro., SUL., *Sul. ac.*, Sum., *Tab.*, **Tar.**, **Thuj.**, VERAT. A., *Verat. v.*, Verb., Zinc.

—Externally.—Acon., *Agar.*, Ambr., *Am. m.*, Ant. t., **Arn.**, Ars., Asar., *Bar. c*, **Bell.**, Bor., Bov., *Bry.*, Calc. c., Camph., *Cannab. s.*, Canth., Caps., Carb. v., **Caust.**, **Chel.**, *Chin.*, Cic., *Cocc.*, Coff., Coloc., Con., *Croc.*, Dig., Dulc., Euphorb., **Gam.**, Graph., Hell., Hyos., *Ign.*, Ip., Kre., Lach., *Laur.*, Led., *Lyc.*, Mag. c., Mang., Meny., MERC., *Mez.*, MOS., Mur. ac., Nat. c., Nux m., Oleand., Par., Petrol., *Phos.*, Pho. ac., PLAT., Pb., **Puls.**, *Ran. b. Ran. s.*, *Rhodo.*, RHUS, *Ruta*,

FEVER.

Saba., Sabi., Samb., SEC. C., *Sep.*, Spig., *Spo.*, *Staph.*, Stro., *Sul.*, Thuj., *Valer.*, VERAT. A., Verb., Vio. t.

Coldness, Internally.—Acon., **Agn.**, Alum., **Ambr.**, Ant. cr., *Ant. t.*, Arn., **Ars.**, Asaf., Bar. c., *Bell.*, Bov., BROM., Bry., CALC. C., **Camph.**, **Caps.**, Carb. an., Carb. v., Caust.,*Chel.,Chin.*, **Colch.**,*Coloc.*, Con., Croc., *Crot. tig.*, **Dig.**, **Dros.**, *Elops.*, Graph., **Grat.**, Hell., *Ign.*, Ip., K. carb., *K. nit.*, Kre., Lach., LAUR., **Lyc.**, Mag. c., Mang., **Meny.**, Merc., *Mez.*, Mos., *Nat. c*, NAT. M., Nit. ac., **Nux v.**, *Oleand.*, *Ox. ac.*, **Par.**, **Petrol.**, PHOS., *Pho. ac.*, Plat., Pb., PULS., *Rhus*, Ruta, Saba., Sars., **Sec. c.**, **Sep.**, Spo., **Sul.**, Sul. ac., *Tab.*, Valer., *Verat. a*, Zinc.

—**One-sided.**—Alum., Ambr., Anac., Ant. t., Arn., *Bar. c.*, **Bell.**, *Bry.*, **Caust.**, Cham., *Chin.*, Cocc., **Con.**, Croc., Dig., Ign., K. carb., *Lyc.*, Nat. c., **Nux v.**, Par., *Phos.*, Pho. ac., Plat., PULS., RHUS, Ruta., *Saba.*, Sars., **Sil.**, Spig., Stan., Stram., *Sul.*, Sul. ac., *Thuj.*, Verb.

—**Shivering in General.**—*Ab. c.*, **Acon.**, **Agar.**, Alum., *Am. carb.*, Am. m., Anac., Ant. cr., *Arg*, Arn., ARS., Asaf., *Asar.*, *Aur.*, Bar. c., BELL., *Bor.*, Bov., *Brom*, Bry., Calad., **Calc. c.**, **Calc. ph.**, *Cannab. s.*, Canth., CAPS., Carb. an., Carb. v., **Caust.**, *Ced.*, Cham., *Chel.*, **Chin.**, *Cimic*, *Cina*, *Clem.*, COCC., *Coc. c*, *Coff.*, Colch., *Coloc.*, Con., Croc., **Cup.**, *Cyc.*, Dig., Dros., Dulc., Euphorb., Fer., *Graph.*, Guai., *Hell.*, *Hep.*, Hyos., *Ign.*, **Ip.**, **K. carb.**, K. nit., Kre., Lach., Laur., Led., Lyc., Mag. c., *Mag. m.*, Mang., *Meny.*, MERC., **Mez.**, *Mos.*, Mur. ac., **Nat. c.**, *Nat. m*, Nit. ac., **Nux v.**, Oleand., Op., Par., PHOS., **Pho. ac.**, **Plat.**, Pb., PULS., Ran. b., *Rheum*, Rhodo., RHUS, *Ruta*, **Saba.**, *Sabi.*, Samb, *Sars.*, Sec. c., Seneg., **Sep.**, SIL., *Spig.*, Spo., Squ., Stan., **Staph.**, STRAM., Stro., Sul., Sul. ac., Tar., **Thuj.**, Valer., VERAT. A., Verb., Vio. o., *Zinc.*

—**Of Special Parts.**—Acon., Am. carb., Arg., *Arn.*, **Ars.**, Asaf., Aur., Bar. c., BELL., Bor., Bov., **Bry.**, *Camph.*, *Cannab. s.*, Canth., Caps., *Carb. ac.*, Carb. v., **Caust.**, **Cham.**, *Chel.*, **Chin.**, *Cina*, *Clem.*, **Cocc.**, *Coff.*, Coloc., Croc., Dig., Euphorb., Graph., Guai., Hell., Hep., *Ign.*, *K. carb*, K. nit., Lach., Laur., Led., Mag. m., Mang., *Meny.*, Merc., Mez., Mos., Nat. c., Nat. m., *Nux v.*, **Par.**, Phos., Pho. ac., *Plat.*, PULS., *Ran. b.*, *Rhodo.*, Rhus, *Ruta*, *Saba.*, *Sabi.*, Samb., *Sang.*, Seneg., Sep., Sil., Spig., Spo., STAPH., Stram., Stro., *Sul.*, Thuj., Valer., *Verat. a.*, Zinc.

—**Of One Side.**—Alum., Ambr., Anac., Ant. t., Arn., *Bar. c.*, **Bell.**, *Bry.*, **Caust**, *Cham.*, *Chin.*, **Cocc.**, Croc., Dig, *Ign*, K. carb, Lyc., Nat. c., Nux v., Par., Phos., Pho. ac., *Plat.*, PULS., RHUS, Ruta, *Saba.*, Sars., *Spig.*, Stan., Stram., *Sul.*, Sul. ac., Thuj., Verb.

Sweat in General.—ACON., *Aconin.*, *Agar.*, Agn., Alum., **Ambr.**, Am. carb., *Am. m.*, Anac., Ant. cr., **Ant. t.**, Arg., Arn., **Ars.**, Asaf.,

FEVER.

Asar., Asc. c., Aur., *Bar. c.*, BELL., *Benz. ac.*, Bor., Bov., **Bry.**, *Cact.*, Calad., **Calc. ac.**, CALC. C., *Calc. iod.*, *Calc. ph.*, Camph., *Cannab. i.*, Cannab. s., **Canth.**, *Caps.*, **Carb. ac.**, *Carb. an.*, **Carb. v.**, *Caust.*, CHAM., **Chel.**, CHIN., Cic., Cina, *Cinnab.*, *Clem.*, Cocc., Coc. c., *Coff.*, *Colch.*, *Coloc.*, Con., **Conv.**, Corn. c., Croc., **Crot. tig.**, Cup., Cyc., **Dig.**, *Dros.*, Dulc., Euphorb., Euphr., Fer., *Fer. ph.*, **Graph.**, Guai., **Hell.**, HEP., *Hyos.*, Ign., Iod., Ip., *Jab.*, *K. bi.*, *K. carb.*, *K. nit.*, Kre., Lach., Laur., **Led.**, Lyc., Mag. c., *Mag. m.*, Mang., Meny., MERC., Mez., Mos., Mur. ac., *Nat. c.*, **Nat. m.**, NIT. AC., NUX V., OP., Par., *Petrol.*, **Phos.**, **Pho. ac.**, Plat., Pb., PSO., **Puls.**, Ran. b., **Ran. s.**, Rheum, *Rhodo.*, RHUS, Ruta, **Saba.**, *Sabi.*, **Samb.**, Sars., Sec. c., SELE., Seneg., SEP., SIL., *Spig.*, **Spo.**, Squ., **Stan.**, *Staph.*, *Stram.*, *Stro.*, SUL., *Sul. ac.*, Tar., Thuj., *Valer.*, VERAT. A., **Verat. v.**, Vio. o., Vio. t., Zinc.

Sweat, Special Parts.—Acon., Agar., *Agn.*, *Ambr.*, Am. carb., Am. m., Anac., *Ant. t.*, **Arg.**, Arn., **Ars.**, Asaf., Asar., Aur., **Bar. c.**, **Bell.**, *Benz. ac.*, **Bor.**, Bov., **Bry.**, Calad., CALC. C., Camph., **Cannab. i.**, *Cannab. s.*, **Canth.**, Caps., *Carb. ac.*, Carb. an., Carb. v., **Cham.**, Chel., **Chin.**, Cic., *Cimic.*, *Cina*, Clem., **Cocc.**, Coc. c., **Coff.**, *Coloc.*, Con., Croc., **Crot. tig.**, Cup., Cyc., Dig., *Dros.*, *Dulc.*, Euphorb., Euphr., Fer., **Graph.**, Guai., Hell., *Hep.*, Hyos., Ign., Iod., **Ip.**, *K. carb.*, K. nit., Kre., **Lach.**, *Laur.*, **Led.**, **Lyc.**, Mag. m., Mang., **Merc.**, MERC. C., Mez., Mos., Nat. c., *Nat. m.*, Nit. ac., Nux v., Op., Par., **Petrol.**, **Phos.**, *Pho. ac.*, Plat., **Pb.**, Pso., **PULS.**, **Ran. s.**, Rheum, *Rhodo.*, Rhus, Ruta, Saba., *Sabi.*, Samb., *Sang.*, **Sars.**, Sec. c., SELE., SEP., SIL., *Spig.*, Spo., *Squ.*, *Stan.*, Staph., Stran., Stro., SUL., Sul. ac., Tar., **Thuj.**, *Valer.*, *Verat. a.*, Vio. t., Zinc.

—On One Side.—Alum., Ambr., Anac., *Ant. t.*, Arn., BAR. C., Bell., **Bry.**, *Caust.*, **Cham.**, *Chin.*, Cocc., Croc., Dig., Ign., K. carb., **Lyc.**, Nat. c., NUX V., Par., *Phos.*, Pho. ac., Plat., **PULS.**, **Rhus**, Ruta, *Saba.*, Sars., *Spig.*, Stan., **Sul.**, Sul. ac., Thuj., Verb.

—Anterior Parts.—*Agar.*, Anac., **Arg.**, Arn., Asar., *Bell.*, Bov., CALC. C., Canth., Cocc., *Dios.*, Dros., *Euphr.*, Graph., Hydras., *K. nit.*, **Merc.**, Pb., *Rhus*, Saba., Sec. c., SELE., *Sep.*

—Posterior Parts.—Acon., CHIN., *Coc. c.*, Coff., *Dulc.*, Ip., Led., **Nux v.**, Par., *Petrol.*, **Puls.**, Sabi., **Sep.**, *Sil.*, Stan., Stram., SUL., *Thuj.*

—On Upper Parts.—*Agn.*, Anac., **Ant. t.**, **Arg.**, ARS., **Asar.**, *Benz. ac.*, **Bov.**, *Bry.*, Camph., *Cannab. i.*, **Caps.**, **Carb. ac.**, Carb. v., *Carb. sul.*, CHAM., **Chin.**, Cic., Cina, *Cocc.*, **Crotal.**, Dig., Dros., Dulc., Guai., **Hell.**, *Ign.*, K. carb., Laur., **Lob. i.**, MERC. C., **Mez.**, Mos., *Nit. ac.*, Nux v., OP., Par., **Phyt.**, Plat., **Puls.**, **Ran. s.**, RHEUM, *Ruta*, **Samb.**,

FEVER.

Sang., **Sars.**, Sec. c., *Sele.*, **Sep.**, **SIL.,** *Spig.*, Spo., *Squ.*, *Stan.*, *Stram.*, Stro., **SUL.**, **Sul. ac.**, **TAB.**, **Valer.**, Verat. a., Vio. t.

Sweat, Lower Parts.—*Am. carb.*, *Am. m.*, **Ars.**, **Bar. c.**, Bor., *Bry.*, Chel., *Cimic.*, *Coff.*, *Cyc.*, Euphorb., Fer., *Iod.*, **Lach.**, **NIT. AC.**, *Nux v.*, Petrol., *Puls.*, *Sabi.*, **SIL.**, *Squ.*, *Sul.*, Tar., **Thuj.**, Zinc.

—**With Thirst.**—*Acon.*, Am. m., Anac., Ant. cr., *Arn.*, *Ars.*, Bar. c., Bell., Bism., Bor., Bov., *Bry.*, *Calc. c.*, Canth., Caps., Carb. v., Caust., **CHAM.**, **CHIN.**, Cic., *Cina*, Coff., *Colch.*, Con., Croc., *Cup.*, *Dros.*, Dulc., Hep., *Hyos.*, Ign., *Iod.*, K. carb., Kre., Lach., Laur., *Mag. m.*, **Merc.**, Mez., *Nat. c.*, **Nat. m.**, Nit. ac., Nux v., Pho. ac., Pb., Puls., *Ran. s.*, *Rhus*, *Ruta*, Saba., **Sec. c.**, Sep., *Sil.*, Spo., *Stan.*, Staph., *Stram.*, Stro., *Sul.*, Sul. ac., *Tar.*, Thuj., Valer., **VERAT. A.**, Verb.

—**Without Thirst.**—*Agn.*, Ambr., *Am. m.*, Ant. cr., **Ant. t.**, *Ars.*, *Asaf.*, **Bell.**, Bry., Calad., *Camph.*, Canth., *Caps.*, Carb. v., *Caust.*, Chel., Chin., Cocc., Coff., Con., *Cyc.*, Dig., **Euphorb.**, **HELL.**, Hep., *Ign.*, *Ip.*, K. nit., Led., *Mang.*, Meny., Merc., Mos., Mur. ac., Nit. ac., **Nux m.**, Nux v., Op., **Phos.**, Pho. ac., **Puls.**, Rhodo., Rhus, **Saba.**, *Sabi.*, **SAMB.**, Sars., *Sep.*, **SPIG.**, Squ., *Staph.*, Stram., Sul., Tar., Thuj., Verat. a.

—**With Inclination To Uncover.**—**ACON.**, Ars., *Asar.*, Aur., Bor., Bry., **Calc. c.**, Carb. v., *Cham.*, *Chin.*, Coff., **Fer.**, *Ign.*, Iod., Lach., *L d.*, Lyc., Merc., Mos., **Mur. ac.**, Nit. ac., Nux v., **Op.**, *Phos.*, *Plat.*, *Puls.*, Rhus, Sec. c., *Seneg.*, Sep., Spig., Staph., *Sul.*, *Thuj.*, Verat. a.

—**With Dread of Uncovering.**—Acon., *Agar.*, Ant. cr., *Arg.*, Arn., Ars., Asar., Aur., *Bell.*, Bor., Bry., *Camph.*, Canth., Caps., *Carb. an.*, Cham., Chin., Cic., **Clem.**, *Cocc.*, Coff., **Colch.**, **Con.**, *Graph.*, Hell., Hep., Ign., *Kre.*, *Lach.*, Led., **Mag. c.**, *Mag. m.*, Meny., *Merc.*, Mur. ac., Nat. c., *Nat. m.*, Nux m., **NUX V.**, Phos., Pho. ac., *Puls.*, Rheum, Rhodo., Rhus, *Saba.*, **SAMB.**, Sep., Sil., Staph., **SQU.**, *Stram.*, **STRO.**, Thuj.

—**Anxious.**—Acon., Anac., Ant. cr., *Arn.*, **Ars.**, Bar. c., Bell., *Bry.*, **CALC. C.**, Carb. v., Caust., **Cham.**, Cocc., Croc., *Fer.*, *Graph.*, *Ign.*, K. nit., Kre., Lyc., *Mang.*, Merc., Mez., Mur. ac., *Nat. c.*, Nux v., **PHOS.**, *Pho. ac.*, **Pb.**, **PULS.**, *Rhus*, Saba., **SEP.**, Sil., *Spo.*, Stan., Staph., *Stram.*, SUL., Thuj., Verat. a.

—**Bloody.** (See **Skin, Blood-Sweating.**)—Acon., *Aconin.*, Am. carb., Anac., **Ant. t.**, *Apis*, Arn., **ARS.**, *Brom.*, Bry., Calc. c., **CANNAB.** I., *Carb. ac.* *Carb. sul.*, **Cham.**, Chin., *Colch.*, *Corn. f.*, *Crotal.*, Dig., *Dios.*, Fer., **Hell.**, Hep., **Iod.**, **LYC.**, **Merc.**, Mos., Nux v., **PHOS.**, **Pho. ac.**, Pb., Sec. c., Spig., *Stan.*, **TAB.**, *Verat. a.*

Sweat, Cold.—*Ac. ac.*, **Acon.**, Ambr., Am. carb., **ANT. T.**, *Arn.*, ARS., Asaf., *Bell.*, *Benz. ac.*, **Brom.**, Bry., **Cact.**, Calc. c., *Camph.*, **Cannab. s.**, Canth., *Caps.*, *Carb. ac.*, *Carb. v.*, Cham., *Chin.*, Cimic., CINA, Cinnab., Cocc., *Coff.*, Colch., Croc., *Crotal.*, Cup., Dig., Dios., Dros., Dulc., Euphorb., Fer., Graph., **Hell.**, HEP., *Hyos.*, Ign., IP., Lach., **Lob. i.**, **Lyc.**, Mag. m., Mang., *Merc.*, **Merc. cy.**, Mez., *Nat. c*, Nit. ac., *Nux v.*, OP., Petrol., Phos., Pho. ac., **Phyt.**, **Pb.**, **PULS.**, **Rheum**, *Rhus*, Ruta, Saba., Sec. c., *Sep.*, Sil., Spig., Squ., **Stan.**, **Staph.**, Stram., **Sul.**, Sul. ac., TAB., **Ter.**, Thuj., VERAT. A., **Verat. v.**

—**Easy.**—*Agar.*, *Ambr.*, Anac., **Ant. t.**, Ars., Asar., *Bell.*, Brom., BRY., **Calc. c.**, *Canth.*, **Carb. an.**, Carb. v., Caust., *Chin.*, Cocc., Coloc., Con., *Dios.*, Dulc., **Fer.**, **Graph.**, Guai., *Hep.*, Ign., *Iod.*, Ip., K. carb., Kre., *Lach*, **Led.**, **Lyc.**, Mag, c., **Mag. m.**, *Merc.*, NAT. C., **Nat. m.**, Nit. ac., *Nux v.*, Op., Petrol., Phos., Pho. ac., *Pso.*, Puls., *Rheum*, Rhodo., *Rhus*. Saba., Sars., **Sele.**, Seneg., SEP., *Sil.*, *Spig.*, Spo., *Stan*, Staph., *Stram.*, SUL., **Sul. ac.**, Valer., *Verat. a.*, Zinc.

—**Exhausting.**—Acon., Ambr., *Anac.*, Ant. cr., Arn., **Ars.**, **Ars.**, **iod.**, Bor., **Bry.**, **Calc. c.**, Canth., *Carb. an.*, **Caust.**, **Chin.**, Cocc., Croc., **Dig.**, **Fer.**, Graph., Hyos., **Iod.**, Ip., K. nit., Kre., **Lyc.**, *Merc.*, **Nat. m.**, Nit. ac., *Nux v.*, PHOS., PSO., Puls., Rheum, Rhodo., Saba., **Samb.**, Sep., Sil., **Stan.**, **Sul.**, Tar., *Verat. a.*

—**Greasy.**—*Agar.*, Aur., Bry., Calc. c., **Chin.**, **Mag. c.**, MERC., *Nat. m.*, Pb., *Sele.*, *Stram.*

—**Hot.**—Am. m., Ant. cr., *Bell.*, Bry., Camph., Canth., *Caps.*, **Cham.**, Chin., Cina, Con., Dros., *Hell.*, Hep., *Ign.*, Ip., Led., *Merc.*, Nat. c., *Nux v.*, OP., Par., **Phos.**, *Pho. ac.*, Pb., Puls., *Rhus*, Saba., **Sep.**, Spig., Spo., Stan., *Staph.*, Stram., Sul., Tar., Valer., *Verat. a.*, Vio. t.

—**Odorous.**—Acon., Ambr., *Arn.*, Ars., *Asar.*, *Bar. c.*, **Bell.**, Bov., *Bry.*, Camph., **Canth.**, Carb. an., Carb. v., Caust., *Cham.*, Coloc., Con., Cyc., *Dulc.*, Euphr., Fer., *Graph.*, Guai., **Hep.**, Hyos., Ign., *Iod.*, Ip., K. carb., Led., LYC., **Mag. c.**, Merc., Mos., Nat. m., NIT. AC., **Nux v.**, Phos., Pb., Puls., *Rheum*, *Rhodo.*, RHUS, SEP., **Sil.**, Spig., Stan., Staph., *Stram.*, Sul., Thuj., **Verat. a.**, Zinc.

— —**Acrid.**—Rhus.

— —**Bitter.**—Verat. a.

— —**Bloody.**—Lyc.

— —**Burnt.**—Bell.

— —**Of Camphor.**—Camph.

— —**Of Cheese.**—*Pb.*

— —**Elderberries.**—Sep.

FEVER. 265

Sweat, Odorous, Of Honey.—Thuj.

— —**Of Mush.**—Mos., Puls., *Sul.*

— —**Musty.**—Nux v., *Puls.*, Rhus, Stan.

— —**Offensive.**—Ars., BAR. C., *Canth.*, *Carb. ac.*, Carb. an., Con., Cyc., **Dios.**, DULC., *Euphr.*, Fer., **Graph.**, *Guai.*, HEP., *Hydras.*, **K. carb.**, Led., Lyc., *Mag. c.*, MERC., **Merc. c.**, **Nit. ac.**, *Nux v.*, *Petrol.*, Phos., **Puls.**, *Rhodo.*, *Rhus*, **Sep.**, SIL., Spig., **Staph.**, Stram., SUL., Thuj., Verat. a., Zinc.

— —**Of Onions.**—*Bov.*, **Lyc.**

— —**Of Rhubarb.**—Rheum.

— —**Sour.**—Acon., *Arn.*, **Asar.**, *Bell.*, BRY., *Carb. v.*, Caust., Cham., Clem., Graph., Hep., Hyos., Ign., Iod., Ip., K. carb., *Led.*, **Lyc.**, **Mag. c.**, Merc., Nat. m., **Nit. ac.**; Nux v., Rheum, *Rhus*, SEP., Sil., Sul., Verat. a.

— —**Spicy.**—*Rhodo.*

— —**Sulphurous.**—Phos.

— —**Sulphuretted Hydrogen.**—*Sul.*

— —**Sweetish-sour.**—*Bry.*

— —**Urinous.**—Canth., Coloc., **Nit. ac.**

—**Staining.**—*Arn.*, **Ars.**, Bell., *Calc. c.*, Carb. an., Cham., Chin., Clem., Dulc., **Graph.**, *Lach.*, *Lyc.*, Mag. c., **Merc.**, Nux m., **Nux v.**, Rheum, **Sele.**

— —**In Spots.**—*Merc.*, Sele.

— —**Red.**—Arn., *Calc. c.*, Cham., Chin., Clem., *Crotal.*, **Dulc.**, Lach., *Lyc.*, Nux m., Nux v.

— —**Yellow.**—*Ars.*, Bell., Carb. **an.**, GRAPH., *Lach.*, Mag. c., MERC., Rheum.

—**Lack Of.** See **Skin, Dryness.**

Sweat with Associated Symptoms.—Acon., Ambr., Anac., *Ant. cr.*, **Ant. t.**, *Arn.*, ARS., Bar. c., *Bell.*, BRY., *Calc. c.*, Camph., Cannab. s., Carb. v., CAUST., CHAM., Chel., Chin., *Cina, Cocc., Coff., Coloc.*, Con., Croc., *Dig.*, Dros., Dulc., *Fer.*, Graph., *Hyos.*, Ign., Ip., K. nit., Kre., Led., Lyc., **Mang.**, MERC., Mez., Mos., Mur. ac., **Nat. c.**, Nat. m., **Nit. ac.**, NUX V., OP., *Par.*, **Phos.**, *Pho. ac.*, Pb., **Puls.**, *Ran. b.*, *Rhodo.*, RHUS, **Saba.**, Sabi., *Samb., Sele.*, SEP., Spo., Stan., Staph., STRAM., *Stro.*, SUL., Tar., *Thuj.*, Valer., VERAT. A.

Compound Fever in General.—Acon., Agn., Alum., Ambr., *Am. carb., Am. m.*, Anac., Ant. cr., *Ant. t.*, Arn., ARS., *Asar.*, Aur., Bar. c., BELL., *Bor.*, Bov., BRY., Calad., **Calc. c.**, Camph., Canth., **Caps.**, *Carb. an., Carb. v., Caust.*, **Cham.**, Chel., **Chin.**, *Cina*, Clem., *Cocc., Coff.*, Coloc., Con.,

Croc., Cyc., *Dig.*, *Dros.*, Dulc., Euphorb., **Graph.**, Guai., **Hell.**, **Hep.**, Hyos., **Ign.**, Iod., *Ip.*, K. carb., K. nit., Kre., *Lach.*, Laur., *Led.*, Lyc., Meny., **Merc.**, Mez., *Mos.*, Nat. c., *Nat. m.*, *Nit. ac.*, Nux m., NUX V., Oleand., *Op*, Petrol., **Phos.**, *Pho. ac.*, Plat., Pb., **Puls.**, Ran. s., Rheum, Rhodo., RHUS, **Saba.**, Sabi., Samb., Sec. c., Sele., *Sep.*, *Spig.*, Spo., Squ., Stan., **Staph.**, *Stram.*, Stro., SUL., Tar., *Thuj.*, Valer., **Verat. a.**, Zinc.

Chill then Heat.—ACON., Alum., Ambr., Am. carb., Am. m., Ant. cr., Ant. t., *Arn.*, Ars., Asar., Bar. c., **Bell.**, *Bor.*, Bry., Canth., Caps., Carb. an., Carb. v., Caust., Cham., *Chin.*, *Cina*, Coff., **Corn. c.**, Croc., *Cyc.*, Dros., Dulc., Graph., Guai., Hell., **Hep.**, *Hyos.*, Ign., Ip., K. carb., *K. nit.*, Kre., Lyc., Meny., Merc., NAT. M., Nit. ac., Nux. m., **Nux v.**, Op., Petrol., *Phos.*, *Pho. ac.*, PULS., **Rhus**, Saba., SANG., **Sec. c.** Sep., **Spig.**, Squ., Staph., Stram., **Sul.**, Valer., VERAT. A.

—**Then Sweat.**—*Am. m.*, Bry., Caps., *Carb. an.*, CAUST., Cham., Chel., Dig., Hell., Hep., *Lyc.*, Nat. m., Nux v., Op., *Petrol.*, Phos., Pho. ac., Rhus, Saba., Sep., Spig., *Thuj.*, **Verat. a.**

—**Then Heat, then Chill.**—Sul.

—**Then Heat, then Sweat.**—Am. m., **Ars.**, **Bry.**, *Caps.*, Caust., Cham., *Chin.*, *Cina*, Cocc., Dig., Dros., **Graph.**, *Hep.*, **Ign.**, Ip., K. carb., *Lyc.*, Nat. m., *Nit. ac.*, Nux v., Op., Pb., **Puls.**, **Rhus**, Saba., *Sabi.*, Samb., Sep., Spo., *Staph.*, **Sul.**, Verat. a.

—**Then Heat with Sweat.**—Acon., Ant. t., **Bell.**, Bry., *Caps.*, CHAM., *Chin.*, Cina, Con., Dig., Graph., *Hell.*, Hep., Ign., Ip., K. carb., Merc., Nit. ac., *Nux v.*, OP., **Phos.**, Puls., **Rhus**, Saba., Spig., Stan., Staph., Stram., Sul., Valer., Verat. a.

—**And Heat at the Same Time.**—ACON., Alum., **Anac.**, Ant. t., *Apis*, ARS., Bar. c., **Bell.**, *Bov.*, **Bry.**, CALC., Camph., Canth., Carb. v., *Ced.*, Cham., **Chel.**, *Chin.*, *Cina*, *Cocc.*, *Coff.*, Coloc., **Dros.**, *Euphorb.*, **Fer.**, Graph., Hell., IGN., *Iod.*, *K. carb.*, *Lach.*, **Led.**, Lyc., **Merc.**, *Mez.*, Mos., Nat. c., **Nit. ac.**, Nux v., Oleand., *Petrol.*, Phos., Plat., Pb., **Puls.**, Rhus, Saba., Samb., **Sang.**, Sep., Spig., Spo., *Squ.*, **Stram.**, SUL., Thuj., Verat. a., *Zinc.*

—**With Sweat.**—*Ars.*, Calc. c., *Euphorb.*, Led., Lyc., Nux v., *Puls.*, Saba., Sang., Sul., Thuj.

—**With Heat and Sweat.**—*Jab.*, **Mez.**, Nux v.

—**Externally with Heat Internally.**—*Acon.*, Agar., Am. m., **Anac.**, **Arn.**, *Ars.*, Asar., Bar. c., *Bell.*, *Bry.*, Calad., *Calc. c.*, Camph., Cannab. s., *Canth.*, Carb. v., *Caust.*, Cham., **Chel.**, *Chin.*, Cic., Cocc., Con., Croc., Cup., Dig., Dulc., Euphorb., Graph., *Hell.*, Ign., **Ip.**, K. carb., **Laur.**,

FEVER.

Lyc., Mag. c., Mag. m., Mang., *Merc., Mez.*, MOS., **Mur. ac.**, Nat. c., Nit. ac., *Nux v., Phos.,* **Pho. ac.,** *Plat.,* **Puls.,** Ran. b,. Ran. s., Rhodo., **Rhus,** Ruta, *Saba.,* Samb., Sars., **Sec. c.,** *Sep.,* **Sil.,** Spig., *Spo.,* Squ., *Stan.,* Staph., Sul., Valer., **Verat. a.,** *Zinc.*

Chill Internally and Heat Externally.—Acon., Agar., *Agn.,* Alum., Ambr., **Anac.,** Arg., **Arn., Ars.,** Asaf., Bar. c., **Bell.,** Bism., *Bry.,* Calad., **CALC. C.,** Camph., Cannab. s., **Caps.,** Carb. an., *Carb. v.,* Caust., *Cham.,* Chel., Chin., Cic., *Cocc.,* **Coff.,** Colch., Coloc., Cup., Cyc., *Dig.,* Dros., Dulc., *Euphorb.,* Hell., Hep., Hyos., **Ign.,** Iod., *Ip.,* K. carb., **K. nit.,** Kre., **Lach.,** LAUR., **Lyc.,** Mang., **Meny.,** *Merc., Mez.,* Mur. ac., *Nat. c., Nat. m.,* **NUX. V.,** Oleand., *Op.,* **Par., Phos.,** Pho. ac., *Pb., Puls.,* Ran. b., *Rhus,* Saba., Samb., Sec. c., **Sele., SEP., Sil.,** *Spig.,* Spo., **Squ.,** Stan., Staph., Stram. Sul., Tar., Thuj., Verat. a., Zinc.

—**Alternating with Heat.**—Acon., *Agn., Am. carb., Am. m., Amyl,* Ant. t., **Ars.,** Asar., Aur., *Bor. c.,* **Bell.,** Bor., **BRY., Calc. c.,** Canth., *Caust., Cham.,* Chel., **Chin.,** *Cocc.,* **Coff.,** *Coloc.,* Dros., Graph., Hep., Iod., *K. carb.,* K. nit., **Kalm.,** *Kre.* Lach., Laur., *Lyc.,* **MERC.,** *Mos.,* Nat. m., Nit. ac., **Nux v., Phos., Pho. ac.,** Rheum, *Rhodo.,* **Rhus,** Saba., *Sele., Sep.,* Sil., Spig., *Stram.,* **Sul.,** Verat. a.

—**Alternating with Sweat.**—Phos.

Heat then Chill.—*Bell.,* **Bry.,** Calad., **CALC. C.,** *Caps.,* Caust., Chin., *Coff.,* Dulc., Ign., *Lyc.,* Meny., Merc., Nit. ac., **Nux v.,** Petrol., Phos., Puls., **SEP.,** Stan, *Staph.,* **Sul.,** Thuj.

—**Then Chill, then Heat.**—Stram.

—**Then Chill, then Heat, then Sweat.**—*Rhus.*

—**Then Shivering.**—*Caps.,* Cocc., Hell., Nat. m., **Puls., Rhus,** Sul.

—**Then Sweat.**—*Am. m.,* Ant. cr., *Ant. t.,* **Ars.,** Bell., Bor., Calc. c., *Carb. an.,* **Carb. v.,** Cham., *Chin.,* **Coff.,** Hell., **Ign.** Kre., *Nux v.,* Op., Petrol., Puls., **Ran. s.,** Rhodo., *Samb.,* **Sil.,** Stro.

—**Then Sweat, then Chill.**—Calad.

—**With Shivering.**—Acon., Anac., Arn., *Ars., Asar.,* **BELL.,** Bry., *Calc. c.,* Caps., Cham., *Coff.,* Dros., **HELL.,** *Ign.,* K. carb., *Merc.,* **Mos.,** Nux v., **Puls.,** Rhus, Sep., Spig., Sul., Zinc.

—**With Sweat.**—Acon., Alum., Am. m., Ant. t., *Bell., Bry.,* **Caps.,** Cham., *Chin., Cina,* Con., Dig., Graph., *Hell.,* Hep., *Ign., Ip.,* K carb., Merc., Nit. ac., **Nux v., OP., PHOS.,** Pb, *Puls.,* Rhus, *Saba., Spig.,* Spo., Stan., *Staph.,* Stram., Sul., Tar., *Valer.,* Verat. a., Zinc.

—**With Sweat, then Chilliness.**—Stan.

—**Alternating With Shivering.**—*Acon.,* Am. carb., **ARS.,** Asar., **Bell.,** Bor., **BRY.,** Calc. c., Caust., **Cham.,** Chel., *Chin.,* **Cocc., Coff.,**

268 FEVER—AGGRAVATIONS.

Coloc., Graph., *Hep.*, K. carb., Lach., MERC., *Mos.*, Nux v., Phos., Pho. ac., Rheum, *Rhus*, Saba., **Sang.**, Sep., *Sil.*, Spig., *Sul*, Verat. a.

Heat Alternating With Sweat.—*Bell.*, Led.

Shivering then Chill.—Ars., Bry., Ip., Lach.

—**Then Heat.**—Bell., *Bry.*, Canth., Carb. v., *Cocc.*, Con., Cyc., Graph., Ign., *Lach.*, Laur., Led., Mos., *Nux v.*, **Puls.**, Sep., Sil., *Staph.* Sul.

—**Then Sweat.**—*Bry.*, Caps., *Caust.*, Clem., Dig., *Graph.*, Nat. m., Rhus.

—**With Sweat.**—Acon., Rhus.

Sweat then Chill.—Carb. v., Hep.

—**Then Chill, then Sweat.**—Nux v.

—**Then Heat.**—Nux v., Samb.

Before Fever.—Acon., Ant. cr., Ant. t., **Arn.**, ARS., Bar. c., *Bell.*, Bry., **Calc. c.**, Caps., **Carb. v.**, Caust., CHIN., **Cina**, Cocc., Fer., Graph., *Hep.*, Hyos., *Ign.*, **Ip.**, K. carb., K. nit., Lach., Lyc., **Mag. c.**, Merc., Nat. c., *Nat. m.*, Nit. ac., *Nux v.*, *Phos.*, Pho. ac., PULS., Rhodo., **Rhus**, Ruta, *Saba.*, Sabi., Samb., *Sep.*, *Sil.*, Spig., **Sul.**, Verat. a.

During Fever.—*Acon.*, Agar., Alum., Ambr., *Am. carb.*, Am. m., Anac., **Ant. cr.**, Ant. t., *Arn.*, ARS., Aur., Bar. c., *Bell.*, Bor., Bov., **Bry.**, Calad., **Calc. c.**, Canth., Caps., Carb. v., Caust., **Cham.**, CHIN., *Cina*, Cocc., *Coff.*, Con., Croc., Dig., *Dros.*, Dulc., Euphorb., **Fer.**, Graph., Hell., *Hep.*, Hyos., *Ign.*, Iod., **Ip.**, **K. carb.**, K. nit., Kre., Lach., Laur., Led., Lyc., Mang., Mar., Meny., Merc., Mez., Mos., Mur. ac., Nat. c., **Nat. m.**, Nit. ac., Nux m., NUX V., **Op.**, Petrol., **Phos.**, *Pho. ac.*, Plat., **Puls.**, Ran. b., Rheum, *Rhodo.*, Rhus, Ruta, *Saba.*, Samb., Sars., Sec. c., SEP., Sil., Spig., Staph., *Stram.*, *Stro.*, Sul., Sul. ac., Tar., Thuj., Valer., *Verat. a.*, Zinc.

After Fever.—Ant. cr., *Ant. t.*, Arn., ARS., Bell., Bry., *Carb. v.*, CHIN., *Cina*, Dig., Hep., *K. carb.*, *Nat. m.*, **Nux v.**, Phos., *Puls.*, Sep., Sil., Verat. a.

Febrile Symptoms—Left Side.—Agar., *Agn.*, Ambr., *Ant. cr.*, Arn., Bar. c., Caust., Cham., Chin., Dig., *Lyc.*, *Par.*, **Plat.**, Puls., RHUS, Ruta, *Spig.*, STAN., *Sul.*, Thuj., Verb.

—**Right Side.**—Ambr., Bell., Bry., *Caust.*, Chin., Cocc., *Fl. ac.*, Nat. c., Nux v., PHOS., PULS., Ran. b., *Sabi.*, Spig., Verb.

Aggravations.

During the Day.—*Am. m.*, *Cimic.*, **Fer.**, *Nat. a.*, *Nat. c.*, **Nat. m.**, Nit. ac., Puls., Rhus, Sang., SEP., SUL.

AGGRAVATIONS.

Morning.—Ab. n., *Abrot., Abs.* Acon., Agar., Agn., **Aloe**, Alum., Ambr., *Am. carb.*, AM. M., Anac., Ant. cr., Ant. t., ARG., **Arg**, n., Arn., **Ars.**, ARS. IOD., Asaf., Asar., AUR., Bap., *Bar. c., Bell.*, Benz. ac., Bism., **Bor., Bov.**, BRY., *Calad.*, CALC. C., **Calc. ph.**, Cannab. s., Canth., **Caps.,** *Carb. an.*, CARB. V., *Caust.,* Cham., CHEL., *Chin.*, **Chrom. ac.,** *Cic., Cimic.,* CINA, *Clem.,* **Coca,** *Cocc., Coc. c., Cod.,* **Coff.,** *Colch.,* Coloc., **Con.,** Corn. c., CROC., *Crot. tig.,* Cup., Cyc., **Dig., Dios.,** Dros., **Dulc., Eup. per.,** *Euphorb.,* Euphr., Fer., *Fer. ph.,* Form., Gam., Gel., *Gran., Graph., Grat.,* Guai., *Hell.,* **Hep.,** Hydras., *Hyos.,* **Ign.,** *Iod., Ip.,* K. BI., **K. carb., K. iod., K. NIT.,** Kalm., **Kre.,** LACH., Laur., **Led.,** *Lyc.,* **Mag. c.,** *Mag. m*, Mang., *Mar.,* Meny., **Merc., Merc. c., Merc. i. f.,** *Menth., Mez.,* Mos., Mur. ac., *Nat. ars.,* **Nat. c., NAT. M., Nat. s., NIT. AC., Nux m., NUX V.,** *Oleand.,* ONOS., *Op., Par., Parei.,* PETROL., PHOS., PHO. AC., **Phyt.,** *Plant.,* Plat., *Pb.,* **POD., Pso.,** PULS., **Ran. b.,** Ran. s., Rheum, RHODO., RHUS, RUMEX, Ruta, Saba., **Sabi., Sal. ac.,** Samb., **Sang.,** *Sars.,* Sec. c., **Sele., Senec., Seneg., SEP., Sil.,** SPIG., Spo., **SQU., Stan., Staph.,** Stram., Stro., **SUL.,** *Sul. ac.,* **Tab., Tar.,** *Thuj.,* VALER., **Verat. a., Verat. v., Verb.,** *Vio. o.,* **Vio. t.,** Zinc.

Forenoon.—*Aloe, Alum.,* Ambr., Am. carb., *Am. m., Ant. cr*, Ant. t., *Aran.,* **Arg.,** Ars., Asaf., Aur., Bar. c., Bell., Bor., Bov., **Bry.,** *Cact., Calc. c.,* **CANNAB. S.,** *Canth.,* Carb. an., **Carb. v.,** Caust., *Ced.,* Cham., Chel., Chin., Cocc., *Coloc.,* Con., Cup., Cyc., Dros., **Dulc.,** Euphorb. Euphr., Fer., Graph., **Guai.,** Hell., **Hep.,** *Ign.,* Ip., K. carb., K. nit., Kre., Lach., **Laur.,** Lyc., Mag. c., Mag. m., **Mang.,** Mar., Merc., Mez., Mos., Mur. ac., *Nat. ars.,* NAT. C., NAT. M., Nit. ac., Nux m., *Nux v., Par.,* Petrol., *Phos., Pho. ac.,* Plat., Pb., **POD., Puls.,** Ran. b., Rhodo., Rhus, *Rumex,* **SABA.,** *Sars.,* Sec. c., Sele., *Seneg.,* **SEP., Sil.,** Spig., Spo., **STAN., Staph.,** Stro., **SUL., SUL. AC.,** Tar., **Valer.,** Verat. a., *Verb.,* **Vio. t.,** Zinc.

At Noon.—*Apis,* ARG., Nux m., *Pœo.,* **Valer.**

Afternoon.—*Acon.,* Agar., *All. c.,* Aloe, ALUM., Ambr., **Am. carb., Am. m.,** Anac., Ant. cr., Ant. t., **Apis,** Arg., Arg. n., Arn., **Ars.,** Asaf., Asar., Aur., Bar. c, BELL., Bism., *Bor.,* Bov., **Brom., Bry.,** *Cact.,* Calad., *Calc. c.,* **Calc. ph.,** *Camph.,* Cannab. s., **Canth.,** Caps., Carb. an., Carb. v., *Carb. sul.,* Caust., *Ced.,* Cham., **Chel.,** Chin., **Cic., Cimic.,** Cina, *Cocc., Coc. c., Coff., Colch.,* **Coloc.,** *Con.,* Croc., Cyc., **Dig.,** Dios., Dros., Dulc., Euphr., *Fer., Gel.,* Graph., Hell., Hep., Hyos., **Ign.,** *Iod., Ip.,* K. BI., K. carb., K. NIT., *Kre., Lach.,* Laur., **Led.,** LYC., Mag. c., Mag. m., Mang., Mar., *Meli.,* Meny., Merc., Mez., **Mos., Mur.**

ac., *Nat. c.*, *Nat. m.*, **Nit. ac.**, Nux m., **Nux v.**, Op., *Par.*, Petrol., **Phos., Pho. ac.**, Plat., *Pb.*, **PULS.**, Ran. b., *Ran. s.*, Rheum, Rhodo., **RHUS, Rumex**, *Ruta*, Saba., Sabi., *Sal. ac.*, **Sang.**, Sars., **Sele.**, Seneg., **SEP., SIL., SIN.**, *Spig.*, Spo., Squ., **Stan., Staph.**, Still., *Stro.*, **SUL., Sul. ac.**, Tar., **THUJ., Valer.**, Verat. a., **Verb., Vio. t.**, ZINC.

Evening.—*Abrot.*, **Acon.**, Agar., *Agn.*, **All. c.**, *Aloe*, Alum., **AMBR., AM. CARB., Am. m.**, *Anac.*, **ANT. CR., ANT. T.**, *Apis*, **Arg., Arg. n., ARN., Ars.**, Asaf., **Asar.**, Aur., **Bap.**, Bar. c., **BELL.**, Bism., **Bor.**, *Bov.*, **Brom., BRY.**, Calad., **Calc. c., Calc. ph.**, Camph., Cannab. s., **Canth., CAPS., Carb. an.**, *Carb. v.*, *Carb. sul.*, **CAUST.**, *Ced.*, **Cham., Chel., Chin.**, Cic., **Cimic.**, Cina., **Clem., Cocc., Coff., COLCH., Coloc., Com., Con., Croc.**, *Cup.*, **CYC.**, *Dig.*, *Dirca*, *Dros.*, **Dulc., EUPHR., Fer., Gam.**, *Graph.*, **Guai., HELL., Hep., HYOS., Ign., Iod., Ip., Jat., K. bi., K. carb., K. NIT.**, Kalm., Kre., **LACH., Laur., Led., LYC., MAG. C., Mag. m., Mang.**, *Mar.*, **MENY., MERC., Merc. i. r., MEZ.**, *Mos.*, **Mur. ac., Nat. c., Nat. m., NIT. AC., Nux m., Nux v.**, Oleand., **Op., Par.**, Petrol., **PHOS., Pho. ac.**, *Phyt.*, **PLAT., PB., PULS., Ran. b., RAN. S.**, Rheum, **Rhodo.**, Rhus, **RUMEX., RUTA**, *Saba.*, **Sabi.**, *Sal. ac.*, **Samb., Sang.**, Sars., *Sele.*, **Seneg., SEP., SIL., SIN.**, *Spig.*, Spo., Squ., **STAN., Staph.**, *Stict.*, **STRO., SUL., SUL. AC., Tab.**, Tar., **Thuj., VALER.**, Verat. a., *Verb.*, *Vib. op*, Vio. o., **Vio. t., ZINC.**

Night.—*Ac. ac.*, **ACON.**, Agar., *Agn.*, *Aloe*, Alum., Ambr., **Am. b., Am. carb., Am. m., Ammc.**, Anac., **Ant. cr., Ant. t., Apoc. c., Aral., Arg.**, *Arg. n.*, **ARN., ARS.**, Ars. iod., Asaf., **Asar.**, Aur., Bar. c., **Bell.**, Benz. ac., *Bism.*, **Bor., Bov., Bry.**, Cact., *Calad.*, **Calc. c.**, *Calc. i.*, **Calc. ph.**, Camph., Cannab. i., **Cannab. s., Canth., Caps.**, *Carb. ac.*, **Carb. an.**, *Carb. v.*, **Caust.**, *Ced.*, **CHAM., Chel., CHIN.**, *Cic.*, *Cinnab.*, **Cina., Clem., Cocc.**, Coc. c., Cod., **Coff., COLCH., Coloc., CON., Croc.**, Crotal., **Cup.**, *Cyc.*, **Dig.**, *Dios.*, **Dol., Dros., DULC.**, *Elaps.*, *Eucal.*, **Euphr.**, Equis., **FER.**, Fl. ac., **Gam., GRAPH.**, *Guai.*, **Hell., HEP., HYOS., Ign., IOD., IP., K. br., K. carb., K. iod.**, K. nit., *Kre.*, **LACH.**, Laur., **Led.**, Lit. t., **Lyc., MAG. C., MAG. M., MANG.**, Mar., Meny., **MERC., Merc. c., Merc. i. f., Mez.**, *Mos.*, **Mur. ac., Nat. c.**, Nat. m., **Nat. s., NIT. AC.**, *Nux m.*, **Nux v.**, Oleand., **Op., Ox. ac.**, *Par.*, **Petrol., PHOS.**, *Pho. ac.*, **Phyt., Pic. ac., Plat., PB., PULS.**, *Ran. b.*, *Ran. s.*, Rheum, *Rhodo.*, **RHUS, RUMEX**, Saba., *Sabi.*, *Sal. ac.*, **Samb.**, *Sang.*, Sars., **Sec. c., Sele.**, *Senec.*, **Seneg., SEP., SIL.**, *Sin.*, **Spig.**, Spo., Squ., **Stan., Staph.**, *Stict.*, Stram., **STRO., SUL., Sul. ac.**, Tar., *Tarent.*, **TELL., Thuj.**, Valer., *Verat. a.*, **Vio. t., ZINC.**

AGGRAVATIONS.

Forepart of Night.—Alum., Ambr., *Am. m.*, *Anac.*, **Ant. t.**, *Apis*, **ARG. N.**, *Arn.*, **ARS.**, Asar., **Bell.**, *Brom.*, **Bry.**, *Calad.*, *Cannab. s.*, **CARB. V.**, **Caust.**, **Cham.**, Chel., Chin.,**COFF.**, *Colch.*, **Cup.**, Cyc., Dulc., Fer., **Graph.**, *Hep.*, Ign., K. carb., **Lach.**, **LED.**, **LYC.**, **Mang.**, Mar., **Merc.**, **Mez.**, Mos., **Mur. ac.**, Nat. m., **Nit. ac.**, Nux v., *Osm.*, Petrol., **PHOS.**, *Phyt.*, Plat., **PULS.**, **Ran. b.**, **RAN. S.**, Rhodo., **Rhus.** RUMEX, Ruta, SABA., Samb., **Sep.**, Spig., **Spo.**, STAN., Staph., Stro., Sul., Thuj., **Valer.**, Vio. t.

After Midnight.—*Acon.*, Alum., Ambr., *Am. m.*, Ant. cr., *Ant. t.*, ARS., Asaf., *Aur.*, Bar. c., Bor., **Bry.**, Calad., **Calc. c.**, **Cannab. s.**, *Canth*, *Caps.*, *Carb. an.*, Carb. v., *Caust.*, Cham., **Chel.**, Chin., Cocc., Coc. c., *Coff.*, Con., *Croc.*, **Cup.**, DROS., *Dulc.*, Euphr., **FER.**, **Gel.**, *Graph.*, Hell., *Hep.*, Ign., *Iod.*, K. CARB., K. NIT., Lyc., **Mag. c.**, Mang., **Merc.**, **Mez.**, *Mur. ac.*, *Nat. c.*, Nat. m., *Nat. s.*, Nit. ac., NUX V., *Par.*, PHOS., **Pho. ac.**, *Phyt.*, *Plat.*, POD., **Puls.**, Ran. b., **Ran. s.**, *Rhodo.*, RHUS, *Rumex*, Saba., Sabi., **Samb.**, Sars., Seneg., Sep., SIL., Spig., Spo., **Squ.**, *Staph.*, Stram., **Sul.**, *Sul. ac.*, *Tar.*, THUJ., *Vio. o.*

Periodically.—*Acon.*, ALUM., Am. br., **Anac.**, Ant. cr., **Ant. t.**, ARG., *Aran.*, Arn., ARS., **Asar.**, Bar. c., *Bell.*, Bov., *Bry.*, **Cact.**, **Calc. c.**, Cannab. s., **Canth.**, **Caps.**, **Carb. v.**, CED., CHIN., *Cina*, Clem., Cocc., Colch., *Croc.*, Cup., Dros., Fer., Graph., **Ign.**, IP., K. nit., *Lach.*, Lyc., Meny., *Menth.*, Merc., NAT. M., NIT. AC., **Nux v.**, *Petrol.*, Phos., **Pb.**, **Puls.**, Rhodo., Rhus, Saba., *Samb.*, Sec. c., SEP. SIL., Spig., Stan., Staph., Sul., *Valer.*, **Verat. a.**, Zinc.

Alone, When.—Ars., Bor., **Con.**, **Dros.**, *K. carb.*, LYC., *Mez.*, Phos., *Sil.*, STRAM., *Zinc.*

Arsenic Fumes.—Camph., *Ip.*, **Merc.**, *Nux v.*

Ascending.—*Acon.*, *Aloe*, *Alum.*, **Am. carb.**, Anac., Ant. cr., Arg., Arn., ARS., Asar., *Aur.*, **Bar. c.**, *Bell.*, **Bor.**, BRY., CALC. C., **Calc. ph.**, *Cannab. i.*, *Cannab. s.*, Canth., Carb. v., *Carb. sul.*, Caust., Chin., *Coca*, Coff., *Conv.*, **Cup.**, Dig., *Dios.*, **Dros.**, *Dub.*, *Euphorb.*, **Gel.**, **Glon.**, Graph., **Hell.**, Hep., *Hyos.*, *Ign.*, K. carb., **K. iod.**, **K. nit.**, Kalm., *Kre.*, Lach., Led., Lyc., Mag. c., Mag. m., *Meny.*, Merc., Mos., Mur. ac., *Nat. c.*, **Nat. m.**, *Nit. ac.*, Nux m., **Nux v.**, **Ox. ac.**, *Par.*, Petrol., **Phos.**, *Pho. ac.*, Plat., Pb., Ran. b., *Rhus*, **Ruta**, Saba., **Seneg.**, **Sep.**, Sil., Spig., SPO., *Squ.*, **Stan.**, *Staph.*, Sul., Sul. ac., **Tab.**, Tar., Thuj., Verb., Zinc.

—**High.**—Acon., *Bry.*, **Calc. c.**, *Coca*, **Conv.**, *Oleand.*, Spig., *Sul.*

Autumn, In.—*Aur.*, Bry., **Chin.**, *Colch.*, **Merc.**, Nux v., RHUS, Stram., **Verat. a.**

AGGRAVATIONS.

Bathing.—Ant. cr., *Ant. s. au*, **Ars. iod.**, *Bell.*, *Bry.*, *Calc. c.*, *Carb. v.*, *Caust.*, Mang., *Nat. m.*, **Nit. ac.**, Phos., RHUS, Sep., *Sil.*, *Sul.*

—Cold.—Ant. cr., Bell., Caps., *Carb. sul.*, *Mur. ac.*, Nit. ac., *Phos.*, RHUS, Sars., Sep.

—Sea.— *Ars.*, Rhus, *Sep.*

Bending or Turning.—*Aloe*, **Am. m.**, Ant. t., Arn., **Bell.**, **Bov.**, **Bry.**, Calc. c., Camph., Caps., Carb. an., Carb. v., Cham., **Chin.**, **Cic.**, Cocc., **Con.**, **Crot. tig.**, Cyc., *Dros.*, Dulc., Euphorb., *Guai.*, Hep., Ign., Iod., Ip., *Lach.*, Laur., *Mag. c.*, Merc., *Mez.*, Mur. ac., **Nat. m.**, Nit. ac., Nux v., *Petrol.*, **Phos.**, Pho. ac., Plat., *Pb.*, Puls., **Ran. b.**, *Rhodo.*, **Rhus**, Saba., *Sabi.*, Samb., **Sele.**, Spig., **Spo.**, Stan., Staph., **Sul.**, *Thuj.*, Varat. a., *Zinc.*

—Affected Part.—Acon., Am. carb., **Am. m.**, *Anac.*, **Ant. cr.**, Ant. t., Arg., **Arn.**, Asaf., Aur., *Bar. c.*, **Bell.**, Bor., Bov., Bry., CALC. C., Camph., Caps., Carb. an., Carb. v., Caust., Cham., **Chel.**, **Chin.**, **Cic.**, Cimic., Cina, Cocc., **Coff.**, Con., Croc., Cup., Cyc., Dig., *Dros.*, Dulc., Glon., Graph., Hep., Hyos., IGN., Iod., Ip., **K. carb.**, *Lach.*, Laur., Led., **Lyc.**, **Mag. c.**, Mar., Merc., *Mez.*, Mur. ac., **Nat. m.**, *Nit. ac*, **Nux v.**, Oleand., Par., *Petrol.*, **Phos.**, Pho. ac., *Plat.*, Pb., Puls., *Ran b.*, **Rhodo.**, **Rhus**, Ruta., Saba., *Sabi.*, Samb., **Sang.**, **Sele.**, Sep., Sil., Spig., Spo., Stan., Staph., *Sul.*, Tar., *Thuj.*, Valer., Verat. a., *Zinc.*

—Backward.—*Am. carb.*, **Anac.**, **Ant. cr.**, Asaf., Aur., **Bar. c.**, **Calc. c.**, Caps., *Carb. v.*, *Caust.*, **Chel.**, Cina, Coff., **Con.**, Cup., Dig., Dros., Dulc., Ign., K. carb., Mar., Nat. m., **Nit. ac.**, Nux v., **Plat.**, Pb., **Puls.**, *Rhodo.*, Rhus, SEP., Stan., Sul., Thuj., Valer.

—Backward and Forward.—Asaf., Chel., *Coff.*, Nux v., Thuj.

—Forward.—Asaf., *Chel.*, *Cimic.*, **Coff.**, Nux v., *Thuj.*

—Inward.—Am. m., **Ign.**, **Stan.**, *Staph.*, Verat. a.

—Outward.—*Caps.*

—To Right.—*Spig.*

—Sideways.—*Acon.*, Bell., *Bor.*, **Calc. c.**, Canth., *Chel.*, Chin., Cocc., K. carb., *Lyc.*, Nat. m., Pb., Stan., Staph.

—Head Backward.—Bell., *Bry.*, Caust., *Chin.*, **Cic.**, Cup., Cyc., *Dig.*, Dros., K. carb., Puls., Sep., *Spo.*, *Valer.*, Vio. o.

— —Forward.—Carb. ac., *Cimic.*, Rhus, Vio. o.

— —Sideways.—Chin., Spo.

Bent, Holding the Part.—Hyos., Mar., **Spo.**, Valer.

Biting Teeth Together.—*Aloe*, *Alum.*, AM. CARB., *Anac.*, *Bell.*, Bry., Carb. an., Caust., Chin., Coff., *Colch.*, Dig., **Graph.**, Guai., Hell.,

Hep., Hyos, Ip., Lach., Mang., Merc., **Mez.**, *Petrol.*, Puls., Rhus, Sars., Sep., Sil., Spo., *Staph.*, *Sul.*, **Sul. ac.**, **Verb.**

Blowing Nose.—Acon., Agn., *Alum.*, Ambr., Am. carb., Ant. t., Arg., Arn., **AUR.**, *Bar. c.*, **Bell.**, *Bry.*, **Calc. c.**, Cannab. s., **Canth.**, Caps., Carb. an., Carb. v., **Caust.**, *Cham.*, Chel., Chin., Cina, Coff., **Colch.**, **Con.**, Dig., Euphorb., Euphr., **HEP.**, *Hyos.*, Iod., **K. carb.**, K. nit., *Kre.*, Led., Lyc., Mag. c., *Mag. m.*, Mang., *Mar.*, Meny., **MERC.**, Mez., *Nat. m.*, Nit. ac., **Nux v.**, Par., **Pho. ac.**, Phos., **PULS.**, **Ran. b.**, *Sabi.*, Sars., Sele., **Sep.**, *Sil.*, **SPIG.**, Spo., Stan., **Staph.**, Stram., Stro., **SUL.**, Tar., *Thuj.*, *Verat. a.*

Breakfast, After.—Ambr., **Am. m.**, *Anac.*, *Ars.*, Bell., Bor., **Bry.**, **Calc. c.**, Carb. an., *Carb. v.*, **Caust.**, **CHAM.**, Chin., **Con.**, Cyc., **Dig.**, Euphorb., *Form.*, **Graph.**, Hell., Ign., **K. carb.**, K. nit., Laur., *Lyc.*, Mag. c., Mang., **Nat. c.**, **Nat. m.**, *Nit. ac.*, *Nux m.*, **NUX V.**, Par., Petrol., **PHOS.**, *Pho. ac.*, *Pb.*, Puls., Rhodo., *Rhus*, *Sars.*, **Sep.**, Sil., Stro., **Sul.**, *Thuj.*, Valer., *Verat. a.*, **ZINC.**

Breathing.—Acon., Agar., Alum., Am. carb., **Am. m.**, **Anac.**, Ant. cr., *Arg.*, Arn., Ars., *Asaf.*, Asar., *Asc. t.*, Aur., **Bell.**, Bism., Bor., Bov., **BRY.**, **Calc. c.**, **Cannab. s.**, **Caps.**, *Cham.*, Chin., **Cina**, Clem., **COCC.**, **COLCH.**, Coloc., Con., *Croc.*, Cup., Dig., Dros., Dulc., Euphr., Graph., **Hep.**, *Hyos.*, **K. carb.**, *K. nit.*, Led., *Lyc.*, Mag. c., **MERC.**, Mez., Mur. ac., *Nat. c.*, **Nat. m.**, Nit. ac., *Nux v.*, **Phel.**, Pho. ac., *Plat.*, **Puls.**, **RAN. B.**, *Rhodo.*, **Rhus**, **Saba.**, *Sars*, Sele., Seneg., **SEP.**, Sil., **SPIG.**, *Squ.*, **STAN.**, **SUL.**, *Sul. ac.*, Thuj., *Verat. a.*

—**Deep.**—**ACON.**, Agn., *Aloe*, *Am. m.*, Ant. t., Arg., **Arn.**, *Asaf.*, Asc. t., BOR., Brom., **BRY.**, Calad., Calc. c., *Calc. ph.*, **Canth.**, *Caps.*, Carb. an., **Caust.**, *Chel.*, *Cina*, *Coral.*, *Crot. tig.*, **Dig.**, *Dros.* Dulc., *Fer.*, **Graph.**, Hell., *Hep.*, Ign., *Ip.*, **K. carb.**, K. nit., Kre., **Lyc.**, Mag. m., *Mang.*, Meny., **Merc.**, Mos., Nat. c., *Nat. m.*, Nux m., Nux v., Oleand., **Phos.**, *Pb.*, **Puls.**, **Ran. s.**, Rheum, **RHUS**, **Rumex**, Saba., **SABI.**, Sang., Seneg., Sep., **Sil.**, **SPIG.**, Spo., **Squ.**, **Sul.**, Thuj., *Valer.*, Verb.

—**When Not.**—*Asaf.*, *Cina*, Ign., **Merc.**, Spig., *Tar.*

—**Holding Breath.**—Dros., **K. nit.**, *Led.*, Meny., *Merc.*, Spig.

Bruises.—**ARN.**, Cic., Con., *Euphr.*, Hep., Iod., *Puls.*, Ruta, Sul., Sul. ac.

Brushing Teeth.—*Carb. v.*, **Coc. c.**, Lyc., Ruta, Staph.

Burns.—Agar., Alum., Ant. cr., **ARS.**, *Calc. c.*, *Carb. ac.*, **Carb. v.**, **CAUST.**, *Cyc.*, Euphorb., **Kre.**, *Lach.*, Mag. c. Rhus, Ruta, Sec. c., Stram.

Change of Position.—Acon., *Bry.*, **CAPS.**, **Carb. v.**, *Caust.*, Chel.,

Con., EUPHORB., FER., **Lach**., **Lyc**., Petrol., **Phos**., Pho. ac., **Plat**., Pb., PULS., *Ran. b*, Rhodo., *Rhus, Saba*., **Samb**., *Sil*., Thuj.

Change of Temperature.—*Acon*., Alum., ARS., **Carb. v**., Caust., Graph., Lyc., Mag. c., *Nux v*., Phos., **Puls**., RAN. B., Ran. s., *Rhus*, **Sabi**., *Spo*., Sul., Verat. a., VERB.

—**Weather.**—Am. carb., Ars., Bor., **Bry**., *Calc. c*., *Calc. ph*., Colch., Dulc., Euphorb., *Gel*., *Graph*., *Hyper*., **Mang**., *Meli*., *Merc*., Nat. c., Nit. ac., NUX M., Nux v., PHOS., *Ran. b*., *Rheum*, RHODO., RHUS, Sep., SIL., Stro., *Sul*., Verat. a.

Chewing, When.—Acon., **Alum**., AM. CARB., **Am. m**., Anac., **Arg**., **Arg. n**., Arn., Ars, *Aur*., **Bell**., **Bor**., Bov., **Bry**., *Calc. c*., Cannab. s., Carb. an., *Carb. v*., Caust., **Chin**., Cocc., Coff., Colch., Dig., *Euphorb*., Euphr., *Graph*., Guai., HEP., **Hyos**., Ign., *Ip*., K. carb., Lach., Mag. c., Mang., *Mar*., MENY., MERC., Nat. c, **Nat. m**., **Nit. ac**., Nux v., Oleand., Petrol., Phos., Pho. ac., Puls., Ran. b., RHUS, Sabi., Sars., *Seneg*., **Sep**., *Sil*., Spig., *Spo*., Squ., **Staph**., Sul., Sul. ac., Tar., Thuj., *Verat. a*., Verb., Zinc.

—**After.**—Sabi., *Staph*.

Chicken-pox. See under **Skin.**

Children Especially, Remedies For.—Acon., **Aeth**., Agar., **Ambr**., *Ant. cr*., Ant. t., Arn., Ars., Asaf., *Bar. c*., BELL., Bor., *Bry*., CALC. C., Calc. ph., Camph., *Canth*., CAPS., CHAM., *Chin*., **Cic**., *Cina*, **Clem**., Cocc., Con., Croc., *Cup*., Dig., Dros., Euphorb., Fer., Graph., *Hell*., HYOS., Ign., Iod., Ip., K. carb., *Kre*., *Lach*., Laur., Lyc., *Mag. c*., MERC., Mur. ac., *Nat. c*., Nux m., Nux v., Op., Pb., *Pod*., **Puls**., **Rheum**, Rhus, Ruta, *Saba*., Sabi., Sec. c., Seneg., Sep., SIL., Spig., **Spo**., *Squ*., Stan., Staph., Sul., Sul. ac., Thuj., *Verat. a*., Vio. o., *Vio. t*., Zinc.

China (Without Quinine Cachexia) (compare "**Quinine**").—Led., Sele.

Clear Weather.—Bry., *Pb*.

Climateric, During.—*Croc*., LACH., *Sang*., *Vinc*.

Closing Eyes.—*Agar*., Arn., Ars., Bell., BRY., *Calad*., *Calc. c*., Carb. an., *Caust*., Chel., **Chin**., **Clem**., Con., **Croc**., Dig., Dub., Fer., *Fl. ac*., Hell., Hep., Ign., *K. carb*., LACH., **Led**., **Mag. m**., Mang., *Merc*., Nux v., Op., Phos., Pho. ac., Puls., Sars., SEP., Sil., *Spo*., Staph., *Stram*., Sul., Ther., Thuj.

—**Mouth.**—Mez., Nux v.

Cloudy Weather.—*Bry*., Calc. c., **Cham**., **Chin**., Dulc., **Mang**., *Merc*., Nux m., Pb., *Rhodo*., RHUS, Sep., *Sul*., Verat. a.

Clutching Anything.—Acon., **Am. carb**., *Am. m*., Arg., Bell., Bov.,

AGGRAVATIONS. 275

Bry., **Calc. c.,** *Cannab. s.,* **Carb. v.,** CAUST., **Cham.,** Chin., *Dros.,* K. carb., K. nit., Laur., *Led.,* **Lyc.,** Nat. c., Nat. m., Nux m., Nux v., Op., *Plat.,* **Puls.,** Rhus, Saba., Sec. c., **Sil.,** Spig., *Verat. a.*

Coal Gas.—*Arn.,* Bov.

Coition, During.—Anac., Asaf., Bar. c., *Calad.,* **Canth.,** *Fer.,* **Graph.,** **K. carb.,** Lyc., Plat., **Sele.,** *Sep., Thuj.*

—**After.**—AGAR., Agn., Anac., *Arg. n.,* Asaf., Bar. c., Bor., **Bov.,** Calad., CALC. C., *Canth.,* **Chin.,** *Con.,* **Graph.,** K. CARB., Lyc., Mag. m., Mos., **Nat. c.,** Nat. m., Nit. ac., *Nux v.,* **Petrol.,** Phos., *Pho. ac.,* Pb., Rhodo., **Sele.,** SEP., SIL., Staph., *Ther.*

Cold in General.—Acon., **Agar.,** Alum., **Am. carb.,** Anac., Ant. cr., *Arg., Arn.,* **ARS.,** Asar., **Aur.,** **Bar. c.,** **Bell.,** Bor., **Bov.,** Bry., *Cad. s.,* Calc. c., *Calc. ph.,* **CAMPH.,** *Canth.,* **Caps.,** *Carb. an., Carb. v., Carb. sul.,* CAUST., Cham., *Chin.,* **Cic.,** *Cinnab., Clem.,* **Cocc.,** *Coff.,* Colch., Coloc., **Con.,** *Dig.,* DULC., *Fer., Graph.,* **Hell.,** HEP., *Hydras.,* **Hyos., Ign.,** Ip., K. CARB., *Kalm., Kre., Lach.,* Laur., Led., Lyc , **Mag. c.,** *Mag. m.,* **Mang., Menth.,** *Meny.,* Merc., *Mez.,* MOS., *Mur. ac., Nat. c.,* **Nat. m.,** Nit. ac., Nux m., **NUX V.,** **Petrol.,** *Phos.,* Pho. ac., Puls., **Ran. b.,** *Rheum,* Rhodo., RHUS, *Rumex, Ruta,* SABA., *Samb., Sars.,* Seneg., Sep., **Sil.,** Spig., *Spo., Squ.,* **Staph.,** *Stram.,* STRO., *Sul., Sul. ac.,* Thuj., Verat. a., *Verb.,* Vio. t., Zinc.

Cold Air.—Acon., **Agar.,** ALL. C., Alum., **Am. carb.,** Anac., Ant. cr., Arn., **ARS.,** Asar., **AUR.,** **Bar. c.,** **Bell.,** Bor., *Bov.,* Bry., **Calc. c.,** *Calc. ph.,* **CAMPH.,** Canth., **Caps.,** *Carb. an.,* **Carb. v.,** CAUST., *Cham.,* Chin., **Cic.,** *Cina, Cist.,* **Cocc.,** *Coff.,* **Colch.,** *Coloc.,* **Con.,** Dig., DULC., *Fer., Fl. ac.,* Graph., **HELL.,** HEP., **Hyos., Ign.,** Ip., K. bi., K. CARB., Kre., Lach., Laur., **Lyc.,** Mag. c., Mag. m., **Mang.,** *Menth.,* Meny., **Merc.,** *Mez.,* MOS., Mur. ac., *Nat. c., Nat. m.,* Nit. ac., **NUX M., NUX V., Osm.,** Par., **Petrol., Phos.,** *Pho. ac.,* **Plant., Puls.,** Ran. b., RHODO., RHUS, RUMEX, *Ruta,* SABA., Samb., *Sars.,* Seneg., **Sep.,** *Sil.,* Spig., *Spo.,* Squ., **Staph., Stram.,** STRO., **Sul.,** Sul. ac., Thuj., **Verat. a.,** Verb., Vio. t., Zinc.

—**Dry.**—Acon., Alum., *Ars.,* **ASAR.,** *Bell.,* Bor., **Bry.,** *Carb. an., Carb. v.,* **CAUST.,** *Cham.,* **HEP., Ip.,** Laur., Mag. c., Mez., Mur. ac., **NUX V.,** Rhodo., **Saba.,** *Sep., Sil.,* Spig., **Spo.,** Staph., Sul., Zinc.

—**Wet.**—Agar., **AM. CARB.,** Ant. cr., *Aur.,* Bar. c., Bell., *Bor.,* Bov., Bry , CALC. C., *Calc. ph.,* Canth., *Carb. an., Carb. v.,* Cham., *Chin., Clem.,* Colch., Con., *Cup.,* DULC., *Fer.,* Hep , Ip., K. carb., *K. nit.,* **Lach.,** *Laur.,* **Lyc.,** *Mag. c.,* **Mang., Merc.,** Mez., *Mur. ac., Nat. c., Nat. s., Nit. ac.,* NUX M , Nux v., Petrol., *Phos., Phyt.,* **Puls.,** *Rhodo.,* RHUS.,

Ruta, *Sars.*, *Seneg.*, Sep., Sil., *Spig.*, Stan., *Staph.*, **Stro.**, **Sul.**, *Sul. ac.*, Verat. a., *Zinc.*

Cold Entering a Cold Place.—ARS., *Calc. ph.*, *Camph.*, *Carb. v.*, *Caust.*, Con., *Dulc.*, K. carb , *Mos.*, Nux m., **Nux v.**, Phos., **Puls.**, RAN. B., Saba., *Sep.*, Sil., Spo., *Stro.*, **Verb.**

—**Becoming Cold.**—Acon., *Agar.*, *Am. carb.*, Ant. cr., **Arn.**, ARS., *Ars. iod.*, Asar., AUR., *Bar. c.*, **Bell.**, *Bor.*, Bov., **Bry.**, *Calc. c.*, **Camph.**, Canth., *Caps.*, Carb.' an., Carb. v., **Caust.**, *Cham.*, **Chin.**, *Cic.*, **Clem.**, **Cocc.**, *Con.*, Dig., Dulc., Fer., **Graph.**, *Hell.*, Hep., **Hyos.**, *Ign.*, K. CARB., *Kre.*, Lach., **Lyc.**, *Mag c.*, Mag. m., *Mang.*, Meny., *Merc.*, *Merc. i. r.*, Mez., MOS., Mur. ac., *Nat. c*, Nat. m., *Nit. ac.*, *Nux m.*, NUX V., *Petrol.*, **Phos.**, *Pho. ac.*, Ran. b., Rhodo., RHUS, Ruta, SABA., Samb., Sars , Sep., *Sil.*, Spig., *Spo.*, Squ., Staph., Stram., **Stro.**, *Sul.*, Sul. ac.. Thuj., *Verat. a.*, *Verb.*, Vio. t., Zinc.

— —**A Part of Body.**—Bell., *Cham.*, **Hell.**, HEP., Led., *Puls.*, Rhus., Sep., SIL.

After Becoming Cold.—Acon., Agar., *Alum.*, Am. carb., Anac., **Ant. t.**, Arn., Ars., Aur., *Bar. c.*, **BELL.**, Bor., **BRY.**, **Calc. c.**, Calc. ph., *Camph.*, **Carb. v.**, *Caust.*, CHAM., Chin., *Cocc.*, **Coff.**, Coloc., Con., *Croc.*, Cup., **Cyc.**, Dig., Dros., DULC., **Graph.**, Hep., HYOS., *Ign.*, **Ip.**, K. carb., Led., **Lyc.**, Mag. c., **Mang.**, MERC., *Nat. c*, Nat. m., **Nit. ac.**, *Nux m.*, NUX V., *Op.*, Petrol., PHOS., Pho. ac., *Plat.*, PULS., *Ran. b.*, RHUS, Ruta, *Sabi.*, **Samb.**, *Sars.*, *Sele.*, **Sep.**, SIL., SPIG., Stan., *Staph.*, Stro., **Sul.**, *Sul. ac*, *Valer.*, **Verat. a.**

—**In Head.**—BELL., Led., Puls., SEP.

—**In Feet.**—*Cham.*, Puls., SIL.

Combing Hair.—Bry., *Chin.*, Ign., Kre., **Sele.**

— —**Backward.**—Puls., *Rhus.*

Conscious, When Half.—Camph.

Coughing, Before.—Cina, Croc., Led.

—**During.** (See under "**Cough, Associated Symptoms.**")

—**After.**—*Ars.*, Calad., *Chin.*, **Cina**, Croc., *Cup.*, Dros., *Fer.*, **Hyos.**, Ip., Nux v., PHOS., **Sep.**, Squ., Sul.

Copper, Fumes of.—*Camph.*, Ip., Lyc., Merc., *Nux v.*, Op., **Puls.**

Cutting Hair.—BELL., Led., *Puls.*, **Sep.**

Cuts, For.—Arn., Merc., *Nat. c*, Pho. ac., Sil., STAPH., *Sul.*, **Sul. ac.**

Dancing, When.—Bor.

—**After.**—Spo.

AGGRAVATIONS.

Darkness.—Am. m., *Ars., Bar. c.,* **Calc. c.,** *Cannab. i., Carb. sul.,* **Carb. an.,** *Carb. v.,* **Phos.,** Staph., **STRAM.,** *Stro.,* **Valer.**

Descending.—*Acon.,* Am. m., *Arg.,* Bar. c., Bell., **BOR.,** Bry., Canth., **Coff., Con., Fer.,** *Lyc., Meny.,* Nit. ac., Pb., Rhodo., Rhus, Ruta, *Sabi.,* Stan., Sul., Verat. a., Verb.

Disordered Stomach.—Acon., ANT. CR., *Ant. t.,* Ars., Bar. c., Bry., *Calc. c.,* Caps., **Carb. v.,** Caust., *Cham.,* Chin., **Cocc., Coff.,** Colch., *Con.,* Cyc., *Euphorb.,* Fer., *Ign.,* IP., Lyc., **Nat. c.,** Nat. m., Nux m., **NUX V.,** *Phos.,* **PULS.,** Rhus, *Sep., Sil.,* Stan., Staph., *Sul.,* Sul. ac., *Verat. a.*

Distortion of Facial Muscles.—*Bry.,* Oleand., Puls., *Spig.*

Draft.—*Acon.,* Anac., **BELL.,** *Benz. ac.,* Bry., **Calc. c.,** *Calc. ph.,* **Caps.,** *Caust.,* Cham., **Chin.,** Coloc., Graph., **Hep.,** *Ign.,* **K. carb.,** Lach., Led., Merc., Mur. ac., *Nat. c.,* Nit. ac., *Nux v.,* Phos., Puls., *Rhus,* Sars., **Sele.,** Sep., **SIL.,** Spig., **Sul.,** *Valer.,* Verb.

Drawing in the Air.—*Alum.,* **ANT. CR., Bell.,** Bry., *Calc. c.,* **Caust.,** Chin., *Cic., Cina,* Hyos., Ign., Ip., K. nit., **Merc.,** Mez., *Nat. m., Nux m.,* Nux v., Par., *Petrol.,* Phos., Pho. ac., **Puls.,** Saba., **Sabi.,** *Sars.,* **Sele.,** Sep., Sil., Spig., Staph., Sul., Thuj., Verb.

—**Off Boots.**—*Calc. c., Graph.*

—**The Limb Back.**—Mos.

—**Up Limbs.**—*Agar.,* Alum., Am. m., Anac., **Ant. t.,** Asar., *Bell.,* Bor., *Bry.,* Carb. an., Carb. v., Cham., Chel., Chin., Coff., *Coloc.,* Dig., Dros., Dulc., Fer., **Guai.,** Hep., *Ign.,* K. carb., *Mag. c.,* Mez., Mur. ac., *Nat. m.,* Nux m., Nux v., Oleand., Par., Petrol., Plat., **PULS.,** Rheum, *Rhodo.,* **RHUS,** *Saba.,* Sabi., SEC. C., Stan., Staph., Thuj., Verb., Zinc.

Drinkers, for Hard (Old Topers).—Acon., **Agar.,** Alum., Am. m., Anac., **Ant. cr.,** *Arn.,* **Ars., Bell.,** *Bor., Bov., Cad. s.,* **Calc. c.,** Carb. an., *Carb. s., Carb. v.,* Caust., **Chel., Chin., Cocc., Coff.,** Con., Hep., *Hyos.,* Ign., **LACH.,** Laur., Led., Lyc., **Nat. c.,** Nat. m., Nux m., **NUX V., OP.,** Petrol., **Puls., RAN. B.,** Rhodo., Rhus, Ruta, *Saba.,* **Sele.,** Sep., Sil., Spig., Stram., Stro., Sul., Sul. ac., Verat. a., Zinc.

Drinking, When.—*Anac.,* Ars., **BELL.,** Bry., **CANTH.,** Cham., Cina, *Colch.,* Con., Cup., Fer., **Hyos.,** Ign., Iod., Lach., *Laur.,* Merc., Nat. m., **Phos.,** Rhus, *Saba.,* Sabi., Sep., *Squ.,* STRAM.

—**After.**—Acon., *Ambr., Anac.,* Ant. t., Apoc. c., Arg. n., Arn., ARS., *Asaf.,* Asar., *Aur.,* **Bell.,** Bry., Cannab. s., *Canth.,* **Caps.,** Carb. v., Caust., *Cham.,* CHIN., Cic., **COCC.,** Colch., **Coloc., Con.,** Croc., CROT. TIG., **Cup.,** *Dig.,* Dros., **EUP. PER.,** Fer., Graph., Hell., Hep., Hyos., *Ign.,* Ip., K. carb., Lach., **Laur., Lyc.,** Mar., Merc., *Mez.,* Mos., Mur. ac.

Nat. c., **Nat. m.**, **Nit. ac.**, **NUX V.**, Op., Petrol., Phos., Pho. ac., *Pb.*, **Pod.**, **PULS.**, Rhodo., **RHUS**, Ruta., Saba., Sabi., Sec. c., Sele., Sep., **SIL**, Spig., *Squ.*, Staph., Stram., Sul., Sul. ac., **Tar.**, Thuj., **VERAT. A.**

Drinking Fast. — Ars., *Ip.*, *Nat. m.*, NIT. AC., **Nux v.**, SIL., *Sul.*

Driving in a Wagon. — **Arg.**, **Bor.**, Calc. c., *Carb. v.*, **COCC.**, Colch., *Croc.*, Fer., Graph., **Hep.**, **Ign.**, **Iod.**, *K. carb.*, Lach., Lyc., *Mag. c.*, Nat. m., **Nux m.**, Petrol., *Phos.*, **Plat.**, **Rumex**, **Sele.**, **SEP.**, **Sil.**, *Staph.*, **Sul.**, *Thuj.*, Valer.

—**After.**—*Graph.*, K. nit., Nat. c., Nat. m., **Nit. ac.**, **Plat.**, SIL.

Dry Weather.—Acon., Alum., *Ars.*, ASAR., **Bell.**, Bor., **Bry.**, *Carb. an.*, *Carb. v.*, CAUST., *Cham.*, HEP., **Ip.**, Laur., Mag. c., Mez., Mur. ac., NUX V., Rhodo., Saba., *Sep.*, *Sil.*, Spig., **Spo.**, Staph., Sul., Zinc.

Eating, Before.—*Acon.*, *Alum.*, Ambr., Am. carb., *Am. m.*, Anac., Arn., *Ars.*, *Bar. c.*, **Bell.**, **Bov.**, Bry., Calc. c., **Cannab. s.**, *Carb. an.*, *Carb. v.*, *Caust.*, Cham., **Chel.**, **Chin.**, Colch., Croc., Dulc., Euphr., Fer., Graph., Hell., *Hep.*, Ign., IOD., *K. carb.*, Lach., **LAUR.**, *Mag. c.*, Mang., Meny., Merc., *Mez.*, Mos., NAT. C., *Nit. ac.*, *Nux v.*, Oleand., Petrol., PHOS., **Pb.**, Puls., *Ran. b.*, Rhus, **Saba.**, Sabi., Sars., Seneg., Sep., Sil., *Spig.* Squ., Stan., **Stro.**, Sul., Tar., *Valer.*, *Verat. a.*, Verb.

—**When.**—*Aloe*, Alum., *Ambr.*, AM. CARB., Am. m., Ant. cr., *Ant. t*, Arg., *Arn.*, *Ars.*, Aur., **Bar. c.**, *Bell.*, Bism., *Bor.*, *Bov.*, **Bry.**, Calc. c., Cannab. s., **Canth.**, **Carb. ac.**, CARB. AN., CARB. V., **Caust.**, Cham., Chin., **Cic.**, Clem., **Cocc.**, Coff., *Colch.*, CON., Cyc., Dig., Dros., Dulc., *Euphorb.*, Fer., **Graph.**, Hell., Hep., *Ign.*, Iod., K. CARB., K. nit., *Lach.*, Laur., Led., **Lyc.**, *Mag. c.*, **Mag. m.**, Mang., *Mar.*, Merc., Nat. c., **Nat. m.**, NIT. AC., *Nux m.*, Nux v., Oleand., Petrol., **Phos.**, Pho. ac., **Plat.**, **Pb.**, **Puls.**, Ran. b., *Ran. s.*, *Rhodo.*, Rhus, **Rumex**, *Ruta*, Sabi., Samb., *Sars.*, Sec. c., **Sep.**, *Sil.*, Spig., Spo., Squ., **Staph.**, Stram., SUL., Sul. ac., Thuj., Valer., *Verat. a.*, Verb., Zinc.

—**When Eating Fast.**—*Ars.*, **Ip.**, Led., Nux v., Sul.

—**After.**—*Ab. n.*, *Acon.*, *Agar.*, *Agn.*, *All. c.*, ALOE, Alum., *Ambr.*, Am. carb., **Am. m.**, **Anac.**, *Ant. cr.*, *Ant. t.*, Apis, *Apoc. c.*, Arg., **Arg. n.**, *Arn.*, ARS, *Asaf.*, Asar., Aur., *Bar. c.*, **Bell.**, Bism., *Bor*, Bov., BRY., *Buf.*, Calad., CALC. C., *Calc. ph.*, Camph., Cannab. s., Canth., **Caps.**, **Carb. an.**, Carb. v., *Carb. sul.*, CAUST., Cham., Chel., **Chin.**, Cic., Cina, Clem., **Cocc.**, Coc. c., Coff., Colch., COLOC., CON., Croc., Crot. tig., Cyc., *Dig.*, Dros., Dulc., *Eup. per.*, Euphorb., **Euphr.**, Fer., **Gran.**, **Graph.**, Hell., *Hep.*, *Hyos.*, Ign., *Iod.*, Ip., K. BI, K. CARB., K. nit., Kre., LACH., Laur., Led., LYC., *Mag. c.*, **Mag. m.**, **Mang., Mar., Meny., Merc., Mez.**, *Mos.*, ac., Nat. c., NAT. M.,

AGGRAVATIONS.

Nat. s., Nit. ac., *Nux m.*, NUX V., Oleand., *Op.*, **Ox. ac.**, Par., **Petrol.**, **PHOS.**, Pho. ac., *Phyt.*, Plat., Pb., **Pod.**, **PULS.**, Ran. b., Ran. s., Rheum, Rhodo., Rhus, RUMEX, Ruta, Saba., *Sabi.*, Samb, *Sang.*, *Sars.*, Sec. c., *Sele.*, Seneg., SEP., SIL., Spig., Spo., Squ., *Stan.*, Staph., Stro., SUL., *Sul. ac.*, Tar., *Thuj.*, *Trill.*, *Trom.*, Valer., **Verat. a.**, Verb., Vio. t., ZINC.

Eating, After Eating to Satiety.—Bar. c., **Calc. c.**, *Carb. v.*, LYC., *Nat. c.*, Nat. m., Nux v., PULS., *Sep.*, *Sil.*, Sul.

Elevation, When on an.—Sul.

Emissions.—*Agar.*, **Alum.**, Ars., Bor., Bov., Calc. c., Cannab. s., *Carb. an.*, Carb. v., Caust., *Chin.*, *Cob.*, *Dig.*, *Iod.*, K. CARB., Led., Lyc., Merc., Mez., Nat. c., NUX V., Petrol., Phos., *Pho. ac.*, *Pic. ac.*, Pb., Puls., *Ran. b.*, Rhodo., *Saba.*, **Sep.**, Sil., **Staph.**, Thuj.

Eructations.—Agar., Alum., *Am. carb.*, Ant. cr., *Bar. c.*, Bell., *Bry.*, *Calad.*, **Cannab. s.**, *Caps.*, CHAM., **Cocc.**, C. c., *Hep.*, **K. carb.**, **Lach.**, Nux v., Par., **Phos.**, Pb., **Puls.**, *Rhodo.*, Rhus, Sabi., Sep., Sil., Spo., Stan., Staph., Sul., **Verb.**, Zinc.

Eruptions, After Suppression of.—Acon., Alum., Ambr., Am. carb., Ars., **Bell.**, BRY., *Calad.*, Calc. c., Carb. an., *Carb. v.*, **Caust.**, Cham., Con., *Cup.*, *Dulc.*, *Graph.*, **Hep.**, Iod., IP., *K. carb.*, **Lach.**, Lyc., Merc., Mez., **Nat. c.**, Nit. ac., Nux m., *Op.*, *Phos.*, PHO. AC., Puls., Rhus, Sars., *Sele.*, **Sep.**, *Sil.*, **Staph.**, *Stram.*, **Sul.**, Sul. ac., *Thuj.*, *Verat. a.*, Vio. t., Zinc.

Excitement, Emotional.—Acon., Alum., Am. m., Ant. t., **Arg. n.**, Arn., *Ars.*, Asar., **Atrop.**, **Aur.**, Bar. c., **Bell.**, **Bry.**, *Cact.*, *Calc. c.*, **Caps.**, Carb. an., **Caust.**, **Cham.**, Chin., Cic., **Cocc.**, **Coff.**, Colch., **COLOC.**, Con., Croc., *Cup.*, *Cyc.*, *Epiph.*, Fer., **Gel.**, Graph., Hep., **HYOS.**, **IGN.**, Ip., *K. carb.*, Lach., Laur., **Lyc.**, Mag. c., Mag. m., Mar., *Merc.*, Nat. c., **Nat. m.**, Nit. ac., Nux m., **NUX V.**, *Oleand.*, **Op.**, Petrol., **Phos.**, PHO. AC., **Plat.**, Pod., **PULS.**, Ran. b., *Rhus.*, Samb., Sec. c., Sele., Seneg., Sep., *Sil.*, Spo., Stan., **STAPH.**, *Stram.*, Stro., *Sul.*, **Verat. a.**, **Verb.**, Zinc.

—**Contradiction.**—**Aur.**, Bry., Ign., Nux v., *Oleand.*

—**Fright.**—ACON., Anac., **Arg. n.**, **Arn.**, Ars., Aur., **Bell.**, **Bry.**, Calc. c., Carb. v., **Caust.**, *Cham.*, Cic., **Cocc.**, **Coff.**, **Cup.**, **Gel.**, Graph., **Hep.**, **Hyos.**, **IGN.**, *Lach.*, Laur., *Lyc.*, Merc., *Nat. m.*, **Nux v.**, OP., **Phos.**, **Plat.**, **PULS.**, Rhus, *Samb.*, *Sec. c.*, Sep., Spo., Stan., *Stram.*, Sul., **Verat. a.**, Verb., Zinc.

—**Grief and Sorrow.**—Am. m., *Ars.*, Aur., Bell., Calc. c., **Caps.**, Caust., *Cocc.*, **Coloc.**, Con., *Cyc.*, Graph., **Hyos.**, **IGN.**, K. carb.,

Lach., *Lyc.*, Nat. c., *Nux v.*, Phos., **Pho. ac.**, Plat., **Puls.**, Rhus, STAPH., Stram., **Verat. a**.

Excitement, Jealousy.—HYOS., Ign., *Lach.*, Nux v., *Pho. ac.*

—**Joy.**—COFF., Croc., Cyc., Nat. c., *Op.*, **Puls.**

—**Unhappy Love.**—*Aur.*, *Caust.*, **Coff.**, HYOS., IGN., K. carb., Lach , *Nux v.*, Pho ac., Sep., **Staph.**

—**Mortification.**—Acon., Ars., *Aur.*, **Bell.**, *Bry.*, Carb. an., **Cham.**, COLOC., IGN., Ip., *Lyc.*, *Merc.*, NAT. M., *Nux v.*, **Pho. ac.**, *Plat.*, *Puls.*, Seneg., STAPH., Stram., *Sul.*, Verat. a.

—**Reproaches.**—*Coloc.*, **Ign.**, OP., Pho. ac., **Staph.**

—**Rudeness of Others.**—Colch., Staph.

—**Scorn.**—*Acon.*, **Aur.**, *Bell.*, BRY., **CHAM.**, *Coff.*, **Coloc.**, *Fer.*, *Hyos.*, Ip., *Lyc.*, *Nat. m.*, NUX V., *Oleand.*, Phos , *Plat.*, Sep., Stro., Sul., *Verat. a.*

—**Vexation.**—ACON., Alum., **Ant. t.**, Ars., *Aur.*, **Bell.**, Bry., Calc. c., Calc. ph., CHAM., Chin., *Cocc.*, **Coff.**, COLOC., Croc., *Cup.*, *Hyos.*, IGN., Ip., Lyc., Mag. c., Mag. m., Nat. c., *Nat. m.*, Nux m , NUX V., Op., Petrol., Phos., *Pho. ac.*, PLAT., **Puls.**, Ran. b., Rhus, Samb., Sec. c., Sele., Sep., Sil , Stan., STAPH., Stram , Sul., *Verat. a.*, Zinc.

— —**With Anxiety.**—ACON., Alum., ARS., *Aur.*, **Bell.**, *Bry.*, *Calc.* Cham., *Cocc.*, Coff., **Cup.**, Hyos., IGN., *Lyc.*, Nat. c., Nat. m., NUX V., Op., Petrol., Phos., **Plat.**, **Puls.**, *Rhus.*, Samb., Sep., Stan , Stram., *Sul.*, *Verat. a.*

— —**With Fright.**—ACON., **Bell.**, *Calc. c.*, Cocc., Cup., IGN , *Nat. c.*, Nux v., Op., *Petrol.*, **Phos.**, **Plat.**, Puls., Samb., Sep., *Sul.*, Zinc.

— —**With Quiet Grief.**—Alum., Ars., *Aur.*, Bell., **Cocc.**, **Coloc.**, Hyos., IGN., LYC., Nat. c., Nat. m., Nux v., Phos., **Pho. ac.**, Plat., Puls., Staph., Verat. a.

— —**With Indignation.**—COLOC., Ip., **Nux v.**, *Plat.*, STAPH.

— —**With Violence.**—ACON., *Aur.*, *Bell.*, Bry., CHAM., **Coff.**, Hyos., *Lyc.*, Nat. m., NUX V., *Phos.*, Sep., Sul., Verat. a , Zinc.

Exertion, Mental.—*Acon.*, *Aconin.*, *Agar.*, Agn., *Ambr.*, Am. carb., Anac., Arg., Arn., *Ars.*, *Asar.*, *Aur.*, Bell., *Bor.*, Calad., CALC. C., Carb. v., Cham., *Chin.*, *Cina*, **Cocc.**, Coff., Colch., *Cup.*, *Dig.*, *Gel.*, Hell., IGN., Iod., K. carb., *Lach.*, Laur., **Lyc.**, *Mag. c.*, Mag. m., Mang., *Meli.*, *Meny.*, Nat. c., **Nat. m.**, *Nux m.*, NUX V., *Oleand.*, *Par.*, *Petrol* , Phos., **Pho. ac.**, *Pic. ac.*, *Plat.*, Puls., **Pso.**, *Ran. b.*, **Saba.**, *Sel.*, SEP, Sil., Stan., *Staph.*, Sul., Tar., Zinc.

—**Physical.**—*Acon.*, *Aconin.*, **Agar.**, *Alum.*, Ambr., Am. carb., **Am. m.**, Ant. cr., ARN., ARS., Asaf., Asar., Aur., Bor., Bov., BRY., *Calc. c.*,

Calc. ph., **Cannab. s.**, Caust., Chin., Cic., Cina, **Cocc.**, *Coff.*, Colch., Con., *Croc.*, Euphr., Fer., Graph., Hell., *Hep.*, Ign., *Iod.*, *Ip.*, K. nit., Kalm., Kre., Lach., Led., *Lil. t.*, **Lyc.**, **Merc.**, Mur. ac., *Nat. c.*, **NAT. M.**, *Nit. ac.*, **Nux m.**, Nux v., *Oleand.*, **Ox. ac.**, Phos., **Pic. ac.**, **Plat.**, Puls., Rheum, *Rhodo.*, **RHUS**, Ruta, Saba., **Sabi.**, **Sang.**, Sars., Sec. c., **Sep.**, Sil., Spig., *Spo.*, *Squ.*, Staph., **SUL.**, Sul. ac., **Thuj.**, *Verat. a.*, Zinc.

Exertion Of Vision.—*Agar.*, Agn., Alum., Am. carb., Am. m., Anac., *Apis*, Arg., **Asaf.**, Asar., **Aur.**, *Bar. c.*, **Bell.**, *Bor.*, Bry., **CALC. C.**, *Canth.*, **Carb. v.**, **Caust.**, Cham., Chel., Chin., **Cic.**, **CINA**, Cocc., Coff., *Con.*, **CROC.**, Cup., *Dros.*, *Dulc.*, Fer., **Graph.**, Hep., *Ign.*, **K. CARB.**, Kre., Laur., Led., **LYC.**, Mag. c., Mag. m., Mang., Meny., Merc., Mez., Mos., *Mur. ac.*, **Nat. c.**, **NAT. M.**, Nit. ac., Nux m., Nux v., *Oleand.*, Par., *Petrol.*, **Phos.**, Pho. ac., *Phys.*, Plat., *Puls.*, *Ran. b.*, Rheum, **RHODO.**, **Rhus**, **RUTA**, *Saba.*, **Sars.**, Sele., **SENEG.**, **Sep.**, **SIL.**, **Spig.**, Spo. **Staph.**, Stram., Stro., *Sul.*, *Sul. ac.*, Thuj., *Valer.*, Verb., Vio. o., Zinc.

Expanding Abdomen.—Ign.

Expectoration.—*Dig.*, Led., Nux v.

—**After.**—Calad., Chin., *Sep.*, *Sul.*

Expiration.—Agn., Ambr., Anac., Ant. cr., *Ant. t.*, Arg., Ars., *Asaf.*, Aur., *Bry.*, **Cannab. s.**, Carb. v., *Caust.*, Cham., Chel., *Chin.*, Cic., *Cina*, Clem., Coff., **COLCH.**, Dig., **Dros.**, *Dulc.*, Euphr., **Ign.**, **Iod.**, Kre. Laur., Led., *Mang.*, Mur. ac., Nat. c., *Nux v.*, **Oleand.**, *Pho. ac.*, **PULS.**, Rhus, *Ruta*, *Saba.*, **Sep.**, **SPIG.**, Spo., *Squ.*, Stan., **Staph.**, Tar., *Verat. a.*, Vio. o., Vio. t., Zinc.

Fainting, After.—Acon., Ars., *Chin.*, **Mos.**, Nux v., **Op.**, *Sep.*, Stram.

Fasting (Before Breakfast).—Acon., *Aloe*, Alum., *Ambr.*, Am. carb., *Am. m.*, Anac., Ars., **Bar. c.**, Bov., Bry., **CALC. C.**, **Cannab. s.**, Canth., *Carb. an.*, *Carb. ac.*, Carb. v., Caust., **Chel.**, Chin., Cina, Coc. c., **CROC.**, Fer., *Fer. ph.*, *Gran.*, Graph., Hell., *Hep.*, Ign., **IOD.**, K. carb., Lach., *Laur.*, Lyc., Mag. c., Mag. m., Mar., Merc., *Mez.*, Nat. c., Nit. ac., *Nux v.*, *Petrol.*, Phos., **Plat.**, *Pb.*, Puls., **Ran. b.**, Ran. s., *Rhodo.*, Rhus, Rumex, Saba., Sep., Spig., **STAPH.**, *Stro.*, *Sul.*, **Tab.**, Tar., *Valer*, Verat. a., Verb.

Fatigue.—Arn., Ars, *Cannab. s.*, *Chin.*, **Coff.**, *Epiph.*, **RHUS**, *Verat. a.*

Feather-bed.—Cocc., Coloc., *Led.*, *Lyc.*, **MANG.**, Merc., Sul.

Fever, Before, During and After. (See under **Fever.**)

Food and Drink, Alcoholic Stimulants in General.—Acon., **Agar.**,

AGGRAVATIONS.

Alum., Am. m., Anac., Ant. cr., Arg. n., *Arn.*, Ars., Bell., *Bor.*, *Bov.*, Calc. c., Carb. an., *Carb. v.*, Caust., Chel., Chin., *Chloral*, *Cocc.*, Coff., Con., Hep., *Hyos.*, Ign., *K. bi.*, LACH., Laur., Led., Lyc., *Naj.*, Nat. c., Nat. m., Nux m., NUX V., OP., Petrol., Puls., RAN. B., Rhodo., Rhus, Ruta, *Saba.*, Sele., Sep., Sil., Spig., Stram., *Stro*, *Strop*, Sul., Sul. ac., *Tab.*, *Thuj.*, Verat. a., Zinc.

Food and Drink, Beans and Peas.—*Ars.*, BRY., Calc. c., Carb.v., *Chin.*, Cup., Hell., *K. carb.*, LYC., *Nat. m.*, Petrol., Puls., Sep., Sil., Verat. a.

—**Beer.**—Acon., *Ars.*, Asaf., Bell., Bry., *Cad. s.*, *Carb. sul.*, *Chel.*, *Chloral*, Chin., *Coc. c.*, *Coloc.*, *Crot. tig.*, Euphorb., Fer., Ign., Lyc., *Mar.*, *Mez.*, Mur. ac., Nux v., Puls., Rhus, Sep., Sil., Stan., Staph., Stram., Sul., *Verat. a.*

— —**Fresh.**—*Chin.*, Lyc., Mar., *Puls.*

—**Brandy.**—*Agar.*, Ars., Bell., Calc. c., *Chel.*, *Chin.*, *Cocc.*, Hep., Hyos., Ign., Lach., Laur., Led., NUX V., OP., *Puls.*, Ran. b., Rhodo., Rhus, Ruta, Spig., Stram., *Sul.*, *Sul. ac.*, *Verat. a.*, Zinc.

—**Bread.**—BRY., *Carb. an.*, Caust., Chin., Clem., Coff., *Crot. tig.*, K. carb., Mar., Merc., Nat. m., Nit. ac., Nux v., Oleand., Phos., Pho. ac., PULS., Ran. s., Rhus, *Ruta*, Sars., Sec. c., Sep., Staph., Sul., Sul. ac., Zinc.

— —**Black.**—Bry., *Ign.*, K. carb., Lyc., Nat. m., Nit. ac., Nux v., Phos., Pho. ac., Puls., Sul.

— —**And Butter.**—Carb. an., Caust., Chin., *Crot. tig.*, Cyc., Meny., Nat. m., Nit. ac., Nux v., Phos., PULS., Sep., Sul.

—**Buckwheat.**—Ip., PULS., *Verat. a.*

—**Butter.**—Acon., Ant. cr., Ant. t., Ars., *Asaf.*, Bell., Carb. an., CARB. V., Caust., Chin., Colch., Cyc., *Dros.*, Euphorb., Fer., *Hell.*, Hep., Ip., *Mag. m.*, Meny., Nat. c., Nat. m., Nit. ac., Nux v., Phos., PULS., Sep., *Spo.*, *Sul.*, Tar., *Thuj.*

—**Cabbage.**—Ars., BRY., Calc. c., Carb. v., Chin., *Cup.*, Hell., K. carb., LYC., Nat. m., PETROL., Puls., Sep., Sil., Verat. a.

—**Carrots.**—*Calc. c.*, *Lyc.*

—**Cheese, Old.**—Ars., Bry., Pho. ac., *Rhus.*

— —**Strong.**—*Coloc.*

—**Coffee.**—*All. c.*, Ars., *Arum t.*, Bell., Calc. c., CANTH., *Caps.*, *Carb. v.*, CAUST., CHAM., *Cist.*, Cocc., Colch., *Coloc.*, *Form.*, *Glon.*, Hep., IGN., Ip., *K. bi.*, *K. nit.*, Lyc., Mag. c., Mang., Merc., Nit. ac., NUX V., *Ox. ac.*, *Pho. ac.*, *Plat.*, Puls., *Rhus*, Sep., *Stram.*, Sul., Sul. ac.

— —**Odor of,**—*Sul. ac.*

—**Cold.**—*Ac. ac.*, *Agar.*, Alum., *Ant. cr.*, *Arg. n.*, ARS., Bar. c., Bov.,

AGGRAVATIONS. 283

Bry., *Calad.*, Calc. c., *Calc. f.*, *Canth.*, Carb. v., Caust., Cham., *Chel.*, *Coc. c.*, Con., Graph., Hell., *Ign.*, K. carb., *K. nit.*, **Kre.**, LACH., LYC., Mag. c., Mag. m., **Mang.**, *Merc.*, *Mur. ac.*, Nat. c., Nat. m., *Nat. s.*, **Nit. ac.**, Nux m., NUX V., Par., Pho. ac., *Pb.*, Puls., Rhodo., RHUS, *Saba.*, Sep., SIL., Spig., Sul., *Sul. ac.*, Thuj., **Verat. a.**

Food and Drink, Crumbs.—*Nux v.*, Staph.

—**Dry.**—*Agar.*, CALC. C., *Chin.*, *Ip.*, **Lyc.**, **Nat. c.**, Nit. ac., *Nux v.*, Petrol., *Pho. ac.*, Puls., Sars., *Sil.*, Sul.

—**Eggs.**—Colch., *Fer.*

— —**Odor Of.**—Colch.

—**Farinaceous.**—*Sul.*

—**Fat.**—*Acon.*, Ant. cr., Ant. t., **Ars.**, **Asaf.**, Bell., Bry., *Carb. an.*, CARB. V., Caust., Chin., **Colch.**, CYC., Dros., *Euphorb.*, FER., **Hell.**, Hep., *Ip.*, K. carb., *K. m.*, Mag. c., **Mag. m.**, Meny., Merc., *Merc. c.*, Nat. c., *Nat. m.*, **Nit. ac.**, *Nux v.*, *Phos.*, PULS., Ruta, Sep., Sil., Spo., Staph., Sul., TAR., Thuj., Verat. a.

—**Fish.**—*Carb. an.*, *K. carb.*, **Pb.**

— —**Shell.**—**Lyc.**, *Urt.*

— —**Spoiled.**—Ars., Carb. v., *Chin.*, Puls.

—**Flatulent.**—Ars., Bry., *Calc. c.*, Carb. v., *Chin.*, Cup., Hell., *K. carb.*, **Lyc.**, Nat. m., Petrol., *Puls.*, *Sep.*, Sil., Verat. a.

—**Frozen.**—Ars., *Carb v.*, PULS.

—**Fruit.**—ARS., Bor., BRY., Calc. ph., Carb. v., CHIN., COLOC., Cub., Ign., Kre., *Lyc.*, Mag. m., **Nat. c.**, Phos., PULS., Rheum, *Rhodo.*, Ruta, Sele., Sep., Tar., VERAT. A.

—**Garlick, Odor of.**—Saba.

—**Heavy.**—*Bry.*, Calc. c., **Caust.**, Cup., IOD., *Lyc.*, Nat. c., **Puls.**, Sul.

—**Honey.**—Nat. c.

—**Hot.**—*Arum. t.*, Bry., Caps., *Carb. v.*, *Coff.*, Fer., Nat. *s.*, *Phyt.*, Puls., Sep.

—**Hot Cakes.** *K. carb.*, Puls.

—**Iron, Cooked In.**—Sul.

—**Lemonade.**—Sele.

—**Meat.**—Carb. an., Caust., **Colch.**, Fer., K. bi., *Mag. c.*, *Mag. m.*, Merc., Puls., *Ruta*, Sil., Staph., *Sul.*

— —**Bad.**—Carb. v., *Chin.*, Puls.

— —**Fresh.**—Caust.

— —**Odor of Cooking.**—Ars., *Colch.*

—**Milk.**—*Alum.*, Ambr., *Ant. t.*, Ars., Bry., CALC. C., Carb. an., Carb. v., Cham., Chel., CHIN., CON., Cup., Hell., *Ign.*, **K. carb.**,

Lach., **Lyc., Nat. c., Nat. m., NIT. AC.,** Nux m., **Nux v., Phos.,** *Puls.,* Rhus, Sabi , *Samb.,* **SEP.,** *Sil.,* *Spo.,* **SUL.,** *Sul. ac.,* Zinc.

Food and Drink, Odor of, and of the Cooking.—Cocc., **COLCH.,** *Merc. i. f.*

—**Oil.**—Bry., *Canth.,* **Puls.**

—**Onions.**—Thuj.

—**Oysters.**—**Lyc.,** *Sul. ac.*

—**Pan-cakes.**—Bry., Ip., *K. carb.,* **PULS.,** **Verat. a.**

—**Pastry.**—Ars., Carb. v., *K. m., Phos.,* Puls.

—**Pears.**—*Bor.,* Bry., **Verat. a.**

—**Pepper.**—Ars., **Cina,** *Nat. c., Sep.,* Sil.

—**Pork.**—Acon., *Ant. cr.,* Ant. t., *Ars.,* Asaf., Bell., **CARB. V.,** Caust., Colch., *Cyc.,* Ip., **Nat. c., Nat. m., PULS., SEP.,** *Tar.,* **Thuj.**

—**Potatoes.**—Alum., Am. m., *Coloc.,* **Sep., Verat. a.**

—**Raw.**—Ars., *Bry.,* Chin., *Lyc.,* Puls., **RUTA, Verat. a.**

—**Salad.**—*Ars.,* Bry., Calc. c., Carb. v., *Lach.,* Lyc.

—**Salt.**—*Ars.,* *Calc. c.,* **Carb. v., Dros.,** *Lyc.,* Nux v.

—**Sausages, Spoiled.**—Ars., **BELL.,** Bry., Pho. ac., *Rhus.*

—**Sight of.**—*Merc. i. f.,* SUL.

—**Smoked.**—Calc. c., Sil.

—**Sour.**—**ANT. CR., Arg. n., Ars.,** Bell., *Bor., Caust., Cub., Dros.,* Fer., *Fer. ph.,* Kre., *Lach.,* Merc. c., Nat. c., *Nat. m., Nux v.,* Phos , *Pho. ac.,* Ran. b., *Sele.,* Sep., Staph., Sul.

—**Sour Kraut.**—Ars., **BRY., Calc. c.,** Carb. v., **Chin.,** Cup., **Hell.,** Lyc., *Nat. m.,* **PETROL., Phos., Puls.,** Sep , Verat. a.

—**Sour Odors.**—*Dros.*

—**Spices.**—*Phos.*

—**Sweats.**—*Acon.,* Am. carb., **Ant. cr., Arg. n.,** *Calc. c.,* **Cham., IGN., Merc.,** *Nat. c., Ox. ac., Phos.,* **Sele.,** *Spig.,* **Zinc.**

—**Tea.**—*Chin., Coff., Dios.,* **Fer.,** Lach., *Rumex,* SELE , *Strop.,* **Thuj.,** *Verat. a.*

—**Thought of Food She Would Like.**—SEP.

—**Tobacco.**—*Acon.,* Agar., *Alum.,* Ambr., **Ant. cr., Arg., Arg. n.,** Bell., **Bry.,** *Calc. c.,* Camph., Carb. an., *Carb. sul.,* *Chin.,* Cic., **Clem.,** *Coca,* **Cocc.,** *Coc. c., Coloc., Con.,* **Cyc.,** *Dig.,* Euphr., Fer., Gel., Hell., Hep., *Hydras.,* **IGN.,** *Iod.,* Ip., Lach., Mag. c., **Menth., Meny.,** Nat. m., **NUX V.,** *Osm.,* Par., *Petrol.,* **Phos., PULS.,** *Ran. b., Rhus,* Ruta, Saba., *Sabi.,* *Sars.,* **Sele.,** *Sep., Sil.,* **SPIG., SPO.,** *Strop.,* **STAPH.,** *Sul., Sul. ac.,* Tar., Thuj., Verat. a.

— —**Chewing.**—Ars., *Verat. a.*

AGGRAVATIONS. 285

Food and Drink, Turnips.— *Bry.*, **Puls.**

—**Veal.**—*Ars.*, **Calc. c.**, **Caust.**, Chin., IP., **K. NIT.**, Nux v., Sep., *Sul.*, Verat. a., **Zinc.**

—**Vegetables** (Green).—*Ars.*, **Bry.**, *Cup.*, **Hell.**, Lyc., **Nat. c.**, *Verat. a.*

—**Vinegar.**—*Aloe*, ANT. CR., **Ars.**, **Bell.**, *Bor.*, *Caust.*, *Dros.*, **Fer.**, Kre., *Lach.*, Nat. c., *Nat. m.*, *Nux v.*, Phos., *Pho. ac.*, Ran. b., **Sep.**, *Staph.*, **Sul.**

—**Warm.**—Acon., *Agn.*, *All. c.*, Alum., **Ambr.**, *Am. carb.*, **Anac.**, *Ant. t.*, Ars., *Asar.*, **Bar. c.**, **Bell.**, *Bism.*, Bor., BRY., **Calc. c.**, *Canth.*, **Carb. v.**, *Caust.*, **Cham.**, Clem., **Cup.**, Dros., **Euphorb.**, *Fer.*, *Gran.*, *Hell.*, **K. carb.**, LACH., *Laur.*, Mag. c., Mag. m., *Merc.*, **Mez.**, Nat. m., **Nit. ac.**, Nux m., Nux v., Par., PHOS., **Pho. ac.**, PULS., Rhodo., **Rhus**, Sars., Sep., Sil., Spig., Squ., *Stan.*, *Sul.*, Sul. ac., Thuj., Verat. a., Zinc.

—**Water, Cold.**—Agar., **Alum.**, Anac., **Ant. cr.**, *Apis*, **Ars.**, Bell., Bor., Calc. c., *Calc. ph.*, CANTH., *Carb. an.*, Clem., *Cocc.*, *Coloc.*, *Croc.*, FER., *Grat.*, Hyos., **Ign.**, K. carb., **Lyc.**, Mang., **Mar.**, Merc., Mur. ac., *Nat. c.*, *Nux m.*, **Nux v.**, *Pho. ac.*, *Puls.*, **Rhodo.**, RHUS, Sars., Sil., Spig., Stram., **Sul.**, *Sul. ac.*, *Thuj.*, *Verat. a.*

—**Wine.**—Acon., Am. m., **Ant. cr.**, Arn., ARS., Bell., **Bor.**, *Bov.*, Bry., **Calc. c.**, Carb. an., *Carb. v.*, *Carb. sul.*, *Chloral.*, *Coc. c.*, **Coff.**, *Coloc.*, Con., **Lach.**, Led., LYC., *Naj.*, **Nat. c.**, **Nat. m.**, Nux m., NUX V., OP, Petrol., **Puls.**, RAN. B., **Rhodo.**, Rhus, *Ruta*, **Saba.**, Sele., SIL., Stro., Verat. a., ZINC.

— —**Containing Lead.**—Alum., Ars., **Bell.**, Chin., *Nux v.*, **Op.**, *Plat.*, **Sul.**, Sul. ac.

— —**Containing Sulphur.**—*Ars.*, Chin., **Merc.**, PULS., *Sep.*

— —**Sour.**—ANT. CR., **Ars.**, *Fer.*, Sep., *Sul.*

Glanders.—Ars., Calc. c., *Pho. ac.*, Sul.

Gargling.—Carb. v.

Grasping Anything Tightly.—*Coff.*, RHUS. Spig.

Hang Down, Letting Limbs.—Alum., **Am. carb.**, CALC. C., *Caust.*, Cina, Dig., Hep., *Ign.*, *Lyc.*, Nat. m., Nux v., *Ox. ac.*, Par., *Phos.*, Pho. ac., *Phyt.*, Plat., *Pb.*, Puls., *Ran. s.*, *Ruta*, **Sabi.**, Stan., Stro., Sul., Sul. ac., *Thuj.*, Valer., **Vip.**

Heated, Becoming.—Acon., Am. carb., ANT. CR., **Bell.**, BRY., *Caps.*, **Carb. v.**, Coff., **Dig.**, Hep., *Ign.*, Ip., **K. CARB.**, Mez., *Nat. m.*, Nux m., Nux v., Oleand., **Op.**, PULS., Sep., *Sil.*, Staph., **Thuj.**, **Zinc.**

—**By the Fire.**—Ant. cr., *Bry.*, **Con.**, Euphorb., Mag. m., **Merc.**, Puls., Zinc.

AGGRAVATIONS.

Hiccough.—Acon., AM. M., *Bell.*, Bor., **Bry.**, *Cic.*, **Cocc.**, *Cup.*, **Cyc.**, **Hyos.**, Ign., Lyc., *Mag. m.*, **Mar.**, Merc., Nat. c., **Nux m.**, **Nux v.**, Par., *Puls.*, *Ran. b.*, Ruta, Sars., Spo., Staph., Stram., Stro., Sul., *Verat. a.*, Verb.

Holding Together Parts.—Ign., Staph.

House, In the.—*Abrot.*, Acon., *Agar.*, **Agn.**, **All. c.**, **Aloe**, **ALUM.**, *Ambr.*, Am. carb., *Am. m.*, Amyl, Anac., **Ant. cr.**, *Apis*, **Arg.**, *Arn.*, ARS., **Asaf.**, Asar., Atrop., *Aur.*, *Bar. c.*, *Bell.*, Bor., *Bov.*, **Bry.**, **Cact.**, *Caj.*, Calc. c., Camph., CANNAB. I., Cannab. s., Canth., Caps., *Carb. ac.*, Carb. an., Carb. v., *Carb. sul.*, *Caust.*, **Chel.**, Chlorum, *Cic.*, **Cimic.**, Cina, *Clem.*, *Coca*, *Coc. c.*, **Coff.**, *Colch.*, *Coloc.*, *Com.*, **Con.**, CROC., *Dig.*, **Dios.**, Dulc., *Euphr.*, **Gam.**, *Gel.*, *Gr. ph.*, **Hell.**, Hep., **Hyd. ac.**, Hyos., Ign., *Iod.*, Ip., K. bi., K. carb., *K. iod.*, K. nit., *Lach*, *Laur.*, Lyc., MAG. C., **Mag. m.**, Mang., **Meli.**, *Meny.*, Merc., *Merc. i. r.*, **Mez.**, *Mos.*, Mur. ac., *Myr.*, *Naph.*, Nat. c., *Nat. m.*, *Nat. s.*, Nit. ac., *Nux v.*, *Op.*, **Osm.**, Phos., *Pho. ac.*, **Phyt.**, *Pic. ac.*, *Plat.*, *Pb.*, PULS., *Ran. b.*, **Ran. s.**, *Rat.*, *Rhodo.*, RHUS, Ruta, SABA., SABI., *Sal. ac.*, *Sang.*, *Sars.*, Sele., **Seneg.**, Sep., Spig., **Spo.**, *Stan.*, Staph., *Stro.*, *Sul.*, Sul. ac., **Tab.**, *Tar.*, Tell., *Thuj.*, *Trill.*, *Verat. a.*, *Verb.*, **Vib. op.**, Vio. t., **Zinc.**

Hunger.—*Aur.*, *Cact.*, Canth., *Caust.*, *Graph.*, Hell., Iod., K. carb., *Oleand.*, Plat., *Rhus*, **Sil.**, **Spig.**, Verat. a.

Idleness.—*Alum.*, Bar. c., **Con.**, *Croc.*, Fer., **Ign.**, Lyc., Mag. m., Nat. c., Nat. m., **Nux v.**, Petrol., *Pb.*, SEP., *Sil.*, Tar., *Verat. a.*

Injuries (Including Blows, Falls and Bruises).—ARN., Bor., Bry., Calc. c., Canth., Carb. v., *Cham.*, Chin., *Cir.*, CON., Croc., **Dulc.**, *Euphr*, HEP., Hyos., **Iod.**, K. carb., Kre., **Lach.**, *Led.*, Laur., Lyc., Merc., Mez., Nat. c., Nat. m., Nit. ac., Nux v., Par., **Phos.**, Pho. ac., Plat., Pb., PULS., RHUS, **Ruta**, *Samb.*, Sec. c., Seneg., *Sil.*, Staph., **Sul.**, SUL. AC., Verat. a., Zinc.

—**Bleeding Profusely.**—Arn., **Carb. v.**, Croc., *Hep.*, Kre., LACH., Merc., Nat. m., PHOS., *Pho. ac.*, Puls., Rhus, **Sul.**, *Sul. ac.*, Zinc.

—**With Extravasations.**—ARN., *Bry.*, Cham., Chin., **Con.**, *Dulc.*, Euphr., Fer., Hep., *Lach.*, **Laur.**, *Nux v.*, Par., Pb., Puls., *Rhus*, Ruta, Sec. c., Sul., SUL. AC.

—**Of Soft Parts.**—ARN., Cham., **Con.**, Dulc., Euphr., *Lach.*, **Puls.**, *Samb.*, Sul., Sul. ac.

Inspiration.—ACON., Agar., Agn., Alum., Am. carb., *Am. m.*, Anac., Arg., Arn., Ars., *Asaf.*, **Asar.**, Aur., *Bar. c.*, **Bor.**, Bov., BRY., Calc. c., *Camph.*, Cannab. s., *Canth.*, **Caps.**, **Carb. an.**, Carb. v., **Caust.**, **Cham.**, **Chel.**, *Chin.*, Cic., *Cimic.*, **Cina**, Clem., Cocc., Colch., Coloc.,

Con., *Croc.*, *Cup.*, *Oyc.*, Dros., *Dulc.*, *Euphr.*, Guai., *Hell.*, *Hyos.*, Ign., Iod., Ip., K. carb., K. nit., Kre., Laur., Led., Lyc., Mag. c., Mag. m., Mar., Menth., Meny., Merc., Mez., *Mos.*, Mur. ac., Nat. c., Nat. m., Nit. ac., *Nux m.*, Nux v., *Oleand.*, *Op.*, Osm., Par., Phos., *Pho. ac.*, *Plat.*, *Pb.*, Puls., RAN. B., *Ran. s.*, Rhodo., RHUS, Ruta, Saba., SABI., *Sars.*, Sele., Seneg., Sep., Sil., SPIG., Spo., SQU., Stan., Stro., Sul., *Sul. ac.*, Tar., Valer., *Verat. a.*, Verb., Vio. t., Zinc.

Inspection Of Cold Air.—Alum., Ant. cr., Ars., Aur., Bell., Bry., Calc. c., *Camph.*, CAUST., Cham., *Cina*, Dulc., Hep., HYOS., K. carb., MERC., *Mos.*, Nat. m., Nux m., NUX V., Par., *Petrol.*, Phos., Puls., Rhodo., Rhus, SABA., *Sars.*, Seneg., Sep., *Sil.*, *Spig.*, Staph., Stro., Sul., Thuj., *Verat. a.*

Intoxication, After.—Acon., *Agar.*, Am. m., Arg., *Bell.*, Bry., Carb. v., *Chin.*, Cocc., Coff., *Ip.*, K. carb., *K. nit.*, *Kre.*, Laur., Mar., Nat. m., Nux m., NUX V., OP., Pho. ac., Puls., *Rheum*, Samb., Spo., Squ., Stram., *Valer.*

Jar.—Acon., Arg. n., ARN., Bell., Bry., CIC., *Glon.*, Hep., *Ign.*, Lil. t., Nux v., *Pho. ac.*, Onos., Rhus, *Ruta.*

Jumping.—*Spig.*

Kneeling.—Cocc., Mag. c., *Sep.*

Labor, Manual.—Am. m., Bov., Fer., *K. carb.*, Lach., Mag. c., *Merc.*, NAT. M., *Nit. ac.*, Sil., Verat. a.

Laughing.—*Acon.*, Arg., Ars., Aur., Bell., BOR., Carb. v., Chin., Coloc., Con., *K. carb.*, Laur., Mang., Mez., *Mos.*, *Mur. ac.*, Nat. m., Nux v., PHOS., Pb., Stan., Sul., Zinc.

Leaning (Against Anything).—Arg., *Arn.*, Bell., Cannab. s., *Cyc.*, Hep., Nit. ac., SAMB., Staph.

—After.—Coloc.

—Backward.—*Nit. ac.*, Staph.

—Against a Sharp Point.—Agar., Samb.

—To One Side.—Meny.

Licking Lips.—Valer.

Lifting.—Alum., *Ambr.*, Arn., *Bar. c.*, Bor., Bry., CALC. C., *Carb. an.*, Carb. v., *Caust.*, Chin., Cocc., Coloc., Con., *Croc.*, Cupr., Dulc., Fer., Graph., *Iod.*, K. carb., Lach., Lyc., Merc., *Mur. ac.*, Nat. c., *Nat. m.*, Nit. ac., *Nux v.*, Oleand., *Phos.*, Pho. ac., Plat., Rhodo., RHUS, Ruta, Sep., Sil., Spig., *Stan.*, Staph., *Sul.*, Sul. ac., Thuj., *Valer.*

Light in General.—Acon., Agar., *Agn.*, Alum., Am. carb., *Am. m.*, Anac., Ant. cr., Arn., Ars., *Asar.*, Bar. c., BELL., *Bor.*, *Bry.*, *Cact.*, CALC. C., Camph., Carb. an., *Caust.*, Cham., Chin., Cic., *Cina*, Clem.,

Cocc., *Coff.*, Colch., CON., **Croc.**, Cup., *Dig.*, **Dros.**, EUPHR., *Glon.*, GRAPH., *Hell*, Hep., *Hyos.*, Ign., K. carb., K. nit., Lach., *Laur.*, Lyc., Mag. c., *Mag. m.*, *Mang.*, **Merc.**, Mez., Mur. ac., **Nat. c.**, Nat. m., *Nit. ac.*, Nux m., **Nux v.**, Petrol., PHOS., **Pho. ac.**, Plat., **Puls.**, Rhodo., Rhus, Ruta, Samb., *Sars.*, Sele., *Seneg.*, **Sep.**, **Sil.**, *Spig.*, Stan., Staph., Stram., **Sul.**, Sul. ac., Tar., Thuj., Valer., Verat. a., Zinc.

Light, Candle or Lamp.—Agn., Am. m., Anac., **Bar. c.**, **Bell.**, *Bor.*, CALC. C., Carb. an., *Caust.*, *Cina*, *Com.*, CON., Croc., DROS., Graph., Hep., Ign., K. carb., *Laur.*, LYC., Mang., MERC., Mez., *Nit. ac.*, Nux m., Petrol., PHOS., **Pho. ac.**, Plat., *Puls.*, RUTA., *Sars.*, *Seneg.*, SEP., **Sil.**, **STRAM.**, *Sul.*

—**Day.**—Am. m., **Ant. cr.**, **Calc. c.**, CON., Dros., EUPHR., GRAPH., *Hell.*, HEP., *Hyos.*, Mag. c., Mang., *Merc.*, Nit. ac., NUX V., Petrol., PHOS., *Pho. ac.*, *Rhodo.*, Samb., *Sars.*, **Sep.**, SIL., *Stram.*, *Sul.*, Thuj.

—**Of Fire.**—**Ant. cr.**, *Bry.*, Euphorb., Mag. m., MERC., *Puls.*, Zinc.

—**Sun.**—*Acon.*, Agar., **Ant. cr.**, Ars., *Asar.*, **Bar. c.**, *Bry.*, CALC. C., *Camph*, Chin., CON., EUPHR., GRAPH., Ign., *Lach.*, Mag. m., **Nat. c.**, Nux v., PHO. AC., **Puls.**, *Sele.*, Seneg., Stan., *Stram.*, Sul., *Valer.*, Verat. a., Zinc.

Looking Around.—*Calc. c.*, **Cic.**, CON., *Ip.*, K. carb.

—**At Distant Objects.**—*Euphr.*, Ruta.

—**Downward.**—*Acon.*, Calc. c., Oleand., *Phyt.*, **Spig.**, SUL.

—**Straight Forward.**—Oleand.

—**Over a Large Surface.**—Sep.

—**At a Bright Light.**—Am. m., Bell., **Bry.**, Calc. c., *Caust.*, *Chel.*, Colch., Ign., *K. carb.*, Kre., **Mag. m.**, **Merc.**, *Nux v.*, Phos., *Pho. ac.*, Saba., Sep., Zinc.

—**Long at Anything.**—Aur., *Cic.*, *Gel.*, Kre., **Nat. m.**, Rheum, Ruta, Spig.

—**At Running Water.**—*Arg.*, BELL., Fer., **Hyos.**, Stram., *Sul.*

—**At Shining Objects.**—BELL., Canth., **Hyos.**, Lach., *Phos.*, Stram.

—**Sideways.**—Bell., *Oleand.*, Spig.

—**At Something Turning Around.**—Lyc.

—**Upward.**—Alum, Ars., CALC. C., *Caps.*, Carb. v., Caust., **Chel.**, **Cup.**, Graph., Petrol., **Phos.**, Plat., *Pb.*, Puls., Saba., Sabi., **Sele.**, Sep., *Sil.*, *Spig.*, **Thuj.**, Zinc.

—**At White Objects.**—*Cham.*, Graph., K. carb., *Nat. m.*, Stram.

AGGRAVATIONS.

Loss of Fluids.—*Agar.*, Alum., Anac., Ant. cr., Ant. t., *Arg.*, Arn., **Ars.**, *Bell.*, Bor., *Bov.*, Bry., **Calad.**, CALC. C., Cannab. s., Canth., Caps., Carb. an., **Carb. v.**, Caust., Cham., CHIN., *Cina*, Coff., **Con.**, Dig., Dulc., *Fer.*, Graph., Hep., *Ign.*, Iod., Ip., **K. carb.**, Led., *Lyc.*, Mag. m., **Merc.**, Mez., Mos., *Nat. c.*, *Nat. m.*, Nit. ac., Nux m., **Nux v.**, Petrol., **Phos.**, PHO. AC., *Pb.*, PULS., *Ran. b.*, Rhodo., Rhus, Ruta, Saba., Samb., *Sele.*, SEP., **Sil.**, *Spig.*, **Squ.**, Stan., STAPH., **Sul.**, Thuj., Valer., Verat. a., *Zinc.*

Lying.—*Ab. n.*, **Acon.**, *Agar.*, Agn., *Alum.*, **Ambr.**, **Am. carb.**, **Am. m.**, Anac., *Ant. cr.*, *Ant. t.*, **Apis**, *Aral.*, **Arg.**, Arn., ARS., **Asaf.**, Asar., AUR., **Bap.**, Bar. c., **Bell.**, *Bism.*, *Bor.*, *Bov.*, **Bry.**, *Cact.*, Calad., Calc. c., *Calc. ph.*, Camph., *Cannab. i.*, Cannab. s., Canth., CAPS., Carb. an., *Carb. v.*, *Carb. sul.*, Caust., CHAM., Chel., Chin., Cic., Cina, *Clem.*, Cocc., Coff., Colch., *Coloc.*, CON., Croc., *Crot. tig.*, *Cup.*, **Cyc.**, Dig., *Dios.*, DROS., Dulc., EUPHORB., **Euphr.**, FER., **Glon.**, Graph., *Grind.*, Guai., **Hell.**, Hep., HYOS., *Ign.*, Iod., Ip., **K. bi.**, **K. br.**, *K. carb.*, **K. nit.**, Kre., *Lach.*, *Laur.*, Led., LYC., **Mag. c.**, **Mag. m.**, Mang., *Mar.*, MENY., Merc., Mez., **Mos.**, **Mur. ac.**, *Naj.*, **Nat. c.**, Nat. m., NAT. S., *Nit. ac.*, Nux m., **Nux v.**, Oleand., *Op.*, Par., Petrol., *Phel.*, PHOS., Pho. ac., PLAT., Pb., PULS., *Raph.*, **Ran. b.**, Rheum, **Rhodo.**, RHUS, RUMEX, Ruta, Saba., Sabi., *Sul. ac.*, SAMB., SANG., Sars., Sec. c., Sele., Seneg., **Sep.**, **Sil.**, Spig., *Spo.*, Squ., *Stan.*, Staph., *Stict.*, Stram., Stro., Sul., Sul. ac., TAR., *Thuj.*, **Valer.**, Verat. a., **Verb.**, *Vio. o.*, Vio. t., *Zinc*, Zing,

After Lying Down.—*Acon.*, Agar., Agn., *Alum.*, AMBR., **Am. carb.**, Am. m., *Ant. cr.*, *Ant. t.*, **Arg.**, Arn., ARS., **Asaf.**, Asar., AUR., Bar. c., **Bell.**, *Bism.*, *Bor.*, Bov., Bry., Calad., Calc. c., Canth., **Caps.**, Carb. an., Carb. v., *Caust.*, **Cham.**, Chel., *Chin.*, **Clem.**, Cocc., Coff., Colch., *Coloc.*, Con., Croc., Cup., **Cyc.**, *Dros.*, DULC., **Euphorb.**, **Euphr.**, **Fer.**, Graph., Guai., Hell., Hep., **Hyos.**, *Ign.*, Ip., **K. carb.**, *K. nit.*, Lach., *Laur.*, *Led.*, LYC., **Mag. c.**, **Mag. m.**, Mang., *Mar.*, **Meny.**, Merc., *Mez.*, Mos., *Mur. ac.*, Nat. c., *Nit. ac.*, Nux m., Nux v., Oleand., *Op.*, Par., Petrol., Phos., *Pho. ac.*, PLAT., **Pb.**, **PULS.**, Ran. b., Ran. s., Rhodo., RHUS, *Ruta*, **Saba.**, Sabi., SAMB., Sars., Sele., Seneg., **Sep.**, Sil., Spig., *Stan.*, Staph., STRO., **Sul.**, **Sul. ac.**, **Tar.**, Thuj., *Valer.*, Verat. a., **Verb.**, *Vio. o.*, Vio. t., Zinc.

—In Bed.—*Acon.*, Agar., *Agn.*, *Aloe*, *Alum.*, AMBR., **Am. carb.**, **Am. m.**, Anac., Ans. cr., **Ant. t.**, **Arg.**, Arn., *Arn.*, **Asaf.**, *Asar.*, **Aur.**, Bar. c., Bell., Bism., **Bor.**, *Bov.*, **Bry.**, *Calad.*, **Calc. c.**, Camph., Cannab. s., Canth., *Caps.*, **Carb. an.**, **Carb. v.**, Caust., **Cham.**, *Chel.*, **Chin.**, Cic.,

Cina, **Clem.**, Cocc., *Coff.*, Colch., **Coloc.**, *Con.*, Croc., *Cyc.*, **Dig.**, *Dios.*, **Dros.**, *Dulc.*, **Euphorb.**, *Euphr.*, **Fer.**, *Graph.*, Guai., *Hell.*, Hep., *Hyos.*, *Ign.*, IOD., **K. carb** , *K. iod.*, *K. nit.*, **Kalm.**, Kre., LACH., *Laur.*, Led., Lil. t., Lith., **LYC.**, **Mag. c.**, Mag. m., **Mang.**, *Mar.*, *Meny.*, MERC., **Merc. i. f.**, **Mez.**, *Mos.*, *Mur. ac.*, *Nat. c.*, **Nat. m.**, Nit. ac., Nux m., **Nux v.**, Oleand., *Op.*, Ox. ac., *Par.*, *Petrol.*, PHOS., **Pho. ac.**, *Phyt.*, **Plat.**, **Pb.**, **PULS**, *Ran. b.*, *Rheum*, **Rhodo.**, Rhus, RUMEX, *Ruta*, Saba., *Sabi.*, *Samb.*, SANG., **Sars.**, *Sec. c.*, **Sele.**, *Seneg.*, SEP., SIL., **Spig.**, Spo., Squ., **Stan.**, Staph., Stict., Stram., **Stro.**, SUL., *Sul. ac.*, Tar., **Tell.**, *Thuj*, *Valer.*, **Verat. a.**, *Verb.*, *Vio. o.*, Vio. t., **Zinc**.

Lying On Back.—*Acon.*, Aloe., Alum., Am. carb., Am. m., Arn., **Ars.**, Bar. c., Bell., Bor., Bry., *Cact.*, *Calc. ph.*, Canth., **Caust.**, **Cham.**, *Chin.*, Cina, Clem., Colch., **Coloc.**, **Cup.**, Dulc., *Eup. per.*, *Euphorb.*, *Ign.*, Iod., K. carb., **K. nit.**, Lach., Mag., m., *Merc.*, Nat. c., Nat. m., **NUX V.**, Par., PHOS., Plat., *Puls.*, Ran. b., Rhus, **Sep.**, **Sil.**, *Spig.*, Spo., *Stro.*, Sul., *Thuj*.

— **With Head Low.**—Ant. t., Arg., ARS., *Cannab. s.*, **Caps.**, **Chin.**, *Clem.*, Colch., *Glon.*, Hep., **K. nit.**, *Lach.*, *Nux v.*, *Petrol.*, Phos., PULS., *Samb.*, **Spig.**, *Spo.*, Stro., *Sul*.

— **On Side.**—ACON., Am. carb., Am. m., ANAC., Arn., Bar. c., Bell., Bor., BRY., **Calad.**, CALC. C, Canth., CARB. AN., Caust., Chin., **Cina**, Clem., Colch., **Con.**, Fer., Ign., **Ip.**, K. CARB., **Kre.**, Lach., LYC., Mag. m., **Merc.**, Merc. c., Mos., *Nat. c.*, Nat. m., *Nux v.*, **Par.**, *Phos.*, Plat., **Puls.**, *Ran. b.*, RHUS, *Saba.*, **Seneg.**, Sep., Sil., Spig., Spo., **STAN.**, Sul., Thuj., Verat. a., *Vio. t*.

— — **Left.**—Acon., Am. carb., Anac., *Ant. t.*, Arn., Bar. c., Bell., *Bry.*, **Cact.**, Calc. c., Canth., Carb. an., Chin., Colch., Con., *Ip.*, *K. carb.*, Kre., Lyc., Merc., **Nat. c.**, **Nat. m.**, Nat. s., *Op.*, Par., PHOS., Plat., **PULS**, *Rhus*, Seneg., **Sep.**, *Sil.*, Spig., *Stan.*, **Sul.**, Thuj.

— — **Right.**—*Acon.*, Am. m., Anac., Benz. ac., Bor., Bry., *Buf.*, Calc. c., Carb. an., *Caust.*, Cina, Clem., Con., *Crotal.*, Ip., *K. carb.*, Kre., Lach., Lyc., Mag. m., MERC., Nat. c., **Nux v.**, Phos., *Pso.*, Puls., Ran. b., Rumex., *Seneg.*, Spig., *Spo.*, *Stan.*, Sul., *Sul. ac.*, Thuj.

— — **Painful.**—Acon., *Agar.*, *Ambr.*, Am. carb., Am. m., Anac., Ant. cr., Arg., Arn., **Ars.**, Bap., BAR. C., *Bell.*, **Bry.**, CALAD., *Calc. c.*, *Calc. f.*, *Cannab. s.*, *Caps.*, Carb. an., *Carb. v.*, *Caust.*, **Chin.**, **Cina**, Clem., Croc., Cup., **Dros.**, Graph., *Guai.*, HEP., Hyos., *Ign.*, IOD., *K. carb.*, *K. nit.*, Lach., Led., **Lyc.**, **Mag. c.**, **Mag. m.**, Mang., Mar., **Merc.**, Mez., **Mos.**, Mur. ac., Nat. m., **Nit. ac.**, **NUX M.**, Nux v., Oleand., **Par.**, *Petrol.*, Phos., **Pho. ac.**, Plat., *Puls.*, Ran. b., Ran. s., **Rheum**,

Rhodo., **Rhus**, **Rumex**, **RUTA**, Saba., Sabi., Samb., Sars., *Sele.*, *Sep.,*
SIL., Spo., *Staph.*, Stram., Sul., Tar., *Thuj.*, Valer., Verat. a., Verb.

Lying On Side Painless.—Ambr., **Arg.**, *Arn.*, Bell., **BRY.**, **Calc. c.,**
Cannab. s., Carb. v., **Caust.**, **CHAM.**, **COLOC.**, Ign., **K. carb.**, Lyc.,
Nux v., **PULS.**, Rhus, Sep., Stan., Vio. o., **Vio. t.**

Lying-in-Women. (The Puerperal State.)—*Acon.*, *Ant. cr.*, Ant. t.,
Arn., Asaf., Asar., Aur., **BELL.**, Bor., Bov., **Bry.**, **Calc. c.**, Camph.,
Canth., **Carb. an.**, Carb. v., Caust., CHAM., *Chin.*, Cina, *Cocc.*, **Coff.,**
Colch., Coloc., *Con.*, **Croc.**, Cup., Dros., *Dulc.*, *Equis.*, **Fer.**, *Gel.,*
Glon., Graph., *Helo.*, Hep., **Hyos.**, *Ign.*, Iod., **Ip.**, **K. carb.**, *Kre.*, Lach.,
Lyc., Mag. c., Mag. m., Merc., *Mos.*, Mur. ac., Nat. c., *Nat. m.*, Nit. ac.,
Nux m., Nux v., *Op.*, **Phos.**, Pho. ac., **Plat.**, **PULS.**, Rheum, **RHUS**,
Ruta, Saba., **SABI.**, **SEC. C.**, **SEP.**, Sil., Stan., *Stram.*, **Sul.**, Sul. ac.,
Thuj., Verat. a., *Verat.v.*, Zinc.

Measles During, see **Skin, Measles.**

—**After.**—*Ant. cr.*, **Bell.**, Bry., *Cham.*, Chin., **Hyos.**, Ign. *Mos.*, Nux
v., **PULS.**, Rhus, *Sul.*

Menstruation, see under **Sexual Organs.**

Mercury, Abuse of.—Acon., **Agn.**, **Ant. cr.**, **Arg.**, *Ath.*, Ars., **Asaf.,**
AUR., **Bell.**, *Bry.*, *Calad.*, **Calc. c.**, **CARB. V.**, **Chin.**, Cic., Cina, **Clem.**,
Cocc., **Coff.**, Colch., **Cup.**, Dig., *Dulc.*, Euphorb., Euphr., Fer., *Graph.,*
Guai., **HEP.**, Iod., **LACH.**, Laur., **Led.**, **Mez.**, Nat. m., **NIT. AC.,**
Nux v., *Op.*, Pho. ac., **Plat.**, Puls., Rheum, *Rhodo.* Rhus, Saba., **Sars.,**
Sele., *Sep.*, **Sil.**, Spo., **STAPH.**, Stram., Stro., **SUL.**, *Thuj.*, *Valer.*, Verat.
a., Vio. t., *Zinc.*

—**Fumes of.**—Carb. v., **Chin.**, *Puls.*, Stram.

Micturition, see under **Urinary Organs.**

Moon, New.—Alum., **Am. carb.**, Calc. c., **Caust.**, Cup., *Lyc.*, Saba.,
Sep., Sil.

—**Full.**—Alum., *Calc. c.*, *Cyc.*, **Graph.**, Mar., *Nat. c.*, Saba., **Sep.**, *Sil.,*
Spo., Sul.

—**Waning.**—*Dulc.*

Moonlight.—*Ant. cr.*

Motion.—Acon., *Agar.*, **Agn.**, *Aloe.*, Alum., Ambr., *Am. carb.*, *Am. m.,*
Anac., Ant. cr., Ant. t., **Apis.**, *Apoc. c.*, **Arg.**, **Arn.**, Ars., **Ars. iod.**, **Asaf.,**
Asar., Aur., *Bap.*, *Bar. c.*, **BELL.**, *Berb.*, **BISM.**, *Bor.*, Bov., **BRY.,**
Buf., **Cact.**, Calad., *Calc. c.*, **Camph.**, *Cannab. i.*, **Cannab. s.**, *Canth.,*
Caps., **Carb. an.**, Carb. v., *Carb. sul.*, Caust., Cham., **Chel.**, Chin. *Cic.,*
Cimic., Cina, Clem., **COCC.**, **Coff.**, **COLCH.**, Coloc., *Con.*, **Croc.**, *Crotal.,*
Crot. tig., **Cup.**, Cyc., **Dig.**, **Dros.**, *Dulc.*, **Eup. per.**, Euphorb., Fer.,

Gel., **Glon.**, **Graph.**, *Guai.*, **Hell. Hep.**, Hyos., Ign., **Iod.**, **Ip.**, K. carb., K. nit., Kalm., *Kre.*, Lach., Laur., **LED.**, Lil. t., Lyc., Mag. c., **Mag. m.**, *Mang.*, Mur., **Meli.**, **Meny.**, **MERC.**, *Merc. c.*, *Mez.*, Mos., Mur. ac., Nat. c., **Nat. m.**, **Nat. s.**, **Nit. ac.**, *Nux m.*, **NUX V.**, Oleand., **Onos.**, **Op.**, *Osm.*, **Ox. ac.**, *Par.*, *Petrol.*, **Phos.**, *Pho. ac.*, Plat., *Pb.*, **PULS.**, RAN. B., Ran. s., **Rheum**, Rhodo., Rhus, *Rumex*, Ruta, Saba., **SABI.**, Samb., **Sang.**, Sars., *Sec. c.*, Sele., *Senec.*, Seneg., Sep., **SIL.**, **SPIG.**, *Spo.*, Squ., Stan., **Staph.**, *Stram.*, Stro., **SUL.**, *Sul. ac.*, Tar., **Ther.**, Thuj., *Trill.*, Valer., **Verat. a.**, *Verb.*, Vio. o., Vio. t., Zinc.

Motion, At Beginning Of.—Asar., Bry., Cact., Calc. c., **CAPS.**, **Carb. v.**, Caust., Chin., Cina, Cocc., CON., Cup., Dros., **EUPHORB.**, **FER.**, Graph., *Lach.*, Led., **LYC.**, Mag. c., Nit. ac., *Petrol.*, **Phos.**, *Plat.*, Pb., **PULS.**, *Rhodo.*, **RHUS**, *Ruta*, **Saba.**, Sabi., **Samb.**, Sars., Sil., **Ther.**, Thuj., *Valer.*

—**After.**—**AGAR.**, *Am. carb.*, **Anac.**, *Arn.*, **ARS.**, *Aspar.*, *Calad.*, Camph., **CANNAB. S.**, **Carb. v.**, *Caust.*, *Cocc.*, **Coff.**, **Croc.**, *Dros*, **Hyos.**, Iod., K. carb., Laur., Merc., *Nit. ac.*, *Nux v.*, Oleand., *Phos.*, Pb., **PULS.**, **RHUS**, Ruta, Sabi., Sep., *Spig.*, **SPO.**, **STAN.**, *Staph.*, **Stram.**, Sul. ac., **VALER.**, Zinc.

—**False.**—Ars., Bry., *Lyc.*, SPIG.

—**Of Affected Part.**—Acon., Aesc., *Agar.*, *Am. carb.*, Anac., Ant. t., **ARN.**, Ars., *Asaf.*, *Asar.*, Bar. c., **Bell.**, **BRY.**, *Camph.*, **Cannab. s.**, Caps., *Caust.*, **CHAM.**, *Chel.*, **Chin.**, Cic., *Cimic.*, *Clem.*, **Cocc.**, **Coff.**, Coloc., **Com.**, Con., *Croc.*, **Cup.**, *Dig.*, **Form.**, **Gel.**, **Glon.**, *Guai.*, Hep., Ign., Iod., K. carb., **Kalm.**, **LED.**, *Mag. c.*, **Mang.**, **Meny.**, **Merc.**, **Mez.**, Nat. c., Nat. m., *Nux m.*, **Nux v.**, *Oleand.*, Petrol., **Phos.**, *Phyt.*, Plat., **Puls.**, Ran. b., **Rheum**, *Rumex*, **RHUS**, *Ruta*, *Saba.*, **Sabi.**, **Samb.**, Sang., Sars., *Sele.*, Sep., **SPIG.**, **Stan.**, *Staph*, Sul., *Thuj.*, Zinc.

—**Of Head.**—*Acon.*, *Am. carb.*, **Arn.**, Bar. c., **Bell.**, Bry., **Calc. c.**, Cannab. s., **Caps.**, Carb. v., *Chin.*, Cocc., Coloc., **Cup.**, *Euphorb.*, Graph., **Hell.**, Ip., K. carb., **LACH.**, **Lyc.**, Mang., Mez., **Mos.**, Nat. c., Nat. m., *Pho. ac.*, Plat., *Puls.*, Rhodo., **Rhus**, **Samb.**, Sep., Sil., Spig., Stan., Staph., Sul., Sul. ac., Verat. a., Vio. o.

—**Of Eyes.**—Acon., *Agn.*, Alum., Arn., Ars., **Bell.**, **BRY.**, Camph., **Caps.**, Carb. v., **Cham.**, *Chin.*, Clem., *Coloc.*, *Con.*, **Cup.**, *Dig.*, Dros., *Gel.*, Hep., Ign., *Mang.*, Merc., Mos., *Mur. ac.*, Nat. m., **NUX V.**, Oleand., Op., Pb., *Puls.*, *Ran. s.*, *Rhus*, *Saba.*, Sabi., Seneg., Sep., **Si'**, Spig., Spo., Stan., Stro., **Sul.**, **Valer.**, Zinc.

—**Of Eyelids.**—Coloc., Mos.

—**Of Arms.**—Acon., *Am. m.*, **Anac.**, *Ant. cr.*, **Asc. t.**, Bar. c., Bor.,

AGGRAVATIONS.

Bry., *Camph.*, *Chel.*, **Dig.**, *Fer.*, **Led.**, Nux m., Pb., *Puls.*, **Ran. b.**, Rhus, *Seneg.*, Sep., *Spig.*, *Spo.*, **Sul.**, Thuj., Vio. t.

Music.—Acon., *Ambr.*, Bry., *Calc. c.*, Carb. an., **Cham.**, *Coff.*, **Dig.**, Ign., *K. carb.*, Kre., Lyc., NAT. C., NUX V., *Phos.*, **Pho. ac.**, *Puls.*, Sabi., SEP., **Stan.**, Staph., *Thuj.*, **Vio. o.**, Zinc.

Narcotics.—Acon., Agar., *Ars.*, Aur., BELL., *Bry.*, Calc. c., Canth., *Carb. v.*, Caust., CHAM., Chin., COFF., *Colch.*, Croc., *Cup.*, **Dig.**, Dulc., Euphorb., Fer., **Graph.**, Hep., **Hyos.**, Ign., **Ip.**, LACH., **Lyc.**, *Merc.*, *Mos.*, Nat. c., Nat. m., Nit. ac., Nux m., NUX V., **Op.**, *Phos.*, Pho. ac., Plat., Pb., **Puls.**, *Rhus*, Seneg., Sep., *Staph.*, Sul., **Valer.**, *Verat. a.*, Zinc.

Narrating Her Symptoms.—Calc. c., *Cic.*, Ign., **Mar.**

Nasal Catarrh During. (See **Nose, Accompanying Symptoms of Nasal Discharges.**)

—**Suppression Of.**—*Ambr.*, **Am. carb.**, Am. m., *Ars.*, BRY., *Calad.*, CALC. C., *Carb. v.*, Caust., Cham., **Chin.**, Cina, **Con.**, **Dulc.**, *Graph.*, Hep., **Ip.**, *K. carb.*, Kre., Lach., Laur., *Lyc.*, Mag. c., Mag. m., Mang., *Mar.*, Merc., Nat. c., *Nat. m.*, Nit. ac., *Nux m.*, NUX V., Par., *Petrol.*, *Phos.*, **Puls.**, *Rhodo.*, Saba., *Samb.*, Sars., Sep., **Sil.**, Spig., Spo., Stan., Stram., *Sul.*, Sul. ac., Thuj., Verat. a., Zinc.

Noises.—ACON., Alum., Am. carb., *Anac.*, **Arn.**, Aur., *Bap.*, Bar. c., **BELL.**, *Bor.*, Bry., *Cact.*, *Calad.*, **Calc. c.**, Cannab. s., Caps., Carb. an., Caust., **Cham.**, *Chin.*, COFF., Colch., **Con.**, **Fer.**, Ign., Iod., *Ip.*, K. carb., Lyc., *Mang.*, Merc., Nat. c., Nit. ac., NUX V., **Pho. ac.**, **Plat.**, Puls., *Saba.*, Sep., *Sil.*, Spig., Stan., **Ther.**, *Zinc.*

Nursing Children.—*Acon.*, Agn., *Ars.*, **Bell.**, BOR., Bry., CALC. C., *Calc. ph.*, Carb. an., *Carb. v.*, **Cham.**, Chel., **Chin.**, Cina, **Con.**, *Crot. tig.*, Dulc., Fer., Graph., Ign., *Iod.*, Ip., *K. carb.*, Lach., Lyc., Merc., Nat. c., Nat. m., *Nux v.*, *Phel.*, *Phos.*, **Pho. ac.**, *Phyt.*, PULS., *Rheum*, Rhus, Samb., Sec. c., Sele., SEP., *Sil.*, Spig., *Squ.*, Stan., **Staph.**, Stram., *Sul.*, Zinc.

Odors, Strong.—Acon., Agar., Anac., Asar., AUR., *Bar. c.*, **BELL.**, Bry., Calc. c., Canth., **Cham.**, **Chin.**, *Cocc.*, COFF., COLCH., *Con.*, *Cup.*, **Graph.**, *Hep.*, IGN., K. carb., LYC., Mag. c., Nat. c., NUX V., Petrol., PHOS., Pb., Puls., Saba., *Sele.*, Sep., Spig., **Sul.**, Valer.

Odor of Wood.—*Graph.*.

Onanism.—Agar., Alum., *Anac.*, **Arg.**, Ars., Bov., *Calad.*, CALC. C., **Carb. v.**, CHIN., *Cina*, CON., Dulc., Fer., Ign., **Iod.**, *K. carb.*, **Lyc.**, **Merc.**, Mos., Nat. c., **Nat. m.**, Nux m., *Nux v.*, Petrol., **Phos.**, PHO. AC., Pb., **Puls.**, Sele., SEP., *Sil.*, **Spig.**, Squ., STAPH., **Sul.**

AGGRAVATIONS.

Open Air.—Acon., Agar., Ign., Alum., Ambr., *Am. carb., Am. m.,* Anac., Ant. cr., **Ant. t.**, Arn., **Ars.**, Aur., Bar. c., *Bell.,* Bor., Bov., **Bry.**, *Cact., Calad., Calc. c., Calc. ph.,* Camph., *Cannab. s.,* Canth., **Caps., Carb. an., Carb. v.**, Caust., *Ced.,* **Cham., Chel., Chin.,** Cic., *Cina,* Clem., **COCC., Coff.,** *Coloc.,* **Con.,** *Crot. tig,* Dig., *Dros.,* Dulc., *Euphorb.,* **Fer.,** *Form.,* Graph., GUAI , Hell., **Hep.,** *Hyos., Ign.,* Iod., *Ip.,* **K. carb.,** *K. nit.,* **Kre.,** Lach., Laur., *Led.,* Lyc., Mag. c., Mag. m., Mang., **Mar.,** Meny., **Merc.,** *Mez., Mos.,* **Mur. ac.,** *Nat. c,* **Nat. m.,** *Nit. ac.,* **NUX M., NUX V.,** *Oleand., Op., Par.,* **Petrol.,** Phos., *Pho. ac., Phyt.,* Plat., Pb., **Poly.,** *Pso.,* Puls., Ran. b., *Rheum,* Rhodo., **Rhus, RUMEX,** *Ruta, Saba.,* Sabi., Sars., **Sele.,** Seneg., Sep., SIL., Spig., Spo., Stan., **Staph.,** **Stram.,** Stro., **Sul.,** *Sul. ac.,* Tar., *Thuj.,* **Valer.,** Verat. a., Verb., *Vio. t.,* Zinc.

—**Evening.**—Am. carb., *Carb. v.,* Merc., Nit. ac., *Sul.*

Opening Eyes.—Acon., Arn., **Aur.,** *Atrop.,* **Bell.,** *Bor.,* **Bry., Calc. c.,** *Calc. f.,* Canth., **Chel.,** *Chin.,* Cic., **Clem.,** Coff., **Con.,** Croc., Euphorb., *Euphr., Fer.,* **Gel., Ign.,** Lyc., Mag. m., *Meli.,* **Nux v.,** Phos., Plat., SENEG., **SIL.,** Spig., **Verat. v.,** Zinc.

—**Mouth.**—*Am. m.,* Bry., Caust., Cham., Cocc., Dros., Hep., MERC., Nux v., Petrol., **Phos.,** Puls., *Rhus,* **Saba.,** Sabi., Sil., **Spig.,** *Spo.,* Sul. ac., Thuj., Verat. a.

Organ, Playing The.—*Lyc.*

Persuasion.—*Bell.,* Chin., **Ign., Nat. m.,** Nux v., *Plat.,* **Sep , Sil.**

Piano, Playing The.—*Anac.,* **Calc. c.,** K. carb., **Nat. c., Sep.,** *Zinc.*

Picking Teeth.—K. carb., **Puls.**

Pregnancy.—*Acon.,* Alum., Ambr., Am. m., *Arn.,* **Ars.,** *Asaf.,* **Asar.,** Bar. c., **BELL., Bry., Calc. c.,** *Calc. ph.,* **Caps.,** *Carb. ac.,* **Caust.,** *Cereum,* **CHAM., Chin.,** Cic., **COCC.,** Coff., *Col., Coloc.,* **Con.,** CROC., Cup., Dulc., *Equis.,* **Fer.,** *Glon.,* Graph., **Hyos.,** *Ign.,* **Ip.,** *Jab.,* **K. br., K. carb..** Kalm., Kre., Lyc., Mag. c., Mag. m., Mang., **Merc.,** *Merc. i. f., Mill., Mos.,* **Mur. ac.,** *Nat. m.,* **Nux m.,** *Nux v., Petrol.,* Phos., **Plat., PULS.,** *Raph.,* **Rhus,** SABI., *Sang.,* **Sec. c.,** *Sele.,* **SEP., Sil.,** *Spig.,* **Staph., Sul.,** *Sul. ac.. Tab., Valer., Verat. c*

Pressure, External.—Acon., **AGAR.,** Alum., Ambr., Am. carb., Am. m., Anac., *Ant. cr.,* APIS, *Arg., Arn.,* **Ars.,** Asaf., **Bap., BAR. C., Bell.,** Bism., Bor., Bov., **Bry.,** *Cact.,* **Calad.,** Calc. c., *Calc. ph.,* Camph., **Cannab. s., Canth., Caps.,** *Carb. an., Carb. sul.,* **Carb. v.,** *Card. m.,* Caust., **Chel.,** Chin., CINA, *Coc. c., Coloc., Crot. tig., Cup.,* Dig., Dros., Dulc., Guai., Hell., **HEP.,** *Hyos.,* Ign., IOD., Ip., **K. bi., K. carb., K. iod.,** K. nit., **LACH.,** Laur., Led., **Lil. t., LYC., Mag. c., Mag. m.,**

Mang., **Mar.**, Meny., **Merc.**, **MERC. C.**, *Mez.*, **Mos.**, *Mur. ac.*, **Nat. c.**, **Nat. m.**, **Nat. s.**, **Nit. ac.**, *Nux m.*, **Nux v.**, Oleand., **Op.**, *Ox. ac.*, *Phos.*, Pho. ac., **Plat.**, Puls., Ran. b., **Ran. s.**, Rhus, **Ruta**, *Saba.*, **Sabi.**, Samb., *Sars.*, **Sele.**, *Seneg.*, Sep., **SIL.**, Spig., Spo., **Stan.**, **Staph.**, **Stram.**, Stro., Sul. Sul. ac., **Thuj.**, **Valer.**, Verat. a., Verb., Zinc.

Pressure Of Clothes.—*Am. carb.*, Arn., *Asar.*, **Bry.**, **CALC. C.**, **Caps.**, Carb. v., **Caust.**, Chin., *Coff.*, **Hep.**, LACH, Lil. t., **LYC.**, **NUX V.**, Oleand., Op., Puls., *Ran. b.*, **Sars.**, Sep., *Spo.*, **Stan.**, Sul.

—Of Hat.—Agar., *Alum.*, *Arg.*, Carb. an., **Carb. v.**, *Hep.*, K. nit., Lach., *Laur.*, Led., *Lyc.*, Mez., **Nit. ac.**, **Sil.**, Stro., Sul., **Valer.**

—On Painless Side.—Ambr., Arn., Bell., **BRY.**, **Calc. c.**, *Cannab. s.*, Carb. an., **Carb. v.**, **Caust.**, **Cham.**, Coloc., **IGN.**, **K. carb.**, Lyc., Nux v., **PULS.**, Rhus, Sep., **Stan.**, Vio. o., **Vio. t.**

Punctures.—Carb. v., *Cic.*, Hep., **NIT. AC.**, *Pb.*, Sil., *Sul.*

Pustule, Malignant.—ARS.

Putting Out The Tongue.—Cocc.

Quinine, Abuse Of. (Compare **"China."**)—Am. carb., **Ant. t.**, ARN., **Ars.**, *Asaf.*, **Bell.**, *Bry.*, **Calc. c.**, *Caps.*, **CARB. V.**, Cham., Cina, Cup., Cyc., Dig., **FER.**, *Gel.*, Hell., **IP.**, **Lach.**, *Merc.*, **NAT. M.**, Nux v., Phos., **Pho. ac.**, Pb., **PULS.**, Samb., **Sep.**, Stan., **Sul.**, *Sul. ac.*, Verat. a.

Raising Eyes.—Ars., Bell., **Bry.**, *Caps.*, Chin., *Puls.*, Sabi.

—Arms.—Acon., *Anac.*, *Ant. cr.*, **Bar. c.**, Bor., Bry., Caps., Chin., **CON.**, **Cup.**, **Fer.**, *Graph.*, Lach., **Led.**, Pb., *Ran. b.*, *Rhus*, *Sul.*, Thuj.

—Affected Limb.—Acon., *Am. m.*, Anac., Ant. cr., Arg., **Arn.**, *Asar.*, Bar. c., **Bell.**, Bor., **Bry.**, Calc. c., Camph., Caps., Caust., Chin., Cic., Cina, **Cocc.**, Coff., Colch., Coloc., **CON.**, *Cup.*, Dros., Euphorb., **Fer.**, Graph., Hep., Ign., Iris v., K. carb., *Kre.*, Lach., **Led.**, Lyc., Mag. c., Mag. nt., Mar., Merc., *Mez.*, **Nat. c.**, Nat. m., Nit. ac., Nux v., Oleand., Petrol., Phos., Pb., Puls., *Ran. b.*, **Rhus**, **Ruta**, Sil, **Stan.**, Sul., Sul. ac., Thuj., Verat. a., Verb.

Reading.—Acon., *Agar.*, **Agn.**, Alum., *Am carb.*, Apis, *Arg.*, **Arn.**, **Ars.**, **Asaf.**, *Asar.*, Aur., **Bar. c.**, **Bell.**, Bor., Bry., **CALC. C.**, Canth., **Carb. ac.**, Carb. v., *Carb. sul.*, **Caust.**, Chin., **Cina**, **Cocc.**, *Coff.*, **Con.**, Croc., *Cup.*, Dros., Dulc., Graph., Hep., *Ign.*, **K. carb.**, Lil. t., **Lyc.**, *Mag. m.*, Mang., Meny., Merc., *Mez.*, Mos., *Na.. c.*, **NAT. M.**, *Nit. ac.*, Nux m., **Nux v.**, Oleand., Op., *Petrol.*, **Phos.**, Pho. ac., Plat., **Puls.**, Rhodo., **RUTA**, *Saba.*, Sars., Sele., **SENEG.**, **SEP.**, **SIL.**, Staph., **Stram.**, **SUL.**, **Sul. ac.**, Tar., Thuj., Valer., **Verb.**, Vio. o., Zinc.

Reading Aloud.—CARB. V., *Cocc.,* **Mang.,** Menth., Nit. ac., **Par.,** PHOS., *Sele , Seneg., Sul.,* **Verb.**

Rest.—Acon., *Agar.,* **Aloe.,** *Alum., Ambr.,* Am. carb., **Am. m.,** *Anac., Ant. cr., Ant. t., Arg.,* Arn.. ARS, *Asaf.,* Asar., **Atrop.,** AUR., Bar. c., **Bell.,** *Benz. ac., Bism.,* Bor., *Bov.,* Brom., **Bry.,** Calc. c., *Calc. ph., Canth.,* CAPS., *Carb. ac.,* Carb. an., Carb. v., Caust., *Cham.,* Chin., Cic., *Cina,* **Coca, Cocc.,** Colch., **Coloc.,** *Com.,* CON., Cup., CYC., **Dios.,** Dros., DULC., EUPHORB., *Euphr.,* FER., **Fl. ac.,** Gam., *Gel.,* Guai., Hep., Hyos., Ign., K. carb., *K. nit.,* Kre., *Lach.,* Laur., *Lith., Lob. i.,* LYC., Mag. c., **Mag. m.,** Mang., Mar., **Meny.,** Merc., **Merc. c.,** Merc. i. f., Mez., **Mos.,** *Mur. ac., Nat. c.,* Nat. m., Nit. ac., Nux m., Oleand., *Op., Oxyt., Par., Petrol., Phos.,* **Pho. ac., Plat.,** Pb., PULS., *Rat.,* RHODO., RHUS, **Ruta,** SABA., Sabi., SAMB., Sars., Sele., Seneg., Sep., *Sil.,* Spig., Spo., Stan., Staph., *Stro.,* SUL., Sul. ac., TAR., *Thuj.,* VALER.. *Verat. a.,* **Verb.;** Vib. op., Vio. t., Zinc.

Retching.—Asar., Oleand.

Retracting Abdomen.—Acon., *Ambr.,* Ant. cr., **Ant. t.,** Asaf., **Asar.,** Bar. c., **Bell.,** Bov., Calc. c., *Chel.,* Lyc., **Nux v.,** Phos., *Valer.,* Zinc.

Reveling, Night.—*Ambr.,* Bry., *Colch.,* Ip., **Laur.,** Led., **Nux v.,** Puls., *Rhus, Sabi.*

Riding Horseback.—Ars., Bry., *Graph.,* Lil. t., Mag. m., **Nat. c.,** SEP., Sil., *Spig.,* Sul. ac., Valer.

Riding One Leg Over The Other.—*Agar.,* Alum., Arn., Asaf., *Aur.,* Bell., *Bry.,* Dig., K. nit., Laur., Mur. ac., Nux v., Phos., Plat., Rheum, *Rhus,* Squ., *Valer.,* Verb.

Ringing of Bell.—*Ant. cr.*

Rising Up.—ACON., Alum., **Am. m.,** *Anac.,* Ant. t., Arg., **Arn.,** Ars., *Asar.,* Bar. c., BELL., *Bov.,* BRY., *Cact., Calad.,* Cannab. i., **Cannab. s.,** *Caps.,* Carb. an., Caust., **Cham.,** Chel., *Chin.,* Cic., COCC., Colch., Coloc., **Con.,** Croc., DIG., Dros., **Fer.,** Hell., *Hep.,* Ign., K. carb., *Lach., Laur.,* **Lyc.,** Mag. m., *Mang.,* Meny., Merc., **Mur. ac.,** Nat. m., Nit. ac., NUX V., OP., Osm., Phos., *Pho. ac,* Plat., Pb., Puls., *Ran. b.,* RHUS, *Rumex, Saba.,* **Sang.,** *Sars.,* Seneg., Sep., SIL., Spo., Squ., Stan., *Staph.,* Stram., SUL., *Sul. ac.,* Tar., *Verat. a., Verat. v.,* **Vio. t.,** Zinc.

—**From Bed.**—Acon., **Aloe,** Am. m., Ant. cr., *Ant. t.,* Ars., *Asar.,* Aur., **Bell.,** Bor., *Bov.,* BRY., Calad., **Calc. c.,** Caps., *Carb. an.,* CARB. V., Caust., **Cham.,** Chel., *Chin.,* Cic., **Cina,** Clem., COCC., CON., *Croc., Crot. tig.,* Dig., **Dulc.,** Fer., Graph., *Guai.,* Hell., Hep., Hyos., **Ign.,** K. **carb.,** Kre., LACH., *Led.,* Lyc., Mag. c., Mag. m., Meny., Merc., Mos.,

Nat. m., *Nit. ac.*, Nux v., Oleand., Par., *Petrol.*, PHOS., **Pho. ac.**, Plat., Pb., PULS., Ran. b., Rhodo., RHUS, Ruta, Sabi., **Sal. ac.**, Samb., **Sele.**, Sep., Sil., Spig., *Squ.*, *Stan.*, Staph., *Stram.*, *Sul.*, Sul. ac., Thuj., *Trom.*, *Valer.*, *Verat. a.*, **Verat. v.**

Rising From Bed, After.—Acon., *Aloe*, Am. carb., **AM. M.**, Anac., Ant. cr., Ant. t., Arg., *Ars.*, Bar. *c.*, Bell., Bor., Bov., **BRY., Calc. c.**, Camph., Cannab. s., *Canth.*, Caps., Carb. an., **Carb. v.**, Caust., **Cham.**, CINA, *Col c.*, Con., Croc., *Dulc.*, Euphorb., Graph., **Guai., Hell.**, *Hep.*, *Hyos.*, **Ign.**, Ip., *K. carb.*, K. nit., LACH., Laur., Led., Lyc., *Mag. c.*, *Mag. m.*, Mang., Meny., Mez., Mur. ac., Nat. c., **Nat. m.**, *Nat. s.*, *Nit. ac.*, Nux m., **Nux v.**, Oleand., *Par.*, Phos., Pho. ac., Plat., Puls., Ran. b., Rhodo., RHUS, Ruta, Saba., *Sars.*, Sep., *Sil.*, Spig., *Spo.*, Squ., **Stan., Staph.**, Stram., SUL., Sul. ac., *Thuj.*, *Valer.*, Verat. a., Verb.

—**From a Seat.**—Acon., Ambr., *Anac., Ant. cr.*, **Ant. t., Arn., Apis**, Ars., *Asar., Aur.*, **Bar. c., Bell.**, Bov., **BRY.**, *Cact., Calc. c., Calc. ph.*, Cannab. s., Canth., **CAPS.**, *Carb. an.*, **Carb. v.**, Caust., *Cham.*, **Chin.**, Cic., **Cocc.**, CON., Croc., **Dig.**, Dros., Euphorb., Fer., *Graph.*, K. carb., K. nit., Lach., Laur., Led., LYC., *Mang.*, Merc., Mur. ac., *Nat. c.*, **Nat. m., Nit. ac.**, Nux v., Oleand., Petrol., **PHOS., Pho. ac.**, Plat., PULS., Ran. b., Rhodo., RHUS, Ruta, Saba., Sang., Sep., *Sil.*, SPIG., Staph., Stram., Stro., SUL., Thuj., **Verat. a., Verat. v.**, *Zinc.*

—**After.**—*Alum.*, Bry., Carb. v., Laur., Oleand., *Puls.*, RHUS, Verat. a.

Room Full of People.—*Ambr.*, Ars., Bar. *c.*, Carb. an., Con., **Hell.**, Lyc., Mag. c., *Nat. c.*, Nat. m., Petrol., **Phos., Pb.**, Puls., Sep., *Stan.*, Stram., Sul.

Rubbing.—Am. m., ANAC., Arn., *Ars.*, Bism., Bor., **Calad., Calc. c.**, Cannab. s., *Canth.*, **Caps.**, Carb. an., **Caust.**, Cham., Chel., **Coff.**, CON., Cup., Dros., *Guai.*, Kre., **Led.**, Mag. c., Mang., *Merc.*, **Mez.**, Mur. ac., Nat. c., Par., Phos., Pho. ac., PULS., Seneg., **SEP., Sil.**, *Spig., Spo.*, Squ., Stan., *Staph.*, Stram., STRO., SUL.

—**Gently** ("Stroking".)—Mar.

Running.—Alum., Arg., **Arn.**, ARS., *Aur.*, **Bell.**, *Bor.*, **BRY., Calc. c.**, **Cannab. s.**, Caust., Chel., *Chin., Cina, Cocc.*, Coff., Croc., **Cup.**, Dros., Hep., Hyos., **Ign.**, *Iod.*, Ip., **K. carb.**, Laur., **Led.**, Lyc., Merc., Mez., Nat. c., **Nat. m.**, Nit. ac., Nux m., Nux v., Oleand., *Phos.*, Rheum, **Rhodo.**, Rhus, Ruta, *Sabi.*, Seneg., *Sep.*, Sil., Spig., Spo., *Squ.*, Staph., SUL., Sul. ac., Verat. a., *Zinc.*

Scratching.—Am. m., ANAC., Arn., ARS., **Bism.**, Bov., **Calad., Calc. c.**, Cannab. s., *Canth.*, CAPS., Carb. an., **Caust.**, Cham., Chel., *Coff.*,

Con., Cup., *Dols.*, Dros., *Guai.*, Kre., **Led.**, Mag. c., Mang., *Merc.*, **Mez.**, Mur. ac., Nat. c., Par., *Phos.*, Pho. ac., *Phyt.*, PULS., *Rhus*, *Seneg.*, *Sep.*, Sil., *Spig.*, *Spo.*, Squ., Stan., Staph., Stram., **Stro.**, SUL.

Scratching On Linen, Noise of.—Asar.

Scarlet Fever, During. (See Skin, Scarlet Fever.)

—**After.**—AM. M., Aur., *Bar. c.*, **BELL.**, **Bry.**, CHAM., *Dulc.*, Euphorb., Hep., *Hyos.*, **Lach.**, *Lyc.*, **Merc.**, *Nit. ac.*, Rhus, Sul.

Sewing.—*Lach.*, **Nat. m.**, *Petrol.*, *Ruta*, Sul. ac.

Sexual Excesses.—Acon., **Agar.**, Agn., Alum., *Anac.*, Ant. cr., **Arn.**, *Ars.*, Asaf., Aur., Bar. c., Bell., Bor., **Bov.**, Bry., *Calad.*, **CALC. C.**, Cannab. s., Canth., Caps., Carb. an., **Carb. v.**, Caust., Cham., **Chin.**, *Cina*, Cocc., Coff., **Con.**, *Dulc.*, *Fer.*, Graph., *Ign.*, **Iod.**, Ip., **K. carb.**, Led., *Lyc.*, Mag. m., **Merc.**, Mez., *Mos.*, **Nat. c.**, *Nat. m.*, Nit. ac., **Nux v.**, Op., Petrol., **Phos.**, PHO. AC., Plat., *Pb.*, **Puls.**, *Ran. b.*, Rhodo., Rhus, Ruta, Saba., Samb., *Sele.*, SEP., **Sil.**, Spig., *Squ.*, Stan., **STAPH.**, Sul., Thuj., Valer., Zinc.

— **Desire, Suppression of.**—CON.,

— **Excitement.**—Bufo., LIL. TIG., Sars.

Shaking Head.—Acon., *Agn.*, Am. carb, Anac., Ant. cr., Ant. t., *Apis*, **Arn.**, *Asar.*, Bar. c., **BELL.**, Bor., **Bry.**, *Calad.*, Calc. c., **Camph.**, Cannab. i., *Cannab. s.*, Canth., *Carb. ac.*, *Carb. an.*, Carb. v., Caust., Cham., *Chel.*, Chin., Cic., *Cocc.*, *Coff.*, **Colch.**, *Coral.*, *Croc.*, Cup., *Dig.*, **GLON.**, *Graph.*, Guai., *Hell.*, **Hep.**, *Iod.*, *Ip.*, Kre., **Led.**, Mang., *Merc.*, Mez., *Nat. m.*, Nit. ac, **Nux m.**, **NUX V.**, Par., Petrol., *Phos.*, Pb., Puls., *Ran. b.*, *Rheum*, Rhus, *Ruta.*, Samb., *Sars.*, Sec. c., *Sele.*, Sep., Sil., Spig., Spo., *Squ.*, **Staph.**, Stram., *Sul.*, Sul. ac., Thuj., Verat. a.

Shaving.—Carb. an.

Shipboard, On.—Ars., Bell., COCC., **Colch.**, *Croc.*, *Euphorb.*, **Fer.**, Nux m., PETROL., Sec. c.

Shooting.—*Bor.*

Shrugging Shoulders.—Calc. c., Cyc.

Singing; When.—*Agar.*, **Am. carb.**, **Arg.**, *Asc. t.*, *Carb. an.*, **CARB. V.**, Cocc., Dros., Mang., Nit. ac., **NUX V.**, *Osm.*, Par., PHOS., Sars., Sele., *Spo.*, **STAN.**, **Sul.**, Verb., *Wye.*

—**After.**—*Agar.*, Hep., *Hyos.*

Sitting, When.—*Acon.*, **Agar.**, Agn., **Aloe**, *Alum.*, **Ambr.**, *Am. carb.*, **Am. m.**, Anac., Ant. cr., Ant. t., **Arg.**, Arn., **Ars.**, **Asaf.**, Asar., Aur., Bar. c., Bell., *Bism.*, *Bor.*, **Bov.**, Bry., *Cact.*, Calad., Calc. c., Camph., Cannab. s., Canth., **CAPS.**, Carb. an., Carb. v., *Caust.*, Cham., **Chel.**, Chin., Cic., **Cina**, Clem., **Cocc.**, Coff., Colch., Coloc., **CON.**, Croc., *Cup.*,

AGGRAVATIONS. 299

CYC., *Dig.*, **Dros.**, **DULC.**, **EUPHORB.**, **Euphr.**, **Fer.**, **Gam.**, *Graph*, *Guai.*, **Hell.**, Hep., Hyos., Ign., Iod., Ip., **K. bi.**, **K. carb.**, *K. nit.*, Kre., Lach., *Laur.*, Led., LYC., *Mag. c.*, **Mag. m.**. Mang., *Mar.*, **Meny.** Merc., Mez., **Mos.**, **Mur. ac.**, **Nat. c.**, Nat. m., Nit. ac., Nux m., Nux v., *Oleand.*, Op., F..., Petrol., Phos., **Pho. ac.**, **PLAT.**, Pb., **Pru.**, **PULS.**, Ran. b., Ran. s., Rheum, **Rhodo.**, **RHUS**, **Ruta**, **Saba.**, *Sabi.*, Samb., Sars., Sec. c., *Sele.*, Seneg., **SEP.**, *Sil.*, Spig., *Spo.*, Squ., *Stan.*, Staph., Stram., *Stro.*, SUL., *Sul. ac.*, **Tar.**, **Thuj.**, **VALER.**, *Verat. a.*, VERB., *Vio. o.*, VIO. T., Zinc.

Sitting Down, On First.—Agn., Alum., AM. M., **Ant. t.**, Arg., *Aur.*, Bar. c., Bov., Bry., Caust., **Chel.**, Chin., **Coff.**, Croc., *Cyc.*, Graph., **Hell.**, **Ip.**, *Iris. v.*, **K. carb.**, *Lyc.*, **Mag. c.**, *Mang.*, Merc., *Murex.* Nit. ac., Phos., Pho. ac., ***Puls.***, *Rhus*, Ruta, *Sabi.*, **Samb.**, *Sars.*, SPIG., **Spo.**, Squ., Thuj., **Valer.**, *Verat. a.*, Vio. t.

—**Bent Over.**—Acon., Agn., *Alum.*, **Am. m.**, **ANT. T.**, Arg., **Ars.**, Asaf., Bar. c., Bor., Bov., Bry., Caps., Carb. v., Caust., Cham., Chel., *Chin.*, **Cic.**, CON., *Crot. tig.*, DIG., *Dulc.*, Fer., Grind., *Hell.*, HYOS., Kalm., *Lach.*, Meny., NAT. S., *Nux v.*, *Phel.*, Phos., Pb., PULS., *Rhodo.*, Rhus, **Sabi.**, Samb., Sang., Sep., Spig., Spo., **Squ.**, **Stan.**, Sul., *Verb.*, Vio. t., *Zinc,* Zing.

—**Upright.**—*Acon.*, *Aloe*, Anac., Ars., Bar. c., **Bell.**, Bor., Bry., Calad., *Calc. ph.*, *Carb. v.*, Caust., Cham., *Chel.*, Chin., Cina, **Colch.**, **Coloc.**, **Con.**, Dig., Ign., K. CARB., Kre., Lyc., Mang., **Merc.**, **Mez.**, Mos., Nux m., Nux v., Op., Puls., **Rheum**, Rhus, *Saba.*, Sars., *Spig.*, *Spo.*, *Staph.*, Sul., Tar., Verat. a., Verb., *Vio. t.*

Sleep, Before.—Acon., Agar., **Agn.**, Alum., Am. br., Am. carb., *Am. m.*, Anac., Ant. cr., *Arn.*, ARS., Asar., *Aur.*, Bar. c., **Bell.**, Bism., *Bor.*, BRY., **Calad.**, CALC. C., Camph., Canth., *Caps.*, **Carb. an.**, CARB. V., Caust., Cham., Chel., **Chin.**, Clem., *Cocc.*, **Coff.**, Coloc., Con., Cyc., Dig., *Dulc.*, Euphorb., Euphr., **Graph.**, *Guai.*, Hep., Ign., *Ip.*, **K. carb.**, K. nit., Kre., Lach., *Laur.*, Led., Lyc., Mag. c., *Mag. m.*, Mang., *Mar.*, MERC., Mez., Mos., Mur. ac., *Nat. c.* Nat. m., Nit. ac., Nux m., *Nux v.*, Par., Petrol., PHOS., *Pho. ac.*, Plat., Pb., PULS., *Ran. b.*, Rheum, Rhodo., RHUS, Saba., *Sabi.*, Samb., **Sars.**, *Sele.*, Seneg., SEP., Sil. Spig., *Spo.*, Stan., *Staph.*, *Stro.*, SUL. Sul. ac., Tar., Thuj., Verat. a., Verb., Vio. t., Zinc.

—**At Beginning of.**—*Agn*, Am. m., *Aral.*, Arn., ARS., Aur., *Bap.*, Bar. c., **BELL.**, Bor., **BRY.**, *Calad.*, **Calc. c.**, **Caps.**, **Carb. an.**, *Carb. v.*, Caust., *Chin.*, Cocc., *Coff.*, *Con.*, *Dulc.*, **Graph.**, Grind., Guai., Hep., *Ign.*, Ip., *K. carb.*, Kre., Lach., Laur., Lyc., Mag. c., Mag. m., Mez.

AGGRAVATIONS.

Merc., *Mur. ac.*, Nat. c., Nat. m., Nux v., **Phos.**, Pho. ac., **PULS., Ran.** b., Rhus, Sabi., *Sars.*, Sele., SEP., *Sil.*, Spo., Staph., Stro., **Sul.**, Tar., *Thuj.*, Verat. a.

Sleep, During.—Acon., Agn., *Alum.*, Ambr., *Am. carb.*, Am. m., *Anac.*, Ant. cr., **Ant. t.,** Apis, ARN., ARS., Aur., **Bar. c., BELL.,** Bism., BOR., *Brom.*, BRY., **Calad.,** Calc. c., Camph., **Cannab. i.,** Cannab. s., Canth., Caps., *Carb. ac.*, *Carb. an.*, Carb. v., *Carb. sul.*, *Caust.*, CHAM., Chel., Chin., Cic., *Cina,* Clem., Cocc., Coff., Colch., Coloc., **Con.,** Croc., Cup., Cyc., *Dig.,* Dros., *Dulc.,* Euphorb., Fer., *Graph.,* Guai., Hell., HEP., HYOS., Ign., *Ip.,* K. br., **K. carb.,** K. nit., Kre., Lach., Laur., *Led.,* Lyc., Mag. c., Mag. m., Mang., Mar., Meny., MERC., Mez., Mos., **Mur. ac.,** *Nat. c.,* **Nat. m.,** *Nit. ac.,* **Nux m.,** *Nux v.,* OP., Par., Petrol., **Phos.,** Pho. ac., Plat., Pb., PULS., Ran. b., Ran. s., Rheum, Rhodo., *Rhus, Ruta,* Sabi., **Samb.,** Sars., Sele., Seneg., **Sep.,** SIL., Spig., Spo., Squ., *Stan.,* Staph., STRAM., Stro., SUL., Sul. ac., *Thuj..* Valer., Verat. a., Verb., Vio. t., ZINC.

—**After.**—Acon., *Ambr.,* Am. m., *Anac.,* **Apis,** Arn., Ars., *Asaf., Bell., Bor.,* Bov., *Bry.,* Calad., *Calc. c.,* **Camph., Carb. v., Caust.,** *Cham.,* Chel., Chin., *Cina, Cocc.,* **Coff., Con.,** Dig., Euphr., **Fer.,** *Graph.,* **Hep.,** Hyos., *Ign.,* **K. carb.,** Kre., LACH., Lyc., Mag. c., *Naj.,* '*Nux m., Nux v.,* Oleand., OP., *Pæo.,* **Phos.,** *Pho. ac.,* Puls., **Rheum,** *Rhus,* **Saba.,** Samb., Sele , Sep., Spig., Spo., Squ. Stan., Staph., STRAM., SUL , Thuj., **Verat. a.**

—**After Afternoon.**—Anac., Bry., Chin., Lach., *Phos.*, **Puls., STAPH.,** Sul.

—**After Long.**—Ambr., Anac., *Arn.,* Asaf., Bell., Bor., Bry., **Calc. c.,** *Carb. v.,* Caust., Cocc., Con., Dig., Euphr., **Graph., Hep.,** Hyos., Ign., K. carb., Kre., *Lyc.,* Mag. c., **Nux v.,** Pho. ac., Puls., Rhus, Spig., Stram., SUL., *Verat. a.*

Small-pox, see under **Skin.**

Smoke.—Calc. c., Caust., Euphr., *Nat. m.,* Nux v., Oleand., **Sep.,** SPIG., *Sul.*

Sneezing.—*Acon.,* Am. carb., **Am. m.,** Ant. t., Arn., **Ars.,** Bar. c., **Bell.,** Bor., Bry., *Calc. c., Canth.,* **Carb. v.,** *Caust.,* **Cham.,** Chin., *Cina,* Con., Dros., Euphorb., *Graph.,* Hell., *Hep.,* K. *carb.,* Lach., Led., **Lyc.,** *Mag. c.,* Mag. m., **Merc.,** *Mez.,* Nat. c., Nat. m., **Nit. ac., Nux v.,** Phos., Pod., Puls., Rhus, **Saba..** Sec. c., *Seneg.,* **Sep.,** Sil., **Spig.,** Squ., Staph., SUL.

Snow-air.—Calc. c., *Caust. Cic.,* CON., Lyc., Mag. m., Merc., **Nat. c.,** *Nux v.,* Phos., **Pho. ac., Puls.,** *Rhus,* SEP., Sil., **Sul.**

AGGRAVATIONS.

Society.—*Ambr.*, **Bar. c.**, Carb. an., Con., *Fer.*, **Hell.**, **Lyc.**, *Mag. c.*, *Nat. c.*, Nat. m., Petrol., *Phos.*, **Pb.**, SEP., *Stan.*, Stram., *Sul.*

Spectacles.—Bor.

Splinters.—**Carb. v.**, *Cic.*, Colch., *Hep.*, **Nit. ac.**, *Petrol.*, Plat., Ran. b., Sil., *Sul.*

Sprains. See under **Sensations.**

Spring, In.—Acon., Ambr., *Aur.*, **Bell.**, *Bry.*, **Calc. c.**, *Carb. v.*, Dulc., *K. bi.* Lach., **Lyc.**, **Nat. m.**, Nux v., **Puls.**, **Rhus**, Sep., Sil., **Sul.**, **Verat. a.**

Squatting Down.—Calc. c., *Coloc.*, Graph.

Standing.—*Acon.*, *Agar.*, Agn., *Aloe*, *Alum.*, Ambr., **Am. carb.**, Am. m., *Arg.*, Arn., Ars., *Asaf.*, Asar., *Aur.*, Bar. c., **Bell.**, Bism., *Bor.*, **Bry.**, *Cact.*, Calc. c., Camph., Cannab. s., **Canth.**, **Caps.**, Carb. an., Carb. v., *Carb. sul.*, *Caust.*, Cham., Chel., Chin., Cic., *Cina*, Cocc., Coff., **Coloc.**, CON., Croc., Cup., **CYC.**, **Dig.**, *Dros.*, *Dulc.*, Euphorb., **Euphr.**, **Fer.**, Graph., Guai., Hell., Hep., *Ign.*, *K. bi.*, **K. carb.**, *K. nit.*, Lach., Laur., Led., **LIL. T.**, *Mag. c.*, *Mag. m.*, *Mang.*, Mar., *Meny.*, Merc., Mez., *Mos.*, Mur. ac., *Nat. c.*, Nat. m., Nit. ac., Nux m., Nux v., *Oleand.*, Op., Par., *Petrol.*, Phos., **Pho. ac.**, **Plat.**, Pb., **Puls.**, Ran. b., **Rheum**, *Rhodo.*, **Rhus**, **Ruta**, Saba., Sabi., Samb., Sars., Sep., Sil., Spig., Spo., *Stan.*, Staph., Stram., *Stro.*, **Sul.**, Sul. ac., Tar., *Thuj.*, **VALER.**, **Verat. a.**, **Verb.**, *Vio. t.*, **Zinc.**

Stepping Hard.—*Alum.*, Ambr., *Am. carb.*, **Anac.**, **Ant. cr.**, *Arg.*, Arn., Ars., Asar., *Bar. c.*, **Bell.**, Bor., BRY., Calad., **Calc. c.**, Camph., Canth., **Caust.**, Cham., Chel., **Chin.**, *Cocc.*, Coff., CON., Dros., Dulc., Euphr., Fer., Graph., **Hell.**, K. carb., K. nit., Lach., Led., **Lyc.**, Mag. c., **Mag. m.**, Meny., Merc., **Nat. c.**, **Nat. m.**, *Nit. ac.*, Nux m., **Nux v.**, Par., Petrol., **Phos.**, *Plat.*, Pb., *Puls.*, Rhodo., RHUS, *Ruta*, **Saba.**, *Sabi.*, Seneg., Sep., SIL., *Spig.*, *Spo.*, Stan., Staph., **Sul.**, *Thuj.*, **Verb.**, *Vio. t.*

Stings of Insects. See under **Skin.**

Stone Cutters, For.—CALC. C., *Ip.*, **Lyc.**, *Nat. c.*, Nit. ac., Pho. ac., Puls., SIL., Sul.

Stool, Before, During and After. See under **Stool.**

Stooping.—Acon., AESC., *Agar.*, *Aloe*, **Alum.**, **AM. CARB.**, *Am. m.*, Anac., *Ant. cr.*, Ant. t., *Apis*, **Arg.**, *Arn.*, Ars., *Asaf.*, *Asar.*, Aur., Bap., **Bar. c.**, Bell., *Berb.*, Bor., *Bov.*, BRY., *Cact.*, **Calc. ac.**, CALC. C., *Calc. i.*, *Calc. ph.*, Camph., Cannab. s., *Canth.*, **Caps.**, Carb. ac., Carb. an., *Carb. v.*, *Carb. sul.*, Caust., **Cham.**, *Chel.*, Chin., Cic., *Cimic.*, Cina, **Clem.**, **Cocc.**, **Coff.**, **Coloc.**, Con., Coral., Croc., *Cup.*, *Cyc.*, *Dig.*, Dios., **Dros.**,

Dulc., Fer., *Form.*, Glon., Graph., *Hell.*, Hep., *Hyos.*, Ign., **Ip.**, **K. carb.**, K. nit., *Kre.*, Lach., *Laur.*, Led., Lith., Lyc., Mag. m., **MANG., Mar.**, Meny., **MERC.**, *Mos.*, Mur. ac., *Nat. c*, *Nat. m.*, Nit. ac., Nux m., Nux v., Oleand., Op., Par., Petrol., Phos., *Pho. ac.*, *Phyt.*, *Plat.*, **Pb.**, Puls., RAN. B., *Rheum*, Rhodo., Rhus, *Rumex*, Ruta, Sabi., Samb., Sang., Sars., Seneg., SEP., Sil., SPIG., Spo., Stan., Staph., **Stro., SUL.**, *Sul. ac.*, Tar., Thuj., VALER., Verat. a., Verb., Vio. t., *Zinc.*

Stooping, Prolonged.—Alum., Asar., Bov., Cannab. s., **Caust., Hep.,** *Hyos.*, Meny., Nat. m., Plat., *Vio. t.*

Strangers, When Among.—*Ambr.*, Bar. c., Lyc., Petrol., Sep., Stram.

Stretching of Limbs.—*Acon.*, *Agar.*, Alum., Am. carb., Am. m., Anac., **Ant. cr.**, *Arg.*, Arn., Aur., Bar. c., Bell., Bov., Bry., **CALC. C.,** Cannab. s., Caps., *Carb. v.*, *Caust.*, *Cham.*, **Chin.**, *Cina*, Clem., *Colch.*, Con., Croc., Dig., Dros., Dulc., Fer., Graph., Guai., Hep., Ign., K. carb., *Laur.*, *Lyc.*, **Mang.**, *Meny.*, Merc., MERC. C., Mur. ac., Nat. m., Nux v., Petrol., Phos., *Plat.*, Pb., Puls., RAN. B., Rheum, Rhus, Ruta, Sabi., Sele., SEP., *Spig.*, Spo., Stan., Staph., SUL., THUJ., Valer., Verat. a.

Storm, Approach of a.—*Bry.*, *Hyper.*, *Meli.*, RHODO.

—During Thunder Storm.—*Bry.*, Caust., *Lach.*, **Nat. c.**, Nat. m., Nit. ac., Petrol., *Phos.*, Rhodo., Sil.

Stumbling.—Bar. c., Bry., Carb. v., **Caust., Hep.,** Puls., Sep., *Sil.*, Spig., Valer.

Sucking Gums.—Bov., *Carb. v.*, K. carb., **Nit. ac., Nux m., Nux v.,** Sil., Zinc.

Summer, In.—Ant. cr., Bar. c., **Bell., Bry.,** Carb. v., Cham., Graph., *Lyc.*, **Nat. c.**, *Nat. m.*, Nux v., Puls., *Sele.*, Thuj.

Sun, In The.—Agar., ANT. CR., Bar. c., *Bell.*, Bry., *Calc. c.*, **Camph.**, *Clem.*, **Euphr.**, *Glon.*, *Graph.*, Ign., *Iod.*, *Ip.*, Lach., Mag. m., NAT. C., Nux v., PULS., Sele., Stan., *Sul.*, Valer., Zinc.

Sun-burn.—Acon., BELL., *Camph.*, Clem., **Hyos.**

Sunrise, After.—Cham., Nux v., Puls.

Sunset, After.—Bry., Ign., Puls., *Rhus.*

Supporting a Limb.—*Am. m.*, Arg., Arn., *Asar.*, Bell., *Camph.*, Caust., *Cina*, Con., Croc., Graph., K. carb., Mag. m., *Mur.*, Nux m., Phos., Rhus, Ruta, Sabi., Samb., Sil., Spo., Squ., Stan., Sul., *Thuj.*, Valer., *Verb.*

Swallowing.—Acon., *Aconin.*, Aesc., *Aloe.*, Alum., Ambr., Am. carb., Am. m., Anac., Ant. t., APIS, *Arg.*, **Ars.**, *Asaf.*, **Atrop.**, Aur., Bar. c., BELL., Bor., *Bov.*, BROM., BRY., *Calc. c.*, *Camph.*, **Canth., Caps.**, Carb. an., Carb. v., *Carb. sul.*, Caust., *Chin.*, Chin., Cic., *Cinnab.,*

Cocc., *Coff., Colch., Con.,* **Croc.,** *Crotal., Crot. tig.,* Cup., Dig., **Dol.,** *Dros., Elaps,* Euphorb., *Fer.,* Gel., Graph., *Hell.,* HEP., **Hydras.,** HYOS., Ign., Iod., Ip., *K. br., K. carb.,* K. chl., *K. nit., Kre.,* LACH., Laur., Led., *Lyc., Mag. c.,* Mag. m., Mang., *Meny.,* MERC., **Merc. c., Merc. d.,** MERC. I. F., *Mez.,* **Mur. ac.,** Nat. n., *Nat. m.,* NIT. AC., Nux v., *Op.,* Par., **Petrol.,** Phos., Pho. ac., **Phyt.,** *Plat.,* **Pb.,** Puls., *Ran. b., Rhodo.,* Rhus, *Ruta,* Saba., Sabi., **Sang.,** *Sars.,* Seneg., **Sep., Sil.,** *Spig.,* Spo., Stan., Staph., STRAM., Stro., SUL., **Sul. ac.,** Tar., Thuj., *Verat. a.,* **Wye.,** Zinc.

Swallowing, Empty.—Arg., **Bar. c.,** Bell., Bor., Bov., Bry., Caps, COCC., Colch., *Croc.,* Graph., **Hep.,** LACH., Mang., **Merc.,** Mez., *Nux v.,* Plat., **Puls.,** Rhus, *Ruta, Saba.,* Sabi., Spig., *Sul.,* Thuj., Zinc

—**Of Food.**—*Alum.,* Ambr., Ars., **Bar. c.,** BRY., Carb. v., Cham., Chin., Colch., Euphorb., HEP., Ign., *Iod.. Lach.,* **Nit. ac., Nux v.,** Petrol., Phos., *Pho. ac.,* Ran. b., **Rhus, Sep.,** SUL., *Zinc.*

— —**After.**—Ambr., Ars., *Bar. c.,* **Bry.,** Carb. v., Cham., Chin., Colch., Euphorb., **Hep.,** Ign., *Iod., Nit. ac.,* NUX V., *Petrol.,* **Phos.,** Puls., Ran. b, **Rhus,** *Sep.,.* **Sul.,** ZINC.

—**Liquids.**—BELL., **Canth.,** *Cina,* Cup., *Hyos., Ign.,* **Iod.,** LACH., Merc., Merc. c., Nat. m., PHOS., Stram.

—**When Not.** See **Amel., Swallowing.**

Sweat, During. See **Fever, Sweat With Associated Symptoms.**

—**After.**—*Ars.,* Bell., Bry., **Calc. c.,** *Carb. v.,* CHIN., *Con.,* Ign., *Iod., K. carb.,* Lyc., **Merc.,** Nat. c., Nat. m., Nux v., Petrol., *Phos.,* PHO. AC., Puls., Sele.. SEP., *Sil.,* Spig., *Squ.,* Staph., Sul.

—**Suppression Of.**—*Acon.,* Am. carb., Arn., *Ars.,* BELL., **Bry.,** CALC. C., Cannab. s., CHAM., CHIN., *Coff., Colch., Coloc., Dulc., Graph.,* Hyos., Iod., Ip., *K. carb., Led.,* **Lyc.,** Mag. c., *Mar ,* Merc., Nat. c., Nit. ac., *Nux m.,* **Nux v.,** *Oleand.,* Op., **Phos.,** *Pho. ac.,* Plat., *Puls.,* **Rhus,** *Saba., Sec. c., Seneg.,* **Sep.,** *Sil.,* Spo., Squ., Staph., SUL., *Verb.,* Vio. o.

Swinging (Rocking).—Bor., *Carb. v.*

Talking.—Acon., *Alum.,* Ambr., Am. carb., *Am. m.,* ANAC., **Arg.,** Arn., *Ars., Asc. t.,* **Arum. t.,** Aur., Bar. c., **Bell.,** *Bor.,* **Bry.,** *Calad.,* CALC. C., *Calc. ph.,* CANNAB. S., Canth., Caps., **Carb. v.,** *Caust.,* **Cham.,** CHIN., Cic., **Cimic.,** *Coca,* COCC., *Coff.,* Con., Croc., Cup., Dig., Dros., Dulc., *Euphr.,* **Fer.,** Graph., Hell., **Hep.,** *Hyos., Ign ,* Iod., **Ip.,** K. bi., K. carb., **Led.,** Lyc., *Mag. c.,* **Mag. m.,** MANG., *Mar.,* Menth., Merc., Mez., *Mur. ac.,* NAT. C., NAT. M., Nux m., *Nux v.,* Par., Petrol. **Phos.,** PHO. AC., *Plat.,* **Pb.,** Puls., Ran. b., RHUS, Sars., SELE.,

304 AGGRAVATIONS.

Sep., Sil., Spig., Squ., STAN., *Staph.*, *Stram.*, Stro., SUL., *Sul. ac.*, Verat. a., *Wye.*

Talking of Other People.—*Am. carb.*, Ars., Cact., *Chin.*, Colch., *Fer.*, Mang., Nat. c., Nux v., *Rhus*, Sep., Sil., Stram., *Verat. a.*, *Zinc.*

—**About Disagreeable Things.**—Calc. c., *Cic.*, Ign., **Mar.**

Thinking of His Disease.—*Agar.*, Bar. c., *Calc. ph.*, Dros., Hell., Nux v., Oleand., *Oxyt.*, *Piper.*, Pb., Ran. b., Saba., *Spig.*, Spo., Staph.

—**Of Something Else.**—Camph., Cic., **Hell.**

Touch.—Acon., Aesc., *Agar.*, Agn., *Aloe*, Ambr., Am. carb., Am. m., *Anac.*, Ant. cr., Ant. t., APIS, *Arg.*, **Arn.**, Ars., Asar., Aur., Bar. c., BELL., *Bor.*, Bov., BRY., Calad., Calc. c., *Calc. ph.*, Camph., **Cannab. s.**, Canth., **Caps.**, *Carb. an.*, Carb. v., Caust., CHAM., *Chel.*, Chin., Cic., Cina, *Clem.*, *Cocc.*, Coff., COLCH., Coloc., Con., *Croc.*, *Crot. tig.*, CUP., *Cyc.*, *Dig.*, Dros., Dulc., Euphorb., Euphr., Fer., *Graph.*, *Guai.*, Hell., HEP., HYOS., Ign., *Iod.*, Ip., K. bi., K. carb., **K. iod.**, K. nit., Kre., LACH., Laur., Led., LYC., **Mag. c.**, **Mag. m.**, Mang., *Mar.*, *Menth.*, Meny, **Merc.**, **Merc. c.**, Mez., *Mos.*, Mur. ac., Nat. c., **Nat. m.**, NIT. AC., *Nux m.*, NUX V., *Oleand.*, **Op.**, *Osm.*, Par., Petrol., Phos., Pho. ac., *Plat.*, Pb., **Puls.**, RAN. B., Ran. s., RHODO., RHUS, *Ruta*, Saba. SABI., *Sal. ac.*, Sang., Sars., Sec. c., Seneg., SEP., SIL., SPIG., Spo. *Squ.*, Stan., STAPH., Stram., Stro., SUL., Sul. ac., Tar., **Thuj.**, *Valer.*, Verat. a., *Verb.*, Vio. o., Vio. t., Zinc.

—**Slight.**—*Ars.*, BELL., CHIN., Colch., Ign., *Lach.*, Mag. m. MERC., **Mez.**, NUX V., Phos., *Pho. ac.*, Stan.

—**Anything.**—Acon., *Am. carb.*, Am. m., Arg., *Arn.*, Bell., Bov., **Bry.**, Calc. c., Cannab. s., **Carb. v.**, Caust., CHAM., Chin., *Dros.*, K. carb., K. nit., Led., *Lyc.*, Merc., Nat. c., Phos., *Plat.*, **Puls.**, Sec. c., **Sil.**, Spig., Verat. a.

—**Cold Things.**—Hep., Merc., **Nat. m.**, Rhus, *Sil.*, *Thuj.*

—**Hair.**—Ambr., Ars., Bell., *Chin.*, **Fer.**, *Ign.*, Nux v., Phos., *Pho. ac.*, Puls., Rhus, SELE., *Stan.*

—**Throat.**—*Apis*, Bell., LACH.

Turning Around.—Agar., *Aloe*, Calc. c., Cham., **Ip.**, *K. carb.*, Merc., Nat. m., *Par.*, Phos., *Sil.*

—**Over in Bed.**—Acon., Agar., Am. m., Anac., *Ars.*, Asar., **Bor.**, Bry., Calc. c., Cannab. s., Caps., Carb. v., *Caust.*, Chin., Cina, Cocc., Con., Cup., Dros., Euphorb., Fer., Graph., Hep., *K. carb.*, Kre., Lach., Led., Lyc., Mag. c., Merc., **Nat. m.**, Nit. ac., **Nux v.**, Petrol., *Phos.*, Plat., Pb., PULS., Ran. b., Rhodo., *Rhus*, Ruta, *Saba.*, Sabi., Samb., Sars., Sil., Staph., Sul., Thuj., Valer.

AGGRAVATIONS. 305

Turning Head.—Am. m., Anac., *Ant. cr.*, **Arn.**, *Asar.*, Bar. c., **Bell.**, Bov., Bry., CALC. C., Camph., Cannab. s., Canth., *Carb. an.*, *Carb. v.*, Caust., Cham., *Chin.*, CIC., Cocc., Coff., *Coloc.*, Cup., *Dros.*, Dulc., *Glon.*, **Hep.**, Hyos., Ign., *Ip.*, **K. carb.**, Lach., Lyc., *Mag. c.*, Mez., **Nat. c.**, Nat. m., Nit. ac., **Nux v.**, Par., Petrol., Phos., Pho. ac., Plat., **Puls.**, Rhus, Sba., Sabi., *Samb.*, **Sang.**, Sars, **Sele.**, Sep., *Spig.*, SPO., *Stan.*, Staph., *Sul.*, Thuj., Verat. a., Vio. t., Zinc.

—**Eyes.**—Bry., *Caps.*, Cup., Lyc., *Nux v.*, Puls., Rhus, **Sang.**, Sep., **Sil.**, **Spig.**

—**Neck.**—Bell., Bry., Hep.

Twilight.—Am. m., **Ars.**, **Calc. c.**, Dig., Nat. m., Pb., PULS., *Rhsn*, *Staph.*, Sul. ac., *Valer.*

Uncleanliness.—CAPS., Chin., Puls., *Sul.*

Uncovering.—Acon., *Acon. f.*, Agar., *Ant. cr.*, **Arg.**, **Arn.**, **Ars.**, Asar., Atrop., Aur., *Bell.*, *Benz. ac.*, Bor., **Bry.**, *Camph.*, *Canth.*, Caps., Carb. an., *Cham.*, *Chin.*, Cic., **Clem.**, Cocc., Coff., **Colch.**, Con., *Dios.*, Dulc., *Graph.*, Hell., HEP., *Hyos.*, Ign., *Kre.*, *Lach.*, Led., *Mag. c.*, *Mag. m.*, Meny., **Merc.**, Mur. ac., *Nat. c.*, *Nat. m.*, **Nux m.**, Nux v., Phos. Pho. ac., Puls., Rheum, **Rhodo.**, RHUS, **Rumex**, *Saba.*, SAMB., Sep., SIL., SQU., Staph., *Stram.*, STRO., Thuj.

—**After.**—Am. m., ARS., **Cocc.**, DROS., Hep., Mag. c., *Mez.*, NUX V., Oleand., Puls., RHUS, Sep., *Sil.*, Spo., Stan.

—**One Part.**—Bry., Hep., Nat. m., RHUS, Sil., *Squ.*, Stro., Thuj.

—**Head.**—Acon., Agar., Ant. cr., Arg., Arn., *Ars.*, **Aur.**, Bell., Camph., Canth., *Cham.*, Chin., *Cic.*, *Clem.*, Cocc., Coff., **Colch.**, Con., Graph., HEP., **Hyos.**, Ign., Kre., Lach., Led., *Mag. c.*, Mag. m., Merc., Nat. c., Nat. m., Nux m., NUX V., Pho. ac., Puls., Rhodo., RHUS, Saba., **Samb.**, Sep., SIL., Squ., Staph., Stram., **Stro.**

Unnatural Position.—*Staph.*, **Tar.**

Vaults (Cellars, etc.).—ARS., **Bry.**, *Calc. c.*, **Carb. an.**, Caust., Lyc., PULS., Sep., Stram.

Vertigo, During.—ACON., Agar., *Alum.*, Ambr., *Am. carb.*, Am. m., Anac., *Ant. cr.*, *Ant. t.*, **Arg.**, Arn., **Ars.**, Asaf., Aur., Bar. c., **Bell.**, Bov., Bry., Calad., CALC. C., Camph., *Canth.*, **Carb. an.**, Carb. v., Caust., Cham., Chel., *Chin.*, Cic., Cina, **Cocc.**, Coff., Coloc., Con., *Croc.*, Cup., Dig., Dulc., Fer., Graph., Hell., *Hep.*, *Hyos.*, *Ign.*, Iod., *Ip.*, K. carb., K. nt., **Lach.**, Laur., Led., *Lyc.*, *Mag. c.*, *Mag. m.*, **Merc.**, Mez., Mos., Nat. c., *Nat. m.*, *Nit. ac.*, *Nux m.*, NUX V., Oleand., Op., Par., *Petrol.*, PHOS., Pho. ac., Plat., Pb., PULS., Ran. s., Rhodo., *Rhus*, Ruta, *Saba.*, *Sabi,*

14

Sars., Sec. c., Sele., Seneg., *Sep.*, Sil., *Spig.*, Spo., Squ., Stan., Staph., STRAM., *Stro.*, *Sul.*, **Verat. a.**, Verb., Zinc.

Violin, Playing the.—Calc. c., **K. carb.**, Vio. o.

Vomiting.—Acon., **Ant. t.**, *Arn.*, ARS., *Asar.*, Bell., Bry., **Calc. c.**, *Caps.*, Cham., *Chin.*, Cina, Cocc., **Colch.**, *Coloc.*, Con., CUP., *Dig.*, **Dros.**, Fer., *Graph.*, **Hyos.**, Iod., IP., Lach., Lyc., Mez., Mos., *Nat. m.*, Nux v., *Op.*, **Phos.**, Pb., PULS., Ran. s., Ruta, Sabi., **Sars.**, *Sec. c.*, **Sep.**, *Sil.*, Stan., SUL., **Verat. a.**

Waking.—*Acon.*, *Agar.*, Agn., *Alum.*, AMBR., **Am. carb.**, AM. M., Anac., **Ant. cr.**, Ant. t., **Arn.**, ARS., Aur., *Bar. c.*, *Bell.*, **Benz. ac.**, Bism., Bor., Bov., Bry., *Cact.*, Calad., CALC. C., *Calc. ph.*, Cannab. s., Canth., **Caps.**, **Carb. an.**, **Carb. v.**, CAUST., *Cham.*, **Chel.**, **Chin.**, Cic., Cina, Clem., **Cocc.**, *Coc. c.*, *Coff.*, *Colch.*, *Con.*, *Corn. c.*, *Croc.*, *Crot. tig.*, *Cup.*, Cyc., **Dig.**, **Dros.**, Dulc., Euphorb., *Euphr.*, Fer., *Form.*, **Graph.**, Guai., HEP., Hydras., HYOS., Ign., Ip., K. bi., **K. carb.**, *K. iod.*, K. nit., Kre., LACH., Laur., Led., **Lyc.**, *Mag. c.*, *Mag. m.*, Mang., Mar., Meny., **Merc.**, **Merc. i. f.**, Mez., Mos., *Mur. ac.*, *Naj.*, *Nat. c.*, **Nat. m.**, NIT. AC., *Nux m.*, NUX V., Op., ONOS., *Petrol.*, PHOS., *Pho. ac.*, Phyt., Plat., *Pso.*, PULS., Ran. b., Ran. s., Rheum., Rhodo., **Rhus**, *Ruta*, *Saba.*, *Sabi.*, Samb., Sang., *Sars.*, Sele., Seneg., SEP., Sil., *Spig.*, Spo., *Squ.*, **Staph.**, *Stram.*, *Stro.*, SUL., Sul. ac., *Tar.*, *Thuj.*, VALER. *Verat. a.*, Vio. o., *Vio. t.*, Zinc.

—Being Awake at Night.—*Ambr.*, Bry., *Chin.*, COCC., **Colch.**, *Ip.*, NUX V., *Pho. ac.*, *Puls.*, Ruta, Sabi., **Sele.**, Sep.

Walking.—*Acon.*, AESC., *Agar.*, **Agn.**, *Aloe*, Alum., Ambr., *Am. carb.*, Am. m., *Anac.*, Ant. cr., **Ant. t.**, *Apis*, Arg., **Arn.**, *Ars.*, Asaf., **Asar.**, Atrop., Aur., **Bap.**, *Bar. c*, BELL., *Bor.*, **Bov.**, BRY., **Cact.**, *Cad. s.*, Calad., CALC. C., **Camph.**, **Cannab. s.**, *Canth.*, Caps., **Carb. ac.**, **Carb. an.**, Carb. v., *Carb. sul.*, Caust., Cham., **Chel.**, Chin., *Cic.*, Cina, *Clem.*, **Cocc.**, Coff., COLCH., **Coloc.**, Con., *Conv.*, Croc., *Cup.*, Cyc., **Dig.**, Dios., Dros., Dulc., Euphorb., Euphr., **Fer.**, *Form.*, **Gel.**, Glon., Gran., **Graph.**, *Guai.*, Hell., Hep., *Hyos.*, Ign., Iod., **Ip.**, K. carb., K. nit., *Kre.*, Lach., Laur., LED., **Lil. t.**, Lyc., Mag. c., Mag. m., *Mang.*, Mar., Meny., **Merc.**, Mez., Mos., Mur. ac., Nat. c., **Nat. m.**, **Nat. s.**, Nit. ac., *Nux m.*, NUX V., Oleand., Op., *Pæo* , *Par.*, Petrol., PHOS., Pho. ac., Phyt., Plat., *Pb.*, *Pso.*, Puls., Ran. b., Ran. s., Rheum., Rhodo., RHUS, **Ruta**, Saba., **Sabi.**, Samb., Sars., *Sec. c.*, Sele., Seneg., SEP., Sil., SPIG., *Spo.*, Squ., Stan., **Staph.**, *Stram.* Stro., SUL., *Sul. ac.*, Tar., **Tarent.**, Thuj., Valer., Verat. a., **Verat. v.**, Verb., Vio. o., Vio. t., **Zinc.**

Walking, Beginning of.—*Acon., Ambr., Am. carb.,* Anac., Ant. cr., Ant. t., Arn., Ars., Asar., Aur., Bar. c., **Bell.,** Bov., **Bry.,** *Cact.,* **Calc. c.,** Cannab. s., Canth., CAPS., *Carb. an.,* **Carb. v., Caust.,** Cham., *Chin.,* Cic., Cina, *Cocc.,* CON., Croc., Cup., *Cyc.,* Dig., *Dros.,* EUPHORB., FER., *Graph.,* K. carb., K. nit., *Lach., Laur., Led.,* LYC., Mag. c., Mang., Merc., Mur. ac., Nat. c., *Nat. m., Nit. ac.,* Nux v., Oleand., *Petrol.,* **Phos.,** *Pho. ac., Plat.,* Pb., PULS., Ran. b., *Rhodo.,* Rhus, **Ruta, Saba.,** Sabi., **Samb.,** Sars., *Sep.,* Sil., *Spig.,* Staph., Stram., Stro., *Sul.,* **Thuj.,** *Valer., Verat. a.*

—**Bent Over.**—Bry.

—**Fast.**—Alum., Arg., **Arn.,** ARS., *Aur.,* BELL., *Bor.,* BRY., **Calc. c., Cannab. s.,** Caust., Chel., *Chin., Cina, Cocc.,* Coff., Croc., **Cup.,** Dros., Hep., Hyos., Ign., *Iod.,* Ip., **K. carb.,** Laur., **Led.,** Lyc., **Merc.,** Mez., Nat. c., **Nat. m.,** Nit. ac., Nux m., **Nux v.,** Oleand., PHOS., *Rheum,* Rhodo., Rhus, Ruta, *Sabi.,* **Seneg.,** Sep., **Sil., Spig.,** Spo., *Squ.,* Staph., SUL., Sul. ac., Verat. a., *Zinc.*

—**On a Level.**—Ran. b.

—**In Open Air.**—*Acon.,* Agar., *Agn.,* Alum., Ambr., *Am. carb.,* Am. m., Anac., Ant. cr., Arg., *Arn.,* ARS., *Asar.,* Aur., Bar. c., **Bell.,** Bor., Bov., **Bry.,** *Calad., Calc. ac., Calc. c.,* **Camph., Cannab. s.,** *Canth.,* Caps., **Carb. ac., Carb. an., Carb. v.,** **Caust.,** *Cham.,* **Chel.,** *Chin.,* Cic., **Cina,** Clem., COCC., **Coff.,** Colch., Coloc., **Con.,** *Croc.,* Dig., Dros., Dulc., Euphorb., **Euphr.,** *Fer.,* **Graph., Guai.,** Hell., Hep., Hyos., Ign., *Iod., Ip.,* K. carb., K. nit., *Kre., Lach.,* Laur., **Led.,** Lyc., Mag. c., Mag. m., Mang., *Mar.,* Meny., **Merc.,** *Merc. c.,* Mez., Mos., Mur. ac., Nat. c., *Nat. m., Nit. ac.,* **Nux m.,** NUX V., Oleand., Op., Par., *Petrol.,* **Phos.,** Pho. ac., **Plant.,** Plat., Pb., Pso., **Puls.,** *Ran. b.,* **Ran. s.,** *Rheum,* Rhodo., Rhus, Ruta, *Saba.,* Sabi., *Sars.,* SELE., **Seneg., Sep.,** Sil., SPIG., Spo., Stan., *Staph.,* **Stram.,** Stro., SUL., *Sul. ac.,* Tar., Thuj., *Valer.,* Verat. a., Verb., Vio. t., Zinc.

—**On a Narrow Bridge.**—Bar. c., *Fer.,* Sul.

—**Sideways.**—Caust.

—**On a Stone Pavement.**—Ant. cr., Con., Hep.

—**Over Water.**—Fer., Sul.

—**In the Wind.**—Acon., *Ars.,* Asar., Aur., BELL., **Carb. v.,** Cham., *Chin.,* Con., *Euphr., Graph., Lach.,* Lyc., **Mur. ac., Nat. c.,** Nux m., NUX V., Phos., Plat., *Puls.,* SEP., *Spig.,* Thuj.

Warmth in General.—*Acon.,* Agar., *Agn.,* **All. c.,** Alum., Ambr., Anac., *Ant. cr.,* **Ant. t., Apis,** Arn., *Ars., Asar.,* Aur., Bar. c., **Bell.,** Bism., Bor., **Bry.,** *Calad.,* Calc. c., Cannab. s., *Canth.,* **Carb. v., Caust.,** Cham., Chin., *Cina,* Cocc., Coc. c., *Colch., Coloc., Croc., Dig.,* **Dros.,** Dulc.,

308   AGGRAVATIONS.

Euphorb., Euphr., Fer., Gel., Glon., Graph., Hell., Hep., Ign., IOD., *Ip.,*
K. br., K. carb., Lach., Laur., **Led.,** *Lyc., Mar.,* Merc., *Mez.,* Mur. ac.,
Nat. c., **Nat. m.,** Nit. ac., Nux m., Nux v., *Op., Phos.,* Pho. ac., *Plat.,*
PULS., *Rhus,* Saba., *Sabi.,* SEC. C., *Sele.,* **Seneg.,** *Sep.,* Sil., Spig., Spo.,
Staph., **Sul.,** *Tab., Thuj.,* Verat. a

Warmth Of Air.—Agn., *Aloe,* Ambr., Anac., **Ant. cr.,** Ant. t., **Asar.,**
Aur., *Bry.,* Calad., Calc. c., Cannab. s., *Carb. v.,* Cham., Cina, **Cocc.,**
Colch., Croc., *Dros.,* Euphorb., *Fer.,* Ign., IOD., Ip., *K. bi., Lach.,* **Led.,**
Lyc., Mar., Merc., **Mez.,** Nat. m., *Nit. ac., Nux m.,* Nux v., Op., **Phos.,**
Pic. ac., *Plat., Pod.,* PULS., Rhus, Sabi., *Sars.,* SEC. C., *Sele.,* Seneg.,
Sep., Sul., Thuj., *Xan.*

—**Of Open Air.**—Acon., Agn., Alum., Ambr., Anac., Ant. cr., Asar.,
Aur., Bar. c., Bell., *Bov.,* BRY., Calad., Calc. c., Cannab. s., Carb. v.,
Caust., Cham., Chin., Cina, Cocc., Coff., Colch., Coloc., Croc., *Dros.,*
Dulc., Euphorb., Graph., *Ign.,* IOD., Ip., K. carb., **Lach.,** *Led.,* LYC.,
Mang., Mar., Merc., Mez., Nat. c., Nat. m., *Nit. ac.,* Nux m., Nux v.,
Oleand., Op., *Petrol* Phos., Pho. ac., Plat., PULS., Rhus, **Saba.,** Sabi.,
Sec. c., Sele., *Seneg.,* Sep., *Sil.,* **Spig.,** Spo., *Staph.,* Sul., Thuj., *Verat. a.*

—**Of Bed.**—Agn., **Alum.,** Ambr., Anac., Ant. cr., *Ant. t.,* Apis, Arn.,
Asar., Aur., Bar. c., Bov., Bry., Calad., *Calc. c.,* Cannab. s., **Carb. v.,**
Caust., Ced., CHAM., Chin., Cina, *Clem.,* **Cocc.,** **Coc. c.,** Colch., Croc.,
DROS., *Dulc.,* Euphorb., *Goss.,* **Graph.,** Hell., Ign., Iod., Ip., *K. carb.,*
Lach., LED., **Lyc.,** Mar., MERC., Mez., Mur. ac., Nat. c., *Nat. m.,*
Nit. ac., Nux m., *Nux v.,* Op., *Phos.,* **Pho. ac.,** *Phyt.,* Plat., *Pso.,* PULS.,
Rhus, Saba., SABI., Sars., SEC. C., Sele., *Seneg.,* Sep., Spig., **Spo.,**
Staph., *Stram.,* SUL., **Thuj., Verat. a.**

—**Of Room.**—*Acon.,* Agn., **Alum.,** *Ambr.,* **Anac., Ant. cr.,** Arn.,
Asar., Aur., Bar. c., Bell., Bor., **Brom.,** Bry., Calc. c., *Calc. ph.,* Cannab.
s., *Carb. ac.,* Carb. v., Caust., *Cina,* **Coc. c.,** *Colch.,* CROC., Dulc., Graph.,
Hell., Hep., Ign., IOD., *Ip.,* K. carb., *Laur.,* **Lil. t.,** *Lyc.,* Merc., *Mez.,*
Mos., Mur. ac., *Nat. a.,* **Nat. c.,** *Nat. m.,* Nit. ac., Nux v., *Op., Oxyt.,*
Phos., Pho. ac., Pic. ac., *Plat.,* PULS., *Ran. b.,* Rhus, SABI., *Sele.,*
Seneg., *Sep.,* Spig., Spo., Staph., *Sul., Thuj.,* Verat. a.

Warm Wraps.—Acon., Ars., Asar., Aur., Bor., *Bry.,* **Calc. c.,** Carb.
v., *Cham., Chin.,* Coff., Fer., *Ign.,* Iod., Lach., Led., LYC., Merc., Mos.,
Mur. ac., Nit. ac., Nux v., *Op., Phos., Plat.,* PULS., Rhus, *Sec. c., Seneg.,*
Sep., Spig., *Staph.,* SUL., *Tab., Thuj.,* **Verat. a.**

—**On Head.**—Acon., *Asar.,* Aur., Bor., Bry., **Calc. c.,** *Carb. v., Cham.,*
Chin., Fer., *Ign.,* IOD., Lach., Led., LYC., Merc., Mur. ac., Nit. ac.,

AGGRAVATIONS.

Op., *Phos.*, *Plat*, **Puls.**, *Sec. c.*, *Seneg.*, Sep., **Spig.**, *Staph.*, *Sul.*, *Thuj.*, **Verat. a.**

Water (and Washing).—AM. CARB., Am. m., ANT. CR., *Ant. s. aur.*, **Ars. iod.**, Bar. c., **Bell.**, *Bor.*, Bov., *Bry.*, CALC. C., **Canth.**, **Carb. v.**, *Caust.*, **Cham.**, CLEM., *Con.*, *Dulc.*, *K. carb.*, **K. nit.**, Laur., Lyc., Mag. c., Mang., **Merc.**, *Mez.*, Mur. ac., Nat. c., *Nat. m.*, **Nit. ac.**, *Nux m.*, Nux v., Phos., **Puls.**, RHUS, Sars., SEP., *Sil.*, Spig., Stan., Staph., **Stro.**, SUL., *Sul. ac.*, Zinc.

Weeping.—*Ant. t.*, **Arn.**, **Bell.**, Bor., Canth., **Cham.**, **Croc.**, Cup., Hep., Lach., **Mar.**, *Nit. ac.*, Stan., **Verat. a.**

Wet Applications.—AM. CARB., Am. m., ANT. CR., Bar. c., **Bell.**, *Bor.*, Bov., *Bry.*, CALC. C., **Canth.**, **Carb. v.**, Cham., CLEM., *Con.*, *Dulc.*, *K. carb.*, **K. nit.**, *Laur.*, Lyc., Mag. c., **Merc.**, *Mez.*, Mur. ac., Nat. c., *Nit. ac.*, *Nux m.*, Nux v., Phos., Puls., RHUS, *Sars.*, Sep., *Sil.*, Spig., Stan., *Staph.*, **Stro.**, SUL., *Sul. ac.*, Zinc.

Wet, Getting.—Am. carb., *Ant. cr.*, Ant. t., *Ars.*, **Bell.**, *Bor.*, **Bry.**, CALC. C., *Calc. ph.*, *Camph.*, Carb. v., *Caust.*, **Colch.**, **Dulc.**, *Euphorb.*, Hep., **Ip.**, *Lach.*, Lyc., *Nit. ac.*, **Nux m.**, *Phos.*, Puls., RHUS, Sars., *Sec. c.*, SEP., *Sul.*, Verat. a., Zinc.

—**Head.**—Bar. c., BELL., *Led.*, **Puls.**

—**Feet.**—Cham., Merc., *Nat. c.*, *Nat. m.*, **Phos.**, Puls., *Rhus*, Sep., SIL., Xan.

—**With Sweat.**—Acon., *Calc. c.*, Dulc., RHUS, Sep.

Wet Weather.—Agar., AM. CARB., *Ant. cr.*, Aran., *Aur.*, Bar. c., **Bell.**, *Bor.*, Bov., Bry., CALC. C., *Calc. ph.*, Canth., *Carb. an.*, *Carb. v.*, Cham., *Chin.*, *Clem.*, Con., **Cup.**, DULC., *Fer.*, Hep., *Hyper.*, Ip., K. carb., *K. nit.*, Lach., *Laur.*, Lyc., *Mag. c.*, **Mang.**, *Meli.*, Merc., Mez., *Mur. ac.*, Nat. c., *Nat. s.*, *Nit. ac.*, NUX M., Nux v., *Pœo.*, Petrol., Phos., **Phyt.**, *Puls.*, *Ran. b.*, RHODO., RHUS, **Ruta**, Sars., *Seneg.*, Sep., *Sil.*, *Spig.*, Stan., *Staph.*, **Stro.**, Sul., *Sul. ac.*, **Verat. a.**, Zinc.

Wind.—Acon., Ars., *Asar.*, *Aur.*, **Bell.**, Bry., Calc. c., *Calc. ph.*, *Carb. v.*, CHAM., Chin., *Con.*, **Euphr.**, *Graph.*, Lach., LYC., Mur. ac., *Nat. c.*, Nux m., NUX V., PHOS., *Plat.*, PULS., RHODO., Spig., Sul., *Sul. ac.*, *Thuj.*

—**East (In Germany, Dry, From The Continent, Like Our West Wind).**—*Acon.*, Ars., Asar., Bell., *Bry.*, Carb. an., **Carb. v.**, Caust., Cham., HEP., *Ip.*, NUX V., *Saba.*, Sep., *Sil.*, SPO.

—**North.**—*Acon.*, Ars., **Asar.**, Bell., *Bry.*, Carb. an., Carb. v., **Caust.**, Cham., Hep., *Ip.*, **Nux v.**, *Saba.*, **Sep.**, Sil., SPO.

—**Windy (and Stormy) Weather.**—Acon., *Ars.*, *Asar.*, Aur., *Bell.*

Bry., *Carb. v.*, **Cham.**, **Chin.**, Con., *Euphr.*, Graph., **Lach.**, *Lyc.*, **Mur. ac.**, *Nat. c.*, NUX M., **Nux v.**, *Petrol.*, Phos., Plat., **Pso.**, Puls., RHODO., *Rhus*, Ruta, *Spig.*, *Sul.*, *Sul. ac.*, Thuj.

Winter, In.—Acon., *Agar.*, **Am. carb.**, Arg., Ars., AUR., *Bar. c.*, Bell., Bov., Bry., *Calc. c*, **Camph.**, *Caps.*, Carb. an., *Carb. v.*, **Caust.**, *Cham.*, Cic., Cina, *Cocc.*, Colch., *Con.*, Dulc., Fer., **Hell.**, **Hep.**, *Hyos.*, *Ign.*, *Ip.*, **K. carb.**, *Lyc.*, Mag. c., *Mang.*, Merc., *Mez.*, **Mos.**, Nat. c., Nat. m., **Nux m.**, NUX V., Petrol., *Phos.*, Pho. ac., Puls., *Rhodo.*, RHUS, Ruta, **Saba.**, Sars., Sep., Sil., Spig., Spo., **Stro.**, *Sul.*, Verat. a., *Vio. t.*

Women, For.—*Agar.*, Ambr., **Am. m.**, Ant. t., Arn., Asaf., BELL., Bor., **Bry.**, CALC. C., Camph., Canth., CAPS., Caust., CHAM., *Chin.*, Cic., *Clem.*, COCC., **Con.**, CROC., Cup., Dig., Euphorb., Fer., Graph., Hell., **Hyos.**, Ign., *Iod.*, Ip., K. carb., Lach., Laur., *Led.*, Mag. c., *Mang.*, Merc., Mos., Mur. ac., Nat. c., **Nux m.**, Op., PLAT., Pb., PULS., Rheum, Rhus, Saba., SABI., **Sec. c.**, **Sele.**, *Seneg.*, SEP., Sil., Spig., *Spo.*, *Sul.*, Sul. ac., Thuj., **Valer.**, Verat. a., Vio. o.

Worms. (See under **Stool.**)

Writing.—*Acon.*, Agar., Alum., Am. carb., **Am. m.**, Anac., Ant. cr., Arn., **Asaf.**, Asar., Aur., *Bar. c.*, Bor., **Bry.**, Calad., CALC. C., Cannab. s., Canth., *Carb. v.*, Caust., Cham., *Chel.*, *Chtn.*, Cic., **Cimic.**, Cina, Cocc., Coloc., Croc., Dros., Euphorb., Fer., *Graph.*, *Hep.*, *Ign.*, K. CARB., Laur., Led., **Lil. t.**, **Lyc.**, Meny., Mez., **Mur. ac.**, *Nat. c.*, NAT. M., Nit. ac., Nux m., **Nux v.**, Oleand., Par., Petrol., **Phos.**, Pho. ac., Plat., Puls., *Ran. b.*, Rheum, Rhodo., Rhus, Ruta, *Saba.*, Sabi., Samb., *Sars.*, **Seneg.**, Sep., SIL., Spig., *Spo.*, Stan., Staph., Stro., *Sul.*, *Sul. ac.*, Thuj., *Valer.*, ZINC.

Yawning.—Acon., Agar., *Am. carb.*, **Am. m.**, Anac., Ant. t., Arg., **Arn.**, Ars., Aur., Bar. c., Bell., *Bor.*, Bry., Calad., Calc. c., Canth., Caps., Carb. an., **Caust.**, **Chel.**, Chin., CINA, *Cocc.*, Croc., Cyc., Dig., Fer., Graph., Hep., IGN., Ip., *K. carb.*, KRE., Laur., **Lyc.**, *Mag. c.*, Mag. m., Mang., Mar., **Meny.**, Mez., **Mur. ac.**, Nat. c., Nat. m., NUX V., **Oleand.**, Op., Par., Petrol., Phos., Pho. ac., Plat., **Puls.**, RHUS, Ruta, Saba., SARS., Sep., *Sil.*, *Stan.*, Staph., Sul., Sul. ac., Thuj., Verat. a., *Vio. o.*, Zinc.

—**After.**—*Am. m.*, Croc., **Nux v.**

Ameliorations.

Alone, When. (See **Agg., Society.**)

Ascending.—*Am. m.*, *Arg.*, Bar. c., Bell., Bry., Canth., Coff., **Con.**,

Fer., *Lyc.*, Meny., Nit. ac., Pb., **Rhodo.**, Rhus, *Ruta*, *Sabi.*, Stan., Sul., **Valer.**, Verb.

Attention, Paying.—Camph., Cic., **Hell.**

Bathing.—*Acon.*, *Agar.*, *Alum.*, **Am. m.**, Ant. t., **Apis**, *Ars.*, ASAR., Bor., *Bry.*, *Cannab. i.*, **Caust.**, Cham., **Chel.**, Euphr., *Form.*, *K. chl.*, Laur., *Mag. c.*, Mez., Mur. ac., *Nux v.*, *Phyt.*, **Pic. ac.**. Pso., PULS., *Rhodo.*, *Saba.*, Sep., **Spig.**, Staph., Zinc.

—**Face.**—Asar., Mez., *Saba.*

Bending or Turning Affected Part.—Acon., Am. m., Arg., BELL., *Calc. c.*, *Cannab. s.*, Cham., **Chin.**, Guai., *Hep.*, K. carb., *Lach.*, Mang., *Mar.*, *Meny.*, Mur. ac., Nux v., Petrol., **Puls.**, *Rheum*, Rhus, Saba. *Sabi.*, Squ., Thuj., Verat. a.

Bending Backward.—*Acon*, **Bell.**, Cannab. s., **Cham.**, *Chin.*, **Cocc.**, K. carb., Lach., *Nux v.*, *Petrol.*, *Puls.*, **Rhus**, Saba., *Sabi.*, SENEG., Thuj., Verat. a.

—**Inward.**—Am. m., Bell., Sabi.

—**Sideways.**—*Meny.*, Puls.

—**Head Backward.**—*Bell.*, *Cact.*, **Cham.**, *Gel.*, **Hep.**, Rhus, Thuj., Verat. a.

—**Head Sideways.**—*Puls.*, Sep.

—**Holding Part Bent.**—*Puls.*, Rhus, **Squ.**

Biting.—Ars., Chin., *Cocc.*, Coff., Euphorb., Mag. m., Staph.

Blinking Eyes.—Asaf., Euphr., *Croc.*, *Oleand.*, Stan.

Blowing Nose.—Mang., *Merc.*, Sil., Stan.

Boring In With The Finger (Ear or Nose).—Bell., **Chel.**, Lach., NAT. C., *Par.*, Phos., Rheum, *Rhus*, Spig., *Sul.*, Thuj., Zinc.

Breakfast. (See Agg., Eating Before.)

Breathing, Deep.—Acon., Asaf., Bar. c., **Cannab. i.**, *Chin.*, Colch., Cup., *Dig.*, Dros., Ign., Iod., Lach., *Meny.*, *Oleand.*, *Osm.*, *Puls.*, Seneg., Sep., Spig., STAN., Staph., Vio. t.

Breath, Holding The.—Bell.

Carrying The Child in The Arms.—Ant. t., **Bell.**, **Cham.**, Merc.

Change of Position.—*Agar.*, Ars., *Cham.*, IGN., Mar., **Meli.**, Pho. ac., *Puls.*, **Valer.**, *Zinc.*

Chewing.—*Bry.*, Seneg.

Closing Eyes. (See **Agg., Opening Eyes.**)

Cloudy Weather. (See **Agg., Clear Weather.**)

Cold, In the. (See **Agg., Warmth in General.**)

—**Air.** (See **Agg., Warm Air.**)

—**Being.**—Acon., Agn., Alum., Ambr., Anac., Ant., cr., 'Ant. t., Arn.,

AMELIORATIONS.

Asar., Aur., Bar. c., Bell., Bov., Bry., Calad., Calc. c., Cannab. s., *Carb. v.,* Caust., Cham., Chin., Cina, Clem., *Cocc.,* Coff., Colch., Coloc., Croc., Dros., *Dulc.,* Euphorb., *Graph.,* Hell., Ign., IOD., Ip., K. carb., Led., LYC., Mang., Mar., Merc., Mez., Mur. ac., Nat. c., Nat. m., Nit. ac., *Nux m.,* Nux v., Oleand., Op., Petrol., Phos., *Pho. ac.,* Plat., PULS., Rhus, *Saba.,* Sabi., Sars., Sec. c., Sele., *Seneg.,* Sep., Sil., *Spig., Spo.,* Staph., Sul., *Thuj.,* Verat. a.

Crossing Limbs.—SEP.

Damp Weather. (See **Agg., Dry Weather.**)

Dancing.—Caust., Ign., Nat. m., SEP., *Sil.,* Stan.

Darkness.—Acon., Agar., *Agn.,* Am. carb., *Am. m.,* Anac., Ant. cr., Arn., *Ars., Asar.,* Bar. c., Bell., *Bor.,* Bry., CALC. C., Camph., Carb. an., *Caust.,* Cham., Chin., Cic., *Cina, Clem.,* Cocc., *Coff.,* Colch., CON., Croc., *Dig.,* Dros., EUPHR., GRAPH., *Hell.,* Hep., *Hyos.,* Ign., K. carb., K. nit., Lach., *Laur.,* Lyc., Mag. c., *Mag. m.,* Mang., Merc., Mez., Mur. ac., Nat. c., Nat. m., *Nit. ac.,* Nux m., Nux v., Petrol., PHOS., Pho. ac., Puls., Rhodo., Rhus, Ruta, *Sars.,* Sele., *Seneg.,* Sep., **Sil.,** Spig., Staph., Stram., Sul., Tar., Thuj., Valer., Verat. a., Zinc.

Descending. (See **Agg., Ascending.**)

Drawing in the Affected Part.—*Sabi.*

Drawing Up the Limb. (See **Agg., Stretching of Limbs.**)

Drinking, After.—*Acon., Aloe, Ars.,* Brom., Bry., *Carb. an., Cist., Crot. tig., Cup.,* Fer., *Graph.,* Ip., LOB. I., Mos., *Nux v., Oleand.,* **Op.,** *Pœo.,* Phos., *Rhus,* Sil., *Spig.,* SPO., *Tar.*

Driving in a Wagon.—*Bry.,* Graph., *K. nit.,* NIT. AC.

Dry Weather. (See **Agg., Wet Weather.**)

Eating, On.—*Aloe,* Alum., Ambr., Am. m., ANAC., Arn., Aur., Bell., *Cad. s., Calc. ph., Cannab. i.,* **Caps.,** Carb. an., Carb. v., Cham., Chel., Chin., Cocc., Croc., Dig., Dros., Fer., Graph., IGN., Iod, LACH., Laur., *Led.,* Lyc., Mag. c., *Mang.,* Merc., **Mez.,** Nat. c., Nit. ac., *Nux v., Par.,* Phos., *Pho. ac.,* Plat., Puls., *Rheum,* Rhodo., Rhus, *Saba.,* Sabi., Sep., Sil., Spig., *Spo.,* Squ., *Stan.,* Staph., Sul., Sul. ac., *Tar.,* ZINC.

—After.—*Acon., Aloe,* Alum., *Ambr.,* Am. carb., Am. m., **Anac.,** Arn., *Ars.,* Bar. c., Bov., *Brom.,* Bry., Calc. c., Cannab. s., Carb. an., *Carb. sul.,* Caust., *Cham.,* Chel., Chin., *Dios.,* Fer., *Gam.,* Graph., Hell., Ign., IOD, *K. bi., K. br.,* K. carb., Lach., Laur., *Lith.,* Mag. c., *Mang.,* Meny., Merc., *Mez.,* Mos., NAT. C., Nux v., *Pœo., Petrol.,* PHOS., Plant., Puls., *Ran. b.,* Rhodo., Rhus, **Saba.,** Sars., SEP., Sil., *Spig.,* SPO., *Squ.,* Stan., Stro., *Verat. a.*

—To Satiety.—Ars., Iod., *Phos.*

Eructations.—*Acon.*, *Agar.*, **Aloe**, **Alum.**, **All. c.**, *Ambr.*, **Am. m.**, **ANT. T.**, **Arg. n.**, *Aur.*, **Bar. c.**, *Bor.*, **Bry.**, Camph., *Cannab. s.*, **Canth.**, **CARB. V.**, *Carb. sul.*, **Chel.**, **Cocc.**, *Coc. c.*, *Colch.*, *Coloc.*, **Dig.**, Dios., GRAPH., IGN., *Iod.*, K. CARB., *Lach.*, Laur., LYC., Mag. c., Mag. m., *Mos.*, **Nat. c.**, **Nit. ac.**, **Nux v.**, Oleand., *Op.*, *Par.*, Petrol., *Phos.*, **Plat.**, Pb., *Rhodo.*, *Rumex*, Saba., *Sabi.*, SANG., Sars., **Sep.**, **Sil.**, Stro., **Sul.**, *Sul. ac.*, Zinc.

Exerting Body.—Canth., Ign., Nat. m., RHUS, SEP., *Sil.*, Stan. *Trill.*

—**Mind.**—*Croc.*, Fer., **Nat. c.**

Expiration.—ACON., *Agar.*, **Am. m.**, Anac., *Arg.*, *Arn.*, Asaf., *Asar.*, Bar. c., **Bor.**, BRY., *Calc. c.*, Camph., Canth., *Caps.*, Carb. an., Caust., *Cham.*, *Chel.*, Chin., Cina, Clem., Croc., Cyc., Euphr., *Guai.*, Hell., Hep., *Ip.*, K. carb., *K. nit.*, Kre., *Lyc.*, **Meny.**, *Merc.*, Mos., Nux m., Oleand., Op., *Ox. ac.*, Plat., Pb., *Ran. b.*, Ran. s., RHUS, *Saba.*, SABI., Sars., *Sele.*, *Seneg.*, Sep., Spig., *Spo.*, **Squ.**, Stan., Sul., Sul. ac., Tar., *Valer.*, Verat. a.

Fasting (Before Breakfast).—Agar., Alum., Ambr., Am. m., Anac., Ant. cr., Arn., **Ars.**, Asaf., Bar. c., **Bell.**, *Bor.*, **Bry.**, Calc. c., Caps., Carb. an. Carb. v., **Caust.**, CHAM., **Chin.**, Cocc., CON., *Cyc.*, **Dig.**, Euphorb., Fer., *Graph.*, Hell., Hep., Hyos., Ign., Iod., **K. carb.**, *K. nit.*, Lach., Laur., *Lyc.*, Mag. c., Mang., *Nat. c.*, NAT. M., *Nit. ac.*, **Nux m.**, *Nux v.*, Par., Petrol., *Phos.*, **Pho. ac.**, Pb., Puls., Rhodo., Rhus, Sabi., Sars., *Sele.*, Sep., **Sil.**, *Stan.*, Stro., *Sul.*, *Sul. ac.*, *Thuj.*, Valer., Verat. a., **Zinc.**

Flatulent Emissions.—*Acon.*, **All. c.**, **Aloe**, Ambr., Anac., Ant. t., Arn., Asaf., Asar., *Aur.*, Bism., Bor., Bry., *Calc. ph.*, Canth., Caps., **Carb. v.**, Cham., *Chel.*, Chin., Cic., **Cocc.**, Coff., Colch., Coloc., *Con.*, *Crot. tig.*, Graph., Guai., Hep., *Hyos*, **Ign.**, *K. carb.*, Lach., Laur., LYC., *Mar.*, Meny., Mez., Nat. m., Nit. ac., *Nux m.*, **NUX V.**, **Phos.**, **Pho. ac.**, Plat., Pb., **PULS.**, *Rheum*, **Rhodo.**, Rhus, Ruta, Sabi., SANG., Sele., Sep., Sil., Spig., Spo., *Squ.*, STAPH., Stram., SUL., Thuj., **Verat. a.**, Verb., Zinc.

Food and Drink, Bacon.—Ran. b., *Ran. s.*

—**Bread.**—Caust., *Laur.*, Nat. c., Phos.

—**Coffee.**—*Acon.*, *Agar.*, **Ars.**, *Cannab. i.*, Canth., CHAM., *Coloc.* Eucal., *Euphr.*, Hyos., *Op.*, Phos.

—**Cold.** (See **Agg., Food and Drink, Warm.**)

—**Fruit.**—*Lach.*

—**Hot.** (See **Agg., Food and Drink, Cold.**)

Food and Drink, Meat.—Verat. a.

—**Milk.**—Ars., *Mez.*, *Ruta*, Verat. a.

—**Salt.**—Mag. c.

—**Tea.**—*Carb. ac.*, *Dig.*, Fer.

—**Tobacco.**—Bor., *Carb. ac.*, **Coloc.**, **Hep.**, *Merc.*, *Nat. c.*, **Sep.**, Spig.

—**Vinegar.**—Asar., Bry., *Ign.*, Meny., *Op.*, Puls., *Stram.*

—**Water, Cold.**—Acon. f., *All. c.*, Anac., **Ant. t.**, Ars., **Asar.**, Bor., **BRY.**, Calc. c., **CAUST.**, Cham., **Clem.**, *Coc. c.*, **Cup.**, K. carb., *Laur.*, **PHOS.**, Puls., SEP., *Thuj.*, Verat. a., *Zinc.*

—**Water, Warm.**—Ars., **Lyc.**, Mang., Nux m., **Nux v.** Rhus, *Verat. a.*

—**Wine.**—Acon., Ars., *Agar.*, Bell., *Brom.*, *Bry.*, **Canth.**, **Carb. ac.**, *Chel.*, Cocc., **Con.**, *Glon.*, Graph., *Lach.*, *Mez.*, **Nux v.**, **Op.**, *Osm.*, **Phos.**, *Sele.*, *Sul.*, **Sul. ac.**, *Thea.*

Grasping.—Spig.

Hæmorrhage.—Bov., Sars., *Sele.*

Hand, Laying, On Part.—Bell., *Calc. c.*, **Canth.**, **Croc.**, *Dros.*, **Mang.**, Meny., *Mur. ac.*, Nat. c., Oleand., *Par.*, Phos., *Rhus*, Saba., Sep., *Spig.*, Sul., *Thuj.*

Hang Down, Letting Limbs. (See **Agg., Raising Affected Limb.**)

House, In the. (See **Agg., Open Air.**)

Inspiration.—Acon., **Ant. t.**, *Asaf.*, Bar. c., Bry., Cannab. s., Caust., Chin., Cina, **COLCH.**, **Cup.**, Dig., *Dros.*, Dulc., **IGN.**, *Iod.*, **Lach.**, Mang., Meny., **Nux v.**, Oleand., *Osm.*, Pho. ac., Puls., Ruta, Saba., Seneg., Sep., **SPIG.**, Squ., Stan., Staph., Tar., Verat. a., *Vio. o.*, *Vio. t.*

Kneeling.—*Euphorb.*

Knitting.—Lyc.

Leaning Against Anything.—Bell., **Carb. v.**, Dros., **FER.**, *K. carb.*, Mang., Merc., Nux v., Rhodo., Rhus, *Saba.*, **Sabi.**, **Seneg.**, **Sep.**, Spig., *Staph.*

—**Against Anything Hard.**—*Bell.*, Rhus, Sep.

—**Head on Anything.**—Bell., *Fer.*, *K. carb.*, **Merc.**, Rhodo., *Saba.*, Sabi., Seneg., *Spig.*

—**Head on One Side.**—Meny.

—**Head on a Table.**—*Fer.*, **Ign.**, Saba.

Licking with the Tongue.—Mang.

Light.—Am. m., Anac., Ars., Bar. c., *Calc. c.*, **Carb. an.**, **Carb. v.**, Con., **Plat.**, **Staph.**, *Stram.*, **STRO.**, *Valer.*

—**Bright.**—Am. m., Anac., *Ars.*, *Bar. c.*, **Calc. c.**, **Carb. an.**, *Carb. v.*, Con., **Plat.**, **Staph.**, *Stram.*, **STRO.**, *Valer.*

AMELIORATIONS. 315

Looking Downward.—Saba.
—**Intently.**—*Agar.*, *Agn.*, **Fer.**, **Nat. c.**, Petrol., Pho. ac.
—**Sideways.**—Oleand.
—**Straight Ahead.**—Bell., *Oleand.*, Spig.

Loosening Clothes.—*Am. carb.*, Arn., *Asar.*, Bry., CALC. C., **Cannab. i.**, Caps., **Carb. v.**, **Caust.**, Chin., *Coff.*, **Hep.**, LACH., LYC., NUX V., Oleand., Op., Puls., *Ran. b.*, **Sars.**, Sep., *Spo.*, **Stan.**, Sul.

Lying.—Acon., Agar., *Agn.*, Alum., Ambr., Am. carb., **Am. m.**, *Anac.*, Ant. cr., Ant. t., **Arg.**, **Arn.**, Ars., **Asar.**, Bar. c., **Bell.**, Bor., BRY., *Calad.*, **Calc. c.**, **Calc. ph.**, *Camph.*, *Cannab. s.*, **Canth.**, Caps., *Carb. ac.*, **Carb. an.**, Carb. v., *Caust.*, Cham., *Chel.*, Chin., *Cic.*, Cina, *Clem.*, *Cocc.*, *Coff.*, Colch., Coloc., Con., *Conv.*, Croc., *Cup.*, *Dig.*, *Dios.*, Dros., Dulc., Euphorb., FER., **Glon.**, Graph., Guai., *Hell.*, *Hep.*, Hyos., **Ign.**, *Iod.*, *Ip.*, K. carb., K. nit., *Kalm.*, *Kre.*, Lach., Laur., **Led.**, Lyc., Mag. c., Mag. m., Mang., Mar., *Merc.*, **Mez.**, Mur. ac., Nat. c., **Nat. m.**, Nit. ac., *Nux m.*, NUX V., *Oleand.*, Op., Par., Petrol., *Phos.*, Pho. ac., Pb., *Ran. b.*, *Rheum*, Rhus, Ruta, Saba., Sabi., *Sars.*, Sec. c., Sele., Seneg., *Sep.*, *Sil.*, **Spig.**, Spo., **Squ.**, *Stan.*, **Staph.**, *Stram.*, **Sul.**, Sul. ac., Thuj., **Verat. a.**, Zinc.

—**After.**—Acon., Agar., Agn., Ambr., *Am. m.*, *Anac.*, Ant. cr., Ant. t., Arg., *Arn.*, ARS., *Asaf.*, Aur., *Bar. c.*, **Bell.**, Bov., BRY., *Caj.*, Calad., CALC. C., *Calc. f.*, *Camph.*, *Cannab. s.*, **Canth.**, Caps., Carb. an., **Carb. v.**, Caust., Cham., *Chel.*, Chin., *Cic.*, **Cina**, Cocc., Coff., Colch., Coloc., Con., **Croc.**, *Crotal.*, Cup., *Dig.*, *Dios.*, Dros., Dulc., Euphr., **Graph.**, *Guai.*, Hell., **Hep.**, Hyos., Ign., **Iod.**, Ip., K. carb., K. nit., *Kre.*, **Lach.**, Laur., Led., Lyc., Mag. c., Mag. m., *Meli.*, **Merc.**, Nat. c., NAT. M., NIT. AC., Nux m., NUX V., **Oleand.**, *Pall.*, Par., *Petrol.*, Phos., *Pho. ac.*, PULS., Ran. b., *Rheum*, Rhodo., Rhus, Sabi., Samb., *Sars.*, Sec. c., Sele., **Sep.**, Sil., *Sin.*, **Spig.**, Spo., SQU., Stan., **Staph.**, Stram., **Sul.**, Sul. ac., Tar., Thuj., Valer., Verat. a., Verb.

—**In Bed.**—Acon., *Agar.*, Ambr., *Am. m*, *Anac.*, Ant. cr., **Ant. t.**, Arg., *Arn.*, Ars., Asar., Aur., Bar. c., **Bell.**, Bov., BRY., Calad., Calc. c., *Camph.*, *Cannab. s.*, **Canth.**, Caps., Carb. an., Carb. v., **Caust.**, Cham., Chel., Chin., Cic., *Cina*, *Clem.*, **Cocc.**, Coc. c., Coff., *Colch.*, Coloc., **Con.**, **Croc.**, Cup., *Dig.*, Dulc., Fer., Graph., *Guai.*, Hell., **Hep.**, *Hyos.*, Ign., Iod., Ip., K. carb., K. nit., Kre., **Lach.**, Laur., Led., **Lyc.**, Mag. c., *Mag. m*, Merc., Mez., Mur. ac., Nat. c., *Nat. m.*, *Nit. ac.*, *Nux m.*, NUX V., *Oleand.*, Par., Petrol., *Phos.*, Pho. ac., **Puls.**, Ran. b., Rheum, Rhodo., **Rhus**, *Saba.*, Sabi., Samb., *Sars.*, Sec. c., Sele., *Sep.*, **Sil.**, *Spig.*, Spo.,

SQU., STAN., Staph., Stram., *Stro.*, *Sul.*, Sul. ac., Tar., Thuj., Valer., *Verat. a.*, Verb., Vio. t.

Lying on Hard Bed.—*Bell.*, Rhus.

—On Back.—Acon., Am. carb., Am. m., **Anac.**, *Arn.*, Bar. c., *Bell.*, Bor., BRY., *Calad.*, CALC. C., *Canth.*, **Carb. an.**, Caust., Chin., *Cina*, Clem., *Colch.*, *Con.*, *Conv.*, *Fer.*, *Ign.*, *Ip.*, **K. carb.**, *Kre.*, Lach., **Lyc.**, Mag. m., *Merc.*, MERC. C., Mos., Nat. c., *Nat. m.*, Nux v., *Ox. ac.*, *Par.*, Phos., Plat., PULS., Ran. b., RHUS, Saba., **Sang.**, *Seneg.*, Sep., Sil., Spig., Spo., **Stan.**, *Sul.*, Thuj., Verat. a., Vio. t.

—Bent Up.—Colch., COLOC., *Puls.*, Rheum., Rhus.

—With Head High. (See Agg., Lying With Head Low.)

—Horizontally.—*Arn.*, *Spo.*

—On Side.—Acon., Alum., Am. carb., *Am. m.*, *Arn.*, *Ars.*, Bar. c., *Bell.*, Bor., Bry., *Calc. ph.*, *Canth.*, *Caust.*, *Cham.*, Chin., Cina, Clem., COCC., Colch., *Coloc.*, *Cup.*, Dulc., Euphorb., Ign., *Iod.*, K. carb., *K. nit.*, Lach., Mag. m., Merc., Nat. c., Nat. m., NUX V., Par., **Phos.**, Plat., *Puls.*, Ran. b., *Rhus*, Sep., *Sil.*, Spig., Spo., Stro., Sul., Thuj.

— —Left. (See Agg., Lying On Right Side.)

— —Right. (See Agg., Lying On Left Side.)

— —Painful.—*Ambr.*, *Arn.*, *Bell.*, BRY., **Calc. c.**, Cannab. s., Carb. v., *Caust.*, Cham., Coloc., *Ign.*, K. carb., Lyc., *Nux v.*, **Puls.**, *Rhus*, Sep., Stram., Vio. o., Vio. t.

— —Painless.—Acon., Agar., Ambr., *Am. carb.*, Am. m., Anac., Ant. cr., Arg., *Arn.*, *Ars.*, **Bap.**, **Bar. c.**, *Bell.*, *Bry.*, **Calad.**, Calc. c., *Calc. f.*, Cannab. s., Caps., *Carb. an.*, Carb. v., Caust., *Chin.*, Cina, Clem., Croc., Cup., *Dros.*, *Graph.*, Guai., **Hep.**, Hyos., Ign., **Iod.**, K. carb., K. nit., Lach., Led., *Lyc.*, *Mag. c.*, *Mag. m.*, Mang., Mar., Merc., **Mez.**, **Mos.**, Mur. ac., Nat. m., *Nit. ac.*, **Nux m.**, **Nux v.**, Oleand., *Par.*, Petrol., *Pho.*, *Pho. ac.*, Plat., *Puls.*, Ran. b., Ran. s., *Rheum*, Rhodo., Rhus, **Rumex**, Ruta, *Saba.*, Sabi., Samb., Sars., Sele., Sep., **Sil.**, **Spo.**, Staph., Stram., Sul., Tar., Thuj., Valer., Verat. a., Verb.

Mesmerism.—Acon., *Bar. c.*, Bell., Chin., *Con.*, CUP., *Graph.*, Ign., Iod., Mar., *Nat. c.*, Nux v., PHOS., Sabi., *Sep.*, Sil., Sul., *Vio. o.*

Moistening Affected Part.—*Alum.*, Am. m., Ant. t., *Ars.*, ASAR., Bor., Bry., Caust., Cham., **Chel.**, Euphr., Laur., *Mag. c.*, Mez., Mur. ac., *Nux v.*, PULS., *Rhodo.*, *Saba.*, Sep., **Spig.**, Staph., Zinc.

Motion in General. (See Agg., Rest.)

Continued.—*Agar.*, Ambr., Am. m., Bry., CAPS., Carb. v., *Caust.*, Chin., Cina, CON., **Cyc.**, Dros., EUPHORB., FER., K. carb., **Lyc.**,

AMELIORATIONS.

Plat., *Pb.*, **PULS.**, Rhodo., *Rhus,* **Ruta, Saba.,** Sabi., **SAMB.,** *Sep.,* **Sil.,** *Tar.,* **Thuj., Valer.,** Verat. a.

Motion Of Affected Part.—*Abrot.,* Acon., Agn., **Am. m., Arn., Ars.,** Asaf., *Asar.,* **Aur.,** Calc. c., **CAPS.,** *Cham.,* **Chin.,** *Cina,* **Con.,** Croc., **DULC., Euphorb., FER., K. bi., K. carb.,** Lyc., **Mag. c., Mag. m.,** *Meny.,* **Mos., Mur. ac.,** *Nat. c.,* **Pho. ac.; PULS.,** Rhodo., **RHUS,** Saba., Samb., Sep., Squ., Stan., *Stro.,* **SUL.,** Tar., *Thuj.,* **Valer.,** *Verb.,* **Vio. t.**

Open Air. (See **Agg., House, In The.**)

Opening Eyes. (See **Agg., Closing Eyes.**)

Pressure, External.—*Ab. c.,* Acon., *Agar.,* **Agn.,** *Alum.,* Ambr., **Am. carb., Am. m.,** *Anac.,* **Ant. cr., Apis, Arg., Arg. n., Arn., Ars., Asaf., Aur.,** *Bell.,* Bism., Bor., *Bov.,* **Bry.,** *Cact.,* **Calc. c.,** *Calc. f.,* Camph., **Canth.,** *Carb. ac.,* **Caust., Chel.,** Chin., *Cina, Cinnab.,* **Clem., Cocc., COLOC., CON., Croc.,** *Crot. tig.,* Dig., Dios., **DROS., Dulc.,** Form., Glon., **Graph.,** Guai., Hell., *Ign.,* Ip., **K. carb., K. iod.,** *Kre.,* Laur., Led., **LIL. T.,** Mag. c., **MAG. M., Mang., MENY., Merc.,** Mez., Mos., Mur. ac., **NAT. C.,** Nat. m., Nat. s., **Nit. ac., Nux m.,** *Nux v.,* Oleand., **Par.,** *Phos.,* **Pt.o. ac., PB., PULS.,** Rhus, Ruta, Saba., Sabi., *Sang.,* Sep., **SIL., Spig.,** *Stan.,* **Sul.,** *Sul. ac.,* **Thuj., Trill.,** Verat. a., **Verb.,** Zinc.

Raising Limbs. (See **Agg., Hang Down, Letting Limbs.**)

Reading.—**Fer., Nat. c.**

Rest. (See **Agg., Motion.**)

Retracting Abdomen. Ign., Sabi.

Rising Up.—Acon., *Alum.,* **AM. CARB., Am. m., Ant. t., ARS.,** Asaf., **Aur., Bar. c.,** *Bell.,* Bor., Bov., **Bry., CALC. C.,** *Cannab. s.,* **Canth., Carb. v.,** Caust., **Cham., Chel.,** *Chin.,* Cic., **Coloc., Con., Cup., Dig., Fer.,** Hell., **Hep., Hyos., Ign., K. carb.,** Laur., **Lyc.,** Mag. c., *Mang.,* Mar., Merc., Mos., *Naj.,* Nat. c., *Nat. m.,* Nux m., Nux v., *Oleand.,* Petrol., *Phos.,* **Puls.,** Rhus, **Sabi., SAMB., SEP., Sil.,** *Spig.,* Squ., Stan., **Sul.,** Sul. ac.

—**From Bed.**—*Am. m., Arg.,* **Ars., AUR., Caps.,** Carb. an., Caust., *Chin.,* Cic., **Con.,** Dig., **DULC., Fer.,** Hell., **Hyos., Ign.,** *K. nit.,* Kre., Laur., **Led., Lyc.,** Mag. c., *Mar.,* Merc., **Mos.,** Nat. c., Par., **Plat.,** Pb., **PULS., Rhus,** Sabi., **Samb., SEP.,** Stan., Sul., Sul. ac., *Tar.,* **Verat. a.,** Zinc.

— —**After.** (See **Agg., Lying in Bed.**)

—**From a Seat.**—Am. m., Arg., **Aur., Bar. c.,** Caust., *Chin.,* Cyc., **Dulc.,** Ign., **K. carb.,** *Lyc.,* **Mag. c.,** *Mang.,* Mar., Merc., *Nat. c.,* Phos., **Plat., Puls.,** *Rhus,* Samb., **Sep.,** Spig., *Spo.,* Valer., **Verat. a.,** Vio. t.

AMELIORATIONS.

Rising From a Seat, After.—Acon., **Agar.**, Agn., *Alum.*, **Ambr.**, Am. carb., Am. m., Anac., *Ant. cr.*, *Ant. t.*, **Arg.**, *Ars.*, **Asaf.**, Asar., *Aur.*, **Bar. c.**, Bell., *Bism.*, Bor., *Bov.*, Calc. c., Cannab. s., Canth., **CAPS.**, Carb. v., *Caust.*, Cham., Chel., *Chin.*, Cic., **Cina**, Cocc., CON., *Cup.*, CYC., *Dig.*, **Dros.**, DULC., Euphorb., *Euphr.*, **Fer.**, *Graph.*, *Guai.*, Hell., Hep., Hyos., **Ign.**, Iod., K. carb., *K. nit.*, Kre., **Lach.**, *Laur.*, Led., LYC., *Mag. c.*, **Mag. m.**, Mang., *Mar.*, **Meny.**, Merc., Mez., **Mos.**, **Mur. ac.**, **Nat. c.**, Nat. m., Nit. ac., *Oleand.*, *Op.*, Par., Petrol., Phos., **Pho. ac.**, PLAT., Pb., PULS., Rhodo., RHUS, Ruta, Saba., *Sabi.*, *Samb.*, Sars., *Sele.*, Seneg., SEP., *Sil.*, Spig., *Spo.*, **Stan.**, Staph., *Stro.*, Sul., Sul. ac., **Tar.**, **Thuj.**, **Valer.**, *Verat. a.*, VERB., *Vio. o.*, VIO. T., Zinc.

Rubbing.—Acon., Agar., Agn., **Alum·**, Ambr., Am. carb., **Am. m.**, Anac., *Ant. cr.*, Ant. t., **Arn.**, Ars., Asaf., Bell., *Bor.*, Bov., *Bry.*, CALC C., Camph., Cannab. s., CANTH., *Caps.*, CARB. AC., *Carb. an.*, Caust., *Ced.*, *Chel.*, *Chin.*, Cic., *Cina*, Colch., **Cyc.**, *Dios.*, **Dros.**, Guai., *Ham.*, Hep., **Ign.**, K. carb., *K. nit.*, Kre., *Laur.*, *Lil. t.*, *Mag. c.*, **Mag. m.**, Mang., *Meny.*, **Merc.**, *Mos.*, **Mur. ac.**, NAT. C., Nit. ac., **Nux v.**, Oleand., *Osm.*, *Pall.*, PHOS., *Pho. ac.*, Plat., PB., Ran. b., *Rhus,* **Ruta**, Saba., Sabi., Samb., Sars., *Sec. c.*, *Sele.*, Seneg., Spig., Spo., *Stan.*, *Staph.*, **Sul.**, Sul. ac., *Tar.*, Thuj., *Valer.*, Vio. t., Zinc.

Running.—Caust., **Ign.**, Nat. m., SEP., *Sil.*, Stan.

Scratching.—Agar., *Agn.*, *Alum.*, Ambr., *Am. carb.*, Am. m., *Anac.*, Ant. cr., *Ant. t.*, *Apis*, Arn., *Ars.*, ASAF., Bar. c., **Bell.**, Bor., Bov., **Brom.**, **Bry.**, CALC. C., Camph., Cannab. s., **Canth.**, *Caps.*, Carb. an., *Caust.*, Chel., Chin., *Cic.*, Cina, Clem., Coloc., *Con.*, Crot. tig., CYC., Dig., **Dros.**, *Form.*, Guai., Hep., *Hydras.*, Ign., Jug. c., K. carb., *K. nit.*, Kre., *Laur.*, Led., *Mag. c.*, Mag. m., **Mang.**, *Meny.*, Merc., Mez., *Mos.*, MUR. AC., NAT. C., Nit. ac., Nux v., *Oleand.*, PHOS., Pho. ac., Plat., **Pb.**, *Pru.*, Ran. b., *Rhus*, **Ruta**, Saba., *Sabi.*, *Sal. ac.*, Samb., Sars., Sec. c., *Sele.*, Seneg., *Sep.*, Spig., Spo., Stan., Staph , *Squ.*, **Sul.**, Sul. ac., *Tar.*, **Thuj.**, Valer., Vio. t., Zinc.

Sexual Suppression.—Calad.

Shaking Head.—Chin., *Cina*, Lach.

Shrugging Shoulders.—Calc. c., Cyc.

Silence. (See **Agg., Noise.**)

Sitting Down.—*Acon.*, Ambr., *Anac.*, *Ant. cr.*, Ant. t., Arn., Ars., *Asar.*, Aur., **Bar. c.**, Bell., Bov., *Bry., Calc. c.*, Cannab. s., Canth., CAPS., **Carb. an.**, Carb. v., Caust., *Cham.*, *Chin.*, Cic., Cocc., CON., Croc., Dig., Dros., Euphorb., Fer., *Graph.*, K. carb., K. nit., Lach., **Laur.**, Led., Lyc., Mang., Merc., Mur. ac., *Nat. c.*, **Nat. m.**, *Nit. ac.*, Nux v., Oleand.,

AMELIORATIONS. 319

Petrol., Phos., *Pho. ac.*, Plat., *Puls.*, Ran. b., Rhodo., Rhus, Ruta, Saba., Sep., *Sil.*, Spig., Staph., Stram., Stro., **Sul.**, *Thuj.*, Verat. a.

While Sitting.—Acon., *Agar.*, Agn., Alum., Am. carb., Am. m., *Anac.*, Ant. t., *Arn.*, Ars., Asaf., *Asar.*, Aur., Bar. c., *Bell.* Bor., **BRY.**, *Cad. s.*, **Calad.**, *Calc. c.*, Camph., *Cannab. s.*, Canth., Caps., Carb. an., Carb. v., Caust., Cham., Chel., Chin., *Cic.*, Cina, Clem., Cocc., **Coff.**, **COLCH.**, **Coloc.**, Con., Croc., Cup., Cyc., Dig., *Fer.*, *Gel.*, **Glon.**, Graph., Guai., *Hell.*, Hep., *Hyos.*, Ign., *Iod.*, *Ip.*, K. carb., K. nit., Kre., *Laur.*, Led., Mag. c., Mag. m., Mang., *Meny.*, **Merc.**, *Mez.*, Mos., Nat. c., *Nat. m.*, Nit. ac., *Nux m.*, **NUX V.**, Op., Par., *Petrol.*, **Phos.**, Pho. ac., Pb., **Puls.**, *Ran. b.*, Ran. s., **Rheum**, Rhus, Saba., Sabi., Samb., Sars., Sec. c., Sele., Sil., Spig., Spo., **Squ.**, Stan., *Staph.*, *Stram.*, Sul., Sul. ac., Tar., Thuj., Valer., Verat. a., Zinc.

—**Bent Over.** (See **Agg., Sitting Upright.**)

—**Upright.** (See **Agg., Sitting Bent Over.**)

Sleep, During.—*Am. m.*, Calad., *Hell.*, Phos., Samb.

—**After.**—Acon., *Agar.*, Ambr., Am. m., *Apis*, **Ars.**, Bry., **Calad.**, Calc. c., Cham., *Chin.*, Cocc., **Colch.**, Con., *Fer.*, *Hell.*, Ign., *Ip.*, Kre., Lach., **Merc.**, Nat. c., **Nux v.**, *Oxyt.*, **PHOS.**, Pho. ac., *Puls.*, Ruta, Sabi., *Samb., Sang.*, Sele., **Sep.**, Spig., Thuj.

—**On Falling Asleep.**—**Merc.**

—**When Half Asleep.**—**Sele.**

Sneezing.—Mag. m.

Society. (See **Agg., Alone, When.**)

Standing.—Agar., *Agn.*, Am. carb., *Anac.*, *Ant. t.*, *Arn.*, **Ars.**, **Asar.**, Bar. c., **BELL.**, *Bor.*, *Bry.*, Calad., *Calc. c.*, *Camph.*, **Cannab. s.**, *Canth.*, Carb. an., Carb. v., *Chel.*, Chin., *Cic.*, Cina, *Cocc.*, *Coff.*, **Colch.**, Coloc., Croc., Cup., *Dig.*, Dios., Euphorr., **Fl. ac.**, Graph., *Guai.*, *Hell.*, Hep., Ign., Iod., Ip., *Kre.*, **Led.**, Mang., Meny., Merc., Mez., *Mur. ac.*, *Naj.*, *Nat. m.*, Nit. ac., Nux m., **Nux v.**, Par., *Petrol.*, **Phos.**, Pb., Ran. b., *Rheum*, Rhus, *Ruta*, Sars., Sec. c., **Sele.**, Spig., *Spo.*, **Squ.**, Stan., *Staph.*, Stram., Sul. ac., Tar., *Tarent.*, Thuj.

Stepping Hard.—Caps.

Stool, After.—Acon., *Agar.*, All. c., **Aloe**, Am. m., Ant. cr., Ant. t., *Apis*, *Apoc. c.*, **Ars.**, **Asaf.**, Aur., Bar. c., Bism., *Bor.*, *Bov.*, **BRY.**, *Calc. ph.*, *Canth.*, Caps., *Carb. sul.*, *Cham.*, *Cina*, Coff., **COLCH.**, **Coloc.**, **Con.**, **Corn. c.**, Croc., *Crotal.*, *Crot. tig.*, *Cup.*, Cyc., *Dulc.*, Fer., *Gam.*, Guai., Hep., *Hydras.*, Ip., Kre., **Lept.**, Mang., Meny., *Nc. c.*, Nat. m., Op., **Oxyt.**, Par., **Puls.**, Rheum, **RHUS**, Saba., *Seneg.*, Sep., **SPIG.**, Squ., **Sul.**, *Thuj.*, Verat. a.

Stooping.—*Acon., Anac.,* **Ant. t.,** *Arn., Ars.,* **Asc. t.,** *Bar. c., Bell., Bry.,* **Cannab. s.,** *Carb. an., Caust., Chin., Cina,* COLCH., COLOC., **Con.,** *Dig., Hell.,* HYOS., *Ign., Iris v., Lach., Laur., Lyc., Mar g.,* **Mar.,** *Meny., Mez., Mos., Mur. ac., Nat. m, Nit. ac., Nux v., Petrol., Phos., Pho. ac.,* **PULS., Ran. b., Rheum,** *Rhus, Sabi., Sang., Sars., Spo.,* **Staph.,** *Sul., Tar., Valer., Verat. a., Verb.,* **Vio. t.**

Stretching Limbs. (See **Agg., Drawing Up Limbs.**)

Sucking With Tongue.—Mang.

Sunlight.—*Anac., Con.,* **Plat.,** *Stram.,* STRO.

Supporting the Limb.—*Alum.,* **Am. carb., Calc. c.,** *Caust., Dros., Hep., Ign., Nux v., Phos.,* **Puls.,** *Ruta, Sabi.,* **Staph.,** *Sul.,* Thuj.

Swallowing.—*Alum.,* **Ambr., Am. m., Arg., Arn., Bell., Caps.,** *Carb. v., Chel., Chin., Cocc., Dig., Dros., Graph.,* IGN., Iod., Ip., Lach., *Laur.,* **Led.,** *Mag. c., Mang., Merc., Mez.,* **Nat. c., Nit. ac., Nux v.,** *Oleand., Par., Phos., Pho. ac.,* **Plat.,** *Puls., Rheum, Rhus, Ruta, Saba., Sabi.,* Spig., *Spo., Squ., Stan., Staph., Sul., Sul. ac, Tar., Zinc.*

Sweat, During.—Ars., Bov., Bry., **Calad., Calc. c.,** CUP., *Lyc., Nat. c.,* Rhus.

—**After.**—Acon., *Aesc.,* Ambr., Am. m., Ant. t., Bar. c., Bell., Bov., Bry., **Calad., Canth.,** CHAM., *Chel., Clem,* Cocc., *Coloc.,* "**Gel.,** Graph., *Hell.,* **Hep.,** Hyos., Ip , K. nit., Led., *Lyc.,* Mag. m., *Nat. m., Nit. ac., Nux v.,* Oleand., Op., Puls., Rhodo., RHUS, Saba., Sabi., Samb., *Sele.,* Spo., Stram., **Stro., Sul.,** Sul. ac., Tar., **Thuj.,** Valer., **Verat. a.**

—**Cold.**—Nux v.

Talking.—Fer.

Touch.—Agar., *Alum.,* **Am. carb.,** Am. m., *Anac.,* **Ant. cr., Arn., Ars.,** **ASAF., Bell., Bism., Bry., CALC. C.,** *Canth.,* **Caust.,** Chel., Chin., **Coloc., Con.,** CYC., *Dros.,* Euphorb., Euphr., Hep., K. carb., Lyc., **Mang., Meny.,** MUR. AC., *Nat. c.,* Nat. m., Oleand., Petrol., **Phos.,** *Pho. ac., Pb.,* Sep., Spo., *Sul.,* Tar., **THUJ.,** Vio. t.

Turning at a Lathe.—Sep.

Twilight, In the.—*Bry.,* Phos.

Tying Up the Hair.—*K. nit.*

Uncovering. (See **Agg., Warm Wraps.**)

Vomiting.—Acon., *Agar.,* Ars., *Carb. sul.,* **Coc. c.,** Colch., **Dig.,** *Hyos. Nux v.,* Op., Puls., Sang., Sec. c.

Waking.—Ambr., Am. m., **Ars.,** Bry., **Calad., Calc. c., Cham.,** *Chin.,* Cocc., **Colch.,** *Hell.,* Ign., Ip., Kre., Lach., Nat. c., **Nux v., Onos.,** PHOS., Pho. ac., *Puls.,* Ruta, Sabi., *Samb.,* Sele., SEP., Spig., Thuj.

Walking.—Acon., *Agar.,* Agn., *Alum.,* Ambr., **Am. carb., Am. m.,** Anac., **Ant. cr., Ant. t** *Apoc c., Arg.,* **Arn., Ars.,** *Asaf.,* Asar., AUR.,

Bar. c., **BELL.**, *Bism., Bov., Brom.,* **Bry.,** *Calc. ac.,* Calc. c., *Canth.,* **CAPS.,** Carb. v., **Caust.,** *Cham.,* Chin., Cic., *Cina,* Cocc., *Coloc.,* CON., *Crotal.,* Cup., CYC., *Dios.,* **Dros.,** DULC., EUPHORB., *Euphr.,* FER., Fl. ac., *Glon.,* Graph., Guai., Hep., Hyos., Ign., *K. bi.,* K. carb., *K. nit.,* Kre., *Lach.,* Laur., Lyc., Mag. c., **Mag. m.,** Mang., Mar., Meli., **Meny.,** Merc., Mez., Mos., *Mur. ac., Nat. c.,* **Nat. m.,** Nit. ac., Nux m., Oleand., *Op., Par., Petrol., Phos.,* **Pho. ac., Plat.,** Pb., PULS., *Raph.,* **Ran. b.,** Rhodo., RHUS, **Ruta,** SABA, *Sabi.,* SAMB., Sars., Sele., Seneg., **Sep.,** Sil., Spig., Spo., Stan., Staph., *Stro.,* SUL, Sul. ac., TAR., *Thuj.,* VALER., *Verat. a.,* **Verb., Vio. t.,** Zinc.

Walking In Open Air.—*Acon.,* Agar., ALUM., Ambr., Am. carb., *Am. m., Anac., Ant. cr., Arg.,* Arn., Ars., *Asaf., Asar.* **Aur.,** *Bap.,* Bar. c., Bell., Bism., Bor., Bov., **Bry.,** Calc. c., *Caps., Carb. ac.,* Carb. v., Caust., Cic., Cina, **Con.,** Dulc., *Gam.,* Graph., Hep., Hyos., Ign., K. carb., K. nit., Laur., Lyc., **Mag. c., Mag. m.,** Mang., *Meny.,* Merc., **Merc. i. r.,** *Mez., Mos., Mur. ac.,* Nat. c., Nat m., Nit. ac., Op., *Ox. ac., Par., Petrol., Phos., Pho. ac.,* **Plat.,** Pb., PULS., *Naj., Rhodo.,* RHUS, Ruta, **Sabi.,** Sang., Sars., Sele., Seneg., **Sep.,** Spig., *Spo.,* Stan., Staph., *Stro.,* **Sul.,** Sul. ac., **Tar.** Thuj., Verat. a., *Verb., Vio. t.,* Zinc.

—**Bent Over.**—*Coloc.,* **CON., Hyos., Lyc.,** Nux v., **Rhus,** Sabi., *Sul.,* **Vio. t.**

—**Rapidly.**—Canth., *Carb. ac.,* **Ign.,** Nat. m., *Petrol.,* SEP., *Sil.,* Stan.

Warm. (See **Agg., Cold, Becoming.**)

Warm Wraps. (See **Agg., Uncovering.**)

Warmth in General. (See **Agg., Cold in General.**)

—**Of Bed.**—*Agar.,* Am. carb., Arn., ARS., *Aur.,* Bar. c., Bell., BRY., *Camph., Canth.,* **Caust.,** *Cic.,* Cocc., **Coloc.,** Con., Dulc., *Graph.,* Hep., *Hyos.,* K. carb., Lach., LYC., *Mos.,* Nit. ac., *Nux m*, NUX V., Phos., Pho. ac., *Rhus,* **Rumex,** Saba., *Sep., Sil.,* Spo., Squ., Staph., Stram., *Stro.,* Sul., Verat. a.

—**Of the Stove.**—Acon., Agar., Am. carb., ARS., *Aur., Bar. c.,* Bell., Bor., *Camph.,* Canth., Caps., *Caust., Cic.,* Cocc., Con., *Conv.,* Dulc., Hell., *Hep.,* Hyos., IGN., *K. carb.,* Mag. c., Mang., *Mos*, Nux m., **Nux v.,** Petrol., Ran. b., Rhodo., **Rhus,** *Saba.,* Sil., **Stro.,** *Sul.*

Weeping.—*Anac.. Dig.,* Ign., **Lyc.,** *Phos.*

Wiping with the Hand.—Alum., Arn., **Asaf.,** Bism., CALC., Canth., **Caps.,** Carb. an., **Cina,** Croc., CYC., **Dros.,** Guai., Ign., Mang., Meny., Merc., *Mur. ac.,* NAT. C., **Phos.,** Pb., *Puls., Ruta,* Sul., *Thuj.,* Zinc.

Wrapping Up Head. (See **Agg., Uncovering Head.**)

Writing, When.—*Fer.,* Nat. c.

Yawning.—Croc., **Staph.**

RELATIONSHIPS OF REMEDIES.

NOTE.—In preparing the chapter of *Relationships of Remedies*, according to the various sub-divisions of this work, the Editor has followed as closely as possible the original methods of Bœnninghausen. Twenty-one new drugs have been added. The aggravations, according to time, have been united to those according to circumstances; and, following the original, no separate section of the relationships of the ameliorations has been deemed necessary.

Aconitum.

Mind.—*Anac., Aloe., Apis, Arg. n., Ars.,* **Bap., Bell.,** *Bry.,* **Cact.,** Calc. c., Camph., CANNAB. I., Canth., *Carb. ac.,* Cham., *Chel.,* Cic., **Cimic.,** *Cocc.,* Con., **Croc.,** *Crotal.,* Cup., **Dig., Glon.,** Graph., *Hyd. ac., Hyos.,* Ign., Ip., *Lach., Lil. t.,* Lob. i., *Lyc., Meli., Merc.,* Mos., *Nat. m., Nux v.,* Onos., Op., *Phos., Phyt., Pso.,* **Puls.,** Rhus, Sal. ac., **Sec. c.,** *Sep., Stram.,* Sul., *Ther., Verat. a., Verat. v.,* Zinc.

Localities.—Aesc., *All. c., Aloe,* APIS, *Apoc. c.,* ARG. N., Arn., *Ars., Arum. t., Bap.,* BELL., Berb., **Bry.,** *Cact.,* **Calc. c., Cannab. i.,** Canth., *Carb. ac., Carb. v.,* (Caul.), Caust., (Ced)., **Cham., Chin.,** Cimic., Cocc., Con., Crotal., Dig., (Dios.), Dros., Dulc., Eup. per., (Fl. ac)., **Gel., Glon.,** Graph., *Hep.,* (Hyd. ac.), *Hyos.,* **Ign.,** *Ip.,* (Iris v.), K. BI., K. carb., Kalm., Lil. t., Lith., **Lyc.,** Meli., *Merc.,* Nat. c., *Nat. m.,* Nit. ac., NUX V., Op., Petrol., **Phos.,** Pho. ac., *Phyt.,* Plat., Pb., *Pod.,* Pso., PULS., **Rhus,** Ruta, Saba., **Sang.,** Sec. c., SEP., *Sil., Spig.,* Stan., Staph., Stram., SUL., **Verat. a., Verat. v.,** Zinc.

Sensations.—*Aesc.,* (All. c.), (Aloe), **Apis,** *Arg. n., Arn.,* **Ars.,** Arum. t., Asaf., **Bap.,** Bar. c., BELL., *Berb.,* **Bry.,** Cact., **Calc. c.,** *Cannab. i.,* Canth., Carb. v., Caust., *Cham., Chin.,* **Cimic.,** Cocc., (Crotal.), Fer., **Gel.,** *Glon.,* Hyos., *Ign.,* Iris v., **K. bi.,** *K. carb.,* Lil. t., **Lyc.,** *Merc.,* Nat. c., *Nat. m.,* Nit. ac., NUX V., **Phos.,** Pho. ac., (*Phyt.*)., Plat., Pod., Pso., **Puls.,** RHUS, **Sang.,** SEP., *Sil., Spig.,* Staph., Stram., SUL., Verat. a., Verat. v.

Glands.—Bell., Bry., Lyc., **Merc.,** Phos., Puls., *Sul.*

Bones.—*Bell.,* Calc. c., Lyc., **Merc.,** Phos., *Puls.,* Sul.

(322)

RELATIONSHIPS.—ACON.—ÆSC. 323

Skin.—Am. carb., **Apis**, Arn., *Ars.*, **Bell.**, **Bry.**, Caust., Cham., Dulc., Hep., Ip., K. carb., Lach., *Lyc.*, MERC., Mez., Nit. ac., Nux v., *Phos.*, Pho. ac., **Puls., Rhus**, Sec. c., Sep., *Sil.*, **Staph., Sul.**

Sleep and Dreams.—Anac., (Apis), Arg. n., *Ars.*, (Bap.), *Bell.*, **Bry.**, *Calc. c.*, Cannab. i., Caust., Cham., *Cham.*, (Cimic.), Con., (Gel.), Graph., *Hep., Ign., K. carb.*, Lach., Lyc., Merc., Nat. c., *Nux v.*, Op., **Phos.**, Pho. ac., (Pod.), *Puls., Rhus, Sep., Sil.*, **Sul.**

Blood, Circulation and Fever.—(Aloe), (Apis), Arg. n., Arn., *Ars.*, **Bell.**, (Berb.), BRY., Cact., *Calc. c.*, Cannab. i., Carb. v., *Cham.*, Chin., (Crotal.), Cup., Fer., (Gel.), *Glon., Hep.*, Hyos., Ign., Iod., Ip., K. carb., Kre., *Lyc.*, **Merc.**, *Nat. m.*, Nit. ac., NUX V., *Op.*, **Phos.**, *Pho. ac.*, Pod., *Puls.*, **Rhus**, Samb., *Sang.*, Sec. c., *Sep., Sil.*, Stan., *Stram., Sul., Verat. a.*, Verat. v.

Aggravations: Time and Circumstances.—Aesc., (All. c.), (Aloe) Anac., Ant. cr., Ant. t., *Apis, Arg. n.,* **Arn.**, *Ars.*, (Bap.), Bar. c., **Bell.**, Bor., BRY., (Cact.), **Calc. c.**, Cannab. i., Caps., Carb. an., Caust., *Cham.*, (Cimic.,) *Croc.*, (Crotal.), Dulc., (Gel)., (Glon.), *Hep., Ign.*, Iod., *K. bi.*, K. carb., Lil. t., **Lyc.**, Mag. c., Mang., Merc., Nit. ac., **Nux v.**, *Phos.*, Phyt., Pb., Pod., *Puls.*, **Rhus**, Saba., *Sabi.*, Samb., **Sang.**, Sep., Sil., Staph., Squ., Sul., Verat. a., (Verat. v.).

Other Remedies.—Aesc., (All. c.), (Aloe), Anac., **Apis, Arg. n.,** Arn., **Ars.**, (Arum t.), Bap., BELL., (Berb.), BRY., *Cact.*, **Calc. c., Cannab. i.**, Carb. v., Caust., *Cham.*, Chin., *Cimic.*, Cocc., (Crotal.), Dulc., Gel., Glon., Graph., *Hep.*, Hyos., *Ign.*, Ip., *K. bi., K. carb.*, Lach., (Lil. t.), **Lyc.**, MERC., Nat. c., *Nat. m.*, Nit. ac., **Nux v.**, Op., PHOS., Pho. ac., Phyt., Pod., PULS., RHUS, *Sang.*, Sec. c., **Sep.**, *Sil.*, Spig., Staph., Stram., SUL., *Verat. a.*, Verat. v.

Antidote.—*Acetum*, Cham., *Coff.*, Nux v., Verat. a., *Vinum.*

Æsculus.

Mind.—*Agn. n., Aloe,* **Bell., Bry.,** *Calc. c.*, **Cham., Cimic.,** Con., *Gels.,* Hep., *Ign., Lyc.,* Merc., Merc. c., Mur. ac., *Nat. c.*, Nit. ac., *Nux v.*, Phos., Pho. ac., **Puls.,** *Rhus, Sep.,* SULPH., *Verat. v.,* Zinc.

Localities.—Acon., Agar., (Agn.), All. c., *Aloe*, Alum., Ambr., (Am. carb.), Am. m., Anac., Ant. c., *Ant. t.,* Apis, Apoc. c., (Arg.), *Arg. n.,* Arn., **Ars.**, (Arum t.), (Asaf.), Asar., Aur., Bap., *Bar. c.,* **Bell.,** (Berb.), Bism., (Bor.), BRY., (Calad.), **Calc. c.,** Camph., (Cannab. i.), *Canth.,* Caps., Carb. ac., Carb. an., Carb. v., *Caust., Cham., Chel.,* **Chin.,** Cimic., Cina, (Clem.), Cocc., (Coff.), **Colch., Coloc.,** Con., (Crotal.), Cup., (Cyc.), **Dig.,** (Dios.), Dros., Dulc., (Eup. per.), Euphorb., **(Euphr.)**, Fer., (Fl.

RELATIONSHIPS.—ÆSC.

ac.), (Gels.), *Graph.*, Hell., Hep., Hyos., **Ign.**, Ip., Iod., Iris v., *K. bi*, **K. carb.**, (K. nit.), Kalm., Kre., Lach., *Lil. t.*, (Lith.), *Lyc.*, (Mag. c., *Mag. m.*, (Mar.), (Meli.), Meny, **Merc.**, (Mez.), (Mos.), (Mur. ac.), Nat. c., **Nat. m.**, **Nit. ac.**, (Nux m.), **NUX V.**, Op., *Petr.*, **PHOS.**, Pho. ac., (Plat.), Pb., (Phyt.), Pod., (Pso.), **PULS.**, Ran. b., Rheum, (Rhodo.), **Rhus**, Ruta, Saba., Sabi., (Samb.), Sang., (Sars.), (Sec. c.), (Sele.), Seneg., **Sep.**, *Sil.*, Spig., (Spo.), Squ., Stan., Staph., (Stram.), (Stro.), **SUL.**, (Sul. ac.), (Ther.), (Thuj.), (Valer.), **Verat. a.**, (Verat. v.), (Verb.), *Zinc.*

Sensations.—*Acon.*, Agar., Alum., (Anac.), Ant. t., (Apis), (Arg.), *Arg. n.*, Arn., Ars., (Arum. t.), (Asaf.), (Asar.), Bap., Bar. c., *Bell.*, (Berb.), *Bry.*, Cact., Calc. c., (Camph.), (Cannab. i.), Canth., (Carb. v.), Caust., (Cham.), (Chel.), *Chin.*, (Cimic.), Cocc., (Colch.), *Coloc.*, Con., (Cup.), Dig., (Dros.), (Eup. per.). Fer., (Gel.), (Hep.), Hyos., (Ign.), (Ip.), (Iod.), K. bi., (K. carb.), (Kre.), *Lach.*, (Laur.), (Led.), (Lil. t.), Lyc., Merc., Mez., (Mur. ac.), Nat. c., *Nat. m.*, **Nit. ac.**, Nux m., **Nux v.**, Op., Par., **Phos.**, *Pho. ac.*, (Phyt.), (Plat.), Pb., Pod., **Puls.**, Ran. b., (Rhodo.), *Rhus*, (Saba.), (Sabi.), Sang., Sars., (Sec. c.), Seneg., **Sep.**, *Sil.*, Spig., (Spo.), (Squ.), *Stan.*, (Staph.), Stram., **Sul.**, Sul. ac., (Tar.), Thuj., *Verat. a.*, (Verat. v., Zinc.

Glands.

Bones.

Skin.

Sleep and Dreams.—(Caust.), (Chel.), (Cina.), (Croc.), (Ign.), (Kre.), (Nux v.), (Rhus).

Blood, Circulation and Fever

Aggravations : Time and Circumstances.—(Acon.), (Agn.), (Apis), (Ant. t.), (Arn.), (Ars.), (Bap.), (Bar. c.), Bell., Bry., Calc. c., (Cannab. s.), (Canth.), (Caps.), (Cham.), (Chel.), Cocc., (Coff.), (Colch.), (Coloc.), (Croc.), (Fer.), (Glon.), (Graph.), (Hell.), Hep., (Hyos.), (Ip.), (Iod.), (Lach.), Led., (Mag. m.), (Mang.), Merc., (Mez.), (Nat. m.), (Nit. ac.), Nux v., (Petrol.), (Phos.), (Pho. ac.), (Phyt.), (Pb.), Puls., Ran. b., (Rhodo.), Rhus, (Ruta), (Sabi.), (Sang.), (Sars.), (Sep.), (Sil.), (Spig.), (Stan.), (Staph.), (Stram.), (Stro.), Sul., (Thuj.), (Valer.), (Verat. a.), (Zinc).

Other Remedies.—Acon., (Agar.), Agn., Aloe., (Alum.), Ant. t., (Apis), Arg. n., Arn., *Ars.*, Bap., Bar. c., **BELL.**, **BRY.**, **Calc. c.**, Camph. Canth., Caust., Cham., Chel., Chin., *Cimic.*, Cocc., Colch., *Coloc.*, Con., (Dig.), Fer., Gel., (Graph.), Hep., Hyos., *Ign.*, (Ip.), (Iod.), K. bi., K. carb., (Kre.), Lach., (Lil. t., *Lyc.*, (Mag. m.), **Merc.**, (Mez.), (Mur. ac.), Nat. c., *Nat. m.*, **Nit. ac.**, **NUX V.**, (Op.), (Petrol.), **Phos.**, *Pho. ac.*

RELATIONSHIPS.—ÆSC.—AGAR. 325

Puls., Ran. b., **Rhus**, (Sabi.), Sang., (Sars.), (Seneg.), Sep., Sil., Spig., Stan., Staph., (Stram.), SUL., (Thuj.), *Verat. a.*, Verat. v., Zinc.

Agaricus Muscarius.

Mind.—Ant. cr., **Bell.**, Bry., Cannab. s., Gel., Glon., Hyos., *Lach.,* Nux v., **OP., Phos.**, Stram., Verat. a.

Localities.—Aesc.. (All. c.), Aloe, Alum., Apis, (Apoc. c.), *Arg. n.,* (Arum. t.), Aur., (Bap.), **Bell.**, (Berb.), Bry., Cact., **CALC. C**, Cannab. i., Canth., (Carb. ac.), Carb. v., *Caust.*, **Chin.**, Cimic., Con., (Crotal.), (Dios.), (Eup. per.), (Gel.), (Glon.), Hep., Ign., (Iris v.), K. bi., *K. carb.,* (Kalm.), (Lil. t.), Mang., (Meli.), MERC., Mez., Nat. m., **Phos., Pho. ac.**, (Phyt.), Pod., **Puls.**, Rhus, Sabi., Sang., Sars., **Sep.**, *Sil.,* Spig., Spo., *Staph.*, Stram., *Sul.*, (Ther.), (Verat. v.), Zinc.

Sensations.—Acon., (Aesc.), (Aloe.), Apis, Arg. n., Ars., (Arum. t.), (Bap.), Bar. c., **BELL.**, Berb., *Bry.*, (Cact.), **Calc. c.**, Cannab. i., Canth., Caust., Cham., *Chin.*, Cimic., **Cocc.**, Con., (Crotal.), Cup., (Dios.), Gel., (Glon.), Hyos., *Ign.*, Iris v., **K. bi.**, K. carb., (Kalm.), (Lil. t.), (Lith.), Lyc., *Merc.*, Nat. m., **Nux v.**, *Phos.*, Pho. ac., (Phyt.), (Pod.), Puls., *Sang.,* Sep., *Sil.*, Stan., *Sul.*, Zinc.

Glands.

Bones.—Am. m., Bell., Caust., *Cocc.*, Hep., Merc., Phos., Puls., *Ruta*, **Skin.**—Ant. cr., *Bry.*, **Calc. c.**, *Chin.*, Lach., *Led., Lyc.*, Mag. c., Merc., Nat. m., Nit. ac., Petrol., Phos., *Pho. ac.*, Puls., **Rhus**, Sele., Sep., *Sil., Sul.*, Verat. a.

Sleep and Dreams.—Acon., Anac., Ant. cr., Cyc., *Lach.*, Nux v., *Phos.*, Sul.

Blood, Circulation and Fever.—Bell., *Bry.*, (Cannab. i.), **Chin.**, Graph., *Hep.*, Lach., *Merc.*, **Nat. m.**, *Rhus*, Samb., (Sang.), Sele., Sep., Stram., Sul.

Aggravations: Time and Circumstances.—(All. c.), (Aloe), Apis, (Arg. n.), *Ars.*, (Bap.), Bar. c., Bov., *Calc. c.*, Cannab. s., Caps., Carb. v., Chel., *Chin.*, Con., *K. bi., K. carb., K. nit.*, **Lach.**, *Lyc.*, **Nat. c.**, Nux m., Nux v., (Pod.), **PULS.**, Ran. b., Rhodo., RHUS, *Ruta*, (Sang.), **Sele.**, Sep., Sil., Spig., Stram., **Valer.**, Zinc.

Other Remedies.—(Aesc.), (All. c.), (Aloe.), Ant. cr., Apis, Arg. n., Ars., (Bap.), **Bell.**, (Berb.), *Bry.*, (Cact.), **Calc. c.**, Cannab. i., Carb. v., Caust., Chin., Cimic., *Cocc.*, Con., (Crotal.), Hep., Gel., (Glon.), **Ign.**, *K. bi., K. carb.*, **Lach.**, (Lil. t.), *Lyc.*, **Merc.**, *Nat. m., Nux v.*, Op., **Phos.**,

Pho. ac., (Phyt.), Pod., **Puls.**, RHUS, *Sang.*, *Sele*, **Sep.**, **Sil**., *Stram.*, *Sul.*, Valer., Zinc.

Antidotes.—Camph., Coff., Puls., Vinum.

Agnus.

Mind.—Abs., Acon., Alum., Anac., Arn., Ars., Aur., Bar. c., **Bell.**, *Calc. c.*, Caust., *Cham.*, Cimic., Cocc., Con., Croc., Graph., Glon., *Hyos.*, IGN., LYC., Merc., Mez., Nat. c., *Nat. m.*, Nux m., *Nux v.*, Oleand., Op., *Pho. ac.*, *Plat.*, **Puls.**, *Rhus*, *Sep.*, Sil., Stram., SUL., Thuj., *Verat. a.*, Zinc.

Localities.—Arn., Ars., Calad., Calc. c., Canth., Chin., Con., Cyc., Gel., *Graph.*, *Hep.*, *Ign.*, *K. carb.*, (Kalm.), **Lyc.**, **Merc.**, *Nux v.*, *Pho. ac.*, **Puls.**, Rhodo., *Rhus*, Sabi., *Sele.*, Sep., Staph., **Sul.**, Thuj., Zinc.

Sensations.—*Arn.*, Bar. c., **Bell.**, **Bry.**, **Calc. c.**, **Caust.**, Chin., Con., Graph., Ign., *K. carb.*, K. nit., Led., *Lyc.*, *Merc.*, Nat. c., Nat. m., Nux v., *Phos.*, **Puls.**, Rhodo., **Rhus**, *Sep.*, Spo., Staph., **Sul.**

Glands.—Arn., **Bell.**, BRY., Calc. c., *Carb. an.*, Chin., Clem., **Con.**, Graph., K. carb., **Lyc.**, *Merc.*, **Phos.**, **Puls.**, *Rhus*, Sil., Spo., **Sul.**

Bones.—*Chin.*, Cup.

Skin.—Arn., Asaf., Bar. c., **Bry.**, *Calc. c.*, *Caust.*, Con., Cyc., Euphorb., Graph., *Lach.*, *Led.*, LYC., Merc., Mez., *Oleand.*, Phos., *Plat.*, **Puls.**, Ran. s., Rhus, *Sil.*, *Spo.*, **Staph.**, *Sul.*

Sleep and Dreams.—Ant. t., Bry., *Croc.*, Nux m., Op., Verat. a.

Blood, Circulation and Fever.—Acon., Ant. t., (Apis), ARS., **Bell.**, *Bry.*, *Calc. c.*, *Chin.*, Cocc., (Gel.), *Hell.*, *Ip.*, Lyc., **Merc.**, Nit. ac., *Nux m.*, **Nux v.**, **Phos.**, **Puls.**, Rhus, *Saba.*, *Sep.*, **Spig.**, **Sul.**, Thuj., Verat. a.

Aggravations: Time and Circumstances.—Acon., (Aesc.), Ant. cr., Ant. t., (Apis), Arn., Asar., **Bell.**, *Bry.*, (Cact.), (Cannab. i.), Carb. an., Chel., (Cimic.), Croc., Dig., Euphr., (Glon.), Graph., *Hell.*, Hep., (K. bi.), (Lil. t.). Lyc., Merc., Nat. m., Nit. ac., **Nux v.**, **Phos.**, (Phyt.), **Puls.**, *Rhus*, *Sabi.*, Sang., Squ., Sul.

Other Remedies.—Apis, *Arn.*, Ars., **Bell.**, **Bry.**, Calc. c., *Caust.*, *Chin.*, Cimic., *Con.*, Croc., Gel., Glon., *Graph.*, Hell., *Ign.*, K. carb., LYC., **Merc.**, Nat. m., Nux m., *Nux v.*, **Phos.**, PULS., Rhus, (Sang.), *Sep.*, Sil., Spo., Staph., SUL., Verat. a.

Antidote.—Camph.

Allium Cepa.

Mind.

Localities.—*Acon.*, (Aesc.), Agar., (Aloe), (Ambr.), *Am. m.*, (Ant. c.), Apis, Apoc. c., **Arg.**, **Arg. n.**, Arn., **Ars.**, *Arum. t.*, (Asaf.), Aur., (Bap.),

Bar. c., **Bell.**, (Bism.), (Bor.), *Bry.*, (Calad.), *Calc. c.*, (Camph,), Cannab. i.), Canth., Caps., Carb. v., (Caust.), Cham., (Chel.), Chin., (Cic.), Cimic., Cina, (Cocc.), (Coff.), (Colch.), Coloc., Con., (Croc.), (Cup.), (Cyc.), **Dig.,** (Dios.), Dros., (Dulc.), (Euphorb.), *Euphr.*, (Fer.), (Gel.), Graph., **(Hell.),** (Hep.), (Hyos.), (Hyper.), (Ign.) ,(Ip.), *Iod.*, K. bi., (K. carb.), (K. nit.), (Kalm.), Kre., *Lach.*, (Laur.), (Led.), (Lil. t.), (Lyc.), (Mag. m.), (Mang.), (Mar.), (Meli.), **Merc.**, *Mez.*, (Mur. ac.), Nat. c., Nat. m., *Nit. ac.*, (Nux m.), **Nux v.**, (Par.), Petrol., *Phos.*, Pho. ac., (Phyt.), (Pb.), (Pod.), (Pso.), **PULS.**, (Ran. b.), **Rhus**, Ruta, Saba., (Sabi.), (Samb.), *Sang.*, (Sars.), (Sele.), Seneg., *Sup.*, Sil., *Spig.*, Spo., *Squ.*, Stan., Staph., *Stram.*, **Sul.**, (Sul. ac.(, Thuj., *Verat. a.*, (Verat. v.), (Verb.), Zinc.

Sensations.—(Acon.), (Ars.), (Asar.), (Bry.), (Caps.), (Lach.), **Merc.**, (Nit. ac.), (Nux v.), (Par.), (Phos.), (Puls.), (Sep.), (Squ.), Sul.

Glands.

Bones.

Skin.

Sleep and Dreams.

Blood, Circulation and Fever.

Aggravations: Time and Circumstances.—(Acon.), (Agar.), (Am. carb.), (Ant. cr.), (Ant. t.), (Arg.), (Ars.), (Asaf.), (Asar.), (Bell.), Bry., (Calc. c.), (Caps.), (Caust.), (Cimic.), (Cocc.), (Colch.), (Con.), (Croc.), (Dulc.), (Hell.), (Hep.), (Hyos.), (Ign.), (Iod.), (K. bi.), (K. carb.), (Led.), (Lyc.), (Mag. c.), (Mag. m.), (Mang.), (Merc.), (Mez.), (Nat. m.), (Nux m.), (Petrol.), (Phos.), Puls., (Ran. s.), (Rhodo.), (Rhus), (Saba.). (Sabi.), (Seneg.), (Sep.), (Stro.), (Sul.), (Zinc).

Other Remedies.—*Acon.*, (Agar.), (Ant. cr.), Arg., *Ars.*, Arum. t., (Asaf.), (Asar.), Bell., Bry., Calc. c., Caps., (Caust.), Cimic., (Cocc.), (Colch.), Con., (Croc.), (Dulc.), *Euphr.*, (Hell.), (Hep.), (Hyos.), (Ign.), *Iod.*, K. bi., (K. carb.), Kre., Lach., (Led.), (Lyc.), (Mag. m.), (Mang.), **Merc.**, Mez., Nat. m., Nit. ac., (Nux m.), **Nux v.**, (Par.), Petrol., Phos., **PULS.**, *Rhus.*, Saba., (Sabi.), *Sang.*, Seneg., Sep., *Sil.*, Squ., **Sul.**, Zinc.

Aloe.

Mind.—*Acon.*, Aesc., Ant. c., Arn., Ars., *Aur.*, *Bap.*, **Bell.**, Bry., *Calc. c.*, Cannab. i., Cannab. s., **Canth.**, Carb. ac., Caust., Chel., Cocc., **Con.**, Hyos., Ign., **Lyc.**, Meli., Merc., *Nat. m.*, **Nux v.**, *Op.*, **Phos.**, **Pho. ac.**, Plat., **Puls.**, Ran. b., Rhus t., *Sep.*, Sil., *Stram.*, **Sulph.**, Verat. a., *Verat. v.*, Zinc.

Localities.—*Acon.*, **Aesc.**, *Agar.*,(Agn.,)(All. c.), Alum.,(Ambr.),(Am. carb.), Am. m., (Anac.), **Ant. cr.**, Ant. t., *Apis*, Apoc. c., **Arg. n.**, **Arn.**,

ARS., (Arum. t.), *Asaf.*, (Asar.), Aur., Bap., *Bar.* c., **BELL.**, (Berb.), Bism., Bor., **BRY.**, (Cact.), (Calad.), **Calc.** c., (Camph.), (Cannab. i.), (Cannab. s.), **Canth.**, *Caps.*, Carb. ac., *Carb. an.*, **Carb. v.**, *Caust.*, **Cham.**, **Chel.**, **Chin.**, (Cic.), (Cimic.), (Cina), (Clem.), **Cocc.**, *Colch.*, COLOC., *Con.*, (Croc.), (Crotal.), Cup., (Dig.), *Dios.*, (Dros.), Dulc., Fer., (Fl. ac.), (Gel.), *Graph.*, (Hell.), Hep., *Hyos.*, *Ign.*, Ip., (Iod.), Iris v., *K. bi.*, **K. carb.**, (K. nit.), (Kalm.), (Kre.), Lach., Laur., **Lil. t.**, **Lyc.**, Mag. m., (Mar.), (Meny.), MERC., (Mez.), Mur. ac., (Nat. c.), **Nat. m.**, *Nit. ac.*, (Nux m.), NUX V., (Oleand.), Op., Petrol., PHOS., *Pho. ac.*, (Phyt.), (Plat.), (Pb.), POD., Pso., PULS., (Ran. b.), (Ran. s.), Rheum, (Rhodo.), *Rhus*, (Ruta), Saba., (Sabi.), (Sang.), (Sars.), Sec. c., SEP., **Sil.**, (Spig.), (Squ.), (Stan.), Staph., (Stram.), SUL., (Sul. ac.), (Tar.), Thuj., (Valer.), *Verat. a.*, (Verb.), Zinc.

Sensations.—Acon., (Agar.), (Alum.), (Arg. n.), Arn., (Arum. t.), (Asaf.), (Bar. c.), Bell., (Bism.), *Bry.*, Calc. c., (Cannab. i.), (Canth.), (Carb. v.), (Caust.), (Chel.), *Chin.*, (Cic.), Cimic., Cocc.), Coloc., (Con.), (Cup.), (Dig.), (Eup. per.), Graph., (Hep.), Ign., (K. bi.), (K. carb.), Lach., (Lil. t.), (Lyc.), (Meny.), *Merc.*, Mez., Mur. ac., Nat. m., (Nit. ac.), *Nux v.*, (Op.), (Petrol.), *Phos.*, Phyt., (Plat.), (Pb.), *Puls.*, Ran. b., (Rhodo.), *Rhus*, (Ruta), (Saba.), Sabi., Sang, (Sec. c.), (Seneg.), *Sep.*, Sil., Spig., Spo., (Squ.), Stan., (Staph.), *Sul.*, (Tar.), Thuj., Valer., Zinc.

Glands.

Bones.

Skin.—(Ambr.), (Am. m.), (Ars.), (Aur.), (Bell.), (Bry.), (Canth.), (Carb. v.), (Cham.), (Chel.), (Chin.), Crotal., (Fer.), (Ign.), (Lyc.), (Nit. ac.), Nux v., (Op), (Phos.) Pb., Sep., (Spig.), (Sul.).

Sleep and Dreams.—(Ant. cr.), (Ant. t.), (Apis), (Cannab. i.), (Croc.), (Nux m.), (Nux v.), (Op.), (Phos.), (Pho. ac.), (Pod.), (Puls.), (Sul.), (Thuj.).

Blood, Circulation and Fever.—Acon., (Apis), (Arn.), Bell., (Bry.), Cact., (Calc. c.), (Camph.), (Chin.), (Fer.), (Glon.), (Hell.), (Laur.), (Lyc.), (Merc.), (Nit. ac.), (Nux v.), (Phos.), (Pod.), (Puls.), (Sep.), (Sil.), Sul., (Vio. o.).

Aggravations: Time and Circumstances.—(Acon.), (Agar.), Alum, (Ambr.), (Am. m.), (Anac.) (Ant. cr.), (Arg.), (Arg. n.), Ars., (Asaf.), (Asar.), Aur., (Bell.), (Bor.), Bry., (Calc. c.), (Caps.), (Carb. v.), (Chel.), (Cimic.), (Cina), (Cocc.), (Coff.), (Coloc), Con., (Croc.), (Dig.), (Dros.), Dulc., (Fer.), (Hep.), (Ign.), K. bi., (K. nit.), (Lach.), (Lyc.), (Mag. m.), (Merc.), (Mos.), (Mur. ac), (Nat. m.), (Nit. ac.), (Nux v), Phos., Pho. ac., (Phyt.), Pod., Puls., (Ran. b.), (Rhodo.), Rhus, (Saba.), (Sabi.),

RELATIONSHIPS.—ALOE.—ALUM.

(Samb.), (Sang.), (Sele.), (Seneg.), Sep., (Sil.), (Spig.), (Staph.), Sul., (Tar.), (Thuj.), (Valer.), (Verat. v.), (Verb.), (Vio. t.), (Zinc).

Other Remedies.—Acon., Aesc., Agar., Alum., (Am. m.), Ant. cr., Apis, Arg. n., *Arn.*, **Ars.**, Asaf., *Aur.*, Bap., (Bar. c.), BELL., BRY., **Calc. c.**, Cannab. i., *Canth., Chel., Chin.,* (Cimic.), *Cocc., Coloc., Con.,* (Dulc.), Fer., Graph., (Hep.), Hyos., *Ign.,* K. bi., K. carb., (Lach.), **Lyc.**, **Merc.**, (Mur. ac.), **Nat. m.**, *Nit. ac.*, NUX V., *Op.*, PHOS., Pho. ac., (Phyt.), Pod., PULS., Ran. b., Rhus, (Saba.), (Sabi.), (Sang.), SEP., Sil., Spig., (Staph.), (Stram.), SUL., Thuj., (Valer.), Verat. a., (Verat. v.), *Zinc.*

Alumina.

Mind.—Anac., *Aur.*, Bell., Carb. an., Crotal., Cyc., *Fer., Graph.*, Hyos. Ign., *Lyc.*, Naj , Nat. m., Phos., **Plat.**, Puls., *Sul., Sul. ac., Zinc.*

Localities.—Aesc., (All. c.), (Aloe), Anac., Apis, (Arg. n.), *Arn.,* Ars., (Arum. t.), (Bap.), **Bell.**, (Berb.), Bry., CALC. C., (Carb. ac.), Carb. an., **Carb. v.**, **Caust.**, Cham., *Chin.,* Cocc., *Con.,* Fer., (Gel.), *Graph.,* Ign., (Iris v.), (K. bi.), **K. carb.**, *Kre.,* (Lil. t.), **Lyc.**, Mag. m., MERC., Nat. c., *Nat. m.*, *Nit. ac.*, **Nux v.**, Petrol., **Phos.**, Pho. ac., Plat., Pb., **Puls.**, *Rhus*, Ruta, *Saba.,* (Sang.), SEP., **Sil.**, *Spig.,* Stan., *Staph.,* SUL., *Sul. ac.,* Thuj., Verat. a., *Zinc.*

Sensations.—Acon., (Aesc.), (Apis), Arg. n., *Arn.*, Arum. t., *Asaf.,* Bap., **Bell.**, Berb., Bry., (Cact.), CALC. C., Cannab. i., **Caust.**, Cham., *Chin.,* (Cimic.), *Cocc.,* Con., Dros., (Eup. per.), (Gel.), (Glon.), Graph. Ign., K. bi., K. carb., (Kalm.), Laur., (Lil. t.), (Lith.), Lyc., *Merc.,* Mez., *Nat. c., Nat. m.,* NUX V., Par., **Phos.**, *Pho. ac.,* (Phyt.), *Plat.,* Pb., (Pod.), PULS., Rhus, Saba., *Sang.,* Sars., **Sep.**, Sil., Spig., Spo., *Stan.,* Staph., SUL., *Sul. ac.,* Tar., Thuj., Verat. a., (Verat. v.), *Zinc.*

Glands.—Bell., Con., Merc., *Phos.*, Puls., Spo., Sul.

Bones.—

Skin.—Ant. cr., Aur., Bry., **Calc. c.**, *Cic.,* (Cimic.), Con., *Dulc.,* (Eup per.), GRAPH., Hep., Lach., Led., *Lyc.*, Mang., Merc., *Nat. m.,* Nit. ac., Petrol., **Puls.**, Rhus, *Saba.,* Sars., SEP., **Sil.**, Staph., **Sul.**, Verat. a., *Zinc.*

Sleep and Dreams.—(Arg. n.), Ars., Bell., Bry., **Calc. c.**, (Cannab. i)., **Caust.**, Cham., *Con.,* Euphr., (Gel.), *Graph.,* Ign., Mag. m., Merc., *Nat. c.*, NUX V., *Phos.*, Pho. ac., Puls., *Rhus,* Saba., **Sep.**, Sil., Staph., SUL.

Blood, Circulation and Fever.—Agn., **Ars.**, Bell., Bov. **Bry.**,

(Cact.), *Calc. c.*, Caps., *Cham.*, *Chin.*, **Hell.**, *Hep.*, *Ign.*, Ip., *Kre.*, **Lyc.**, Merc., Mez., Nat. m., **Nux m.**, **Nux v.**, Phos., **Puls.**, Ran. b., *Rhus*, Saba., Sep., Sil., *Spig.*, *Sul.*, *Verat. a.*

Aggravations: Time and Circumstances.—(Aesc.), Aloe, Am. carb., Anac., Ant. cr., (Apis), (Arg. n.), Ars., Bell., Bry., Cact., **Calc. c.**, (Cannab. i.), Canth., Chin., Cimic., **Croc**, Hep., *Ign.*, **K.** bi., K. carb., *Lyc.*, Mang., Merc., Nat. m., **Nux v.**, Phos., **Puls.**, Ruta, **Sabi.**, (Sang.), SEP., Spig., Staph., Sul., *Thuj.*, Zinc.

Other Remedies.—Aesc., (Aloe), Anac., Ant. cr., Apis, (Arg. n), Arn., Ars., (Arum. t.), Aur., (Bap.), *Bell.*, (Berb.), *Bry.*, (Cact.), **Calc. c.**, Cannab. i., Carb. v., *Caust.*, Cham., *Chin.*, Cimic., Cocc., Con., Croc., Fer., (Gel.), *Graph.*, Hep., **Ign.**, K. bi., K. carb., Kre., **Lyc.**, *Merc.*, Nat. c., *Nat. m.*, Nit. ac., **Nux v.**, Petrol., **Phos.**, Pho. ac., Plat., PULS., *Rhus*, Saba., Sabi., (Sang.), SEP., *Sil.*, Spig., Spo., Stan., Staph., SUL., Sul. ac., Thuj., Verat. a., *Zinc.*

Antidotes.—*Bry.*, (Camph.), Cham., Ip., Puls.

Ambra Grisea.

Mind.—Bap., Chel., Cic., Cimic., Cocc., Con., Crotal., Gel., Glon., Hell., Hyd. ac., *Ign.*, **Lyc.**, Op., Pic. ac., Pho. ac., Puls., Rhus, *Sil.*, Staph., Stram., Sul., Tab., Ther.

Localities.—(Aesc.), (All. c.), (Aloe.), (Apis), Ant. cr., (Arg. n.), (Arum. t.), Bell., (Berb.), Bry., Calc. c., Canth., Carb. v., Caust., *Chin.*, (Cimic.), (Dios.), (Fl. ac.), Ign., K. bi., K. carb., (Lil. t.), (Lith), *Lyc.*, (Meli.), *Merc.*, Nat. m., Nit. ac., Nux v., *Phos.*, (Pso.), Puls., Rhus, (Sang.), Sep., Sil., *Sul.*, Verat. a.

Sensations.—Arg. n., Arn., Bell., Bry., (Cact.), *Calc. c.*, *Carb. v.*, *Caust.*, Cham., Chin., Fer., (Gel.), **Ign.**, K. carb., (Lil. t.), *Lyc.*, *Merc.*, **Nat. m.**, **Nux v.**, Petrol., *Phos.*, *Puls.*, Rhus, (Sang.), *Sep.*, Sil., **Sul.**, (Verat. v.), Zinc.

Glands.—*Ars.*, **Bell.**, Bry., Calc. c., *Carb. an.*, **Clem.**, **Con.**, Dulc., Graph., Hep., *Luc.*, *Merc.*, Nit. ac., *Phos.*, Puls., Rhus, *Sil.*, *Sul.*

Bones.

Skin.—Anac., Ars., Bell., Bry., (Carb. ac.), Carb. v., *Caust.*, Con., (Crotal.), Hep., LYC., *Merc.*, Oleand., Rhus, Sec. c., *Sep.*, Sil., Sul.

Sleep and Dreams.—Bry., *Calc. c.*, *Caust.*, Con., Hep., *Ign.*, Lyc., Nit. ac., Nux v., Phos., Puls., Rhus, Sep., Sil., Staph., Sul.

Blood, Circulation and Fever.—(Arg. n.), *Arn.*, Bry., Calc. c., Caust., (Glon.), Graph., Hep., K. carb., **Lyc.**, **Nux v.**, *Phos.*, **Puls.**, Rhus, (Sang.), Sep., **Sul.**, Thuj.

Aggravations: Time and Circumstances.—(All. c.), (Aloe), Ant. cr., Ant. t., (Apis), (Arg. n.), Arn., *Ars.*, (Bap.), Bry., **Calc.** c., Caps., Caust., *Cham.*, Chin., (Cimic.), Dulc., Euphr., Fer., Ign., Iod., K. bi., K. carb., K. nit., Lyc., Mag. m., *Nat. c.*, Nit. ac., Nux v., *Phos.*, (Phyt.), Plat., (Pod.), PULS., Rhus, Saba., Samb., *Sang.*, SEP., Stro., *Sul.*, Tar., Vio. t.

Other Remedies.—(All. c.), (Aloe), Ant. cr., (Apis), Arg. n., Arn., *Ars.*, Bap., *Bell.*, *Bry.*, Calc. c., Carb. an., Carb. v., **Caust.**, Cham., Chin., Cimic., Clem., *Con.*, (Crotal.), Dulc., Fer., (Gel.), (Glon,), Graph., Hep., Ign., (K bi.), K. carb., (Lil. t.), LYC., Merc., Nat. c., Nat. m., Nit. ac., Nux v., Phos., **Puls.**, Rhus, Sang., SEP., Sil., Staph., SUL.

Antidotes.—(Camph.), Coff., *Nux v.*, *Puls.*, Staph.

Ammonium Carbonicum.

Mind.—Bar. c., Cannab. i., Carb. sul., Cham., Cocc., Glon., K. bi., Lyc., Merc., Sep.

Localities.—(Aesc.), (Apis), (Berb.), Bry., *Calc. c.*, Carb. an., Carb. v., Caust., *Chin.*, (Eup. per.), Graph., Ign., K. carb., *Lyc.*, Merc., **Nat. c.**, *Nat. m.*, Nit. ac., *Nux v.*, Petrol., PHOS., Puls., Sang., **Sep.**, Sil., Staph., *Sul.*, Sul. ac., Verat. a., Zinc.

Sensations.—Acon., (Arg. n.), Arn., Bar. c., BELL., Bry., CALC. C., Canth., Carb. an., Carb. v., Caust., Cham., Chin., Croc., Fer., *Graph.*, Hep., *Ign.*, K. carb., **Lyc.**, *Merc.*, Nat. c., Nat. m., *Nux v.*, Op., Petrol., *Phos.*, **Puls.**, *Rhus*, Sars., Sep., Sil., Spo., Stan., Staph., Stro., *Sul.*, Thuj.

Glands.—*Arn.*, *Bell.*, Bry., Calc. c., *Carb. an.*, Carb. v., Chin., Graph., K. carb., *Lyc.*, *Merc.*, Phos., **Puls.**, Rhus, Sil., *Spig.*, Spo., Staph., *Sul*

Bones.—Asaf., Bell., *Calc. c*, Hep., Lyc., *Merc.*, Nit. ac., Phos., **Puls.**, Ruta, Sep., Sil., Sul.

Skin.—Acon., Ant. cr., (Apis), Arn., *Ars.*, BELL., *Bry.*, *Calc. c.*, (Carb. ac.), Caust., Clem., Cyc., *Dulc.*, *Graph.*, Hep., K. carb., Kre., *Lach.*, Led., **Lyc.**, Mag. c., **Merc.**, Mez., Nat. c., Nit. ac., Oleand., **Phos.**, Pho. ac., *Puls.*, Ran. b., RHUS, Saba., Sep., Sil., Squ., *Staph.*, SUL.

Sleep and Dreams.—Arn., **Ars.**, Calc. c., Carb. v., *Caust.*, Cocc., Graph., Hep., Ign., Ip., K. carb., Lyc., Mag. c., Nat. m., **Nux v.**, Phos., *Puls.*, *Rhus*, Saba., Sep., *Sil.*, Staph., Sul.

Blood, Circulation and Fever.—(Arg. n.), *Arn.*, *Ars.*, Bell., Bov., **Bry.**, **Calc. c.**, Cham., **Chin.**, Croc., *Fer.*, (Glon.), Graph., Hep., Iod., K. carb., Kre., *Lyc.*, Merc., *Nat. m.*, *Nux v.*, Op., PHOS., Pho. ac., *Puls.*, *Rhus*, Sars., *Sep.*, Sil., **Sul.**, Thuj.

Aggravations: Time and Circumstances.—(Aesc.), Ant. cr., (Arg.

n.), *Ars.,* (Bap.), *Bar. c.,* Bell., *Bry.,* CALC. C., *Carb. v.,* Caust., *Cham.,* Clem., Cocc., *Dulc.,* (Glon.), Graph., **Hep.,** Hyos., Ign., K. bi., **K. carb.,** *K. nit.,* (Lith.), **Lyc.,** Mag. c., Mag. m., Mang., **Merc.,** Nat. m., Nit. ac., *Nux m.,* Nux v., Phos., (Phyt.), Puls., Ran. s., RHUS, Ruta, Sang., SEP., Sil., Spig., Stro., SUL., Verat. a., Zinc.

Other Remedies.—Acon., (Aesc.), Ant. cr., (Apis.), (Arg. n.), *Arn.,* **Ars.,** Bar. c., **Bell.,** Bry., CALC. C., Carb. an., *Carb. v., Caust., Cham., Chin.,* Clem., Cocc., Croc., Dulc., Fer., (Glon.), **Graph.,** Hep., *Ign.,* K. bi., **K. carb.,** K. nit., Kre., Lach., LYC., Mag. c., **Merc.,** *Nat. c., Nat. m., Nit. ac.,* Nux m., **Nux v.,** Op., Petrol., PHOS., Pho. ac., PULS., Rhus, Ruta, Saba., Sang., Sars., SEP., **Sil.,** Spig., Spo., *Staph., Stro.,* SUL., Thuj., Verat. a., Zinc.

Antidotes.—Arn., *Camph.,* Hep.

Injurious.—Lach.

Ammonium Muriaticum.

Mind.—Aur., Caust., Cham., Con., Glon., *Ign.,* **Lyc.,** Phos., Puls., Sep., Sul.

Localities.—Acon., (Aesc.), All. c., (Aloe), (Apis.), Apoc. c., *Arg. n.,* Ars., Arum t., *Aur.,* (Bap.), *Bell.,* (Berb.), Bry., (Cact.), Calc. c., (Carb. ac.), Cham., Chin., (Cimic.), Cocc., Dios., Fl. ac., (Gel.), Hyos., *Ign.,* (Iris v.), *K. bi.,* Lyc., Merc., Nat. c., *Nat. m.,* Nit. ac., **Nux v.,** Phos., Phyt., Pod., Puls., *Rhus, Sang.,* Sep., **Sil.,** Sul., *Sul. ac.,* **Verat. a.,** (Verat. v.)

Sensations.—(Aloe.), (Arg, n.), (Arum. t.), *Asaf.,* Bar. c., **Bell.,** (Berb.), Bry., (Cact.), **Calc. c.,** Cannab. i., Carb. v., **Caust.,** *Chin.,* Cocc., (Gel.), (Glon.), **Graph.,** (Iris v.), K. bi., **K. carb.,** Laur., (Lil. t.), (Lith.), Lyc., *Merc.,* Mur. ac., *Nat. c., Nat. m.,* Nit. ac., Nux v., **Phos.,** (Pso.), *Puls.,* Rhodo., **Rhus,** Ruta, Saba., Sabi., (Sang.), SEP., Sil., *Spig.,* Spo., Stan., Staph., **Sul.,** Tar., *Zinc.*

Glands.—(Arum. t.), *Asaf.,* Bell., *Bry.,* Calc. c., Caust., Cocc., Con., Graph., *Ign.,* **K. carb.,** MERC.. *Nat. m.,* Nit. ac., PHOS., **Puls.,** Ran. s., *Rhus,* Saba., *Sep., Sil ,* Spig., **Sul.**

Bones.—Agar., Bry., *Cocc., Hep.,* Ign., Ip., Led., Phos., PULS., Rhus, **Ruta,** Sul., Verat. a.

Skin.—Acon., Am. carb., Ars., *Bell.,* **Bry.,** Calc. c., Caust., Chin., Clem., Euphorb., *Graph., Lach., Led.,* Lyc., *Mez.,* **Oleand.,** Phos., PULS., Rhus, Sep., Staph., Sul.

Sleep and Dreams.—Arn., *Ars.,* Bell., Bry., *Calc. c., Chin.,* **Graph.,** Hep., Ign., *K. carb.,* Lach., *Lyc.,* Merc., *Nux v., Phos.,* Puls., Sele., *Sil.,* **Sul.,** (Verat. v.)

RELATIONSHIPS.—AM. MUR.—ANAC. 333

Blood, Circulation and Fever.—Ars., (Berb.), Bry., *Calc. c.*, Caust., Euphorb., (Gel.), *Merc.*, Phos., Puls., Ran. s., *Rhus*, Sec. c., Verat. a.

Aggravations: Time and Circumstances.—(Aloe), (Apis), Arg. n., *Ars.*, Aur., (Bap.), Bell., **Bry.**, *Calc. c.*, Caps., *Carb. v.*, Caust., *Cham.*, Chel., Chin., Cic., (Cimic.), Cocc., *Con.*, Croc., Cyc., Euphr., Fer., (Gel.), Graph., Hep., Ign., Iod., *K. bi.*, K. carb., K. nit., Lach., *Lyc.*, Mag. m., Meny., Merc., Mur. ac., Nat. c., **Nat. m.**, Nit. ac., **Nux v.**, Phos., Pho. ac., (Phyt.), Pod., PULS., Rhodo., RHUS, Saba., Samb., *Sang.*, **Sep.**, Sil., *Spig.*, Squ., Spo., *Sul.*, Valer., Verb., (Verat. v.)

Other Remedies.—(Aloe), (Apis), Arg. n., *Ars.*, Arum. t., Asaf., Aur., (Bap.), *Bell.*, (Berb.), Bry., (Cact.), **Calc. c.**, Carb. v., *Caust.*, Cham., *Chin.*, (Cimic.), *Cocc.*, Con., Gel., (Glon.), *Graph.*, Hep., *Ign.*, *K. bi.*, *K. carb*, Lach., Led., *Lyc.*, *Merc.*, Nat. c., *Nat. m.*, Nit. ac., *Nux v.*, Oleand., PHOS., (Phyt.), Pod., PULS., RHUS, Ruta, Saba., *Sang.*, **Sep.**, *Sil.*, Spig., *Sul.*, Verat. a., (Verat. v.)

Antidotes. -(Camph.), *Coff.*, (Hep.), Nux v.

Anacardium.

Mind.—Acon., Aloe., Ars., Aur., Bap., **Bell.**, Bry., Calc. c., *Cannab. i.*, Chel., Cimic., Con., Crotal., Dios., **Glon.**, Graph., Hell., **Hyos.**, *Hyper.*, Ign., K. bi., LYC., *Meli.*, *Merc.*, Nat. c., Nat. m., Nux v., Op., Petrol., Phos., *Pho. ac.*, *Pic. ac.*, Plat., *Puls.*, Rhus, Sep., **Stram.**, **Sul.**, Tell., **Ther.**, *Verat. a.*

Localities.—Alum., (Apis), (Arg. n.), Arn., *Bell.*, (Berb.), (Cact.) **Calc. c.**, (Cannab. i.), Chin., Cimic., Cocc., (Gel.), Graph., Ign., (Iris v.), **K. carb.**, Kre., **Lyc.**, Merc., *Nat. m*, *Nux v.*, Petrol., *Phos.*, **Pho. ac.**, (Phyt.), Plat., Pb., (Pod.), PULS., Rhus, Ruta, (Sang.), Sec. c., *Sep.*, *Sil.*, Spig., Staph., **Sul.**, *Verat. a.*

Sensations.—(Aesc.), (Aloe), Arg. n., Arn., Ars., *Asaf.*, Asar., (Bap.), **Bell.**, Bry., (Cact.), **Calc. c.**, (Cannab. i.), Cannab. s., Carb. v., *Caust.*, Chin., Cimic., *Cocc.*, *Con.*, (Crotal.), *Dulc.*, Gel., (Glon.), Ign., K. carb., (Kalm.), (Lil. t.), (Lith.), **Lyc.**, Nat. m., *Nit. ac.*, *Nux v.*, *Oleand.*, Phos., Pho. ac., (Phyt.), **PLAT.**, (Pod.), **Puls.**, Rhus, Ruta, (Sang.), Sars., *Sep.*, *Stan.*, Staph., **Sul.**, *Sul. ac.*, Verat. a.

Glands.—Calc. c., Caust., *Con.*, Phos., **Plat.**, Sil., Spo.

Bones.—Bell., Merc., Puls., *Ruta.*

Skin.—*Ars.*, Bell., *Bry.*, *Caust.*, Cocc., **Con.**, Hep., K. carb., **LYC.**, Merc., *Mez.*, *Oleand.*, Op., *Pho. ac.*, *Puls.*, Sec. c., **Sil.**, Sul.

Sleep and Dreams.—Acon., (Apis), Bell., Bry., (Cannab. i.), Con., Croc., **Nux v.**, Op., *Phos.*, Pho. ac., (Pod.), Puls., **Sul.**

Blood, Circulation and Fever.—Ars., *Calc. c.*, *Cham.*, Lyc., **Nux v.**, *Sep.*, Verat. a.

Aggravations: Time and Circumstances.—Acon., (Aloe), (Arg. n.), Bell., *Bry.*, (Cact.), **Calc. c.**, (Cannab. i.), Caps., **Carb. v.**, Cham., Chin., (Cimic.), *Con.*, Ign., K. bi., **K. carb.**, Led., *Lyc.*, Mez., *Nat. c.*, *Nat. m.*, Nux v., Phos., Pho. ac., (Phyt.), (Pod.), PULS., Rhodo., *Rhus*, Saba., *Sep.*, Sil., Stan., Staph., *Sul.*, Zinc.

Other Remedies.—Acon., Aloe, (Apis), Arg. n., *Ars*, (Bap.), **Bell.**, *Bry.*, (Cact.), **Calc. c.**, *Cannab. i.*, *Carb. v.*, *Caust.*, Cham., *Chin.*, *Cimic.*, *Cocc.*, **Con.**, (Crotal.), (Gel.), (Glon.), Hyos., Ign., *K. carb.*, LYC., Merc., Mez., Nat. c., *Nat. m.*, *Nux v.*, Oleand., Op., *Phos.*, **Pho. ac.**, (Phyt.), *Plat.*, Pod., PULS., *Rhus*, Ruta, (Sang.), *Sep.*, *Sil.*, Stan., Staph., Stram., **Sul.**, *Varat. a.*

Antidotes.—*Coff.*, Jug.

Antimonium Crudum.

Mind.—Agar., Apis., Bell., Canth., *Hyos.*, LACH., Lyc., *Op.*, **Phos.**, Plat., Puls., Stram., Sul. ac., Verat. a.

Localities.—Acon., (Aesc.), (All. c.), Aloe, Apis, Arg. n., Arn., *Ars.*, Arum. t., Bap., *Bell.*, *Bry.*, (Cact.), **Calc. c.**, Canth., *Carb. v.*, *Caust.*, Cham., *Chin.*, (Cimic.), (Dios.), Dulc., Eup. per., Fer., (Fl. ac.), (Gel.), *Graph.*, Hep., Hyos., *Ign.*, (Iris v.), *K. bi.*, K. carb., Kre., Lyc., **Merc.**, **Nat. m.**, *Nit. ac.*, *Nux v.*, Petrol., **Phos.**, Pho. ac., Phyt., Plat., *Pod.*, Pso., **Puls.**, *Rhus*, Sang., SEP., **Sil.**, *Staph.*, SUL., *Verat. a.*, Verat. v.

Sensations.—Aloe, Arn., Ars., Asaf., *Bell.*, Bry., *Calc. c.*, Caps., Chin., Croc., Cup., Fer., Led., *Lyc.*, Merc., *Nux v.*, **Puls.**, *Rhus*, Sep., *Sul.*

Glands.—Acon., Arn., **Bell.**, *Bry.*, Carb. an., Con., Hep., Lyc., Merc., Phos., Puls., Rhus, Sil., *Sul.*

Bones.—Asaf., Aur., *Chin.*, *Merc.*, **Pho. ac.**, Puls., *Sil.*, Staph.

Skin.—Acon., **Apis**, **Ars.**, Bell., *Bry.*, *Calc. c.*, Caust., Dulc., Graph., Hep., (K. bi.), Lach., Led., *Lyc.*, Merc., Nit. ac., Phos., PULS., Ran. b., Rhus, Sep., *Sil.*, Staph., SUL.

Sleep and Dreams.—(Aloe), *Ant. t.*, Apis, Ars., Bry., Calc. c., Cannab. i., Carb. v., *Croc.*, *Ign.*, Nat. c., Nux m., **Nux v.**, *Op.*, **Phos.**, *Pho. ac.*, Pod., PULS., Rhus, Saba., *Sep.*, Sul., Verat. a.

Blood, Circulation and Fever.—Ars., Bry., *Hep.*, Nat. m., Nux v., *Rhus*.

Aggravations: Time and Circumstances.—(All. c.), (Aloe), Arg. n., Arn., Ars., (Bap.), **Bell.**, *Bry.*, (Cact.), CALC. C., (Cannab. i.), Canth., Caps., Carb. v., *Chin.*, (Cimic.), Clem., Con., Euphr., (Gel.), Graph.,

RELATIONSHIPS.—ANT. CR.—ANT. TART.

Hep., Ign., Ip., K. bi., (Lil. t.), *Lyc.*, *Merc.*, **Nat.** c., Nat. m., Nit. ac., **Nux v.**, *Phos.*, (Phyt.), (Pod.), PULS., **Rhus**, Sang., **Sep.**, *Sil.*, Spig., Staph., SUL.

Other Remedies.—Acon., (All. c.), Aloe, *Apis*, Arg. n., Arn., *Ars.*, Asaf., (Bap.), **Bell.**, *Bry.*, (Cact.), *Calc. c.*, (Cannab. i.), Canth., Carb. v., Caust., Chin., (Cimic.), Con., Croc., (Gel.), Graph., Hep., **Hyos.**, Ign., K. bi., Lach., *Lyc.*, *Merc.*, Nat. m., Nit. ac., *Nux v.*, Op., **Phos.**, Pho. ac., (Phyt.), Pod., PULS., Rhus, **Sep.**, Sang., *Sil.*, Staph., **Sul.**, Verat. a.

Antidotes.—Hep., Merc.

Antimonium Tart.

Mind.—*Ars.*, Bar. c., **Bell.**, Bry., Calc. c., Glon., Hep., **Hyos.**, Ign., Laur., *Merc.*, Nat. c., Nux v., Phos., Puls., Rhus, Sil., Sul.

Localities.—Aesc., Aloe, *Apis*, Apoc. c., **Arg. n.**, *Arn.*, Ars., Bap., *Bell.*, (Berb.), **Bry.**, Cact., Calc. c., Cannab. i., Carb. ac., *Carb. v.*, Caust., Cham., *Chin.*, Cimic., Cocc., Con., (Dios.), Eup. per., (Fl. ac.), Gel., (Glon.), Hyos., *Ign.*, **K. bi.**, K. carb., Kalm., Lil. t., (Lith.), **Lyc.**, (Meli.), Nat. m., NUX V., PHOS., (Phyt.), Pb., Pod., (Pso.), PULS., Rhus, Sang., *Sep.*, *Sil.*, Staph., **Sul.**, (Ther.), **Verat. a.**, Verat. v.

Sensations.—Acon., (Aesc.), Alum., (Apis), Arg. n., Arn., Ars., Asaf., (Bap.), Bell., (Berb.), (Cact.), *Calc. c.*, (Cannab. i.), Cannab. s., Caust., Cimic., Con., (Crotal.), Gel., Glon., Graph., Hep., Iod., Ip., Kre., Lach., (Lil. t.), *Merc.*, Mos., *Nux v.*, Phos., (Phyt.), **Puls.**, Sang., Spig., *Sul.*, Verat. a., (Verat. v.).

Glands.—Bell., Phos., Sul.

Bones.

Skin.—*Ant. cr.*, Ars., *Bell.*, Carb. v., K. bi., Lyc., **Merc.**, **Puls.**, Rhus, *Sul.*, Verat. a.

Sleep and Dreams.—(Aloe.), Apis., Ars., **Bry.**, *Cannab. i.*, Con., *Croc.*, Cup., *Ign.*, Laur., Nux m., Nux v., **Op.**, Phos., Pho. ac., Pod., PULS., Rhus, Verat. a.

Blood, Circulation and Fever.—*Ars.*, Bell., Bry., (Cact.), Cannab. i., Chin., (Gel.), Graph., Hep., K. carb., Lyc., *Merc.*, **Nux v.**, Phos., (Phyt.), PULS., *Rhus*, (Sang.), *Sep.*, Sul., Verat. a., Verat. v.

Aggravations: Time and Circumstances.—Acon., Aesc., (All. c.), Apis, Arg. n., *Ars.*, (Bap.), Bell., Bry., (Cannab. i.), Carb. v., Caust., Chin., (Cimic.), Colch., **Dig.**, (Gel.), (Glon.), Ign., Iod., K. bi., K. carb., Lach., Led., (Lil. t.), *Lyc.*, Mez., Nit. ac., *Nux v.*, Phos., (Phyt.), (Pod.), **PULS.**, *Ran. s.*, Rhus, *Sang.*, Sep., Spig., Stro., **Sul.**, *Verat. a.*, **(Verat. v.).**

Other Remedies.—Aesc., (Aloe), *Apis*, *Arg. n.*, Arn., *Ars.*, Bap., Bell., (Berb.), *Bry.*, Cact., Calc. c., *Cannab. i.*, Carb. v., Caust., Chin., Cimic., Con., Dig., Gel., Glon., Hep., Ign., K. bi., K. carb., (Lil. t.), *Lyc.*, *Merc.*, Nux m., Nux v., Op., **Phos.**, (Phyt.), Pod., PULS., **Rhus**, Sang., Sep., Sil., Spig., Sul., *Verat. a.*, **Verat. v.**

Antidotes.—Cocc., *Ip.*, *Op*, Puls., Sep.

Apis.

Mind.—Acon., Agar., Ant. t., *Arn.*, Ars., *Aur.*, Bap., Bar. c., Bell., Bry., Calc. c., *Camph.*, **Cannab. i.**, *Canth.*, Caust., Chin., Cimic., Cocc., Con., Crotal., Cup., Dig., GELS., Glon., Graph., *Hyd. ac.*, *Hyos.*, Ign., Ip., **Lach.**, Laur., *Lyc.*, Meli., *Merc.*, Mur. ac., Nat. c., *Nat. m.*, Nux m., Nux v., **OP.**, *Petrol.*, **Phos.**, Pho. ac., *Phyt.*, Pic. ac., Pb., **PULS.**, **Rhus t.**, **Sep.**, Sil., *Stram.*, **Sul.**, **Verat. a.**, *Verat. v.*, Vio. t.

Localities.—Acon., Aesc., Agar., (Agn.), (All. c.), Aloe, Alum., (Ambr.), (Am. carb.), Am. m., (Anac.), (Ant. cr.), Ant. t., Apoc. c., Arg., **Arg. n.**, Arn., ARS., Arum t., *Asaf.*, (Asar.), Aur., Bap., *Bar. c.*, BELL., (Berb.), (Bism.), Bor., (Bov.), BRY., (Cact.), (Calad.), **Calc. c.**, (Camph.), Cannab. i., Cannab. s., **Canth.**, *Caps.*, Carb. ac., (Carb. an.), *Carb. v.*, (Caul.), *Caust.*, (Ced.), **Cham. Chel.**, CHIN., (Cic.), Cimic., (Cina), (Clem.), Cocc., (Coff.), Colch., Coloc., Con., Croc., Crotal., Cup., (Cyc.), Dig., (Dios.), Dros., Dulc., (Eup. per.), (Euphorb.), (Euphr.), Fer., (Fl. ac.), **Gel.**, (Glon.), *Graph.*, (Guai.), Hell., **Hep.**, **Hyos.**, Ign., *Ip.*, *Iod.*, K. bi., K. CARB., (K. nit.), Kre., *Lach.*, Laur., (Led.), (Lil. t.), (Lith.), *Lyc.*, (Mag. c.), (Mang.), (Mar.), (Meli.), Meny., MERC., Mez., (Mos.), Mur. ac., Nat. c., **Nat. m.**, Nit. ac., NUX V., Oleand., *Op.*, Par., Petrol., PHOS., **Pho. ac.**, Phyt., Plat., Pb., **Pod.**, (Pso.), PULS., Ran. b., (Ran. s.), (Rheum), (Rhodo.), Rhus, *Ruta*, *Saba.*, Sabi., (Samb.), Sang., (Sars.), *Sec. c.*, (Sele.), Seneg., SEP., SIL., Spig., *Spo.*, Squ., *Stan.*, *Staph.*, *Stram.*, (Stro.), SUL., Sul. ac., **(Tar.)**, Thuj., (Valer.), **Verat. a.**, Verat. v., (Verb.), **Zinc.**

Sensations.—Acon., (Aesc.), Agar., Alum., (Ant. cr.), Ant. t., (Arg.), (Arg. n.), Arn., **Ars.**, Arum t., (Asaf.), Asar., Aur., Bap., *Bar. c.*, **Bell.**, Berb., Bism., **Bry.**, (Cact.), (Calad.), *Calc. c.*, (Camph.), (Cannab. i.), **Canth.**, (Carb. v.), *Caust.*, Cham., Chel., **Chin.**, (Cic.), (Cimic.), **(Clem.)**, *Cocc.*, *Colch.*, *Coloc.*, *Con.*, (Crotal.), (Cup.), (Dig.), Dros., (Dulc.), (Eup. per.), (Euphr.), Fer., Gel., (Glon.), (Graph.), Hell., Hep., Hyos., Ign., (Ip.), Iod., Iris v., K. bi., *K. carb.*, *Lach.*, Laur., Led., (Lil. t.), **Lyc.**, **Merc.**, **Mez.**, Mos., Mur. ac., *Nat. c.*, *Nat. m.*, **Nit. ac.**, Nux m., Nux v., **(Oleand.), Op., (Petrol.), Phos.**, *Pho. ac.*, Phyt., **(Plat.)**, **Pb.**, (Pod.),

(Pso.), **PULS.**, *Ran. b.*, (Ran. s.), Rhodo., **Rhus**, Ruta, *Saba.*, *Sabi.*, (Samb.), Sang., (Sars.), Sec. c., Seneg., SEP., Sil., (Spig.), *Spo.*, (Squ.), *Stan.*, Stram., SUL., Sul. ac., Thuj., Valer., *Verat. a.*, (Verat. v.), *Zinc.*

Glands.

Bones.

Skin.—Acon., Agar., Alum., *Ant. cr.*, Arn., ARS., Bar. c., **BELL.**, (Bor.), **Bry.**, **Calc. c.**, (Carb. an.), **Caust.**, Cham., *Chin.*, Cic., (Clem.), (Coff.), Con., **Dulc.**, *Euphorb.*, (Fer.), Graph., **Hep.**, (Hyos.), (Ip.), (Iod.), (Kre.), **Lach.**, Led., **Lyc.**, Mag. c., Mang., MERC., Mez., (Mos.), (Mur. ac.), *Nat. m.*, Nit. ac., (Nux m.), Nux v., *Petrol.*, Phos., Pho. ac., Plat., Pb., **Puls.**, (Ran. s.), RHUS, Ruta, Sabi., Samb., Sec. c., (Sele.), Sep., *Sil.*, (Spig.), (Squ.), (Staph.), SUL., *Thuj.*, Verat. a., (Verat. v.).

Sleep and Dreams.—(Aloe), (Anac.), Ant. cr., Ant. t., (Ars.), (Asaf.), (Bell.), (Bry.), (Calc. c.), (Camph.), Cannab. i., (Carb. v.), (Caust.), (Chel.), (Con.), (Cyc.), (Fl. ac.), (K. carb.), (Laur.), (Mos.), (Nat. c.), (Nat. m.), Nux m., Nux v., Op., Phos., Pho. ac., Pod., Puls., (Rhus), (Saba.), (Samb.), (Sep.), (Sil.), (Stram.), Sul., (Sul. ac.), Thuj., (Verat. a.).

Blood, Circulation and Fever.—*Acon.*, (Agn.), (Aloe), (Arn.), *Ars.*, (Asaf.), Bell., (Bry.), Cact., (Calc. c.), Camph., Caps., (Carb. v.), (Caust.), Chin., (Cup.), (Dros.), (Fer.), Gel., Glon., (Graph.), *Hell.*, (K. nit.), (Lach.), (Lyc.), (Mang.), Meny., (Merc.), (Mur. ac.), (Nit. ac.), Nux m., Nux v., (Oleand.), *Phos.*, Pho. ac., *Puls.*, (Ran. b.), (Rhus), Saba., (Samb.), (Sec. c.), Sep., (Sil.), Spig., (Squ.), (Stram.), Sul., (Tar.), (Thuj.), (Verat. a.), (Vio. o.).

Aggravations: Time and Circumstances.—Acon., (Aesc.), Agar., (Agn.), (Alum.), (Ambr.), (Am. carb.), (Am. m.), Ant. t., (Arg.), Arn., Ars., (Asaf.), (Asar.), (Aur.), (Bap.), Bar. c., *Bell.*, (Bism.), *Bry.*, (Calad.), (Camph.), (Cannab. s.), (Canth.), Caps., (Carb. v.), Cham., (Chel.), (Chin.), (Cimic.), (Cina), Cocc., (Colch.), Con., (Croc.), (Dig.), (Dros.), (Dulc.), (Euphorb.), (Euphr.), Fer., (Glon.), (Graph.), (Hell.), **Hep.**, Hyos., (Ign.), (Ip.), Iod., (K. bi.), (K. nit.), *Lach.*, (Laur.), Led., (Lil. t.), *Lyc.*, (Mag. c.), (Mag. m.), (Mar.), *Merc.*, (Mos.), (Mur. ac.), Nat. m., Nia ac., (Nux m.), Nux v., (Oleand.), Op., (Petrol.), Phos., **Pho. ac.**, (Plat.), **Puls.**, Ran. b., (Rheum), (Rhodo.), Rhus, (Ruta), (Saba.), Sabi., (Samb.), Sang., (Sars.), (Sec. c.), (Sele.), (Seneg.), Sep., *Sil.*, Spig., (Spo.), (Stan.), *Staph.*, Stram., (Stro.), **Sul.**, (Tar.), Thuj., (Valer.), Verat. a., (Verb.), (Vio. t.), (Zinc.).

Other Remedies.—Acon., (Aesc.), **Agar.**, (Agn.), (Aloe), *Alum.*, (Am. m.), *Ant. cr.*, **Ant. t.**, (Arg.), Arg. n., ARN., ARS., (Arum. t.),

Asaf., (Asar.), *Aur.*, *Bap.*, **Bar. c.**, BELL., (Berb.), (Bism.), (Bor.), BRY., (Cact.), **Calc. c.**, *Camph.*, *Cannab. i.*, (Cannab. s.), **Canth.**, *Caps.*, *Carb. v.*, **Caust.**, **Cham.**, *Chel.*, CHIN., Cic., Cimic., (Clem.), **Cocc.**, Colch., Coloc., **Con.**, (Croc.), Crotal., Cup., Dig., Dros., *Dulc.*, Euphorb., (Euphr.), **Fer.**, **Gel.**, Glon., **Graph.**, *Hell.*, **Hep.**, (Hyd. ac.), **Hyos.**, *Ign.*, *Ip.*, *Iod.*, K. bi., *K. carb.*, (K. nit.), LACH., *Laur.*, Led., (Lil. t.), LYC., (Mag. c.), (Mang.), (Meli.), (Meny.), MERC., Mez., Mos., *Mur. ac.*, *Nat. c.*, NAT. M., **Nit. ac.**, Nux m., NUX V., Oleand., OP., **Petrol.**, PHOS., PHO. AC., Phyt., Plat., *Pb.*, *Pod.*, PULS., *Ran. b.*, (Ran. s.), (Rhodo.), RHUS, *Ruta*, **Saba.**, *Sabi.*, Samb., Sang., (Sars.), *Sec. c.*, (Sele.), Seneg, SEP., SIL., *Spig.*, *Spo.*, (Squ.), **Stan.**, **Staph.**, **Stram.**, **SUL.**, Sul. ac., (Tar.), *Thuj.*, (Valer.), **Verat. a.**, *Verat. v.*, (Vio. t.), **Zinc.**

Argentum.

Mind.—Acon., **Bell.**, Bry., **Calc. c.**, Gel., *Laur.*, **Nux v.**, Op., *Phos.*, *Puls.*, Rhus, *Stram.*, Verat. a.

Localities.—(Aesc.), (All. c.), Alum, Apis, (Arg. n.), (Bap.), **Bell.**, *Bry.*, (Berb.), CALC. C., Cannab. i., (Carb. ac.), **Chin.**, Cimic., (Gel.), (Iris v.), K. bi., *K. carb.*, Kre., Lil. t., Lyc., (Meli.), *Merc.*, Nat. m., Nit. ac., Phos., (Phyt.), (Pod.), *Puls.*, Saba., (Sang.), Sep., Spig., Stan., Sul., Sul. ac.

Sensations.—(Aesc.), Alum., (Apis), (Arg. n.), (Arum. t), **Asaf.**, *Aur.*, (Bap.), **Bell.**, *Bry.*, Calc. c., **Caust.**, Chin., Cocc., Con., Cyc., (Eup. per.), Ign., (K. bi.), **K. CARB.**, (Lith.), **Lyc.**, **Merc.**, *Mez.*, Nat. c. Nat. m., Nux v., *Oleand.*, *Phos.*, Pho. ac., Plat., (Pod.), **Puls.**, Rhodo., *Rhus*, Ruta, Sabi., (Sang.), *Sep.*, Sil., *Spig.*, Spo, *Stan.*, *Staph.*, *Stro.*, **Sul.**, Sul. ac., Tar., Zinc.

Glands.—Arn., Ars., *Bell.*, Bry., Calc. c, Carb. an., Cic., Con., Ign., *Lyc.*, Merc., Phos., Puls., Rhus, Ruta, **Sep.**, *Spo.*, Sui.

Bones.—Asaf., Bell., Bism., Cup., **Cyc.**, (Eup. per.), Lyc., Phos., Ruta, Sabi., *Staph.*

Skin.—*Asaf.*, Bell., *Bry.*, Calc. c., Cocc., *Cyc.*, *Hep.*, K. carb, *Lyc.*, MERC., Mez., *Phos.*, **Puls.**, *Rhus*, Sabi., Sep., SIL., Spig., *Staph.*, **Sul.**, Zinc.

Sleep and Dreams.

Blood, Circulation and Fever.—Ars., *Cham.*, Chin., Nux m., *Nux v.*, Puls., Rhus, Samb., Sep., Sil., Spig., Verat. a.

Aggravations: Time and Circumstances.—*Acon.*, (Aesc.), (All. c.), (Aloe), Ambr., Ant. cr., (Apis), (Arg. n.), Ars., *Asaf.*, *Aur.*, (Bap.), *Bor.*, Bry., (Cact.), **Calc. c.**, (Cannab. i). Caps., (Cimic.), **Con.**, Dros., Dulc.,

RELATIONSHIPS.—ARGENTUM.—ARG. NIT. 339

Euphorb., Fer., (Gel.), *Hep.*, *K. bi.*, K. carb., Lach., Laur., **LYC.**, Mag. m., Mar., Meny., *Merc.*, Phos., Nat. c., (Phyt.), Plat., Pod., **PULS.**, *Rhodo.*, Rhus, Ruta, *Saba.*, *Sang.*, *Sep.*, *Sil.*, Staph., **Stro.**, *Sul. ac.*, **Valer.**, Vic. t., (Verat. v.).

Other Remedies.—Acon., (Aesc.), (All. c.), Apis, (Arg. n.), Ars., Asaf., Aur., (Bap.), Bell., *Bry.*, CALC. C., (Cannab. i.), Caust., *Chin.*, (Cimic.), *Con.*, *Cyc.*, Gel., Hep., K. bi., *K. carb.*, Laur., **Lyc.**, **Merc.**, Mez., Nat. m., Nux v., Phos., (Phyt.), (Pod.), **PULS.**, Rhodo., **Rhus**, Ruta, Saba., Sabi., Sang., SEP., **Sil.**, Spig., Spo., Stan., *Staph.*, **Stro.**, *Sul.*, Sul. ac., Zinc.

Antidotes.—*Merc.*, Puls.

Argentum Nitricum.
Mind.
Localities.—ACON., *Aesc.*, Agar., (All. c.), Aloe, Alum., (Ambr.), (Am. carb.), *Am. m.*, (Anac.), Ant. cr., **Ant. t.**, Apis, Apoc. c., **Arg.**, Arn., *Arum. t.*, ARS., *Asaf.*, Asar., *Aur.*, *Bap.*, Bar. c., BELL., (Berb.), (Bism.), Bor., (Bov.), BRY., Cact., (Calad.), CALC. C., Camph., Cannab. i., (Cannab. s.), *Canth.*, *Caps.*, *Carb. ac.*, Carb. an., **Carb. v.**, **Caust.** (Ced.), **Cham.**, **Chel.**, CHIN., Cic., Cimic., (Cina), Clem., *Cocc.*, (Coff.), *Colch.*, *Coloc.*, **Con.**, (Croc.), Crotal., *Cup.*, Cyc., *Dig.*, Dios., Dros., *Dulc.*, (Eup. per.), (Euphorb.), (Euphr.), Fer., (Fl. ac.), Gel., (Glon.), *Graph.*, Hell., *Hep.*, (Hyd. ac.), *Hyos.*, *Ign.*, Ip., *Iod.*, (Iris. v.), *K. carb.*, K. BI., (K. nit.), (Kalm.), (Kre.), Lach., Laur., (Led.), Lil. t., (Lith.,) LYC., (Mag. c.), Mag. m., (Mang.), (Mar.), (Meli.), (Meny.), MERC., Mez., (Mos.), (Mur. ac.), *Nat. c.*, **Nat. m.**, **Nit. ac.**, (Nux m.), **NUX V.**, (Oleand., *Op.*, Par., *Petrol.*, PHOS., *Pho. ac*, Phyt., (Pic. ac.), Plat., *Pb.*, **Pod.**, Pso., PULS., Ran. b., (Ran. s.). Rheum, Rhodo., *Rhus*, (Ruta), Saba, (Sabi.), Samb., *Sang.*, (Sars.), *Sec. c.*, (Sele), Seneg., SEP., SIL., Spig., *Spo.*, Squ., *Stan.*, Staph., *Stram.*, (Stro.), SUL., Sul. ac., (Tar.), (Ther.), Thuj., Valer., **Verat. a.**, Verat. v., (Verb.), Zinc.

Sensations.—Acon., Aesc., Agar., Alum., (Ambr.), (Am. m.), Anac., *Ant t.*, (Apis), *Arn.*, **Ars.**, Arum. t., (Asaf.), (Asar.), (Aur.), Bar. c., **Bell.**, Berb., (Bism.), (Bor.), **Bry.**, Cact., (Calad.), **Calc. c.**, *Camph.*, Cannab. i., Cannab. s., Canth., Caps., Carb. v., **Caust.**, *Cham.*, *Chel.*, **Chin.**, Cic., Cimic., Cina, *Cocc.*, *Colch.*, *Coloc.*, **Con.**, (Croc.), Crotal., **Cup.**, *Dig.*, Dros., Dulc., *Fer.*, Gel., Glon., Graph., (Hell.), (Hep.), *Hyos.*, *Ign.*, Ip., *Iod.*, *K. bi.*, K. carb., (Kalm.), Kre., Lach., Laur., Led., Lil. t., *Lyc.*, Meny., **Merc.**, *Mez.*, Mos., (Mur. ac.), Nat. c., **Nat. m.**, **Nit. ac.**, Nux m., **NUX V.**, Oleand., *Op.*, Par., Petrol., **Phos.**, **Pho. ac.**, (Phyt.), Plat., *Pb.*, (Pod.), (Pso.), **PULS.**, Ran. b., (Ran. s.), *Rhodo.*, **RHUS**, (Ruta), *Saba.*, Sabi.,

(Samb.), Sang., Sars., **Sec. c.**, *Seneg.*, **SEP., SIL.,** *Spig.,* Spo., Squ. Stan., (Staph.), *Stram.,* (Stro.), SUL., (Sul. ac.), **Tar.,** *Thuj.,* **(Valer.), Verat. a., Verat. v., Zinc.**

Glands.
Bones.
Skin.

Sleep and Dreams.—*Acon.,* (Alum.), Arn., Ars., Bap., (Bell.), (Bor.), *Bry.,* Calc. c., Cannab. i., (Canth.), (Caps.), (Caust.), **Cham.,** *Chin.,* (Cic.), (Cimic.), (Cocc.), Coff., Con., *Graph.,* **Hep.,** Hyos., Ign., *K. carb.,* Kre., Lach., (Led.), *Mag. c.,* **Merc.,** Nat. c., Nat. m., **Nit. ac.,** *Nux v.,* Op., **Phos.,** Pho. ac., Pb., *Puls.,* Ran. b., **Rhus,** Saba., Sele., *Sep.,* **Sil.,** Stan., **Staph.,** *Sul., Thuj.*

Blood, Circulation and Fever.—*Acon.,* (Ambr.), (Am. carb.), (Arn.), (Ars.), Aur., Bell., (Bov.), Bry., Calc. c. (Carb. v.), (Caust.,), (Croc.), (Cup.), Fer., Glon., (Hep.), (Iod.), (K. carb.), Kre., (Lach.), *Lyc.,* (Meny.), (Merc.), Nat. m., (Nux m.), (Nux v.), (Op.), (Petrol.), (Phos.), (Pho. ac.), Rhus, (Samb.), (Sars.), (Seneg.), (Sep.), **Sil.,** Spo., (Stan.), Stram., *Sul.,* (Thuj.), Verat. a.

Aggravations: Time and Circumstances.—Acon., (Agar., (Aloe), (Alum.), (Ambr.), (Am. carb.), Am. m., Ant. cr., Ant. t., (Arg.), Arn., *Ars.,* (Asaf.), (Asar.), (Aur.), (Bap.), *Bell.,* (Bor.), *Bry.,* (Calc. c.), (Caps.), (Carb. v.), Caust., Cham., (Chel.), (Chin.), (Cic.), (Cimic.), (Cocc.), (Coff.), Coloc., Con., (Croc.), (Dig.), (Dulc.), (Euphr.), (Fer.), (Guai.), Hep., Hyos., *Ign.,* (K. bi.), (K. carb.), K. nit., (Lach.), (Laur.), Led., Lyc., (Mang.), (Mar.), (Meny.), Merc., (Mez.), (Mur. ac.), (Nat. c., Nat. m., Nit. ac., (Nux m.), *Nux v.,* (Op.), (Petrol.), Phos., Pho. ac., (Plat.), (Pod.), *Puls.,* Ran. b., (Ran. s.), Rhodo., *Rhus,* (Ruta), (Sabi.), (Sang.), (Sars.), (Sele.), (Seneg.), *Sep.,* Sil., Spig., (Stan.), Staph., (Stram.), (Stro.), Sul., (Tar.)., (Thuj.), Valer., Verat. a., (Verb.), Zinc.

Other Remedies.—ACON., Aesc., *Agar.,* Aloe., Alum., (Ambr (Am. carb.), Am. m., (Ant. cr.), Apis, Arg., **Arn.,** Arum. t., ARS., Asaf., (Asar.), *Aur.,* Bap., Bar. c., **BELL.,** Bor., BRY., (Cact.), **Calc. c.,** Camph., Cannab. i., Canth., *Caps.,* **Carb. v., Caust., Cham.,** *Chel.,* Chin., Cic., Cimic., *Cocc.,* (Coff.), Colch., *Coloc.,* **Con.,** (Croc.), (Crotal.), *Cup., Dig.,* (Dros.), Dulc., *Fer.,* Gel., (Glon.), *Graph.,* **Hep., Hyos., Ign.,** Ip., *Iod., K. bi., K. carb., Kre.,* **Lach.,** Laur., Led., (Lil. t.), **Lyc.,** (Mag. c.), Meny., MERC., Mez., (Mur. ac.), *Nat. c.,* **Nat. m., Nit. ac.,** Nux m., **NUX V., Op.,** (Par.), *Petrol.,* PHOS., Pho. ac., Pod., Plat., *Pb.,* PULS., *Ran. b.,* (Ran. s.), *Rhodo.,* RHUS, (Ruta), *Saba.,* (Sabi.), (Samb.), Sang., Sars., Sec. c., (Sele.), *Seneg.,* SEP., SIL., *Spig., Spo.,* Squ., **Stan.,** *Staph.,*

Stram., (Stro.), SUL., (Sul. ac.), (Tar.), *Thuj.*, **Verat. a.**, (Verat. v.), **Zinc.**

Arnica.

Mind.—Acon., Aesc., Aloe, *Apis*, Arum. t., Bar. c., *Bell.*, Bry., *Camph.*, *Cannab. i.*, Carb. ac., Cham., Cic., *Crotal.*, Gel., *Glon.*, Hyd. ac., Lach., Lyc., Nat. m., *Nux v.*, Puls., Rhus, *Sep.*, Stram., Sul., *Verat. a.*, *Verat. v.*

Localities.—*Acon.*, Aesc., All. c., *Aloe*, Alum., APIS, *Apoc. c.*, **Arg. n.**, Ars., Arum. t., *Bap.*, Bar. c., **Bell.**, Berb., *Bry.*, Cact., *Calc. c.*, *Cannab. i.*, Canth., Carb. ac., Carb. v., Caust., *Cham.*, **Chin.**, Cimic., Cocc., Colch., *Con.*, Crotal., Dios., Eup. per., (Fl. ac.), (Gel.), (Glon.), Graph., Hep., (Hyd. ac.), Hyos., *Ign.*, (Iris v.), K. Bi., K. carb., Kalm., Lil. t., *Lyc.*, Meli., **Merc.**, *Nat. m.*, Nit. ac., **Nux v.**, *Phos.*, Phyt., *Pod.*, *Pso.*, PULS., *Rhus*, Ruta, Saba., Sang., **Sep.**, *Sil.*, Spig., Stan., *Staph.*, Stram., Sul., Thuj., *Verat. a.*, Verat. v.

Sensations.—*Acon.*, (Aesc.), (Aloe), Alum., Apis, *Arg. n.*, Ars., Arum. t., Asaf., Asar., (Bap.), Bar. c., **BELL.**, *Berb.*, **Bry.**, (Cact.), CALC. C., Cannab. i., Canth., *Caust.*, **CHIN.**, Cimic., Cocc., *Con.*, Croc., (Crotal.), (Dios.), Eup. per., Fer., Gel., (Glon.), Graph., Hep., Ign., (Iris v.), *K. bi.*, *K. carb.*, (Kalm.), (Lil. t.), (Lith.), *Lyc.*, (Meli.), **Merc.**, Mez., Nat. c., *Nat. m.*, Nit. ac., Nux m., **Nux v.**, PHOS., Pho. ac., Phyt., *Plat.*, PULS., RHUS, Ruta, Sang., **Sep.**, *Sil.*, Spig., Stan., SUL., Thuj., Verat. a., Verat. v., Zinc.

Glands.—*Acon.*, Ars., Asaf., Bar. c., BELL., BRY., *Calc. c.*, **Carb. an.**, Carb. v., Caust., **Chin.**, Clem., CON., Dulc., Graph., *Hep.*, Iod., K. carb. Lyc., Merc., Nat. c., Nux v., PHOS., Plat., PULS., RHUS., *Sep.*, *Sil.*, Spig., *Spo.*, Sul., Thuj.

Bones.—Arg., Chin., Cyc.

Skin.—Acon., **Apis**, *Ars.*, Asaf., *Bell.*, *Bry.*, *Calc. c.*, *Caust.*, Chin., *Con.*, Graph., **Hep.**, Hyos., K. carb., **Lach.**, Led., Lyc., **Merc.**, Nit. ac., Nux v., Petrol., **Phos.**, Pho. ac., PULS., **Rhus**, Sec. c., **Sep.**, *Sil.*, *Staph.*, Stro., SUL., *Sul. ac.*

Sleep and Dreams.—Arg. n., *Ars.*, (Bap.), Bell., *Bry.*, Calc. c., (Cannab. i.), Chin., *Graph.*, *Ign.*, K. carb., Lyc., *Mag. c.*, Merc., NUX V., PHOS., Puls., Rhus, Sep., *Sil.*, Sul., Sul. ac., Thuj.

Blood, Circulation and Fever.—Acon., (Aloe.), (Apis), (Arg. n.), Bell., (Berb.), Bry., (Cact.), *Calc. c.*, Carb. v., Chel., *Chin.*, Fer., Glon., *Graph.*, Hep., Hyos., Ip., K. carb., Merc., Nit. ac., **Nux v.**, Phos., (Pod.), *Puls.*, *Rhus*, Sang., Sep., Sil., **Sul.**, Thuj., Verat. a.

Aggravations: Time and Circumstances.—*Acon.*, (Aesc.), (All. c.), Ambr., Ant. cr., Ant. t., Apis, **Arg. n.**, ***Ars.***, (Bap.), BELL., **Bry.**,

(Cact.), **Calc. c.**, (Cannab. i.), Cannab. s., *Caps.*, *Carb. v.*, Caust., Cham., **Chin.**, (Cimic.), Cocc., Colch., **Con.**, (Crotal.), Fer., Glon., Graph., **Hep.**, *Ign.*, Ip., K. bi., K. carb., Lach., *Led.*, Lil. t., *Lyc.*, Mag. c., Merc., Nat. c., **Nat. m.**, *Nit. ac.*, Nux v., *Phos.*, Pho. ac., Phyt., (Pod.), **Puls.**, Ran. s., RHUS, Ruta, *Sang.*, *Sep.*, **Sil.**, *Spig.*, Staph., SUL., Sul. ac., Verat. a., (Verat. v.)

Other Remedies.—*Acon.*, Aesc., (All. c.), Aloe, APIS. **Arg. n.**, *Ars.*, Arum. t., Asaf., Bap., Bar. c., **Bell.**, Berb., Bry., Cact., **Calc. c.**, *Cannab. i.*, Carb. an., *Carb. v.*, *Caust.*, Cham., **Chin.**, Cimic., Cocc., Colch., Con., *Crotal.* Fer., Gel., *Glon.*, *Graph.*, **Hep.**, Hyos., *Ign.*, **K. bi.**, *K. carb.*, Lach., Led., Lil. t., **Lyc.**, Mag. c., *Merc.*, Nat. c., *Nat. m.*, *Nit. ac.*, **Nux v.**, Phos., Pho. ac., Phyt., Plat., Pod., PULS., Rhus, Ruta, *Sang.*, Sep., Sil., *Spig.*, Stan., Staph., **Sul.**, Sul. ac., Thuj., *Verat. a.*, *Verat. a.*

Antidotes.—Am. carb., *Camph.*, Chin., Cic., Fer., Ign., *Ip.*, Seneg.

Injurious.—(Vinum.)

Arsenicum Album.

Mind.—*Acon.*, Anac., *Apis*, Arum. t., Aur., Bap., BELL., Bry., **Calc. c.**, *Cannab. i.*, Carb. ac., Cimic., Cup., Gel., *Glon.*, Graph., *Hyd. ac.*, *Hyos*, Laur., LYC., **Meli.**, Merc. c., Nat. c., Nat. m., Nux v., *Op.*, Phos., Pho. ac., Pic. ac., PULS., *Rhus*, Sep., STRAM., Sul., Verat. a., *Verat. v.*

Localities.—*Acon.*, Aesc., *All. c.*, Aloe, APIS, Apoc. c, ARG. N., Arn., *Arum. t.*, Bap., Bar. c., **Bell.**, Berb., **Bry.**, Cact., *Calc c.*, Cannab. i., Carb. ac., *Carb. v.*, Caust., *Cham.*, **Chin.**, *Cimic.*, Cocc., Con., Crotal., Cup., Dig., Dios., Dulc., Fer. Eup. per., (Fl. ac.), *Gel.*, (Glon.), Graph., **Hep.**, (Hyd. ac.), Hyos., (Hyper.), *Ign.*, *Ip.*, Iris v., K. BI., *K. carb.*, Kalm., Lil. t., **Lyc.**, Meli., **Merc.**, Nat. c., *Nat. m.*, *Nit. ac.*, Nux v., Op., **Phos.**, *Pho. ac.*, **Phyt.**, Pb., POD., *Pso.*, *Puls.*, *Rhus*, *Sang.*, Sec. c., **Sep.**, *Sil.*, Spig., Staph., Stram., SUL., (Ther.), **Verat. a.**, Verat. v.

Sensations.—Acon., Aesc., Anac., *Apis*, **Arg. n.**, *Arn.*, Arum. t., Bap., Bar. c., **Bell.**, *Berb.*, **Bry.**, Cact., **Calc. c.**, *Cannab. i.*, Cannab. s., Canth., *Carb. v.*, *Caust.*, *Cham.*, **Chin.**, *Cimic.*, Cocc., **Con.**, Crotal., *Cup.*, Dig., (Dios.), Dulc., *Fer.*, Gel., *Glon.*, Graph., Hyos., *Ign.*, Iod., (Iris v.), **K. bi.**, *K. carb.*, (Kalm.), Lil. t., **Lyc.**, **Merc.**, *Nat. m.*, *Nit. ac.*, **Nux v.**, Op., *Phos.*, Pho. ac., (Phyt.), Plat., Pod., (Pso.), **Puls.**, *Rhus*, *Sang.*, Sec. c., **Sep.**, *Sil.*, Spig., Squ., *Stan.*, Staph., *Stram.*, Stro., SUL., *Verat. a.*, Verat. v., Zinc.

Glands.—(Arum. t.), **Bell.**, **Con.**, Hep., Merc., *Phos.*, *Sil.*, *Sul.*

Bones.—Asaf., *Calc. c.*, Merc., Staph., Sul.

Skin.—Acon., Ant. cr., *Apis, Asaf., Bell., Bry.,* Calc. c., (Carb. ac.), Carb. an., *Carb. v., Caust.,* Chin., (Cimic.), Con., (Crotal.), Cyc., Dulc., (Eup. per.), Graph., *Hep.,* Hyos., K bi., Kre., LACH., **Lyc., Merc.,** Mez., Nit. ac., *Phos.,* Pho. ac., Pb., Puls., Rhus, *Sec. c., Sep.,* SIL., Squ., Staph., Sul., Verat. a.

Sleep and Dreams.—(Apis), Arg. n., (Bap.), *Bell., Bry.,* Calc. c., Cannab. i., Carb. v., Cham., Chin., (Cimic.), (Gel.), *Hep.,* Ign., **K. carb.,** (Lil. t.), Lyc., Mag. c., Merc., Mur. ac., **Nux v.,** Op., *Phos.,* Pho. ac., (Pod.), **Puls.,** *Rhus, Sep.,* **Sil.,** *Sul.*

Blood, Circulation and Fever.—Acon., Apis, (Arg. n.), (Bap.), **Bell.,** Berb., BRY., (Cact.), Calc c., *Cannab. i.,* Cham., CHIN., (Cimic.), Cocc., (Crotal.), Gel., Glon., Lach., (Lil. t.), Lyc., **Merc.,** Nux m., **NUX V.,** Op., *Phos.,* Pho. ac., Phyt., (Pod.), Puls., Rhus, Saba., Samb., *Sang., Sep.,* Sil., *Spig.,* Squ., Staph., Stan., Sul., *Verat. a.,* (Verat. v.)

Aggravations: Time and Circumstances.—Acon., (Aesc.), (All. c.), Aloe, Apis, *Arg. n.,* Arn., Aur., Bap., Bell., **Bry.,** (Cact.), Calc. c., (Cannab. i.), *Carb. v., Caust., Cham.,* Chin., (Cimic.), Colch., (Crotal.), Dros. Dulc., *Fer.,* (Gel.), (Glon.), *Hep.,* Ign., Ip., *K. bi.,* K. carb., (Lil. t.), *Lyc.,* Mag. c., Mang., *Merc.,* Mos., Nat. m., Nit. ac., Nux m., **NUX V.,** *Phos.,* Phyt., Pb., Pod., PULS., Rhus, Saba., Samb., *Sang., Sep., Sil.,* Stram., *Stro., Sul.,* Thuj., Verat. a.

Other Remedies.—*Acon.,* Aesc., All. c., Aloe, Anac., APIS, (Apoc. c.), Arg. n., Arn. *Arum. t.,* Asaf., **Bap., Bell.,** Berb., **Bry., Calc. c.,** Cact., Cannab. i., *Carb. v.,* Caust., *Cham.,* Chin., Cimic., Cocc., Con., *Crotal.,* Cup., Dulc., Fer., Gel., Glon., Graph., *Hep.,* Hyos., Ign., Ip., **K. bi.,** *K. carb.,* Lach., *Lil. t.,* Lyc., Merc., Nat. m., Nit. ac., **Nux v.,** Op., Phos., *Pho. ac., Phyt.,* Pb., Pod., PULS., Rhus, Sang., Sec. c., **Sep.,** Sil., Spig., Squ., Staph., *Stram.,* Stro., Sul., *Verat. a.,* **Verat. v.**

Antidotes.—Carb. v., Chin., Fer., Graph., *Hep.,* Iod., *Ip.,* Lach., *Nux v.,* Samb., Verat. a.

Arum Triphyllum.

Mind.

Localities.—Acon., Aesc., Agar., All. c., (Aloe), (Alum), Am. m., Ant. cr., Apis, (Apoc. c.), (Arg.), Arg. n., Arn., *Ars.,* (Asaf.), (Aur.), Bap., Bar. c., *Bell.,* (Bism.), Bor., (Bov.), *Bry., Calc.* c., Camph., (Cannab. i.), (Canth.), Caps., (Carb. ac.), (Carb. an.), Carb. v., (Caust.), *Cham.,* Chel., (Chin.), (Cic.), (Cimic.), (Cina) (Cocc.), (Coff.), (Colch.), Coloc., Con., (Crotal.), (Cup.), (Dig.), Dros., (Dulc.), Euphr., (Fer.), (Fl. ac.), (Gel.), Graph., (Hep.), (Hyos.), Ign., (Ip.), Iod., *K. bi.,* K. carb., (K. nit.), Kre., Lach., (Laur.), (Lyc.) (Mag. m.), (Mar.), (Meli.), *Merc.,*

Mez., (Mos.), Mur. ac., Nat. c., Nat. m., Nit. ac., (Nux m.), Nux v., Op., Par., Petrol., **Phos.**, Pho. ac., Phyt., (Plat.), (Pb.), Pod., (Pso.), **Puls.**, (Ran. b.), (Rheum), (Rhodo), Rhus, (Ruta), Saba., (Samb.), **Sang.**, (Sars.), (Sec. c.), Seneg., *Sep.*, *Sil.*, *Spig.*, Spo., (Squ.), Stan., Staph., (Stram.), **Sul.**, (Sul. ac.), (Tar.), (Thuj.), Verat. a., (Verat. v.), (Verb.), Zinc.

Sensations.—Acon., (Aesc.), (Agar.), Alum., Apis, Arg. n., Arn., *Ars.*, (Aur.), (Bap.), Bar. c., *Bell.*, Berb., *Bry.*, Calc. c., (Cannab. i.), Canth., Carb. v., Caust., Chel., Chin., Cimic., Cocc., Coloc., (Con.), (Cup.), (Dros.), (Euphr.), (Fer.), Graph., (Hyos.), Ign., (Iod.), (Iris v.), K. bi., (K. carb.), Lach., (Laur.), Lil. t., Lyc., *Merc.*, Mez., Nat. m., Nit. ac., Nux v., Op., (Petrol.), **Phos.**, Pho. ac., Phyt., (Pb.), (Pod.), (Pso.), Puls., (Ran. b.), *Rhus*, Saba., Sang., Sec. c., Seneg., *Sep.*, Sil., Spig., Spo., *Stan.*, (Stram.), *Sal.*, (Sul. ac.), (Tar.), (Thuj.), (Valer.), Verat. a., Zinc.

Glands.—(Am. m.), (Ars.), Bar. c., Bell., (Canth.), (Carb. an.), (Cham.), (Clem.), Con., (Dulc.), (Graph.), (Hep.), (K. carb.), Lyc., Merc., (Nat. c.), Nit. ac., (Nux v.), Phos., (Puls.), Rhus, Sul., (Thuj.)

Bones.

Skin.

Sleep and Dreams.

Blood, Circulation and Fever.

Aggravations: Time and Circumstances.—(Anac), (CALC. C.), (Cannab. s.), (Chin.), (Cocc.), (Mang.), (Nat. c.), (Nat. m.), (Pho. ac.), Rhus, (Sele.), (Stan.), (Sul.).

Other Remedies.—Acon., (Aesc.), (Agar.), (Alum.), (Am. m.), Apis, Arg. n., Arn., *Ars.*, (Bap.), *Bar. c.*, *Bell.*, **Bry.**, **Calc. c.**, Canth., (Carb. v.), (Caust.), Cham., (Chel.), Chin., (Cimic.), Cocc., Coloc., Con., (Dros.), (Euphr.), Graph., Ign., K. bi., K. carb., Lach., Lyc., *Merc.*, Mez., Nat. c., Nit. ac., *Nux v.*, Op., (Petrol.), **Phos.**, Pho. ac., Phyt., (Pod.), **Puls.**, Rhus, Saba., Sang., (Sec. c.), Seneg., Spo., **Sul.**, (Thuj.), Verat. a., (Zinc.)

Asafœtida.

Mind.—*Alum.*, Aur., *Ign.*, Lyc., Phos., *Plat.*, Puls., Sul., Sul. ac., Zinc.

Localities.—(All. c.), Aloe, Apis, (Apoc. c.), Arg. n., Arn., Ars., (Arum t.), Aur., (Bap.), Bor., Bry., *Calc. c.*, Carb. ac., **Carb. v.**, (Caul.), *Caust.*, Cham., CHIN., (Cimic.), Con., (Crotal.), (Dios.), (Gel.), *Ign.*, K. bi., Laur., (Lil. t.), *Lyc.*, Merc., **Nit. ac.**, Nux v., Phos., Plat., Pb., Pod., (Pso.), PULS., Ran. b., Sang., Sele., Sep., Sil., Spig., Staph., *Sul.*, **Thuj.**, Valer., Verat. a., *Zinc.*

Sensations.—Acon., (Aloe), Alum., Anac., (Apis), Arg., Arg. n., Arn., (Arum t.), Asar., **Bell.**, Berb., *Bry.*, **Calc. c.**, Cannab. i., *Caust.*, Cimic., *Cocc.*, Con., Cup., (Dios.), Dulc., Fer., (Gel.), Glon., Graph., *Ign.*, Iod., (Iris v.), *K. bi.*, *K. carb.*, (Lith.), *Lyc.*, *Merc.*, Mez., *Mos.*, Nat. c., Nat. m., Nux m., **Nux v.**, Oleand., *Phos.*, (Phyt.), *Plat.*, (Pso.), PULS, Rhus, Sabi., Sang., *Sep.*, Sil., **Spig.**, Spo., *Stan.*, *Staph.*, Stro., **Sul.**, Tar., Thuj., *Valer.*, Zinc.

Glands.—Am. m., Bell., *Bry.*, **Calc. c.**, Cocc., *Con.*, Ign., *Merc.*, Nat. m., **Phos.**, **Puls.**, Ran. s., Rhus, Sep., Spo., **Sul.**

Bones.—Bell., **Calc. c.**, Chin., (Cimic.), Eup. per., Hep., *Lyc.*, MERC., Mez., Nit. ac., Phos., **Pho. ac.**, **Puls.**, Ruta, Sep., SIL., *Staph.*, **Sul.**

Skin.—Acon., Ars., Bell., Bry., *Calc. c.*, Carb. v., *Caust.*, **Hep.**, *Lach.*, *Lyc.*, **Merc.**, Nit. ac., Phos., Pho. ac., Pb., PULS., Rhus, Sec. c., Sep., SIL., Staph., **Sul.**, Thuj.

Sleep and Dreams.—(Apis), Ars., Bry., (Cannab. i.), K. carb., Nat. c., Nux m., Nux v., Phos., (Pod.), *Puls.*, Sep.

Blood, Circulation and Fever.—(Apis), *Ars.*, Cocc., (Gel.), Phos., *Puls.*, Samb., Spig.

Aggravations: Time and Circumstances.—(All. c.), (Aloe), (Apis), Arg., Arg. n., Arn., Ars., Aur., (Bap.), Bell., *Calc. c.*, (Cannab. i.), Caps., Carb. v., *Chin.*, Cimic., Cina, Cocc., Con., **Cyc.**, Dros., Dulc., Euphorb. Euphr., *Fer.*, (Glon.), Hep., K. bi., K. carb., K. nit., Lach., (Lil. t.) Lyc., Mag. m., Merc., Mur. ac., Nat. c., Nat. m., Nux v., *Phos.*, (Phyt.) PULS., Rhodo., Rhus, *Ruta*, Saba., Sang., **Sep.**, Sil., **Sul.**, *Tar.*

Other Remedies.—(All. c.), Aloe, Alum, Apis, Arg. n., Arn., *Ars.*, (Arum t.), Aur., (Bap.), *Bell.*, *Bry.*, **Calc. c.**, Cannab. i., *Carb. v.*, *Caust.*, *Chin.*, Cimic., Cocc., Con., Cyc., Fer., (Gel.), (Glon.), Hep., *Ign.*, *K. bi.*, K. carb., Lach., (Lil. t.), **Lyc.**, **Merc.**, Nat. c., Nat. m., Nit. ac., Nux v., **Phos.**, Pho. ac., (Phyt.), Plat., (Pod.), PULS., Rhus, Ruta, Sang., **Sep.** Sil., Spig., Staph., **Sul.**, Tar., Thuj., Valer., Zinc.

Antidotes.—Camph., Caust., *Chin.*, *Merc.*,—Electric.

Asarum.

Mind.—*Cocc.*, Con., Ign., Lyc., Mez., Nat. m., Op., *Pho. ac.*, PULS., Rhus, Sep., SIL., Stram.

Localities.—Acon., Aesc., (Aloe), Arg. n., Arn., (Bap.), *Bell.*, Bry., *Calc. c.*, Caust., Cham., *Chin.*, (Cimic.), Con., Graph., K. bi., *K. carb.*, Kre., *Lyc.*, **Merc.**, Nat. m., Nit. ac., **Nux v.**, *Phos.*, (Phyt.), (Pod.), PULS., (Sang.), *Sep.*, Sil., *Spig.*, *Sul.*, Verat. a., (Verat. v.).

Sensations.—Acon., (Aesc.), Alum., Anac., (Apis), (Arg. n.), *Arn.,* Asaf., Aur., (Bap.), *Bell.,* (Berb.), Bry. (Cact.), Calc. c., (Cannab. i.), Canth., **Chin.,** (Cimic.), **Cocc.,** Coff., Con., Cup., (Gel.), Glon., *Ign.,* Iod., (K. bi.), K. carb., Lyc., Mez., Mos., Nat. m., *Nux m.,* **Nux v.,** Phos., (Phyt.), *Plat.,* PULS., Rhus, (Sang.), *Sep.,* Sil., Spig., *Stan.,* Staph., *Sul.,* Sul. ac., Valer., **Verat. a.**

Glands.—Hyos.

Bones.

Skin.—*Caust.,* Chin., Merc., Phos., *Plat., Puls.,* Rhus, Spig., *Sul.*

Sleep and Dreams.—Bry., Calc. c., (Cannab. i.), (Gel.), Ign., K. carb., Nux v., Sul.

Blood, Circulation and Fever.—Acon., Bell., Calc. c., **Cham.,** Merc., Nux v., Rhus, Spig., Sul., *Verat. a.*

Aggravations: Time and Circumstances.—*Acon.,* (Aesc.), Agn., (All. c.), (Aloe), Anac., Ant. cr., (Apis), (Arg. n.), Arn., (Bap.), *Bell.,* **Bry.,** (Cact.), Calc. c., (Cannab. i.), CAUST., Cham., Chel., Chin., (Cimic.), Colch., Con., Croc., Euphr., Fer., (Glon.), **Hep.,** *Iod.,* Ip., (K. bi.), K. carb., Led., (Lit. t.), *Lyc.,* Merc., Mez., **Nux v., Phos.,** (Phyt.), Plat., PULS., Rhus, Saba., (Sang.), Sep., Sil., *Spig., Spo.,* Sul., Valer.

Other Remedies.—Acon., Aesc., (Aloe), (Apis), (Arg. n.), Arn., (Bap.), *Bell.,* Bry., (Cact.), Calc. c., (Cannab. i.), *Caust.,* Cham., *Chin.,* (Cimic.), Cocc., Con., (Gel.), (Glon.), Hep., Ign., Iod., K. bi., K. carb., *Lyc.,* Merc., Mez., Nat. m., **Nux v.,** *Phos.,* (Phyt.), Plat., PULS., *Rhus,* (Sang.), Sep., *Sil., Spig., Sul.,* Verat. a.

Antidotes.—Acetum, Camph.

Aurum Foliatum.

Mind.—*Aloe,* Apis, *Anac.,* Ars., **Bap.,** BELL., *Bor.,* Bry., *Cact.,* Calc. c., **Cannab. i.,** Caust., Cham., *Cimic.,* Coff., *Crotal.,* Dig., Gel., *Glon., Graph., Hyd. ac.,* **Hyos.,** *Ign.,* LYC., *Meli.,* Nat. c., Nux v., Op., Phos., *Plat.,* **Puls.,** Rhus, Sec. c., Sep., *Stram.,* **Sul.,** *Sul. ac. Ther.,* **Verat. a., Verat. v.**

Localities.—(Aesc.), Agar., All. c., Aloe, Am. carb., Am. m., Apis, Arg. n., *Arn.,* Ars., (Arum t.), Asaf., (Bap.), **Bell.,** (Berb.), *Bry.,* (Cact.), CALC. C., (Cannab. i.), Canth., (Carb. ac.), Carb. an., *Carb. v.,* **Caust.,** *Cham.,* Chin., Cimic., Clem., *Con.,* (Crotal.), Gel., (Glon.), *Graph.,* Hep., *Hyos.,* Ign., K. bi., **K. carb.,** (Kalm.), (Lil. t.), **Lyc.,** (Meli.), **Merc.,** *Nat. c., Nat. m., Nit. ac.,* **Nux v.,** Op., **Phos.,** *Pho. ac.,* (Pic. ac.), Plat., *Pb.,* (Pod.), PULS., *Rhus,* Ruta, Sabi., Sang., Sec. c.,

RELATIONSHIPS.—AURUM FOL.

SEP., Sil., *Spig.*, *Staph.*, Stram., Sul., Sul. ac., *Thuj.*, *Verat. a.*, Verat. v., *Zinc.*

Sensations.—*Acon.*, (Aesc.), (Aloe), Ambr., Anac., Apis, *Arg.*, Arg. n., *Arn.*, (Arum. t.), Asaf., Asar., (Bap.), **Bell.**, Berb., *Bry.*, **Calc. c.**, Cannab. i., Canth., (Carb. ac.), Carb. v., *Caust.*, Cham., CHIN., (Cimic.), Cocc., Coff., *Con.*, *Fer.*, (Gel.), (Glon.), *Graph.*, Hep., Ign., (K. bi.), *K. carb.*, K. nit., (Kalm.), (Lil. t.), LYC., Mag. c., **Merc.**, Mez., *Nat. c.*, **Nat. m.**, *Nit. ac.*, **Nux v.**, **Phos.**, Plat., PULS., Rhus, Sabi, (Sang.), Seneg., Sep., *Sil.*, *Spig.*, *Stan.*, Staph., Stro., **Sul.**, Tar., Valer., Verat. a., *Zinc.*

Glands.—Arn., **Bell.**, Carb. an., Iod., Lyc., Merc., Phos., *Puls.*, Rhus, Sil., Spo., Sul.

Bones.—*Asaf.*, Bell., Calc. c., Chin., Cyc., (Eup. per.), Lyc., MERC., Mez., Nit. ac., Phos., *Pho. ac.*, Puls., Ruta, Sep., **Sil.**, Staph., Sul.

Skin.—Alum., Ars., Bell., *Bry.*, **Calc. c.**, Caust., Cic., Clem., Con., (Crotal.), Dig., Graph., *Hep.*, *Lyc.*, MERC., Nat. m., Nit. ac., Petrol., *Phos.*, Pho. ac., **Puls.**, *Rhus*, **Sep.**, *Sil.*, Spig., Staph., **Sul.**, *Verat. a.*, Zinc.

Sleep and Dreams.—Ars., Bell., Calc. c., Coff., Dulc., Fer., *K. carb.* Lyc., Mag. c., *Nat. c.*, **Nux v.**, Phos., Puls., **Sep.**, **Sil.**, *Sul.*

Blood, Circulation and Fever.—ACON., Arg. n., Arn., *Ars.*, *Bell.*, *Bry.*, (Cact.), **Calc. c.**, Carb. v., *Chin.*, Con., Fer., Glon., Hep., K. carb., *Lyc.*, Mag. c., Nat. m., Nit. ac., Nux m., **Nux v.**, *Phos.*, *Puls.*, RHUS, Samb., (Sang.), *Sep.*, *Sil.*, Stram., *Sul.*

Aggravations: Time and Circumstances.—Acon., (Aesc.), (Aloe), Am. carb., (Apis), (Arg. n.), Arn., **Ars.**, (Bap.), **Bell.**, Bry., Calc. c., *Caps.*, *Caust.*, Cham., Cocc., Colch., **Con.**, Croc., Cyc., Dros., **Dulc.**, *Euphorb.*, *Fer.*, (Gel.), (Glon.), **Hep.**, *Hyos.*, Ign., *Iod.*, (K. bi.), *K. carb.*, K. nit., Lil. t., **Lyc.**, Mag. c., Mag. m., Merc., *Mos.*, Nat. m., Nit. ac., Nux m., **Nux v.**, Phos., Pho. ac., (Phyt.), *Plat.*, (Pod.), PULS., *Rhodo*, RHUS, Saba., Samb., Sang., **Sep.**, Sil., Squ., Staph., Stro., Sul., *Tar.*, Valer., Verat. a., (Verat. v.).

Other Remedies.—Acon., (Aesc.), *Aloe*, Apis, *Arg. n.*, Arn., *Ars.*, (Arum. t.), Asaf., *Bap.*, BELL., (Berb.), Bry., Cact., **Calc. c.**, *Cannab. i.*, Carb. v., *Caust.*, Cham., *Chin.*, Cimic., *Con.*, Crotal., Dulc., *Fer.*, Gel., *Glon.*, Graph., **Hep.**, *Hyos.*, Ign., K. bi., *K. carb.*, Lil. t., LYC., Mag. c., Merc., Nat. c., *Nat. m.*, *Nit. ac.*, **Nux v.**, **Phos.**, Pho. ac., Plat., (Pod.), PULS., Rhus, Samb., Sang., SEP., **Sil.**, Spig., Staph., Stram., Stro., SUL., *Verat. a.*, *Verat. v.*, Zinc.

Antidotes.—Bell., *Camph.*, Chin., *Coff.*, *Cup.*, *Merc.*, Puls., Spig.

Baptisia.

Mind.—Acon., Anac., Ant. t., Apis, Arn., Ars., Aur., Bar. c., **BELL.,** Bry., Cact., Camph., *Cannab. i.*, Canth., Caust., Chel., *Cic.*, **Cocc.**, Con., Crotal., Cup., *Dig.*, Dros., Gels., *Hell.*, Hyd. ac., *Hyos.*, Ign., Ip., Lach., LYC., **Merc. c.**, Nat. c., **Op.**, Petrol., Phos., Pho. ac., Pic. ac., Plat., *Pb.*, Puls., Rhus t., Sec. c., Sep., Sil., Staph., **Stram.**, Sul., Sul. ac., *Verat. a.*, Verat. v.

Localities.—Acon., (Aesc.), Agar., (Aloe.), (Alum.), Am. m., (Ant. cr), Ant t., Apis, (Apoc. c.), (Arg.), Arg. n., *Arn.*, *Ars.*, (Arum. t.), Asaf., (Asar.), (Aur.), Bar. c., *Bell.*, (Berb.), (Bism.), Bor., (Bov.), *Bry.*, (Calad.), *Calc. c.*, (Cannab. i.), *Canth.*, (Caps.), (Carb. ac.), (Carb. an.), Carb. v., (Caust.), *Cham.*, Chel., *Chin.*, (Cic.), (Cimic.), (Cina.), (Clem.), Cocc., (Coff.), Colch., Coloc., Con., (Croc.), (Crotal.), Cup., (Cyc.), Dig., (Dios.), Dros., (Dulc.), (Eup. per.), Fer., (Fl. ac.), (Gel.), (Glon.), (Graph.), (Hell.), Hep., Hyos., *Ign.*, Ip., Iod., (Iris v.), *K. bi.*, K. carb., (K. nit.), (Kre.), Lach., (Laur.), (Led.), (Lil. t.), *Lyc.*, (Mag. m.), (Meli.), **Merc.**, (Mez.), (Mos.), (Mur. ac.), (Nat. c.), Nat. m, *Nit. ac.*, (Nux m.), **Nux v.**, (Op.), Petrol., **Phos.**, Pho. ac., **Phyt.**, (Plat.), Pb., Pod., (Pso.), **Puls.**, (Ran. b.), (Rheum), (Rhodo.), *Rhus*, (Ruta), *Saba.*, (Sabi.), (Samb.), (Sang.), Sec. c., (Sele.), Seneg., **Sep.**, Sil., Spig., (Spo.), (Squ.), Stan., (Staph.), Stram., (Stro.), SUL., Sul. ac., (Tar.), Thuj., (Valer.), Verat. a., (Verat. v.), (Verb.), Zinc.

Sensations.—Acon., (Aesc.), (Agar.), Anac., (Ant. t.), Apis, Arg., (Arg. n.), Arn., *Ars.*, (Arum. t.), (Asar.), (Aur.), Bar. c., **Bell.**, Berb., (Bor.), *Bry.*, (Cact.), (Calad.), *Calc. c.*, (Cannab. i.), *Canth.*, (Carb. v.), Caust., (Cham.), Chel., Chin., Cic., Cimic., Cocc., (Colch.), Coloc., Con., Cup., (Dig.), (Dros.), (Eup. per.), (Fer.), (Gel.), (Hell.), (Hep.), Hyos., *Ign.*, (Ip.), Iod., (Iris v.), K. bi., (K. carb.), *Lach.*, (Led.), (Lil. t.), *Lyc.*, (Mag. m.), *Merc.*, (Mez.), (Mos.), (Mur. ac.), (Nat. c.), *Nat. m.*, (Nit. ac.) Nux m., **Nux v.**, Oleand., Op., (Petrol.), *Phos.*, Pho. ac., (Phyt.), Plat., Pb., (Pod.), **Puls.**, (Ran. b.), (Ran. s.), Rhodo., *Rhus*, Ruta, Saba., (Sabi.), (Sang.), Sars., Sec. c., (Seneg.), **Sep.**, **Sil.**, (Spig.), (Spo.), Squ., Stan., (Staph.), Stram., *Sul.*, Sul. ac., (Thuj.), Verat. a., Verat. v., Zinc.

Glands.

Bones.

Skin.—(Arn.), (Ars.), (Bar. c.), (Bell.), Caust., (Coloc.), (Con.), (Cup.), Dig., Lach., Nux v., Op., (Phos.), (Plat.), (Puls.), (Rhus), (Sec. c.), (Spig.), (Stram.), Stro., (Sul.), Verat. a., (Vio. o.).

Sleep and Dreams.—Acon., Arg. n., (Arn.), Ars., (Bell.), Bry., (Calc. c.), (Cham.), (Chin.), (Coff.), Graph., Hep., (Hyos.), (Ign.), K.

carb., (Kre.), (Led.), (Mag. c.), Merc., (Nat. m.), Nux v., *Phos.*, (Pb.), *Puls., Rhus,* Sep., *Sil., Sul.,* Thuj.

Blood, Circulation and Fever.—(Ars.), (Bell.), (Bor.), (Bry.), (Fer.), (Merc.), (Nux v.), (Op.), (Phos.), (Pho. ac.), (Puls.), (Ruta), (Sang.), (Sil.), (Spo.), (Stram.), (Sul.).

Aggravations : Time and Circumstances.—Acon., (Aesc.), (Agar.), (Ambr.), (Am. carb.), (Am. m.), (Ant. cr.), (Ant. t.), (Apis), Arg., (Arg. n.), (Arn.,), Ars., (Asaf.), (Asar.), (Aur.), (Bar. c.), (Bell.), (Bor.) (Bov.), *Bry.*, Calad., Calc., c., (Cannab. s.), Caps., (Carb. an.), (Carb. v.), (Cham.), (Chel.), (Cina), (Cocc.), (Coff.), (Colch.), (Coloc.), Con., Croc., (Cyc.), (Dig.), Dros., (Dulc.), (Euphr.), Fer., (Glon.), (Graph.), (Guai.), (Hell.), Hep., (Hyos.), (Ign.), (Ip.), Iod., (K. bi.), (K. carb.), K. nit., (Lach.), (Led.), (Lil. t.), Lyc., (Mag. c.), Mag. m., (Mang.), (Mar.), (Meny.), Merc., (Mez.), (Mos.), (Nat. c.), Nat. m., Nit. ac., (Nux m.), Nux v., (Oleand.), (Par.), Petrol., Phos., Pho. ac., (Phyt.), (Plat.), (Pb.), Puls., *Ran. b.*, Ran. s., Rheum, (Rhodo.), Rhus, Ruta, (Saba.), (Sabi.), (Samb.), Sang., (Sars.), (Séle.), (Seneg.), Sep., Sil., (Spig.), (Spo.), (Squ.), Stan., (Staph.), (Stro.), Sul., (Tar.), (Thuj.), Valer., (Verat. a.), (Verat. v.), (Verb.), (Zinc).

Other Remedies.—*Acon.*, (Aesc.), Agar., (Am. m.), Anac., Ant. t., *Apis*, Arg., Arg. n., **Arn., Ars.**, (Asaf.), (Asar.), Aur., *Bar. c.*, **BELL.,** (Berb.), Bor., **BRY.,** (Cact.), Calad., *Calc. c.,* Cannab. i., *Canth.,*. Caps., Carb. v., *Caust.*, Cham., *Chel.*, Chin., Cic., (Cimic.), *Cocc.*, Colch., Coloc., Con., (Croc.), *Cup., Dig., Dros.*, Fer., Gel., Graph., Hell., *Hep., Hyos.*, Ign., Ip., Iod., K. bi., K. carb., (K. nit.), **Lach.,** Led., (Lil. t.), **Lyc.,** Mag. m., Merc., (Mez.), (Mos.), Nat. c., *Nat. m., Nit. ac.,* Nux m., NUX V., (Oleand.), **Op.,** *Petrol.*, PHOS., *Pho. ac.*, Phyt., *Plat.*, **Pb.,** (Pod.), PULS., Ran. b., (Ran. s.), (Rheum), Rhodo., RHUS, Ruta, Saba., (Sabi.), Sang., (Sars.), *Sec. c.*, Seneg., **Sep.,** Sil., Spig., Spo., Squ., Stan., Staph., **Stram.,** Stro., SUL., Sul. ac., Thuj., (Valer.), **Verat. a.,** Verat. v., Zinc.

Baryta Carbonica.

Mind.—*Acon.*, Anac., *Apis*, **Arn.,** *Ars., Bap., Bell.,* Bor., Bry., *Cact., Cannab. i.,* Caust., Cham., Cimic., Cocc., *Dig., Gel., Glon., Hell.,* Hyd. ac., Hyos., Ign., K. carb., *Lyc.,* Nux v., Op., *Puls., Rhus,* Sep., *Stram., Sul., Verat. a.*

Localities.—*Aesc.*, Aloe, Alum, *Apis*, Apoc. c., *Arg. n.*, Arn., *Ars.*, Arum. t., Bap., **Bell.,** Berb., Bry., Cact., CALC. C., Cannab. i., Carb. ac., Carb. v., *Caust., Chin.*, Cimic., Con., Crotal., Dios., (Fl. ac.), Gel., (Glon.), *Graph.,* Hep., Ign., Iris v., **K. bi., K. carb.,** (Kalm.), Kre., Lil. t., **Lyc.,**

(Meli.), **Merc.**, Mez., Nat. c., *Nat. m., Nit. ac., Nux v.*, Oleand., Par., Petrol., **Phos.**, Phyt., Pod., Pso., *Puls., Rhus*, Ruta, *Saba.*, Sang., *Sep.*, Sil., Spig., *Staph.*, Sul., *Verat. a.*, Verat. v.

Sensations.—*Acon.*, (Aesc.), Agn., (Aloe), Apis, (Arg. n.), *Arn.*, (Arum. t.), Ars., Asaf., (Bap.), **Bell.**, (Berb.), *Bry.*, (Cact.), *Calc. c.*, (Cannab. i.), Canth., Carb. v., Caust., *Cham.*, **Chin.**, (Cimic.), Cocc., Con., Croc., Cup., Cyc., Fer., (Gel.), (Glon.), *Graph.*, Hyos., Ign., (Iris v.), (K. bi.), *K. carb.*, (Lil. t.), **Lyc.**, **Merc.**, Mez., *Nat. c., Nat. m.*, Nux v., **Phos.**, Pho. ac., (Phyt.), Plat., **PULS.**, Rhus, Sabi., (Sang.), Sep., *Sil.*, Spig., Spo., Stan., Staph., *Stro.*, **SUL.**, Thuj., Verat. a., (Verat. v.), Zinc.

Glands.—Arum. t., ***Bell.***, *Bry.*, Carb. an., Caust., Cham., Clem., CON., Graph., *Lyc.*, Merc., Nux v., **PHOS.**, **PULS.**, *Rhus*, Sil., *Spo.*, Sul.

Bones.—Cocc., Ruta.

Skin.—Apis, Arn., (Bap.), Bry., **Calc. c.**, *Caust.*, Cham., Con., *Cyc.*, Dulc., *Graph.*, **Hep.**, *Led., Lyc.*, **Merc.**, *Nit. ac.*, Oleand., Petrol., Phos., *Plat.*, **Puls.**, RHUS, Saba., SEP., SIL., Spig., *Spo.*, **Staph.**, SUL., Verat. a., Vio. t.

Sleep and Dreams.—Ars., Calc. c., **Chin.**, (Cimic.), (Gel.), K. carb., *Nat. c.*, Nux v., **Phos.**, Puls., Rhus, Sep., Sil., SUL., Vio. t.

Blood, Circulation and Fever.—Acon., Arn., Bell., *Bry.*, Calc. c., Caust., Chin., Graph., K. carb., **Lyc.**, **Nux v.**, *Phos., Puls.*, Rhus, *Sep., Sul.*, Thuj.

Aggravations: Time and Circumstances.—*Acon.*, (Aesc.), Agar., *Am. carb.*, Apis, Arn., *Ars.*, (Bap.), *Bell., Bry.*, (Cact.), Calc. c., Caps., Carb. v., Caust., *Cham.*, Chin., Cic., Cocc., **Con.**, Dulc., Fer., (Glon.), Graph., **Hep.**, *Ign.*, Iod., (K. bi.), **K. carb.**, K. nit., Led., (Lil. t.), **Lyc.**, Merc., Mos., Nat. m., Nit. ac., *Nux v.*, Petrol., **Phos.**, Pho. ac., (Phyt.), Plat. Pb., **Puls.**, Ran. b., Rhodo., *Rhus*, Ruta, *Saba.*, (Sang.), SEP., SIL., Spig., Staph., **Sul.**

Other Remedies.—Acon., Aesc., (Aloe), *Apis*, *Arn.*, *Ars.*, Arum. t., *Bap.*, **Bell.**, (Berb.), *Bry.*, *Cact.*, **Calc. c.**, Cannab. i., Carb. v., *Caust.*, *Cham.*, *Chin.*, Cimic., Cocc., *Con.*, Cyc., Fer., *Gel.*, Glon., *Graph.*, Hep., Ign., K. bi., *K. carb.*, Led., Lil. t., **Lyc.**, **Merc.**, Nat. c., Nat. m., Nit. ac., **Nux v.**, Petrol., PHOS., Pho. ac., Phyt., Plat., **PULS.**, Rhus, Ruta, Saba., Sang., **Sep.**, Sil., Spig., Spo., *Staph.*, SUL., Verat. a., (Verat. v.), Vio. t.

Antidotes.—Ant. t., Bell., *Camph.*, Dulc.

Belladonna.

Mind.—*Acon.*, Ail., *Aloe*, Anac., Apis, Arg. n., **Aur.**, **Bap.**, Bar. c.,

RELATIONSHIPS.—BELLADONNA.

Bry., Cact., CANNAB. I., *Carb. ac.*, Cham., *Cic.*, *Cimic.*, Coff., *Crotal.*, Cup., Dig., Dios., **Gel.**, **Glon.**, **Hyd. ac.**, HYOS., **Hyper.**, Ign., K. bi., Kalm., Lil. t., Lyc., Meli., Nat. m., Nux v., **Op.**, Phos., *Pho. ac,*, *Phyt.*, Pic. ac., Plat., *Pso.*, **Puls.**, Rhus, Sang., *Sec. c.*, Sep., *Still*, **Stram.**, *Sul.*, *Ther.*, **Verat. a.**, **Verat. v.**

Localities.—*Acon.*, **Aesc.**, All. c., **Aloe**, Ant. cr., **APIS**, Apoc. c., ARG. N., Arn., *Ars.*, *Arum. t.*, *Aur.*, **Bap.**, Bar. c., **Bry.**, *Cact.*, CALC. C., *Cannab. i.*, *Canth.*, Caps., *Carb. ac.*, Carb. v., *Caust.*, *Cham.*, *Chin.*, Cic., CIMIC., Cocc., *Con.*, Crotal., Cup., Dios., Dros., Eup. per., Euphr., Fl. ac., **Gel.**, Glon., *Graph.*, *Hep.*, (Hyd. ac.), Hyos., *Ign.*, Ip., *Iris v.*, K. BI., *K. carb.*, Kalm., Kre., *Lil. t.*, Lith., Lyc., Meli., **Merc.**, Nat. c., *Nat. m.*, **Nit. ac.**, Nux v., Oleand., *Op.*, Petrol., **Phos.**, Pho. ac., Phyt., (Pic. ac.), Plat., Pb., *Pod.*, Pso., PULS., *Rhus*, Ruta, Saba., **Sang.**, Sec. c., Sep., Sil., *Spig.*, Stan., *Stap.*, *Stram.*, SUL., Ther., *Verat. a.*, **Verat. v.**, Zinc.

Sensations.—*Acon.*, *Aesc.*, Aloe, **Apis**, ARG. N., *Arn.*, *Ars.*, *Arum. t.*, *Asaf.*, *Bap.*, *Berb.*, *Bry.*, Cact., CALC. C., *Cannab. i.*, *Canth.*, *Caust.*, *Cham.*, *Chin.*, *Cic.*, **Cimic.**, Cocc., *Con.*, (Crotal.), *Cup.*, (Dios.), Dulc., (Eup. per.), *Fer.*, **Gel.**, **Glon.**, Hyos., *Ign.*, Iris v., K. BI., *K. carb.*, Kalm., *Lil. t.*, Lith., **Lyc.**, (Meli.), **Merc.**, Nat. c., *Nat. m.*, Nit. ac., NUX V., *Op.*, *Phos.*, Phyt., *Plat.*, Pb., Pod., Pso., **PULS.**, Rhus, Sabi., **Sang.**, Sec. c., SEP., *Sil.*, *Spig*., Stan., *Staph.*, *Stram.*, Stro., SUL., Thuj., *Verat. a.*, *Verat. v.*

Glands.—Acon., **Arn.**, Arum. t., **Bry.**, Calc. c., Carb. an., *Chin.*, Clem., *Con.*, Hyos., Iod., LYC., MERC., PHOS., **Puls.**, Rhus, Sep., *Sil.*, Spo., Sul.

Bones.—Arg., Asaf., **Calc. c.**, Caust., Chin., Cimic., Con., Cup., Cyc., Dros., Hell., Hep., K. carb., *Lyc.*, MERC., Nit. ac., *Phos.*, **Puls.**, Ruta, Sabi., Sars., Sep., *Sil.*, Spig., Staph., Sul.

Skin.—Acon., *Am. carb.*, **Apis**, **Ars.**, Asaf., *Bry.*, *Calc. c.*, (Carb. ac.), Caust., Chin., Con., Crotal., Dulc., *Fer.*, Graph., *Hep.*, Hyos., (K. bi.), *K. carb.*, *Lach.*, **Lyc.**, MERC., Mez., Nit. ac., Oleand., *Phos.*, **PULS.**, RHUS, (Sang.), Sec. c., **Sep.**, *Sil.*, Staph., **Sul.**, Verat. a., (Verat. v.).

Sleep and Dreams.—(Apis), (Arg. n.), *Ars.*, (Bap.), Bry., Calc. c., Cannab. i., Cham., Chin., (Cimic.), (Gel.), Graph., **Hep.**, Hyos., Ign., K. carb., Led., Lyc., *Merc.*, *Nux v.*, **Phos.**, Pho. ac., (Pod.), PULS., Rhus Sep., Sil., Spig., Stram., **Sul.**

Blood, Circulation and Fever.—ACON., Aloe., Apis, Arg. n., **Ars.**, (Bap.), (Berb.), Bry., Cact., Calc. c., *Cham.*, *Chin.*, Cocc., (Crotal.), Fer. *Glon.*, Graph., *Hep.*, **Hyos.**, Ign., Iod., (Lil. t.), **Merc.**, Nat. m., Nit. ac.

NUX V., *Phos.*, Pho. ac., Pod., PULS., Rhus, Saba., *Sang.*, *Sep.*, Sil., Stram., Sul., Thuj., Verat. a., Verat. v.

Aggravations: Time and Circumstances.—*Acon.*, Aesc., (All. c.), (Aloe), Ant. cr., Ant. t., *Apis*, *Arg. n.*, *Arn.*, *Ars.*, (Bap.), Bar. c., BRY., Calc. c., (Cannab. i.), Canth., Caps., Carb. v., Caust., Cham., *Chin.*, Cimic., *Colch.*, *Con.*, Croc., Cup., Fer., Glon., Hep., Hyos., *Ign.*, Ip., K. bi., *K. carb.*, K. nit., Lach., *Led.*, Lil. t., *Lyc.*, *Merc.*, Mez., Nat. m., Nux m., Nux v., *Op.*, *Phos.*, Pho. ac., (Phyt.), (Pod.), PULS., Ran. s., Rhus, *Sang.*, SEP., *Sil.*, *Spig.*, Stram., Stro., Sul., (Verat. v.).

Other Remedies.—*Acon.*, Aesc., (All. c.). Aloe., APIS., ARG. N., Arn., *Ars.*, *Arum. t.*, Asaf., Aur., Bap., Bar. c., Berb., Bry., Cact., Calc. c., Cannab. i., Canth., *Caust.*, *Cham.*, *Chin.*, Cic., CIMIC., Cocc., *Con.*, *Crotal.*, Cup., Fer., Gel., Glon., Graph., *Hep.*, Hyos., *Ign.*, K. bi., *K. carb.*, Lach., Led., Lil. t., Lith., Lyc., Merc., Nat. m., Nit. ac., *Nux v.*, *Op.*, Phos., Pho. ac., *Phyt.*, Plat., *Pod.*, PULS,, Rhus, SANG., Sec. c., Sep., *Sil.*, Spig., Staph., *Stram.*, Stro., Sul., Verat. a., VERAT. V.

Antidotes.—*Coff.*, Hep., *Hyos.*, Op., Puls., Vinum.

Injurious.—Acetum., Dulc.

Mind.

Berberis.

Localities.—Acon., Aesc., (Agar.), Aloe, (Alum.), (Amb.), (Am. carb.), (Am. m.), (Anac.), (Ant. cr.), (Ant. t.), Apis, (Apoc. c.), (Arg.), (Arg. n.), Arn., Ars., Aur., Bap., (Bar. c.), Bell., (Bor.), Bry., Calc. c., Cannab. i., (Cannab. s.), Canth., (Caps.), (Carb. ac.), (Carb. an.), (Carb. v.), (Caust.), (Cham.), Chel., Chin., (Cina), (Clem.), (Cocc.), Colch., Coloc., Con., (Crotal.), (Cup.), Dig., (Fer.), (Graph.), (Hell.), (Hep.), (Ign.), (Ip.), (Iod.), (Iris v.), (K. bi.), K. carb., (K. nit.), (Kre.), (Lach.), (Laur.), (Lith.), *Lyc.*, Merc., (Mez.), Nat. m., (Nit. ac.), *Nux v.*, (Op.), Petrol., Phos., (Pho. ac.), (Phyt.), (Pb.), (Pod.), (Pso.), *Puls.*, (Rhodo.), Rhus, (Ruta), (Saba.), (Sars.), (Sec. c.), (Sele.), *Sep.*, Sil., (Spig.), (Spo.), (Stan.), (Staph.), Sul., (Sul. ac.), (Thuj.), (Valer.), Verat. a., Zinc.

Sensations.—*Acon.*, (Aesc.), Agar., Alum., (Ant. t.), *Apis*, Arg. n., Arn., *Ars.*, *Arum. t.*, Asaf., (Aur.), Bap., Bar. c., Bell., (Bor.), Bry., (Calad.), *Calc. c.*, Cannab. i., *Canth.*, Caps., (Carb. v.), Caust., (Cham.), *Chel.*, Chin., (Cic.), (Cimic.), (Clem.), (Cocc.), *Coloc.*, Con., (Dios.), Dulc., (Eup. per.), (Euphr.), Glon., Graph., Hyos., *Ign.*, Iris v., *K. bi.*, *K. carb.*, Lach., (Laur.), (Lil. t.), Lyc., Merc., Mez., (Mur. ac.), Nat. c., Nat. m., *Nit. ac.*, (Nux m.), Nux v., Oleand., Op., Par., (Petrol.), Phos., *Pho. ac.*, Phyt., (Plat.), (Pb.), PULS., *Ran. b.*, (Rheum), (Rhodo.), Rhus, Saba., (Sabi.), Sang., Sec. c., Seneg., Sep., Sil., *Spig.*, (Spo.), (Squ,), *Stan.*,

(Staph.), Stram., Stro., **Sul.**, (Tar.), (Thuj.), (Valer.), *Verat. a.,* (Verat. v.), **Zinc.**

Glands.

Bones.

Skin.

Sleep and Dreams.

Blood, Circulation and Fever.—(Acon.), (Am. m.), (Arn.), Ars., (Bell.), (Bor.), Bry., (Calc. c.), (Canth.), (Caps,), (Cham.), (Chin.), (Cocc.) (Colch.), (Fer.), (Gel.), (Graph.), (Hep.), (Ign.), (Kre.), (Lach.), (Led.), Lyc., (Meny.), Merc., (Mez.), (Nat. m.), Nux v., (Op.), Phos., (Pho. ac.) Puls., Rhus, (Ruta), Sang., Sep., *Sil.,* Spig., (Spo.), (Stan.), (Stram.) *Sul.,* (Verat. a.)

Aggravations: Time and Circumstances.

Other Remedies.—*Acon.,* (Aesc.), (Agar.), (Alum.), Apis, (Arg. n.), Arn., *Ars.,* (Arum. t.), (Aur.), Bap., (Bar. c.), *Bell.,* (Bor.), **Bry.,** *Calc. c.,* Cannab. i., *Canth.,* Caps., (Caust.), (Chel.), Chin., (Cocc.), (Colch.), Coloc., Con., Graph., Ign., (Iris v.), K. bi., K. carb., Lach., **Lyc., Merc.,** Mez., *Nat. m.,* Nit. ac., **Nux v.,** Op., **Phos.,** Pho. ac., (Phyt.), PULS., (Ran. b.), Rhus, (Saba.), Sang., (Sec. c.), **Sep., Sil.,** *Spig.,* Stan., (Stram.), **Sul.,** *Verat. a.,* **Zinc.**

Bismuthum.

Mind.—Alum., Aur., Bell., Carb. an., *Fer.,* Glon., Graph., Ign., Plat., *Zinc.*

Localities.—*Acon.,* (Aesc.), Aloe, (Apoc. c.), Arg. n., Arn., *Ars.,* (Arum. t.), (Bap.), **Bell.,** Bry., Calc. c., Cannab. i., Cham., *Chin.,* (Cimic.), Cocc., (Dios.), (Eup. per.), (Fl. ac.), Gel., (Glon.), Hell., **Ign.,** (Iris v.), (K. bi.), (Lil. t.), (Lith.), *Lyc.,* (Meli.), *Merc.,* **Nux v.,** Phos., Pho. ac., (Pso.), **Puls.,** (Sang.), Sec. c., *Sep.,* Spo., Stan., *Sul.,* Verat. a., (Verat. v.)

Sensations.—Apis, Arg. n., Ars., (Arum. t.), (Bap.), BELL., (Berb.), *Bry.,* (Cact.), Calc. c., (Cannab. i.), *Caust.,* **Chin.,** (Cimic.), Colch., Dulc., Gel., (Glon.), (Iris v.), (K. bi.), K. carb., (Lith.), *Lyc.,* Merc., Nat. m., **Nux v.,** Oleand., *Puls., Rhus,* Sabi., Sang., Sep., Sil., Stan., Staph., Sul.

Glands.

Bones.—Arg., Cyc.

Skin.—Acon., Arn., Ars., *Bell.,* Bry., *Calc. c.,* Caps., Caust., K. carb., *Lach.,* **Led.,** *Lyc., Merc.,* Mez., Nux v., *Op.,* Phos., Plat., **Puls.,** *Rhus,* Sep., **Sil.,** Spo., *Staph.,* Sul.

Sleep and Dreams.—Ant. cr., Bry., **Calc. c.**, Cannab. s., Carb. an., Carb. v., Chin., Graph., Hep., *Ign.*, K. carb., Lach., *Lyc.*, Nat. c., **Nux v.**, Phos., *Puls.*, Rhus, Saba., **Sep.**, *Sil.*, Staph., Sul.

Blood, Circulation and Fever.—Acon., Arn., Ars., Bell., *Carb. v.* Cham., *Cocc.*, Hyos., *K. carb.*, Lyc., Merc., Nux v., Op., *Phos.*, Sep., Sil., Stan., Sul.

Aggravations: Time and Circumstances.—(Aloe), Alum, Ant. cr., (Apis), (Arg. n.), Asaf., Aur., *Bell.*, Canth., **CAPS.**, (Cimic.), **Con., Cyc.**, Dros., *Dulc., Euphorb., Fer.*, Ign., (K. bi.), K. nit., *Lyc., Mag. m.*, **Meny.**, Mos., Nit. ac., Pho. ac., *Plat.*, **PULS.**, Rhodo., *Rhus, Saba.*, Samb., (Sang.), Sele., **Sep.**, *Stro.*, Sil., Staph., *Stro. Tar., Thuj.*, Valer., Verb., Vio. t.

Other Remedies.—Acon., (Aloe), (Apis), Arg. n., **Arn., Ars.**, (Arum. t.), (Bap.), BELL., *Bry.*, **Calc. c.**, (Cannab. i.), *Caps.*, Carb. v., *Caust., Chin.*, (Cimic.), Cocc., Con., Cyc., Dulc., Fer., Gel., Glon., **Ign.**, (K. bi.), **K. carb.**, Lach., Led., (Lith.), *Lyc.*, Meny., *Merc.*, **Nux v.**, Op., *Phos.*, Plat., PULS., Rhus, Saba., Sang., SEP., **Sil.**, Stan., *Staph.*, **Sul.**

Antidotes.—*Calc. c.*, Caps., (Nux v.),

Borax.

Mind.—Bell., Calc. c., Glon., Lyc., Nat. m., *Nux v.*, Phos., Rhus, *Sep.*, Sul.

Localities.—(Aesc.), (All. c.), Aloe., Alum., Apis, (Apoc. c.), *Arg. n.*, Arn., Ars., Arum. t., Asaf., Aur., Bap., Bar. c., *Bell.*, (Berb.), *Bry.*, **CALC. C.**, Cannab. i., *Carb. v.*, *Caust., Cham., Chin.*, Dios., Dulc., (Fl. ac.), Gel., (Glon.), *Graph.*, Hep., Ign., *K. bi., K. carb.*, Lach., (Lil. t.), *Lyc.*, **Merc.**, Mez., *Nat. m.*, Nit. ac., **Nux v.**, *Petrol., Phos.*, (Phyt.), (Pic. ac.), Pb., Pod., Pso., **Puls.**, *Rhus*, Ruta, Sang., **Sep.**, *Sil., Spig., Staph., Sul.*, (Verat. v.).

Sensations.—Acon., (Aloe), (Apis), (Arg. n.), Arn., *Ars.*, Asaf., (Bap.), *Bell.*, (Berb.), *Bry.*, **CALC. C.**, (Cannab. i.), *Carb. v.*, Cham., Chin., (Cimic.), Gel., (Glon.), *Graph.*, Hell., Ign., (Iris v.), (K. bi.), K carb., (Lil. t.), *Lyc.*, **Merc.**, Nat. m., *Nux v.*, **Phos., Puls.**, Rhus, (Sang.), *Sep.*, Sil., Stan., Staph., **Sul.**, Zinc.

Glands.—*Bell.*, Bry., *Ign.*, Iod., Merc., Nux v., Phos., Puls., Sul.

Bones.

Skin.—Apis, Bar. c., Bry., *Calc. c.*, Cham., *Graph.*, *Hep.*, *Lyc.*, Merc., Nit. ac., Petrol., *Rhus, Sep.*, Sil., Squ., Staph., *Sul.*

Sleep and Dreams.—(Arg. n.), **Ars.**, Calc. c., Ign., **K. carb.**, Mur. ac., Nux v., Puls., *Ran. b.*, Sep., *Sil.*

Blood, Circulation and Fever.—Acon., (Apis), (Bap.), Bell., (Berb.), *Bry.*, *Calc. c.*, Cham., Glon., *Hep.*, (Lil. t.), Nat. m., *Nux v.* *Rhus*, (Sang.). *Verat. a.*

Aggravations: Time and Circumstances.—*Acon.*, (Aesc.), (Aloe), Am. carb., (Arg., n.), *Ars.*, (Bap.), Bell., *Bry.*, **Calc. c.**, Caps., Cocc., Fer., (Glon.), Graph., *Ign.*, Iod., (K. bi.), **K. carb.** *K. nit.*, LYC., *Mang.*, Merc., NUX V., Phos., Pho. ac., (Pod.), **Puls.**, Rhus, Saba., Sang., Sep., Sil., Spig., Stro., **Sul.**, Thuj., **Verat. a.**

Other Remedies.—Acon., (Aesc.), Aloe, Apis, Arg. n., *Ars.*, Bap., *Bell.*, (Berb.), **Bry.**, CALC. C., (Cannab. i.), Carb. v., Cham., Chin., Gel., Glon., *Graph.*, Hep., *Ign.*, K. bi., *K. carb.*, (Lil. t.), **Lyc.**, **Merc.**, Nat. m., NUX V., Petrol., *Phos.*, (Pod.), **Puls.**, Rhus, Sang., **Sep.**, Sil., Spig., Staph., **Sul.**, Verat. a.

Antidotes.— Cham., Coff.
Injurious.—*Acetum*, Vinum.

Bovista.

Mind.—Alum., Apis, Bell., Caj., Calad., *Calc. c.*, Cannab. i., Carb. ac., Carb. sul., Cic., Cocc., Gel., Glon., Hell., Hyd. ac., Hyos., *Ign.*, **Lyc.**, Meli., Merc., Nat. m., *Nux v*, *Op.*, **Puls.**, Rhus, Sep., Sil., *Sul.*, Ter., **Verat. a.**

Localities.—*Ant. cr.*, *Bell.*, Bry., *Calc. c.*, **Caust.**, K. bi., *Kre.*, Lach., Led., Nat. c., *Nat. m.*, Nux v., Phos., *Pho. ac.*, Plat., RHUS, SEP., Sil., Spig., **Staph.**, *Sul.*, Verat. a.

Sensations.—Acon., Am. m., Arn., Aur., *Bell.*, *Bry.*, *Calc. c.*, (Cannab. i.), *Caust.*, Chin., (Gel.), **K. carb.**, Laur., Lyc., Mag. m., *Nat. m.*, *Phos.*, Pb., Puls., *Rhus*, Sars., **Sep.**, Spig., **Stan.**, Staph., *Sul.*, Zinc.

Glands.—Phos., Sul.

Bones.—Agar., Am. m., *Cocc.*, *Hep.*, Phos., Puls., *Ruta*, Verat. a.

Skin.—Ars., Bar. c., Calc. c., *Carb. v.*, *Clem.*, Cup., *Dulc.*, **Graph.**, *Ip.*, K. carb., Kre., Lach., Led., Lyc., Mag. c., Merc., Petrol., Phos., Puls., Rhus, Sele., SEP., Sil., **Staph.**, Sul., *Verat. a.*

Sleep and Dreams.—K. carb., Sil.

Blood, Circulation and Fever.—Acon., (Arg. n.), Arn., Bell., *Bry.*, CALC. C., **Cham.**, (Glon.), Hep., Ign., *Lyc.*, *Merc.*, *Nat. m.*, Nux v., Rhus, *Sep.*, Sul., *Verat. a.*

Aggravations: Time and Circumstances.—(Aesc.), Ant. cr., Arn., (Bap.), CALC. C., Cannab. s., **Carb. v.**, **Chin.**, Con., Ign., Iod., (K. bi.), K. carb., (Lil. t.), Merc., *Nat. c.*, **Phos.**, Pho. ac., (Phyt.), (Pod.), **Puls.**, Rhus, Sep., Sil., Staph., Sul., (Verat. v.).

Other Remedies.—Acon., Ant. cr., Arn., *Bell.*, *Bry.*, CALC. C., (Cannab. i.), *Carb. v.*, *Caust.*, Cham., Chin., Cocc., (Gel.), (Glon.), **Graph.**, Hep., Ign., Iod., (K. bi.), *K. carb.*, Kre., *Lyc.*, Merc., Nat. c, *Nat. m.*, Nux v., **Phos.**, Pho. ac., **Puls.**, RHUS, SEP., *Sil.*, **Staph.**, **Sul.**, **Verat. a.**

Antidote.—Camph.

Bryonia.

Mind.—Aesc., *Aloe*, **Apis**, Arum. t., **Bap.**, BELL., Calc. c., *Cannab. i.*, Carb. ac., *Cimic.*, Crotal., **Gel.**, Glon., **Hyd. ac.**, *Hyos.*, Lyc., Meli., **Merc. c.**, Nat. m., *Nux v.*, Op., Pic. ac., Rhus, Sep., Stram., *Sul.*, Tab., Ter., Thea., *Verat. a.*, **Verat. v.**, *Zinc.*

Localities.—*Acon.*, AESC., All. c., ALOE, APIS, Apoc. c., ARG. N., Arn., **Ars.**, *Aur.*, Arum. t., **Bap.**, BELL., Berb., Bor., Cact., Calc. c., *Cannab. i.*, Canth., *Carb. ac.*, *Carb. v.*, (Caul.), *Caust.*, **Cham.**, *Chin.*, Cimic., Con., *Crotal.*, Dig., *Dios.*, Eup. per., (Fl. ac.), *Gel.*, Glon., Graph., Hep., *Hyos.*, *Ign.*, Iris v., K. BI., *K. carb.*, Kalm., Kre., Lil. t., Lith., *Lyc.*, Meli., MERC., Nat. c., *Nat m.*, Nit. ac., NUX V., Petrol., *Phos.*, Pho. ac., *Phyt.*, (Pic. ac.), Pb., POD., *Pso.*, **PULS.**, *Rhus*, Saba., SANG., SEP., Sil., *Spig.*, *Staph.*, **Sul.**, **Verat. a.**, *Verat. v.*, Zinc.

Sensations.—*Acon.*, *Aesc.*, (All. c.), *Aloe*, **Apis**, **Arg. n.**, Arn., Ars., Arum. t., Asaf., *Bap.*, BELL., **Berb.**, *Cact.*, **Calc. c.**, *Cannab. i.*, Canth., Carb. v., *Caust.*, Cham., *Chin*, Cimic., Con., (Crotal.), (Dios.), Eup. per., **Gel.**, *Glon.*, Graph., *Ign.*, *Iris v.*, **K. bi.**, K. carb., Kalm., *Lil. t.*, Lith., Lyc., (Meli.), **Merc.**, Mez., *Nat. m.*, Nit. ac., **Nux v.**, **Phos.**, *Phyt.*, Pod., *Pso.*, PULS., RHUS, **Sang.**, SEP., *Sil.*, *Spig.*, Stro., SUL., *Verat. v.*

Glands.—BELL., Calc. c., *Con.*, Lyc., *Merc.*, PHOS., *Puls.*, Rhus, Sul.

Bones.—*Arg.*, *Asaf.*, Bell., Calc. c., Chin., Cup., *Cyc.*, Ign., *Lyc.*, **Merc.**, Mez., *Nit. ac.*, *Phos.*, Pho. ac., *Puls.*, *Rhodo.*, **Rhus**, *Ruta*, Sabi., Sil., **Staph.**, SUL., Thuj.

Skin.—*Acon.*, Ant. cr., **Apis**, Arn., **Ars.**, Asaf., Bar. c., *Bell.*, Calc. c., (Carb. ac.), *Caust.*, Chin., Cic., (Cimic.), Con., (Crotal.), (Eup. per.), *Graph.*, *Hep.*, Ip., K. carb., Lach., Led., **Lyc.**, *Merc.*, Mez., Nat. m., Nux v., *Phos.*, PULS., Rhus, *Sep.*, **Sil.**, Spig., Spo., *Staph.*, **Sul.**, Vio. t.

Sleep and Dreams.—Acon., Ant. t., (Apis), Arg. n., Ars., (Bap.), Bell., *Calc.* c., Cannab. i., Caust., *Chin.*, Cic., **Con.**, Croc., (Gel.), Hep., **Ign.**, (Lil. t.), Lyc., Mag. c., Merc., Nat. c., Nux m., **Nux v.**, **Op.**, PHOS., *Pho. ac.*, (Pod.), PULS., Rhus, Saba., *Sep.*, *Sil.*, SUL.

Blood, Circulation and Fever.—Acon., (Aloe), (Apis), Arg. n., **Ars.**, (Bap.), *Bell.*, Berb., Cact., *Calc.* c., Cham., **Chin.**, (Crotal.), Chin., Dig., *Fer.*, (Gel.), *Glon.*, Graph., Hep., **Hyos.**, Iod., Ip., K. carb., (Lit.

t.), **Lyc.**, *Merc., Nat. m.,* NUX V., **Phos.**, Pho. ac., Pod., PULS., *Rhus, Sang.,* **Sep.**, Sil., Spig., Stram., SUL., Verat. a., (Verat. v.).

Aggravations: Time and Circumstances.—*Acon.,* Aesc., (All. c.), Aloe, *Apis, Arg. n.,* Arn., *Ars., Bap.,* **Bell.,** (Cact.), **Calc. c.,** (Cannab. i.), Caps., *Carb. v., Caust., Cham., Chin.,* Cimic., Cocc., Colch., Coloc., Con., Gel., Glon., *Hep.,* Hyos., Ign., Ip., *K. bi.,* K. carb., Lach., Led., *Lil. t.,* (Lith.), **Lyc.,** Nat. c., Nux v., Op., *Phos.,* Phyt., Pod., PULS., Rhus, Sabi., **Sang.,** Sep., *Sil.,* Spig., Stan., Stram., **Sul.,** Verat. a., *Verat. v.*

Other Remedies.—*Açon.,* **Aesc.,** (All. c.), **Aloe,** APIS, ARG. N., Arn., *Ars.,* Arum. t., Asaf., BAP., **Bell.,** *Berb., Cact.,* **Calc. c.,** Cannab. i., Canth., Carb. v., *Caust.,* Cham., Chin., **Cimic., Con.,** Crotal., GEL., Glon., Graph., Hep., Hyos., *Ign.,* Ip., **K. bi.,** K. carb., Lil. t., Lith., **Lyc., Merc.,** Mez., Nat. c., *Nat. m.,* Nit. ac., **Nux v.,** Op., **Phos.,** Pho. ac., *Phyt.,* Pod., PULS., Rhus, SANG., **Sep.,** *Sil.,* Spig., Staph., Stram., SUL., Verat. a., **Verat. v.**

Antidotes.—*Acon.,* Alum., *Camph., Cham.,* Clem., *Coff.,* Ign., Mur. ac., Nux v., Puls., *Rhus,* Seneg.

Cactus.

Mind.—*Acon.,* Arn., *Ars.,* Aur., Bap., Bar. c., *Bell., Cannab. i.,* Cina, Cocc., *Dig.,* Ign., Lil. t., **Lyc.,** Merc., Nit. ac., Puls., *Rhus t., Sec. c., Sep.,* Sil., Spo., Stan., *Stram., Sul., Sul. ac.,* **Verat. a.**

Localities.—Acon., Agar., (Aloe), (Ambr.), (Am. m.), Anac., Ant. t., (Apis), *Apoc. c.,* (Arg.), *Arg. n.,* Arn., *Ars.,* Aur., (Bap.), Bar. c., *Bell.,* (Bor.), (Bov.), *Bry.,* Calc. c., Cannab. i., (Canth.), (Caps.), Carb. v., Caust., Cham., (Chel.), *Chin.,* (Cic.), Cimic., (Cina), Cocc., Colch., Con., (Croc.), (Crotal.), Cup., Dig., Dros., (Dulc.), Fer., (Fl. ac.), Gel., (Glon.), (Graph.), (Guai.), (Hell.), Hep., (Hyd. ac.), (Hyos.), Ign., Ip., Iod., (K. bi.), K. carb., K. nit., Kalm., (Kre.), Lach., (Laur.), (Led.), Lyc., (Mang.), (Meli.), Merc., (Mez.), Mos., Nat. c., **Nat. m.,** Nit. ac., (Nux m.), *Nux v.,* (Op.), (Petrol.), *Phos.,* Pho. ac., (Phyt.), (Plat.), Pb., *Puls.,* (Ran. s.), (Rhodo.), Rhus, (Ruta), (Saba.), (Sabi.), (Samb.), (Sang.), (Sars.), Sec. c., (Seneg.), Sep., Sil., Spig., (Spo.), (Squ.), Stan., Stram., *Sul.,* (Sul. ac.), (Tar.), (Thuj.), (Valer.), Verat. a., Verat. v., (Verb.), (Vio. t.), Zinc.

Sensations.—*Acon.,* Aesc., (Agar.), (Alum.), (Anac.), Ant. t., Arg. n., Arn., Ars., (Asaf.), (Asar.), (Bap.), *Bell.,* (Bor.), *Bry.,* Calc. c., (Cannab. i.), Canth., (Cham.), Chel., Chin., Cocc., *Coloc.,* Con., (Croc.), (Crotal.), (Cup.), (Dig.), (Dros.), Fer., (Glon.), (Graph.), (Hyos.), Ign., Ip., Iod.,

(K. carb.), (Kre.), Lach., (Laur.), (Led.), (Lyc.), Merc., Nat. m., *Nit. ac.*, Nux v., Op., (Par.), *Phos.*, Pho. ac., Plat., Pb., *Puls.*, (Ran. b.), Rhus, (Saba.), (Sabi.), (Sec. c.), *Sep.*, Sil., Spig., (Spo.), (Squ.), (Stan.), (Stram.), *Sul.*, (Sul. ac.), (Thuj.), (Verat. a.), (Zinc).

Glands.

Bones.

Skin.

Blood, Circulation and Fever.—*Acon.*, Aloe, (Alum.), (Ant. t.), Apis, Arn., Ars., (Aur.), Bell., (Bor.), Bry., (Calc. c.), (Camph.), (Canth.), (Carb. v.), (Caust.), Chin., (Cina), (Con.), (Dig.), Fer., Glon., (Graph.), Hell., (Hep.), (Hyos.), Ip., (Lach.), (Lyc.), (Meny.), Merc., (Nat. c.), (Nat. m.), (Nit. ac.), Nux v., (Op.), (Petrol.), Phos., *Puls.*, (Ran. b.), Rhus, Sec. c., (Seneg.), Sep., Sil., (Spo.), Stram., *Sul.*, (Valer.), Verat. a. Vio. o.

Aggravations: Time and Circumstances.—(Acon.), (Agn.), (Alum.), (Anac.), (Ant. cr.), (Arg.), (Arn.), (Ars.), (Asar.), (Bar. c.), (Bry.), (Calc. c.), (Chel.), (Coff.), (Colch.), (Con.), (Croc.), (Hell.), (Ip.), (Mez.), (Nat. c.), (Nat. m.), (Nux v.), (Phos.), (Phyt.), Puls., (Rhus), (Saba.), (Sabi.), Sep., (Sil.), (Spig.), (Staph.), (Sul.), (Zinc.).

Other Remedies.—Acon., (Agar.), (Aloe), (Alum.), Anac., Ant. t., (Apis), (Apoc. c.), Arg. n., *Arn.*, **Ars.**, (Asar.), Aur., Bap., Bar, c., **Bell.**, *Bry.*, *Calc. c.*, Cannab i., Canth., (Carb. v.), (Caust.), (Cham.), Chel., *Chin.*, Cina, *Cocc.*, (Colch.), Con., (Croc.), (Crotal.), (Cup.), *Dig.*, (Dros.), Fer., (Glon.), (Graph.), Hell., (Hep.), (Hyos.), Ign., *Ip.*, Iod., (K. carb.), (Kalm.), (Kre.), Lach., (Laur.), (Led.), *Lyc.*, *Merc.*, (Mez.), Nat. c., *Nat. m.*, *Nit. ac.*, Nux v., Op., Pb., (Petrol.), *Phos.*, Pho. ac., (Phyt.), (Plat.), *Puls.*, (Ran. b.), (Ran. s.), *Rhus*, (Saba.), (Sabi.), Sec. c., (Seneg.), Sep., *Sil.*, Spig., Spo., (Squ.), Stan., *Stram.*, **Sul.**, Sul. ac., (Thuj.), (Valer.), *Verat. a.*, Zinc.

Caladium.

Mind.—*Cocc.*, *Ign.*, **Lyc.**, PULS., Sil., Verat. a.

Localities.—Acon., (Apis), (Arg. n.), Arn., *Ars.*, (Arum. t.), (Bap.), Bry., Calc. c., Carb. v., Cham., *Chin.*, *Cocc.*, Con., Dulc., Hell., Hyos., (K. bi.), Lyc., Mag. m., *Merc.*, Nat. c., *Nat. m.*, Nit. ac., **Nux v.**, Oleand., Op., Petrol., *Phos.*, PULS., Rhus, Saba., Sep., Sil., Spig., Staph., **Sul.**, *Verat. a.*

Sensations.—ACON., **Ars.**, Bar. c., **Bell.**, (Berb.), *Bry.*, Calc. c., (Cannab. i.), Canth., Carb. v., *Cham.*, Chel., Cocc., (Dios.), Guai., *Ign.*, (**K. bi.**), K. carb., K. nit., *Lyc.*, *Merc.*, Mez., Mur. ac., Nat. m, Nux m.,

NUX V., Par., *Phos.*, (Pod.), **Puls.**, *Rhus*, Saba., (Sang.), Sars., Seneg., Sep., Sil., Stan., Stram., **Sul.**, *Verat. a.*, (Verat. v.)

Glands.

Bones.

Skin.—Acon., Ant. t., Ars., *Bell.*, *Bry.*, Carb. v., CAUST., Con., Hep., Ign., K. carb., Lach., Led., Lyc., *Merc.*, **Mez.**, Nit. ac., Nux v., Phos., *Puls.*, Ran. b., Rhus, *Sep.*, Sil., Squ., Staph., Sul.

Sleep and Dreams.—Ars., **Bell.**, Bry., *Calc. c.*, Carb. v., Chin., Con., *Graph.*, Hep., Ign., K. carb., Led., *Lyc.*, Mar., Merc., Nux v., Phos., Puls., *Rhus*, Sele., *Sep.*, *Sil.*, *Sul.*

Blood, Circulation and Fever.—Ars., *Bry.*, (Cact.), *Calc. c.*, (Cannab. i.), Cham., *Merc.*, Mez., *Nux v.*, Phos., Puls., Rhus, Sep., Sul.

Aggravations: Time and Circumstances.—(Aesc.), Agar., Ant. t., Apis, Ars., Bap., *Bell.*, **Bry.**, *Calc. c.*, *Cannab. s.*, Carb. an., Carb. v., Caust., *Chin.*, (Cimic.), Cocc., Coff., Colch., Con., (Glon.), *Graph.*, Hep., *Iod.*, Ip., (K. bi.), K. carb., Lach., *Led.*, (Lil. t.), *Lyc.*, Merc., Nat. m., Nux v., PHOS., PULS., Ran. *s.*, Rhus, (Sang.), Sele, SEP., *Sil.*, Staph., Stro.

Other Remedies.—Acon., (Apis), *Ars.*, (Bap.), *Bell.*, **Bry.**, *Calc. c.*, (Cannab. i.), Carb. v., Caust., Cham., Chin., Cocc., Con., Graph., Hep., *Ign.*, (K. bi.), K. carb., Led., **Lyc.**, **Merc.**, Mez., Nat. m., Nux v., Phos., PULS., *Rhus*, (Sang.), Sep., *Sil.*, Staph., Sul., Verat. a.

Antidotes.—(Camph.), Caps.

Calcarea Carbonica.

Mind.—Aesc., **Aloe**, *Apis*, Arg. n., Ars. iod., *Bap.*, **Bell.**, Cact., Cannab. i., Carb. ac., Cimic., *Gel.*, Glon., Hyd. ac., Hyper., Lil. t., *Lyc.*, Meli., Merc. c., Nux v., *Op.*, Phyt., Pic. ac., Pso., Puls., Rhus, Sep., *Stram.*, Sul., Ther., Verat. a., Verat. v.

Localities.—Acon., *Aesc.*, All. c., *Aloe*, Am. carb., Anac., *Ant. cr.*, **Apis**, Apoc. c., ARG. N., Arn., *Ars.*, *Arum. t.*, *Aur.*, *Bap.*, Bar. c., BELL., Berb., *Bry.*, Cact., *Cannab. i.*, Canth., Caps., Carb. ac., Carb. an., *Carb. v.*, *Caust.*, Cham., *Chin.*, Cimic., Cina, Clem., Cocc., *Con.*, Croc., Crotal., Dios., Eup. per., Euphr., Fl. ac., *Gel.*, Glon., *Graph.*, Hep., (Hyd. ac.), *Hyos.*, *Ign.*, Ip., Iris v., K. BI., *K. carb.*, Kalm., *Kre.*, Lil. t., Lith., **Lyc.**, Mag. m., **Merc.**, Mez., *Nat. c.*, **Nat. m.**, *Nit. ac.*, Nux v., Oleand., Par., Petrol., **Phos.**, Phyt., *Pod.*, Pso., PULS., *Rhus*, *Ruta*, Saba., *Sang.*, Sec. c., **Sep.**, SIL., *Spig.*, Stan., **Staph.**, SUL., Sul. ac. Thuj., *Verat. a.*, *Verat. v.*, *Zinc.*

Sensations.—*Acon.*, (Aesc.), (Aloe.), Alum, Ant. cr., *Apis*, ARG N.,

Arn., *Ars.*, (Arum. t.), *Bap.*, BELL., *Berb.*, *Bry.*, (Cact.), *Cannab. i.*, Canth., Caps., Carb. v., *Caust.*, *Cham.*, *Chin.*, *Cimic.*, Cina, *Cocc.*, *Con.*, Crotal., *Cup.*, Dios., Eup. per., Fer., (Fl. ac.), Gel., *Glon.*, *Graph.*, Hyos., *Ign.*, Iod., Ip., Iris v., **K. bi.**, *K. carb.*, Lil. t., Lith., LYC., Merc., Mez., Nat. c., *Nat. m.*, *Nit. ac.*, **Nux v.**, Petrol., *Phos.*, *Phyt.*, Plat., Pb., (Pod.), **Puls.**, Rhodo., Rhus, Sang., Sec. c., SEP., **Sil.**, *Spig.*, Spo., Stan., Staph., *Stram.*, Stro., SUL., Verat. v., Zinc.

Glands.—Bell., *Bry.*, Clem., Con., Dulc., K. carb., Lyc., MERC., Nat. m., **Phos.**, *Puls.*, Rhodo., Sil., *Spo.*, Staph., SUL.

Bones.—Asaf., *Bell.*, (Eup. per.), Hep., *Lyc.*, **Merc.**, Mez., *Nit. ac.*, *Phos.*, Pho. ac., **Puls.**, *Sep.*, **Sil.**, Staph., Sul.

Skin.—Ant. cr., *Apis*, Arn., Ars., Asaf., Bar. c., *Bell.*, *Bry.*, Carb. v., Caust., Chin., (Cimic.), Clem., *Con.*, *Dulc.*, (Eup. per.), *Graph.*, Hep., Lach., Led., **Lyc.**, Merc., Mez., Nat. c., Nat. m., *Nit. ac.*, Petrol., *Phos.*, Pho. ac., **Puls.**, Rhus, (Sang.), SEP., SIL., *Staph.*, SUL., Verat. a., Vio. t.

Sleep and Dreams.—(Apis), Arg. n., Ars., (Bap.), *Bell.*, *Bry.*, (Cannab. i.), Carb. v., Caust., Chin., *Con.*, *Graph.*, Ign., K. carb., (Lil. t.), *Merc.*, **Nat. c.**, NUX V., **Phos.**, Pho. ac., (Pod.), PULS., Rhus, SEP., Sil., Sul.

Blood, Circulation and Fever.—Acon., (Aloe), Anac., (Apis), Arg. n., *Ars.*, *Bell.*, (Berb.), **Bry.**, Cact., (Cannab. i.), *Cham.*, Chin., Fer., Glon., Hep., Ign., K. carb., Lyc., **Merc.**, *Nat. m.*, Nit. ac., **Nux v.**, Phos., (Pod.), *Puls.*, Rhus, Sang., *Sele.*, SEP., Spig., SUL., *Verat. a.*, (Verat. v.).

Aggravations : Time and Circumstances.—Aesc., (All. c.), (Aloe), Am. carb., Anac., Arg. n., Ars., Aur., Bap., Bell., *Bry.*, (Cact.), Caps., Carb. v., Caust., Cham., *Chin.*, Cimic., *Con.*, Croc., (Gel.), (Glon.), Graph., *Ign.*, Iod., *K. bi.*, *K. carb.*, K. nit., (Lil. t.), **Lyc.**, Merc., *Nat. c.*, *Nat. m.*, Nux m., *Nux v.*, *Phos.*, Pho. ac., Phyt., Plat., Pod., **Puls.**, *Rhus*, Saba., Sang., Sele., SEP., *Sil.*, *Spig.*, Squ., Stan., Staph., **Sul.**, Verat. v.

Other Remedies.—Acon., *Aesc.*, **Aloe**, Anac., Ant. cr., Apis, ARG. N., Arn., *Ars.*, Arum. t., Asaf., Aur., **Bap.**, Bell., Berb., *Bry.*, *Cact.*, **Cannab. i.**, Caps., Carb. v., Caust., Cham., *Chin.*, *Cimic.*, Clem., Cocc., *Con.*, Croc., Crotal., Dulc., **Gel.**, Glon., *Graph.*, Hep., Hyos., *Ign.*, *K. bi.*, *K. carb.*, *Lil. t.*, Lith., **Lyc.**, Merc., Mez., *Nat. c.*, *Nat. m.*, *Nit. ac.*, **Nux v.**, Petrol., **Phos.**, Pho. ac., *Phyt.*, *Pod.*, PULS., Rhus, **Sang.**, Sele., SEP., **Sil.**, Spig., Spo., Stan., *Staph.*, Stram., SUL., Verat. a., **Verat. v.**, Zinc.

Antidotes.—Bry., Camph., Chin., **Nit. ac.**, *Nux v.*, Sul., Spir. nit. dulc.

Camphora.

Mind.—Ail., **Apis**, Ars., Aur., *Bap.*, BELL., *Cannab. i.*, Con., *Crotal.*, Cup., *Gel.*, *Glon.*, **Hyd. ac.**, **Hyos.**, Lyc., *Meli.*, Merc. c., **Nat. m.**, Op., Petrol., Puls., *Rhus*, *Stram.*, *Verat. a.*, *Verat. v.*

Localities.—Acon., Aesc., All. c., (Aloe), Alum., Anac., (Apis), (Apoc. c.), Arg. n., **Ars.**, (Arum t.), BELL., Bry., (Cact.), (Cannab. i.), (Carb. ac.), *Cham.*, Chin., *Cic.*, Con., Cup., (Gel.), Hep., (Hyd. ac.), *Hyos.*, **Ign.**, K. bi., *K. carb.*, (Kalm.), (Lil. t.), Lyc., Merc., Nux v., Op., (Pod.), *Puls.*, Rhus, Sep., Staph., Stram., *Sul.*, **Verat. a.**

Sensations.—Acon., (Aesc.), Arg. n., Arn., Ars., BELL., Bry., (Cact.), *Calc. c.*, Caust., Cham., *Chin.*, Cic., (Cimic.), COCC., Con., *Cup.*, Gel., (Glon.), *Hyos.*, **Ign.**, Ip., Laur., (Lil. t.), *Lyc.*, Merc., Mos., Nux m., Nux v., Op., Phos., (Phyt.), Plat., (Pod.), *Puls.*, Rhus, (Sang.), Sec. c., Sep., Sil., Stan., *Stram.*, **Sul.**, Thuj., **Verat. a.**, (Verat. v.).

Glands.—Bar. c., *Bell.*, Bry., Carb. an., Clem., Con., Graph., Lyc., Merc., Nux v., Phos., Puls., Sil., Sul.

Bones.

Skin.—Acon., (Apis), Arn., *Ars.*, Bell., Bry., Calc. c., Dulc., Hep., Lyc., *Merc.*, Nit. ac., Nux v., Phos., Pho. ac., *Puls.*, **Rhus**, Sec. c., Sep., *Sil.*, **Sul.**, Verat. a.

Sleep and Dreams.—Ant. t., (Apis), Bry., (Cannab. i.), Con., **Croc.**, Cup., Nux m., **Op.**, Pho. ac., (Pod.), Puls., *Verat. a.*

Blood, Circulation and Fever.—*Acon.*, (Aloe), Apis, ARS., **Bell.**, (Cact.), Calc. c., Cannab. i., Chin., *Con.*, (Gel.), Hell., K. nit., Laur., Merc., Nux m., **Nux v.**, Phos., Pho. ac., Pod., *Puls.*, *Rhus*, **Saba.**, *Samb.*, Sep., Spig., Sul., **Verat. a.**

Aggravations: Time and Circumstances.—Acon., (Aesc.), Agar., (Apis.), *Arn.*, **Ars.**, *Aur.*, *Bell.*, **Bry.**, Carb. an., Carb. v., **Caust.**, Chel., *Cocc.*, Coff., *Colch.*, *Con.*, Dig., *Dulc.*, (Glon.), Graph., *Hell.*, HEP., Hyos., **K. carb.**, Led., (Lil. t.), Lyc., Merc., *Mos.*, *Nux m.*, NUX V., *Phos.*, (Phyt.), Puls., Ran. b., Rheum, RHUS, **Saba.**, Sele., Sep., Sil., Spig., Squ., Staph., Stram., **Sto.**

Other Remedies.—*Acon.*, Aesc., (Aloe), Ant. t., Apis, Arg. n., Arn., ARS., Aur., BELL., *Bry.*, (Cact.), Calc. c., *Cannab. i.*, Caust., Cham., Chin., Cic., *Cocc.*, **Con.**, Croc., *Cup.*, Dulc., *Gel.*, Glon., Hell., *Hep.*, Hyos., *Ign.*, Ip., *K. carb.*, (Lil. t.), **Lyc.**, **Merc.**, Mos., Nat. m., *Nux m.*, Nux v., Op., *Phos.*, Pho. ac., (Phyt.), Pod., **Puls.**, **Rhus**, *Saba.*, Sec. c., **Sep.**, **Sil.**, *Stram.*, Stro., **Sul.**, VERAT. A., Verat. v.

Antidotes.—Op., Spir. nit. dul.
Injurious.—(K. nit.).

Cannabis Indica.

Mind.—Acon., Ambr., Anac., Ant. t., *Apis*, Arn., *Ars., Aur., Bap.,* Bar. c., BELL., *Bry.,* Cact., Camph., Canth., Caust., *Cic., Cocc., Coff., Con., Croc.,* Crotal., Cup., Dig., Gels., *Glon.,* Hell., *Hyd. ac.,* **Hyos.**, Ign., *Lach.*, Lil. t., **Lyc.**, Meli., *Merc.,* Mur. ac., Nat. c., *Nat. m.,* **Nit. ac.**, *Nux m., Nux v.,* OP., *Petrol.,* **Phos.**, *Pho. ac.,* Plat., Pb., *Puls.,* Pso., Rhus t., Sec. c., *Sep.,* Sil., Spig., STRAM., **Sul.,** Sul. ac., Valer., **Verat. a.**, *Verat. v.*, Viola o., Zinc.

Localities.—Acon., (Aesc.), *Agar.,* (Agn.), (All. c.), (Aloe), (Alum.), (Ambr.), (Am. carb.), Am. m., (Anac.), *Ant. t.,* Apis, (Apoc. c.), *Arg.* Arg. n., *Arn.,* **Ars.**, (Arum. t.) Aur., BELL., (Berb.), Bism., Bor., *Bry.,* Cact., *Calc. c.,* Camph., Cannab. s., *Canth.,* Caps., (Carb. ac.), Carb. v., *Caust.,* Cham., Chel., *Chin.,* (Cic.), (Cimic.), Cina, Clem., Cocc., (Coff.), Colch., Coloc., *Con.,* (Croc.), (Crotal.), Cup., Dig., Dros., (Dulc.), (Eup. per.), (Euphr.), Fer., (Fl. ac.), Gel., (Glon.), Graph., (Guai.), (Hell.), Hep., (Hyd. ac.), Hyos., *Ign.,* (Ip.), Iod., K. bi., K. carb., K. nit., (Kalm.), (Kre.), Lach., (Laur.), (Led.), (Lil. t.), *Lyc.,* Meli., (Meny.), **Merc.**, (Mez.), (Mos.), (Mur. ac.), Nat. c., *Nat. m.,* Nit. ac., (Nux m.), **Nux v.**, (Oleand.), Op., Petrol., **Phos.**, *Pho. ac.,* (Pic. ac.), (Plat.), *Pb.,* **Puls.**, (Rhodo.), *Rhus,* (Ruta), Saba., Sabi., Samb., (Sang.), Sars., Sec. c., Sele., (Seneg.), **Sep.**, *Sil., Spig.,* Spo., *Squ.,* Stan., Staph., *Stram.,* **Sul.**, (Tar.), *Thuj.,* (Valer.), *Verat. a.,* (Verat. v.), Verb., (Vio. o.), (Vio. t.), Zinc.

Sensations.—Acon., Agar., Aloe, Alum., (Am. m.), (Ant. t.), (Apis), *Arg. n.,* Arn., *Ars.,* (Arum. t.), Asaf., (Aur.), Bar. c., **Bell.**, Berb., (Bism.), Bor., **Bry.**, (Calad.), *Calc. c.,* Canth., (Caps.), (Carb. v.), (Caust.), Chel., Chin., Cic., (Cimic.), (Clem.), *Cocc.,* (Colch.), *Coloc., Cm.,* Cup., (Dig.), (Dros.), Fer., Gel., Glon., Graph., (Hell.), (Hyos.), Ign., K. bi., (K. carb.), *Lach.,* Laur., (Lit. t.), (Lith.), Lyc., (Mag. c.), Meny., *Merc.,* Mez., (Mur. ac.), (Nat. c.), *Nat. m., Nit. ac.,* Nux m., **Nux v.**, (Oleand.), Op., (Par.), Petrol., **Phos.**, Pho. ac., (Phyt.), *Pb.,* (Pso.), **Puls.**, Ran. b., (Rhodo.), Rhus, *Saba.,* Sabi., *Sang.,* (Sars.), Sec. c., *Seneg.,* **Sep.**, *Sil., Spig.,* Spo., Squ., *Stan.,* (Staph.), Stram., **Sul.**, (Tar.), *Thuj.,* (Valer.), Verat. a., (Verat. v.), **Zinc.**

Glands.
Bones.
Skin.

Sleep and Dreams.—Acon., (Aloe), (Anac.), Ant. cr., *Ant. t.*, Apis, Arg. n., (Arn.), Ars., (Asaf.), (Bell.), Bry., Calc. c., (Camph.), Carb. v., Caust., (Chel.), (Chin.), Con., (Croc.), (Cup.), (Cyc.), (Fl. ac.), (Hyos.) *Ign*, (K. carb.), Laur., (Led.), Mag. c., (Merc.), (Mos.), Nat. c., Nat. m., *Nux m.*, **Nux v.**, Op., **Phos.**, *Pho. ac.*, Pod., **Puls.**, (Rhodo.), Rhus, Saba., (Samb.), (Sec. c.), (Seneg.), Sep., *Sil.*, (Staph.), (Stram.), Sul., (Sul. ac.), Thuj., Verat. a. (Vio. t.).

Blood, Circulation and Fever.—Acon., (Agar.), (Ant. t.), *Ars*, (Bell.), (Calad.), (Calc. c.), Camph., (Canth.), (Caps.), (Caust.), (Cham.), (Chel.), (Chin.), (Con.), (Cup.), Dig., (Gel.), Hell., (Ip.), (Iod.), (K. nit.), (Kalm.), (Lach.), (Laur.), (Led.), Lyc., (Meny.), Merc., (Nat. c.), (Nit. ac.), (Nux m.), (Nux v.), Op., (Petrol.), Phos., (Pho. ac.), (Pb.), Puls., (Ran. b.), (Ran. s.), Rhus, (Sang.), Sec. c., (Sele.), Sep., Sil., (Spig.), Stram., Sul., (Thuj.), Verat. a., (Verat. v.).

Aggravations: Time and Circumstances.—(Acon.), (Arn.), (Ars.), (Bell.), (Bry.), (Cham.), (Chel.), (Con.), (Ign.), (Lyc.), (Mur. ac.), (Nat. m.), Op., (Phos.), Puls., Rhus, Sil., (Stram.), Sul., (Zinc).

Other Remedies.—ACON., Agar., Aloe, (Alum.), (Ambr.), (Am. m.), Anac., *Ant. t.*, *Apis*, Arg. n., *Arn.*, **Ars.**, (Asaf.), Aur., Bar. c., BELL., Berb., (Bism.), Bor., **Bry.**, Cact., (Calad.), *Calc. c.*, *Camph.*, Canth., (Caps.), (Carb. v.), Caust., (Cham.), *Chel.*, *Chin.*, Cic., (Cimic.), (Clem.), *Cocc.*, Coff., Colch., Coloc., **Con.**, Croc., (Crotal.), *Cup.*, *Dig.*, (Dros.), Fer., (Fl. ac.), *Gel.*, Glon., Graph., Hell., Hyd. ac., *Hyos.*, **Ign.**, (Ip.), (Iod.), K. bi., K. carb., (K. nit.), *Lach.*, Laur., (Led.), Lil. t., **Lyc.**, (Mag. c.), Meli., Meny., **Merc.**, (Mez.), (Mos.), Mur. ac., *Nat. c.*, **Nat. m.**, *Nit. ac.*, *Nux m.*, NUX V., OP., *Petrol.*, **Phos.**, Pho. ac., (Plat.), *Pb.*, (Pso.), PULS., (Ran. b.), (Rhodo.), RHUS, *Saba.*, Sabi., (Samb.), Sang., (Sars), *Sec. c.*, (Sele.), Seneg., **Sep.**, **Sil.**, *Spig.*, Spo., Squ., Stan., **Staph.**, **Stram.**, SUL., (Sul. ac.), (Tar.), *Thuj.*, **Verat. a.**, Verat. v., (Vio. o.), (Vio. t.), *Zinc*.

Cannabis Sativa.

Mind.—Acon., Aur., **Bell.**, Calc. c., Chel., *Cocc.*, *Con.*, Gel., Glon. Hyos., *Ign.*, LYC., Merc., *Nat. c.*, Nux v., OP., *Phos.*, **Pho. ac.**, *Plat.* **Puls.**, *Rhus*, Sep., *Sil.*, STRAM., Sul., **Verat. a.**

Localities.—(Aloe), Ant. t., Apis, (Apoc. c.), Arg. n., Arn., (Arum. t.), *Bell.*, Berb., Bry., (Cact.), *Calc. c.*, Cannab. i., **Caust.**, Chin., (Cimic.), *Con.*, (Crotal.), Dulc., Euphr., (Fl. ac.), **Hep.**, *Ign.*, K. bi., K. carb., Lil. t., (Lith.), Lyc., *Merc.*, *Nux v.*, **Phos.**, (Phyt.), PULS., Rhus, Ruta, Sep., Sil., Staph., **Sul.**, Sul. ac., Verat. a, (Verat. v.), Zinc.

Sensations.—*Acon.*, Anac., (Arg. n.), Arn., *Ars.*, BELL., *Bry.*, **Calc. c.**, Cannab. i., Canth., Caust., Cham., Chin., *Cocc.*, Con., Dulc., Gel. Glon., Graph., Hyos., *Ign.*, Ip., Laur., Lyc., *Merc.*, Nux m., NUX V., Phos., *Plat.*, *Puls.*, *Rhus*, (Sang.), *Sep.*, Sil., Spig., Spo., Stan. *Sul.*, Sul. ac., **Verat. a.**

Glands.—Bell., Phos.

Bones.—*Cocc.*, Hep., Puls., *Ruta.*

Skin.—Acon., Arn., *Ars.*, Bell., *Bry.*, Calc. c., Carb. an., *Caust.*, Chin., Cocc., Graph., K. carb., Kre., *Lyc.*, Merc., Mez., Nit. ac., Nux v., *Phos.*, Plat., *Puls.*, Rhus, Saba., Sec. c., Sep., Sil., Staph., *Sul.*, Verat. a.

Sleep and Dreams.—Bism., Chin., Hep., *Nat. c.*, Nux v., Saba., Sep., Sil.

Blood, Circulation and Fever.—*Acon.*, Ars., Bry., Merc., **Puls.**, Rhus, Sul. VERAT. A.

Aggravations: Time and Circumstances.—Acon., Aesc., Agar., Ant. t., Apis, **Arn.**, *Ars.*, (Bap.), *Bell.*, Bry., Calad., Caps., Carb. v., Caust., *Cham.*, Chin., (Cimic.), *Cocc.*, Colch., Con., Fer., (Glon.), *Hep.*, *Ign.*, Iod., (K. bi.), K. carb., Led., (Lil. t.), **Lyc.**, *Mang.*, Merc., Nat. c., **Nat. m.**, Nit. ac., **Nux v.**, Oleand., *Phos.*, Pho. ac., (Phyt.), (Pod.), PULS., *Ran. b.*, RHUS, Saba., Sang., Sele., *Sep.*, *Sil.*, *Spig.*, Stan., Staph., Sul., Sul. ac., Vio. t.

Other Remedies.—*Acon.*, (Aesc.), Ant. t., Apis, (Arg. n.), *Arn.*, *Ars.*, **Bell.**, Bry., *Calc. c.*, Cannab. i., Carb. v., *Caust.*, Cham., *Chin.*, (Cimic.), **Cocc.**, Colch., *Con.*, Dulc., Fer., Gel., Glon., Graph., *Hep.*, Hyos., *Ign.*, Iod., (K. bi.), K. carb., Led., (Lil. t.), **Lyc.**, Mang., **Merc.**, Mez., Nat. c., Nat. m., Nit. ac., **Nux v.**, Op., **Phos.**, Pho. ac., (Phyt.), *Plat.*, PULS., Ran. b., Rhus, Ruta, Saba., (Sang.), Sep., Sil., Spig., Stan., Staph., Stram., Sul., Sul. ac., **Verat. a.**

Antidote.—Camph.

Cantharis.

Mind.—*Apis*, Arum. t., Aur., Bap., *Bell.*, Cic., *Cimic.*, Crotal., Cup., Gel., *Glon.*, Hyos., Ign., Lach., **Lyc.**, Merc. c., Op., Phos., *Plat.*, Puls., Sil., **Stram.**, Sul., *Verat. a.*, Verat. v.

Localities.—Acon., *Aesc.*, All. c., *Aloe*, Alum, Ambr., Ant. cr., **Apis**, Apoc. c., *Arg. n.*, *Arn.*, Ars., Arum. t., Aur., *Bap*, Bar. c., BELL., Berb., *Bry.*, (Cact.), **Calc. c.**, Cannab. i., Caps., Carb. ac., *Carb. v.*, *Caust*, *Cham.*, *Chin.*, (Cimic.), Cocc., Colch., Con., Crotal., (Dios.), (Eup. per.), (Fl. ac.), Gel., (Glon.), Graph., *Hep.*, Hyos., *Ign.*, Ip., Iris v., **K. bi.**, K. carb., Kalm., Lach., Laur., *Lil. t.*, Lith., **Lyc.**, Meli., **Merc.**, Mez., Nat. c.,

RELATIONSHIPS.—CANTH.

Nat. m., *Nit. ac.*, **Nux** v., Op., *Phos.*, Pho. ac., Phyt., (Pic. ac.), *Pb.*, Pod., (Pso.), PULS., Ran. b., *Rhus, Saba.*, Sabi., Sang., Sars., SEP., **Sil.**, *Staph.*, Stram., SUL., Thuj., **Verat. a.**, Verat. v., *Zinc.*

Sensations.—*Acon.*, (Aesc.), (Aloe), Alum., **Apis**, *Arg. n.*, *Arn.*, Ars., *Arum. t.*, Asar., Bap., BELL., *Berb.*, *Bry.*, (Cact.), *Calc. c.*, Cannab. i., Carb. v., *Cham.*, **Chin.**, (Cimic.), Cocc., Con., (Crotal.), Cup., (Dios.), Dros., Fer., (Gel.), (Glon.), Hell., Hyos., *Ign.*, Ip., (Iris v.), *K. bi.*, *K. carb.*, Laur., Lil. t., (Lith.), *Lyc.*, *Merc.*, Mos., Nat. c., Nit. ac., **Nux v.**, **Phos.**, Pho. ac., Phyt., Plat., (Pod.), Pb., PULS., *Rhus*, Ruta, Saba., Sabi., *Sang.*, Sars., **Sep.**, Sil., Spig., Stan., Staph., **Sul.**, *Verat. a.*, Verat. v., Zinc.

Glands.—Acon., Arn., (Arum. t.), BELL., Bry., Con., *Merc.*, **Phos.**, Puls., Rhus, *Sil.*, *Sul.*

Bones.—*Arg.*, Aur., *Bell.*, Calc. c., Caust., *Chin.*, Cocc., Con., *Cup.*, Cyc., Dros., K. carb., Lyc., *Merc.*, Phos., Pho. ac., Puls., Rhodo., Rhus, Ruta, *Sabi.*, Sep., *Staph.*

Skin.—Acon., Am. m., Arn., *Ars.*, *Bell.*, **Bry.**, Calc. c., Carb. v., *Caust.* Chin., (Crotal.), Cyc., Graph., Hep., K. carb., Lach., Led., *Lyc.*, *Merc.*, Mez., Nit. ac., Nux v., Oleand., *Phos.*, Pho. ac., **Puls.**, Rhus, *Sep.*, Sil., Spo., *Staph.*, SUL., Thuj., Vio. t.

Sleep and Dreams.—(Arg. n.), Lach., Nat. c., *Nux v.*, Phos., Sep. Sil., Staph.

Blood, Circulation and Fever.—*Acon.*, (Aloe), Arn., **Ars.**, BELL., (Berb.), **Bry.**, (Cact.), *Calc. c.*, Camph., Cannab. i., *Cham.*, Chin., (Gel.), Hell., *Hep.*, Laur., Lyc., *Merc.*, Nit. ac., Nux m., **Nux v.**, **Phos.**, Pho. ac., Pod., Puls., *Rhus*, Saba., Sang., SEP., Sil., Spig., *Sul.*, *Verat. a.*, (Verat. v.).

Aggravations: Time and Circumstances.—(Aesc.), Alum., Ant. cr., Apis, Arn., **Bell.**, **Bry.**, **Calc. c.**, *Carb. v.*, *Caust.*, *Cham.*, Clem., Cocc., Colch., *Con.*, Graph., **Hep.**, *Ign.*, Iod., (K. bi.), K. carb., Lach., (Lil. t.), **Lyc.**, MERC., Nat. c., **Nux v.**, **Phos.**, (Phyt.), **Puls.**, **Rhus**, (Sang.), *Sep.*, *Sil.*, *Spig.*, Squ., *Staph.*, *Stro.*, **Sul.**, *Thuj.*

Other Remedies.—*Acon.*, Aesc., Aloe, Alum., **Apis**, *Arg. n.*, *Arn.*, Ars., *Arum. t.*, Aur., *Bap.*, BELL., Berb., **Bry.**, (Cact.), **Calc. c.**, Cannab. i., Carb. v., Caust., *Cham.*, *Chin.*, Cimic., Cocc., Con., Crotal., Cup., Gel., Glon., Graph., *Hep.*, Hyos., *Ign.*, *K. bi.*, K. carb., Lach., Laur., Lil. t., (Lith.), **Lyc.**, **Merc.**, Nat. c., Nit. ac., **Nux. v.**, PHOS., Pho. ac., Phyt., Plat., *Pod.*, **Puls.**, Rhus, Saba., Sabi., *Sang.*, **Sep.**, **Sil.**, Spig., Staph., Stram., SUL., Thuj., *Verat. a.*, *Verat. v.*, Zinc.

Antidotes.—Acon., *Camph.*, Laur., *Puls.*
Injurious.—Coff.

Capsicum.

Mind.—*Anac.*, Ars., Aur., **Bell.**, Calc. c., Caust., Cham., Cocc., Con., Croc., *Hyos.*, *Ign.*, LYC., Merc., *Nat. c.*, **Nat. m.**, *Op.*, Phos., *Pho. ac.*, Puls., Sep., Sil., Staph., *Stram.*, Sul., Sul. ac.

Localities.—Acon., Aesc., (All. c.), Aloe, Apis, Apoc. c., *Arg. n.*, *Ars.*, (Arum. t.), Bap., **Bell.**, Berb., *Bry.*, (Cact.), *Calc. c.*, Cannab. i., *Canth.*, Caust., *Cham.*, (Cimic.), (Crotal.), Dios., (Eup. per.), (Fl. ac.), Hep., Hyos., Ign., (Iris v.), *K. bi.*, K. carb., Lil. t., *Lyc.*, (Meli.), **Merc.**, Mez., Nat. c., NUX V., Op., Phos., Pho. ac., (Phyt.), *Pod.*, (Pso.), PULS., *Rhus*, Sang., *Sep.*, Sil., *Staph.*, **Sul.**, Verat. a., Verat. v.

Sensations.—*Acon.*, Arg. n., Ars., (Arum. t.), BELL., Berb., **Bry.**, (Cact.), **Calc. c.**, (Cannab. i.), Caust., *Cham.*, Chin., (Cimic.), *Cocc.*, Con., Croc., (Gel.), *Glon.*, Hyos., Ign., (Iris v.), (K. bi.), K. carb., *Laur.*, *Lyc.*, *Merc.*, **Nux v.**, Oleand., **Phos.**, (Phyt.), **PULS.**, **Rhus**, Saba., Sang.), *Sep.*, *Sil.*, Spig., **Sul.**, Verat. a.

Glands.—Bell., Bry., Calc. c., *Clem.*, Con., Lyc., Puls., Rhus, *Sul.*

Bones.—Asaf., Aur., Calc. c., Chin., Con., (Eup. per.), Hep., *Lyc.*, Merc., Mez., Phos., *Pho. ac.*, Puls., *Ruta*, Sep., *Sil.*, Staph., Sul.

Skin.—Acon., Ars., Asaf., Bell., *Bry.*, *Calc. c.*, Caust., Chin., Cocc., Lach., Lyc., **Merc.**, Mez., Oleand., Phos., PULS., Rhus, Sep., SIL., *Spig.*, Staph., *Sul.*

Sleep and Dreams.—(Arg. n.), **Ars.**, Aur., *Coff.*, Hep., **K. carb.**, Nat. c., *Nux v.*, Sep., **Sil.**

Blood, Circulation and Fever.—*Acon.*, Apis, *Ars.*, (Berb.), **Bry.**, *Calc. c.*, (Cannab. i.), **Cham.**, *Chin.*, (Gel.), (Glon.), *Hep.*, **Ign.**, Lach., Lyc., Merc., Nat. m., **Nux v.**, Op., Phos., Puls., **Rhus**, Saba., Samb., Sang., *Sep.*, Spig., Sul., *Verat. a.*

Aggravations: Time and Circumstances.—*Acon.*, (Aesc.), (All. c.), (Aloe), Ant. cr., Ant. t., Apis., (Arg. n.), Arn., *Ars.*, Aur., Bap., Bar. c., *Bell.*, Bor., **Bry.**, *Calc. c.*, Cannab. s., Canth., *Carb. v.*, *Caust.*, *Cham.*, Chin., (Cimic.), Cina., Cocc., **Con.**, Cyc., Dros., Dulc., *Euphorb.*, (Glon.), *Fer.*, **Hep.**, *Ign.*, *K. bi.*, K. carb., K. nit., Lach., Led., Lil., t., **Lyc.**, *Mag. c.*, Mag. m., Mang., Meny., Merc., Mos., Nat. m., *Nux v.*, Phos., Pho. ac., (Phyt.), Plat., (Pod.), PULS., Ran. s., Rhodo., **Rhus**, Ruta, *Saba.*, *Samb.*, *Sang.*, Sele., **Sep.**, *Sil.*, *Spig.*, Staph., Stro., *Sul.*, Sul. ac., Tar., Thuj., *Valer.*, Verat. a., (Verat. v.), Verb.

Other Remedies.—*Acon.*, (Aesc.), (All. c.), (Aloe), Apis, *Arg. n.*,

Ars., (Arum. t.), Asaf., Aur., Bap., **Bell.**, Berb., **Bry.**, (Cact.), **Calc. c.**, Cannab. i., Caust., *Cham.*, (Cimic.), Cocc., Con., (Gel.), Glon., *Hep.*, Hyos., *Ign.*, *K. bi.*, K. carb., Lil. t., **LYC.**, **Merc.**, Nat. c., Nat. m., **Nux v.**, Op., *Phos.*, Pho. ac., (Phyt.), Pod., **PULS.**, **Rhus**, Saba., Samb., *Sang.*, **Sep.**, **Sil.**, Spig., Staph., **Sul.**, Verat. a., (Verat. v.).

Antidotes.—Calad., Camph., Chin., *Cina.*

Carbo Animalis.

Mind.—Alum., Aur., Bell., Coff., Croc., *Fer.*, Graph., **Ign.**, *Lach.*, Mez., *Mos.*, Naj., **Nat. c.**, *Op.*, Petrol., *Phos.*, *Plat.*, Seneg., Sep., Sil., Spig., Stram., Sul., Sul. ac., Thuj., Vert. a., **Zinc.**

Localities.—Aesc., Aloe, *Alum*, Am. carb., Ant. cr., (Apis), Arg. n., Aur., (Bap.), Bar. c., Bell., (Berb.), Bry., (Cact.), **Calc. c.**, (Cannab. i.), (Carb. ac.), CARB. V., **Caust.**, Chel., Chin., (Cimic.), Con., Cyc., (Dios.), (Gel.), *Graph.*, *Ign.*, (K. bi.), *K. carb.*, Lil. t., *Lyc.*, Mag. m., **Merc.**, Nat. c., *Nat. m.*, Nit. ac., **Nux v.**, Op., *Petrol.*, *Phos.*, Pod., Pb., *Puls.*, Rhus, Ruta, Saba., Sang., **SEP.**, **Sil.**, Staph., **Sul.**, Sul. ac., Thuj. Verat. a., Verb.

Sensations.—(Aloe), Am. carb, Ars., Asaf., Bar. c., **Bell.**, Bry., *Calc. c.*, *Carb. v.*, Caust., Cham., Chin., Cocc., Coloc., (Gel.), **GRAPH.**, Hep., *Ign.*, **K. carb.**, (Lil. t.), **Lyc.**, Mag. m., *Merc.*, Mur. ac., Nat. c., *Nat. m.*, Nit. ac., **Nux v.**, Oleand., Op., Petrol., *Phos.*, Plat., Puls., Rhus, Ruta, *Sabi.*, (Sang.), **Sep.**, *Sil.*, Stan., *Staph.*, Stro., **Sul.**, Thuj., Zinc.

Glands.—*Arn.*, (Arum. t.), **BELL.**, Bry., Con., Graph., Hep., Iod., Lach., *Lyc.*, **Merc.**, *Phos.*, **PULS.**, **SIL.**, *Sul.*, Thuj.

Bones.—*Asaf.*, Cocc., *Ruta.*

Skin.—Ant. cr., (Apis.), Arn., **ARS.**, Bell., *Bry.*, (Carb. ac.), Carb. v. Caust., Clem., Con., Dulc., Graph., *Hep.*, **Lach.**, *Lyc.*, *Merc.*, Nit. ac., Phos., Puls., Ran. b., *Rhus*, *Sep.*, Sil., Staph., **SUL.**, *Thuj.*

Sleep and Dreams.—Ars., Calc. c., Chin., *Graph.*, Hep., Ign., K. carb., Lach., Lyc., Merc., Nux v., *Phos.*, **Puls.**, Ran. b., Rhus, **Sep.**, *Sil.*, Sul.

Blood, Circulation and Fever.—Ant. t., Ars., Bry., Calc. c., Graph., Hep., *K. carb.*, Lyc., Nat. m., Nux v., *Phos.*, Rhus, **SEP.**, *Sul.*

Aggravations: Time and Circumstances.—(Aesc.), *Am. carb.*, Am. m., Anac., (Apis), (Arg. n.), Arn., *Ars.*, (Bap.), *Bell.*, **BRY.**, **Calc. c.**, **Carb. v.**, Chin., (Cimic.), Cocc., Colch., *Con.*, (Glon.), *Graph.*, Fer., Hep., Ign., (K. bi.), **K. carb.**, K. nit., Led., (Lil. t.), **Lyc.**, *Mag. c.*, Mang., Merc., *Nat. m.*, *Nit. ac.*, **Nux v.**, Phos., (Phyt.), **PULS.**, *Rhus*, (Sang.), Sele., *Sep.*, *Sil.*, Spig., Stan., Stro., **Sul.**

Other Remedies.—(Aesc.), (Aloe), Alum., Am. carb., (Apis), (Arg. n.), Arn., *Ars.*, Asaf., *Bell.*, *Bry.*, *Calc. c.*, *Carb. v.*, Caust., Chin., (Cimic.), Cocc., Con., Fer., (Gel.), **Graph.**, Hep., *Ign.*, (K. bi.), *K. carb.*, Lach., Lil. t., Lyc., **Merc.**, Nat. c., Nat. m., Nit. ac., *Nux v.*, Op., Petrol., PHOS., Plat., **Puls.**, *Rhus*, Ruta, Sang., SEP., **Sil.**, **Staph.**, Stro., SUL., Thuj., Zinc.

Antidotes.—Ars., Camph., Nux v., Vinum.

Carbo Vegetabilis.

Mind.—Acon., Anac., *Aur.*, **Bell.**, Bry., Calc. c., **Cham.**, Cocc., *Ign.*, Lyc., Nux v., Phos., Puls., Rhus, Sul., *Verat. a.*

Localities.—Acon., Aesc., All. c., *Aloe*, Alum., Am. carb., Ant. t., *Apis*, Apoc. c., *Arg. n.*, *Arn.*, *Ars.*, Arum. t., Asaf., Aur., Bap., *Bell.*, (Berb.), *Bry.*, Cact., **Calc. c.**, Cannab. i., Canth., Carb. ac., *Carb. an.*, *Caust.*, *Cham.*, **Chin.**, Cimic., Clem., Cocc., Con., Crotal., Dios., Dulc., (Eup. per.), Fl. ac., Gel., Glon., *Graph.*, Hep., *Ign.*, (Iris v.), **K. bi.**, *K. carb.*, Kre., Led., Lil. t., **Lyc.**, (Meli.), **Merc.**, *Nat. c.*, *Nat. m.*, **Nit. ac.**, NUX V., *Petrol.*, **Phos.**, Pho. ac., Phyt., Pb., *Pod.*, (Pso.), PULS., Ran. b., Rhodo., *Rhus*, Saba., *Sang.*, SEP., **Sil.**, **Staph.**, SUL., Tell., Thuj., *Verat. a.*, Verat. v., Zinc.

Sensations.—*Acon.*, (Aesc.), (Aloe), Ambr., (Apis), Arg. n., Arn., *Ars.*, (Arum. t.), Bar. c., *Bell.*, (Berb.), *Bry.*, **Calc. c.**, (Cannab. i.), Canth., Carb. an., *Caust.*, Cham., Chel., *Chin.*, Cimic., Cocc., Con., Dulc., Fer., Gel., (Glon.), **Graph.**, Ign., (Iris v.), (K. bi.), *K. carb.*, Kre., Laur., (Lil. t.), Lyc., (Meli.), *Merc.*, Mez., Nat. c., *Nat. m.*, Nit. ac. Nux v., Op., Petrol., *Phos.*, Pho. ac., (Phyt.) Plat., (Pso.), **Puls.**, Ran. b., Rhodo., **Rhus**, Sang., Sars., Seneg., SEP., **Sil.**, Spig., Spo., Stan., *Staph.*, Stram., SUL., Verat. a., *Zinc.*

Glands.—Arn., **Bell.**, *Bry.*, Carb. an., Graph., **Lyc.**, Merc., Phos., Puls., Sul.

Bones.—Asaf., Merc., Pho. ac., Ruta, Sul.

Skin.—Ant. t., *Ars.*, Asar., Bell., Bry., Calc. c., (Carb. ac.), Carb. an., *Caust.*, Chin., Clem., Con., Crotal., *Graph.*, Hep., Ip., K. carb., Kre., Lach., LYC., *Merc.*, Mez., *Nit. ac.*, Nux v., Petrol., *Phos.*, Pho. ac., *Puls.*, Rhus, Sele., *Sep.*, **Sil.**, Staph., Sul., Verat. a.

Sleep and Dreams.—(Apis), Bell., Bry., *Calc. c.*, (Cannab. i.), *Graph.*, Ign., K. carb., Merc., Nux v., Phos., (Pod.), **Puls.**, *Rhus*, SEP., Sil., Sul.

Blood, Circulation and Fever.—ACON., (Aloe), (Apis), (Arg. n.), Arn., **Ars.**, *Bell.*, *Bry.*, (Cact.), *Calc. c.*, *Cham.*, Chin., Cocc., Cup., (Gel.),

RELATIONSHIPS.—CARBO V.—CAUST. 369

Glon., Hep., Ign., Ip., K. carb., Lyc., Merc., Nat. m., Nit. ac., Nux v.,
Op., Phos., Pho. ac., (Pod.), Puls., Rhus, Sang., Sep., Sil., Stan., Stram.,
Sul., Verat. a., (Verat. v.).

Aggravations: Time and Circumstances.—(Aloe), Apis, Arg. n.,
Ars., (Bap.), Bell., Bry., Calc. c., Caps., Carb. an., Caust., Cham., Chin.,
Cocc., Colch., Con., Euphorb., Fer., (Gel.), Graph., Hep., Ign., K. bi.,
K. carb., Lach., (Lil. t.), Lyc., Merc., Nat. c., Nat. m., Nit. ac., Nux v.,
Phos., Pho. ac., (Phyt.), Pod., PULS., Rhodo., Rhus, Saba., Sang.
Sele., SEP., Sil., Spig., Staph., Stram., Sul., Verat. a., (Verat. v.).

Other Remedies.—Acon., (Aesc.), Aloe, Apis, Arg. n., Arn., Ars.,
(Arum. t.), Asaf., Aur., (Bap.), Bell., (Berb.), Bry., (Cact.), Calc. c.,
Cannab. i., Carb. an., Caust., Cham., Chin., Cimic., Cocc., Con., Crotal.,
Gel., Glon., Graph., Hep., Ign., K. bi., K. carb., Kre., Lach., Lil. t., LYC.,
Merc., Nat. c., Nat. m., Nit. ac., Nux v., Petrol., Phos., Pho. ac.,
Phyt., Pod., PULS., Rhodo., Rhus, Saba., Sang., SEP., Sil., Spig., Staph.,
Stram., SUL., Verat. a., Verat. v., Zinc.

Antidotes.—Ars., Camph., Coff., Lach., Spir. nit. dul.

Causticum.

Mind.—Aesc., Aloe, Bap., Bar. c., Cact., Calc. c., Cannab. i., Carb.
ac., Cham., Con., Ign., Lyc., Meli., Pso., Puls., Rhus, Sec. c., Sep.,
Verat. v.

Localities.—Acon., Aesc., All., c., Aloe, Alum., Ant. cr., Apis, (Apoc.
c.), ARG. N., Arn., Ars., Arum. t., Aur., Bap., Bar. c., Bell., Berb.,
Bov., Bry., Cact., CALC. C., Cannab. i., Cannab. s., Canth., Carb. ac.,
Carb. v., Caul., Cham., Chin., Cimic., Clem., Con., (Crotal.), Dios., (Eup.
per.), (Fl. ac.), Gel., Glon., Graph., Hep., (Hyd. ac.), (Hyper.), Ign., (Iris
v.), K. BI., K. carb., Kalm., Kre., Led., Lil. t., Lith., Lyc., Merc., Nat. c.,
Nat. m., Nit. ac., Nux v., Op., Par., Petrol., Phos., Pho. ac., Phyt.,
(Pic. ac.), Pb., Pod., Puls., Rhus, Ruta, Saba., Sang., SEP., Sil., Spig.,
Staph., SUL., Thuj., Verat. a., Verat. v., Zinc.

Sensations.—Acon., (Aesc.), (Aloe), Alum., Apis, Arg. n., Arn., Ars.,
Arum. t., Asaf., Aur., Bap., Bell., Berb., Bry., CALC. C., Cannab. i., Carb.
v., Cham., Chin., Cic., Cimic., Cocc., Coloc., Con., Croc., Crotal., Dulc., Eup.
per., Gel., Glon., Graph., Hep., Ign., Iod., (Iris v.), K. bi., K. carb.,
(Kalm.), Kre., (Lil. t.), Lith., LYC., Mag. c., Merc., Nat. c., Nat. m.,
Nit. ac., Nux v., Petrol., Phos., Pho. ac., Phyt., Plat., (Pod.), PULS.,
Rhodo., RHUS, Saba., Sang., Sars., Sec. c., Seneg., SEP., Sil., Spig.,
Spo., Stan., Staph., Stram., Stro., SUL., Tar., Thuj. Valer., Verat. a.,
Zinc.

Glands.—Bell., Bry., Calc. c., *Con.*, K. carb., Lyc., Merc., **Phos.**, *Puls.*, Rhus, Sil., Spo., **Sul.**

Bones.—*Bell.*, *Calc. c.*, Chin., Con., Dros., Hell., Lyc., *Merc.*, Pho. ac., *Puls.*, *Ruta*, Sep.

Skin.—Apis, Arn., **Ars.**, *Asaf.*, (Bap.), Bry., Calc. c., Carb. ac., *Carb. v.*, Chin., Con., Dulc., Graph., *Hep.*, *Lach.*, Led., Lyc., **Merc.**, *Mez.*, *Nit. ac.*, Phos., **PULS.**, Ran. b., Ran. s., **RHUS**, *Sep.*, **Sil.**, *Staph.*, *Stro.*, Sul., Thuj.

Sleep and Dreams.—(Apis), (Arg. n.), Bell., Bry., **Calc. c.**, (Cannab. i.), Con., *Graph.*, Ign., Merc., Nat. c., **Nux v.**, *Phos.*, Pho. ac., Pod.), *Rhus*, Sep., *Sil.*, Staph., Sul.

Blood, Circulation and Fever.—Acon., (Apis), (Arg. n.), *Arn.*, Ars., Bell., Bry., (Cact.), *Calc. c.*, (Cannab. i.), (Glon.), Graph., K. carb., Lyc., Merc., Nux v., Phos., Puls., **RHUS**, *Sep.*, *Sul.*, **Verat. a.**

Aggravations: Time and Circumstances.—All. c., Acon., Ant. cr., (Apis), Arg. n., *Ars.*, **Asar.**, (Bap.), Bell., *Bry.*, *Calc. c.*, Carb. v., *Cham.*, (Cimic.), Con., **Hep.**, Ign., K. bi., K. carb., Lach., (Lil. t.), *Lyc.*, Mez., Nux v., *Phos.*, (Phyt.), (Pod.), **PULS.**, *Rhus*, Saba., (Sang.), **SEP.**, Sil., Sul.

Other Remedies.—Acon., *Aesc.*, All. c., *Aloe*, Apis, Arg. n., Arn., *Ars.*, Arum. t., Asaf., Asar., *Bap.*, *Bell.*, Berb., *Bry.*, Cact., **Calc. c.**, **Cannab. i.**, *Carb. v.*, Cham., Chin., *Cimic.*, **Con.**, (Crotal.), Gel., Glon., Graph., Hep., Ign., *K. bi.*, *K. carb.*, Lach., Lil. t., Lith., Lyc., Merc. Mez., Nat. c., Nat. m., Nit. ac., *Nux v.*, **Phos.**, Pho. ac., Phyt., Pod., **PULS.**, **RHUS**, Ruta, Saba., Sang., **SEP.**, *Sil.*, Spig., Staph., Stro., **SUL.**, Thuj., Verat. a., Verat. v., Zinc.

Antidotes.—Asaf., Coff., Coloc., Nux v., *Spir. nit. dulc.*

Injurious.—Acetum, Coff., Phos.

Chamomilla.

Mind.—ACON., Aesc., Aloe, Anac., *Ars.*, Ars. iod., Aur., Bell., Calc. c., Cannab. i., Carb. ac., *Caust.*, Cimic., Crotal., Graph., Ign., Lil. t., **LYC.**, Merc., Nat. m., **NUX V.**, *Phos.*, Plat., **PULS.**, Sep., Stram., *Sul.*, Thea, Verat. a.

Localities.—Acon., Aesc., All. c., *Aloe*, Alum., Apis, Apoc. c., **ARG. N.**, *Arn.*, Ars., *Arum. t.*, Bap., Bell., (Berb.), Bry., (Cact.), *Calc. c.*, Cannab. i., Canth., Caps., Carb. ac., *Carb. v.*, *Caust.*, Chin., Cimic., Cocc., Con., Croc., Crotal., *Dig.*, Dios., Dulc., (Eup. per.), (Fl. ac.), Gel., (Glon.), *Graph.*, *Hep.*, (Hyd. ac.), *Hyos.*, Ign., *Ip.*, Iris v., K. bi., *K. carb.*, Lach., Lil. t., Lyc., (Meli.), **MERC.**, Nat. c., *Nat. m.*, Nit. ac., **NUX V.**, Petrol.,

Phos., *Pho. ac*, *Phyt.*, *Pb.*, *Pod.*, *Pso.*, PULS., Rhus, Saba., Sang., Sec. c., Sep., *Sil.*, *Spig.*, Stan., Staph., Stram., SUL., *Verat. a. Verat. v.*, Zinc.

Sensations.—Acon., Agar., Alum., Ambr., Apis, Arg. n., Arn., Ars., Aur., (Bap.), *Bar. c.*, BELL., Berb., Bry., (Cact.), Calc. c., (Cannab. i.), Canth., Caps., Carb. v., *Caust.*, Chin., *Cic.*, Cimic., *Cocc.*, *Coff.*, Con., Croc., (Crotal.), *Cup.*, *Fer.*, Gel., Glon., Graph., Hyos., Ign., Iod., *Ip.*, K. bi., K. carb., Lyc., (Meli.), Merc., Mos., Nat. c., Nat. m., Nit. ac., NUX V., *Op.*, *Petrol.*, Phos., Pho. ac., Phyt., *Plat.*, (Pod.), Puls., Rhus, Sabi., (Sang.), *Sec. c.*, SEP., *Sil.*, Spig., Spo., Stan., Staph., *Stram.*, Sul., *Verat. a.*, Verat. v., Zinc.

Glands.—(Arum. t.), *Bell.*, Bry., *Con.*, K. carb., *Lyc.*, Merc., *Phos.*, Puls., *Sil.*, *Sul.*

Bones.—Arg., Bell.

Skin.—Acon., Apis, Ars., Asaf., Bell., Bry., Calc. c., Caust., Con., (Crotal.), Graph., Hep., Lach., Lyc., Merc., *Nit. ac.*, *Petrol.*, PULS., Rhus, Sep., SIL., Staph., SUL.

Sleep and Dreams.—Arg. n., Ars., (Bap.), Bell., Bry., Calc. c., Chin., Hep., *K. carb.*, (Lil. t.), Merc., *Nux v.*, Phos., Pho. ac., PULS., *Rhus*, Saba., Sep., Sil., *Sul.*

Blood, Circulation and Fever.—Acon., Ars., Bell., (Berb.), Bry., Calc. c., (Cannab. i.), *Chin.*, *Hep.*, Ign., Laur., Lyc., Merc., Nat. m., NUX V., *Op.*, *Phos.*, Pho. ac., (Phyt.), (Pod.), Puls., Rhus, Sang., Sec. c., Sep., Sil., Stram., Sul., Verat. a., (Verat. v.),

Aggravations: Time and Circumstances.—*Acon.*, (Aesc.), (Aloe), Ambr., Am. carb., Apis, Arg. n., Arn., *Ars.*, (Bap.), (Bell., BRY., Calc. c., (Cannab. i.), *Caps.*, Carb. v., *Caust.*, Chin., (Cimic.), *Cocc.*, Coff., Coloc., Con., (Crotal.), (Glon.), *Graph.*, Hep., Hyos., Ign., Ip., K. bi., *K. carb.*, *Lach.*, Led., (Lil. t.), Lyc., Mang., *Merc.*, Nat. c., Nat. m., Nux m., NUX V., Op., Phos., *Pho. ac.*, (Phyt.), Plat., (Pod.), PULS., Rhus, Sabi., Sang., Sep., *Sil.*, Spig., Staph., Stram., Stro., Sul., *Verat. a.*

Other Remedies.—Acon., Aesc., Aloe, Apis, Arg. n., Arn., *Ars.*, Arum. t., Aur., *Bap.*, BELL., Berb., Bry., (Cact.), Calc. c., *Cannab. i.*, Caps., Carb. v., *Caust.*, Chin., *Cimic.*, Cocc., Con., *Crotal.*, Gel., (Glon.), Graph., *Hep.*, Hyos., *Ign.*, Ip., *K. bi.*, K. carb., Lach., Lil. t., Lyc., Merc., Nat. m., Nit. ac., NUX V., Op., Petrol., Phos., Pho. ac., *Phyt.*, Plat., Pod., PULS., Rhus, *Sang.*, Sec. c., Sep., Sil., Spig., Staph., Stram., SUL., Verat. a., Verat. v.

Antidotes.—*Acon.*, Alum., Bor., Camph., Cocc., *Coff.*, Coloc., *Ign.*, *Nux v.*, Puls.

Chelidonium.

Mind.—Acon., Apis, Bap., *Bell.*, Calc. c., Con., *Gel.*, *Nat. m.*, Nux v., Phos., Pho. ac., Pic. ac., Puls., Rhus, Sep., Stram., Verat. a.

Localities.—Aesc., (All. c.), Aloe, Alum., Anac., **Apis**, Apoc. c., A;g. n., Arn., Ars., Arum. t., Aur., Bap., *Bell.*, *Berb.*, Bor., Bry., (Cact.), Calc. c., Cannab. i., Carb. ac., Carb. v., Caust., Cham., Chin., Cimic., Cocc., Con., (Crotal.), Dios., Eup. per., (Fl. ac.), Gel., (Glon.), Graph., Hep., Ign., (Iris v.), K. bi., K. carb., (Kalm.), (Lil. t.), Lith., Lyc., Mag. m., Merc., Mez., Nat. m., *Nux v.*, Oleand., Petrol., **Phos.**, Pho. ac., Phyt., (Pic. ac.), Pb., *Pod.*, Pso. **Puls.**, Rhus, Ruta, Saba., *Sang.*, SEP., *Sil.*, Spig., Staph., Stram., **Sul.**, Sul. ac., Thuj., *Verat. a.*, Verat. v., Verb., Zinc.

Sensations.—Acon., Aesc., Aloe, Alum., Apis, Arg. n., Arn., **Ars.**, Arum. t., Bap., Bar. c., *Bell.*, *Berb.*, Bry., Cact., *Calc. c.*, Cannab. i., Canth., (Carb. ac.), Carb. v., *Caust.*, Cham., Chin., (Cimic.), **Cocc.**, Con., Cyc., Dios., Dulc., (Gel.), (Glon.), Graph., Guai., *Ign.*, Iris v., K. bi., K. carb., Laur., Lil. t., (Lith.), LYC., Merc., Mez., Mos., *Nat. c.*, Nat. m., NUX V., Phos., *Pho. ac.*, (Phyt.), Plat., Pb., (Pso.), Puls., *Rhus*, Ruta, Saba., Sang., Sec. c., **Sep.**, Spig., Spo., Stan., Staph., **Sul.**, Tar., Verat. a., Verat. v., *Zinc.*

Glands.—Ars., Bell., *Chin.*, *Cocc.*, Dig., Merc.

Bones.

Skin.—Arn., Bar. c., Bell., Bor., Bry., *Calc. c.*, Canth., *Caust.*, *Cham.*, Chin., Con., (Crotal.), **Graph.**, Hep., Lyc., *Merc.*, **Nit. ac.**, Nux v., Petrol., Phos., **Puls.**, Rhus, Saba., **Sep.**, Sil., Squ., Staph., SUL., Vio. t.

Sleep and Dreams.—(Apis), (Cannab. i.), Mur. ac., **Nux v.**, Phos., (Pod.), Rhus, Sul.

Blood, Circulation and Fever.—ACON., *Arn.*, Ars., Bell., Bry., Calc. c., Camph., (Cannab. i.), Caust., *Chin.*, Dig., Fer., (Glon.), Hyos., Ip., K. nit., Nit. ac., Nux v., Phos., *Puls.*, *Rhus*, Saba., (Sang.), Sep., Spig., Stram., Sul., Thuj., Verat. a., (Verat. v.).

Aggravations: Time and Circumstances.—(Aesc.), (Aloe.), (Apis), (Arg. n.), Arn., (Bap.), *Bell.*, Bry., (Cact.), Calc. c., Camph., (Cannab. i.), Cannab. s., Carb. an., Cham., *Chin.*, (Cimic.), Cocc., Coff., Con., Croc., (Gel.), (Glon.), Graph., Ign., Iod., K. bi., K. carb., K. nit., *Lach.*, Led., (Lil. t.), Lyc., *Nat. c.*, Nat. m., Nux m., **Nux v.**, *Phos.*, Phyt., Pod., **Puls.**, *Ran. b.*, *Rhus*, Saba., *Sang*, **Sele.**, Sep., Sil., SPIG., Staph., Stram., (Verat. v.).

Other Remedies.—Acon., Aesc., Aloe, Apis, Arg. n., Arn., Ars., Arum. t., *Bap.*, Bar. c., **Bell.**, Berb., *Bry.*, Cact., **Calc. c.**, Cannab. i., Caust., Cham., *Chin.*, Cimic., *Cocc.*, Con., (Crotal.), *Gel.*, Glon., Graph., *Ign.*, *K. bi.*, K. carb., Lil. t., (Llth.), *Lyc.*, *Merc.*, Nat. c., Nat. m., Nit. ac., **NUX V.**, **Phos.**, Pho. ac., Phyt., Pod., Puls., Rhus, Saba., *Sang.*, **Sele.**, **Sep.**, Sil., *Spig.*, Staph., Stram., **Sul.**, Verat. a., Verat. v., Zinc.

Antidotes.—Camph., Coff.

China.

Mind.—Acon., Anac., Apis, Ars., Bell., Calc. c., Caust., Cham., Chel., Cocc., Con., Gel., Glon., Graph., Ign., Lach., *Lyc.*, Meli., Merc., Nat. c., *Nat. m.*, Nux v., *Phos.*, Pho. ac., Phyt., Pic. ac., Plat., **PULS.**, Rhus, Sep., *Sil.*, Staph., Sul.

Localities.—Acon., *Aesc.*, (All. c.), *Aloe*, Anac., Ant. cr., Ant. t., **APIS**, Apoc. c., **ARG. N.**, *Arn.*, **Ars.**, Arum. t., Aur., *Bap.*, Bell., *Berb.*, *Bry.*, Cact., **Calc. c.**, *Cannab. i.*, Canth., **Carb. ac.**, *Carb. v.*, Caust., (Ced.), *Cham.*, Cimic., Cocc., *Con.*, Crotal., Dios., Dulc., Eup. per., *Fer.*, Fl. ac., Gel., Glon., Graph., Hep., (Hyd. ac.), Hyos., *Ign.*, Ip., Iris v., **K. BI.**, *K. carb.*, (Kalm.), Kre., Lil. t., *Lyc.*, Meli., **Merc.**, Nat. c., *Nat. m.*, *Nit. ac.*, **NUX V.**, **PHOS.**, Pho. ac., *Phyt.*, Pic. ac., Pb., Pod., *Pso.*, **PULS.**, *Rhus*, *Sang.*, Sec. c., Sep., *Sil.*, Spig., Stan., Staph., Stram., **SUL.**, Verat. a., *Verat. v.*

Sensations.—Acon., Aesc., (Aloe), Apis, Arg. n., *Arn.*, Ars., (Arum. t.), Bap., Bar. c., **Bell.**, Berb., *Bry.*, Cact., **Calc. c.**, Cannab. i., Canth., Carb. v., Cham., Cimic., Cocc., Colch., Con., (Crotal.), Dig., (Eup. per.), *Fer.*, Gel., (Glon.), Graph., Hell., Hyos., Ign., Ip., (Iris v.), K. bi., *K. carb.*, (Kalm.), (Lil. t.), (Lith.), *Lyc.*, Mar., (Meli.), *Merc.*, Nat. c., Nat. m., Nit. ac., Nux v., *Phos.*, Pho. ac., (Phyt.), Pb., (Pod.), **PULS.**, Rhus, *Sang.*, **Sep.**, Sil., Spig., Stan., Staph., **SUL.**, Thuj., Verat. a., (Verat. v.), Zinc.

Glands.—Arn., **BELL.**, Bry., Calc. c., Iod., Lyc., Merc., Phos., **Puls.**, *Sul.*

Bones.—Asaf., (Eup. per.), **MERC.**, **Pho. ac.**, Puls., Rhodo., Rhus, *Ruta*, Sil.

Skin.—Ant. cr., Apis, *Arn.*, Ars., *Asaf.*, *Bell.*, Bry., *Calc. c.*, Carb. v., Caust., Con., (Crotal.), Dulc., Fer., *Graph.*, *Hep.*, Lach., Led., Lyc., *Merc.*, Nat. m., Nit. ac., Nux v., Petrol., Phos., *Pho. ac.*, Puls., Rhus, (Sang.), Sele., **Sep.**, Sil., Staph., **SUL.**, Thuj., Verat. a.

Sleep and Dreams.—Acon., Arg. n., *Ars.*, (Bap.), Bell., *Bry.*, *Calc. c.*, (Cannab. i.), Carb. an., Cham., (Cimic.), (Gel.), Graph., Hep., Ign., K.

carb., Lach., (Lil. t.), Lyc., Merc., Nat. c., **Nux v., Phos.**, **Pho. ac.,** Puls., Ran. b., Rhus, Sep., *Sil.*, SUL.

Blood, Circulation and Fever.—Acon., (Aloe), (Apis), **Ars., BELL.,** (Berb.), **Bry.,** Cact., *Calc. c.*, (Cannab. i.), *Cham.,* (Cimic.), Con., *Dig.,* Fer., (Gel.), (Glon.), Graph., Hep., Hyos., *Ip*, *Merc.,* **Nat. m., Nux v.,** Phos., Pho. ac., PULS., *Rhus*, Saba., Samb., (Sang.), Sele., **Sep.,** Sil., Spig., Staph., Stram., SUL., *Thuj.,* Verat. a., (Verat. v.).

Aggravations: Time and Circumstances.—Acon., Alum., Ant. cr., (Apis), (Apoc. c.), Arg. n., Arn., *Ars.,* (Arum. t.), **Bell., Bry.,** (Cact.), Calc. c., (Cannab. i.), Caps., *Carb. v., Cham.,* (Cimic.), Cocc., Colch., *Con.,* (Crotal.), Fer., Graph., *Hep.,* Ign., Iod., Ip., (K. bi.), **K. carb.,** Lach., Led., (Lil. t.), *Lyc.,* Mang., *Merc.,* Nat. c., *Nat. m.,* Nit. ac., Nux m., **Nux v.,** Phos., *Pho. ac.,* (Phyt.), (Pod.), PULS., *Rhus,* Ruta, (Sang.), *Sele.,* **Sep.,** *Sil.,* Spig., Stan., *Staph.,* SUL., Thuj., Verat. a.

Other Remedies.—*Acon.,* Aesc., Aloe, **Apis,** (Apoc. c.), **Arg. n.,** *Arn.,* **Ars.,** Arum. t., Asaf., Bap., **Bell.,** Berb., **Bry.,** *Cact.,* **Calc. c.,** *Cannab. i.,* Carb. v., Caust., *Cham., Cimic.,* Cocc., *Con.,* Crotal., *Fer., Gel.,* Glon., Graph., Hep., *Ign.,* Ip., *K. bi.,* K. carb., Lil. t., **Lyc., Merc.,** Nat. c., *Nat. m.,* Nit. ac., **Nux v., Phos., Pho. ac.,** *Phyt.,* Pod., PULS., **Rhus,** *Sang.,* Sele., **Sep.,** *Sil.,* Spig., Staph., SUL., Thuj., Verat. a., Verat. v.

Antidotes.—*Arn.,* **Ars.,** *Bell.,* Calc. c., **Carb. v.,** *Fer.,* **Ip.,** Merc., Nat. c., Nat. m., Puls., Sep., *Sul.,* Salvia off., **Thea., Verat. a.**

Injurious.—Dig., Led., Sele.

Cicuta.

Mind.—*Aloe,* Anac., Arum. t., Aur., *Bap.,* Bar. c., **Bell.,** *Cannab. i.,* Caust., *Cimic.,* Cup., *Gel.,* **Glon.,** Hell., **Hyd. ac., Hyos.,** Hyper., *Lyc.,* Meli., Merc. c., Nat. m., Op., Phos., Pho. ac., Plat., Pso., **Puls.,** Rhus, Sil., *Stram.,* Sul., Ter., Ther., Verat. a., Verat. v.

Localities.—Anac., Apis, Arg. n., **Ars.,** (Arum. t.), (Bap.), **BELL.,** Bry., Calc. c., *Camph.,* Cham., Chin., Cocc., *Cup.,* Cyc., Dig., Fer., Gel., (Glon.), Graph., Hep., Hyos., **Ign.,** (K. bi.), *Lyc.,* (Meli.), *Merc.,* Nat. m., **Nux v.,** Oleand., Op., Phos., Pho. ac., **Puls.,** Rhus, Ruta, Saba., Sec. c., *Sep.,* Sil., Spig., Stram., Sul., Thuj., *Verat. a., Verat. v.*

Sensations.—Anac., (Apis), *Arg. n., Arn.,* Ars., (Bap.), **BELL.,** (Berb.), *Bry.,* Calc. c., Camph., (Cannab. i.), Carb. v., **Caust., Cham.,** (Cimic.), Cocc., Con., **Cup.,** Dros., (Gel.), (Glon.), Graph., **Hyos.,** Ign., *Ip.,* (K. bi.), K. carb., Lyc., *Merc.,* Mez., Mos., Nat. m., Nux v., Oleand., **OP.,** Petrol., Phos., Phyt., **Plat.,** Pb., Ruta, (Sang.), **Sec. c.,** Sep., Sil., Stan., **Stram., Sul.,** *Sul. ac.,* Verat. a., Zinc.

Glands.—Arn., Carb. an., Con., Sep.

Bones.

Skin.—Ant. cr., Apis, Bry., *Calc. c*, Carb. ac., (Cimic.), *Clem.*, **Dulc.**, (Eup. per.), **Graph.**, Hep., K. carb., Kre., Lach., *Lyc.*, *Merc.*, Nat. c., Petrol., Phos., Puls., Ran. b., RHUS, SEP., Sil., *Staph.*, Sul.

Sleep and Dreams.—(Arg. n.), **Bell.**, **Bry.**, Chin., Ign., Lyc., **Nux v.**, Phos., **Puls.**, Rhus, *Sul.*

Blood, Circulation and Fever.—(Pod.), Rhus.

Aggravations: Time and Circumstances.—*Acon.*, (Aesc.), Am. m., Ant. cr., (Arg. n.), *Arn.*, *Ars.*, Aur., *Bell.*, *Bry.*, *Calc. c*, Canth., Carb. v., Caust., Cham., Cocc., Colch., Con., Croc., Graph., HEP., Ign., Ip., (K. bi.), *K. carb.*, Lyc., Nat. m., Nit. ac., Nux m., Nux v., Phos., Puls., Rhodo., RHUS, Ruta, Samb., Sang., Sele, Sep., Sil., *Spig.*, *Spo.*, *Squ*, Staph., *Stro*, Sul., Thuj.

Other Remedies.—Anac., Apis, *Arg. n.*, Arn., Ars., (Arum. t.), Bap., BELL., Bay., *Calc. c*, Camph., Cannab. i., Caust., Cham, Cimic., *Cocc.*, Con., *Cup.*, Dulc., Gel., Glon., *Graph.*, Hep., *Hyos.*, Ign., Ip., (K. bi.), K. carb., Lyc., Merc., *Nat. m.*, Nux v., Op., Phos, Plat., PULS., Rhus, Ruta, (Sang.), Sec. c., Sep., Sil., Spig., Staph., *Stram.*, Sul., Verat. a., Verat. v.

Antidotes.—*Arn.*, Op., Tab.

Cimicifuga.

Mind.—*Acon.*, Agn., *Ars.*, *Aur.*, Dig., Gels., Hyos., *Ign.*, *Lil. t.*, Lyc., Merc., Mez., Nat. c., Phos., Plat., Puls., Sep., Sil., Stan., Stram., *Sulph.*, Verat. a.

Localities.—*Acon.*, Aesc., *Agar.*, (All. c.), (Aloe), (Ambr.), Am. m., (Anac.), (Ant. cr.), (Ant. t.), Apis, (Apoc. c.), (Arg.), Arg. n., *Arn.*, *Ars.*, (Arum. t.), (Asaf.), (Asar.), Aur., Bap., Bar. c., **Bell.**, (Bism.), (Bor.), *Bry.*, Cact., Calc. c., (Cannab. s.), Canth., (Caps.), Carb. ac., (Carb. an.), Carb. v., Caust., Cham., *Chel.*, *Chin.*, Cina, (Clem.), (Cocc.), (Coff.), (Colch.), (Coloc.), Con., (Croc.), (Cup.), (Cyc.), Dig., (Dios.), (Dros.), (Dulc.), (Eup. per.), (Euphr.), (Fer.), (Fl. ac.), Gel., (Glon.), (Graph.), (Guai.), (Hell.), (Hep.), (Hyos.), (Hyper.), Ign., Ip., Iod., (Iris v.), (K. bi.), *K. carb.*, (K. nit.), (Kalm.), (Kre.), Lach., (Laur.), (Lil. t.), Lyc., (Mag. c.), (Mag. m.), Merc., Mos., (Mur. ac.), Nat. c., *Nat. m.*, Nit. ac., (Nux m.), *Nux v.*, Op., Petrol., *Phos.*, (Pho. ac.), (Phyt.), (Plat.), Pb, (Pod.), Puls., (Ran. b.), (Rheum.), Rhus, (Ruta), (Saba.), Sabi., (Samb.), (Sang.), (Sars.), Sec. c., *Seneg.*, *Sep.*, **Sil.**, *Spig.*, Spo., (Squ.), **Stan.**, (Staph.),

(Stram.), (Stro.), Sul., (Sul. ac.), (Ther.), Thuj., (Valer.), Verat. a., (Verat. v.), (Verb.), Zinc.

Sensations.—Acon., (Aesc.), Agar., (Aloe), (Am. m.), Anac., Ant. t., (Apis), Arg. n., *Arn.*, *Ars.*, Arum. t., Asaf., (Asar.), (Bap.), Bar. c., **Bell.**, (Berb.), (Bor.), Bry., *Calc. c.*, Canth., (Caps.), Carb. v., *Caust.*, (Cham.), Chel., Chin., Cic., Cocc., Colch., *Coloc.*, (Con.), Cup., (Cyc.), (Dig.), Dros., (Eur. per.), Fer., (Gel.), (Glon.), Graph., (Hell.), (Hep.), Hyos., Ign., (Iod.), (K. bi.), K. carb., (Kalm.), *Lach.*, Led., (Lil. t.), *Lyc.*, **Merc.**, *Mez.*, Mos., (Mur. ac.), (Nat. c.), *Nat. m.*, Nit. ac., Nux m., **Nux v.**, (Oleand.), *Op.*, (Petrol.), **Phos.**, Pho. ac., (Phyt.), *Plat.*, *Pb.*, Pod., **Puls.**, Ran. b., (Rhodo.), **Rhus**, Ruta, (Sabi.), Sang., Sec. c., (Seneg.), Sep., Sil., Spig., Spo., *Stan.*, Staph., *Stram.*, Sul., Sul. ac., (Thuj.), Valer., Verat. a., (Verat. v.), Zinc.

Glands.

Bones.—(Asaf.), Bell., (Con.), (Merc.), (Nit. ac.), (Ruta), (Sul.), (Valer.).

Skin.—Alum., Ars., Bry., Calc. c., Cic., Dros., *Eup. per.*, Glon., Graph., Hep., Ign., Nat. m., Nit. ac., Nux v., Petrol., Plat., Puls., Rhus, Sep., Sul., *Zinc.*

Sleep and Dreams.—(Acon.), (Ars.), (Bar. c.), (Bell.), (Chin.), (Puls.), (Rhus), (Sil.), (Sul.).

Blood, Circulation and Fever.—(Ars.), (Chin.), (Dig.), (Nat. m.), (Pho. ac.), (Stram.).

Aggravations: Time and Circumstances.—(Acon.), (Agn.), (All. c.), (Aloe), Alum., Ambr., (Am. carb.), (Am. m.), (Anac.), Ant. cr., (Apis), Arg., (Arg. n.), Arn., Ars., Asaf., Asar., *Bell.*, (Bism.), Bry., (Calad.), Calc. c., (Cannab. s.), (Caps.), (Carb. an.), (Cham.), (Chel.), Cocc., (Coff.,), Colch., (Coloc.), (Con.) Croc., (Dig.), (Dulc.), (Fer.), (Graph.), Hell., (Hep.), (Ign.), (Ip.), (Iod.), K. bi., (K. carb.), K. nit., (Laur.), Led., Lyc. Mag. c., (Mag. m.), (Mang.), Merc., (Mez.), (Nat. c.), Nat. m., Nit. ac., Nux v., Phos., Pho. ac., *Puls.*, Ran. b., (Ran. s.), (Rhodo.), Rhus, (Ruta), Sabi., (Sang.), Sars., Sele., Seneg., *Sep.*, Sil., (Spig.), Stan., (Staph.), *Sul.*, (Thuj.), (Verat. a.), Zinc.

Other Remedies.—Acon., (Aesc.), Agar., (All. c.), (Aloe), Alum., (Ambr.), Am. m., Anac., (Ant. cr.), (Ant. t.), Apis, (Arg.), Arg. n., *Arn.*, Ars., (Arum. t.), Asaf., Asar., (Bap.), Bar. c., **Bell.**, (Bism.), (Bor.), Bry., *Calc. c.*, Canth., (Caps.), (Carb. an.), Carb. v., Caust., Cham., Chel., *Chin.*, Cic., Cocc., (Coff.), Colch., Coloc., Con., (Croc.), (Cup.), (Cyc.), Dig., Dros., (Dulc.), Eup. per., Fer., (Gel.), Glon., Graph., Hell., Hep., (Hyos.), *Ign.*, (Ip.), Iod., K. bi., K. carb., (K. nit.),

(Kalm.), Lach., Led., (Lil. t.), *Lyc.*, (Mag. c.), (Mag. m.), *Merc.*, *Mez.*, Mos., (Mur. ac.), Nat. c., **Nat. m.**, *Nit. ac.*, (Nux m.), **Nux v.**, **Op.**, Petrol., *Phos.*, Pho. ac., (Phyt.), **Plat.**, **Pb.**, (Pod.), **Puls.**, Ran. b., (Rhodo.), Rhus, Ruta, Sabi., Sang., (Sars.), Sec. c., (Seneg.), *Sep.*, **Sil.**, Spig., Spo., *Stan.*, Staph., Stram., **Sul.**, (Sul. ac.), Thuj., Valer., Verat. a., (Verat v.), Zinc.

Cina.

Mind.—Cham., Ign., Lil. t., Lyc., Plat., *Puls.*, *Sul. ac.*

Localities.—Acon., Aesc., All. c., Anac., (Apis), (Apoc. c.), Arg., Arg. n., *Ars.*, (Arum t.), Aur., (Bap.), **Bell.**, (Berb.), *Bry.*, **CALC. C.**, Cannab. i., **CHIN.**, (Carb. ac.), (Cimic.), Cocc., Con., *Cup.*, (Dios.), (Eup. per.), *Fer.*, Gel., Hyos., **IGN.**, *K. bi.*, K. carb., (Lil. t.), Lyc., (Meli.), Merc., Nat. m., Nux v., Oleand., Phos., *Pho. ac.*, (Phyt.), *Plat.*, (Pod.), Pso., **Puls.**, Rhus, Saba., *Sang.*, Sec. c., Sep., Sil., Spig., Stan., Staph., *Sul.*, Sul. ac., *Verat. a.*, Verat. v., Verb., Zinc.

Sensations.—Alum., Anac. Arg. n., Arn., Asaf., **Bell.**, **CALC. C.**, Caust., Cham., Chin., Cocc., *Dulc.*, (Eup. per.), (Gel.), (Glon.), Ign., K. carb., Lyc., Merc., Nat. c., Nat. m., Nit. ac., *Nux v.*, **PLAT.**, Puls., *Sabi.* Sep., Sil., Spig., Sul. ac.

Glands.—Merc.

Bones.

Skin.—Acon., *Ars.*, Asaf., *Bell.* Bry., Hep., Lach., *Lyc.*, **Merc.**, **PULS.**, Rhus, *Sil.*, Sul.

Sleep and Dreams.—Ars., Caust., Ign., *Kre.*, **NUX V.**, **RHUS**, Sars.

Blood, Circulation and Fever.—Acon., Bry., (Cact.), *Cham.*, Chin., Hep., Ip., Nat. m., (Phyt.), (Sang.), Verat. a., (Verat. v.).

Aggravations: Time and Circumstances.—Acon., (Aloe.), Ant. cr., Apis, (Arg. n.), Arn., **Ars.**, Asaf., Bap., Bar. c., *Bell.*, Bry., **CALC. C.**, Canth., *Caps.*, Carb. v., **Chin.**, Fer., (Gel.), Graph., *Hep.*, Ign., K. bi., K. carb., Lach., (Lil. t.), **Lyc.**, **Nat. m.**, Nux v., Oleand., Pb., *Phos.*, (Phyt.), Plat., (Pod.), Puls., *Rhodo.*, *Rhus*, *Ruta,* Saba., (Sang.), **Sep.**, **SIL.**, *Spig.*, Staph., **Sul.**, (Verat. v).

Other Remedies.—Acon., (Apis), Arg. n., Arn., *Ars.*, Asaf., (Bap.), *Bell.*, Bry., **CALC. C.**, Caps., Cham., Chin., Fer., Gel., Hep., Ign., K. bi., K. carb., Lil. t., **Lyc.**, Merc., *Nat. m.*, Nux v., Phos., (Phyt.), **Plat.**, (Pod.), **PULS.**, *Rhus*, Saba., Sang., Sep., Sil., Spig., *Sul.*, Sul. ac., Verat. a., Verat. v.

Antidotes.—Camph., Caps., *Chin.*, (Ip.), Piper nig.

Clematis.

Mind.—Calc. c., Cocc., Ign., Merc., *Pho. ac.*, Puls., Sil., *Sul.*, Zinc.

Localities.—(Aloe.), Alum., **Apis**, *Arg. n.*, Ars., (Bap.), Bell., *Berb.*, Bry., CALC. C., *Cannab. i.*, Carb. v., *Caust.*, Cham., (Cimic.), Cocc., Gel., Hep., K. bi., K. carb., (Lil. t.), **Lyc**, **Merc.**, Nat. m., Nit. ac., *Nux v.*, Petrol., Phos., *Pho. ac.*, (Phyt.), *Puls.*, RHUS, **Sep.**, **Sil.**, *Spig.*, Staph., Sul., Sul. ac., **Thuj.**, Verat. a.

Sensations.—(Aesc.), Alum., Arn., (Arum. t.), *Bell.*, Berb., Bry., *Calc. c.*, (Cannab. i.), Cham., Chin., Cocc., (Gel.), Graph., Ign., (Iris v.), K. bi., Lyc., Merc., Mez., Nat. c., Nux v., Phos., Plat., (Pso.), *Puls.*, *Rhus*, (Sang.), Sep., Spo., *Sul.*, Sul. ac.

Glands.—(Arum. t.), **Bell.**, *Bry.*, **Calc.** c., Carb. an., **Con.**, Merc., Phos., *Puls.*, Sil., **Sul.**

Bones.—Asaf., Calc. c., *Puls.*

Skin.—Am. carb. Am. m., Ant. cr., (Apis), **Ars.**, Bell., Bov., Calc. c., Carb. an., Carb. v., Caust., Con., Dulc., *Graph.*, Hep., (K. bi.), **K. carb.**, Kre., *Lach.*, Led., *Lyc.*, Mag. c., **Merc.**, *Nit. ac.*, Petrol., *Phos.*, Puls., Rhus, SEP., SIL., **Staph.**, **Sul.**, Vio. t.

Sleep and Dreams.—*Calc. c.*, Nux v., *Phos.*, Sil., *Sul.*

Blood, Circulation and Fever.—(Sang.).

Aggravations: Time and Circumstances.—Acon., (Aesc.), **Am. carb.**, Ant. cr., Arn., Ars., *Aur.*, **Bell.**, **Calc. c.**, Cocc., Colch., Con., Dulc., (Gel.), **Hep.**, (Lith.), *Lyc.*, Merc., Nat. m., Nit. ac., Nux m., *Nux v.*, Phos., **Puls.**, RHUS, Samb., (Sang.), Sep., *Sil.*, Spig., Stro., *Sul.*

Other Remedies.—(Aesc.), Am. carb., Ant. cr., (Apis), Ars., (Arum. t.), Aur., *Bell.*, Berb., Bry., CALC. C., Cannab. i., Caust., Cocc., *Con.*, Gel., Graph., *Hep.*, K. bi., *Lyc.*, **Merc.**, Nit. ac., Nux v., *Phos.*, Pho. ac., **Puls.**, **Rhus**, (Sang.), **Sep.**, **Sil.**, Spig., Staph., Stro., SUL., Thuj.

Antidotes.—Bry., Camph.

Cocculus.

Mind.—Acon., Aloe, Bap., *Bell.*, Calc. c., Cannab. i., Cimic., *Gel.*, *Glon.*, Hell., Hyos., **Ign.**, *Lyc.*, *Meli.*, Nux v., Op., Petrol., Phos., *Pho. ac.*, Phyt., *Pic. ac.*, PULS., Rhus, Sep., Sil., Stram., Sul., *Ther.*, Verat. a.

Localities.—Acon., Aesc., *Aloe.*, Alum., Anac., *Apis*, (Apoc. c.), **Arg. n.**, *Arn.*, Ars., (Arum. t.), Aur., *Bap.*, **Bell.**, (Berb.), Bry., Cact., **Calc. c.**, (Cannab. i.), Canth., Caps., Carb. ac., *Carb. v.*, Caust., *Cham.*, **Chin.**, Cimic., *Con.*, (Crotal.), Cup., Dios., (Eup. per.), (Fl. ac.), Gel., Glon., Graph., Hep., *Hyos.*, Ign., Iris v., *K. bi.*, K. carb., (Kalm.), Lil. t., **LYC.**, **Merc.**, Nat. c., *Nat. m.*, Nit. ac., NUX V., *Op.*, Petrol., *Phos.*,

Phyt., Pb., Pod., Pso. **PULS.**, **Rhus**, *Saba.*, *Sang.*, *Sep.*, **Sil.**, Spig., *Stan.*, Staph., Stram., **Sul.**, *Sul. ac.*, *Thuj.*, **Verat. a.**, Verat. v., Zinc.

Sensations.—*Acon.*, Aesc., Aloe. Alum., Anac., *Apis*, **Arg. n.**, Arn., Ars., (Arum. t.), Asaf., Asar., Bap., BELL., (Berb.), *Bry.*, Cact., **Calc. c.**, Camph., *Cannab. i.*, *Caust.*, *Cham.*, Chel., *Chin.*, Cic., Cimic., *Con.*, (Crotal.), (Dios.), (Eup. per.), Fer., **Gel.**, *Glon.*, Graph., Hell., *Hyos.*, IGN., Ip., K. bi., *K. carb.*, Lach., Laur., Lil. t., (Lith.), **Lyc.**, *Merc.*, Mez., Mos., *Nat. m.*, Nit. ac., NUX V., Oleand., Op., Petrol., *Phos.*, Pho. ac., *Phyt.*, *Plat.*, Pb., Pod., PULS., RHUS, Ruta, **Sang.**, Sec. c., **Sep.**, **Sil.**, Spig., Spo., *Stan.*, Staph., Stram., **Sul.**, Sul. ac., Thuj., **Verat. a.**, Verat. v., Zinc.

Glands.—*Ars.*, **Bell.**, Bry. Calc. c., *Con.*, Merc., *Phos.*, Sul.

Bones.—Chin., Cyc., (Eup. per.), Hep., *Puls.*, *Ruta*, Sabi., Sil., Staph.

Skin.—Acon., Arn., *Ars.*, Bar. c., *Bell.*, Bry., Calc. c., **Caust.**, Con., Dulc., Hep., K. carb., Lach., **Lyc.**, **Merc.**, Nat. m., Nit ac., *Phos.*, Pho. ac., PULS., Rhus, Saba., Sep., Sil., Spo., Squ., Staph., SUL., Thuj.

Sleep and Dreams.—(Arg. n.), Bell., Con., Nux v., Phos., Puls., Sep., Sil.

Blood, Circulation and Fever.—*Acon.*, Arn., ARS., **Bell.**, (Berb.) *Bry.*, Calc. c., Carb. v., Caust., *Cham.*, Chin., Hep., Ip., *K. carb.*, Kre. *Lyc.*, **Merc.**, **Nux v.**, Op., *Phos.*, **Puls.**, Rhus, Sang., Sec. c., *Sep.*, *Sil.*, Spig., Stan., *Staph.*, *Sul.*, *Verat. a.*

Aggravations: Time and Circumstances.—Aesc., (All. c.), (Aloe), *Am. carb.*, *Ant. cr.*, Apis, (Apoc. c.), (Arg. n.), Arn., *Ars.*, (Arum. t.), Asaf., Asar., Aur., (Bap.), **Bell.**, **Bry.**, Calc. c., *Camph.*, (Cannab. i.), Cannab. s., Caps., Carb. an., *Carb. v.*, Caust., Cham., Chel., Chin., Cic., (Cimic.), Coff., Colch., Coloc., **Con.**, Dulc., (Gel.), (Glon.), *Graph.*, **HEP.**, **Ign.**, Ip., K. bi., *K. carb.*, *K. nit.*, Lach., Laur., Led., (Lil. t.), **Lyc.**, Mang., Merc., *Nat. m.*, *Nit. ac.*, Nux m., NUX V., Petrol., *Phos.*, (Phyt.), (Pod.), **Puls.**, Ran. b., Rhodo., Rhus, Saba., *Sang.*, Sele., Sep., SIL., Spig., Squ., Staph., *Stro.*, Sul., *Thuj.*, Valer., (Verat. v.), *Zinc.*

Other Remedies.—Acon., Aesc., *Aloe*, Am. carb., *Apis*, **Arg. n.**, Arn., *Ars.*, (Arum. t.), Bap., **Bell.**, (Berb.), *Bry.*, Cact., *Calc. c.*, Camph., *Cannab. i.*, Carb. v., Caust., *Cham.*, Chin., *Cimic.*, *Con.*, (Crotal.), **Gel.**, *Glon.*, Graph., Hep., Hyos., Ign., Ip., *K. bi.*, *K. carb.*, Lach., Lil. t., **Lyc.**, *Merc.*, Nat. m., Nit. ac., **Nux v.**, Op., Petrol., **Phos.**, Pho. ac., *Phyt.*, Pod., PULS., Rhus, Ruta, Saba., Sang., Sele., *Sep.*, Sil., Spig., Stan., Staph., Stram., *Sul.*, Sul. ac., Thuj., Verat. a., Verat. v., Zinc.

Antidotes.—*Camph.*, Cham., Cup., Ign., *Nux v.*

Injurious.—Coff.

Coffea.

Mind.—*Aur.*, *Bell.*, *Cannab. i.*, Hyos., *Lach.*, Nux m., Nux v., OP., Phos., Pic. ac., Stram., Sul. ac., *Thea*, Verat. a., Vio. o.

Localities.—Acon., (All. c.), (Apis), (Arg. n.), Arn., (Arum. t.), AUR., (Bap.), BELL., *Bry.*, Calc. c., (Cannab. i.), Cham., Chin., (Cimic.), Con., (Fl. ac.), (Gel.), Graph., Hep., (K. bi.), LYC., Merc., Nux v., *Phos.*, Puls., Sep., Spig., Stram., Sul., Verat. v.

Sensations.—Acon., (Arg. n.), Arn., *Asar.*, Aur., Bell., Bry., Calc. c., Canth., *Cham.*, Chin., Cocc., Con., Fer., Gel., Hyos., Ign., Lyc., Mar., Nat. c., Nux m., NUX V., Op., Petrol., Phos., *Puls.*, Rhus, Sep., *Sil.*, Stram., Sul., Verat. a.

Glands.

Bones.

Skin.—Acon., Arn., Ars., Bell., *Bry.*, Calc. c., Hyos., Ip., K. carb., Led., Lyc., Merc., Nux v., Op., Phos., Pho. ac., Puls., *Rhus*, Sep., Sil., Squ., Sul.

Sleep and Dreams.—Arg. n., *Ars.*, (Bap.), Calc. c., *K. carb.*, (Lil. t.), Nux v., Puls., *Sep.*, *Sil.*

Blood, Circulation and Fever.—Ars., Bry., Calc. c., Lyc., Nux v., *Puls.*, Sep.

Aggravations: Time and Circumstances.—Acon., (Aesc.), (Aloe), (Apis), Arg. n., Arn., (Bap.), Bell., Bry., (Cact.), Calad., Calc. c., Camph., (Cannab. i.), Carb. an., *Carb. v.*, Cham., Chel., Chin., (Cimic.), *Cocc.*, Colch., Con., Dros., (Glon.), Graph, Hep., Hyos., Ign., Ip., K. bi., K. carb., K. nit., Lach., Led., (Lil. t.), *Lyc.*, Merc., Nat. m., Nux m., NUX V., Op., Phos., Pho. ac., (Phyt.), (Pod.), Puls., Rhus, (Sang.), Sele., *Sep.*, *Sil.*, Spig., Squ., Staph., Stram., (Verat. v.).

Other Remedies.—*Acon*, (Apis), Arg. n., Arn., *Ars.*, *Aur.*, (Bap.), BELL., Bry., *Calc. c.*, Cannab. i., *Cham.*, Chel., *Chin.*, (Cimic.), Cocc., Con., (Gel.), *Hyos.*, Ign., (K. bi.), K. carb., (Lil. t.), Lyc., Merc., NUX V., *Op.*, *Phos.*, Puls., Rhus, Sele., Sep., *Sil.*, Spig., Stram., Sul., Verat. a., (Verat. v.).

Antidotes.—Acon., Cham., Ign., *Nux v.*, Puls.

Injurious.—Canth., Caust., Cocc., Ign.

Colchicum.

Mind.—Bell., Calc. c., Caust., Con., Ign., *Lyc.*, Merc., *Nat. c.*, Op., Pho. ac., Puls., *Rhus*, Sep., *Sil.*

Localities.—Acon., *Aesc.*, (All. c.), *Aloe*, Alum., Ant. cr., Apis, Apoc. c., *Arn.*, *Arg. n.*, Ars., (Arum. t.), Aur., **Bap.**, Bell., Berb., *Bry.*, **Calc.**

c., Cannab. i., Canth., Carb. ac., Caust., Cham., Cimic., (Crotal.), Dig., (Dios.), Eup. per., (Fl. ac.), Gel., Hep., *Ign.*, Iris v., *K. bi.*, *K. carb.*, Lil. t., (Lith.), *Lyc.*, Mag. m., MERC., Nat. c., *Nat. m.*, Nit. ac., Nux v., (Phyt.), Pod., Pso., **Puls.**, *Rhus*, Sang., SEP., Sil., *Spig.*, *Staph.*, Sul., *Verat. a.*, Verat. v.

Sensations.—Acon., (Aesc.), Ant. cr., Apis, (Apoc. c.), *Arg. n.*, *Arn.*, Ars., (Arum. t.), (Bap.), **Bell.**, (Berb.), Bry., *Calc. c.*, Cannab. i., Caust., Cham., Chin., Cimic., Cocc., Coloc., (Crotal.), Dig., (Dios.), (Gel.), (Glon.), Hell., Ign., (Iris v.), (K. bi.), **K. carb.**, (Kalm.), (Lil. t.), (Lith.), Lyc., *Merc.*, Nat. c., **Nux v.**, Phos., Pho. ac., (Phyt.), **Plat.**, (Pso.), **Puls.**, Rhodo., RHUS, Sang., Sec. c., **Sep.**, Spig., Spo., Squ., Sul., Zinc.

Glands.

Bones.—Bell., *Calc. c.*, Chin., *Puls.*, Rhus, Sep.

Skin.—Acon., Ars., Bell., Bry., *Calc. c.*, Caust., Ip., *Led.*, Lyc., *Merc.*, PULS., Rhus, Sil., Spo., Sul.

Sleep and Dreams.

Blood, Circulation and Fever.—*Ars.*, (Berb.), (Cact.), Calc. c., Cham., (Gel.), (Glon.), Hep., Nat. m., *Nux v.*, *Rhus*, (Sang.), *Sil.*, Sul.

Aggravations: Time and Circumstances.—Aesc., (All. c.), Apis, (Arg. n.), Arn., Ars., Asar., Aur., (Bap.), **Bell.**, **Bry.**, (Cact.), *Calad.*, Calc. c., Cannab. s., (Cimic.), *Cocc.*, *Coff.*, *Con.*, (Crotal.), Glon., Hep., Hyos., *Ign.*, Iod., Ip., K. bi., *Led.*, Lil. t., *Lyc.*, Mag. c., *Merc.*, Nat. m., *Nit. ac.*, *Nux m.*, NUX V., Phos., Phyt., Puls., Ran. b., Rheum, Rhus, Sang., Sars., Sele., *Sep.*, Sil., Spig., *Squ.*, Staph., Stro., *Sul.*, (Verat. v.).

Other Remedies.—Acon., Aesc., (All. c.), (Aloe), Apis, (Apoc. c.), *Arg. n.*, Arn., *Ars.*, (Arum. t.), Bap., **Bell.**, Berb., **Bry.**, (Cact.), Calc. c., Cannab. i., Caust., Cham., Chin., Cimic., Cocc., Con., (Crotal.), Gel., Glon., *Hep.*, *Ign.*, K. bi., K. carb., Led., Lil. t., (Lith.), Lyc., Merc., Nat. c., Nat. m., Nit. ac., Nux v., Phos., Plat., (Pod.), PULS., RHUS, *Sang.*, SEP., *Sil.*, *Spig.*, Squ., Staph., **Sul.**, (Verat. v.).

Antidotes.—Bell., Camph., Cocc., *Nux v.*, *Puls.*

Colocynthis.

Mind.—Anac., Aur., *Cup.*, Hyos., Lyc., Stram., Verat. a.

Localities.—*Aesc.*, All. c., *Aloe*, Apis, *Apoc. c.*, **Arg. n.**, Arn., Arum. t., Bap., Bell., Berb., *Calc. c.*, *Cannab. i.*, Canth., Carb. ac., Carb. v., Chin., (Cimic.), (Crotal.), Dios., (Eup. per.), (Fl. ac.), Gel., (Glon.), Ign., Iris v., *K. bi.*, K. carb., (Kalm.), Lil. t., (Lith.), *Lyc.*, (Meli.), Merc., Nat. m., Nit. ac., **Nux v.**, Petrol., *Phos.*, **Pho. ac.**, (Phyt.), Pod., Pso.,

382 RELATIONSHIPS.—COLOC.—CON.

PULS., *Rhus*, Sang., **Sep., Sil., Spig.**, Sul., Thuj., Valer., Verat. **a,** (Verat. v.).

Sensations.—Aesc., Aloe, Apis, Arg. n., Arn., Arum. t., Asaf., Bap., *Bell., Berb.,* Cact., *Calc. c., Cannab. i.,* **Caust.,** Chin., *Cimic.,* Cocc., Con., (Dios.), (Eup. per.), Gel., *Glon.,* **Graph.,** *Ign., Iris* v., *K. bi., K. carb.,* (Kalm.), *Lil. t.,* Lith., *Lyc.,* Merc., Nat. m., Nit. ac., *Nux v.,* Petrol., Phos., Pho. ac., Phyt., **Plat.,** *Pod., Puls., Rhus,* Sang., **Sep., Sil.,** Spig., Spo., Stro., *Sul.,* Sul. ac., Thuj., Verat. a., Verat. v.

Glands.—*Bell.,* Carb. an., Con., Lyc., Phos., Puls., Sul.

Bones.—Arg., Bell., Pho. ac., Puls., Staph.

Skin.—Acon., *Arn., Bell., Phos.,* **Puls.,** Rhus, Sul.

Sleep and Dreams.—Bell., *Nux v.,* Puls.

Blood, Circulation and Fever.—Acon., Ars., *Bell.,* **Bry.,** Canth., Chin., Hyos., Merc., Nux v., Phos., Stram., Sul.

Aggravations: Time and Circumstances.—Aesc., Aloe, (Apis), Arg. n., Ars., Asaf., Aur., (Bap.), *Bell., Bry.,* Calc. c., **Cham.,** (Cimic.), Con., Dros., *Fer.,* (Glon.), Hep., **Ign.,** K. bi., K. carb., Lil. t., (Lith.), *Lyc.,* Mang., *Merc.,* Nat. m., Nit. ac., **Nux v.,** Phos., Pho. ac., (Phyt.), Plat., (Pod.), PULS., Rhodo., *Rhus,* Sang., Sep., Sil., Spig., **Staph.,** Sul., Verat. a., Zinc.

Other Remedies.—Aesc., *Aloe,* Apis, Arg. n., Arn., Arum. t., Bap., **Bell.,** Berb., Bry., Calc. c., Caust., Cham., Chin., Cimic., Con., Gel., Glon., Graph., *Ign., K. bi.,* K. carb., *Lil. t.,* Lith., **Lyc.,** Merc., Nat. m., Nit. ac., **Nux v.,** *Phos.,* Pho. ac., Phyt., Plat., *Pod.,* PULS., *Rhus, Sang.,* Sep., Sil., Spig., Staph., *Sul.,* Verat. a., (Verat. v.).

Antidotes.—*Camph.,* (Caust.), (Cham.), Coff., *Staph.*

Conium.

Mind.—Aloe, Anac., Apis, Bap., *Bell.,* Bry., *Calc. c.,* **Cannab. i.,** Cannab. s., Carb. ac., Caust., *Cimic.,* Crotal., Gel., *Glon.,* Graph., Hell., Hyd. ac., Hyper., *Hyos., Ign.,* Laur., Lyc., Meli., Merc. c., Nat. c., Nat. m., Nux m., Nux v., Op., Petrol., *Phos.,* Pho. ac., Phyt., *Pic. ac.,* Pso., PULS., Rhus, Sep., Sil., STRAM., Sul., Tab., Ter., Ther., **Verat. a., Verat. v.**

Localities.—Acon., Aesc., All. c., Aloe, *Apis,* Apoc. c., ARG. N., *Arn,* Ars., Arum. t., Aur., Bap., **Bell.,** Berb., *Bry.,* (Cact.), **Calc. c., Cannab. i.,** Cannab. s., (Carb. ac.), *Caust., Cham.,* Chin., Cimic., Cocc., (Crotal.), Dios., (Eup. per.), Euphr., Fl. ac. Gel., (Glon.), *Graph.,* Hep., *Hyos., Ign.,* (Iris v.), K. bi., K. carb., (Kalm.), Lil. t., Lyc., (Meli.), **Merc.,** *Nat. m.,* Nit. ac., **Nux v.,** Oleand., Op. *Petrol.,* **Phos.,** Pho. ac., (Phyt.), (Pic.

RELATIONSHIPS.—CON.

ac.), Pod., *Pso.*, PULS., *Rhus, Saba., Sang.*, **Sep.**, **Sil.**, Spig., *Staph., Stram.*, Sul , *Verat. a., Verat. v.*

Sensations.—Acon., Aesc., (Aloe), Alum., Anac., Apis, (Apoc. c.), *Arg. n., Arn., Ars.,* (Arum. t.), Asaf., Aur., Bap., BELL., Berb., *Bry.,* Cact., **Calc.** c., *Cannab. i.,* (Carb. ac.), *Caust.,* Cham., **Chin.**, Cimic., *Cocc.,* (Crotal.), Cup., (Dios.), *Gel., Glon.,* Graph., *Ign.,* Iod., Iris v., K. bi., *K. carb.*; Lil. t., Lith., **Lyc.**, *Merc.,* Mos., Nat. c., Nat. m., Nit. ac., **Nux v.**, Oleand., Op., *Phos.,* Pho. ac., Phyt., Plat., (Pod.), (Pso.), **Puls.**, *Rhus, Sang.*, **Sep.**, *Sil., Spig.,* Spo., Stan , Staph., Stram., Stro., **Sul.**, Valer., (Verat. v.).

Glands.—*Ars.,* Arum. t., **Bell.**, Bry., Carb. an., Cham., Clem., Hep., Lyc., Nit. ac., PHOS., Puls., *Rhus,* **Sep.**, Sil., Spo., **Sul.**

Bones.—Asaf., Bell., *Calc. c.,* (Cimic.), (Eup. per.), Lyc., **Merc.**, **Nit. ac.**, PULS., Ruta, *Sep.,* Sil., Staph., **Sul.**

Skin.—(Aloe), *Arn., Ars.,* Bar. c., *Bell.,* Bry., **Calc.** c., (Carb. ac.), Carb. v., Caust., Clem., Crotal., Dulc., *Graph., Hep.,* K. carb., Lach., **Lyc.**, *Merc.,* Mez., Nit. ac., Nux v., Petrol., Phos., Pho. ac., **Puls.**, Rhus, Sep., SIL., Staph., Stro., SUL , Sul. ac., Vio. t.

Sleep and Dreams.—Ant. t., (Apis), Arg. n., Bell., Bry., **Calc.** c. Cannab. i., Caust. Croc., **Graph.**, Hep., Ign., Merc., *Nat. c.,* Nux m. NUX V., **Op.**, Phos., *Pho. ac.,* (Pod.), Puls., *Sep.,* Sil., **Sul.**

Blood, Circulation and Fever.—**Ars.**, Aur., Bell., (Cact.), Camph., (Cannab. i.), Chin., Nux v., Phos., Puls., RHUS, Sep., Sul., Verat. a.

Aggravations: Time and Circumstances.—*Acon.,* (Aesc.), (All. c.), Aloe, Apis, Arg. n., *Arn.,* Ars., *Aur.,* Bap., Bar. c., Bell., Bry., (Cact.), **Calc.** c., (Cannab. i.,), **Caps.**, *Carb. v.,* Caust., Cham., Chin , (Cimic.), Cocc., Croc., (Crotal.),Cyc., *Dros., Dulc., Euphorb.,* Euphr., **Fer.**, (Gel.), (Glon.), Graph., *Hep.,* Ign., K. bi., *K. carb.,* Lil. t., LYC., Merc., Nat. c., *Nat. m.,* Nux v., **Phos.**, *Pho. ac.,* (Phyt.) Plat., (Pod.), PULS., Rhus, Saba., *Samb.,* Sang., **Sep.**, **Sil.**, Spig., **Sul.**, Tar., Valer., Verat. v., Vio. t.

Other Remedies.—Acon., Aesc., (All. c.), *Aloe,* **Apis**, (Apoc. c.), **Arg., n.**, *Arn., Ars.,* Arum. t., Aur., **Bep.**, **Bell.**, Berb., *Bry.,* Cact., **Calc.** c., CANNAB. I., Caps., Carb. v., *Caust.,* Cham., **Chin**, *Cimic.,* Cocc., *Crotal.,* Dulc., Fer., **Gel.**, *Glon.,* Graph., *Hep.,* Hyos., *Ign.,* K. bi., K. carb., Lil. t., **Lyc.**, *Merc ,* Nat. c., *Nat. m.,* **Nit. ac.**, **Nux** v., Op., Petrol., **Phos.**, *Pho. ac.,* Phyt., Pod., PULS., **Rhus**, Saba., *Sang.,* **Sep.**, **Sil.**, Spig., Staph., Stram., SUL., Verat. a.; **Verat. v.**

Antidotes.—Coff., Nit. ac., *Spir. nit. dul.*

Crocus.

Mind.—Anac., Aur., **Bell.**, Carb. an, *Hyos.*, Lach., *Lyc.*, Merc. c., Nat. c., Op., Plat., *Stram.*, **Verat. a.**, *Verat. v.*, Zinc.

Localities.—Acon., *Apis*, (Bap.), **Bell.**, Bry., (Cact.), **Calc. c.**, Caust., Cham., Chin., (Cimic.), *Con.*, Gel., Hep., Hyos., Lyc., *Merc.*, NUX V., **Phos.**, Pho. ac., *Puls.*, Rhus, (Sang.), *Sep.*, *Spig.*, *Sul.*, Verat. a., (Verat. v.), Zinc.

Sensations.—Acon., Alum., (Arg. n.), **Arn.**, Asar., Aur., (Bap.), *Bell.* Bry. Calc. c., (Cannab. i.). Carb. v., Caust., *Chin.*, Cocc., Fer., G ., Graph., Hyos., Ign., K. carb., (Kalm.), *Lyc.*, **Merc.**, Nat. m., N . ac. Nux v., Phos., Plat., PULS., Rhodo., **Rhus**, *Sep.*, Sil., Spig., SUL.

Glands.

Bones.

Skin.—Asaf., Bar. c., Calc. c., Carb. v., *Cham.*, Chin., Hep., K. carb., Lyc., *Merc.*, Nit. ac., Petrol., **PULS.**, Rhus, *Sep.*, **Sil.**, Spig., SUL.

Sleep and Dreams.—(Aloe), **Ant. t.**, Apis, Ars., Bry., *Cannab. i.*, *Con.*, Cup., Ign., Lach., Laur., *Nux m.*, *Nux v.*, **Op.**, **Phos.**, Pho. ac., Pod., *Puls.*, Rhus, Sil., Staph., Verat. a.

Blood, Circulation and Fever.—(Arg. n.), *Bell.*, Bry., (Glon.), Hep., *Sul.*

Aggravations: Time and Circumstances.—(Aesc.), (Aloe), *Alum.*, Anac., (Apis), (Arg. n.), Arn., Asar., (Bap.), **Bell.**, Bry., (Cact.), **Calc. c.**, (Cannab. i.), Cannab. s., Caps., Cham., *Chel.*, (Cimic.), *Cocc.*, Dros., (Gel.), (Glon.), Graph., Hep., *Ign.*, **Iod.**, (K. bi.), K. carb., K. nit., (Lil. t.), Lyc., Merc., Nat m., **Nux v.**, *Phos.*, Pho. ac., Phyt., (Pod.), PULS., Rhus, Ruta, Sabi., Sang., Seneg., *Sep.*, Sil., *Spig.*, Squ., Staph., Sul., (Verat. v.).

Other Remedies.—(Aloe), Alum., Ant. t., Apis, (Arg. n.), Arn. (Bap.), Bell., *Bry.*, (Cact.), **Calc. c.**, Cannab. i., Cham., Chin., (Cimic.), Cocc., Con., Gel., (Glon.), *Hep.*, Hyos., *Ign.*, Iod., K. carb., Lyc., Merc. Nux v., *Op*, Phos., Pho. ac., (Pod.), PULS., *Rhus*, Sabi., (Sang.), **Sep.**, *Sil.*, *Spig.*, Sul., *Verat. a.*, Verat. v.

Antidotes.—Acon., *Op.*

Crotalus.

Mind.—Anac., Apis, Ars., Aur., *Bap.*, *Bell.*, Bry., Camph., Cannab. i., Canth., Cic., Cocc., *Con.*, Cup., Gels., Hell., *Hyd. ac.*, *Hyos.*, Ip., *Lach.*, Lyc., Merc., Merc. c., Nat. c., *Nat. m.*, Nux m., Oleand., *Op.*, *Petrol.*, Phos., Pho. ac., *Rhus t.*, Sele., Sil., Spig., *Stram.*, Sul., *Verat. a.*, Verat. v.

Localities.—Acon., (Agar.), (Aloe.), (Alum.), (Am. m.), (Ant. t.),

RELATIONSHIPS.—CROTAL. 385

(Apis), (Apoc. c.), (Arg. n.), Arn., Ars., (Asaf.), (Aur.), (Bap.), Bar. c., Bell., (Berb.), *Bry.*, (Cact.), Calc. c., (Cannab. i.), (Cannab. s.), (Canth.), (Caps.), (Carb. ac.), (Carb. an.), Carb. v., (Caust.), Cham., Chel., Chin., (Clem.), (Cocc.), (Colch.), (Coloc.), (Con.), (Croc.), Cup., (Dig.), Dros., (Dulc.), (Fer.), (Gel.), (Hep.), (Hyos.), Ign., Ip., (Iod.), (K. bi.), (K. carb.), (K. nit.), (Kalm.), Lach., (Led.), (Lil. t.), Lyc., Merc., (Mos.), (Mur. ac.), Nat. c., Nat. m., Nit. ac., *Nux v.*, (Op.), (Petrol.), *Phos.*, (Pho. ac.), (Plat.), (Pb.), (Pod.), *Puls.*, (Rhodo.), Rhus, (Ruta.), (Saba.), (Sabi.), (Sang.), (Sec. c.), (Sele.), (Seneg.), Sep., (Sil.), (Spig.), (Spo.), (Stan.), Stram., Sul., (Thuj.), (Valer.), Verat. a., (Verat. v.), Zinc.

Sensations.—(Ant. t.), Arg. n., (Arn.), Ars., Bell., Bry., Calc. c., (Canth.), Caust., (Chin.), (Cic.), (Con.), (Cup.), (Fer.), (Gel.), Iod., (K. carb.), Lach., (Led.), Lyc., Merc., (Mur. ac.), Nat. m., (Nit. ac.), Nux v., (Op.), Phos, (Pho. ac.), (Plat.), (Pb.), Puls., (Ran. b.), (Rhodo.), Rhus, (Sabi.), (Sec. c.), Sep., Sil., (Spo.), (Stan.), (Stram.), Sul., (Sul. ac.), Verat. a.).

Glands.

Bones.

Skin.—Aloe, Ambr., Am. m., (Ant. t.), Ars., Aur., Bell., Bry., (Camph.), Canth., (Caps.), Carb. v., (Caust.), Cham., Chel., Chin., Con., Dig., (Dios.), Fer., (Hyd. ac), Ign., Lyc., (Mez.), Nit. ac., (Nux m.), *Nux v.*, Op., Phos., Pb, Rhus, (Samb.), Sec. c., **Sep.**, Spig., *Sul.*, Verat. a.

Sleep and Dreams.

Blood, Circulation and Fever.—(Ars.), (Bell.), (Bry.), (Dig.), (Iod.), (Merc.), (Phos.), (Pho. ac.), (Sec. c.), (Sil.), (Stan.), (Stram.), (Sul.),

Aggravations: Time and Circumstances.—(Acon.), (Arn.), (Ars.), (Cham.), (Chin.), (Colch.), (Con.), (Dulc.), (Fer.), (Graph.), (Hep.), (Hyos.), (Ip.), (Iod.), (Lach.), (Mag. c.), (Mag. m.), (Mang.), (Merc.), (Nit. ac.), (Phos.), (Pb.), (Puls.), (Rhus), (Sep.), (Sil.), (Stro.), (Sul.), (Zinc).

Other Remedies.—(Acon.), (Aloe), (Am. m.), (Ant. t.), (Apis), (Arg. n.) Arn., **Ars.**, Aur., Bap., Bell., **Bry.**, Calc. c., (Camph.), (Cannab. i.), Canth., Carb. v., Caust., Cham., Chel., Chin. (Cic.), (Cocc.), (Colch.), *Con.*, Cup., Dig., (Dulc.), Fer., Gel., (Hep.), Hyd. ac., Hyos., Ign., Ip., Iod., (K. carb.), *Lach.*, (Led.), *Lyc.*, *Merc.*, (Mur. ac.), Nat. c., *Nat. m.*, Nit. ac., (Nux m.), *Nux v*, *Op.*, Petrol., **Phos.**, Pho. ac., (Plat.), Pb., Puls., (Rhodo.), **Rhus**, (Sabi.), Sec. c., (Sele.), *Sep.*, *Sil.*, (Spig.), (Spo.), (Stan.), *Stram.*, **Sul.**, *Verat. a.*, (Verat. v.) (Zinc).

Cuprum.

Mind.—Anac., Apis, *Ars.*, *Aur.*, *Bap.*, **Bell.**, *Cannab. i.*, Cic., *Cimic.*, Crotal., Gel., Glon., *Hyd. ac.*, **Hyos.**, *Lyc.*, Meli., Merc. c., Nat. m., Nux v., *Op.*, Rhus, STRAM., *Ter.*, **Verat. a.**, Verat. v.

Localities.—Acon., Aesc., (All. c.), Aloe., Apis, Apoc. c., *Arg. n.*, Ars., (Arum t.), Aur., (Bap.), BELL., *Bry.*, Cact., Camph., Cannab. i., Carb. ac., Cham., *Chin.*, Cic., (Cimic.), Cina., Cocc., Con., Crotal., Dios., (Eup. per.), (Fl. ac.), (Gel.), (Glon.), Hep., (Hyd. ac.), Hyos., Ign., Ip., (Iris v.), *K. bi.*, *Lyc.*, Merc., Nit. ac., **Nux v.**, *Op.*, Phos., Pho ac., Phyt., Pod., Pso., *Puls.*, Rhus, Sang., Sec. c., *Sep.*, Sil., Stan., *Stram.*, Sul., VERAT. A., Verat. v.

Sensations.—Acon., (Aesc.), (Aloe.), (Apis), **Arg. n.**, *Ars.*, Arum t.), (Bap.), Bar. c., BELL., Bry., Cact., **Calc. c.**, Cannab. i., Caust., **Cham.**, *Chin.*, *Cic.*, Cimic., Cocc., *Con.*, (Crotal.), (Dios.), Gel., (Glon.), Hyos., *Ign.*, Ip., (Iris v.), (K. bi.), Lach., Lil. t., (Lith.), *Lyc.*, *Merc.*, **Nux v**, **Op.**, Phos., Pho. ac., (Phyt.), Puls., Sang., **Sec. c.** *Sep.*, *Sil.*, Stan., *Stram.*, Sul., *Verat. a.*, (Verat. v.).

Glands.—Ars., Bell., Bry., Carb an., Con., Merc., Phos., Rhus, Sep., *Sul.*

Bones.—Arg., *Chin.*, (Eup. per.), Sabi., Staph.

Skin.—Am. m., Ant. cr., Ars., *Bell.*, **Calc. c.**, Clem., Dulc., Hep., Mag. c., *Merc.* Phos., Puls., Rhus, Sep., Sil., Verat. a.

Sleep and Dreams.—Ant. t., (Cannab. i.), Croc., Ign., Op., Puls.

Blood, Circulation and Fever.—Acon., (Apis), Bell., Camph., Cannab. i., **Carb. v.**, Dig., (Gel.), (Glon.), Guai., Hyos., Laur., Merc., Op., (Sang.), Sil., *Stram.*, VERAT. A., (Verat. v.).

Aggravations: Time and Circumstances.—(Aesc.), (Apis), (Arg. n.), Arn., *Ars.*, Bell., Bry., *Calc. c.*, Carb. v., Caust., Cham., Chin., Colch., Fer., Graph., Ign., **Lyc.**, *Merc.*, **Nux v.**, *Phos.*, (Pod.), PULS., Rhus, Sep., Sil., *Spig.*, Sul., Verat. a.

Other Remedies.—Acon., Aesc., (Aloe), *Apis*, *Arg. n.*, **Ars.**, (Arum t.), Aur., Bap., BELL., *Bry.*, *Calc. c.*, *Cannab. i.*, Carb. v., Cham., *Chin.*, Cic., Cimic., *Con.*, Crotal., Gel., Glon., **Hyos.**, *Ign.*, Ip., K. bi., *Lyc.*, *Merc.*, **Nux v.**, Op., Phos., Pho. ac., (Phyt.), (Pod.), *Puls.*, Rhus, Sang., Sec. c., **Sep.**, *Sil.*, *Stram.*, Sul., VERAT. A., *Verat. v.*

Antidotes.—Aur., Bell., *Camph.*, Chin., Cocc., Dulc., *Hep.*, Ip., Merc., Nux v., Saccharum.

Cyclamen.

Mind.—Anac., *Aur.*, *Bell.*, Con., Crotal., Graph., Hyos., *Ign.*, Lyc., Nux m., Op., Pho. ac., Plat., Puls., Rhus, Sep., *Stram.*, Sul., Verat. a.

Localities.—(Aesc.) (All. c.), *Alum.*, Anac., (Apis), Arg. n., Ars., *Bell.*, *Bry.*, **Calc. c.**, (Carb. ac.), Caust., **Chin.**, (Cimic.), Con., (Dios.), (Fl. ac.), Gel., Hyos., Ign., K. bi., K. carb., **Lyc.**, *Merc.*, **Nux v.**, Petrol. Phos., Pho. ac., **PULS.**, Rhus, *Sep.*, Sil., *Spig.*, Staph., **Sul.**, Thuj., *Verat. a.*, (Verat. v.), Verb.

Sensations.—*Acon.*, Anac., *Arn.*, *Ars.*, *Bar. c*, *Bell.*, Calc. c, **Carb. v.**, Caust., Cham., Chel., *Chin.*, (Cimic.), **Cocc.**, Guai., Ign., (Iris v.), (K. bi.), K. carb., *Lyc.*, Nat. m., *Nux m.*, *Nux v.*, Oleand., **PHOS.**, *Pho. ac.*, Plat., *Puls.*, Rhus, *Ruta*, Sabi., Sep., **Staph.**, *Sul.*, Sul. ac., **Tar.**, Zinc.

Glands.—Bell., Bry., Calc. c., *Cocc.*, Con., Lyc., Sul.

Bones.—*Arg.*, Phos.

Skin.—Arn., **Ars.**, Asaf., Bar. c., *Bry.*, **Calc. c.**, Carb. v., Caust., Cocc., Con., Graph., Hep., Lach., *Lyc.*, **Merc.**, *Nit. ac.*, Petrol., Phos., PULS., RHUS, SEP., *Sil.*, Spo., Staph., SUL., Thuj., Vio. t.

Sleep and Dreams.—(Apis), Ars., Calc. c., (Cannab. i.), K. carb., Nux v., (Pod.).

Blood, Circulation and Fever.—Acon., (Apis), **Ars.**, **Bell.**, Euphorb., (Gel.), Hell., Ign., Nux m., *Nux v.*, Phos., **Puls.**, *Rhus*, *Saba.* SEP., *Spig.*, Sul.

Aggravations: Time and Circumstances.—(Aloe), Am. m., Ant. t., (Apis), (Arg. n.), Ars., *Asaf.*, Aur., (Bap.), Bell., Bry., Calc. c, **Caps.**, Carb. v., Caust., Cham., **Con.**, *Dros.*, *Dulc.*, Euphorb., Euphr., **Fer.**, (K. bi.), Lach., Led., (Lil. t.), **Lyc.**, Mag. m., Meny., Mez., Mur. ac., Nat. c., Nit. ac., Phos., Pho. ac., *Plat.*, PULS., *Ran. s.*, Rhus, Ruta, *Saba.*, *Samb.*, (Sang.), Sep., Stro., Sul., **Tar.**, *Valer.*, *Verb.*, Vio. t.

Other Remedies.—Acon., Anac., Apis, (Arg. n.), Arn., *Ars.*, Asaf., Aur., Bar. c., **Bell.**, Bry., *Calc. c.*, Caps., Carb. v., Caust., Chin., (Cimic.), Cocc., Con., Euphorb., Fer., (Gel.), Ign., K. bi., K. carb., **Lyc.**, Merc., Nit. ac., Nux m., *Nux v.*, Phos., Pho. ac., Plat., PULS., Rhus, Ruta, Saba., **Sep.**, Sil., Spig., Staph., **Sul.**, Tar., Valer., Verat. a., Verb., Vio. t.

Antidotes.—Camph., *Coff.*, Puls.

Digitalis.

Mind.—Acon., Anac., Ars., Aur., Bell., Calc. c., *Graph.*, Ign., **Lyc.**, PULS., Rhus, Stram., Sul.

Localities.—*Acon.*, Aesc., (All. c.), (Aloe), *Apis*, Apoc. c., **Arg. n.**, *Ars.*, (Arum. t.), Bap., BELL., (Berb.), *Bry.*, *Calc. c.*, Cannab. i., Canth., (Carb. ac.), *Cham.*, *Chin.*, Cic., (Cimic.), Clem., Cocc., *Con.*, (Crotal.)

(Eup. per.), Euphr., (Fl. ac.), Gel., (Glon.), *Hep.*, *Hyos.*, Ign., (Iris v.), *K. bi.*, K. carb., Kalm., (Lil. t.), (Lith.), *Lyc.*, (Meli.), **Merc.**, Nat. m., Nux v., Op., **Phos.**, *Pho. ac.*, Phyt., (Pic. ac.), Pod., (Pso.), **PULS.**, *Rhus*, *Ruta*, Sang., Sec. c., **Sep.**, *Sul.*, Spig., Stan., Staph., SUL., Thuj., **Verat. a.**, *Verat. v.*

Sensations.—*Acon.*, (Aesc.), (Aloe), Alum., (Apis), *Arg. n.*, Arn., *Ars.*, Aur., (Bap.), **Bell.**, Bry., (Cact.), *Calc. c.*, (Cannab. i.), Canth., Carb. v., Caust., Cham., CHIN., Cimic., *Cocc.*, Colch., *Con.*, Cup., Fer., (Gel.), Glon., Hell., *Ign.*, Iod., K. carb., (Kalm.), Lach., (Lil. t.), *Lyc.*, *Merc.*, Mez., Nat. m., Nit. ac., NUX V., Oleand., Op., Phos., *Pho. ac.*, Phyt., Plat., Pb., (Pod.), *Puls.*, Rhus, Sang., Seneg., **Sep.**, Spig., Stan., Staph., SUL., *Verat. a.*, (Verat. v.)

Glands.—Bry., Con., Puls.

Bones.

Skin.—Acon., Ant. cr., Arn., *Ars.*, Aur., Bar. c., **Bell.**, Bry., *Calc. c.*, *Caust.*, Cham., Chel., **Chin.**, Cocc., Graph., Hell., *Lach.*, Led., LYC., **Merc.**, Mez., *Nit. ac.*, Nux v., *Oleand.*, Op., Phos., Plat., PULS., Rhus, *Sep.*, Sil., Spo., Squ., Staph., SUL., VERAT. A.

Sleep and Dreams.—Ars., Puls.

Blood, Circulation and Fever.—Acon., Ars., **Bell.**, Bry., (Cact.), Cannab. i., Chel., CHIN., (Cimic.), (Crotal.), Gel., Glon., Hep., *Hyos.*, *K. nit.*, Nat. m., *Pho. ac.*, Sang., *Sep.*, **Stram.**, *Sul.*, Verat. a., Verat. v.

Aggravations: Time and Circumstances.—(Aesc.), (Aloe), Acon., Am. m., **Ant. t.**, (Apis), (Arg. n.), *Arn.*, *Ars.*, (Bap.), **Bell.**, Bry., Calc. c., Cannab. s., Carb. an., Carb. v., Caust., Cham., *Chin.*, Cic., (Cimic.), Cocc., *Colch.*, Con., (Glon.), *Graph.*, *Hep.*, Ign., Iod., Ip., K. bi., **K. carb.**, Led., Lil. t., Lyc., Merc., Nat. c., *Nat. m.*, NUX V., **Phos.**, (Phyt.), (Pod.), **Puls.**, Ran. b., *Rhus*, Sabi., Samb., *Sang.*, *Sep.*, Sil., *Spig.*, Squ., Staph., Sul., (Verat. v.), Zinc.

Other Remedies.—*Acon.*, Aesc., (Aloe), Anac., Ant. t., Apis, *Arg. n.*, Arn., *Ars.*, Aur., Bap., **Bell.**, Bry., (Cact.), *Calc. c.*, Cannab. i., Caust., Cham., **Chin.**, Cimic., Cocc., Colch., *Con.*, *Gel.*, Glon., Graph., Hep., Hyos., *Ign.*, K. bi., K. carb., Lach., Lil. t., **Lyc.**, *Merc.*, Nat. m., Nit. ac., Nux v., Oleand., Op., **Phos.**, Pho. ac., Phyt., Pod., PULS., *Rhus*, Sang., Sep., Sil., Spig., *Staph.*, Stram., SUL., Verat. a., Verat. v.

Antidotes.—*Camph.*, Nux v., Op., Serpentaria.

Injurious.—Chin., Spir. nit. dul.

Drosera.

Mind.—Bar. c., Bell., *Caust.*, *Cic.*, Lyc., *Puls.*, **Sul. ac.**, Zinc.

RELATIONSHIPS.—DROS.

Localities.—Acon., Aesc., All. c., (Aloe), Alum., *Apis*, *Arg. n.*, **Arn.**, *Ars.*, Arum. t., Bap., **Bell.**, **Bry.**, (Cact.), CALC. C., Cannab. i., **Canth.**, **Caps.**, (Carb. ac.), Carb. v., *Caust.*, Cham., Chin., (Cimic.), Cocc., Con., Crotal, (Eup. per.), Gel., Hep., *Hyos.*, **Ign.**, Ip., *K. bi.*, *K. carb.*, Led., *Lyc.*, **Merc.**, Nat. c., *Nat. m.*, Nit. ac., **Nux v.**, Par., Phos., Phyt., Pso., **Puls.**, *Rhus*, Saba., *Sang.*, **Sep.**, **Sil.**, Spig., Staph., Stram., **Sul.**, *Verat. a.*, Verat. v.

Sensations.—Acon., (Aesc.), *Alum.*, **Apis**, Arg., (Arg. n.), *Arn.*, Arum. t., Asaf., (Bap.), **Bell.**, (Berb.), Bry., (Cact.), **Calc. c.**, (Cannab. i.), *Canth.*, Carb. v., Caust., Cham., **Chin.**, Cic., Cimic., *Cocc.*, Con., (Glon.), **Ign.**, Ip., (Iris v.), K. bi., *K. carb.*, Laur., Led., (Lith.), Lyc., Mar., *Merc.*, Mez., Mos., Mur. ac., Nat. c., Nat. m., Nit. ac., *Nux v.*, Par., **Phos.**, Pho. ac., (Phyt.), *Plat.*, (Pso.), **Puls.**, *Ran. s*, *Rhus*, **Ruta**, Sabi., Sang., Sars., *Sep.*, Sil., Spig., Spo., Stan., *Staph.*, **Sul.**, *Sul. ac.*, Verat. a., Zinc.

Glands.

Bones.—Arg., Bell., Chin., Cup., Merc., *Rhus*, Ruta, Sabi., Staph., Sul.

Skin.—*Agn.*, Arn., *Bar. c.*, Bell., **Bry.**, *Calc. c.*, Caust., (Cimic.), *Cyc.*, (Eup. per.), *Graph.*, Hep., *Led.*, Lyc., Merc., Mez., *Nat. c.*, Nat. m., *Nit. ac.*, *Oleand.*, Petrol., *Plat.*, PULS., Ran. s., *Rhus*, Sep., Sil., Spo., Staph., SUL., Thuj., Vio. t., Zinc.

Sleep and Dreams.—Calc. c., *Nux v.*, Sil.

Blood, Circulation and Fever.—(Apis), **Ars.**, Cham., Chin., (Gel.), (Glon.), Nux v., *Rhus,* (Sang.), *Sul.*

Aggravations: Time and Circumstances.—(Aesc.), (Aloe), Am. m. (Apis), Arg., *Ars.*, Asaf., (Bap.), Bry., *Calc. c*, *Caps.*, Carb. v., Cham., *Con.*, *Cyc.*, Dulc., Euphorb., *Fer.*, (Gel.), (Glon.), Graph., Hep., Ign., *Iod.*, (K. bi.), K. carb., *K. nit.*, Led., (Lil. t.), (Lith.), **Lyc.**, *Mag. m.*, Meny., Merc., Mos., Nat. c., *Nux v.*, **Phos.**, *Pho. ac.*, (Phyt.), Plat., Pod., PULS., Rhodo., *Rhus*, Ruta, Saba., Samb., Sang., SEP., *Sul.*, Tar., Valer., Verat. a., Verb., Vio. t.

Other Remedies.—Aesc., (Aloe), Alum., *Apis*, Arg., Arg. n., Arn., *Ars.*, Arum. t., Bap., Bar. c., *Bell.*, *Bry.*, (Cact.), **Calc. c.**, (Cannab. i), Canth., Caps., Carb. v., *Caust.*, Cham., *Chin.*, Cic., Cimic., Cocc., Con., Cyc., Gel., (Glon.), Graph., Hep., *Ign.*, K. bi., K. carb., Led., (Lith.), Lyc., *Merc.*, Nat. c., Nat. m., Nit. ac., **Nux v.**, Par., *Phos.*, Pho. ac., (Phyt.), Plat., PULS., Ran. s., Rhus, Ruta, *Sang.*, Sep., *Sil.*, Spo., Staph., SUL., Sul. ac., Verat. a., Zinc.

Antidote.—Camph.

Dulcamara.

Mind.—Ars., Bell., Lach., *Lyc.*, Plat., Stram., *Verat. a.*

Localities.—(Aesc.), (All. c.), Aloe, Ant. cr., *Apis*, Apoc. ., **Arg. n.**, Arn., **Ars.**, Bap., *Bell.*, Bry., (Cact.), Calc. c., (Cannab. i.), (Carb. ac.), Carb. v., Caust., *Cham., Chin.,* (Cimic.), (Crotal.), *Dios.,* (Eup. per.), Gel., Graph., Hyos., Ign., Ip., Iris v., *K. bi.,* K. carb., Laur., Lil. t., Lyc., **Merc.**, Nat. c., Nat. m., *Nit. ac., Nux v.,* Oleand., *Phos.,* Pho. ac., Plat., Pb., *Pod.,* Pso., PULS., Rhus, Sang., *Sep.,* Sil., Spig., Stan., Staph. *Sul.*, Sul. ac., (Ther.), Verat. a., Verat. v.

Sensations.—*Acon.,* Anac., (Apis), Arg. n., Arn., *Ars.,* (Arum t.), *Asaf.,* **BELL.**, Berb., Bism., *Bry.,* CALC. C., Carb. v., Caust., *Chin.,* (Cimic.), Cina, Cocc., Con., (Crotal.), (Dios.), Gel., (Glon.), Graph., Hell., Hyos, (Iris v.), K. bi., K. carb., Laur., (Lith.), *Lyc., Merc.,* Mez., Mur. ac., *Nat. c.,* Nat. m., *Nit. ac., Nux v.,* Oleand., Phos., Plat., (Pso.), Puls., Rhodo., **Rhus**, Ruta, (Sang.), Sele., Sep., *Sil.,* Spig., *Stan.,* Staph., Sul., Verat. a., Zinc.

Glands.—Ars., (Arum t.), **Bell.**, Bry., *Con.,* Hep., Lyc., *Sil.,* **Sul.**

Bones.—Calc. c., Merc., Puls.

Skin.—Acon., Am. carb., *Ant. cr., Apis, Ars., Bell.,* Bov., *Bry.,* **Calc. c.**, *Caust.,* Chin., Con., Graph., Hep., K. carb., *Lach.,* Led., Lyc., Mag. c., **Merc.**, Mez., Nat. c., *Nit. ac.,* Oleand., Petrol., *Phos.,* Pho. ac., *Puls.,* RHUS, Sec. c., SEP., *Sil.,* Staph., Sul., Verat. a.

Sleep and Dreams.—Aur., Sep., Sil., Sul. ac.

Blood, Circulation and Fever.—Arn., Bry., Lyc., *Sep.,* Staph.

Aggravations: Time and Circumstances.—(All. c.), (Aloe), Am. carb., (Apis), (Arg. n.), *Ars.,* **Aur.**, (Bap.), Bry., Calc. c., Camph., Cannab s., **Caps.**, Caust., Cham., (Cimic.), *Con., Cyc.,* Dros., Euphorb., *Fer.,* Graph., *Hep.,* Ign., K. bi., *K. carb.,* Lyc., Mag. c., **Mang.**, Merc., Mos., Nux m., *Nux v.,* Phos., (Phyt.), Plat., **Puls.**, RHUS, **Saba.**, *Samb.,* Sang., *Sep.,* Sil., *Stro.,* Sul., Tar., Thuj., Verat. a., (Verat. v.), Verb.

Other Remedies.—Acon., (All. c.), (Aloe), Ant. cr., *Apis,* Arg. n., Arn., *Ars.,* (Arum t.), Aur., (Bap.), **Bell.**, Bry., *Calc. c.,* Caps., Caust., Cham., Chin., (Cimic.), *Con.,* (Crotal.), Fer., Gel., Graph., Hep., *K. bi., K. carb.,* Lach., LYC., *Merc.,* Mez., Nat. c., *Nit. ac.,* Nux v., Oleand., Phos., Plat., (Pod.), **Puls.**, Rhus, Saba., Samb., (Sang.), SEP., *Sil.,* Spig., Stan., Staph., Sul., *Verat. a.,* (Verat. v.).

Antidotes.—*Camph.,* Cup., Ip., Merc.

Injurious.—Bell., Lach.

Euphorbium.

Mind.—Cannab s., *Cocc.*, Con., Led., Lyc., Puls., Sep., Sil., Sul. ac., Thuj.

Localities.—Acon., Aesc., (Apis), (Arg. n.), Arn., Ars., Asaf., **Bell.**, *Bry.*, **Calc. c.**, Caps., Carb. v., *Caust*, *Chin.*, Cocc., Colch., Con., (Gel.), (Glon.), Graph., Hell., Hep., *Ign.*, *K. carb.*, Led., **Lyc.**, Merc., Mez., Nat. c., *Nat. m.*, Nit. ac., *Nux v.*, *Phos.*, **Puls.**, *Rhodo.*, Rhus, Ruta, Sabi., SEP., *Sil.*, Spig., Spo., *Staph.*, Stro., SUL., Verat. a., (Verat. v.), Zinc.

Sensations.—Acon., Anac., Arn., Ars., Asar., *Bell.*, *Bry.*, **Calc. c.**, Canth., Caps., Carb. v., Caust., Chin., Colch., Croc., (Dios.), Ign., (Iris v.), (K. bi.), *K. carb.*, Lach., **Lyc.**, *Merc.*, Mez., Mur. ac., Nat. m., Nit. ac., *Nux v.*, *Phos.*, Plat., *Puls.*, Rhodo., *Rhus*, Saba., (Sang.), *Sep.*, Sil., Stan., Stro., SUL., *Sul. ac.*, Verat. a.

Glands.—Bell., Bry., Calc. c., Merc., Phos., Sul.

Bones.—Asaf., Pho. ac., Sul.

Skin.—*Apis*, *Ars.*, Asaf., Bry., Calc. c., Caust., LACH., **Led.**, **Lyc.**, Merc., Mez., Oleand., PULS., Sec. c., **Sil.**, Spo., Sul.

Sleep and Dreams.—Calc. c., *Chin.*, Ign., Lach., Phos., Rhus, Sul.

Blood, Circulation and Fever.—Acon., Ars., Bell., *Bry.*, Calc. c., Cham., Cyc., Ign., Merc., Nux v., *Phos.*, (Pod.), PULS., Rhus, *Saba.*, *Sep.*, Spig., *Sul.*

Aggravations: Time and Circumstances.—Ambr., Apis, Arg., Ars., Asaf., *Aur.*, Bar. c., Bell., Bry., **Caps.**, *Carb. v.*, Cham., **Con.**, *Cyc.*, Dros., *Dulc.*, FER., (K. bi.), K. carb., (Lil. t.), Lyc., *Mag. m.*, Meny., Mos., Nat. m., Phos., Pho. ac., *Plat.*, PULS., *Rhodo.*, *Rhus*, Ruta, *Saba.*, Samb., Sang., *Sep.*, Sil., Stro., Sul., *Tar.*, *Valer.*, Verat. a., (Verat. v.), Verb.

Other Remedies.—Acon., Apis, *Ars.*, Asaf., Bell., *Bry.*, **Calc. c.**, Caps., Carb. v., Caust., Chin., Cocc., Con., Cyc., Fer., Ign., (K. bi.), K. carb., *Lach.*, Led., **Lyc.**, *Merc.*, Mez., Nat. m., Nux v., *Phos.*, Plat., PULS., Rhodo., *Rhus*, Saba., (Sang.), Sep., *Sil.*, Spig., SUL., Sul. ac., Verat. a., (Verat. v.),

Antidotes.—Camph., Succus. citri.

Euphrasia.

Mind.—Bell., Ign., Phos., Puls., Sep., Sil., Sul.

Localities.—*Acon.*, *All. c.*, Apis, Arg. n., Arum. t., **Bell.**, **Calc. c.**, Cannab. i., Cannab. s., *Caust.*, Chin., (Cimic.), Clem., **Con.**, Dig., Gel., **Hep.**, Hyos., *K. bi.*, (Kalm.), (Lil. t.), *Lyc.*, (Meli.), *Merc.*, Nat. m., Nit. ac., *Nux v.*, *Phos.*, (Pso.), PULS., Rhus, Ruta, Sang., *Sep.*, **Sil.**, Spig., Staph., Stram., SUL., Tell., Verat. v.

Sensations.—Agar., Ars., (Arum. t.), **Bell.**, **Calc. c.**, Caust., Cham., Chin., Cocc., Con., Dros., (Gel.), *Graph.*, *Ign.*, (Iris. v.), K. bi., K. carb., Lyc., *Merc.*, Nat. m., Nit. ac., *Nux v.*, **Phos.**, *Puls.*, Rhus, (Sang.), *Sep.*, *Sil.*, Spig., Spo., *Stan.*, Staph., **Sul.**

Glands.

Bones.

Skin.—Bry., Merc., Pho. ac., Staph., Sul., Thuj.

Sleep and Dreams.—*Calc. c.*, *Con.*, **Graph.**, Nat. c., **NUX V.**, *Phos.*, *Sep.*, Sil., Sul.

Blood, Circulation and Fever.

Aggravations: Time and Circumstances.—Am. m., Ant. cr., (Apis), (Arg. n.), Arn., Asar., (Bap.), *Calc. c.*, Caps., Caust., Cham., Chin., CON., Cyc., Dros., Euphorb., Fer., (Gel.), *Graph.*, *Hep.*, Ign., (K. bi.), (Lil. t.), *Lyc.*, Mag. c., *Meny.*, Nat. c., Nit. ac., *Nux v.*, **Phos.**, *Pho. ac.*, (Phyt.), Plat., **Puls.**, *Rhus*, Ruta, *Saba.*, (Sang.), Sep., *Sul.*, Tar., Valer., Verb.

Other Remedies.—Acon., (Apis), (Arg. n.), (Arum t.), *Bell.*, **Calc. c.**, Caust., Cham., Chin., **Con.**, Dros., Gel., *Graph.*, *Hep.*, Ign., K. bi., (Lil. t.), Lyc., Meny., Merc., Nat. c., Nat. m., Nit. ac., **Nux v.**, PHOS, Pho. ac., **Puls.**, *Rhus*, Ruta, Saba., (Sang.), **Sep.**, *Sil.*, Spig., Stan., Staph., SUL.

Antidote.—Camph.

Ferrum.

Mind.—Acon., Aur., Coff., *Glon.*, Nux v., Plat., Zinc.

Localities.—Acon., Aloe, *Apis*, Apoc. c., Ant. cr., *Arg. n.*, Arn., **Ars.**, Arum. t., Bap., **Bell.**, *Bry.*, Cact., *Calc. c*, Cannab. i., Canth., Caps., (Carb. ac.), Carb. v., *Cham.*, CHIN., (Cimic.), Cina, Crotal., (Dios.), (Eup. per.), Gel., (Glon.), Graph., Hep., *Hyos.*, Ign., *Ip.*, (Iris v.), K. bi., K. carb., (Kalm.), Lil. t., (Lith.), Lyc., Meli., **Merc.**, Nat. m., *Nit. ac.*, **Nux v.**, **PHOS.**, Pho. ac., Phyt., *Plat.*, Pod., Pso., **Puls.**, *Rhus*, Saba., *Sang.*, **Sep.**, *Sil.*, Spig., Stan., Stram., SUL., Verat. a., Verat. v.

Sensations.—*Acon.*, (Aesc.), (Aloe), Ambr., Apis, (Apoc. c.), *Arg. n.*, Arn., *Ars.*, (Arum. t.), Asaf., Aur., Bar. c., **Bell.**, *Bry.*, Cact., **Calc. c.**, Cannab. i., Canth., Caps., *Carb. v.*, Caust., *Cham.*, CHIN., *Cimic.*, Cocc., Con., (Crotal.), Cup., (Eup. per.), Gel., *Glon.*, Graph., *Hyos.*, Ign., Iod., Ip., (Iris v.), (K. bi.), *K. carb.*, (Kalm.), (Lil. t.), (Lith.), **Lyc.**, (Meli.), *Merc.*, Nat. m., Nit. ac., **Nux v.**, Op., *Phos.*, Pho. ac., Phyt., (Pod.), (Pso.), PULS., *Rhus*, Sabi., *Sang.*, Sec. c., **Sep.**, *Sil.*, Spig., Stan., **Sul.**, Verat. a., (Verat. v.).

RELATIONSHIPS.—FER.—GEL. 393

Glands.—Bell., Bry., Lyc.

Bones.—*Asaf.*, **Calc. c.**, *Lyc.*, Merc., Nit. ac., *Phos.*, Puls., **Sil.**, *Sul.*

Skin.—Ars., *Bell.*, Bry., **Calc. c.**, *Chin.*, (Crotal.), **Lyc.**, Merc., Nat. m., Phos., Pho. ac., Puls., Rhus, *Sep.*, Spig., **Sul.**, Verat. a.

Sleep and Dreams.—Ars., Bell., Chin., *Sil.*, Sul.

Blood, Circulation and Fever.—ACON., (Aloe), (Apis), Arg. n., Ars., (Bap.), *Bell.*, (Berb.), Bry., Cact., *Calc. c.*, CHIN., Glon., Hyos., *Iod.*, (Lil. t.), LYC., Phos., *Puls.*, *Sang.*, *Sep.*, *Sul.*, Verat. a.

Aggravations: Time and Circumstances.—*Acon.*, (Aesc.), (Aloe), Am. m., Apis, Arg. n., Arn., *Ars.*, *Aur.*, Bap., Bar. c., Bell., Bry., Calc. c., **Caps.**, *Carb. v.*, Caust., Cham., *Chin.*, (Cimic.), Cina, Cocc., CON., *Cyc.*, Dros., Dulc., **Euphorb.**, Euphr., (Gel.), (Glon.), Ign., K. bi., K. carb., Lach., Led., Lil. t., (Lith.), **Lyc.**, Mag. c., Mag. m., Mang., Mar., Meny., Merc., Nat. c., Nat. m., *Nux v.*, *Phos.*, Pho. ac., (Phyt.), *Plat.* Pod., PULS., Rhodo., Rhus, Saba., *Samb.*, *Sang.*, Sele., *Sep.*, *Sil*, Spig., *Sul.*, Tar., Thuj., *Valer.*, Verat. a., (Verat. v.).

Other Remedies.—*Acon.*, (Aesc.), Aloe, *Apis*, (Apoc. c.), **Arg. n.**, Arn., Ars., (Arum. t.), Aur., Bap., **Bell.**, *Bry.*, Cact., **Calc. c.**, Cannab. i., Caps., Carb. v., Cham., CHIN., Cimic., Con., Crotal., Gel., *Glon.*, Hyos., Ign., Ip., K. bi., K. carb., Lil. t., (Lith.), LYC., *Merc.*, Nat. m., Nit. ac., *Nux v.*, **Phos.**, Pho. ac., Phyt., Plat., Pod., **Puls.**, *Rhus*, Saba., *Sang.*, **Sep.**, Sil., Spig., SUL., Tar., Verat. a., Verat. v.

Antidotes.—Ars., *Chin.*, Ip., *Puls.*, *Thea*, Verat. a.

Gelsemium.

Mind.—Apis, Bap., *Bell.*, Bry., Calc. c., Cannab. i., Cannab. s., Chel., Cic., Cimic., Cocc., *Con.*, Crotal., Dig., Glon., Hyd. ac., Hyos., Ign., K. carb., Laur., Meli., Merc., Mez., Mur. ac., Nat. c., Nat. m., Nux m., Nux v., **Op.**, Petrol., Phos., *Pho. ac.*, Phyt., *Puls.*, Rhus t., *Sep.*, **Sil.**, Spig., Stram., Sul., Tab., Thuj., Zinc.

Localities.—Acon., (Aesc.), Agar., Agn., (All. c.), (Aloe), Alum., Am m., (Anac.), Ant. cr., Ant. t., *Apis*, Apoc. c., Arg., Arg. n., **Arn.**, **Ars.**, Arum. t., Asaf., (Asar.), Aur., (Bap.), Bar. c., BELL., Bism., Bor., *Bry.*, (Cact.), *Calc. c.*, Camph., Cannab. i., (Cannab. s.), Canth., (Caps.), (Carb. ac.), (Carb. v.), *Caust.*, Cham., *Chel.*, Chin., Cic., Cimic., (Cina), (Clem.), Cocc., (Coff.), Colch., Coloc., *Con.*, Croc., (Cup.), Cyc., Dig., (Dios.), (Dros.), (Dulc.), Euphorb., Euphr., Fer., (Fl. ac.), (Glon.), (Guai.), Hell., Hep., Hyos., Ign., (Ip.), Iod., K. bi., K. carb., K. nit., (Kalm.), (Kre.), Lach., (Laur.), Lil. t., Lyc., (Mag. c.), (Mang.), Meli., (Meny.), *Merc.*, (Mez.), Mos., Mur. ac., Nat. c., **Nat. m.**, *Nit. ac.*, Nux m., *Nux v.*,

Oleand., *Op.*, (Par.), (Petrol.), PHOS., *Pho..ac.*, (Phyt.), Plat., **Pb.**, Pod., (Pso.), **Puls.**, (Rhodo.), **Rhus**, Ruta, Saba., Sabi., Samb., (Sang.), Sars., Sec. c., Seneg., *Sep.*, Sil., *Spig.*, Spo., Squ., (Stan.), Staph., Stram., **Sul.**, (Sul. ac.), (Tar.), (Thuj.), (Valer.), *Verat. a.*, Verat. v., Verb., (Vio. o.), Zinc.

Sensations.—Acon., (Aesc.), Agar., (Aloe), (Alum.), (Anac.), (Ant. t.), Apis, Arg. n., Arn., **Ars.**, Asaf., Asar., (Bap.), (Bar. c.), **BELL.**, (Bism.), *Bry.*, (Calad.), *Calc. c.*, (Camph.), Cannab. i., (Cannab. s.), Canth., (Caps.), (Carb. an.), Carb. v., *Caust.*, Cham., (Chel.), Chin., (Cic.), (Cimic.), *Cocc.*, (Colch.), Coloc., *Con.*, Croc., (Crotal.), Cup., (Dig.) Dulc., (Euphr.), Fes., *Hyos.*, (Ign.), (Ip.), Iod., (K. bi.), K. carb., *Lach.*, Laur., (Led.), (Lil. t.), *Lyc.*, (Meny.), *Merc.*, Mez., Mur. ac., (Nat. c.), **Nat. m.**, *Nit. ac.*, *Nux m.*, Nux v., Oleand., Op., Petrol., *Phos.*, Pho. ac., Plat., **Pb.**, Pod., **Puls.**, (Ran. b.), *Rhoda.*, Rhus, Ruta, (Saba.), Sabi., Sang., *Sec. c.*, *Seneg.*, **Sep.**, Sil., Spo., (Squ.), *Stan.*, (Staph.), *Stram.*, SUL., (Sul. ac.), (Thuj.), (Valer.), *Verat. a.*, (Verat. v.), *Zinc.*

Glands.

Bones.

Skin.

Sleep and Dreams.—(Acon.), (Ars.), (Asar.), (Bar. c.), (Bell.), (Bry.), (Chin.), (Ign.), (Nux v.), (Puls.), Rhus, (Sil.), Sul.

Blood, Circulation and Fever.—Acon., (Agn.), (Am. m.), Ant. t., Apis, Ars., (Asaf.), (Bell.), (Berb.), (Bry.), (Camph.), (Cannab. i.), (Canth.), (Caps.), (Carb. v.), (Chin.), (Colch.), Cup., Dig., (Dros.), Hell., (Hep.), (Ign.), (K. nit.), (Kalm.), (Kre.), (Lach.), (Lyc.), (Mang.), Meny., (Merc.), Mur. ac., (Nat. m.), Nux m., Nux v., (Oleand.), Op., Phos., (Pho. ac.), *Puls.*, (Rhus), (Saba.), (Samb.), (Sang.), Sep., Sil. *Spig.*, (Squ.), Stram., Sul., (Tar.), (Thuj.), Verat. a., (Verat. v.).

Aggravations: Time and Circumstances.—(Acon.), (Am. m.), (Ant. cr.), (Ant. t.), (Apis), (Arg.), Ars., (Aur.), (Bell.), Bry., Calc. c., (Carb. v.), Chel., (Cina), (Clem.), (Cocc.), (Con.), Croc., (Dros.), (Euphr.), (Fer.), (Hep.), (Hyos.), Ign., (K. bi.), (K. carb.), K. nit., Lach., Merc., (Nat. m.), Nit. ac., *Nux v.*, (Petrol.), Phos., (Pho. ac.), (Phyt.), Pod., Puls., (Rhodo.), Rhus, (Sang.), (Sele.), (Seneg.), (Sep.), Sil., Spig., (Spo.), (Squ.), (Stan.), (Staph.), (Stram.), Sul., (Tar.), (Thuj.), (Valer.), (Verat. v.).

Other Remedies.—Acon., (Aesc.), Agar., (Agn.), (Aloe), (Alum.), Am. m., (Anac.), (Ant. cr.), Ant. t., **Apis**, (Arg.), Arg. n., Arn., **Ars.**, Asaf., Asar., (Aur.), Bap., Bar. c., **BELL.**, (Bism.), **Bry.**, *Calc. c.*, Camph., Cannab. i., Cannab. s., Canth., (Caps.), Carb. v., Caust., Cham.,

Chel., Chin., Cic., Cimic., (Cina), (Clem.), *Cocc.*, Colch., Coloc., *Con.*, Croc., (Crotal.), Cup., *Dig.*, (Dros.), (Dulc.), Euphr., Fer., (Glon.), Hell., Hep., *Hyos.*, *Ign.*, (Ip.), Iod., K. bi., *K. carb.*, K. nit., (Kalm.), (Kre.), *Lach.*, Laur., (Lil. t.), Lyc., (Mang.), Meli., (Meny.), **Merc.**, Mez., *Mur. ac.*, Nat. c., **Nat. m.**, *Nit. ac.*, *Nux m.*, **Nux v.**, Oleand., *Op.*, (Par.), Petrol., **Phos.**, **Pho. ac.**, Phyt., Plat., Pb., Pod., PULS., Rhodo., RHUS, Ruta, Saba., Sabi., (Samb.), Sang., Sec. c., Seneg., **Sep.**, Sil., *Spig.*, Spo., Squ., Stan., Staph., *Stram.*, SUL., (Sul. ac.), (Tar.), Thuj., (Valer.), *Verat. a.*, Verat. v., Zinc.

Glonoine.

Mind.—*Acon.*, Ambr., Anac., Arn., Ars., Aur., Bap., Bar. c., **Bell.**, Bry., Calc. c., Camph., **Cannab. i.**, *Cic.*, Cimic., Cocc., Con., Cup., Gels., Hell., Hyd. ac., *Hyos.*, K. carb., Lyc., Meli., *Merc.*, Mos., Mur. ac., Nat. m., Nux v., *Op.*, *Petrol.*, Phos., *Pho. ac.*, Plat., Puls., *Rhus t.*, Saba., Sec. c., Seneg., Sep., Sil., Spig., **Stram.**, *Sul.*, Thuj., Valer., *Verat. a.*, Zinc.

Localities.—Acon., (Agar.), (Ant. t.), (Apis), (Arn.), (Ars.), (Aur.), (Bar. c.), Bell., Bry., (Calc. c.), (Canth.), (Carb. v.), (Caust.), (Cham.), (Chel.), (Chin.), (Cic.), (Cocc.), (Colch.), (Con.), (Croc.), (Cup.), (Dig.), (Euphorb.), (Fer.), (Gel.), (Hell.), (Hep.), (Hyos.), Ign., (Ip.), (Iod.), (K. bi.), (K. carb.), (Lach.), Lyc., (Mar.), (Meny.), Merc., (Mez.), (Nat. c.), Nat. m., (Nit. ac.), Nux v., Op., (Petrol.), Phos., (Pho. ac.), (Pb.), Puls., (Ran. b.), (Rhus), (Saba.), (Sars.), (Sec. c.), Sep., Sil., Spig., (Spo.), (Squ.), (Stan.), (Staph.), Stram., Sul., (Tar.), (Thuj.), Verat. a., (Zinc).

Sensations.—*Acon.*, (Agar.), (Alum.), (Am. m.), (Anac.), *Ant. t.*, (Apis), Arg. n., Arn., Ars., Asaf., Asar., (Aur.), (Bar. c.), **Bell.**, Berb., (Bism.), (Bor.), *Bry.*, (Cact.), *Calc. c.*, (Camph.), Cannab. i., (Cannab. s.), Canth., Caps., (Carb. v.), Caust., Cham., (Chel.), Chin., Cic., (Cimic.), (Cina), *Cocc.*, (Colch.), **Coloc.**, *Con.*, Cup., Dig., (Dros.), *Fer.*, Graph., Hell., (Hyos.), *Ign.*, (Ip.), *K. carb.*, Lach., Laur., *Lyc.*, (Meny.), *Merc.*, Mos., Nat. m., *Nit. ac.*, (Nux m.), *Nux v.*, Oleand., Op., Par., Petrol., **Phos.**, Pho. ac., Phyt., Plat., Pb., (Pod.), **Puls.**, Ran. b., (Ran. s.), Rhus, (Ruta), Saba., Sang., Sec. c., Seneg., **Sep.**, *Sil.*, *Spig.*, Spo., (Squ.), *Stan.*, (Staph.), Stram., (Stro.), **Sul.**, (Sul. ac.), (Tar.), Thuj., (Valer.), Verat. a., Zinc.

Glands.
Bones.
Skin.—(Alum.), (Ars.), (Bry.), (Calc. c.), (Cic.), Cimic., (Dros.),

(Graph.), Hep., (Ign.), (Nat. m.), (Nit. ac.), (Nux v.), (Petrol.), **(Plat.),** (Puls.), (Rhus.), Sep., (Sul.), Zinc.

Sleep and Dreams.

Blood, Circulation and Fever.—ACON., (Aloe.), (Ambr.), (Am. carb.), (Apis), Arg. n., Arn., Ars., Aur., BELL., Bor., (Bov.), *Bry.*, Cact., Calc. c., (Caps.), Carb. v., (Caust.), (Chel.), (Chin.), (Colch.), (Croc.), Cup., Dig., (Dros.), *Fer.*, (Graph.), (Hell.), (Hep.), Hyos., Iod., (K. carb.), (K. nit.), Kre., (Lach.), Lyc., Merc., (Mos.), Nat. m., (Nit. ac.), (Nux m.), Nux v., Op., (Petrol.), *Phos.*, *Pho. ac.*, Puls., Rhus, Ruta), (Saba.), (Sabi.), (Samb)., (Sang.), (Sars.), (Sec. c.), (Seneg.), Sep., Sil., (Spig.), Spo., Stran., *Stram.*, Sul., (Thuj.), Verat. a., (Vio. o.).

Aggravations: Time and Circumstances.—(Acon.), Aesc., (Agn.), (Am. carb.), (Ant. t.), (Apis), (Arg.), (Arn.), Ars., (Asaf.), (Asar.), Aur., (Bap.), (Bar. c.), **Bell.**, (Bor.), **Bry.**, (Calad.), Calc. c., (Camph.), (Cannab. s.), Caps., (Carb. an.), Cham., (Chel.), Cocc., (Coff.), Colch., (Coloc.), (Con.), (Croc.), (Dig.), (Dros.), Fer., (Graph.), (Hell.), (Hep.), (Hyos.), (Ip.), (Iod.), (K. nit.), Led., (Lil. t.), (Lyc.), (Mag. m.), (Mang.), (Meny.), *Merc.*, (Nat. m.), (Nit. ac.), **Nux v.**, (Petrol.), Phos., (Pho. ac.), (Plat.), *Puls.*, Ran. b., (Rheum), (Rhodo.), *Rhus*, Ruta, Sabi., (Samb.), Sang., (Sars.), (Sele.), (Seneg.), *Sep.*, Sil., *Spig.*, (Spo.), (Squ.), Stan., (Staph.), (Stro.), *Sul.*, (Tar.), (Valer.), (Verat. a.), (Verb.), (Zinc).

Other Remedies.—Acon., (Agar.), (Alum.), (Ambr.), (Am. carb.), (Anac.), Ant. t., Apis, Arg. n., Arn., *Ars.*, (Asaf.), (Asar.), *Aur.*, (Bap.), Bar. c., BELL., Bor., **Bry.**, (Cact.), **Calc. c.**, Camph., (Cannab. s.), (Canth.), Caps., Carb. v., Caust., Cham., Chel., Chin., *Cic.*, Cimic., *Cocc.*, Colch., Coloc., *Con.*, (Croc.), *Cup.*, Dig., Dros., *Fer.*, (Gel.), Graph., *Hell.*, Hep., *Hyos.*, Ign., (Ip.), Iod., *K. carb.*, (K. nit.), Lach., *Lyc.*, (Meny.), **Merc.**, Mos., **Nat. m.**, *Nit. ac.*, **Nux v.**, *Op.*, *Petrol.*, **Phos.**, *Pho. ac.*, Plat., (Pb.), **Puls.**, Ran. b., **Rhus**, Ruta, Saba., (Sabi.), (Samb.), Sang., (Sars.), Sec. c., Seneg., **Sep.**, Sil., Spig., *Spo.*, (Squ.), *Stan.*, (Staph.), **Stram.**, (Stro.), SUL., (Tar.), Thuj., Valer., *Verat. a.*, Zinc.

Graphites.

Mind.—Bell., Cham., *Cimic.*, IGN., Lil. t., *Lyc.*, *Naj.*, Nat. m., **Nux v.**, **Puls.**, *Rhus*, Sep., Stan., Stram., Sul., Verat. a.

Localities.—Acon., Aesc., All. c., *Aloe*, Alum., *Apis*, **Arg. n.**, Arn., Ars., *Arum. t.*, Aur., (Bap.), Bar. c., BELL., (Berb.), Bor., Bry., (Cact.), CALC. C., Cannab. i., Canth., (Carb. ac.), *Carb. v.*, Caul., **Caust.**, *Cham.*, *Chin.*, Con., Dios., (Fl. ac.), *Hep.*, *Ign.*, (Iris v.), *K. bi.*, *K. carb.*, Lil. t

(Lith.), Lv., **Merc.**, *Nat. m.*, *Nit. ae.*, **Nux v.**, Op., **Petrol.**, *Phos.*, (Phyt.) (Pic. ac.), Plat., Pb., *Pod.*, Pso., **PULS.**, *Rhus*, *Saba.*, *Sang.*, Sec., **Sep.**, **Sil.**, Spig., **Staph.**, SUL., Thuj., *Verat. a.*, Verat. v., Zinc.

Sensations.—Acon., (Aloe), Alum., Am. carb., Am. m., (Apis), Arg. n., *Arn.*, *Ars.*, (Arum. t.), Asaf., Aur., Bar. c., **Bell.**, (Berb.), *Bry.*, (Cact.), CALC. C., Cannab. i., Carb. an., *Carb. v.*, *Caust.*, Cham., *Chin.*, Cimic., *Cocc.*, Coloc., Con., (Eup. per.), Fer., (Gel.), Glon., Hyos., *Ign.*, Iod., K. bi., *K. carb.*, (Lil. t.), (Lith.), LYC., Meny., *Merc.*, Mez., Nat. c., **Nat. m.**, *Nit. ac.*, Nux v., Petrol., *Phos.*, Pho. ac., (Phyt.), Plat., **Puls.**, Rhus, Sang., **Sep.**, *Sil.*, Spig., Spo., Stan., Staph., Stro., Sul., Thuj., Verat. a., (Verat. v.), *Zinc.*

Glands.—(Arum. t.), *Bell.*, **Bry.**, Carb. an., **Con.**, Lyc., Merc., **Phos.**, **PULS.**, Rhus, Spo., Sul.

Bones.—Con., Merc., *Nit. ac.*, *Puls.*, *Sul.*

Skin.—Ant. cr., Apis, Arn., Ars., *Bar. c.*, Bell., *Bry.*, **Calc. c.**, Carb. v., Cham., Chin., Cic., (Cimic.), Clem., *Con.*, Dulc., (Eup. per.), *Hep.*, K. carb., **Lyc.**, *Merc.*, Nat. m., *Nit. ac.*, *Petrol.*, Phos., Pho. ac., *Puls.*, RHUS, Saba., SEP., *Sil.*, Spo., Squ., Staph., **Sul.**, Vio. t.

Sleep and Dreams.—Arg. n., Ars., (Bap.), Bell., Bry., CALC. C., (Cannab. i.), Caust., Chin., Con., Hep., Ign., K. carb., Lach., Lyc., Merc., Nat. c., **Nux v.**, Op., **Phos.**, *Puls.*, **Sep.**, *Sil.*, Sul.

Blood, Circulation and Fever.—Acon., Ant. cr., (Apis), *Arn.*, *Ars.*, Bar. c., *Bell.*, (Berb.), Bry., (Cact.), *Calc. c.*, (Cannab. i.), *Chin.*, (Glon.), Hep., *K. carb.*, **Lyc.**, *Merc.*, Nit. ac., **Nux v.**, Phos., **Puls.**, *Rhus*, Sang., Sep., Sil., Staph., Sul., *Thuj.*

Aggravations: Time and Circumstances.—Acon., (Aesc.), Agn., (Aloe), Am. carb., Am. m., (Apis), (Arg. n.), *Arn.*, *Ars.*, Aur., (Bap.), *Bell.*, Bor., BRY., Calad., CALC. C., Camph., Carb. an., *Carb. v.*, *Caust.*, *Cham.*, Chel., Chin., (Cimic.), Cina, *Cocc.*, Coff., **Con.**, Croc., Dig., Dulc., Euphr., (Glon.), Hell., Hep., Hyos., *Ign.*, Iod., Ip., (K. bi.), **K. carb.**, Kre., Led., (Lil. t.), **Lyc.**, Mag. m., Mang., *Merc.*, Nat. c., **Nat. m.**, NUX V., *Oleand.*, PHOS., Pho. ac., (Phyt.), *Puls.*, Rhodo., **Rhus**, Ruta, *Saba.*, (Sang.), Sars., **Sep.**, Sil., Spig., Squ., *Staph.*, Stro., **Sul.**, Verat. a., (Verat. v.).

Other Remedies.—Acon., (Aesc.), Aloe, *Apis*, *Arg. n.*, *Arn.*, *Ars.*, Arum. t., (Bap.), Bar. c., **Bell.**, (Berb.), **Bry.**, (Cact.), CALC. C., Cannab. i., Carb. an., Carb v., *Caust.*, *Cham.*, *Chin.*, Cimic., Cocc., *Con.*, Glon., *Hep.*, *Ign.*, K. bi., *K. carb.*, Lil. t., (Lith.), LYC., **Merc.**, *Nat. m.*, *Nit. ac.*, **Nux v.**, Petrol., **Phos.**, (Phyt.), PULS., Rhus, Saba., *Sang.*, SEP., *Sil.*, Spig., *Staph.*, SUL., Thuj., Verat. a., Verat. v., Zinc.

Antidotes.—*Ars.*, Nux v., Vinum.

Guaicum.

Mind.—*Anac.*, Bell., *Hyos.*, *Lyc.*, Nat. m., Pho. ac., Plat., *Stram.*, Verat. a.

Localities.—Acon., (Apis), (Apoc. c.), Arn., *Ars.*, *Bell.*, (Cact.), *Calc. c.*, (Cannab. i.), Carb. v., **Caust.**, *Chin.*, (Cimic.), Cocc., Con., Dulc., (Gel.), *Graph*, Hep., *K. carb.*, **Lyc.**, MERC., Nat. c., Nat. m., **Nux v.**, Phos., **Pho. ac.**, Puls., Rhus, *Ruta*, **Sep.**, *Sil.*, Spig., Stan., **Staph.**, Sul., Thuj., Verat. a., *Zinc.*

Sensations.—Acon., Alum., Anac., *Ars.*, Bar. c., *Bell.*, Bry., **Calc. c.**, Caps., Caust., Cham., Chin., *Cocc.*, Graph., Ign., *K. carb.*, *Lyc.*, Merc., Nat. c., *Nat. m.*, **Nux v.**, Petrol., Phos., Pho. ac., Plat., **Puls.**, *Rhus*, *Sep.*, Sil., *Spig.*, Spo., Stan., *Sul.*, Thuj., Verat. a.

Glands.

Bones.—Asaf., Calc. c., Lyc., Merc., Mez., Pho. ac., Sil., *Staph.*, Sul.

Skin.—Asaf., *Bry.*, Calc. c., Caust., *Puls.*, Rhus.

Sleep and Dreams.—*Ars.*, *Bell.*, *Bry.*, **Calc. c.**, *Carb. v.*, Chin., Graph., *Hep.*, *Ign.*, *Lach.*, *Lyc.*, Merc., Nux v., Phos., *Puls.*, *Rhus*, *Sep.*, *Sil.*, Spig., Sul.

Blood, Circulation and Fever.—Acon., Carb. v., Chin., Cup., Laur., Sep., Sil., **Verat. a.**

Aggravations: Time and Circumstances.—Agar., Am. carb., (Apis), (Arg. n.), Arn., Asaf., (Bap.), Bry., *Calc. c.*, Camph., Carb. an., *Carb. v.*, Cham., Chel., Chin., *Cocc.*, Coff., Con., *Hep.*, Ign., Ip., (K. bi.), Kre., *Lach.*, Laur., Lyc., Mar., Mang., Merc., *Nat. c.*, Nat. m., *Nux m.*, *Nux v.*, Oleand., Phos., (Pod.), Puls., Ran. b., *Rhus*, Ruta, (Sang.), *Sele.*, *Sep.*, Sil., Spig., Staph., Stram., Sul., Thuj., Valer., Verb., Zinc.

Other Remedies.—Acon., Anac., (Apis), *Ars.*, Asaf., *Bell.*, *Bry.*, CALC. C., **Carb. v.**, *Caust.*, **Chin.**, *Cocc.*, *Graph.*, *Hep.*, Ign., K. carb., Lach., **Lyc.**, **Merc.**, Nat. c., *Nat. m.*, Nux m., *Nux v.*, Phos., *Pho. ac.*, Puls., *Rhus*, Ruta, Sep., Sil., Spig., *Staph.*, Stram., **Sul.**, Thuj., *Verat. a.*, Zinc.

Antidotes.

Helleborus.

Mind.—Acon., *Anac.*, Apis, Ars., *Bap.*, Bar. c., BELL., Bov., Bry., Cact., *Cannab. i.*, Caust., Cham., *Cic.*, Cimic. Cocc., Con., Crotal., Cyc., *Gel.*, *Glon.*, Graph., *Hyd. ac.*, Hyper., *Hyos.*, *Ign.*, Laur., **Lyc.**, Meli., Meny., Merc., *Merc. c.*, *Nat. m.*, *Nux m.*, Nux v., *Op.*, Phos., *Pho. ac.*, *Pic. ac.*, PULS., Rhus, Sep., Sil., Spig., Staph., *Stram.*, Sul., Verat. a.

Localities.—Acon., Aesc., (All. c.), (Aloe), Ant. cr., Apis, (Apoc. c.), Arg. n., Arn., *Ars.*, (Bap.), **Bell.**, **Bry.**, (Cact.). *Calc. c.*, (Cannab. i.),

Canth., Caps., (Carb. ac.), Carb. v., *Caust.*, Cham., *Chin.*, Cocc., Colch., Cup., (Dios.), Dros., Dulc., Gel., Glon., *Graph.*, Hep., *Hyos.*, Ign., *Ip.*, (Iris v.), K. bi., *K. carb.*, (Kalm.), Led., (Lil. t.), LYC., Mag. m., Merc., Nat. c., Nat. m., *Nux v.*, Oleand., Op., Petrol., Phos., Pho. ac., (Phyt.), Pod., PULS., *Rhus*, Sang., *Sep.*, Sil., Spig., *Staph.*, Stram., Sul., Sul. ac., *Verat. a.*, (Verat. v.), Zinc.

Sensations.—(Aloe), Alum., Ant. cr., Apis, Arg. n., *Arn.*, Ars., Asaf., (Bap.), Bar. c., BELL., Bor., *Bry.*, (Cact.), Calc. c., Canth., *Caust.*, CHIN., (Cimic.), Cocc., Colch., Con., Dig., Dros., *Dulc.*, Gel., Glon., Graph., *Ign.*, Ip., K. carb., Laur., *Lyc.*, Meny., Merc., Mez., Mos., Mur. ac., Nat. c., *Nat. m.*, Nit. ac., Nux m., Nux v., Oleand., Op., *Phos.*, (Phyt.), *Plat.*, Pb., Puls., *Ran. s.*, Rhus, Ruta, Saba., *Sabi.*, (Sang.), *Sars.*, Sep., Sil., *Spig.*, Spo., *Stan.*, Staph., Sul., Sul. ac., *Tar.*, Thuj., Verat. a., *Zinc.*

Glands.—Bell., Calc. c., *Merc.*, Puls., Sep.

Bones.—Bell., Merc., Phos., Puls., Sul.

Skin.—Ant. cr., Arn., Ars., *Bell.*, *Bry.*, Calc. c., Caust., *Chin.*, Cocc., Con., Dulc., Graph., K. carb., Lach., Lyc., Merc., Nat. m., Nit. ac., Nux v., Phos., PULS., Rhus, Samb., *Sec. c.*, Sep., Sil., Spig., Spo., Squ., Stan., Staph., SUL., Verat. a.

Sleep and Dreams.

Blood, Circulation and Fever.—Apis, Ars., BELL., Bry., (Cact.) Calc. c., Camph., Cannab. i., *Cham.*, Gel., (Glon.), Merc., Nux m., *Nux. v.*, Op., Phos., Pho. ac., *Puls.*, Rhus, Saba., Samb., (Sang.), Sep., Spig., *Verat. a.*, (Verat. v.).

Aggravations: Time and Circumstances.—*Acon.*, (Aesc.), *Agn.*, (All. c.), Ant. cr., (Apis), *Arn.*, *Ars.*, *Asar.*, Aur., (Bap.), Bell., BRY., (Cact.), Calc. c., Camph., (Cannab. i.), Cannab. s., Caps., Carb. v., *Caust.*, Chel., Chin., (Cimic.), Cocc., Coff., Colch., Con., Croc., Dulc., (Glon.), *Graph.*, Hep., Ip., K. bi., *K. carb.*, Led., (Lil. t.), Lyc., *Mag. c.*, Mag. m., Merc., Mez., Mos., Nat. m., Nux m., NUX V., Petrol., PHOS., (Phyt.), PULS., *Ran. b.*, Rhus, *Saba.*, Sabi., Sang., Sep., *Sil.*, Spig., Spo., Squ., Staph., *Stro.*, Sul., *Sul. ac.*

Other Remedies.—Acon., (Aesc.), Aloe, Ant. cr., *Apis*, Arg. n., Arn., *Ars.*, Bap., BELL., Bry., Cact., *Calc. c.*, Camph., Cannab. i., *Caust.*, Cham., *Chin.*, Cimic., *Cocc.*, Colch., Con., Dulc., *Gel.*, *Glon.*, *Graph.*, Hep., Hyos., Ign., Ip., K. bi., *K. carb.*, Led., (Lil. t.), Lyc., Mag. c., Mag. m., Merc., *Nat. m.*, Nux m., Nux v., Op., Phos., Pho. ac., (Phyt.), PULS., Rhus, Saba., Sabi., Sang., Sep., Sil., *Spig.*, Spo., Stan., *Staph.*, Stram., Sul., Sul. ac., *Verat. a.*, (Verat. v.), Zinc.

Antidotes.—Camph., *Chin.*

Hepar Sulfuris Calcareum.

Mind.—Aur., Bell., Calc. c., Caust., Con., **Lyc.**, Nat. m., **Phos.**, Puls., Sil., **Sul.**

Localities.—*Acon.*, (Aesc.), All. c., Aloe, Alum., Ant. cr., **Apis.** Apoc. c., **Arg. n.**, *Arn.*, **Ars.**, (Arum t.), Bap., Bar. c., **BELL.**, *Bry.*, (Cact.), **Calc. c.**, Camph., *Cannab. i.*, Cannab. s., *Canth.*, (Carb. ac.), *Carb. v.*, **Caust.**, *Cham.*, *Chin.*, (Cimic.), Clem., Colch., *Con.*, (Crotal.), Cup., Dig., (Dios.), (Eup. per.), Euphr., *Gel.*, (Glon.), *Graph.*, (Hyd. ac.), *Hyos.*, Ign., Ip., (Iris v.), *K. bi.*, *K. carb.*, (Kalm.), Laur., Lil. t., (Lith.), **Lyc.**, (Meli.), MERC., Nat. c., *Nat. m.*, *Nit. ac.*, **Nux v.**, Oleand., *Op.*, *Petrol.*, **Phos.**, *Pho. ac.*, Phyt., Pb., (Pod.), PULS., Rhus, Ruta, Saba., Sang., Sele., Sep., Sil., *Spig.*, *Spo.*, *Staph.*, Stram., SUL., *Thuj.*, *Verat. a.*, *Verat. v.*, Zinc.

Sensations.—Acon., (Aesc.), (Aloe), (Apis), (Arg n.), *Arn.*, Ars., Aur., (Bap.), **Bell.**, *Bry.*, **Calc. c.**, Canth., **Caust.**, *Chin.*, Cocc., (Crotal.), (Eup. per.), (Fl. ac.), Graph., *Ign.*, (K. bi.), *K. carb.*, **Lyc.**, **Merc.**, Nat. c., *Nat. m.*, Nux v., **Phos.**, (Pod.), **Puls.**, *Rhus*, Ruta, **Sep.**, **Sil.**, *Spig.*, Spo., Stan., Stro., **Sul.**, Thuj., Verat. a., *Zinc.*

Glands.—*Ars.*, (Arum. t.), BELL., Con., Dulc., Lyc., *Merc.*, **Phos.**, SIL., Sul.

Bones.—Asaf., *Calc. c.*, (Eup. per.), Lyc., Merc., Nit. ac., Pho. ac., PULS., Sep., **Sil.**, Staph., *Sul.*

Skin.—Acon., Alum., Ant. cr., *Apis*, Arn., **Ars.**, *Asaf.*, Bar. c., *Bell.*, Bor., *Bry.*, **Calc. c.**, (Carb. ac.), Carb. v., *Caust.*, Cham., Chin., Cimic., Clem., *Con.*, Dulc., Eup. per., (Glon.), Graph., *Lach.*, **Lyc.**, **Merc.**, Mez., Nat. m., *Nit. ac.*, Nux v., *Petrol.*, Phos., PULS., Ran. b., **Rhus**, Sep., SIL., Spig., Squ., *Staph.*, SUL , Verat. a., Vio. t., Zinc.

Sleep and Dreams.—Acon., Arg. n., Ars., (Bap.), **BELL.**, Bry., **Calc. c.**, *Cham.*, Chin., Con., Graph., *Ign.*, *K. carb.*, Lyc., **Merc.**, *Nux v.*, Op., **Phos.**, PULS., *Rhus*, SEP., *Sil.*, Sul.

Blood, Circulation and Fever.—Acon., (Arg. n.), Arn., *Ars.*, **Bell.**, (Berb.), Bry., (Cact.), *Calc. c.*, Carb. v., **Cham.**, Chin., Colch., (Gel.), (Glon.), Graph., Ign., Ip., K. carb., Kre., Lyc., *Merc.*, *Nat. m.*, Nit. ac., Nux m., **Nux v.**, Op., Phos., Pho. ac., (Phyt.), *Puls.*, RHUS, Samb., *Sang.*, Sec. c., *Sep.*, Sil., Spig., SUL., Thuj., *Verat. a.*, (Verat. v.).

Aggravations: Time and Circumstances.—Acon., Aesc., (All. c.), (Aloe), Am. carb., Ant. cr., Apis, Arg. n., Arn., *Ars.*, Asar., Aur., Bap., Bar. c., **Bell.**, BRY., Calad., **Calc. c.**, Camph., Cannab. s., Caps., *Carb. v.*, **Caust.**, *Cham.*, *Chin.*, Cic., (Cimic.), *Cocc.*, Colch., *Con.*, Croc., Dulc.,

RELATIONSHIPS.—HEPAR SUL.—HYOS. 401

(Gel.), Glon., *Graph.*, Guai., Hyos., Ign., Iod., **Ip.**, *K. bi.*, K. carb., Lach., Lil. t., **Lyc.**, *Mang.*, **Merc.**, Nat. c., *Nat. m.*, *Nit. ac.*, *Nux m.*, NUX V., **Phos.**, Pho. ac., **Phyt.**, Pod., **Puls.**, RHUS, Ruta, Saba., Samb., *Sang.*, Sars., Sele., SEP., SIL., *Spig.*, Spo., Squ., **Staph.**, *Stro.*, **Sul.**, Thuj., Verat. a., (Verat. v.).

Other Remedies.—*Acon.*, Aesc., (All. c.), Aloe, **Apis**, **Arg. n.**, Arn., *Ars.*, (Arum. t.), Asaf., Bap., **Bell.**, **Bry.**, (Cact.), **Calc. c.**, Carb. v., *Caust.*, *Cham.*, *Chin.*, Cimic., Con., (Crotal.), Gel., Glon., *Graph.*, Ign., Ip., *K. bi.*, K. carb., Lil. t., *Lyc.*, **Merc.**, *Nat. m.*, Nit. ac., *Nux v.*, **Phos.**, Pho. ac., **Phyt.**, Pod., **Puls.**, *Rhus*, *Sang.*, **Sep.**, SIL., Spig., Staph., SUL., Thuj., Verat. a., Verat. v.

Antidotes.—Acetum veget., *Bell.*, Cham., Sil.

Hyoscyamus.

Mind.—Acon., *Anac.*, *Apis*, Ars., Aur., BELL., CANNAB. I., Cic., C.mic., Coff., Crotal., Cup., *Gel.*, **Glon.**, Hell., *Hyd. ac.*, *Hyper.*, Ign., Lach., **Lyc.**, *Meli.*, Merc. c., Nat. c., *Nat. m.*, Nux v., **Op.**, Phos., *Pho. ac.*, Pic. ac., *Plat.*, Puls., Rhus, Sep., STRAM., Sul., Ther., VERAT. A., Verat. v.

Localities.—*Acon.*, Aesc., (All. c.), Aloe, **Apis**, Apoc. c., **Arg. n.**, *Ars.*, Arum. t., Bap., BELL., Bry., *Calc. c.*, Camph., Cannab. i., *Canth.*, (Carb. ac.), Caust., *Cham.*, *Chin.*, (Cimic.), Cocc., *Con.*, (Crotal.), Cup., Dig., (Dios.), Dulc., (Eup. per.), Fer., *Gel.*, Glon., *Hep.*, *Ign.*, Ip., (Iris v.), *K. bi.*, K. carb., (Lil. t.), *Lyc.*, Meli., *Merc.*, *Nat. m.*, Nit. ac., **Nux v.**, *Op.*, **Phos.**, Phyt., (Pod.), (Pso.), PULS., Rhus, Ruta, Sabi., Sang., Sec. c., *Sep.*, *Sil.*, Spig., Spo., **Stram.**, **Sul.**, *Verat. a.*, *Verat. v.*

Sensations.—*Acon.*, (Aesc.), Apis, *Arg. n.*, *Ars.*, (Arum t.), Bap., BELL., Berb., *Bry.*, (Cact.), *Calc. c.*, Camph., (Cannab. i.), Caust., **Cham.**, *Chin.*, Cic., Cimic., Cocc., Con., (Crotal.), *Cup.*, (Dios.), Dulc., Fer., **Gel.**, (Glon.), *Ign.*, *Ip.*, (K. bi.), *Lyc.*, *Merc.*, Nit. ac., Nux m., *Nux v.*, .**Op.**, **Phos.**, (Phyt.), Plat., Pb., (Pod.), **Puls.**, *Rhus*, (Sang.), Sec. c., *Sep.*, *Sil.*, STRAM., *Sul.*, Verat. a., Verat. v.

Glands.—Bell., Bry., Carb. an., Con., Hep., Lyc., Merc., Phos., Sil., Sul.

Bones.

Skin.—Ars., *Bell.*, Bry., Lyc., Merc., Phos., Rhus, Sec. c., *Sul.*

Sleep and Dreams.—Arg. n., (Bap.), **Bell.**, Cannab. i., Ign., (Lil. t.), Merc., *Nux v.*, Op., Puls.

Blood, Circulation and Fever.—Acon., Arn., BELL., Bry.,

(Cact.), Calc. c., Chin., Dig., Fer., (Glon.), Nat. m., Phos., Puls., Rhus, (Sang.), Sil., *Stram.*, *Sul.*, (Verat. v.).

Aggravations: Time and Circumstances.—Acon., (Aesc.), (All. c.), Am. carb., Apis, (Arg. n.), *Ars.*, *Aur.*, (Bap.), BELL., Bry., *Calc. c.*, Caps., *Caust.*, Cham., Cocc., Coff., *Colch.*, Con., Dulc., Graph., Hell., *Hep.*, Ign., Ip., K. bi., *K. carb.*, (Lil. t.), Lyc., Merc., Mez., *Nux m.*, Nux v., *Phos.*, Pho. ac., (Phyt.), Plat., (Pod.), Puls., Rhus, Saba., Sabi., Samb., *Sang.*, Sep., *Sil.*, Staph., *Stro.*, Sul., Sul. ac., Verat. a.

Other Remedies.—*Acon.*, Aesc., (All. c.), Apis, *Arg. n.*, *Ars.*, (Arum t., Bap., BELL., Bry., (Cact.), Calc. c., Cannab. i., Caust., *Cham.*, Chin., Cimic., Cocc., Con., Crotal., Cup., Gel., *Glon.*, Hep., *Ign.*, Ip., K. bi., (Lil. t.), Lyc., Merc., Nat. m., *Nux v.*, Op., Phos., Phyt., Plat., (Pod.), Puls., Rhus, *Sang.*, Sec. c., Sep., Sil., Stram., *Sul.*, Verat. a., *Verat. v.*

Antidotes.—*Bell.*, Camph., Chin., *Stram.*

Ignatia.

Mind.—*Acon.*, Aloe, Apis, *Aur.*, *Bap.*, *Cannab. i.*, Cham., Chel., Cimic., Cocc., Con., Gel., Glon., *Graph.*, LYC., *Meli.*, Merc. c., Naj., Nat. m., *Op.*, Phos., Pho. ac., *Pic. ac.*, *Plat.*, *Pso.*, PULS., *Rhus*, Sep., *Sil.*, Sul., Ther., Verat. v.

Localities.—*Acon.*, *Aesc.*, All. c., *Aloe*, Alum., Ant. cr., *Apis*, Apoc. c., Arg. n., Arn., *Ars.*, *Arum t.*, Asaf., *Bap.*, Bell., (Berb.), *Bry.*, Cact., Calc. c., *Cannab. i.*, *Canth.*, Carb. ac., Carb. v., Caust., *Cham.*, CHIN. Cimic., Cina, Cocc., Con., Crotal., Dios., (Eup. per.), Fer., Fl. ac., *Gel.*, Glon., *Graph*, Hep., (Hyd. ac.), *Hyos.*, Ip., (Iris v.), K. bi., *K. carb.*, (Kalm.), Lil. t., *Lyc.*, Mar., Meli., *Merc.*, Nat. c., *Nat. m.*, Nit. ac., NUX V., Op., Petrol., Phos., Pho. ac., Phyt., Plat., Pb., *Pod.*, (Pso.), PULS., Ran. b., *Rhus*, Saba., Sabi., *Sang.*, Sec. c., Sep., *Sil.*, Spig., Spo., Squ., Stan., *Staph.*, Stram., SUL., Thuj., Verat. a., *Verat. v.*, Zinc.

Sensations.—*Acon.*, (Aesc.), Aloe, Alum., Ambr., Apis, *Arg. n.*, Arn., *Ars.*, Arum t., Asaf., *Bap.*, BELL., *Berb.*, Bry., Cact., CALC. C., Cannab. i., Canth., Carb. v., Caust., *Cham.*, Chel., *Chin.*, Cic., Cimic., Cocc., *Con.*, Croc., Dros., Eup. per., Gel., *Glon.*, Graph., Hyos., Ip., Iris v., K. bi., K. carb., (Kalm.), Laur., (Lil. t.), Lyc., Merc., Mos., Mur. ac., Nat. c., *Nat. m.*, Nit. ac., NUX V., Op., *Petrol.*, Phos., Pho. ac., *Phyt.*, *Plat.*, Pb., Pod., Puls., Ran. b., Rhus, Sang., Sec. c., SEP., *Sil.*, *Spig.*, Stan., Staph., *Stram.*, SUL., Thuj., *Verat. a.*, Verat. v., *Zinc.*

Glands.—*Bell.*, *Con.*, Merc., Puls., Rhus, *Sep.*, Spo., Sul.

Bones.—Pho. ac., Rhus, Ruta.

Skin.—Arn., Bell., Bry., *Calc. c.*, Caust., (Cimic.), (Crotal.), (Eup.

per.), *Hep.*, Lyc., Merc., Mez., Nux v., **Puls.**, **Rhus**, SEP., Sil., **Staph.**, **Sul.**

Sleep and Dreams.—Arg. n., (Bap.), Bell., **Bry.**, *Calc. c.*, Cannab. i., Chin., Cimic., Con., (Gel.), *Graph.*, Hep., Lyc., Merc., Nat. c., NUX V., *Phos.*, **Puls.**, **Rhus.**, *Sep.*, Sil., *Sul.*

Blood, Circulation and Fever.—Acon., Arn., ARS., **Bell.**, (Berb.), **Bry.**, *Calc. c.*, Caps., *Cham.*, *Chin.*, (Gel.), Hep., Lyc., *Merc.*, NUX V., Phos., **Puls.**, RHUS, (Sang.), **Sep.**, Sil., Spig., *Sul.*, *Verat. a.*

Aggravations: Time and Circumstances.—Acon., (All. c.), Aloe, *Ant. cr.*, (Apis), *Arg. n.*, Arn., Ars., (Bap.), *Bell.*, **Bry.**, **Calc. c.**, (Cannab. i.), Caust., *Cham.*, Chel., Chin., (Cimic.), Cocc., Coff., Colch., Coloc., Con., (Gel.), Graph., Hep., Hyos., K. bi., *K. carb.*, K. nit., Lach., LYC., Merc., Nat. c., *Nat. m.*, Nit. ac., NUX V., *Phos.*, Pho. ac., (Phyt.), Plat., (Pod.), PULS., Rhodo., **Rhus**, *Sang.*, Sele., SEP., Sil., *Spig.*, **Staph.**, Sul., Thuj., (Verat. v.).

Other Remedies.—*Acon.*, Aesc., (All. c.), *Aloe*, *Apis*, **Arg. n.**, Arn., *Ars.*, Arum. t., *Bap.*, **Bell.**, Berb., **Bry.**, Cact., **Calc. c.**, **Cannab. i.**, Caust., *Cham.*, *Chin.*, **Cimic.**, Cocc., Con., (Crotal.), Gel., *Glon.*, Graph., Hep., K. bi., *K. carb.*, (Lil. t.), Lyc., *Merc.*, Nat. m., NUX V., *Phos.*, Pho. ac., Phyt., Plat., Pod., PULS., RHUS, **Sang.**, Sep., *Sil.*, Spig., Staph., SUL., Verat. a., *Verat. v.*

Antidotes.—Arn., Camph., Cham., Cocc., *Coff.*, *Nux v.*, *Puls.*

Injurious.—Coff., Tab.

Iodium.

Mind.—Acon., *Aur.*, *Bell.*, Carb. an., Fer., *Graph.*, Ign., *Lyc.*, Nat. c., Nat. m., Phos., Plat., *Puls.*, Rhus, Sul., Verat. v., Zinc.

Localities.—Acon., Aesc., All. c., Ant. t., Apis, (Apoc. c.), *Arg. n.*, Arn., *Ars.*, *Arum t.*, Bap., Bell., (Berb.), *Bry.*, Cact., **Calc. c.**, Cannab. i., (Carb. ac.), *Carb. v.*, Caust., Cham., **Chin.**, Cimic., Cina, (Crotal.), Dros., Gel., (Glon.), Graph., Hep., Hyos., Ign., (Iris v.), **K. bi.**, K. carb., (Kalm.), Lach., Laur., (Lil. t.), LYC., (Meli.), **Merc.**, Nat. c., *Nat. m.*, Nit. ac., **Nux v.**, PHOS., Phyt., (Pod.), Pso., PULS., Rhus, *Sang.*, Seneg., **Sep.**, Sil., Spig., *Spo.*, Stan., Staph., Sul., (Tell.), **Verat. a.**, Verat. v., Zinc.

Sensations.—(Aesc.), Ambr., Anac., *Apis*, *Arg. n.*, *Ars.*, Asaf., Asar., Bap., **Bell.**, Bry., Cact., **Calc. c.**, Caust., Cham., *Chin.*, (Cimic.), Cocc., *Con.*, Crotal., Cup., Fer., Gel., (Glon.), Graph., Ign., *K. carb.*, **Lyc.**, Mar., *Merc.*, Nat. m., Nit. ac., Nux m., **Nux v.**, Op., **Phos.**, Pho., ac., Plat., **Puls.**, Rhus, Sang., Sec. c., Sele., *Sep.*, **Stan.**, Stram., **Sul.**, Verat. a.

Glands.—Arn., *Bell.*, Chin., Nux v., *Puls.*, Rhus.

Bones.—Asaf., Bell., *Calc. c.*, Lyc., **Merc.**, Nit. ac., Puls., Sep., Sil., Sul.

Skin.—Acon., Am. carb., (Apis), Arn., **Ars.**, *Bell.*, **Bry.**, *Calc. c.*, Chin., Con., K. carb., **Lyc.**, *Merc.*, Nit. ac., *Phos.*, *Pho. ac.*, Puls., *Rhus*, *Sil.*, **Sul.**

Sleep and Dreams.—*Ars.*, Aur., *K. carb.*, Mag. c., Nat. c., *Nux v.*, Phos., Sep., Sil., Thuj.

Blood, Circulation and Fever.—ACON., (Arg. n.), Ars., Bell., Bry., Calc. c., (Cannab. i.), Carb. v., Cham., (Crotal.), Fer., Glon., Hep., K. carb., **Lyc.**, **Merc.**, Op., PHOS., Pho. ac., *Sep.*, *Sil.*, **Stan.**, Sul., Verat. a.

Aggravations: Time and Circumstances.—Acon., (Aesc.), (All. c.), Ambr., Apis, Arn., **Ars.**, *Asar.*, (Bap.), Bar. c., Bell., Bor., Bry., *Culad.*, **Calc. c.**, Cannab. s., *Carb. v.*, Cham., Chel., Chin., (Cimic.), *Colch.*, *Croc.*, Dros., Dulc., *Fer.*, (Glon,), Graph., *Hep.*, Ign., (K. bi.), *K. carb.*, K. nit. Lach., *Led.*, Lil. t., **Lyc.**, *Mag. c.*, Mag. m., *Mang.*, *Merc.*, Nat. c., Nat. m., Nit. ac., *Nux v.*, **Phos.**, Pho. ac., (Phyt.), Pb., **PULS.**, Ran. b., *Rhus*, Saba., Samb., (Sang.), *Sele.*, **Sep.**, *Sil.*, **Spig.**, Squ., **Staph.**, Stro., **Sul.**, *Thuj.*, Verat. a.

Other Remedies.—*Acon.*, Aesc., (All. c.), *Apis*, Arg. n., Arn., **Ars.**, Asar., Bap., **Bell.**, *Bry.*, Cact., **Calc. c.**, Carb. v., Cham., *Chin.*, Cimic., Colch., Crotal., Fer., Gel., Glon., Graph., Hep., Ign., K. bi., *K. carb.*, (Lil. t.), LYC., Mag. c., MERC., Nat. c., Nat. m., Nit. ac., **Nux v.**, PHOS., Pho. ac., (Phyt.), PULS., *Rhus*, Sang., Sele., **Sep.**, *Sil.*, Spig., Stan., Staph., **Sul.**, Verat. a., Verat. v.

Antidotes.—*Ars.*, **Bell.**, Camph., Chin., Coff., **Hep.**, *Phos.*, Sul.

Ipecacuanha.

Mind.—Acon., Bell., Cham., Con., Ign., Lyc., *Na.t m.*, Phos., Pho. ac., *Puls.*, Sep., Sil., Sul., Verat. v.

Localities.—*Acon.*, Aesc., (All. c.), Aloe, Ant. cr., *Apis*, (Apoc. c.), **Arg. n.**, Arn., *Ars.*, (Arum t.), *Bap.*, **Bell.**, *Bry.*, Cact., **Calc. c.**, (Cannab. i.), Canth., Caps., Carb. ac., Carb. v., *Cham.*, **Chin.**, Cimic., Cocc., Con., Crotal., Cup., Dios., Dros., Dulc., Eup. per., Fer., (Fl. ac.), Gel., Hep., *Hyos.*, Ign., Iris v., **K. bi.**, K. carb., (Lith.), *Lyc.*, (Meli.), *Merc.*, **Nat. m.**, **Nux v.**, **Phos.**, Phyt., Plat., Pod., Pso. PULS., *Rhus*, Saba., Sabi., *Sang.*, Sec. c., **Sep.**, Sil., Spig., Stan., Staph., Stram., **Sul.**, Verat. a., Verat. v.

RELATIONSHIPS.—IPEC.—KALI B. 405

Sensations.—Acon., Aesc., Alum., Apis, *Arg. n.*, Arn., Ars., (Bap.), **BELL.**, Bry., Cact., **Calc. c.**, *Camph.*, (Cannab. i.), Cannab. s., *Canth.*, Carb. v., Caust., **CHAM.**, *Chin.*, *Cic.*, (Cimic.), **Cocc.**, Con., (Crotal.), *Cup.*, Dios., Dros., Fer., Gel., (Glon.), Hell., **Hyos.**, IGN., (K. bi.), K. carb., Lach., (Lil. t.), Lyc., *Merc.*, **Mos.**, Nat. m., Nit. ac., Nux m., **Nux v.**, Op., Petrol., *Phos.*, Pho. ac., (Phyt.), **Plat.**, Pb., (Pod.), **Puls.**, Rhodo., Rhus, (Sang.), *Sec. c.*, **Sep.**, Sil., **Stan.**, Staph., *Stram.*, **Sul.**, **Verat. a.**, (Verat. v.), Zinc.

Glands.

Bones.—*Hep.*, Puls.

Skin.—Acon., *Ars.*, *Bell.*, BRY., Calc. c., Carb. v., Caust., Chin., (Crotal.), (Hyd. ac.), Lach., *Led.*, *Lyc.*, Merc., Mez., Oleand., Pho. ac., Puls, Rhus, Sil., Spo., *Sul.*, Verat. a.

Sleep and Dreams.—Calc. c., Sul.

Blood, Circulation and Fever.—Acon., Agn., Ars., Bell., Bry., Cact. Calc. c., (Cannab. i.), Carb. v., Caust., *Cham.*, *Chin.*, Cocc., Graph., Hep., Ign., *Lyc.*, *Merc.*, Nit. ac., **Nux v.**, *Phos.*, (Phyt.), Puls., *Rhus*, Saba., Sep., *Sil.*, Sul., Thuj., VERAT. A., (Verat. v.).

Aggravations: Time and Circumstances.—*Acon.*, (Aesc.), Ant. cr., Arn., *Ars.*, *Asar.*, (Bap.), **Bell.**, BRY., (Cact.), Calad., **Calc. c.**, Cannab. s., Carb. an., Carb. v., *Caust.*, Cham., Chel., Chin., (Cimic.), *Cocc.*, Coff., *Colch.*, Croc., Dig., (Glon.), Graph., **Hep.**, Ign., (K. bi.), Led., (Lil. t.), *Lyc.*, Merc., Nat. c., *Nat. m.*, Nit. ac., NUX V., **Phos.**, (Phyt.), PULS., Ran. b., Rhodo., *Rhus*, Saba, (Sang.), Sars., Sele., **Sep.**, Sil., Spig., Spo., Squ., Staph., **Sul.**, Verat. a.

Other Remedies.—*Acon.*, Aesc., Apis, Arg. n., Arn., *Ars.*, Bap., **Bell.**, **Bry.**, Cact., *Calc. c.*, (Cannab. i.), Carb. v., Caust., *Cham.*, *Chin.*, Cimic., Cocc., Crotal., Cup., Gel., (Glon.), Hep., Hyos., *Ign.*, K. bi., (Lil. t.), **Lyc.**, *Merc.*, Nat. m., **Nux v.**, **Phos.**, Phyt., Plat., (Pod.), PULS., *Rhus*, Sang., Sec. c., **Sep.**, Sil., **Sul.**, *Verat. a.*, *Verat. v.*

Antidotes.—Arn., *Ars.*, *Chin.*, Nux v., Tab.

Kali Bichrom.

Mind.—*Bap.*, Bry., Con., Gel., Phos., Pho. ac., *Pic. ac.*, Lyc., Merc., *Nat. c.*, *Nux m.*, Op., Sep.

Localities.—Acon., Aesc., *Agar.*, *All. c.*, Aloe, (Alum), (Ambr.), Am. m., (Anac.), Ant. cr., *Ant. t.*, *Apis*, Apoc. c., Arg., **Arg. n.**, Arn., ARS., *Arum. t.*, Asaf., Asar., Aur., *Bap.*, Bar. c., BELL., (Berb.), Bism., Bor., (Bov.), BRY., **Calc. c.**, Camph., Cannab. i., Cannab. s., **Canth.**, *Caps.*, Carb. ac., **Carb. v.**, **Caust.**, **Cham.**, *Chel.*, **Chin.**, Cic., (Cimic.),

Cina, Clem., *Cocc.*, Coff., *Colch.*, **Coloc.**, *Con.*, (Crotal.), Cup., Cyc., *Dig.*, Dios., *Dros.*, Dulc., Eup. per., (Euphorb.), Euphr., *Fer.*, Fl. ac., Gel. (Glon.), Graph., Hell., Hep., Hyos., *Ign.*, Ip., *Iod.*, *K. carb.*, (K. nit.), (Kalm.), Kre., *Lach.*, Laur., Led., (Lil. t.), Lyc., (Mag. c.), (Mag. m.), Mang., Mar., MERC., Mez., Mur. ac., *Nat. c.*, **Nat. m.**, NIT. AC., (Nux m.), NUX V., (Oleand.), Op., (Par.), *Petrol.*, PHOS., *Pho. ac.*, Phyt., Plat., *Pod.*, Pb., Pso., PULS., Ran. b., Rheum, (Rhodo.), Rhus, Ruta, Saba., (Sabi.), Samb., **Sang.**, *Sec. c.*, Sele., *Seneg.*, SEP., SIL., *Spig.*, Spo., Squ., *Stan.*, Staph., Stram., SUL., Sul. ac., (Tar.), Thuj., Valer., **Verat. a.**, Verat. v., (Verb.), (Vio. t.), **Zinc.**

Sensations.—Acon., Aesc., Agar., (Aloe), Alum., (Ambr.), Am. m., (Apis), (Arg.), Arg. n., *Arn.*, Ars., Arum. t., *Asaf.*, Bap., Bar. c., BELL., *Berb.*, Bor., **Bry.**, (Calad.), **Calc. c.**, Cannab. i., *Canth.*, (Caps.), Carb. v., *Caust.*, (Cham.), *Chel.*, *Chin.*, (Cic.), (Cimic.), (Clem.), Cocc., (Colch.), **Coloc.**, Con., (Dios.), Dros., Dulc., (Eup. per.), (Euphr.), Fer., (Gel.), (Glon.), (Graph.), Hep., *Ign.*, (Ip.), (Iris v.), *K. carb.*, Lach., (Laur.), (Led.), Lil. t., *Lyc.*, Merc., *Mez.*, (Mur. ac.), *Nat. c.*, **Nat. m.**, Nit. ac., (Nux m.), **Nux v.**, (Oleand.), Op., (Par.), Petrol., PHOS., *Pho. ac.*, (Phyt.), Pb., (Pod.), PULS., *Ran. b.*, (Ran. s.), *Rhodo.*, Rhus, Ruta, *Saba.*, Sabi., Sang., (Sars.), (Sec. c.), Seneg., **Sep.**, **Sil.**, Spig., (Spo.), Squ., **Stan.**, (Staph.), Stram., SUL., Tar., *Thuj.*, Valer., Verat. a., Zinc.

Glands.

Bones.

Skin.—(Agar.), (Am. m.), Ant. cr., Ant. t., Ars., (Aur.), (Bar. c.), Bell., Clem., (Hyos.), (Lach.), (Led.), (Mag. c.), Merc., (Oleand.), *Phos.*, (Pho. ac.), (Phyt.), (Puls.), *Rhus*, Sep., (Staph.), Sul.

Blood, Circulation and Fever.

Aggravations: Time and Circumstances.—Acon., *Agar.*, (Agn.), (All. c.), (Aloe), Alum., *Ambr.*, Am. carb., *Am. m.*, Anac., Ant. cr., Ant. t., Apis, *Arg.*, (Arg. n.), Arn., **Ars.**, Asaf., (Asar.), Aur., (Bap.), Bar. c., *Bell.*, (Bor.), **Bry.**, (Calad.), *Calc. c.*, (Camph.), (Cannab. i.), Cannab. s., (Canth.), **Caps.**, (Carb. an.), Carb. v., Caust., Cham., Chel., (Chin.), Cimic., Cina, Cocc., (Coff.), Colch., (Coloc.), Con., Croc., (Cup.), Cyc., (Dig.), (Dros.), *Dulc.*, (Euphorb.), Euphr., Fer., (Gel.), (Graph.), (Guai.), *Hell.*, Hep., *Hyos.*, Ign., (Ip.), (Iod.), K. carb., K. nit., (Kre.), **Lach.**, (Laur.), Led., **Lyc.**, Mag. c., Mag. m., Mang., (Mar.), (Meny.), *Merc.*, Mez., Mos., (Mur. ac.), Nat. c., *Nat. m.*, *Nit. ac.*, (Nux m.), *Nux v.*, (Oleand.), (Par.), Petrol., *Phos.*, *Pho. ac.*, (Phyt.), Plat., (Pb.), (Pod.), **PULS.**, *Ran. b.*, **Ran. s.**, *Rhodo.*, RHUS, Ruta, Saba., *Sabi.*, (Samb.),

Saug., (Sars.), Sele., Seneg., **Sep., Sil.,** Spig., (Spo.), (Squ.), Stan., Staph., (Stram.), Stro., SUL., (Sul. ac.), (Tar.), Thuj., **Valer.,** (Verat. a.), (Verat. v.), Verb., (Vio. t.), *Zinc.*

Other Remedies.—Acon., (Aesc.),*Agar.,* (All. c.), Aloe, Alum., **Ambr., Am. m.,** (Anac.), Ant. cr., *Ant. t.,* Apis, *Arg., Arg. n.,* Arn., **Ars.,** Arum. t., Asaf., (Asar.), Aur., *Bap., Bar. c.,* **Bell.,** (Berb.), Bor., **Bry.,** (Calad.), **Calc. c.,** (Camph.), Cannab. i., Cannab. s., *Canth.,* Caps., *Carb. v., Caust.,* Cham., *Chel., Chin.,* (Cic.), Cimic., Cina, Clem., Cocc., (Coff.), Colch., *Coloc., Con.,* (Cup.), Cyc., (Dig.), (Dios.), Dros., *Dulc.,* (Eup. per.), (Euphorb.), Euphr., *Fer., Gel.,* (Glon.), Graph., Hell., *Hep., Hyos., Ign.,* Ip., (Iod.), *K. carb.,* (K. nit.), (Kre.), **Lach.,** Laur., **Led.,** (Lil. t.), Lyc., Mag. c., Mag. m., (Mar.), **Merc.,** *Mez.,* Mur. ac., *Nat. c.,* **Nat. m., Nit. ac.,** (Nux m.)*, Nux v.,* (Oleand.), Op., (Par.), Petrol., **Phos.,** Pho. ac., Phyt., Plat., Pb., Pod., PULS., *Ran. b.,* (Ran. s.), *Rhodo.,* RHUS, Ruta, *Saba.,* Sabi., (Samb.), *Sang.,* (Sars.), (Sec. c.), Sele., *Seneg.,* Sep., Sil., *Spig.,* Spo., Squ., *Stan.,* Staph., Stram., SUL., (Sul. ac.), **Tar.,** *Thuj., Valer., Verat. a.,* (Verat. v.), (Verb.), (Vio. t.), **Zinc.**

Kali Carbonicum.

Mind.—Acon., Anac., *Bell.,* Calc. c., Cham., Gel., Glon., Graph., *Ign.,* Lyc., Nat. m., *Nux v.,* Op., Pho. ac., Plat., **Puls.,** *Rhus,* Sil., *Stram.,* Verat. a.

Localities.—Acon., **Aesc.,** (All. c.), **Aloe,** Alum., Am. carb., Anac., Ant. cr., **Apis,** (Apoc. c.), *Arg. n., Arn.,* Ars., Arum. t., Aur., Bap., Bar. c., **Bell.,** *Berb.,* Bor., **Bry.,** Cact., **Calc. c.,** *Cannab. i.,* Canth., *Carb. ac.,* Carb. an., Carb. v., (Caul.), **Caust.,** Cham., *Chin., Cimic.,* Cocc., Con., Crotal., Dios., Dros., Dulc., (Eup. per.), Fer., (Fl. ac.), Gel., Glon., **Graph.,** Hep., (Hyd. ac.), Hyos., *Ign.,* Iris v., K. bi., Kalm., Kre., *Lil. t.,* (Lith.), **Lyc.,** Mag. c., Mag. m., **Merc.,** Nac. c., *Nat. m.,* Nit. ac., **Nux v.,** Petrol., **Phos.,** *Pho. ac.,* Phyt., (Pic. ac.), Plat., *Pod.,* Pso., PULS., *Rhus,* Saba., Sabi., *Sang.,* SEP., *Sil.,* Spig., Stan., Staph., **Sul.,** (Tell.), Thuj., Verat. a., Verat. v., Zinc.

Sensations.—*Acon.,* (Aesc.), (Aloe), Alum, *Apis, Arg. n.,* Arn., **Ars.,** (Arum. t.), Asaf., **Bell.,** Berb., *Bry.,* **Calc. c.,** Canth., Carb. an., Carb. v., *Caust.,* Cham., *Chin.,* Cimic., Cocc., Con., (Crotal.), (Eup. per.), Fer., Gel., *Glon.,* Graph., Hep., *Ign.,* Iris v., *K. bi.,* **Lyc.,** Merc., Mez., Nat. c., *Nat. m.,* Nit. ac., *Nux v., Phos.,* Pho. ac., Phyt., Plat., (Pod.), **Puls.,** Rhodo., *Rhus,* Sabi., *Sang.,* SEP., *Sil.,* Spig., Spo., Stan., *Staph., Stro.,* **Sul.,** Tar., Thuj., Verat. a., *Zinc.*

Glands.—(Arum t.), Bell., *Bry., Con.,* Lyc., *Phos.,* Puls., *Sil.,* Spo., *Sul.*

Bones.—Bell., Chin., Merc.

Skin.—Acon., Arn., **Ars.**, Bell., *Bry.*, *Calc. c.*, Caust., *Chin.*, Con., Dulc., *Graph.*, *Hep.*, Lach., Lyc., **Merc.**, Nit. ac., **Phos.**, Pho. ac., **PULS.**, Rhus, Sec. c., **SEP.**, **Sil.**, Spig., Squ., Staph., **SUL.**

Sleep and Dreams.—(Apis), **ARS.**, Arg. n., (Bap.), *Calc. c.*, (Cannab. i.), Coff., Hep., Nat. c., **Nux v.**, (Pod.), *Sep.*, *Sil.*

Blood, Circulation and Fever.—Acon., (Arg. n.), *Arn.*, *Ars.*, Bell., Bry., Calc. c., *Carb. v.*, Caust., Cham., *Chin.*, Cocc., Fer., (Glon.), *Graph.*, Hep., Ign., Lyc., *Merc.*, *Nat. m.*, Nit. ac., **Nux v.**, Op., PHOS., *Pho. ac.*, *Puls.*, Rhus, Samb., (Sang.), SEP., Sil., *Stan.*, Staph., Stram.; SUL., Thuj., Verat. a.

Aggravations: Time and Circumstances.—Acon., (All. c.), (Aloe), Ambr., Am. carb., Anac., (Apis), (Arg. n.), Arn., *Ars.*, Aur., (Bap.), Bar. c., *Bell.*, BRY., **Calc. c.**, Carb. an., Carb. v., *Caust.*, *Cham.*, Chin., (Cimic.), Cocc., *Con.*, Dros., Dulc., Fer., (Gel.), *Graph.*, Hep., Hyos., *Ign.*, K. bi., (Lil. t.), (Lith.), LYC., *Merc.*, Nat. c., *Nat. m.*, Nit. ac., **Nux v.**, *Phos.*, Pho. ac., (Phyt.), Pod., **Puls.**, Rhodo., *Rhus*, Saba., *Sang.*, Sele., Seneg., SEP., **Sil.**, Spig., Stro., **Sul.**

Other Remedies.—*Acon.*, Aesc., (All. c.), Aloe, Anac., Apis, **Arg. n.**, Arn., **Ars.**, Arum t., Bap., **Bell.**, Berb., **Bry.**, **Calc. c.**, (Cannab. i.), Carb. an., Carb. v., *Caust.*, Cham., *Chin.*, Cimic., Cocc., Con., (Crotal.), Fer., *Gel.*, Glon., *Graph.*, Hep., *Ign.*, *K. bi.*, Lil. t., (Lith.), LYC., **Merc.**, Nat. c., *Nat. m.*, Nit. ac., **Nux v.**, Op., **Phos.**, Pho. ac., Phyt., Plat., Pod., **PULS.**, Rhus, **Sang.**, SEP., **Sili**, Spig., Stan., Staph., Stram., Stro., SUL., Thuj., Verat. a., Zinc.

Antidotes.—Camph., Coff., *Spir. nit. dul.*

Kali Nitricum.

Mind.—*Bell.*, Bry., Calc. c., *Nux v.*, Op., Pho. ac., Puls., *Rhus*, Sep., Sil., *Stram.*, Sul., Verat. a.

Localities.—Acon., Ambr., (Apis), Arg., (Arg. n.), Arn., Ars., Asaf., Aur., *Bar. c.*, *Bell.*, *Bry.*, **Calc. c.**, (Cannab. i.), Canth., Carb. v., *Caust.*, Cham., *Chin.*, Colch., *Con.*, Croc., Fer., Gel., *Graph.*, Hep., Hyos., *Ign.*, K. carb., *Kre.*, Led., (Lil. t.), *Lyc.*, Mang., (Meli.), Merc., *Mez.*, Mur. ac., Nat. c., *Nat. m.*, Nit. ac., Nux v., Oleand., **Phos.**, *Pho ac.*, Puls., Rhus, Ruta, Sabi., Sars., Sec. c., Seneg., SEP., *Sil.*, Spig., Squ., Stan., Staph., Stram., **Sul.**, Sul. ac., Thuj., (Verat. v.), Zinc.

Sensations.—Acon., (Aesc.), Arg., *Arn.*, Ars., Asaf., Aur., BELL., (Berb.), **Bry.**, CALC. C., *Canth.*, Carb. v., *Caust.*, Cham., *Chin.*, Cocc., Con., Dros., Graph., *Ign.*, **K. carb.**, Laur., **Lyc.**, **Merc.**, Mos., Nat. c.,

Nat. m., Nit. ac., **Nux** v., Par., **Phos.**, Pho. ac., Plat., PULS., Rhus, Saba., Sabi., Sars., **Sep.**, Sil., *Spig.*, Stan., *Staph.*, **Stro.**, **Sul.**, Sul. ac., Verat. a., *Zinc.*

Glands.—Bell., Puis., Rhus., Spo.

Bones.—*Cyc.*, Phos.

Skin.—Arn., Bell., *Bry.*, Canth., Caust., *Chin.*, Cyc., *Phos.*, Rhus, *Sep.*, *Sul.*

Sleep and Dreams.—Ars., Aur., Bell., Calc. c., Hep., K. carb. Nat. c., Nux v., Phos., Sep., Sil.

Blood, Circulation and Fever.—Acon., (Apis), Arn., Bell., Bry., (Cannab. i.), Chel., Chin., Dig., (Gel.), (Glon.), *Hyos.*, Sep., *Stram.*, (Verat. v.).

Aggravations: Time and Circumstances.—(Aloe.), Am. carb., (Apis), Arg. n., Ars., Bap., Bell., Bor., *Bry.*, **Calc. c.**, *Cham.*, (Cimic.), (Gel.), (Glon.), Ip., K. bi., K. carb., *Lyc.*, **Merc.**, *Nux v.*, Pod., Puls., *Rhus*, Sang., Seneg., **Sep.**, *Spig.*, Stro., Sul., *Thuj.*

Other Remedies.—Acon., (Apis), (Arg. n.), Arn., Ars., BELL., Bry., Calc. c., (Cannab. i.), Canth., Caust., Cham., *Chin.*, Gel., (Glon.), Ign., K. carb, *Lyc.*, *Merc.*, Nat. m., **Nux v.**, *Phos*, Pho. ac., *Puls.*, RHUS, SEP., Sil., Spig., Staph., Stram., Stro., *Sul.*, (Verat. v.).

Antidotes.—Spir. nit. dul.

Injurious.—Camph.

Kreosotum.

Mind.—*Acon.*, *Anac.*, **Bell.**, Bry., Cham., Graph., *Lyc.*, **Nat. m.**, Phos., *Puls.*, Rhus, *Sul.*

Localities.—(Aesc.), All. c., Alum., Anac., **Ant. cr.**, Apis, Arg., Ars., Arum t., Bar. c., BELL., Bov., *Bry.*, (Cact.), CALC. C., (Cannab. i.), *Carb. v.*, *Caust.*, **Chin.**, Fl. ac., Gel., (Glon.), Hep., K. bi., K. CARB., (Kalm.), Led., Lil. t., Lyc., **Merc.**, Nat. c., **Nat. m.**, Nit. ac., *Nux v.*, **Par.**, **Phos.**, **Pho. ac.**, Plat., Puls., RHUS, Saba., (Sang.), SEP., Sil., Spig., Staph., **Sul.**, Sul. ac., Tell., Verat. a., Verb., Zinc.

Sensations.—Acon., (Aesc.), (Arg. n.), Arn., Asaf., **Bell.**, Bry., (Cact.), Calc. c., (Cannab. i.), Carb. v., *Caust.*, Cham., Chin., Cocc., *Fer.*, (Gel.), (Glon.), Hep., Ign., *K. carb.*, Li. t., Lyc., Nat. m., *Nux v.*, Op., *Phos.*, (Pod.), **Puls.**, **Rhus**, Saba., SEP., Sil., *Spig.*, Staph., *Sul.*, Thuj., Zinc.

Glands.—Ars., **Bell.**, *Con.*, *Hep.*, Merc., Phos., Sep., *Sil.*, **Sul.**

Bones.—Ars., *Asaf., Calc. c., Lyc., Merc.,* Mez., NIT. AC., *Phos.,* Pho. ac., *Puls.,* Rhus, Ruta, *Sil., Staph.,* SUL.

Skin.—Ant. cr., ARS., Bell., Calc. c., Carb. an., **Carb. v.,** *Caust.,* Clem., *Graph., Hep.,* K. carb., **Lach.,** LYC., **Merc.,** Oleand., *Petrol.,* Phos., Puls., RHUS, SEP., **Sil.,** Staph., **Sul.**

Sleep and Dreams.—(Arg. n.), Ars., (Bap.), Bry., Cina, **Ign.,** Lyc., Mur. ac., *Nux v.,* Phos., Puls., **Rhus,** Sars., Sep., Sil.

Blood, Circulation and Fever.—Acon., Arg. n., *Ars.,* (Berb.), *Bry., Calc. c., Chin.,* (Gel.), Glon., *Hep.,* Lyc., Merc., *Nux v., Phos.,* Puls., Rhus, Sil.

Aggravations: Time and Circumstances.—Agar., *Ant. cr.,* (Apis), *Ars.,* Bor., Bry., Calc. c., Carb. an., Carb. v., Chel., *Con., Graph.,* Ign., K. carb., (K. bi.), *K. nit.,* Lyc., Merc., Nit. ac., Nux m., **NUX V.,** Phos., (Pod.), Puls., Ran. b., **Rhus,** (Sang.), Sep., Sil., Spig., Staph., Stram., Sul.

Other Remedies.—Acon., (Aesc.), Anac., Ant. cr., (Apis), Arg. n., *Ars.,* Asaf., **Bell.,** Bry, (Cact.), *Calc. c.,* (Cannab. i.), Carb. v., Caust., Chin., Con., Gel., Glon., Graph., *Hep.,* Ign., (K. bi.), K. carb., Lach., (Lil. t.), **Lyc.,** *Merc.,* Nat. m., Nit. ac., **Nux v.,** Par., **Phos.,** Pho. ac., Pod., **Puls.,** RHUS, **Sang., Sep., Sil.,** Spig., *Staph.,* SUL.

Antidote.—*Nux v.*

Lachesis.

Mind.—Acon., Aloe, Apis, *Bap.,* **Bell.,** *Cannab. i.,* Cimic., Coff., *Crotal.,* Hyd. ac., Hyper., **HYOS.,** Lyc., Meli., Nat. m., Nux v., *Op.,* Phos., Plat., Stram., Ter., Ther., **Verat. a.,** Verat. v.

Localities.—Acon., Aesc., *All. c.,* Aloe, Ant. cr., **Apis,** Apoc. c., **Arg. n.,** Ars., *Arum t., Bap.,* Bar. c., **Bell.,** (Berb.), Bor., *Bry.,* Cact., **Calc. c.,** Cannab. i., *Canth.,* (Carb. ac.), Carb. v., *Caust.,* **Cham.,** Chin., (Cimic.), *Con.,* Crotal., (Dios.), (Fl. ac.), *Gel.,* (Glon.), *Graph.,* Hep., *Hyos.,* Ign., Iris v., **K. bi.,** K. carb., (Kalm.), Kre., (Lil. t.), Lyc., Meli., MERC., *Mez.,* Nat. m., *Nit. ac.,* Nux v., Petrol., Phos., *Phyt.,* Pod., Pso., PULS, *Rhus,* Saba., *Sang.,* Sele., Sep., *Sil.,* Spig., Spo., **Staph.,** *Stram.,* SUL., Thuj., *Verat. a., Verat v.,* Zinc.

Sensations.—Acon., *Aesc.,* (Aloe), Am. carb., *Apis,* **Arg. n., Arn.,** Ars., *Arum t., Bap.,* Bar. c., **Bell.,** *Berb.,* Bry., Cact., Calc. c., **Cannab. i.,** Canth., Caust., Cham., **Chin., Cimic.,** *Cocc.,* Crotal., *Cup.,* Dig., *Fer., Gel.,* Glon., Graph., *Hyos.,* Ign., Ip., (Iris v.), **K. bi.,** (Kalm.), Lil. t., (Lith.), Lyc., *Merc.,* Nit. ac., *Nux v.,* **Op.,** *Phos.,* Pho. ac., *Phyt., Pb.,* Pod., (Pso.), **Puls.,** Sang., Sele., *Sep.,* Sil., Spig., Stram., **Sul.,** Verat. a., *Verat. v.*

Glands.—Bell., *Carb. an.*, *Hep.*, Merc., *Sil.*, *Sul.*

Bones.—Bell., Calc. c., Caust., Chin., Dros., Lyc., *Merc.*, Phos., Pho. ac., Puls., *Ruta*, Staph.

Skin.—*Acon.*, Ant. cr., **Apis**, *Arn.*, ARS., *Asaf.*, (Bap.), **Bell.**, *Bry.*, *Calc. c.*, (Carb. ac.), Carb. an., Carb. v., *Caust.*, Cham., Con., Euphorb., Graph., *Hep.*, K. carb., Kre., Led., LYC., *Merc.*, Mez., Op., Petrol., *Phos.*, Pho. ac., PULS., Rhus, Sec. c., Sele., Sep., *SIL.*, *Staph.*, Sul., Verat. a.

Sleep and Dreams.—Acon., Arg. n., **Bry.**, *Calc. c.*, (Cannab. i.), Chin., Graph., Hep., *Ign.*, Lyc., Nux v., Op., **Phos.**, Rhus, Sele., Sil., Sul.

Blood, Circulation and Fever.—*Acon.*, (Apis), (Arg. n.), ARS., Bell., (Berb.), **Bry.**, (Cact.), *Calc. c.*, (Cannab. i.), Caps., (Gel.), (Glon.), Hell., *Lyc.*, Merc., Nux v., Op., *Phos.*, Pho. ac., Puls., *Rhus*, Samb., Sang., Sep., Spig., Squ., Sul.

Aggravations : Time and Circumstances.—(Aesc.), *Agar.*, (All. c.), (Aloe), *Ambr.*, Ant. cr., Ant. t., Apis, *Arg. n.*, Arn., *Ars.*, (Bap.), Bar. c., **Bell.**, *Bry.*, Caps., Caust., **Cham.**, *Chel.*, Chin., Cina, *Cocc.*, Coff., Con., Dulc., *Fer.*, (Gel.), Graph., Hep., Ign., Iod., *K. bi.*, Led., Lil. t., **Lyc.**, Merc., Mez., Nat. c., Nat. m., Nux m., NUX V., Op., Phos., Phyt., Plat., (Pod.), PULS., *Ran. b.*, Rhodo., Rhus, *Ruta*, Saba., Sang., *Sele.*, Sep., *Sil.*, Spig. Staph., Stram., Stro., *Sul.*, **Tar.**, Valer., *Verat. a.*, (Verat. v.), Verb., Zinc.

Other Remedies.—*Acon.*, Aesc., (All. c.), Aloe, Ant. cr., APIS, **Arg. n.**, Arn., *Ars.*, Arum t., **Bap.**, Bar. c., Bell., Berb., *Bry.*, Cact., *Calc. c.*, Cannab. i., Canth., Carb. an., *Cham.*, *Chin.*, *Cimic.*, Cocc., Con., *Crotal.*, Fer., *Gel.*, Glon., Graph., Hep., **Hyos.**, Ign., **K. bi.**, Lil. t., LYC., *Merc.*, Mez., Nat. m., Nit. ac., *Nux v.*, Op., PHOS., Pho. ac., *Phyt.*, Pod., PULS., *Rhus*, Ruta, Saba., **Sang.**, Sele., Sep., *Sil.*, Spig., Staph., Stram., Sul., *Verat. a.*, Verat. v.

Antidotes.—Ars., *Bell.*, *Merc.*, Nux v., Pho. ac., *Acids*, Cerevisia, Vinum.

Injurious.—Am. carb., Dulc., Nit. ac., Pso.

Laurocerasus.

Mind.—Acon., Apis, (Bap.), BELL., *Bry.*, Calc. c., Cannab. s., Cham., Cimic., **Con.**, Crotal., *Gel.*, Hyd. ac., Hyos., Ign., *Lyc.*, Nat. c., *Nat. m.*, Nux v., Op., **Phos.**, Pho. ac., Pic. ac., Puls., *Rhus*, Sep., Sil., **Stram.**, Sul., **Verat. a.**

Localities.—(Aesc.), (All. c.), Aloe, Alum., Ambr., Apis, (Apoc. c.),

Arg. n., Arn., Asaf., (Arum t.), (Bap.), **Bell.**, Bry., Calc. c, **Canth.,** (Carb. ac.), (Carb. v.), *Caust.,* Cham., **Chin.,** Cocc., (Dios.), Dros., Dulc., (Fl. ac.), (Gel.), Graph., *Hep.,* **Hyos.,** Ign., Iod., Ip., Iris v., K. bi., *K. carb.,* (Lil. t.), Lyc., Merc., *Nat. c.,* Nat. m., *Nit. ac.,* **Nux v.,** Op., PHOS., (Phyt.), Pb., Pod., Pso., PULS., Rhus, Ruta, Sang., Sep., Sil., Stan., Staph., Stram., *Sul.,* Verat. a., **Zinc.**

Sensations.—*Acon.,* (Aesc.), (Aloe), *Alum.,* (Apis), *Arg. n., Arn.,* Ars., Arum t., Asaf, **Bell.,** Berb., *Bry.,* (Cact.), **Calc. c.,** Cannab. i., Canth., Caps., Carb. v., Caust., Chel., *Chin.,* Cocc., Con., Dros., Dulc., *Gel.,* Glon., Hell., Hyos., *Ign.,* (K. bi.), K. carb., (Lil. t.), (Lith.), *Lyc., Merc.,* Mos., Nat. c., Nit. ac., Nux m., *Nux v.,* Oleand., *Op.,* Par., *Phos., Pho. ac.,* (Phyt.), *Pb., Puls.,* **Rhus,** *Saba., Sang.,* Sars., *Sep.,* Sil., Spig., Stan., Staph., Stram., **Sul.,** Verat. a., Zinc.

Glands.—Bell., *Phos.,* Spo.

Bones.

Skin.—Bell., *Bry.,* Con., Phos., Puls., *Rhus,* Sep., **Sul.**

Sleep and Dreams.—Ant. t., (Apis), Ars., Cannab. i., Croc., Nux v., Phos., Pho. ac., (Pod.), Sil.

Blood, Circulation and Fever.—Acon., (Aloe), *Ars.,* **Bell.,** Bry., *Calc. c.,* (Cannab. i.), Canth., *Carb. v., Cham., Cup.,* Guai., *Lyc.,* **Merc.,** Nux v., **Phos.,** Pod., (Sang.), *Sep.,* Stram., **Sul.,** Sul. ac., VERAT. A.

Aggravations: Time and Circumstances.—Ant. cr., (Apis), (Arg. n.), Bar. c., *Bell.,* Bry., *Calc. c.,* Carb. v., Caust., Chel., (Cimic.), Coloc., Con., Croc., Fer., Ign., Iod., (K. bi.), *K. nit.,* Lach., *Lyc.,* Merc., Nat. c., Nit. ac., **Nux v.,** PHOS., *Puls.,* Ran. b., Rhus, Saba., (Sang.), **Sep.,** Sil., Spig., Staph., Stro., Sul., Thuj., Valer., Verat. a., Zinc.

Other Remedies.—*Acon.,* (Aesc.), Aloe, Alum., *Apis,* Arg. n., Arn., Ars., (Arum t.), (Bap.), BELL., Bry., **Calc. c.,** Cannab. i., Canth., Carb. v., Caust., Cham., Chin., (Cimic.), Cocc., *Con., Gel., Hyos., Ign.,* K. bi., K. carb., (Lil. t.), **Lyc.,** Merc., *Nat. c.,* Nat. m., Nit. ac., **Nux v.,** Op., PHOS., *Pho. ac.,* (Phyt.), Pb., Pod., **Puls., Rhus,** Saba., *Sang,* **Sep.,** Sil., Staph., *Stram.,* **Sul., Verat. a.,** Zinc.

Antidotes.—Camph., *Coff.,* Ip., *Op.*

Ledum.

Mind.—Cham., Cocc., Ign., Lyc., Merc.

Localities.—Acon., Ambr., (Apis), Arg. n., *Arn.,* Ars., *Bell.,* Bov., Bry., (Cact.), **Calc. c.,** (Cannab. i.), Canth., Carb. v., (Caul.), **Caust.,** Cham., *Chin.,* Con., Croc., (Crotal.), Dros., Fer., Graph., *Hep.,* Hyos., *Ign.,* Ip., K. bi., *K. carb.,* Kre., (Lith.), **Lyc.,** *Merc.,* Nat. c., Nat. m.,

Nit. ac., *Nux v.*, Petrol., *Phos.*, Pho. ac., **Puls., Rhus**, *Ruta*, *Sabi.*, *Sang.*, *Sec. c.*, SEP., *Sil.*, Spig., *Staph.*, Stram., Stro., SUL., Sul. ac., Verat. a., (Verat. v.), *Zinc.*

Sensations.—Acon., (Aesc.), Ant. cr., Apis, Arg. n., Arn., Ars., Bap., Bell., Bry., (Cact.), **Calc. c.**, Caps., *Chin.*, Cimic., Colch., Crotal., Dros., (Eup. per.), Gel., Ign., (K. bi.), K. carb., Kalm., *Lyc.*, Mar., **Merc.**, Nit. ac., **Nux v.**, Petrol., *Phos.*, (Phyt.), Plat., **Puls.**, RHUS, Ruta, Saba, Sabi., (Sang.), **Sep.**, Spig., Spo., Stan., Staph., **Sul.**, Verat. a., Zinc.

Glands.—Bry., Phos., Sul.

Bones.—Asaf., Cocc., Hep., Ign., Ip., Merc., Pho. ac., Puls., *Ruta*, Sil., Verat. a.

Skin.—Acon., Am. m., Ant. cr., *Apis*, Arn., Ars., Bar. c., *Bell.*, BRY., Calc. c., *Caust., Dulc.*, Euphorb., Graph., Hep., Ip., *Lach.*, **Lyc.**, Mag. c., **Merc.**, Mez., *Oleand.*, Petrol., *Phos.*, Pho. ac., Plat., PULS., Rhus, Sec. c., **Sep.**, Sil., Spo., Squ., Staph., SUL., *Verat. a.*

Sleep and Dreams.—Arg. n, Ars., (Bap.), **Bell.**, Bry., Calc. c., (Cannab. i.), Con., *Graph.*, Hep., *Ign.*, Nux m., Nux v., Op., *Phos.*, Puls.

Blood, Circulation and Fever.—ACON., Ars., (Berb.), *Calc. c.*, (Cannab. i.), Chin., Iod., *Ip.*, **Lyc.**, Merc., Mur. ac., Nit. ac., *Nux v.*, Op., *Phos.,* **Puls.**, Rhus, Saba., Samb., Sang., SEP., Sil., Spig., *Sul.*, *Verat. a.*

Aggravations: Time and Circumstances.—Aesc., (All. c.), Ant. t., Apis, Arg. n., **Arn.**, Ars., (Bap.), Bar. c., BELL., BRY., Calad., Cannab. s., *Caps.*, Caust., Cham., Chel., Chin., (Cimic.), Cocc., Coff., *Colch.*, *Con.*, Dros., Fer., (Glon.), Graph., Hell., Hep., Ign., *Iod*, K. bi., K. carb., Lach., Lil. t., (Lith.), *Lyc.*, Mang., **Merc.**, Mez., *Nat. m.*, NUX V., *Phos.*, (Phyt.), **Puls.**, *Ran. b.*, Ran. s., *Rhodo.*, **Rhus**, Saba., *Sang.*, *Sele.*, *Sep.*, *Sil.*, **Spig.**, Staph., Stro., *Sul.*, *Verat. a.*, (Verat. v.),

Other Remedies.—Acon., (Aesc.), *Apis, Arg. n.*, Arn., Ars., Bap., Bell., Bry., (Cact.), **Calc. c.**, Cannab. i., Caust., Cham., Chin., (Cimic.), Con., (Crotal.), Graph., Hep., *Ign.*, Ip., K. bi., K. carb., (Lith.), **Lyc.**, Merc., *Nux v.*, Petrol., *Phos.*, (Phyt.), PULS., Rhus, Ruta, *Sang.*, **Sep.**, *Sil.*, Spig., Staph., Sul., *Verat. a.*, (Verat. v.).

Antidote.—Camph.

Injurious.—Chin.

Lilium Tig.

Mind.—Acon., Agn., Anac., Arg. n., Arn., *Ars.*, *Bor.*, Cact., Calc. c., Cimic., Cina, Cocc., Croc., Dros., Graph., *Ign.*, *Lyc.*, Meli., Merc., **Nat. m.**

Nit. ac., Nux v., *Phos.*, Phyt., *Plat.*, **Puls**., Pso., Rhus t., Sabi., **Sep.**, Stan., *Stram*., *Sul.*, *Thuj.*, *Verat. a.*

Localities.—*Acon.*, *Aesc.*, Agar., (All. c.), **Aloe**, (Alum.), (Ambr.), (Am. m.), (Ant. cr.), Ant. t., (Apis), (Apoc. c.), Arg., Arg. n., Arn., *Ars.*, (Asaf.), Aur., (Bap.), *Bar. c.*, **Bell.**, (Bism.), (Bor.), Bry., Calc. c., (Camph.), (Cannab. i.), (Cannab. s.), *Canth.*, Caps., (Carb. ac.), Carb. an., (Carb. v.), Caust., (Cham.), (Chel.), Chin., Cimic., (Cina), (Clem.), Cocc., Colch., Coloc., *Con.*, (Cup.), (Dig.), (Dros.), Dulc., (Euphr.), Fer., Gel., Graph., (Hell.), Hep., (Hyos.), Ign., (Ip.), (Iod.), (Iris v.), K. carb., (K. bi.), (K. nit.), Kalm., (Kre.), Lach., (Laur.), *Lyc.*, (Mag. m.), (Meli.), (Meny.), *Merc.*, (Mur. ac.), (Nat. c), *Nat. m.*, *Nit. ac.*, **Nux v.**, Op., (Petrol.), *Phos.*, Pho. ac., Plat., (Pb.), (Pod.), (Pso.), **Puls.**, (Ran. b.), (Rheum), (Rhodo.), *Rhus*, Ruta, (Saba.), Sabi., (Samb.), Sars., Sec. c., (Sele.), **Sep.**, Sil., Spig., Squ., (Stan.), *Staph.*, (Stram.), **Sul.**, Thuj., (Valer.), Verat. a., (Verat. v.), (Verb.), (Zinc).

Sensations.—*Acon.*, (Aesc.), (Agar.), (Aloe), (Apis), Arg. n., (Arn.), Ars., Arum. t., (Asaf.), (Bap.), (Bar. c.), *Bell.*, (Berb.), *Bry.*, Calc. c., (Cannab. i.), Canth., (Carb. v.), (Caust.), Chel., Chin., Cimic., Cocc., *Coloc.*, (Con.), Cup., (Dig.), (Dios.), (Eur. per.), (Hep.), Ign., Ip., (Iris v.), K. bi., Lach., (Laur.), Lyc., (Meny.), Merc., Mez., (Nat. c.), Nat. m., Nit. ac., **Nux v.**, Op., Petrol., *Phos.*, Pho. ac., (Phyt.), (Plat.), Pb., Pod., *Puls.*, (Ran. b.), Rhodo., Rhus, (Ruta), (Saba.), (Sabi.), Sang., (Sars.), Sec. c., (Seneg.), *Sep.*, *Sil.*, Spig., (Spo.), (Squ.), Stan., (Stram.), Sul., (Thuj.), Valer., Verat. a., (Verat. v.), Zinc.

Glands.

Bones.

Skin.

Sleep and Dreams.—(Ars.), (Bry.), (Calc. c.), (Cham.), (Chin.), (Coff.), (Hyos.), (Merc.), (Phos.), (Puls.), (Rhus), (Sep.), (Sul.).

Blood, Circulation and Fever.—(Ars.), (Bell.), (Bor.), (Bry.), (Fer.), (Merc.), (Nux v.), (Op.), (Phos.), (Pho. ac.), (Puls.), (Ruta), (Sang.), (Sil.), (Spo.), (Stram.), (Sul.).

Aggravations: Time and Circumstances.—Acon., (Aesc.), (Agar.), (Agn.), (Ambr.), (Ant. cr.), (Ant. t.), (Apis), Arn., (Ars.), (Asaf.), (Asar.), Aur., (Bap.), (Bar. c.), *Bell.*, (Bov.), **Bry.**, (Calad.), Calc. c., (Camph.), Cannab. s., (Canth.), Caps., (Carb. an.), (Carb. v.), (Caust.), (Cham.), (Chel.), (Chin.), (Cic.), (Cimic.), (Cina), (Cocc.), (Coff.), Colch., Coloc., *Con.*, Croc., Cyc., (Dig.), (Dros.), (Dulc.), (Euphorb.), (Euphr.), Fer., (Glon.), Graph., (Hell.), Hep., (Hyos.), (Ign.), Ip., Iod., (K. carb.), Lach., Led., *Lyc.*, Mag. c., (Mag. m.), (Mang.), *Merc.*, (Mez.), Nat. m.,

RELATIONSHIPS.—LIL. T.—LITH. 415

Nit. ac., *Nux v.*, (Oleand.), (Petrol.), *Phos.*, (Pho. ac.), (Phyt.), (Plat.), (Pb.), **Puls.**, Ran. b., Rheum, Rhus, (Ruta), (Saba.), *Sabi.*, (Samb.), (Sang.), Sars., Sele., *Sep.*, *Sil.*, Spig., (Spo.), (Squ.), Stan., Staph., (Stro.), *Sul.*, Valer., (Verat. a.), (Verb.), Zinc.

Other Remedies.—Acon., Aesc., Agar., (Agn.), Aloe, (Ambr.), (Ant. cr.), (Ant. t.), (Apis), Arg. n., *Arn.*, **Ars.**, (Asaf.), Aur., (Bap.), Bar. c., **Bell.**, Bor., **Bry.**, *Calc. c.*, (Camph.), Cannab. i., (Cannab. s.), Canth., Caps., (Carb. an.), (Carb. v.), Caust., (Cham.), Chel., Chin., *Cimic.*, Cina, *Cocc.*, (Coff.), Colch., *Coloc.*, Con., Croc., (Cup.), (Dig.), Dros., (Dulc.), Fer., Graph., (Hell.), Hep., (Hyos.), *Ign.*, Ip., (Iod.), (Iris v.), (K. bi.), (K. carb.), Lach., (Laur.), **Lyc.**, (Mag. m.), (Meny.), **Merc.**, (Mez.), (Nat. c.), **Nat. m.**, *Nit. ac.*, **Nux v.**, Op., Petrol., **Phos.**, Pho. ac., Phyt., Plat., (Pb.), (Pod.), PULS., Ran. b., (Rheum), (Rhodo.), **Rhus**, Ruta, (Saba.), *Sabi.*, (Samb.), Sang., Sars., Scc. c., (Sele.), SEP., *Sil.*, Spig., (Spo.), Squ., *Stan.*, Staph., Stram., SUL., Thuj., **Valer.**, *Verat. a.*, (Verat. v.), (Verb.), Zinc.

Lithium.

Mind.

Localities.—(Acon.), (Ambr.), (Am. m.), (Ant. t.), (Apis), (Arg. n.), (Arn.), Bell., Bry., (Calc. c.), (Canth.), (Caust.), (Chel.), (Colch.), (Coloc.), (Dig.), (Fer.), (Graph.), (Hep.), (Ign.), (Ip.), (K. carb.), (Led.), (Lyc.), (Mag. c.), Merc., (Nat. m.), (Nux v.), (Op.), Phos., Pb., Puls., (Rhodo.), Rhus, Sep., (Sil.), (Staph.), Sul., (Verat. a.).

Sensations.—(Acon.), Alum., (Apis), (Arg.), (Arg. n.), Arn., Ars., (Arum. t.), Asaf., (Aur.), *Bell.*, (Bism.), (Bor.), Bry., Calc. c., (Cannab. i.), (Canth.), (Caps.), (Carb. v.), Caust., Chel., Chin., (Cic.), (Cimic.), (Cocc.), (Colch.), Coloc., Con., (Cup.), Dros., (Dulc.), (Euphorb.), (Fer.), (Graph.), (Ign.), (K. bi.), Lach., (Laur.), (Lil. t.), Lyc., (Meny.), Merc., Mez., (Nat. c.), (Nat. m.), Nit. ac., Nux v., (Op.), (Par.), Phos., Phyt., (Pb.), Puls., Ran. b., (Ran. s.), (Rhodo.), Rhus, (Ruta), Saba., Sabi., Sang., (Sars.), (Sec. c.), Seneg., Sep., Sil., Spig., Spo., (Squ.). Stan., Staph., Sul., Tar., Thuj., (Valer.), (Verat. a.), (Zinc.).

Glands.
Bones.
Skin.
Sleep and Dreams.
Blood, Circulation and Fever.
Aggravations: Time and Circumstances.—(Aesc.), (Ambr.), (Am. carb.), (Arg.), (Aur.), (Bor.), (Bry.), (Calc. c.), (Clem.), (Coloc.), (Dros.),

(Fer.), (Iod.), (K. carb.), (Lach.), (Led.), (Lyc.), (Mang.), Merc., (Nux v.), (Phos.), (Pb.), (Puls.), (Ran. b.), (Rhodo.), (Rhus), (Sang.), Sep., (Sil.), (Spig.), (Stro.), Sul., (Valer.), (Verat. a.).

Other Remedies.—(Acon.), (Ambr.), (Apis), (Arg.), (Arg. n.), (Arn.), (Aur.), Bell., (Bor.), Bry., Calc. c., (Canth.), (Caust.), (Chel.), (Colch.), Coloc., (Dros.), (Fer.), (Graph.), (Ign.), (K. carb.), (Lach.), (Led.), Lyc., Merc., (Nat. m.), Nux v., (Op.), Phos., Pb., Puls., (Ran. b.), (Rhodo.), Rhus, (Sang.), Sep., Sil., (Spig.), (Staph.), Sul., (Valer.), (Verat. a.).

Lycopodium.

Mind.—*Acon.,* Aloe, **Apis**, Anac., Arg. n., *Ars.,* **Aur.**, **Bap.**, Bar. c., **BELL.**, Calc. c., **Cannab. i.**, Carb. ac., Caust., Cham., Cic., *Cimic.,* Cocc., *Crotal.,* Gel., *Glon.,* Graph., Hell., Hyd. ac., Hyper., **HYOS.**, **Ign.**, K. br., Lach., *Meli.,* Merc. c., Nat. c., Nat. m., *Nux v.,* Op., Phos., *Pho. ac.,* Pic. ac., **Plat.**, Pso., **PULS.**, Rhus, *Sep.,* Sil., Still., **STRAM.**, *Sul.,* Ther., **VERAT. A.**, **Verat. v.**

Localities.—Acon., *Aesc.,* Agn., (All. c.), *Aloe,* Alum., APIS, Apoc. c., ARG. N., *Arn.,* **Ars.**, Arum. t., Aur., *Bap.,* Bar. c., **Bell.**, *Berb., Bry., Cact.,* CALC. C., *Cannab. i., Canth.,* Caps., *Carb. ac.,* Carb. v., (Caul.), *Caust., Cham.,* **Chin.**, Cimic., Clem., Cocc., *Con., Crotal.,* Cup., Dios., Dulc., Eup. per., Fer., Fl. ac., *Gel.,* Glon., *Graph., Hep.,* (Hyd. ac.), Hyos., Ign., Ip., Iris v., K. BI., *K. carb.,* Kalm., *Lil. t.,* (Lith.), (Meli.), **Merc.**, Nat. c., *Nat. m.,* Nit. ac., NUX V., Op., Petrol., PHOS., Pho. ac., Phyt., Pic. ac., Pb., *Pod., Pso.,* PULS., *Rhus,* Ruta, Saba., **Sang.**, Sec. c., Sele., SEP., **Sil.**, *Spig.,* Stan., *Staph.,* Stram., SUL., Thuj., *Verat. a., Verat. v.,* Zinc.

Sensations.—*Acon.,* (Aesc.), (Aloe), Anac., **Apis**, *Arg. n.,* Arn., *Ars.,* Arum. t., Asaf., Aur., *Bap.,* Bar. c., **Bell.**, Berb., *Bry.,* (Cact.), CALC. C., Cannab. i., Canth., Caps., Carb. v., **Caust.**, *Cham.,* Chel., **Chin.**, *Cimic.,* Cocc., *Con.,* Crotal., Cup., Dios., (Eup. per.), *Fer.,* Gel., *Glon., Graph., Hyos., Ign.,* Iod., Ip., Iris v., *K. bi., K. carb.,* Lil. t., (Lith.), (Meli.), *Merc.,* Nat. c., *Nat. m., Nut ac.,* **Nux v.**, Oleand., Op., Petrol., *Phos.,* Pho. ac., Phyt., Plat., Pod., **Puls.**, **Rhus**, *Sang.,* Sec. c., SEP., *Sil.,* Spig., Spo., *Stan., Stram ,* Stro., **Sul.**, Verat. v., Zinc.

Glands.—Arn., Arum t., **BELL.**, Bry., Calc. c., Carb. an., *Con.,* Hep., **Merc.**, Nit. ac., *Phos.,* Puls., Rhus, Sep., Sil., Spo., *Sul.*

Bones.—Asaf., Bell., **Calc. c.**, (Eup. per.), Hep., Merc., Mez., **Nit. ac.**, Phos., Pho. ac., *Puls.,* Sep., **Sil.**, *Staph.,* Sul.

Skin.—Acon., Agn., Anac., Ant. cr., **Apis**, Arn., **Ars.**, *Bell.,* **Bry.**,

CALC. C., (Carb. ac.), *Carb. v.*, Caust., Chin., Cocc., *Con.*, Crotal., Dulc., Graph., *Hep.*, *K. carb.*, Lach., Led., *Merc.*, *Nit. ac.*, *Oleand.*, Phos., Pho. ac., Plat., **Puls.**, Rhus, Sec. c., **Sep.**, SIL., *Staph.*, SUL.

Sleep and Dreams.—Arn., *Ars.*, *Bell.*, *Bry.*, *Calc. c.*, Carb. an., Chin., Cic., Graph., Hep., *Ign.*, K. carb., Mar., Merc., Mur. ac., **Nux v.**, Phos., PULS., Ran. b., Rhus, Sele., *Sep.*, *Sil.*, Sul.

Blood, Circulation and Fever.—Acon., (Aloe), (Apis), Arg. n., *Ars.*, Aur., (Berb.), **Bry.**, (Cact)., CALC. C., Cannab. i., Chin., *Fer.*, (Gel.), Glon., Graph., Iod., K. carb., Merc., Nat. m., *Nux v.*, Op., PHOS., (Pod.), **Puls.**, Rhus, *Sang.*, *Sep.*, Spig., *Sul.*, Verat. a., (Verat. v.).

Aggravations: Time and Circumstances.—Acon., (All. c.), *Aloe.*, Alum., Am. carb., *Ant. cr.*, *Apis*, *Arg. n.*, Arn., *Ars.*, Aur., Bap., **Bell.**, Bor., BRY., CALC. C., (Cannab. i.), Canth., Caps., *Carb. v.*, Caust., *Cham.*, Chin., (Cimic.), Cocc., Colch., **Con.**, Dros., Dulc., Euphorb., *Fer.*, Graph., Hep., *Ign.*, Iod., *K. bi.*, *K. carb.*, K. nit., (Lil. t.), *Merc.*, Nat. c., *Nat. m.*, Nit. ac., NUX V., Petrol., **Phos.**, *Pho. ac.*, (Phyt.), Plat., (Pod.), PULS., Ran. b., Rhodo., **Rhus.**, Ruta, Saba., Samb., **Sang.**, Sep., Sil., Spig., *Staph.*, Sul., *Thuj.*, Valer., Verat. a., (Verat. v.),

Other Remedies.—*Acon.*, Aesc., (All. c.), *Aloe*, APIS, **Arg. n.**, Arn., Ars., Arum. t., Aur., **Bap.**, **Bell.**, *Berb.*, *Bry.*, Cact., CALC. C., **Cannab. i.**, Carb. v., Caust., Cham., *Chin.*, *Cimic.*, Cocc., *Con.*, *Crotal.*, Fer., *Gel.*, Glon., Graph., Hep., Hyos., *Ign.*, K. bi., *K. carb.*, Lil. t., (Lith.), **Merc.**, Nat. m., *Nit. ac.*, **Nux v.**, **Phos.**, Pho. ac., Phyt., Plat., *Pod.*, PULS., Rhus, *Sang.*, Sep., Sil., Spig., Staph., Stram., SUL., Verat. a., **Verat. v.**

Antidotes.—Acon., Camp., Cham., *Puls.*

Magnesia Carbonica.

Mind.—*Calc. c.*, Phos.

Localities.—Agn. Am. carb., Am. m., Ant. cr., *Bell.*, Bry., **Calc. c.**, Caust., Cham., (Cimic.), Cocc., *Con.*, Fer., **Graph.**, Hep., Hyos., K. bi., **K. carb.**, Kre., (Lith.), *Lyc.*, **Merc.**, **Nat. m.**, Nit. ac., *Nux v.*, Petrol., **Phos.**, Pho. ac., Pb., PULS., *Rhus*, Ruta, Sabi., (Sang.), SEP., Sil., Stan., Staph., SUL., Zinc.

Sensations.—Alum., Am. m., Arg., (Arg. n.), *Arn.*, Ars., Asaf., Asar., Aur., Bar. c., **Bell.**, Bov., Bry., **Calc. c.**, (Cannab. i.), *Canth.*, Carb. v., CAUST., *Chin.*, Cocc., Con., Dros., Dulc., (Gel.), Graph., Hell., *Hep.*, *Ign.*, **K. carb.**, *Lyc.*, Mag. m., **Merc.**, Mez., Nat. c., **Nat. m.**, *Nit. ac.*, *Nux v.*, **Phos.**, *Pho. ac.*, *Plat.*, **Puls.**, *Rhodo.*, *Rhus*, Ruta, Sars., **Sep.**, *Sil.*, Spig., **Stan.**, Staph., Stro., **Sul.**, Tar., *Zinc.*

Glands.—Con., Lyc., *Phos.*

Bones.—Caust.

Skin.—Am. carb., (Apis), Arn., *Bell.*, Bry., *Calc. c.*, Chin., Clem., Con., Dulc., *Led.*, Lyc., *Merc.*, Nat. m., Nit. ac., Oleand., Petrol., *Phos.*, *Pho. ac.*, Puls., *Rhus*, Sec. c., *Sep.*, **Sil.**, Staph., Sul., *Verat. a.*

Sleep and Dreams.—Arg. n., *Arn.*, **Ars.**, (Bap.), Bry., (Cannab. i.), Graph., K. carb., **Nux v.**, PHOS , Puls., Sep., *Sil.*

Blood, Circulation and Fever.—Ars., Bry., Chin., Colch., Graph., Hep., *Merc.*, Nit. ac., Nux m., Rhus, *Sil.*, Squ.

Aggravations: Time and Circumstances.—*Acon.*, (All. c.), Alum., Am. carb., (Apis), Arn., Ars., *Aur.*, (Bap.), Bell., (Cannab. i.), *Caps.* (Cimic.), Dulc., (Gel.), *Hell.*, Hep., Hyos., Ign., (K. bi.), *K. carb.*, (Lil. t.), **Lyc.**, *Mag. m.*, Mang., Merc., Nit. ac., *Nux v.*, Phos., PULS., (Phyt.), *Rhus*, Saba., Sabi., (Sang.), **Sep.**, Sil., Spo., Stro., Sul.

Other Remedies.—Am. carb., (Apis), (Arg. n.), Arn., *Ars.*, Aur., (Bap.), *Bell.*, Bry., *Calc. c.*, (Cannab. i.), *Caust.*, Chin , (Cimic.), Cocc., *Con.*, Dulc., (Gel.), Graph., Hell., Hep., Ign., (K. bi.), *K. carb.*, Lyc., Mag. m., Merc., *Nat. m.*, Nit. ac., *Nux v.*, PHOS, Pho. ac., **Puls.**, *Rhus*, (Sang.), **Sep.**, Sil., Stan., Staph., Stro., *Sul.*, Zinc.

Antidotes.

Magnesia Muriatica.

Mind.—Calc. c., Ign., Nat. c., Nux v., Pho. ac., *Puls.*, **Sil.**, Sul.

Localities.—Aesc., Aloe, Alum., Am. carb., Arg. n., Ars., (Arum. t.), (Bap.), *Bell.*, *Bry.*, **Calc. c.**, (Carb. ac.), Carb. v., Caust., Cham., **Chin.**, Cocc., Graph., *Ign.*, (Iris v.), K. bi., **K. carb.**, (Lil. t.), *Lyc.*, **Merc.**, Mez., *Nat. c.*, NAT. M., Nit. ac., **Nux v.**, Op., **Phos.**, Pod., *Puls.*, *Rhus*, Sang., *Sep.*, *Sil.*, Staph., **Sul.**, Thuj., Verat. a., Zinc.

Sensations.—(Apis), *Arn.*, *Asaf.*, Aur., (Bap.), (Berh.), BELL., Bov., *Bry.*, **Calc. c.**, Canth., Carb. v., *Caust.*, Cham., *Chin.*, *Cocc.*, Con., Fer., Graph , Hep., *Ign.*, (Iris v.), *K. carb.*, *Lyc.*, *Merc.*, Nat. c , Nat. m., *Nux v.*, *Phos*, Plat., **Puls.**, *Rhus*, Sabi., (Sang.), **Sep.**, **Sil.**, Spig., Stan., Staph., Stro., Sul., Thuj., Verat. a., Zinc.

Glands.—Bell., Bry., Carb. an., Clem., Con., Graph., *Lyc.*, Puls.

Bones.—Bell., *Lyc.*, Merc., Staph.

Skin.—Bry., *Lyc.*, Nat. m., Puls., Sep.

Sleep and Dreams.—Bry., *Calc. c.*, Chin., Con., **Graph.**, Merc., Nux v., PHOS., Pho. ac., *Puls.*, Rhus, Sep., *Sil.*, **Sul.**

Blood, Circulation and Fever.

Aggravations: Time and Circumstances.—*Acon.*, (Aesc.), (All.

RELATIONSHIPS.—MAG. M.—MANG. 419

c.), (Aloe), Ambr., Am. carb., *Am. m.*, (Apis), Arg., Ars., Asaf., *Aur.*, (Bap.), Bar. c., Bell., Bry., Calc. c., **Caps.**, Carb. an., Carb. v., Cham., Chin., (Cimic.), Clem., Cocc., Con., *Cyc.*, Dros., **Dulc.**, *Euphorb.*, **Fer.**, (Glon.), Graph., Hell., Hep., Ign., Iod., K. bi., K. carb., Led., **LYC.**, *Mag. c.*, Mang., Meny., Merc., *Mos.*, *Nat. c.*, Nit. ac., Nux v., *Phos.*, **Pho. ac.**, (Phyt.), Plat., **PULS.**, Rhodo., Rhus, Ruta, **Saba.**, Samb., (Sang.), SEP., Sil., Spo., Sul., **Tar.**, *Valer.*, Verb., Vio. t.

Other Remedies.—(Aesc.), (Aloe), (Apis), (Bap.), *Bell.*, *Bry.*, **Calc. c.**, Cham., *Chin.*, Cocc., Con., Dulc., Fer., *Graph.*, Ign., K. bi., *K. carb.*, LYC., *Merc.*, Nat. c., Nat. m., *Nux v.*, **Phos.**, Pho. ac., PULS., *Rhus*, Sang., SEP., Sil., Sul.

Antidotes.—Camph.

Manganum.

Mind.—Acon., *Anac.*, Ign., *Lyc.*, Merc., Nux v., Pho. ac., **Puls.**, Sil., Sul.

Localities.—(All. c.), Am. carb., Anac., (Apis), (Arg. n.), (Arum. t.), Asaf., Bell., *Bry.*, Calc. c., Canth., *Carl. v.*, **Caust.**, Chin., *Con.*, Dros., (Gel.), Graph., Hep., (K. bi.), *K. carb.*, Kre., Laur., *Lyc.*, **Merc.**, *Nat. m.*, **Phos.**, Pho. ac., Plat., PULS., *Rhus*, Saba., Sabi., Sars., **Sep.**, *Sil.*, Spig., Spo., Stan., Staph., Stro., **Sul.**, Verat. a., Zinc.

Sensations.—Acon., Alum., (Apis), Arn., *Ars.*, (Bap.), **Bell.**, *Bry.*, **Calc. c.**, Canth., *Caust.*, Cham., *Chin.*, Cocc., *Con.*, Dros., Graph., Ign., (K. bi.), *K. carb.*, *Lyc.*, *Merc.*, Mez., Nat. c., Nat. m., Nit. ac., *Nux v.*, *Phos.*, Plat, **Puls.**, *Rhus*, *Sep.*, *Sil.*, Spig., Spo., Stan., Staph., Stro., **Sul.**, Thuj., Verat. a., Zinc.

Glands.—*Bell.*, Carb. an., Lyc., Merc.

Bones.—*Bell.*, *Calc. c.*, Chin., **Merc.**, Phos., **Puls.**, *Ruta*, Sil., *Staph.*

Skin.—Alum., (Apis), *Bry.*, **Calc. c.**, Graph., *Hep.*, *Nat. m.*, *Petrol.*, Phos., PULS., Rhus, Sep., *Sul.*, Zinc.

Sleep and Dreams.—Ars., K. carb., Mag. c., Nat. c., *Nux v.*, *Sep.*, *Sil.*

Blood, Circulation and Fever.—(Apis), Ars., (Gel.), Nux v., Saba., Sep.

Aggravations: Time and Circumstances.—(Aesc.), (All. c.), **Am. carb.**, (Arg. n.), *Ars.*, Aur., (Bap.), Bell., *Bor.*, Bry., **Calc. c.**, Cnam., *Chin.*, (Cimic.), Cocc., Coloc., Con., Dros., *Dulc.*, Graph., *Hep.*, Ign., K. bi.), K. carb., (Lil. t.), (Lith.), Lyc., **Merc.**, Nat. c., **Nux m.**, Nux v., **Phos.**, (Phyt.), (Pod.), *Rhodo.*, RHUS, *Ruta*, (Sang.), **Sep.**, Sil., *Spig.*, *Stro.*, **SUL.**, Thuj., **Verat. a.**

Other Remedies.—(All. c.), Am. carb., Apis, (Arg. n.), Ars., (Bap.), *Bell.*, *Bry.*, Calc. c., Caust., Chin., Con., (Gel.), Graph., Hep., (K. bi.), K. carb., *Lyc.*, **Merc.**, Nat. m., Nux v., **Phos.**, PULS., **Rhus**, Ruta, **Sep.**, *Sil.*, Spig., Staph., Stro. **Sul.**, Verat. a.

Antidote.—Coff.

Marum Verum

Mind.—Anac., Aur., Cham.

Localities.—(All. c.), Aloe, Am. m., (Apis), (Arg. n.), Arn., Aur., (Arum. t.), *Bry.*, Calc. c., (Carb. ac.), *Carb. v.*, Caust., Cham., **Chin.**, (Crotal.), Cyc., Dios., Dulc., (Glon.), *Graph.*, *Ign.*, K. bi., *K. carb.*, Kre., *Lyc.*, **Merc.**, Nit. ac., **Nux v.**, *Phos.*, Pho. ac., *Pb.*, Pod., PULS., Ran. b., Rhus, Ruta, Saba., Sang., Sep., *Sil.*, Spig., Stan., *Staph.*, **Sul.**, Sul. ac., Verat. a.

Sensations.—Ambr., (Apis), Arg., (Arg. n.), Ars., Bell., Bry., *Calc. c.*, Canth., *Carb. v.*, *Caust.*, Cham., CHIN., Cocc., Colch., Con., Cup., *Ign.*, Iod., **K. carb.**, **Lyc.**, **Merc.**, Nat. m., **Nux v.**, **Phos.**, **Pho. ac.**, **Puls.**, Rhodo., Rhus, Ruta, **Sep.**, Sil., Stan., Staph., *Sul.*, Zinc.

Glands.—Con., Ign., *Merc.*, Rhus, *Spo.*

Bones.

Skin.—*Calc. c.*, Dulc., *Graph.*, Led., Lyc., **Merc.**, *Phos.*, Saba., SIL., Staph., Sul.

Sleep and Dreams.—Bell., Bry., Calc. c., Ign., Lyc., Merc., Phos., Puls., Rhus, Sep., Sil., Sul.

Blood, Circulation and Fever.—K. carb., Lyc., Phos., (Sang.), Sul.

Aggravations: Time and Circumstances.—Agar., (Apis), (Arg. n.), (Bap.), Bry., Calc. c., Carb. v., Cham., *Chin.*, Cina, Cocc., *Fer.*, Guai., Hep., *Ign*., (K. bi.), K. nit., Lach., Lyc., Mang., Mur. ac., **Nux v.**, *Petrol.*, (Pod.), Puls., Ran. b., Saba., (Sang.), **Sil.**, *Spig.*, Spo., Staph., **Sul.**, Valer.

Other Remedies.—(Apis), (Arg. n.), Bry., *Calc. c.*, *Carb. v.*, Caust., Cham., Chin., Cocc., Graph., *Ign.*, (K. bi.), K. carb., **Lyc.**, **Merc.**, **Nux v.**, **Phos.**, Pho. ac., (Pod.), **Puls.**, Rhus, Saba., Sang., Sep., SIL., Spig., Spo., *Staph.*, **Sul.**, Valer.

Antidote.—Camph.

Menyanthes.

Mind.—Bap., Bell., Gel., Hell., Hyos., Ign., *Lyc.*, Merc., *Nat. c.*, *Op.*, Phos., Puls., Sil., Staph., *Stram.*, Zinc.

Localities.—(Aesc.), (Aloe), Apis, (Apoc. c.), (Arg. n.), *Bell.*, *Bry.*, (Cact.), *Calc. c.*, (Cannab. i.), Carb. an., Carb. v., *Caust.*, Chel., Chin.,

Con., (Dios.), (Fl. ac.), (Gel.), Graph., Ign., K. carb., (Lil. t)., *Lyc.*, Merc., Mez., Nat. m., Nit. ac., Nux v., Petrol., Phos., PULS., Rhus, **Sep.**, Sil., Spig., Staph., **Sul.**, Verat. a., Zinc.

Sensations.—(Aloe), Alum., (Arg. n.), Arn., *Asaf.*, **Bell.**, Bry., **Calc. c.**, (Cannab. i.), Caust., Chin., (Cimic.), Cocc., (Gel.), (Glon.), Graph., Ign., K. carb., (Lil. t.), (Lith.), Lyc., *Merc.*, Mur. ac., Nat. c., Nat. m., *Nux v.*, *Phos.*, (Phyt.), Plat., *Puls*, *Rhus*, Saba., Sang., *Sep.*, Sil., Spig., Spo., **Stan.**, *Staph.*, **Sul.**, Tar., Thuj., Zinc.

Glands.—Calc. c., Clem., Rhodo., Spo.

Bones.

Skin.—Led., *Lyc.*, *Staph.*

Sleep and Dreams.

Blood, Circulation and Fever.—Apis, (Arg. n.), *Ars.*, Bell., (Berb.), (Cact.), Calc. c., (Cannab. i.), Gel., *Hell.*, Lyc., Nux m., Nux v., *Phos.*, Puls., (Sang.), Sep., Spig., Sul.

Aggravations: Time and Circumstances.—Am. m, Arg., (Arg. n.), Asaf., *Aur.*, (Bap.), *Bell.*, *Bry*, CAPS., Caust., Cham., Con., Cyc., Dros., Dulc., *Euphorb.*, Euphr., *Fer.*, (Glon.), (K. bi.), *Lach.*, Lyc., Mag. m., Mez., *Mos.*, Mur. ac., *Pho. ac.*, *Plat.*, Puls., Ran. s., *Rhodo.*, RHUS, Saba., Samb., Sang., Sep., Stro., **Tar.**, *Valer.*, *Verb.*, Vio. t.

Other Remedies.—(Aloe), Apis, Arg. n., (Bap.), Bell., Bry., **Calc. c.**, (Cannab. i.), Caps., Caust., Gel., (Glon.), Ign., (Lil. t.), LYC., Merc., Nux v., Phos., PULS., *Rhus*, Saba., Sang., **Sep.**, Sil., Spig., Staph., *Sul.*, Tar.

Mercurius Vivus.

Mind.—Acon., Aesc., Aloe, Anac., Apis, Arg. n., **Bap.**, Calc. c., *Cannab. i.*, Carb. ac., Chel., **Cimic.**, Crotal., Gel., Glon., *Hell.*, Hyd. ac., Hyper., *Ign.*, *Lyc.*, Meli., *Merc. c.*, *Nat. c.*, *Nux v.*, Op., Phos., *Pho. ac.*, Phyt., Pic. ac., *Puls.*, *Ran. b.*, *Rhus*, Sep., *Sil.*, Staph., Stram., *Sul.*, Ther., *Thuj.*, Verat. v.

Localities.—Acon., **Aesc.**, **All. c.**, ALOE, Alum., APIS, **Apoc. c.**, ARG. N., Arn., *Ars*, Arum t., Aur., **BAP.**, **Bell.**, **Berb.**, Bor., *Bry.*, *Cact.*, CALC. C., *Cannab. i.*, Canth., **Carb. ac.**, Carb. v., Caul., *Caust.*, Cham., *Chin.*, *Cimic.*, Clem., Con., Crotal., *Dios.*, Eup. per., *Fl. ac.*, **Gel.**, Glon., Graph., *Hep.*, (Hyd. ac.), Iris v., K. BI., K. carb., Kalm., Kre., *Lil. t*, Lith., *Lyc.*, Meli., Nat. c., *Nat. m.*, *Nit. ac.*, Nux v., Petrol., **Phos.**, Pho. ac., *Phyt.*, Plat., Pb., POD., *Pso.*, PULS., Rhus, Ruta, Saba., *Sang.*, Sele., **Sep.**, Sil., *Spig.*, Staph., Stram., SUL., Tell., Thuj., *Verat. a.*, **Verat. v.**

Sensations.—Acon., (Aesc.), (All. c.), *Aloe*, **Apis**, **Arg. n.**, **Arn.**, Ars., *Arum t.*, Asaf., Bap., **Bell.**, **Berb.**, *Bry.*, Cact., **Calc. c.**, **Cannab. i.**, Canth., (Carb. ac.), Carb. v., *Caust.*, Cham., Chin., Cic., **Cimic.**, Cocc., Con., Croc., Crotal., Dios., (Eup. per.), Fer., (Fl. ac.), **Gel.**, *Glon.*, Graph., Hell., Hep., Hyos., *Ign.*, Iris v., **K. bi.**, *K. carb.*, (Kalm.), Lil. t., Lith., *Lyc.*, Nat. c., Nat. m., Nit. ac., **Nux v.**, **Phos.**, Phyt., Plat., (Pod.), (Pso.), PULS, Rhodo., RHUS., Saba., **Sang.**, **Sep.**, *Sil.*, Spig., Staph., SUL., Thuj., Verat. a., Verat. v., Zinc.

Glands.—Arum t., BELL., Bry., Calc. c., *Lyc.*, **Phos.**, Puls., Sil., Spo., **Sul.**

Bones.—ASAF., *Bell.*, **Calc. c.**, Chin., (Cimic.), Eup. per., Hep., *Lyc.*, Nit. ac., Phos., *Pho. ac.*, *Puls.*, *Sep.*, *Sil.*, Staph., *Sul.*

Skin.—Acon., *Apis*, **Ars.**, Asaf., *Bell.*, Bry., *Calc. c.*, Carb. ac., Caust., Dulc., Graph., **Hep.**, (K. bi.), Lach., *Lyc.*, *Nit. ac.*, Phos., Puls., RHUS, (Sang.), **Sep.**, SIL., Staph., SUL., Thuj., Verat. a.

Sleep and Dreams.—Acon., Arg. n., *Ars.*, (Bap.), *Bell.*, **Bry.**, **Calc. c.**, Cannab. i., Caust., Cham., Chin., *Con.*, Graph., *Hep.*, Ign., K. carb., (Lil. t.), Lyc., Nat. c., Nux v., PHOS., *Pho. ac.*, **Puls.**, *Rhus*, SEP., **Sil.**, Sul.

Blood, Circulation and Fever.—Acon., (Aloe), (Apis), (Arg. n.), ARS., (Bap.), **Bell.**, Berb., **Bry.**, Cact., *Calc. c.*, Cannab. i., Carb. v. *Cham.*, Chin., Cocc., (Crotal.), Cup., (Gel.), (Glon.), Graph., *Hep.*, Ign., *Iod.*, Ip., Laur., (Lil. t.), Mos., **Nux v.**, **Phos.**, *Pho. ac.*, Plat., Pod., **Puls.**, Rhus, *Sang.*, *Sec. c.*, Sele., *Sep.*, Sil., *Sul*, Valer., **Verat. a.**, (Verat. v.).

Aggravations: Time and Circumstances.—Acon., Aesc., (All c.), (Aloe), *Am. carb.*, Ant. cr., *Apis*, Arg. n., Arn., *Ars.*, Aur., Bap., **Bell.**, Bor., **Bry.**, **Calc. c.**, Canth., *Carb. v.*, Caust., *Cham.*, Chin., (Cimic.), Cocc., Colch., Coloc., Con., Dros., Fer., (Gel.), Glon., Graph., **Hep.**, *Ign.*, *Iod.*, Ip., *K. bi.*, *K. carb.*, Lach., *Led.*, Lil. t., (Lith.), LYC., *Mag. c.*, *Mang.*, Nat. m., *Nit. ac.*, **Nux v.**, **Phos.**, Pho. ac., *Phyt.*, Pod., PULS., Rhus, Saba., Samb., **Sang.**, Sep., *Sil.*, **Spig.**, Staph., *Stro.*, SUL., Thuj., *Verat. a.*, (Verat. v.).

Other Remedies.—Acon., Aesc., All. c., **Aloe**, APIS, (Apoc. c.), ARG. N., *Ars.*, Asaf., Arum t., BAP., **Bell.**, Berb., *Bry.*, Cact., **Calc. c.**, **Cannab. i.**, Carb. v., Caust., Cham., Chin., **Cimic.**, Con., *Crotal.*, **Gel.**, *Glon.*, Graph., *Hep.*, Ign., Iod., **K. bi.**, K. carb., *Lil. t.*, Lith., *Lyc.*, Mang., Nat. c., Nat. m., Nit. ac., *Nux v.*, **Phos.**, Pho. ac., *Phyt.*, **Pod.**, PULS., Rhus, **Sang.**, Sep., Sil., Spig., Staph., SUL., Thuj., Verat. a., Verat. v.

RELATIONSHIPS.—MERC. VIV.—MEZ.

Antidotes.—Asaf., Aur., *Bell.*, Camph., *Curb. v.*, *Chin.*, **Hep.**, Lach., Mez., **Nit. ac.**, Op., Sars., Sep., Sil., Staph., *Sul.*, Electric.

Mezereum.

Mind.—Acon., Bell., Calc. c., Cham., Cimic., Cocc., *Con.*, Gel., Hell., IGN., *Lyc.*, *Merc.*, Nat. c., Nat. m., Nux v., **Op.**, Phos., **Pho. ac.**, **Puls.**, *Rhus*, Sep., **Sil.**, Staph., Stram.

Localities.—(Aesc.), All. c., (Aloe), Am. carb., (Apis), Arg. n., *Arn.*, *Ars.*, *Arum t.*, (Bap.), Bar. c., *Bell.*, Berb., Bry., **Calc. c.**, Cannab. i., *Canth.*, Caps., (Carb. ac.), Carb. v., *Caust.*, Cham., *Chin.*, *Cocc.*, Con., (Fl. ac.), Gel., Glon., *Graph.*, Hep., *Ign.*, **K. bi.**, *K. carb.*, LYC., **Merc.**, Nat. c., *Nat. m.*, Nit. ac., *Nux v.*, Par., *Petrol.*, PHOS., Pho. ac.. (Pod.), Pso., *Puls.*, *Rhus*, Ruta, Sabi., Sang., SEP., *Sil.*, *Spig.*, Stan., *Staph.*, **Sul.**, *Thuj.*, Verat. a., (Verat. v.), **Zinc**.

Sensations.—Acon., Aesc., Aloe, Alum., Apis, Arg., *Arg. n.*, Arn., Arum. t, *Asaf.*, Bap., **Bell.**, Berb., *Bry.*, **Calc. c.**, Cannab. i., Carb. v., Caust., *Chin.*, **Cimic.**, Cocc., Con., (Eup. per.), *Gel.*, *Ign.*, (Iris v.), **K. bi.**, **K. carb.**, Lil. t., Lith., Lyc., Merc., Nat. c., *Nat. m.*, **Nux v.**, *Phos.*, Phyt., Plat., Pod., (Pso.), Puls., Rhus, Sep., Sang., Spig., Spo., *Stan.*, *Staph.*, Stro., **Sul.**, Thuj., *Zinc*.

Glands.—Bell., *Bry.*, Con., Phos., Sul.

Bones.—Asaf., Calc. c., (Eup. per.), Lyc., *Merc.*, *Pho. ac.*, *Sil.*, Staph., Sul.

Skin.—Acon., Am. carb., Am. m., Ant. cr., Apis, *Ars.*, **Bell.**, **Bry.**, *Calc. c.*, (Carb. ac.), Carb. v., CAUST., Con., Dulc., Euphorb., *Hep.*, Ip., Lach., *Led.*, LYC., **Merc.**, Nux v., *Oleand.*, Petrol., Phos., PULS., Rhus, *Sep.*, **Sil.**, Spo., *Staph.*, **Sul.**, Verat. a.

Sleep and Dreams.

Blood, Circulation and Fever.—Acon., Arn., Ars., **Bell.**, (Berb.), Bry., CALC. C., Canth., Cham., *Chin.*, Hep., *Ign.*, Lyc., Merc., Nat. m., Nit. ac., NUX V., *Phos.*, (Pod.), **Puls.**, Rhus, (Sang.), Sep., Sil., *Sul.*, Verat. a.

Aggravations: Time and Circumstances.—(Aesc.), (All. c), (Aloe), Ambr., **Anac.**, Ant. t., (Apis), (Arg. n), (Bap.), *Bell.*, Bry., (Cact.), *Caps*, Carb. v., Caust., Cham., (Cimic.), Colch., Con., Euphorb., (Glon.), Ign., K. bi., *K. carb.*, Lach., Led., (Lil. t.), Lyc., Mag. m., *Merc.*, Nux v., *Phos.*, (Phyt.), (Pod.), Puls., Sang., Sil., Stro.

Other Remedies.—Acon., Aesc., (All. c.), Aloe, Apis, Arg. n., Arn., *Ars.*, Arum t., Asaf., Bap., **Bell.**, Berb., **Bry.**, **Calc. c.**, Cannab. i., Carb. v., *Caust.*, Cham., Chin., Cimic., Cocc., *Con.*, *Gel.*, (Glon.), **Hep.**,

Ign., *K. bi.*, *K. carb.*, Lach., (Lil. t.), **Lyc.**, MERC., Nat. m., **Nux v.**, Phos., Pho. ac., (Phyt.), Pod., PULS., **Rhus**, *Sang.*, **Sep.**, **Sil.**, *Staph.*, Sul., Verat. a., Zinc.

Antidotes.—*Acetum*, Bry., Camph., *Merc.*, Rhus,

Moschus.

Mind.—Acon., Ars., *Bell.*, Bry., **Calc. c.**, Con., Laur., *Merc.*, *Nat. m.*, **Nux v.**, Op., Phos., Pho. ac., Puls., Rhus, *Sil.*, **Stram.**, Sul., *Verat. a.*, Zinc.

Localities.—*Acon.*, Ant. cr., Arg. n., Ars., **Bell.**, *Bry.*, (Cact.), **Calc. c.**, (Cannab. i.), (Carb. ac.), *Carb. v.*, Caust., Cham., *Chin.*, Cimic., Cocc., Con., *Cup.*, (Fl. ac.), Gel., Hell., Ign., Ip., (Iris v.), K. carb., Lyc., (Meli.), *Merc.*, Nat. c., Nat. m., Nit. ac, **Nux v.**, Oleand., Op., Phos., Pho. ac., Plat., (Pod.), PULS., Sabi., (Sang.), Seneg., SEP., *Sil.*, Spig., Staph., Stram., *Sul.*, Sul. ac., Verat. a., (Verat. v.), Zinc.

Sensations.—Acon., Anac., (Apis), (Apoc. c.), Arg. n., Arn., *Asaf.*, Bap., **Bell.**, (Berb.), Bry., *Calc. c.*, Canth., Carb. v., *Caust.*, Cham., *Chin.*, Cimic., COCC., *Con.*, Dros., (Gel.), (Glon.), Hyos., **Ign.**, *Ip*, *K. carb.*, **Lyc.**, Mag. m., Nat. m., Nux m., **Nux v.**, Oleand., *Op.*, Petrol., **Phos.**, Pho. ac., **Plat.**, (Pod.), **Puls.**, *Rhus*, Sabi., (Sang.), Sec. c., **Sep.**, Sil., Stan., Staph., *Stram.*, *Sul.*, Sul. ac., Valer., *Verat. a.*

Glands.

Bones.

Skin.—Acon., Arn., Bell., **Bry.**, *Calc. c.*, Caust., *Merc.*, **Phos.**, Plat., Puls., Rhus, Sep., *Verat. a.*

Sleep and Dreams.—(Apis), *Bry.*, (Cannab. i.), Con., Hep., Ign., Nux v., *Phos.*, (Pod.), Puls., *Rhus*, Sep., Sul.

Blood, Circulation and Fever.—Acon., *Arn.*, *Ars.*, BELL., BRY., *Calc. c.*, Caust., Cham., *Chel.*, Chin., (Glon.), Hyos., **Merc.**, *Nux v*, Phos., Pho. ac., Plat., Puls., *Rhus*, Sep., Sil., Stan., Stram., *Verat. a.*

Aggravations: Time and Circumstances.—Acon., Agar., (Aloe), (Apis), **Ars.**, Aur., (Bap.), Bar. c., Bell., *Camph.*, **Caps.**, *Caust.*, Cocc., *Con.*, Cyc., Dros., **Dulc.**, Euphorb., Fer., Hell., *Hep.*, Hyos., Ign., K. bi., *K. carb.*, **Lyc.**, *Mag. m.*, Meny., Nux m., **Nux v.**, Phos., *Pho. ac.*, Plat., **Puls.**, Ran. b., *Rhodo.*, Rhus, SABA., (Sang.), Sele., **Sep.**, *Stro.*, Tar., Thuj., *Valer.*, Verb., Vio. t.

Other Remedies.—*Acon.*, (Apis), Arg. n., Arn., *Ars.*, Aur., (Bap.), BELL., Bry., *Calc c.*, (Cannab. i), Caps., Carb. v., *Caust.*, Cham., Chin., Cimic., Cocc., *Con.*, Dulc., (Gel.), (Glon.), Hep., Hyos., Ign., Ip., K. carb., *Lyc.*, Mag. m., *Merc.*, Nat. m., **Nux v.**, **Op.**, PHOS., *Pho. ac.*,

Plat, Puls., Rhus, Saba., (Sang.), **Sep.**, Sil., *Stram.*, Sul., Valer., Verat. a.

Antidote.—Camph.

Muriaticum Acidum.

Mind.—Ign., Pho. ac., Puls., Sil., Sul., Verat. v.

Localities.—(Aesc.), Aloe, Anac., Apis, Ant. cr., Arg., (Arg. n.), Arn., Ars., Arum t., Asaf., (Bap.), *Bar. c.*, **Bell.**, Bry., (Cact.), **Calc. c.**, Camph., (Cannab. i.), Canth., (Carb. ac.), *Carb. v.*, **Caust.**, Cham., **Chin.**, (Cimic.), Gel., *Graph.*, Hep., Hyos., *Ign.*, *K. bi.*, **K. carb.**, Kre., (Lil. t.), **Lyc.**, *Merc.*, Nat. c., *Nat. m.*, *Nux v.*, Oleand., Petrol., **Phos.**, *Pho. ac.*, (Phyt.), (Pod.), **PULS.**, Rhus, Saba., Sabi., **SEP.**, Sil., *Spig.*, Squ., *Staph.*, **SUL.**, Thuj., (Verat. v.), *Zinc.*

Sensations.—Acon., (Aesc.), Aloe, Alum., Am. m., (Apis), (Arg. n.), Arn., Ars., (Arum t.), *Asaf.*, (Bap.), **Bell.**, (Berb.), *Bry.*, **Calc. c.**, (Cannab. i.), *Carb. v.*, **Caust.**, *Chin.*, Cimic., Cocc., *Con.*, (Crotal.), (Dios.), Dros., Dulc., (Eup. per.), Gel., (Glon.), *Graph.*, Hell., Hep., Ign., (Iris v.), K. bi., K. **CARB.**, *Lyc.*, Mar., Meny., **Merc.**, Mez., **Nat. c.**, *Nat. m.*, Nit. ac., **Nux v.**, Phos., Pho. ac., Phyt., Plat., (Pod.), **Puls.**, Rhodo., **Rhus**, Ruta, *Saba.*, Sang., **SEP.**, *Sil.*, **Spig.**, Spo., **Stan.**, **Staph.**, **Sul.**, Tar., Thuj., (Verat. v.), *Zinc.*

Glands.—*Bry.*, *Phos.*, Puls., Rhus.

Bones.

Skin.—Arn., Ars., *Asaf.*, Bar. c., Bell., Bry., **CALC. C.**, Chin., *Con.*, Cyc., Dulc., *Graph.*, Hep., K. carb., **Lyc.**, **Merc.**, Nat. m., Nit. ac., *Phos.*, Pho. ac., *Puls., Rhus,* Saba., Sec. c., *Sep.*, SIL., Staph., SUL., Thuj,

Sleep and Dreams.—Ars., Bell., *Bry.*, Calc. c., Chin., Graph., Hep., *Ign.*, *K. carb.*, Kre., *Lyc.*, Meny., NUX V., **Phos.**, *Puls.*, Ran. b. Rhus, Saba., **Sep.**, Sil., Sul.

Blood, Circulation and Fever.—Acon., (Apis), Bry., Chin., (Gel.), Op., Saba., Samb., **Spig.**, (Verat. v.),

Aggravations: Time and Circumstances.—Am. m., Apis, (Arg. n.), Arn., Ars., **Asaf.**, *Bell.*, Bry., *Calc. c.*, (Cannab. i.), Caps., Cham., Cina, *Con.*, **Cyc.**, Dros., Dulc., Fer., Ign., (K. bi.), Lach., *Lyc.*, Mag. m., Mang., *Meny.*, Nat. c., Nux v., **Phos.**, Pho. ac., *Puls.*, Ran. b., Rhodo., **Rhus**, *Ruta*, Saba., Sang., Sep., *Sul.*, Valer., Vio. t.

Other Remedies.—Acon., (Aesc.), Aloe, Apis, (Arg n.), Arn., Ars., (Arum t.), *Asaf.*, (Bap.), *Bell., Bry.*, **Calc. c.**, (Cannab. i.), Carb. v., Caust., *Chin.*, (Cimic.), Con., Cyc., Gel., Graph., Hep., *Ign.*, K. bi., *K. carb.*, **Lyc.**, Meny., *Merc.*, Nat. c., Nat. m., *Nux v.*, **Phos.**, Pho. ac.,

(Phyt.), (Pod.), PULS., **Rhus**, Saba., Sang., **Sep.**, *Sil.*, *Spig.*, Staph., Sul., (Verat. v.), Zinc.

Antidotes.—Camph., *Bry.*

Natrum Carbonicum.

Mind.—Aloe, *Anac.*, Ars., Aur., Bap., *Bell.*, Calc. c., Cannab. i., Chel., Con., Croc., Hyos., Ign., **Lyc.**, Meli., Merc., Merc. c., **Op.**, Phos., **Pho. ac.**, *Pic. ac.*, Puls., Rhus, Sep., Sil., Staph., *Stram.*, Sul.

Localities.—*Acon.*, (Aesc.), (All. c.), Aloe, Ambr., Am. carb., Am. m., Anac., Apis, (Apoc. c.), *Arg. n.*, Arn., *Ars.*, Arum t., *Aur.*, Bar. c., Bap., *Bell.*, *Bry.*, Cact., **CALC. C.**, Cannab. i., Canth., Carb. ac., *Carb. v.*, **Caust.**, Cham., **Chin.**, Cimic., Con., Crotal., Dios., (Eup. per.), (Fl. ac.), Gel., Glon., *Graph.*, Hep., *Ign.*, (Iris v.), **K. bi.**, **K. carb.**, (Kalm.), *Kre.*, **Lyc.**, **Merc.**, *Nat. m.*, Nit. ac., **Nux v.**, Petrol., *Phos.*, *Pho. ac.*, (Phyt.), Plat., Pb., (Pod.), Pso., **PULS.**, **Rhus**, Saba., Sabi., *Sang.*, Sele., **SEP.**, Sil., *Spig.*, Stan., *Staph.*, **Sul.**, Thuj., *Verat. a.*, (Verat. v.), Zinc.

Sensations.—*Acon.*, (Aesc.), Alum., Anac., **Apis**, Arg. n., *Arn.*, Ars., (Arum t.), *Asaf.*, Aur., (Bap.), Bar. c., **Bell.**, Berb., Bry., **CALC. C.**, Cannab. i., Canth., Carb. v., *Caust.*, Cham., *Chin.*, Cocc., Coff., Con., Cup., Dulc., (Eup. per.), (Gel.), (Glon.), Graph., Hep., *Ign.*, (Iris v.), **K. bi.**, *K. carb.* (Lil. t.), (Lith.), **Lyc.**, **Merc.**, Mez., *Nat. m.*, Nit. ac., **Nux v.**, Petrol., **Phos.**, Pho. ac., Pso., *Plat*, **Puls.**, Rhodo., **Rhus**, *Saba.*, Sang., Sep., *Sil.*, *Spig.*, Spo., *Stan.*, Staph., **Sul.**, Tar., Thuj., Valer., Verat. a., Zinc.

Glands.—Arn., (Arum t.), **Bell.**, *Bry.*, **Calc. c.**, Carb. an., Chin., Clem., *Con.*, K. carb., **Lyc.**, *Merc.*, *Phos.*, **Puls.**, Rhus, *Sep.*, *Sil.*, Spo., *Sul.*

Bones.

Skin.—Am. carb., Ant. cr., Arn., *Ars.*, Bar. c., *Bell.*, Bry., **Calc. c.**, Cham., Clem., Con., **Dulc.**, *Graph*, Hep., **Lyc.**, *Merc.*, **Nit. ac**, Phos., Pho. ac., **Rhus**, Sele., **SEP.**, *Sil.*, Squ., Staph., **Sul.**, Vio. t.

Sleep and Dreams.—(Apis), Arg. n., Ars., Aur., *Calc. c.*, Cannab. i., Cannab. s., Chin., Con., Graph., Hep., Ign., **K. carb.**, **NUX V.**, Op., *Phos.*, (Pod.), Puls., Saba., SEP., *Sil.*, Sul., Sul. ac.

Blood, Circulation and Fever.—(Cact.), (Cannab. i.), *K. carb.*, Lyc., (Sang.), *Sep.*, Sul.

Aggravations: Time and Circumstances.—Acon., (Aloe), Ant. cr., (Apis), (Arg. n.), Arn., Ars., Asaf., (Bap.), Bell., *Bry.*, (Cact.), **CALC. C.**, *Carb. v.*, Caust., Cham., Chel., *Chin.*, (Cimic.), **Con.**, Cyc., Dros., *Graph.*, Guai., Hep., *Ign.*, K. bi., K. carb., (Lil. t.), **Lyc.**, Mag. m., Merc., *Nat.*

RELATIONSHIPS.—NAT. CARB.—NAT. MUR.

m., Nux v., Phos., *Pho. ac.*, Pod., Pb., **Puls.**, *Rhus*, Ruta, Saba., Sang., Sele., SEP., *Sil.*, **Sul.**, Sul. ac., Thuj).

Other Remedies.—Acon., (Aesc.), Aloe, Apis, *Arg. n.*, Arn., *Ars.*, Arum t, Aur., Bap., *Bell.*, Bry., Cact., CALC. C., *Cannab. i*, Carb. v., Caust., *Chin.*, (Cimic.), *Con.*, (Gel.), (Glon.), *Graph*, *Ign.*, *K. bi*, *K. carb.*, (Lil. t.), **Lyc.**, *Merc.*, Nat. m., Nit. ac., *Nux v.*, **Phos.**, *Pho. ac*, Pod., **Puls.**, *Rhus*, Saba., *Sang.*, SEP., **Sil.**, Staph., SUL.

Antidotes.—*Camph.*, Spir. nit. dul.

Natrum Muriaticum.

Mind.—*Acon.*, Aloe, Alum., Anac., **Apis**, Bap., **Bell.**, Bry., Calc. c., *Cannab. i.*, Chel., Cic., Cimic., *Con.*, Crotal., Cup., *Gel.*, *Glon.*, Graph., Hell., *Hyd. ac.*, Hyper., **Hyos.**, *Ign.*, Laur., *Lyc.*, *Meli.*, Nux m., *Nux v.*, Op., Oxyt., Petrol., *Phos.*, Pho. ac., Phyt., Pic. ac., Plat., Pso., *Puls.*, *Rhus*, Sep., Sil., **Stram.**, Sul., Ter., **Verat. a.**

Localities.—Acon., **Aesc.**, All. c., *Aloe*, Anac., Ant. cr., *Apis*, Apoc. c., ARG. N., Arn., Ars., *Arum t.*, Aur., *Bap.*, Bar. c., **Bell.**, *Berb.*, Bry., Cact., CALC. C., *Cannab. i.*, *Carb. ac.*, Carb. v., (Caul.), **Caust.**, *Chin.*, Cimic., Cocc., Con., *Crotal.*, Dios., Dulc., Eup. per., Fer., Fl. ac., **Gel.**, Glon., Graph., Hep., (Hyd. ac.), Hyos., Ign., Iris v., K. BI., **K. carb.**, Kalm., Kre., Led., *Lil. t.*, Lith., **Lyc.**, Meli., *Merc.*, Nit. ac., *Nux v.*, Petrol., **Phos.**, Pho. ac., Phyt., (Pic. ac.), Plat., *Pod.*, *Pso.*, PULS., Rhus, Ruta, **Sang.**, Sec. c., SEP., **Sil.**, Spig., Staph., SUL., Verat. a., *Verat. v.*, Zinc.

Sensations.—Acon., Aesc., Aloe, Ambr., *Apis*, **Arg. n.**, Arn., Ars., Arum. t., Aur., *Bap.*, **Bell.**, **Berb.**, Bry., Cact., **Calc. c.**, *Cannab. i.*, (Carb. ac.), Carb. v., **Caust.**, Cham., Chin., *Cimic.*, Cocc., Con., Crotal., Dios., Eup. per., Fer., **Gel.**, Glon., *Graph.*, *Ign.*, Iris v., **K. bi.**, *K. carb.*, (Kalm.), Lil. t., (Lith.), **Lyc.**, *Merc.*, Mez., Nat. c., Nit. ac., **Nux v.**, Petrol., **Phos.**, (Phyt.), Plat., (Pod.), (Pso.), **Puls.**, Rhodo., **Rhus**, Ruta, **Sang.**, SEP., *Sil.*, *Spig.*, Stan., Staph., SUL., Thuj., Verat. a., *Verat. v.*, Zinc.

Glands.—Bell., Calc. c., Phos., **Puls.**, Sul.

Bones.—Asaf., Aur., Calc. c., Chin., *Lyc.*, Nit. ac., **Puls.**, Sil., *Sul.*

Skin.—Alum., Apis, Ars., Bell., *Bry.*, **Calc. c.**, Chin., (Cimic.), Con., (Eup. per.), Graph., *Hep.*, *K. carb.*, Lyc., **Merc.**, *Nit. ac.*, *Petrol.*, Phos., Pho. ac., Puls., RHUS, *Sele.*, SEP., *Sil.*, SUL., Thuj.

Sleep and Dreams.—(Apis), Arg. n., (Bap.), *Bry.*, *Calc. c.*, Cannab. i., Caust., Chin., Con., Ign., Nux v., *Op.*, *Phos.*, (Pod.), *Sep.*, SIL., **Sul.**

Blood, Circulation and Fever.—Acon., (Arg. n.), Ars., Bell.,

(Berb.), BRY., (Cact.), *Calc. c.,* (Cannab. i.), Cham., **Chin.**, (Cimic.), *Dig., Fer.,* (Gel.), (Glon.), *Hep.,* Hyos., *K. carb., Lyc.,* Nux v., *Op.,* Phos., *Pho. ac.,* Puls., *Rhus,* Samb., *Sang.,* Sec. c., *Sep.,* Stram., Sul.

Aggravations : Time and Circumstances.—Acon., (Aesc.), (All. c.), Aloe, Am. m., Ant. cr., *Apis,* Arg. n., *Arn.,* Ars., (Bap.), **Bell., Bry.,** (Cact.), CALC. C., Cannab. s., *Carb. v.,* Caust., Cham., *Chin.,* Cic., Cimic., Cina, *Cocc., Con.,* Fer., (Gel.), (Glon.), *Graph., Hep., Ign.,* Ip., *K. bj., K. carb.,* Lil. t., **Lyc.,** Merc., *Nat. c.,* Nit. ac., **Nux v.,** Oleand., Phos., *Pho. ac.,* (Phyt.), Pod., *Puls.,* Rhodo., *Rhus,* Ruta, *Sang.,* Sele., **Sep., Sil.,** Spig., Squ., *Staph.,* Sul., (Verat. v.).

Other Remedies.—Acon., Aesc., (All. c.), *Aloe,* APIS, **Arg. n.,** Arn., Ars., **Bap.,** *Bell.,* Berb., **Bry.,** *Cact.,* CALC. C., **Cannab. i.,** Carb. v., Caust., *Chin.,* **Cimic.,** Cocc., Con., Crotal., Fer., **Gel.,** *Glon.,* **Graph.,** Hep., Hyos., Ign., K. bi., *K. carb., Lil. t.,* (Lith.), **Lyc.,** Merc., Nit. ac., *Nux v.,* Op., Petrol., Phos., *Pho. ac.,* Phyt., *Pod ,* PULS., **Rhus, Sang.,** SEP., **Sil.,** Staph., SUL., Verat. a., Verat. v.

Antidote.—Camph., Spir. nit. d.

Nitrum Acidum.

Mind.—Acon., **Anac.,** Ars., Aur., *Bar. c., Bell. c., Calc. c.,* Caust., Cup., Graph., Hell., Hyos., Ign., **Lyc.,** Nat. c., Nat. m., Nux m., Nux v., Pho. ac., **Puls.,** *Rhus, Stram., Sul.*

Localities.—*Aesc. c., All. c., Aloe,* Alum., **Apis,** Apoc. c., ARG. N., Arn., *Ars., Arum t.,* Aur., Bap., **Bell.,** Berb., *Bry.,* Cact., CALC. C., *Cannab. i.,* Canth., Carb. ac., Carb. an., **Carb. v.,** *Caust.,* Cham., *Chin.,* Cimic., Clem., Con., Crotal., Dios., Dulc., (Eup. per.), Fer., Fl. ac., Gel., (Glon.), **Graph.,** *Hep.,* Hyos., Ign., Iris v., K. BI., *K. carb.,* Kalm., Kre., *Lil. t., Lyc.,* MERC., Nat. c., *Nat. m.,* **Nux v.,** PHOS., *Pho. ac., Phyt.,* (Pic. ac.), **Pod.,** Pso., PULS., *Rhus,* Ruta, *Sang.,* **Sep.,** *Sil.,* Spig., Stan., *Staph.,* Stram., SUL., Sul. ac., *Thuj.,* Verat. a., Verat. v., Zinc.

Sensations.—*Acon.,* Aesc., (All. c.), (Aloe), *Anac.,* Apis, (Apoc. c.), *Arg. n., Arn., Ars.,* Arum t., Asaf., Aur., Bap., **Bell.,** *Berb., Bry.,* Cact., **Calc. c.,** Cannab. i., Canth., (Carb. ac.), *Carb. v., Caust.,* Cham., **Chin.,** Cimic., *Cocc., Con.,* (Crotal.), (Dios.), *Dulc.,* (Eup. per.), Fer., (Fl. ac.), *Gel., Glon., Graph.,* Hyos., Ign., (Iris v.), **K. bi.,** *K. carb.,* (Kalm.), Lil. t., (Lith.), **Lyc.,** *Merc.,* Nat. c., **Nat. m., Nux v.,** Petrol., **Phos.,** Pho. ac., Phyt., *Plat.,* Pb., Pod., Pso., PULS., Rhodo., *Rhus,* Ruta, *Sang.,* **Sep.,** *Sil.,* Spig., Spo., Stan., Staph., Stram., Stro., SUL., Verat. a., Verat. v., *Zinc.*

Glands.—Arum t., **Bell.,** Bry., *Calc. c.,* Carb. an., Cham., Chin.,

RELATIONSHIPS.—NIT. AC.—NUX MOS.

Con., Dulc., Ign., K. carb., Lyc., **Merc.**, Nux m., **Phos.**, *Puls., Rhus,* Sil., Spo., SUL.

Bones.—Asaf., Calc. c., (Cimic.), Con., Eup. per., Graph., *Lyc., Merc., Phos.,* **Puls.**, Rhus, Ruta, Sep., *Sil.,* Staph., SUL.

Skin.—Apis, *Ars.,* Asaf., Bar. c., Bell., Bry., *Calc. c., Carb. v.,* Caust., Cham., (Cimic.), Con., Crotal., Dulc., (Eup. per.), Graph., **Hep., Lyc., Merc.**, Petrol., *Phos.,* **Puls.**, Rhus, *Sep.,* Sil., Staph., SUL., Thuj.

Sleep and Dreams.—(Arg. n.), Ars., *Calc. c.,* Caust., Con., Hep., Ign., Phos., Puls., Sep., Sil., *Sul.*

Blood, Circulation and Fever.—Acon., (Aloe), (Apis), *Arn., Ars.,* Bell., Bry., Cact., Calc. c., (Cannab. i.), Carb. v., *Cham., Chin.,* (Glon.), Graph., Hep., Hyos., Ign., *Ip.,* K. carb., Led., *Lyc.,* MERC., Nat. c., Nat. m., **Nux v.**, Op., Petrol., PHOS., Pho. ac., (Pod.), **Puls.**, Ran. b., Rhus, Saba., Sang., **Sep.**, *Sil.,* Spo., Stram., SUL., Verat. a., (Verat. v.).

Aggravations : Time and Circumstances.—Acon., (Aesc.), (Aloe), *Ant. cr., Apis,* Arg. n., *Ars.,* Bap., Bar. c., Bell., **Bry.**, (Cact.), *Calc. c.,* CARB. V., Cham., *Chin.,* (Cimic.), Colch., *Con.,* (Gel.), Graph., **Hep.**, Ign., *K. bi.,* K. carb., K. nit., (Lil. t.), **Lyc.,** *Merc., Nat. m.,* **Nux v., Phos.**, Phyt., Pod., PULS., **Rhus**, *Sang.,* SEP., *Sil.,* Staph., SUL., Verat. a., (Verat. v.).

Other Remedies.—Acon., (Aesc.), (All. c.), Aloe, Anac., **Apis**, Apoc. c., *Arg. n.,* Arn., *Ars., Arum. t.,* Aur., *Bap., Bell.,* Berb., *Bry., Cact.,* **Calc. c.**, Cannab. i., *Carb. v.,* Caust., Cham., *Chin., Cimic., Con.,* Crotal., Dulc., Gel., Glon., *Graph., Hep.,* Hyos., Ign., **K. bi.**, K. carb., Lil. t., **Lyc., Merc.**, Nat. c., *Nat. m., Nux v.,* **Phos.**, Pho. ac., *Phyt., Pod.,* PULS., Rhus, *Sang.,* Sep., Sil., Staph., Stram., SUL., Verat. a., Verat. v.

Antidotes.—Camph., *Hep.,* Mez., Sul.

Injurious.—Lach.

Nux Moschata.

Mind.—Alum., *Apis,* Bap., **Bell.**, Bry., *Cannab. i.,* Cannab. s., Carb. an., Cimic., *Con., Crotal.,* Cyc., *Gel., Glon., Graph.,* **Hell.**, *Hyd. ac.,* **Hyos.**, Ign., K. br., K. carb., Laur., *Lyc., Meli.,* Merc., *Merc. c., Nat. c.,* **Nat. m.**, Nux v., **Op.**, *Phos., Pho. ac.,* Pic. ac., **Plat.**, *Puls.,* **Rhus**, Sep., Sil., Spig., STRAM., Sul. ac., Ter., *Thuj., Verat. a.,* Zinc.

Localities.—(Aloe), Anac., Ant. cr., (Apis), (Apoc. c.), (Arg. n.), Arn., Bell., *Bry.,* **Calc. c.**, (Cannab. i.), *Carb. v.,* Caust., *Cham., Chin.,* Cocc., Con., (Dios.), (Gel.), (Glon.), *Graph.,* Hyos., Ign., Ip., (K. bi.), *K. carb., Kre.,* (Lil. t.), Merc., Nat. c., *Nat. m.,* Nit. ac., **Nux v.**, Op.,

Phos., Pho. ac., Plat., Pb., (Pod.), PULS., Rhus, Ruta, (Sang.), **Sep.**, Sil., Spig., Stan., Staph., Stram., Sul., **Verat. a**.

Sensations.—*Acon.*, (Aesc.), *Apis*, (Apoc. c.), (Arg. n.), *Arn.*, Ars., Asar., Bap., Bar. c., **Bell.**, (Berb.), *Bry.*, (Cact.), *Calc. c.*, Camph., Cannab. i., Canth., Caust., *Cham.*, *Chin.*, Cimic., *Cocc.*, Coff., *Con.*, Cup., (Eup. per.), *Gel.*, Glon., Hyos., *Ign.*, Iod., Ip., (Iris v.), (K. bi.), K. carb., *Laur.*, *Lyc.*, Merc., Mos., *Nat. c*, NUX V., *Oleand.*, *Op.*, *Phos,* Pho. ac., (Phyt.), *Plat.*, (Pod.), (Pso.), **Puls.**, **Rhus**, Ruta, Saba., Sang , *Sep.*, *Sil.*, Spig., Stan., *Stram.*, **Sul.**, *Sul. ac.*, Valer., *Verat. a.*, Verat. v.

Glands.—Bell., Cham., Iod., Puls., Rhus, Sec. c., Spo.

Bones.

Skin.—Arn., **Bell.**, Bry., **Calc. c.**, Chin., *Led.*, LYC., *Nit. ac.*, Nux v., **Phos.**, *Pho. ac.*, *Puls.*, **Rhus**, Sec. c., **Sep.**, *Sil.*, Sul.

Sleep and Dreams.—(Aloe), ANT. T., Apis, Bry., Cannab. i., Con., Croc., K. carb., **Op.**, Phos., Pho. ac , Pod., Puls., Rhus, Verat. a

Blood, Circulation and Fever.—Apis, (Arg. n.), **Ars.**, Bry., (Cannab. i.), Cham , *Chin.*, Colch., Gel., (Glon.), Hep., Lyc , *Nux v.*, Phos., **Puls.**, **Rhus**, Saba., (Sang.), *Sil.*, Spig., Sul.

Aggravations: Time and Circumstances.—Agar., (All. c.), *Am. carb.*, (Arg. n.), **Ars.**, Aur., (Bap.), Bar. c., *Bell.*, Bor., Bry., *Calc. c.*, Camph., Caust., Cham., Chel., Chin., Cic., *Cocc* , Coff., Colch., *Con.*, Dulc., Guai., **Hep.**, Hyos., Ign., (K. bi.), Kre , *Lach.*, *Lyc* , *Mang* , Merc., Nat. c., **Nux v.**, Petrol., Ran. b., *Rhodo.*, **Rhus**, Ruta, Saba., Sele., SIL. Spig., Stram., *Stro.*, Sul., Verat. a.

Other Remedies.—(Aloe), Ant. t., **Apis**, (Apoc. c.), Arg. n., Arn., Ars., Bap., **Bell.**, *Bry.*, *Calc. c* , *Cannab. i.*, Cham., *Chin.*, Cimic., Cocc., Con., *Gel.*, Glon., Graph., Hep., Hyos., Ign., K. bi., K carb., **Lyc.**, Merc., Nat. c., Nat. m., NUX V., *Op.*, **Phos.**, *Pho. ac.*, Plat., Pod., PULS., RHUS, Saba, Sang., *Sep.*, Sil., *Spig.*, *Stram.*, **Sul.**, *Verat. a.*

Antidotes.—Camph., *Sem. carvi.*

Nux Vomica.

Mind.—Acon., *Aloe*, Anac., *Apis*, Ars., Aur., Bap , *Bell.*, Bry., **Calc. c.**, *Cannab. i* , *Cham.*, Cimic., Cocc., *Gel.*, Glon., Gran., Hyos., Hyper., Lyc., *Meli.*, Merc. c., Nat. m., Op., Phos., *Puls.*, Rhus, Sep., *Stram.*, Sul., **Verat. a.**, *Verat. v.*

Localities.—*Acon.*, *Aesc.*, *All. c.*, Aloe., APIS, *Apoc. c.*, ARG. N., Arn., Ars., Arum t., Aur., **Bap.**, Bell., *Berb.*, *Bor.*, **Bry.**, *Cact* , Calc. c., CANNAB. I., Canth., *Carb. ac.*, Carb. v., (Caul.), *Caust.*, (Ced.), **Cham.**, **Chin.**, **Cimic.**, Cocc., Coff., *Con.*, Croc., *Crotal.*, Cup., *Dios.*,

Eup. per., Euphr., Fer., *Fl. ac.*, *Gel.*, Glon., Graph., Hep., (Hyd. ac.), Hyos., (Hyper.), *Ign.*, *Ip.*, *Iris v.*, K. Bl., *K. carb.*, Kalm., Kre., *Lil. t.*, (Lith.), **Lyc.**, Meli., **Merc.**, Nat. c., *Nat. m.*, Nit. ac., Op., Petrol., **Phos.**, Pho. ac., **Phyt.**, (Pic. ac.), Plat., Pb., POD., *Pso.*, PULS., *Rhus*, Sabi., SANG., **Sep.**, *Sil.*, Spig., *Staph.*, Stram., SUL., (Tell.), *Verat. a.*, *Verat. v.*

Sensations.—Acon., Aesc., *Aloe*, Ambr., Apis, ARG. N., *Arn.* Ars., *Arum t.*, Asaf., Aur., *Bap.*, BELL., Berb., *Bry.*, *Cact.*, **Calc. c.**, **Cannab. i.**, Canth., Carb. v., *Caust.*, *Cham.*, **Chin.**, CIMIC., Cina, **Cocc.**, Coff., Con., Crotal., Dios., *Fer.*, *Fup. per.*, GEL., *Glon.*, Graph., Hep., Hyos., *Ign.*, Iod., Ip., *Iris v.*, K. bi., *K. carb.*, (Kalm.), Lil. t., (Lith.), **Lyc.**, Mar., Meli., **Merc.**, Mez., Nat. c., *Nat. m.*, Nit. ac., Petrol., **Phos.**, **Phyt.**, *Plat.*, *Pod.*, *Pso.*, PULS., RHUS, Ruta, Saba., **Sang.**, SEP., *Sil.*, *Spig.*, Spo., *Stan.*, *Staph.*, Stro., **Sul**, *Verat. a.*, Verat. v., Zinc.

Glands.—Arn., (Arum t.), Bell., Bry., Calc. c., *Chin.*, Con., *Ign.*, *Iod.*, Lyc., *Merc.*, Phos., PULS., *Sil.*, Spo., **Sul**.

Bones.—*Chin.*, Cocc., Dros., Merc., Puls., *Ruta*.

Skin.—*Acon.*, Apis, Arn., *Ars.*, (Bap.), *Bell.*, **Bry.**, *Calc. c.*, (Carb. ac.), Carb. v., *Caust.*, (Cimic.), Con., Crotal., (Eup. per.), Hep., Ip., K. carb., Lach., Led., LYC., *Merc.*, Mez., Nit. ac., *Phos.*, **Puls.**, Ran. b., RHUS. Sec. c., SEP., **Sil.**, Squ., Staph., SUL.

Sleep and Dreams.—(Aloe), Ant. t., Apis, *Arg. n.*, *Ars.*, (Bap.), Bell. Bry., **Calc. c.**, *Cannab. i.*, Chin., *Con.*, Croc., (Gel.), Graph., Hep., **Ign.**, K. carb., Kre., *Nat. c.*, Phos., Pod., **Puls.**, RHUS *Sep.*, Sil., Sul.

Blood, Circulation and Fever.—Acon., (Aloe), (Apis), (Arg. n.), ARS., (Bap.), Bar. c., Bell., (Berb.), BRY., Cact., **Calc. c.**, (Cannab. i.), Caps., **Caust.**, **Cham.**, Chin., Dulc., Gel., (Glon.), *Hep.*, Ign., Ip., (Lil. t.), *Lyc.*, *Merc.*, Nat. m., Op., **Phos.**, Pho. ac., (Pod.), PULS., RHUS, Saba., Samb., **Sang.**, Sep., Sil., Spig., **Sul.**, Verat. a., (Verat. v.).

Aggravations: Time and Circumstances.—Acon., Aesc., Aloe, Am. m., *Apis*, *Arg. n.*, *Arn.*, ARS., Asar., Aur., Bap., **Bell.**, BRY., (Cact.), **Calc. c.**, Carb. v., **Caust.**, **Cham.**, *Chel.*, *Chin.*, (Cimic.), *Cocc.*, Coff., Colch., Con., Dros., Fer., Gel., *Glon.*, Graph., **Hep.**, Hyos., *Ign.*, Ip., *K. bi.*, *K. carb.*, K. nit., Lach., Led., Lil. t., (Lith.), **Lyc.**, Merc., Mos., Nat. c., *Nat. m.*, Nit. ac., Nux m., Op., **Phos.**, Phyt., Pod., **Puls.**, Ran b., RHUS, Saba., **Sang.**, Sele., **Sep.**, Sil., *Spig.*, Squ., **Sul.**, *Thuj.*, Verat. v.

Other Remedies.—*Acon.*, Aesc., **Aloe**, APIS, ARG. N., Arn., **Ars.**, Arum t., Aur., **Bap.**, **Bell.**, *Berb.*, Bry., *Cact.*, **Calc. c.**, CANNAB. I., Carb. v., *Caust.* Cham., Chin., Cimic., Cocc., Con., *Crotal.*, Fer., GEL., Glon., Graph., *Hep.*, Hyos., *Ign.*, Ip., K. bi., *K. carb.*, **Lil. t.**, (Lith.),

Merc., Nat. c., Nat. m., Nit. ac., Op., **Phos.**, *Phyt.*, Pod., **PULS.,**
RHUS, **SANG.**, **Sep.**, *Sil.*, Spig., Staph., **Sul.**, Verat. a., **Verat. v.**

Antidotes.—Acon., Camph., Cham., Cocc., *Coff.*, *Ign.*, Puls., Alcohol, Vinum.

Injurious.—*Acetum*, Zinc.

Oleander.

Mind.—Acon., Arn., Bar. c., **Bell.**, *Bry.*, Cannab. s., Cham., Cic., Cocc., CON., *Crotal.*, **Hell.**, *Hyos.*, Ign., *Laur.*, **Lyc.**, Merc., NAT. M., *Nux m.*, Nux v., Op., Phos., **Pho. ac.**, *Puls.*, **Rhus**, SEP., Sil., Stram., Sul., **Verat. a.**

Localities.—Aloe, Anac., Apis, Arg. n., Arn., *Ars.*, Aur., Bar. c., Bell., *Bry.*, **Calc. c.**, (Cannab. i.), Caps., *Caust.*, Chel., *Chin.*, Cic., Cina, Cocc., Con., (Dios.), Fer., (Fl. ac.), Gel., *Graph.*, Hep., Hyos., Ign., Ip., (K. bi.), K. carb., *Lyc.*, *Merc.*, Mez., *Nat. m.*, *Nux v.*, Op., Petrol., **Phos.**, *Pho. ac.*, (Pod.), (Pso.), **Puls.**, *Rhus*, Ruta, *Saba*, Sec. c., *Sep.*, Sil., *Spig.*, Stan., **Staph.**, *Sul.*, Verat. a.

Sensations.—Acon., (Aloe), Alum., *Anac.*, (Apis), Arg., Arg. n., Arn., Ars., *Asaf.*, (Bap.), **Bell.**, Berb., Bism., *Bry.*, **Calc. c.**, (Cannab. i.), Caps., *Caust.*, Cimic., **Cocc.**, **Con.**, (Crotal.), Cup., (Eup. per.), *Gel.*, *Glon.*, Hell., Ign., (Iris v.), (K. bi.), *K. carb.*, *Laur.*, LYC., Merc., Nat. m., *Nux m.*, Nux v., Op., Phos., Pho. ac., (Pod.), **Plat.**, **PULS.**, **RHUS**, *Ruta*, Saba., Sang., **Sep.**, Sil., *Spig.*, Stan., *Staph.*, **Sul.**, *Sul. ac.*, Tar., Thuj., *Verat. a.*, Verb.

Glands.

Bones.

Skin.—*Agn.*, Am. m., Anac., Ars., Bar. c., *Bry.*, Calc. c., Caust., Ip., Lach., *Led.*, LYC., Mez., Pho. ac., *Plat.*, *Puls.*, Rhus, *Sec. c.*, Sil., *Spo.*, Staph., Sul.

Sleep and Dreams.—*Ign.*, Nux v., *Phos.*, *Saba.*

Blood, Circulation and Fever.—Acon., (Apis), **Ars.**, Bell., Bry., *Calc. c.*, (Gel.), Lyc., Nux v., Pho. ac., *Sep.*, *Sul.*

Aggravations: Time and Circumstances.—Acon., (Apis), Arn., Bar. c., *Bell.*, Bry., **Calc. c.**, Caps., Carb. v., Caust., Cham., Chin., Cina, Cocc., Colch., Con., Cup., *Graph.*, *Hep.*, **Ign.**, K. carb., Lach., Led., *Lyc.*, Nat. m., Nit. ac., **Nux v.**, *Phos.*, Puls., Rhodo., **Rhus**, Ruta, (Sang.), *Sep.*, Sil., SPIG., *Staph.*, Sul., Thuj., Verat. a., (Verat. v.).

Other Remedies.—Acon., (Aloe), Anac., Apis, Arg. n., Arn., *Ars.*, Bar. c., **Bell.**, Bry., **Calc. c.**, (Cannab. i.), Caust., Chin., Cocc., *Con.*, Crotal., Gel., Graph., Hell., Hep., *Ign.*, (K. bi.), K. carb., Laur., LYC.,

Merc., *Nat. m.*, Nux m., Nux v., Op., *Phos.*, *Pho. ac.*, Plat., (Pod.), Puls., Rhus, Ruta, Saba, (Sang.), **Sep.**, *Sil.*, *Spig.*, *Staph.*, **Sul.**, Verat. a.

Antidotes.—Camph.

Opium.

Mind.—Acon., *Aloe*, *Apis*, Arn., Ars., *Aur.*, *Bap.*, Bar. c., **BELL.**, **Cannab. i.**, Cimic., Cocc., **Coff.**, Crotal., **Gel.**, *Glon.*, *Hyd. ac.*, **HYOS.**, **Ign.**, *Lach.*, *Lyc.*, *Meli.*, Merc. c., Nat. c., Nat. m., Nux m., Nux v., *Phos.*, Pho. ac., Pic. ac , Puls., Rhus, *Sep.*, Sil., **Stram.**, Ter., **Ther.**, **Verat. a.**, *Verat. v.*

Localities.—*Acon.*, Aesc., Aloe, *Apis*, Apoc. c., **Arg. n.**, Arn., *Ars.*, (Arum t.), (Bap.), BELL., (Berb.), *Bry.*, (Cact.), *Calc. c.*, Camph., Cannab. i., Canth., Caps., Carb. ac., Caust., *Cham.*, *Chin.*, Cimic., Cocc., Con., (Crotal.), *Cup.*, *Dig.*, Dios., Dulc., Gel., Glon., Graph., **Hep.**, (Hyd. ac.), HYOS., *Ign.*, Ip., (Iris v.), *K. bi.*, *K. carb.*, (Kalm.), Laur., Lil. t., (Lith.), *Lyc.*, (Meli.), *Nat. m.*, Nit. ac., **Nux v.**, *Phos.*, Pho. ac., (Phyt.), Pb., *Pod.*, Pso., **Puls.**, Rhus, Ruta, Samb., Sang., Sec. c., *Sep.*, *Sil.*, Spo., Staph., **Stram.**, **Sul.**, *Verat. a.*, *Verat. v.*

Sensations.—*Acon.*, (Aesc.), Anac., Apis, *Arg. n.*, Arn., Ars., Arum t., (Bap.), BELL., Berb., Cact., Calc. c., Camph., Cannab. i., Carb. v., *Cham.*, *Chin.*, *Cic.*, *Cimic.*, **Cocc.**, Coff., *Con.*, (Crotal.), *Cup.*, Dig., (Dios.), Fer., **Gel.**, Glon., HYOS., *Ign.*, Iod., Ip., Iris v., K. bi., K. carb., Lach., *Laur.*, Lil. t., **Lyc.**, Merc., Nux m., *Nux v.*, Oleand., Phos., Pho. ac., (Phyt.), *Plat.*, Pb., (Pod.), *Puls.*, Rhus, Samb., (Sang.), **Sec. c.**, *Sep.*, *Sil.*, Spig., **Stram.**, *Sul.*, *Verat. a.*, (Verat. v.).

Glands.

Bones.

Skin.—*Acon.*, **Arn.**, **Ars.**, (Bap.), BELL., **Bry.**, Calc. c., Chin., Con., (Crotal.), Dig., *Dulc.*, Graph., Hyos., *K. carb.*, *Lach.*, Led., **Lyc.**, **Merc.**, Nux v., Phos., Pho. ac., **Puls.**, *Rhus*, Sec. c., Sep., *Sil.*, Squ., **Sul.**, Verat. a.

Sleep and Dreams.—Acon., (Aloe), ANT. T., Apis, (Arg. n.), Ars., Bell., **BRY.**, Calc. c., *Cannab. i.*, **Con.**, Croc., Hep., Ign., Laur., Nat. c., Nat. m., **NUX M.**, Nux v., *Phos.*, Pho. ac., Pod., *Puls.*, Sep., Staph., Sul., Verat. a.

Blood, Circulation and Fever.—ACON., (Arg. n.), **Ars.**, (Bap.), *Bell.*, (Berb.), *Bry.*, (Cact.), Calc. c., Cannab. i., Caps., *Carb. v.*, **Cham.**, *Chin.*, Cocc., Cup., Dig., Fer., Gel., Glon., Hep., Hyos., Iod., Ip., *K. carb.*, (Lil. t.), *Lyc.*, Merc., *Nat. m.*, *Nux v.*, Phos., *Pho. ac.*, Phyt., Puls., **Rhus**, Samb., Sang., Sec. c., **Sep.**, Sil., Spig., **Stram.**, *Sul.*, **Verat. a.**, Verat. v.

Aggravations: Time and Circumstances.—*Acon.*, Ant. cr., (Apis), (Arg. n.), **Ars.**, *Bell.*, *Bry.*, (Cannab. i), Caust., *Cham.*, Coff., Con., Fer., Hep., *Ign.*, K. carb., Lach., *Lyc.*, Merc., Nat. m., NUX V., Phos., Plat., **Puls.**, *Ran. b.*, *Rhus*, Saba., (Sang.), Sep., Sil., Spig., *Stram.*, *Sul.*, Verat. a., Zinc.

Other Remedies.—Acon., (Aesc.), Aloe, Ant. t., **Apis**, *Arg. n.*, Arn., Ars., (Arum t.), **Bap.**, BELL., Berb., **Bry.**, Cact., Calc. c., **Cannab. i.**, *Cham.*, *Chin.*, Cimic., Cocc., Coff., *Con.*, Crotal., Cup., Dig., **Gel.**, *Glon.*, Hep., **Hyos.**, *Ign.*, K. bi., *K. carb.*, Lach., Laur., Lil. t., **Lyc.**, Merc., Nat. m., Nux m., **Nux v.**, *Phos.*, Pho. ac., Phyt., Pod., **Puls.**, **Rhus**, Sang., Sec. c., *Sep.*, *Sil.*, **Stram.**, **Sul.**, **Verat. a.**, *Verat. v.*

Antidotes.—Camph., Coff., Con., *Ip.*, Merc., Pb., *Vinum*, Vanilla arom.

Paris.

Mind.—*Anac.*, *Bell.*, Cup., **Hyos.**, Lach., **Lyc.**, *Plat.*, **Stram.**, *Verat. a.*

Localities.—Alum., Anac., Ant. cr., (Apis), Arg., (Arg. n.), Arn., *Ars.*, (Arum t.), Bar. c., *Bell*, *Bry.*, CALC. C., *Carb. v.*, **Caust.**, Cham., *Chin.*, Graph., *Hep.*, *K. bi.*, K. carb., Kre., *Lyc.*, *Merc*, Mez., Nat. c., Nat. m., Nit. ac., *Nux v.*, Petrol., PHOS., Pho. ac., Pso., **Puls.**, **Rhus**, Saba., Sabi., (Sang.), Seneg., **Sep.**, Sil., Squ., Stan., **Staph.**, **Sul.**, Thuj., Verat. a., *Zinc.*

Sensations.—Acon., (Aesc..), Alum., Arg., Arg. n., *Arn.*, Ars., Bar. c., **Bell.**, Berb., *Bry.*, **Calc. c.**, (Cact.), (Cannab. i.), Canth., Caust., Cham., *Chin.*, (Cimic.), Cocc., Con., (Dios.), *Dros.*, (Gel.), Glon., Graph., *Ign.*, K. bi., *K. carb.*, *Lyc.*, **Merc.**, Nat. c., Nat. m., **Nux v.**, **Phos.**, Plat., PULS., Rhus, Ruta, (Sang.), Sep., *Sil.*, Spig., Spo., *Stan.*, Staph., *Stro.*, **Sul.**, Tar., Verat. a., Zinc.

Glands.—Merc., Spo.

Bones.—Phos., Ruta.

Skin.—Am. carb., Ars., *Bar. c.*, Bell., **Bry.**, *Calc. c.*, *Caust.*, Cham., Clem., *Con.*, **Graph.**, *Hep.*, K. carb., Lach., Lyc., *Merc.*, Mez., *Nit. ac.*, Oleand., *Petrol.*, Phos., *Puls.*, Ran. b., RHUS, Sep., Sil., Spig., *Squ.*, *Staph.*, Sul., Vio. t.

Sleep and Dreams.—Bry., Ign., *Nux v.*, Phos., Rhus, Sul.

Blood, Circulation and Fever.—Ars., Bell., **Bry.**, *Lyc.*, NUX V., Puls., Rhus, Sep., *Sul.*

Aggravations: Time and Circumstances.—Acon., (Aesc.), *Am. carb.*, Anac., Arn., (Bap.), Bar. c., Bry., *Calc. c.*, Caps., Carb. v., Graph., Hep., *Ign.*, (K. bi.), Lach., Lyc., *Nat. c.*, Nat. m., Nux v., *Phos.*, **Puls.**, (Sang.), *Sep.*, Spig., Spo., **Sul.**

RELATIONSHIPS.—PARIS.—PETR.   435

Other Remedies.—(Aesc.), Anac., (Arg. n.), Arn., Ars., Bar. c., *Bell.*, **Bry.**, **Calc. c.**, Caust., Chin., Graph., Hep., Ign., K. bi., K. carb., **Lyc.**, *Merc.*, Nat. c., **Nux v.**, Phos., Puls., Rhus, (Sang.), SEP., Sil., Spig, *Staph.*, SUL., Verat. a.

Antidotes.—Camph., *Coff.*

Petroleum.

Mind.—Acon., Anac., **Bell.**, *Bry.*, Calc. c., Cannab. i., Con., *Glon.*, Graph., Hell., Hyos., Laur., *Lyc.*, Merc., **Nat. m.**, Nux m., *Nux v.*, Op., Phos., Pho. ac., Puls., **Rhus**, **Sep.**, Sil., Spig., **Stram.**, **Sul.**, *Verat. a.*

Localities.—Acon., Aesc., **All. c.**, Aloe, Ant. cr., *Apis*, (Apoc. c.), **Arg. n.**, *Arn.*, *Ars.*, Arum t., Bap., Bar. c., **Bell.**, (Berb.), Bor., *Bry.*, (Cact.), CALC. C., Cannab. i., Carb. ac., *Carb. v.*, (Caul.), **Caust.**, Cham., Chel., *Chin.*, Cimic., *Con.*, (Crotal.), Dios., Dulc., (Eup. per.), (Fl. ac.), Gel., (Glon.), Graph., Ign., (Iris v.), K. bi., **K. carb.**, (Kalm.), Kre., Led., (Lit. t.), **Lyc.**, **Merc.**, Mez., Mur. ac., Nat. c., *Nat. m.*, Nit. ac., **Nux v.**, Oleand., **Phos.**, Pho. ac., Phyt., (Pic. ac.), *Pod.*, *Pso.*, PULS., Rhus, *Ruta*, Saba., Sabi., *Sang.*, **Sep.**, **Sil.**, *Spig.*, *Staph.*, SUL., (Ther.), Thuj., Verat. a., *Verat. v.*, Zinc.

Sensations.—(Aloe), Ambr., (Apis), Arg. n., *Arn.*, (Arum t.), Aur., (Bap.), *Bell.*, (Berb.), *Bry.*, **Calc. c.**, Cannab. i., *Caust.*, *Cham.*, *Chin.*, Cic., (Cimic.), *Cocc.*, (Crotal.), (Dios.), *Gel.*, (Glon.), *Graph.*, **Ign.**, Ip., (Iris v.), (K. bi.), *K. carb.*, (Lil. t.), (Lith.), **Lyc.**, *Merc.*, Nat. c., **Nat. m.**, Nit. ac., *Nux v.*, Phos., (Phyt.), *Plat.*, (Pod.), (Pso.), Puls., **Rhus**, *Sarg.*, SEP., *Sil.*, Spig., Stan., **Sul.**, Thuj., Verat. a.

Glands.—*Bell.*, Carb. an., **Lyc.**, Merc., Phos., Puls.

Bones.—Asaf., *Calc. c.*, Con., Merc., Nit. ac., PULS., Ruta, Sil., *Sul.*

Skin.—Ant. cr., Apis, Ars., Asaf., Bar. c., Bell., Bov., Bry., **Calc. c.**, Carb. v., Caust., *Cham.*, (Cimic.), Clem., Con., Dulc., (Eup. per.), **Graph.**, Hep., *Kre.*, **Lach.**, Led., **Lyc.**, *Merc.*, Mez., Nat. m., *Nit. ac.*, Oleand., Phos., Pho. ac., *Puls.*, **Rhus**, (Sang.), Sars., SEP., SIL., Squ., **Staph.**, SUL., Verat. a.

Sleep and Dreams.—Bry., *Calc. c.*, Con., Ign., Lyc., Nux v., **Sil.**, Sul.

Blood, Circulation and Fever.—*Acon.*, (Arg. n.), *Arn.*, Ars., Bell., *Bry.*, (Cact.), *Calc. c.*, (Cannab. i.), Carb. v., Cham., Chin., (Glon.), Hep., Ign., Merc., Nit. ac., **Nux v.**, Phos., Pho. ac., Puls., **Rhus**, Sang., *Sep.*, Sil., Stan., **Sul.**

Aggravations: Time and Circumstances.—Acon., (Aesc.), Agar.,

(All. c.), (Aloe.), *Am. carb.*, Ant. t., (Apis), (Arg. n.), Ars., Aur., **(Bap.)**, *Bar. c.*, **Bell., BRY., Calc. c.**, Camph., *Caps., Carb. v., Caust., Chin.*, **Cocc.**, *Con.*, Dulc., Fer., (Gel.), (Glon.), Hell., **Hep.**, Ign., K. bi., *K. carb.*, (Lil. t.), **Lyc.**, Mang., Merc., Mos., Nat. m., Nit. ac., **Nux m., NUX V. Phos.**, (Phyt.), (Pod.), **Puls.**, Ran. b., Rhodo., Rhus, Saba, **Sang., SEP.** *Sil.*, Spig., Stro., *Sul.*, Verat. a., (Verat. v.).

Other Remedies.—Acon., (Aesc.), (All. c.), Aloe, *Apis, Arg. n.*, **Arn.**, Ars., (Arum t.), Bap., Bar. c., **Bell.**, (Berb.), **Bry.**, (Cact.), **CALC. C**, *Cannab. i.*, Carb. v., *Caust.*, Cham., Chin., Cimic., Cocc., *Con.*, (Crotal.), Gel., *Glon., Graph., Hep.*, Ign., *K. bi.*, K. carb., (Lil. t.), **LYC.**, *Merc., Nat. m., Nit. ac.*, **Nux v.**, Phos.,Phyt., Pod., **Puls., Rhus**, *Sang.*, **SEP., Sil.**, Spig., Staph., **SUL.**, Verat. a., Verat. v.

Antidote.—Nux v.

Phosphorus.

Mind.—**Acon.**, Aloe, **Apis, Aur., Bap., Bell.**, Bry., *Calc. c., Cannab. i.*, Carb. ac., Cham., Chel., Cimic., Coff., Con., Crotal., **Gel.,** *Glon.*, Hell., *Hyd. ac., Hyos.*, Ign., Lach., Laur., Lyc., **Meli.**, Merc., **Merc. c.**, Mos., Nat. c., *Nat. m.*, Nux v., *Op.*, **Pho. ac.**, *Pic. ac., Plot.*, **PULS.**, Rhus, *Sep., Sil.*, Staph., **Stram.**, *Sul.*, Ther., Valer., **Verat. a.**, *Verat. v.*, Zinc.

Localities.—*Acon.*, **Aesc.**, *All. c.*, Aloe, Alum., Anac., Ant. cr., **APIS**, *Apoc. c.*, **ARG. N.**, *Arn.*, **Ars., Arum t.**, Aur., **Bap.**, Bar. c., **BELL.**, *Berb., Bry., Cact.*, **CALC. C, Cannab. i.**, *Carb. ac., Carb. v.*, (Caul.), *Caust., Cham.,* Chel., **Chin.**, *Cimic., Con., Crotal., Dios.*, Dros., Eup. per., Fer., *Fl. ac.*, **GEL.,** *Glon.*, Graph., *Hep.*, (Hyd. ac.), Hyos., (Hyper.), Ign., *Ip., Iris v.*, **K. BI.**, *K. carb.*, Kalm., Kre., Led., *Lil. t.*, Lith., **Lyc.**, Meli., **Merc.**, Mez., *Nat. m.*, *Nit. ac.*, **Nux v.**, Oleand., Par., Petrol., *Pho. ac., Phyt.*, (Pic. ac.), Plat., Pb., **Pod.**, *Pso.*, **PULS.**, *Rhus, Ruta*, **SANG., SEP., Sil.**, *Spig.*, Spo., Squ., *Stan.*, **Staph.**, Stram., **SUL.**, Sul. ac., *Verat. a., Verat. v.*, Zinc.

Sensations.—*Acon.*, **Aesc.**, (All. c.), *Aloe*, Alum., **Apis, ARG. N.**, *Arn.*, Ars., **Arum t.**, Asaf., *Bap., Bar. c.*, **Bell**, Berb., **Bry.**, *Cact.*, Calc. c., *Cannab. i., Canth.*, (Carb. ac.), Carb. v., *Caust., Cham.*, **Chin.**, Cimic., Cocc., *Con.*, Crotal., (Dios.), Dros., Eup. per., *Fer.*, **Gel., Glon.**, *Graph.*, **Ign.**, Jod., Ip., Iris v., **K. BI.**, *K. carb.*, (Kalm.), *Lil. t.*, Lith., **Lyc.**, Meli., **Merc.**, Mos., Nat. c., *Nat. m., Nit. ac.*, **NUX V.**, Par., Petrol., Pho. ac., *Phyt.*, Pod., *Pso., Plat.*, **PULS., Rhus,** Ruta, Saba., **SANG., Sep.,** *Sil., Spig.*, Spo., *Stan.*, Staph., *Stro.*, **SUL.**, Sul. ac., Thuj., *Verat. a., Verat. v.*, Zinc.

Glands.—Arn., Arum t, Ars., Bar. c., **BELL., Bry.**, Calc. c., **Carb. an.**, Caust., **Con.**, Hep., *Lyc.*, **Merc.**, Puls., *Rhus*, Sil., Spo., **Sul.**

Bones.—*Asaf.*, Bell., *Calc. c.*, Eup. per., **Lyc.**, **Merc.**, Mez., Nit. ac., Pho. ac., Puls., *Sil.*, Staph., *Sul.*

Skin.—*Acon.*, Am. carb., *Apis*, *Arn.*, **Ars.**, Asaf., *Bell.*, *Bry.*, *Calc. c.*, Carb. an., Carb. v., Caust., Clem., *Con.*, Crotal., Dulc., Graph., Hep., (K. bi.), K. carb., **Lach.**, **Lyc.**, *Merc.*, Nat. c., Nat. m., *Nit. ac.*, Pho. ac., Puls., *Rhus*, *Sep.*, **Sil.**, Staph., Stro., SUL., Thuj.

Sleep and Dreams.—Acon., (Aloe), *Ant. t.*, Apis, *Arg. n.*, Ars., Bap., *Bell.*, **Bry.**, **Calc. c.**, *Cannab. i.*, Caust., Cham., Chin., *Con.*, *Croc.*, *Graph.*, Hep., Ign., K. carb., (Lil. t.), Mag. c., *Merc.*, Nat. m., Nux m., **Nux v.**, Op., Pho. ac., Pod., PULS., Rhus, Sars., SEP., *Sil.*, **Sul.**

Blood, Circulation and Fever.—Acon., (Aloe), Apis, (Arg. n.), Arn., **Ars.**, (Bap.), **Bell.**, Berb., BRY., Cact., *Calc. c.*, Cannab. i., Carb. v., *Cham.*, *Chin.*, Croc., (Crotal.), Fer., Gel., Glon., Graph., Hyos., *Iod.*, K. carb., (Lil. t.), LYC., **Merc.**, Nat. m., **Nux v.**, *Op.*, **Pho. ac.**, Pod., **Puls.**, Rhus, *Sang.*, *Sep.*, *Sil.*, Spig., Stan., *Stram.*, *Sul.*, Thuj., Verat. a., (Verat. v.).

Aggravations: Time and Circumstances.—Acon., (Aesc.), Agn., (All. c.), Aloe, Am. carb., Ant. t., Apis, *Arg. n.*, Arn., *Ars.*, Asaf., Bap., Bar. c., *Bell.*, **Bry.**, Cact., Calad., **Calc. c.**, (Cannab. i.), Cannab. s., *Carb. v.*, Caust., Cham., *Chin.*, Cimic. Cocc., Colch., *Con.*, Dros., Euphr., Gel., Glon., *Graph.*, Hep., Ign., Iod., Ip., *K. bi.*, K. carb., Lach., Lil. t., **Lyc.**, Mang., *Merc.*, Nat. c., Nat. m., Nit. ac., NUX V., Pho. ac., Phyt., Pod., PULS., Rhus, Saba., *Sang.*, Sele., SEP., *Sil.*, Spig., Squ., Staph., **Sul.**, Thuj., Verat. v.

Other Remedies.—*Acon.*, *Aesc.*, All. c., **Aloe**, APIS, ARG. N., Arn., *Ars.*, *Arum t.*, Asaf., **Bap.**, Bar. c., **Bell.**, Berb., **Bry.**, **Cact.**, **Calc. c.**, **Cannab. i.**, **Carb. v.**, Caust., Cham., *Chin.*, Cimic., *Con.*, **Crotal.**, GEL., Glon., Graph., Hep., Ign., Iod., Ip., **K. bi.**, K. carb., Lach., **Lil. t.**, Lith., **Lyc.**, **Merc.**, Nat. c., Nat. m., Nit. ac., **Nux v.**, Op., *Pho. ac.*, *Phyt.*, Plat., **Pod.**, PULS., *Rhus*, **Sang.**, Sep., **Sil.**, Spig., Stan., **Staph.**, Stram., SUL., Thuj., Verat. a., **Verat. v.**

Antidotes.—Camph., Coff., *Nux v.*, Vinum.

Injurious.—Rhus.

Phosphoricum Acidum.

Mind.—Acon., *Aloe*, Anac., *Apis*, Ars., *Bap.*, BELL., Bry., *Calc. c.*, Cannab. i., Cannab. s., Cic., Cocc., *Con.*, Crotal., **Gel.**, Glon., *Hell.*, Hyd. ac., **Hyos.**, *Ign.*, K. carb., *Laur.*, **Lyc.**, **Meli.**, Merc., Merc. c., Mez., *Nat. c.*, *Nat. m.*, Nux m., Nux v., **Op.**, *Phos.*, *Pic. ac.*, Pso., **Puls.**, Rhus, Saba., **Sep.**, **Sil.**, Staph., STRAM., *Sul.*, *Verat. a.*, Verat. v.

Localities.—Acon., (Aesc.), All. c., Aloe, *Alum.*, Anac., *Apis,* **Apoc.** c., Arg., *Arg. n.,* Arn., *Ars.,* Arum t., Aur., Bap., Bar. c., *Bell.,* Berb., *Bry.,* Cact., **Calc. c.,** *Cannab. i., Canth.,* Carb. ac., Carb. v., **CAUST.,** Cham., **Chin.,** (Cimic.), Cocc., Con., Croc., (Crotal.), Cup., Dios., Dros., Dulc., Fer., Fl. ac., Gel., Glon., Graph., *Hep.,* Ign., (Iris v.), *K. bi.,* **K. carb.,** K. nit., (Kalm.), *Kre.,* Led., Lil. t., *Lyc.,* Mag. c., Meli., **Merc.,** Mur. ac., *Nat, c., Nat. m., Nit. ac.,* Nux v., Petrol., **Phos.,** *Phyt.,* (Pic. ac.), Plat., Pb., Pod., Pso., **PULS.,** **Rhus,** *Ruta,* Sang., Sars., Sec. c., Seneg., **SEP.,** *Sil., Spig., Squ.,* Stan., *Staph.,* Stram., **Sul.,** Thuj., *Valer.,* Verat. a., Verat. v., Verb., *Zinc.*

Sensations.—*Acon.,* Aesc., *Alum.,* Ambr., Anac., *Apis,* Arg., *Arg. n., Arn., Ars.,* Arum t., Bap., Bar. c., **Bell.,** *Berb., Bry.,* Cact., **Calc. c.,** *Cannab. i.,* Canth., *Carb. v.,* **Caust.,** Cham., **CHIN.,** (Cimic.), *Cocc.,* Con., (Crotal.), Cup., Dros., (Eup. per.), Fer., *Gel.,* (Glon.), Graph., Ign., Iod., (Iris v.), *K. bi.,* **K. carb.,** (Kalm.), Laur., Lil. t., *Lyc.,* Mag. c., Mar., *Merc.,* Nat. c., Nat. m., Nit. ac., **NUX V.,** Oleand., Op., **Phos.,** (Phyt.), Plat., Pb, (Pod.), (Pso.), **Puls., Rhus,** *Sang, Sars.,* Sec. c., **Sep.,** Sil., Spig., *Stan.,* Staph., Stram., Stro., **SUL.,** Sul. ac., Tar., Thuj., Verat. a., Verat. v., *Zinc.*

Glands.—Bell., **Con.,** *Plat.,* Rhus, **Sep.,** *Spo.,* Sul.

Bones.—Asaf., Calc. c., Eup. per., Merc., Puls., *Sil.,* Staph., *Sul.*

Skin.—Acon., (Apis.), Arn., **Ars.,** Asaf., *Bell.,* Bry., *Calc. c.,* Chin., Con., Dulc., Graph., *Hep., Lach.,* **LYC.,** *Merc., Nit. ac.,* Oleand., Petrol., **Phos.,** *Puls., Rhus,* (Sang.), *Sec. c.,* **Sele., Sep., Sil., Sul.,** Thuj., Verat. a.

Sleep and Dreams.—Acon., (Aloe), Ant. t., Apis, (Arg. n.), Ars., *Bell., Bry.,* Calc. c., *Cannab. i.,* Cham., Chin., **Con.,** Croc., Hep., *Ign.,* K. carb., *Merc.,* Nat. c., Nux m., **Nux v.,** Op., **Phos.,** Po l., **Puls.,** Saba., Sep., *Sil., Sul.*

Blood, Circulation and Fever.—**Acon.,** (Apis), (Arg. n.), ARS., (Bap.), *Bell.,* (Berb.), *Bry.,* Calc. c., (Cannab. i.), Cham., **Chin.,** (Cimic.), Crotal.), Dig., (Gel.), Glon., Hep., Hyos., Ign., Iod., (Lil. t.), **Merc.,** Nat. m., Nux v., Op., **Phos.,** (Pod.), Puls., *Rhus,* Sang., Sec. c., Sep., Sil., Stan., **Stram.,** *Sul.*

Aggravations: Time and Circumstances.—Acon., (Aesc.), Aloe, Am. m., Apis, Arg. n., Arn., Ars., Aur., Bap., Bar. c., *Bell., Bry.,* **Calc. c.,** Caps., *Carb. v., Cham.,* **Chin.,** (Cimic.), Cocc., **Con.,** Cyc., Dros., Dulc., Euphorb., Fer., (Gel.), (Glon.), Graph., Hep., Ign., Iod., *K. bi.,* K. carb., (Lil. t.), **Lyc.,** Mag. m., Meny., Merc., Mos., *Nat. c., Nat. m.,* Nux v., *Phos.,* (Phyt.), Plat., Pod., **PULS.,** Rhodo., *Rhus,* Saba., Samb., *Sang.,* **SEP.,** *Sil.,* Spig., *Staph.,* **Sul.,** Tar., Valer., Verat. a., Verat. v., Verb.

RELATIONSHIPS.—PHOS. AC.—PHYT. 439

Other Remedies.—Acon., Aesc., *Aloe*, Alum., **APIS, Arg.** n., Arn., **Ars.**, Asaf., *Bap.,* **Bell.**, Berb., *Bry.*, Cact., **Calc. c., Cannab.** i., Carb. v., Caust., Cham., **Chin.**, Cimic., Cocc., **Con.**, Crotal., **Gel.,** *Glon.,* Graph., Hep., Hyos., *Ign.*, *K. bi.*, *K. carb.*, Lil. t., **Lyc., Merc.,** *Nat. c., Nat. m.*, Nit. ac., *Nux v.*, Op., Phos., Phyt., Plat., *Pod.*, PULS, **Rhus**, Sang., Sec. c., **SEP.**, *Sil.*, Spig., Stan., Staph., *Stram.*, **SUL**., Verat. a., Verat. v., Zinc.

Antidotes.—Camph., *Coff.*

Phytolacca.

Mind.—Acon., Ars., *Aur.*, Bell., Calc. c., *Cimic.*, Con., Ign., Lil. t., Meli., Merc., *Nat. m.*, Nux v., Phos., Puls., *Rhus t.*, Sang., Sep., Sil., Stram., *Sul.*, **Thuj.**

Localities.—Acon., (Aloe), Am. m., (Ant. cr.), (Ant. t.), Apis, (Apoc. c.), *Arg. n.*, Arn., *Ars.*, Arum t., (Asaf.), (Asar.), Bap., Bar. c., *Bell.*, Bor., *Bry.*, (Cact.), Calc. c., Canth., Caps., (Carb. ac.), (Carb. an.), (Carb. v.), (Caust.), Cham., Chel., Chin., (Cimic.), (Cina), (Clem.), (Colch.), (Coloc.), Con., (Crotal.), Cup., Dig., (Dros.), (Gel.), (Graph.), (Hell.), Hep., Hyos., Ign., *Ip.*, Iod., *K. bi.*, K. carb., Lach., (Laur.), Lyc., **Merc.**, (Mur. ac.), (Nat. m.), *Nit. ac.*, Nux v., Op., Petrol., PHOS., Pho. ac., Pod. (Pso.), *Puls.*, Rhus, (Saba.), (Samb.), (Sang.), Sec. c., (Seneg.), Sep., Sil., Spig., Spo., Stan., Stram., *Sul.*, (Sul. ac.), (Tar.), (Thuj.), Verat. a., (Verat. v.), (Verb.), Zinc.

Sensations.—Acon., (Aesc.), (Agar.), Aloe, Alum., (Ant. t.), Apis, Arg. n., Arn., Ars., Arum t., Asaf., (Asar.), (Bap.), Bar. c., *Bell.*, (Berb.), **Bry.**, *Calc. c.*, (Camph.), Cannab. i., Canth., (Caps.), Carb. v., Caust., (Cham.), Chel., Chin., Cic., Cimic., Cocc., (Colch.), Coloc., Con., Cup., Dig., Dros., (Eup. per.), Fer., (Gel.), Glon., (Graph.), Hell., (Hyos.), *Ign.*, (Ip.), (Iris v.), K. bi., K. carb., *Lach.*, (Laur.), (Led.), (Lil. t.), (Lith.), Lyc., Meny., Merc., Mez., (Mos.), Mur. ac., (Nat. c.), Nat. m., Nit. ac., Nux m., **Nux v.**, (Op.), (Petrol.), *Phos.*, Pho. ac., Plat., (Pod.), Pb., **Puls.**, Ran. b., (Rhodo.), Rhus, (Ruta), Saba., *Sabi., Sang.*, (Sars.), Sec. c., Seneg., **Sep.**, *Sil.*, Spig., Spo., Squ., *Stan.*, (Staph.), Stram., **Sul.**, Sul. ac., (Tar.), *Thuj.*, *Valer.*, Verat. a., (Verat. v.), *Zinc.*

Glands.

Bones.

Skin.—(Agar.), (Bar. c.), (K. bi.), (Lach.), (Phos.), (Pho. ac.), (Rhus), Sul.

Sleep and Dreams.

Blood, Circulation and Fever.—(Ant. t.), Ars., (Cham.), (Cina), (Hell.), (Hep.), (Ip.), Op., Puls., (Rheum), (Sil.), (Sul.), (Verat. a.).

Aggravations: Time and Circumstances.—Acon., (Aesc.), (Agn.), (Aloe), (Alum.), (Ambr.), (Am. carb.), Am. m., (Anac.), Ant. cr., **Ant. t.,** (Apis), Arg., Arn., *Ars.,* (Asaf.), (Asar.), (Aur.), (Bap.), (Bar. c.), Bell., (Bov.), *Bry.,* (Cact.), *Calc. c.,* (Camph.), (Cannab. i.), (Cannab. s.), (Canth.), (Caps.), (Carb. an.), (Carb. v.), (Caust.), (Cham.), Chel., (Chin.), (Cina), (Cocc.), (Coff.), Colch., (Coloc.), Con., *Croc.,* Dig., (Dros.), Dulc., (Euphr.), Fer., (Gel.), Graph., (Hell.), *Hep.,* Hyos., (Ign.), Ip., Iod., (K. b.), (K. carb.), (K. nit.), *Lach.,* (Led.), (Lil. t.), (Lyc.), Mag. c., (Mag. m.), (Mang.), *Merc.,* (Mez.), Nat. m., *Nit. ac.,* (Nux m.), *Nux v.,* Petrol., **Phos.,** (Pho. ac.), (Pb.), (Pod.), **Puls.,** (Ran. b.), (Rheum), Rhodo., **Rhus,** (Ruta), (Saba.) Sabi., (Samb.), (Sang.), (Sars.), (Sele.), (Seneg.), *Sep.,* Sil., Spig., (Spo.) (Squ.), (Stan.), Staph., (Stram.), (Stro.), **Sul.,** (Sul. ac.), (Thuj.), Valer., (Verat. a.), Zinc.

Other Remedies.—*Acon.,* (Aesc.), (Agar.), (Ant. cr.), Ant. t., Apis, Arg. n., Arn., **Ars.,** Arum t., Asaf., (Asar.), Aur., (Bap.), Bar. c., **Bell., Bry.,** (Cact.), **Calc. c.,** (Camph.), (Cannab. i.), Canth., Caps., (Carb. an.), Carb. v., Caust., Cham., Chel., Chin., Cimic., (Cina), (Cocc.), Colch., Coloc., *Con.,* Cup., Dig., Dros., Fer., (Gel.), Graph., Hell., Hep., Hyos., *Ign., Ip.,* Iod., *K. bi.,* K. carb., *Lach.,* (Laur.), (Led.), Lil. t., Lyc., **Merc.,** (Mez.), (Mur. ac.), Nat. m., *Nit. ac.,* (Nux m.), **Nux v.,** Op., Petrol., PHOS., Pho. ac., (Pb.), Pod., PULS., (Ran. b.), (Rheum), (Rhodo.), **Rhus,** (Ruta), Saba., Sabi., *Sang.,* (Sars.), Sec. c., Seneg., **Sep., Sil.,** Spig., Spo., (Squ.), Stan., (Staph.), *Stram.,* SUL., Sul. ac., (Tar.), *Thuj.,* Valer., Verat. a., (Verat. v.), *Zinc.*

Platina.

Mind.—*Aloe,* Alum., *Aur., Bap., Bell., Cannab. i., Cimic.,* Glon., Graph., Hyos., IGN., LYC., *Meli., Naj.,* Phos., *Puls.,* Sil., *Stan.,* **Stram.,** Sul., Ther., *Thuj.,* VERAT A. *Verat. v.,* Zinc.

Localities.—Acon., (Aloe), Alum., Anac., Apis, Arg. n., *Arn.,* Ars., Asaf., Asar., (Bap.), Bar. c., **Bell.,** Bor., Bry., (Cact.), **Calc. c.,** Cannab. i., Canth., (Carb. ac.), *Carb. v., Caust.,* Cham., **Chin.,** Cimic., Cina, Cocc., Coff., Con., Croc., (Crotal.) *Fer.,* (Fl. ac.), Gel., (Glon.), *Graph.,* Hyos., *Ign.,* Ip., (Iris v.), K. bi., **K. carb.,** *Kre.,* Lil. t., *Lyc.,* Mang., (Meli.), **Merc.,** Nat. c., *Nat. m.,* Nux m., **Nux v.,** Op., Petrol., **Phos.,** *Pho. ac.,* (Pic. ac.), Pb., (Pod.), (Pso.), PULS., Rhus, Saba., **Sabi.,** Sang., Sec. c., **Sep.,** *Sil., Spig.,* Stan., Staph., Stram., **Sul.,** Sul. ac., Thuj., **Verat.** a., (Verat. v.), *Zinc.*

Sensations.—*Acon.,* Alum., **Anac.,** (Apis), (Arg. n.), *Arn.,* Ars., **(Arum t.)** *Asaf.,* Asar., Bap., BELL., Bry., Cact., **Calc. c.,** (Cannab. i.),

RELATIONSHIPS.—PLAT.—PB. 441

Cannab. *., (Carb. ac.), *Caust.*, Cham., Chin., *Cic.*, *Cimic.*, Cina, *Cocc.*, Con., (Eup. per.), Gel., Glon., Graph., Hyos., **Ign.**, *Ip.*, *K. carb.*, (Kalm.), (Lil. t.), *Lyc*, *Merc.*, Mez., *Mos.*, Nat. c., (Nat. m.), Nit. ac., Nux m., **Nux v.**, Oleand., Op., Petrol., *Phos.*, (Phyt.), **Puls.**, *Rhus*, Saba., Sang., *Sec. c.*, **Sep.**, *Spig.*, *Stan.*, Staph., *Stram.*, **Sul.**, Sul. ac., Thuj., Verat. a., (Verat. v.), Zinc.

Glands.—Arn., Calc. c., **Con.**, Rhus, **Sep.**, *Spo.*

Bones.

Skin.—Acon., Agn., (Apis), Arn., *Bar. c.*, Bell., Bry., *Calc. c.*, *Caust.*, (Cimic.), Colch., (Eup. per.), Graph., *Led.*, **LYC.**, *Merc.*, *Nit. ac.*, *Nux v.*, Oleand., Pho. ac., Phos., **Puls.**, Ran. s., Rhus, Saba., *Sec. c.*, *Sep.*, Sil., Spig., Spo., **Staph.**, **SUL.**

Sleep and Dreams.—Ign., *Rhus*, Sep.

Blood, Circulation and Fever.—Acon., Ars., Bell., Calc. c., Carb. v., Cham., Cocc., Cup., **Merc.**, Op., Rhus, *Sec. c.*, Sil., **Verat. a.**

Aggravations: Time and Circumstances.—Acon., Am. m., (Apis), (Arg. n.), Ars., **Aur.**, (Bap.), Bar. c., Bell., *Calc. c.*, **Caps.**, Cham., **Con.**, *Cyc.*, Dros., **Dulc.**, *Euphorb.*, Euphr., *Fer.*, Graph., *Ign.*, (K. bi.), Lach., (Lil. t.), **Lyc.**, Mag. m., *Meny.*, Mos., Nat. c., Nit. ac., Nux v., *Pho. ac.*, **PULS.**, Rhodo., *Rhus*, **Saba.**, *Samb.*, (Sang.), SEP., Sil., Spig., Stro., *Sul.*, Sul. ac., **Tar.**, *Valer.*, **Verb.**, *Vio. t.*

Other Remedies.—Acon., (Aloe), Alum., Anac., Apis, Arg. n., *Arn.*, Ars., Aur., *Bap.*, Bar. c., **Bell.**, (Cact.), **Calc. c.**, Cannab. i., Caps., Caust., Cham., Chin., *Cimic.*, Cocc., *Con.*, Fer., Gel., (Glon.), Graph., Hyos., **Ign.**, (K. bi.), K. carb., Lil. t., LYC., **Merc.**, Nit. ac., *Nux v.*, Oleand., *Phos.*, Pho. ac., PULS., RHUS, Saba., (Sang.), *Sec. c.*, SEP., Sil., Spig., Staph., Stram., **Sul.**, *Verat. a.*, Verat. v., Zinc.

Antidote.—Puls.

Plumbum.

Mind.—Apis, Ars., Aur., *Bap.*, *Bell.*, *Cimic.*, *Crotal.*, *Gel.*, *Hyd. ac.*, **Hyos.**, **LYC.**, *Merc. c.*, Nat. c., Op., *Pic. ac.*, *Puls.*, *Stram.*, Sul. ac., Verat. a.

Localities.—Acon., Aesc., Aloe, *Apis*, Apoc. c., *Arg. n.*, Arn., *Ars.*, (Arum t.), Aur., Bap., **BELL.**, Berb., Bry., (Cact.), Calc. c., Cannab. i., *Canth.*, Carb. ac., Caust., *Cham.*, *Chin.*, Cimic., Cocc., Crotal., *Dios.*, *Eup. per.*, (Fl. ac.), Gel., (Glon.), Graph., Hep., (Hyd. ac.), Hyos., Ign., (Iris v.), *K. bi.*, *K. carb.*, Kalm., *Laur.*, Lil. t., Lith., **Lyc.**, *Merc.*, Nat. c., Nit. ac., **Nux v.**, **Op.**, **PHOS.**, Pho. ac., Phyt., Pod., Pso., **PULS.**, *Rhus*, Ruta, Sang., **Sep.**, Sil., Stan, *Staph.*, Stram., **Sul.**, (Ther.), Thuj., *Verat. a.*, Verat. v., Verb., Zinc.

Sensations.—Acon., Aesc., (Aloe), Alum, *Apis, Arg. n.*, Arn., **Ars.**, (Arum t.), Bap., **BELL.**, (Berb.), Bry., Cact., **Calc. c.**, *Cannab. i.*, Canth., *Caust.*, Cham., **Chin.**, Cic., Cimic., *Cocc.*, Con., (Crotal.), Cup., *Gel.*, Glon., Hyos., *Ign.*, K. bi., K. carb., (Kalm.), Lach., Laur., (Lil. t.), *Lyc.*, Merc., Mos., Nat. m., Nit. ac., **Nux v.**, Oleand., *Op., Phos.*, Phyt., (Pod.), *Puls.*, Rhus, Ruta, Sabi., *Sang.*, Sec. c., *Sep., Sil.*, Stram., **Sul.**, *Verat. a.*, Verat. v.

Glands.—Bell., Bry., Con., Merc., Nux v., Phos., **Puls.**, *Sul.*

Bones.—Asaf., *Bell., Calc. c.*, **Lyc.**, MERC., *Nit. ac.*, PHOS., *Puls.*, Sep., **Sil.**, Staph., Sul.

Skin.—(Aloe), ARS., *Asaf. Bell.*, **Bry.**, *Calc. c.*, Carb. v., Cham., *Chin., Con.*, Crotal., Dulc., Fer., Hep., K. carb., Lach., Laur., **Lyc.**, Merc., Nat. m., Nit. ac., Op., *Phos.*, Pho. ac., Puls., (Sang.), **Sec. c.**, *Sep*, SIL., Squ., SUL.

Sleep and Dreams.—Ant. t., Arg. n., (Bap.), Nux m., *Op.*, Verat. a.

Blood, Circulation and Fever.—Acon., (Cannab. i.), Cham., *Op.*, Phos.

Aggravations: Time and Circumstances.—(Aesc.), Arn., Ars., Asaf., (Bap.), **Calc. c.**, Caps., Cham., Cocc., Con., *Cyc.*, Dros., Graph., *Ign.*, (Lil. t.), (Lith.), *Lyc., Mang.*, Nat. c., Nux v., **Phos.**, (Phyt.), *Puls.*, Rhus, Saba., (Sang.), **Sep.**, *Sul*, Thuj., Verat. a.

Other Remedies.—Acon., Aesc., Aloe, *Apis, Arg. n., Ars.*, (Arum t.), Asaf., *Bep.*, **BELL.**, (Berb.), Bry., (Cact.), **Calc. c.**, Cannab. i., Cham., *Chin., Cimic.*, Cocc., Con., *Crotal., Gel.*, (Glon.), Hyos., Ign., K. bi., K. carb., Laur., Lil. t., (Lith.), **Lyc., Merc.**, Nat. c., Nit. ac., *Nux v.*, **Op.**, PHOS., Phyt., (Pod.), PULS., Rhus, Sang., Sec. c., **Sep., Sil.**, Stram., SUL., *Verat. a.*, Verat. v.

Antidotes.—Alum., Bell., Hyos., **Op.**, *Plat.*, Stram, Electric.

Podophyllum.

Mind.

Localities.—Acon., *Aesc.*, Agar., (All. c.), *Aloe*, (Alum.), (Ambr.), (Am. carb.), Am. m., Ant. t., *Apis*, Apoc. c., **Arg. n.**, *Arn.*, **Ars.**, Arum t., Asaf., Asar., (Aur.), Bap., Bar. c., *Bell.*, Berb., Bor., (Bov.), BRY., *Calc. c.*, (Camph.), *Canth.*, Caps., (Carb. ac.), Carb. an., *Carb. v.*, Caust., *Cham., Chel.*, **Chin.**, (Cimic.), (Cina), Cocc., *Colch.*, **Coloc.**, Con., (Crotal.), Cup., Dig., Dios., Dulc., (Eup. per.), Fer., (Gel.), Graph., Hell., (Hep.). (Hyos.), Ign., Ip., (Iod.), Iris v., K. bi., *K. carb.*, (K. nit.), Lach., Laur., (Lit. t), *Lyc.*, Mag. m., (Mar.), **Merc.**, (Mos.), (Nat. c.), Nat. m., *Nit. ac.*, **Nux v.**, Oleand., Op., *Petrol.*, PHOS., *Pho. ac.*, (Phyt.), (Plat.), Pb.,

Pso., **Puls.**, (Ran. b.), Rheum, (Rhodo.), Rhus, (Saba.), Sang., *Sec. c.*, (Sele.), Sep., *Sil.*, (Spig.), (Squ.), (Stan.), Staph., Stram., SUL., Sul. ac., (Tar.), Thuj., (Valer.), *Verat. a.*, (Verat. v), Zinc.

Sensations.—Acon., (Aesc.), (Agar.), Alum., (Apis), (Arg.), (Arg. n.), (Arn.), Ars., (Arum t.), (Asaf.), (Aur.), (Bap.), (Bar. c.), *Bell.*, (Bor.), Bry., Calc. c., (Cannab. i.), Canth., (Carb. v.), (Caust.), (Cham.), (Chin.), Cimic., Cocc., Coloc., Con., (Dig.), (Eup. per.), (Fer.), Gel., Ign., **(K. bi.)**, (K. carb.), Lach., Lil. t., Lyc., (Merc.), (Mez.), Nat. m., Nit. ac., (Nux m.), *Nux v.*, (Op.), Petrol., Phos., (Pho. ac.), (Phyt.), (Pb.), *Puls.*, (Ran. b.), (Rhodo.), Rhus, (Ruta), (Saba.), Sabi, *Sang.*, Sars., Sec. c., (Seneg.), Sep., *Sil.*, (Spig.), (Spo.), Stan., Staph., (Stram.), Sul., (Sul. ac.), (Valer.), Verat. a., (Verat. v.), Zinc.

Glands.

Bones.

Skin.

Sleep and Dreams.—(Acon.), (Aloe), (Anac.), Ant. cr., Ant. t., Apis, (Ars.), (Asaf.), (Bell.), (Bry.), (Calc. c.), (Camph.), Cannab. i., (Carb. v.), (Caust.), (Chel.), (Con.), (Cyc.), (Fl. ac.), (K. carb.), (Laur.) (Mos.), (Nat. c.), (Nat. m.), Nux m., Nux v., Op., Phos, Pho. ac. Puls., (Rhus), (Saba), (Samb.), (Sep.), (Sil.), (Stram.), Sul., (Sul. ac.), Thuj., (Verat. a.).

Blood, Circulation and Fever.—Acon., (Aloe), (Arn.), Ars., Bell., Bry., (Calc. c.), Camph., Canth., (Carb. v.), (Cham.), (Cic.), (Euphorb.), Laur., (Lyc.), Merc., (Mez.), (Nit. ac.), (Nux v.), Phos., (Pho. ac.), Puls., (Ran. b.), (Rhus), (Saba.), Sec. c., (Sep.), (Sil.), Sul., (Verat. a.),

Aggravations: Time and Circumstances.—(Acon.), (Agar.), (Aloe), (Ambr.), Am. m., (Anac.), (Ant. cr.), (Ant. t.), Arg., (Arg. n.), (Arn.), Ars., Aur., (Bap.), (Bor.), (Bov.), *Bry.*, Calc. c., Cannab. s., (Caps.), Carb. v., Chel., Cina, (Coff.), (Con.), Croc., (Cup.), (Dig.), Dros., (Dulc.), (Euphr.), Fer., Gel., Guai., Hep., Ign., K. bi., K. carb., *K. nit.*, (Kre.), Lach., (Laur.), (Mag. c.), Mang., (Mar.), Merc., (Mez.), Nat. c., *Nat. m.*, Nit. ac., (Nux m.), *Nux v.*, Petrol., *Phos.*, Pho. ac., (Phyt.), Puls., Ran. b., (Ran. s.), (Rheum) Rhodo., **Rhus**, Saba., (Sabi), (Samb.), (Sang.), (Sele.), (Seneg.), *Sep.*, *Sil.*, Spig., Squ., Stan., Staph., (Stram.), **Sul.**, Sul. ac., (Tar.), Thuj., Valer., (Verat. a.), (Verat. v.), (Verb.), (Vio. t.).

Other Remedies.—*Acon.*, Aesc., Agar., Aloe, (Alum.), (Ambr.), Am. m., (Anac.), (Ant. cr.), Ant. t., Apis, (Arg.), Arg. n., Arn., *Ars.*, (Arum t.), Asaf., Aur., Bap., (Bar. c.), *Bell.*, Bor., (Bov.), **Bry.**, *Calc. c.*, Camph., (Cannab. i.), *Canth.*, Caps., *Carb. v.*, Caust., Cham., Chel., Chin., (Cimic.), (Cina.), Cocc., Coloc., Con., (Cup.), Dig., (Dulc.), (Eup. per.), Fer., Gel.,

(Hep.), Ign., K. bi., *K. carb.*, K. nit., Lach., Laur., (Lil. t.), Lyc., (**Mar.**), *Merc.*, (Mez.), (Mos.), Nat. c., *Nat. m.*, *Nit. ac.*, **Nux m.**, **Nux v.**, (Op.), *Petrol.*, **Phos.**, *Pho. ac.*, (Phyt.), (Pb.), *Puls.*, Ran. b., (Rheum), Rhodo., *Rhus*, Saba., (Sabi.), (Samb.), Sang., *Sec. c.*, (Sele.), (Seneg.), **Sep.**, *Sil.*, Spig., (Squ.), Stan., Staph., Stram., SUL., Sul. ac., (Tar.), Thuj., Valer., *Verat. a.*, (Verat. **v.**), Zinc.

Pulsatilla.

Mind.—Acon., Aloe, Anac., *Apis*, Arn., *Ars.*, Aur., Bap., Bar. c., **Bell.**, Bry., **Calc. c.**, *Cannab. i.*, Cannab. s., *Caust.*, *Cham.*, Cic., Cimic., **Cocc.**, *Con.*, *Gel.*, Glon., Graph., *Hell.*, Hyd. ac., *Hyos.*, IGN., Lach., Laur., **LYC.**, *Meli.*, Merc., Merc. c., Nat. c., *Nat. m.*, **Nux v.**, Op., **Phos.**, **Pho. ac.**, Phyt., *Pic. ac.*, **Plat.**, *Pso.*, Rhus, *Sep*, **Sil.**, **Stram.**, *Sul.*, Ther., **Verat. a.**, Verat. v.

Localities.—Acon., Aesc., *All. c.*, **Aloe**, APIS, Apoc. c., ARG. N., Arn., *Ars.*, **Arum t.**, Asaf., Bap., *Bell.*, *Berb.*, *Bry.*, *Cact.*, **Calc. c.**, **Cannab. i.**, Cannab. s., Canth., **Carb. ac.**, Carb. v., Caul., *Caust.*, *Cham.*, *Chin.*, **Cimic.**, Cocc., *Con.*, *Crotal.*, Cup., Cyc., *Dios.*, Dulc., Eup. per. Euphr., *Fl. ac.*, **GEL**, Glon., *Graph.*, (Hyd. ac.), Hyos., (Hyper.), Ign., Ip., Iris v., K. BI., *K. carb.*, Kalm., *Lil. t.*, Lith., *Lyc.*, Meli., **Merc.**, (Millef.), Nat. c., *Nat. m.*, Nit. ac., **NUX V.**, Par., Petrol., **PHOS.**, Pho. ac., *Phyt.*, Pic. ac., Plat., Pb., **POD**, **Pso.**, *Rhus*, Saba., Sabi., **SANG.**, Sec. c., **SEP.**, **Sil.**, Spig., Spo., Stan., *Staph.*, SUL., (Ther.), Thuj., Valer., *Verat. a.*, *Verat. v.*

Sensations.—*Acon.*, *Aesc.*, *Aloe*, Anac., APIS, (Apoc. c.), ARG. N., Arn., Ars., **Arum. t.**, *Asaf.*, Aur., *Bap.*, Bar. c., **BELL.**, Berb., **Bry.**, *Cact.*, Calc. c., **Cannab. i.**, *Canth.*, Caps., (Carb. ac.), *Carb. v.*, (Caul.), **Caust.**, *Cham.*, Chin., Cic., **Cimic.**, **Cocc.**, Colch., Con., Croc., Crotal., Cup., Dios., Eup. per., *Fer.*, (Fl ac.), **Gel.**, Glon., *Graph.*, Hyos., *Ign.*, Iod., *Iris v*, K. BI., *K. carb.*, *Kalm*, Kre., Laur., *Lil. t.*, (Lith.), *Lyc*, (Meli.), **Merc.**, Mez, *Nat. m.*, Nit. ac., Nux m., **NUX V.**, Oleand., Par., Petrol., **Phos.**, Phyt., *Plat.*, **Pod.**, *Pso.*, RHUS, Saba., Sabi., SANG., Sec. c, **Sep.**, *Sil.*, Spig., *Stan.*, *Staph.* Stram., Stro., SUL., **Tar.**, *Thuj.*, Verat. a., Verat. v., Zinc.

Glands.—Acon., *Arn.*, (Arum t.), **BELL.**, Bry., Calc. c, *Carb. an.*, Chin., Con., **Lyc.**, **Merc.**, Phos., *Rhus*, Sil., *Spo.*, **Sul.**

Bones.—*Asaf.*, Bell., *Calc. c.*, Con., Eup. per, Hep., *Merc.*, **Nit. ac.**, Sep., *Sil.*, **Sul.**

Skin.—*Acon.*, Am. m., *Apis*, Arn., **Ars.**, **Asaf.**, *Bell.*, **Bry.**, **Calc. c.**, (Carb. ac.), Carb. v., *Caust.*, (Cimic.), Clem., Con., (Eup. per.), Euphorb.,

Graph., **Hep.**, Lach., *Led.*, Lyc., Merc., *Nit. ac.*, Phos., Plat., **Rhus**, Sep., SIL., Spo., Staph., SUL.

Sleep and Dreams.—(Aloe), Ant. t., Apis, *Arg. n.*, *Ars.*, Bap., *Bell.*, BRY., **Calc. c.**, *Cannab. i.*, Carb. v., Cham., Chin., (Cimic.), Con., Croc., (Gel.), Graph., *Hep.*, Ign., Led., (Lil. t.), Merc., Nux m., *Nux v.*, Op., PHOS., *Pho. ac.*, Pod., *Rhus*, Sep., Sil., Stram., *Sul.*, Verat. a.

Blood, Circulation and Fever.—Acon., (Aloe), Apis, (Arg. n.), Arn., ARS., (Bap.), *Bell.*, (Berb.), Bry., Cact., Calc. c., (Cannab. i.), Caust., *Chin.*, Gel., Glon., Hell., Ign., Ip., (Lil. t.), *Lyc.*, *Merc.*, NUX V., **Phos.**, Phyt., (Pod.), Rhus, *Sang.*, Sep., *Spig.*, Staph., *Sul.*, Verat. a., (Verat., v.).

Aggravations: Time and Circumstances.—*Acon.*, Aesc., All. c., Aloe, Ambr., Am. carb., Anac., Ant. cr., *Apis*, *Arg. n.*, Arn., **Ars.**, Aur., Bap., *Bell.*, **Bry.**, Cact., **Calc. c.**, (Cannab. i.), Cannab. s., Canth., **Caps.**, *Carb. v.*, Caust., *Cham.*, Chin., Cimic., Colch., Coloc., **Con.**, Croc., Cup., Cyc., *Dulc.*, *Euphorb.*, **Fer.**, Gel., Glon., Graph., *Hep.*, Hyos., **Ign.**, Iod., Ip., *K. bi.*, K. carb., Led., Lil. t., (Lith.), LYC., Mag. c., Merc., Nat. c., Nat. m., Nit. ac., *Nux v.*, Op., **Phos.**, *Pho. ac.*, Phyt., *Plat.*, Pod., Ran. b., **Rhus**, Saba., Sabi., Samb., **Sang.**, SEP., *Sil.*, Spig., *Staph.*, Stram., Stro., **Sul.**, Tar., Thuj., Valer., Verat. a., Verat. v., Vio. t.

Other Remedies.—*Acon.*, Aesc., All. c., **Aloe**, APIS, (Apoc. c.), ARG. N., Arn., **Ars.**, *Arum t.*, Asaf., **Bap.**, BELL., *Berb.*, Bry., Cact., **Calc. c.**, CANNAB. I., Canth., Caps., Carb. v., *Coust.*, *Cham.*, *Chin.*, Cimic., Cocc., *Con.*, Crotal., Fer., GEL., **Glon.**, Graph., *Hep.*, Hyos., *Ign.*, Iod., K. bi., K. carb., Lach., Lil. t., Lith., LYC., Merc., Nat. m., Nit. ac., **Nux v.**, PHOS., *Pho. ac.*, Phyt., *Plat.*, Pod., RHUS, Saba., SANG., **Sep.**, **Sil.**, Spig., Spo., *Staph.*, Stram., SUL., Thuj., *Verat. a.*, *Verat. v.*

Antidotes.—Cham., *Coff.*, Ign., Nux v., Acetum.

Ranunculus Bulbosus.

Mind.—Bap., Bell., Con., Gel., Laur., *Lyc.*, Merc. c., Nat. c., Phos., *Pho. ac.*, *Sep.*, Sil., Stram., Sul., Verat. v.

Localities.—*Acon.*, Aesc., (Aloe), Apis, (Arg. n.), Arn., (Arum. t.), Asaf., Aur., (Bap.), *Bell.*, BRY., **Calc. c.**, *Canth.*, (Carb. ac.), *Carb. v.*, Caust., **Chin.**, (Cimic.), *Cocc.*, (Dios.), Dulc., (Gel.), Hep., IGN., (Iris v.), K. bi., *K. carb.*, Lach., Laur., (Lil. t.), **Lyc.**, *Merc.*, Mez., Nat. c., Nat. m., **Nux v.**, *Phos.*, (Pod.), **Puls.**, *Rhus*, Saba., Sang., **Sep.**, *Sil.*, **Spig.**, Squ., *Stan.*, Staph., **Sul.**, Thuj. *Verat. a.*, Verat. v., **Zinc.**

Sensations.—*Acon.*, Aesc., (Aloe), Alum., Apis, *Arg. n.*, (Arum t.),

Asaf., Bap., *Bell.*, *Berb.*, **Bry.**, *Calc. c.*, Cannab. i., Canth., Carb. v., *Caust.*, *Chin.*, (Cimic.), Cocc., (Eup. per.), Gel., Glon., **Ign.**, *K. bi.*, K. carb., (Kalm.), Lil. t., (Lith.), Lyc., *Merc.*, Nat. m., **Nux v.**, Par., *Phos.*, Phyt., (Pod.), **Puls.**, RHUS, Saba., *Sang.*, **Sep.**, Sil., *Spig.*, Spo., Stan., Sul., Verat. a., (Verat. v.), Zinc.

Glands.

Bones.

Skin. – Ant. cr., **Ars.**, Bell., *Bry.*, (Carb. ac.), *Caust.*, Clem., Con., Dulc., *Graph.*, Hep., *Lach.*, *Lyc.*, *Merc.*, Phos., Puls., RHUS, *Sep.*, **Sil.**, Staph., **Sul.**, Vio. t.

Sleep and Dreams.—(Arg. n.), **Ars.**, Bell., Bor., Calc. c., Carb. an., Chin., Hep., *Ign.*, K. CARB., Lyc., *Merc.*, Mur. ac., *Nux v.*, *Phos.*, *Puls.*, Rhus, **Sep.**, **Sil.**, *Sul.*

Blood, Circulation and Fever.—Acon., (Apis), Arn., *Ars.*, *Bry.*, (Cact.), Calc. c., (Cannab. i.), *Chin.*, Lyc., Nat. m., Nit. ac., *Nux v*, *Phos.*, (Pod.), **Puls.**, Rhus, Sep., Sil., Spig., *Sul.*, Verat. a.

Aggravations: Time and Circumstances.—Aesc., (Aloe), Ant. cr., Apis, Arg. n., Arn., *Ars.*, Bap., Bar. c., **Bell.**, Calc. c., *Cannab. s.*, *Chel.*, Cimic.), *Colch.*, Glon., Hell., *Hep.*, Ign., *Iod.*, *K. bi.*, K. nit., Lach., *Led.*, Lil. t., Nat. m., Nit. ac., NUX V., (Phyt.), Pod., *Rhus*, Saba., *Sang.*, *Sele.*, Sep., Sil., **Spig.**, **Staph.**, (Verat. v.),

Other Remedies.—Acon., Aesc., (Aloe), Ant. cr., *Apis*, *Arg. n.*, **Ars.**, (Arum t.), *Bap.*, **Bell.**, (Berb.), **Bry.**, *Calc. c.*, (Cannab. i.), Caust., *Chin.*, (Cimic.), Gel., Glon., Hep., **Ign.**, *K. bi.*, *K. carb.*, Lach., Lil. t., **Lyc.**, *Merc.*, Nat. m., NUX V., *Phos.*, (Phyt.), Pod., **Puls.**, RHUS, *Sang.*, SEP., **Sil.**, *Spig.*, *Staph.*, **Sul.**, Verat. a., Verat v., Zinc.

Antidotes.—Bry., *Camph.*, Rhus.

Injurious.—Acetum, Spir. nit. dul., *Spir. vini.*, *Staph.*, Sul., *Vinum.*

Ranunculus Sceleratus.

Mind.—*Acon.*, *Bell.*, Calc. c., Laur., Mos., Nat. m., Nux v., Phos., *Puls.*, Rhus, Stram , Verat. a.

Localities.– Am. carb., (Arg. n.), Aur., Bry., (Cact.), *Calc. c.*, (Carb. ac.), Carb. an., Carb. v., Caust., Chin., (Dios.), Graph., *K. carb.*, *Kre.*, Lyc., Merc., Mez., Nat. m., Nit. ac., PHOS., Pho. ac., (Pso.), Rhus, Sil., Spig., *Sul.*, *Thuj.*, Verat. a., Zinc.

Sensations.—Alum., (Apis), (Arg. n.), *Arn.*, (Bap.), BELL., (Berb.), Calc. c., (Cannab. i.), *Canth.*, Carb. v., Caust., *Chin.*, Cocc., Con., Dros., (Glon.), Graph., Hell., Ign., (Iris v.), (K. bi.), *K. carb.*, Laur., (Lith.), Merc., Mez., Nat. c., Nat. m., Nit. ac., *Nux v.*, Phos., Pho. ac., (Phyt.),

Plat., Puls., *Rhus*, (Sang.), Sars., **Sep.**, Sil., Spig., *Spo.*, Stan., **Staph.**, **Sul.**, Zinc.

Glands.—Bell., Merc., Phos., Puls., *Spo.*

Bones.

Skin.—Ars., Asaf., *Bry.*, Calc. c., *Caust.*, Hep., **Lyc.**, Merc., **Nux v.**, Plat., *Puls.*, RHUS, *Sep.*, SIL., Staph., **Sul.**

Sleep and Dreams.—Ars., Coff., K. carb., Sil.

Blood, Circulation and Fever.—Acon., Ars., Bell., *Bry.*, (Cannab.), *Cham.*, Chin., Hep., Hyos., Nat. m.

Aggravations: Time and Circumstances.—Acon., Agn., (All. c.), Alum., (Arg. n.), (Bap.), (Cimic.), Croc., Hell., (K. bi.), *Mag. c.*, Mang., *Puls.*, Rhus, *Sabi.*, (Sang.), Spo.

Other Remedies.—*Acon.*, Am. carb., (Arg. n.), Ars., (Bap.), **Bell.**, *Bry.*, Calc. c., (Cannab. i.), Caust., Chin., (K. bi.), *K. carb.*, Lyc., Merc., Nat. m., Nux v., *Phos.*, Plat., PULS., Rhus, (Sang.), *Sep.*, Sil., Spig., *Spo.*, Sul., *Zinc.*

Antidote.—Camph.

Rheum.

Mind.—Acon., Ars., **Bell.**, Bry., Calc. c., Con., Gel., Hell., Laur., *Nat. m.*, Nux v., Op., Phos., *Pho. ac.*, Puls, *Rhus*, Sep., Sil., Stram., Sul., Verat. a., Zinc.

Localities.—Aesc., Aloe., Ant. cr., (Apis), (Apoc. c.), Arg. n., Arn., *Ars.*, (Arum t.), Bap., Bell., (Berb.), Bor., **Bry.**, *Calc. c.*, Canth., Carb. v., **Cham.**, Chin., (Dios.), Dulc., Graph., Hep., Ign., (Iris v.), K. bi., K. carb., (Lil. t.), *Lyc.*, **Merc.**, *Nat. c.*, Nat. m., Nit. ac., Nux v., **Phos.**, *Pho. ac.*, (Phyt.), Pod., (Pso.), **Puls.**, RHUS, (Sang.), *Sep.*, Spig., Staph., SUL., *Verat. a.*

Sensations.—Acon., (Arg. n.), Arn., (Arum t.), *Asaf.*, **Bell.**, (Berb.), **Calc. c.**, Caust., Cham., *Chin.*, (Cimic.), Cocc., Colch., Con., (Crotal.), (Gel.), Graph., Ign., Iris v., *K. carb.*, (Lil. t.), *Lyc.*, Merc., Mez., Nat. c., *Nat. m*, **Nux v.**, Phos., Plat., PULS., *Rhus*, **Sep.**, Stan., Staph., Sul., Verat. a.

Glands.—*Bell.*, Calc. c., Merc., *Phos.*, Spo., Sul.

Bones.

Skin.

Sleep and Dreams.- (Cannab. i.).

Blood, Circulation and Fever.—Cham., Chin., Hep., Ip., Merc., (Phyt.), *Sep.*, *Sul.*, **Verat. a.**, (Verat. v.),

Aggravations: Time and Circumstances.—(Aesc.), (Aloe), (Apis),

(Arg. n.), *Arn.*, Ars., (Bap.), **Bell.**, **Bry.**, Calad., Chin., Cocc., **Coff.**, *Colch.*, *Croc.*, Dros., Fer., (Glon.), Graph., *Hep.*, *Ign.*, *Iod.*, (K. bi.), *K. carb.*, K. nit., Led., Lil. t., *Lyc.*, **Merc.**, Nat. m., **Nux v.**, Phos., (Phyt.), (Pod.), Puls., *Rhus*, (Sang.), Sil., Spig., Spo., Squ., *Staph.*, Sul., Thuj., (Verat. v.).

Other Remedies.—(Aesc.), Aloe, (Apis), Arg. n., Arn., Ars., (Arum t.), (Bap.), BELL., (Berb.), *Bry.*, Calc. c., *Cham.*, *Chin.*, (Gel.), Hep., Ign., (K. bi.), K. carb., Lil. t., Lyc., **Merc.**, Nat. m., **Nux v.**, *Phos.*, Pho ac., (Phyt.), (Pod.), **Puls.**, **Rhus**, (Sang.), *Sep.*, Staph., SUL., *Verat. a.*, (Verat. v.).

Antidotes.—Camph., *Cham.*, Coloc., Merc., *Nux v.*, Puls.

Rhododendron.

Mind.—Acon., Ars., **Bell.**, Bov., Bry., Calc. c., Cocc., Con., *Hell.*, Hyos., K. carb., Laur., *Nat. m.*, Nux m., *Nux v.*, *Op.*, Phos., **Pho. ac.**, **Puls.**, *Rhus*, Sep., Sil., *Stam.*, Sul., Verat. a., Zinc.

Localities.—Acon., (Aesc.), (Aloe.), Am. carb., Am. m., Apis, (Apoc. c.), Arg. n., Arn., (Arum t.), Asaf., Aur., Bar. c., (Berb.), *Bry.*, (Cact.), **Calc. c.**, Cannab. i., *Carb. v.*, *Caust.*, Cham., *Chin.*, Clem., Con., (Dios.), Fl. ac., (Gel.), (Glon.), *Graph.*, Hep., *Ign.*, (K. bi.), *K. carb.*, (Lil. t.), (Lith.), *Lyc.*, **Merc.**, Mez., Nat. c., Nat. m., Nit. ac., *Nux v.*, Petrol., **Phos.**, *Pho. ac.*, (Pod.), (Pso.), PULS., Rhus, Sabi., Sang., Sep., Sil., Spig., Stan., **Staph.**, Stro., SUL., Thuj., Verat. a., (Verat. v.), Zinc.

Sensations.—Acon., Alum., Ambr., Apis, Arg., *Arg. n.*, *Arn.*, (Arum t.), Asaf., Bap., *Bell.*, Berb., *Bry.*, CALC. C., Cannab. i., Canth., Carb. v., *Caust.*, Cham., *Chin.*, (Cimic.), Cocc., Con., Croc., (Crotal.), Dros., Dulc., (Eup. per.), *Gel.*, (Glon.), Graph., Hell., *Ign.*, Ip., *K. bi.*, **K. carb.**, (Lil. t.), (Lith.), **Lyc.**, Meny., **Merc.**, Mez., Nat. c., *Nat. m.*, *Nit. ac.*, *Nux v.*, Oleand., *Phos.*, Pho. ac., (Phyt.), *Plat.*, (Pod.), Puls, RHUS, Ruta, Saba., Sang., SEP., *Sil.*, *Spig.*, Spo., *Stan.*, *Staph.*, **Sul.**, Tar., Thuj., Verat. a., (Verat. v.), Zinc.

Glands.—ARN., *Bell.*, Bry., *Calc. c.*, Chin., Clem., CON., Puls., *Spo.*, Sul.

Bones.—Asaf., Bell., *Calc. c.*, *Chin.*, (Eup. per.), MERC., Phos., *Pho. ac.*, **Puls.**, Ruta, *Sil.*, Sul.

Skin.—Ant. cr., Ars., *Bry.*, Calc. c., Caust., Chin., LYC., Merc., **Plat.**, Puls., RHUS, **Sec. c.**, Sep., *Sil.*, Staph., *Sul.*, Verat. a.

Sleep and Dreams.—*Ars.*, Con., *Ign.*, K. carb., Op., *Puls.*, Sep., Sil.

Blood, Circulation and Fever.—ARS., Bry., Calc. c., Caust., *Chin.*,

RELATIONSHIPS.—RHOD.—RHUS. 449

Con., *Merc.*, **Nux v.**, *Phos.*, Pho. ac., Puls., *Rhus*, (Sang.), **Sep.**, Staph., Sul.

Aggravations: Time and Circumstances.—Acon., (Aesc.), (All. c.), (Aloe), Am. carb., Ant. cr., (Apis), Arg. n., Arn., *Ars.*, **Aur.**, Bap., *Bell.*, Bry., *Calc. c.*, **Caps.**, Carb. v., Cham., (Cimic.), *Cina.*, *Cocc.*, **Con.**, Dros., *Dulc.*, *Euphorb.*, *Fer.*, (Gel.), (Glon.), Graph., *Hep.*, *Ign.*, K. bi., **K. carb.**, Led., (Lith.), LYC., Mag. m., *Mang.*, Merc., Mos., *Nat. m.*, *Nux m.*, **Nux v.**, Oleand., *Phos.*, Pho. ac., (Phyt.), Plat., (Pod.), **Puls.**, RHUS, *Ruta*, Saba., Samb., Sang., Seneg., **Sep.**, SIL., Spig., *Stro.*, Sul., Tar., Valer., **Verat. a.**, (Verat. v.), Verb.

Other Remedies.—Acon., (Aesc.), (Aloe), Apis, *Arg. n.*, Arn., *Ars.*, (Arum t.), Asaf., Aur., Bap., *Bell.*, (Berb.), *Bry.*, **Calc. c.**, Cannab. i., Carb. v., Caust., *Chin.*, (Cimic.), Cocc., **Con.**, Gel., (Glon.), Graph., *Ign.*, K. bi., *K. carb.*, (Lil. t.), (Lith.), **Lyc.**, Merc., Nat. m., **Nux v.**, *Phos.*, Pho. ac., (Phyt.), Plat., (Pod.), PULS., RHUS, Ruta, *Sang.*, Sep., Sil., Staph., **Sul.**, Verat. a., (Verat. v.), Zinc.

Antidotes.—Bry., Camph., *Clem.*, Rhus.

Rhus Tox.

Mind.—*Acon.*, Anac., *Apis*, Arn., Ars., *Bap*, BELL., Bry., *Calc. c.*, Cannab. i., Cannab. s., Cic., Cimic., Cocc., **Con.**, Crotal., *Gel.*, Glon., Graph., **Hell.**, *Hyos.*, *Ign.*, K. carb., *Laur.*, **Lyc.**, *Meli.*, Merc. c., Mez., Nat. c., *Nat. m.*, Nux m., Nux v., **Op.**, Petrol., Phos., **Pho. ac.**, Phyt., Pic. ac., Pso., **Puls.**, Sep., *Sil.*, Spig., Staph., STRAM., *Sul.*, Ther., *Verat. a.*, Verat. v.

Localities.—Acon., *Aesc.*, *All. c.*, *Aloe*, Ant. cr., APIS, Apoc. c., Arg., ARG. N., Arn., *Ars.*, *Arum t.*, *Bap.*, Bar. c., *Bell.*, Berb., *Bry.*, Cact., **Calc. c.**, *Cannab. i.*, Carb. ac., Carb. v., Caul., **Caust.**, *Cham.*, *Chin.*, Cimic., Crotal., Dios., Eup. per., Fl. ac., **Gel.**, Glon., Graph., Hep., (Hyo. ac.), Ign., Ip., (Iris v.), K. BI., *K. carb.*, Kalm., *Kre.*, Led., *Lil. t.*, Lith., Lyc., Meli., **Merc.**, Mur. ac., Nat. c., Nat. m., Nit. ac., *Nux v.*, Oleand., Petrol., *Phos.*, *Pho. ac.*, Phyt., (Pic. ac.), Plat., *Pod.*, *Pso.*, **Puls.**, Saba., Sabi., SANG., Sele., SEP., *Sil.*, Spig., Squ., *Staph.*, SUL., Valer., Verat. a., *Verat. v.*, Verb.

Sensations.—Acon., *Aesc.*, *Aloe*, Alum., Am. m., Anac., Ant. cr., **Apis**, Arg., ARG. N., *Arn.*, *Ars.*, *Arum t.*, *Asaf.*, *Bap.*, Bar. c., BELL., *Berb.*, *Bry.*, Cact., **Calc. c.**, *Cannab. i.*, Canth., Caps., Carb. v., (Caul.), *Caust.*, Cham., *Chin.*, Cic., CIMIC., **Cocc.**, Colch., Con., Croc., Crotal., (Dios.), Dros., Eup. per., *Fer.*, (Fl. ac.), **Gel.**, *Glon.*, *Graph.*, Hyos., *Ign.*, Iris v., K. bi., *K. carb.*, Kalm., Kre., Led., Lil. t., Lith., **Lyc.**, Meli., **Merc.**, *Nat. c.*, *Nat. m.*, Nit. ac., Nux m., NUX V., *Oleand.*, Par., Petrol.,

20

Phos., Pho. ac., **Phyt.**, (Pic. ac.), *Plat.*, Pod., *Pso.*, PULS., *Saba.*, Sabi., Sang., Sele., SEP., *Sil.*, **Spig.**, Spo., *Stan.*, *Staph.*, *Stram.*, Stro., SUL., Sul. ac., Thuj., Verat. v., Zinc.

Glands.—Arum t., **Bell.**, *Bry.*, **Con.**, Dulc., Hep., Lyc., *Merc.*, PHOS., PULS., **Spo.**, *Sul.*

Bones.—Arg., **Asaf.**, *Calc. c.*, *Chin.*, (Eup. per.), Lyc., Merc., *Nit. ac.*, Phos., *Pho. ac.*, PULS., *Ruta*, Sil., *Staph.*, Sul.

Skin.—Acon., **Apis**, *Arn.*, **Ars.**, Bar. c., *Bell.*, Bor., *Bry.*, *Calc. c.*, (Carb. ac.), Carb. v., **Caust.**, (Cimic.), Clem., (Crotal.), Dulc., (Eup. per.), GRAPH., (Hyd. ac.), K. bi., K. carb., *Lach.*, Lyc., MERC., Mez., Nat. m., Nit. ac., Phos., Plat., **Puls.**, Ran. b., (Sang.), Sec. c., Sele., SEP., *Sil.*, Spo., Staph., SUL., Verat. a., (Verat. v.), Vio. t.

Sleep and Dreams.—(Apis), *Arg. n.*, Ars., Bap., *Bry.*, *Calc. c.*, *Cannab. i.*, Carb. v., *Chin.*, (Cimic.), (Gel.), Hep., *Ign.*, (Lil. t.), Lyc., Merc., Nux v., *Phos.*, Plat., (Pod.), *Puls.*, Sep., Sul.

Blood, Circulation and Fever.—Acon., (Apis), Arg. n., ARS., Bell., (Berb.), Bry., Cact., *Calc. c.*, Cannab. i., Caps., Caust., **Cham.**, *Chin.*, (Gel.), Glon., Hep., Ign., *Ip.*, **Merc.**, Nit. ac., **Nux v.**, Op., Phos., (Pod.), PULS., Saba., Samb., *Sang.*, Sec. c., Sep., Sil., Spig., Stram., SUL., **Verat. a.**, (Verat. v.).

Aggravations: Time and Circumstances.—Acon., Aesc., Agn., (All. c.), Aloe, *Am. carb.*, Am. m., Ant. t., Apis, *Arg. n.*, Arn., **Ars.**, Aur., Bap., Bell., Bor., BRY., Cact.), *Calc. c.*, (Cannab. i.), Caps., Caust., Cham., Cic., Cimic., Clem., Cocc., *Con.*, Dros., *Dulc.*, Euphorb., *Fer.*, (Gel.), Glon., *Hep.*, *Ign.*, Kali., *K. carb. K. nit.*, Lil. t., (Lith.), **Lyc.**, Merc., Mos., Nat. m., Nit. ac., *Nux m.*, **Nux v.**, *Phos.*, Pho. ac., *Phyt.* Pod., Puls., *Saba.*, Sabi., *Samb.*, SANG., **Sep.**, Sil., Spig., Squ., *Stro.*, Sul., Thuj., Verat. v., Vio. t.

Other Remedies.—Acon., Aesc., All. c., *Aloe*, APIS, ARG. N., Arn., *Ars.*, Arum t., **Bap.**, *Bell.*, Berb., Bry., *Cact*, *Calc. c.*, **Cannab. i.**, Caust., Cham., Chin., **Cimic.**, Con., *Crotal*, Gel., Glon., Graph., Hep., Ign., **K. bi.**, K. carb., Lil. t., Lith., *Lyc.*, *Merc.*, Nat. m., Nit. ac., **Nux v.**, *Phos.*, Pho. ac., **Phyt.**, *Pod.*, PULS., Saba., SANG., **Sep.**, *Sil.*, Spig., Staph., Stram., SUL., Verat. a., **Verat. v.**

Antidotes.—Bell., *Bry.*, Camph., Coff., Sul.

Injurious.—Phos.

Ruta.

Mind.—*Anac.*, Ars., Aur., Bell., *Calc. c.*, Con., *Graph.*, Hell., **Ign.**, LYC., Merc., *Nat. c.*, Nux v., Phos., Pho. ac., PULS., *Rhus*, Sep., *Sil.*, Staph., *Stram.*, *Sul.*

RELATIONSHIPS.—RUTA.—SABA.

Localities.—Acon., Aesc., (All. c.), (Aloe), Alum., Anac., *Apis*, (Apoc. c.), Arg. n., **Arn.**, Ars., Aur., Bar. c., **Bell.**, Bry., CALC. C., (Cannab. i.), *Canth.*, Caps., (Carb. ac.), Carb. v., (Caul.), Caust., *Chin.*, (Cimic.), Cocc., Con., *Dig.*, Dros., (Eup. per.), Euphr., (Fl. ac.), (Gel.), *Graph*, Hep., *Hyos.*, Ign., K. bi., *K. carb.*, (Kalm.), Kre., Led., Lil. t., **Lyc.**, **Merc.**, Nat. m., Nit. ac., Nux v., Op., Petrol, Phos., *Pho. ac.*, Pb., Puls., *Rhus*, Saba., Sars., Sec. c., Seneg., **Sep.**, **Sil.**, Spig., Squ., *Staph.*, Stram., SUL., Tell., Thuj., Verat. a., Zinc.

Sensations.—Acon., (Aloe), Alum., Anac., Apis, Arg., Arg. n., **Arn.**, Bap., *Bell.*, *Bry.*, *Calc. c.*, Canth., Carb. v., CAUST., *Chin.*, Cic., Cimic., **Cocc.**, Con., Cup., *Dros.*, Dulc., Eup. per., Gel., (Glon.), Hell., Hep., *Ign.*, K. bi., *K. carb.*, Kalm., Led., (Lil. t.), (Lith.), *Lyc.*, Mar., *Merc.*, Mez., *Nat. c.*, *Nat. m.*, Nit. ac., Nux m., **Nux v.**, *Oleand.*, **Phos.**, Pho. ac., *Plat.*, Pb., (Pod.), *Puls.*, Rhodo., *Rhus*, Saba., Sang., **Sep.**, Sil., Spig., *Stan.*, *Staph.*, Sul., Sul. ac., *Verat. a.*, Verb., Zinc.

Glands.—Arn., Carb. an., Con., Phos., *Rhus*.

Bones.—Asaf., Bell., *Calc. c.*, *Chin.*, (Cimic.), Dros., Eup. per., Hep., Lyc., **Merc.**, Nit. ac., Phos., PHO. AC., PULS., Sep., Sil., Staph., *Sul.*

Skin.—(Apis), **Arn.**, Ars., Asaf., **Bry.**, Calc. c., Caust., Chin., Dulc., K. carb., Lach., **Led.**, LYC., Mang., *Merc.*, Phos., Pho. ac., **Puls.**, Rhus, Sep., *Sil.*, Staph., Sul.

Sleep and Dreams.

Blood, Circulation and Fever.—Ars., (Bap.), (Berb.), Cham., *Chin.*, (Glon.), (Lil. t.), Merc., Puls., Rhus, Sang., SEP., *Sul.*, Verat. a.

Aggravations: Time and Circumstances.—(Aesc.), Am. carb., (Apis), (Arg. n.), Arn., *Asaf.*, Bap., Bar. c., *Bry.*, CALC. C., *Caps.*, Chin., (Cimic.), Cina, Cocc., Con., Cyc., Dros., Dulc., (Glon.), Hep., (K. bi.), K. carb., *Lach.*, (Lil. t.), LYC., Mang., *Merc.*, *Nat. c.*, **Nat. m.**, Nux m., Nux v., *Phos.*, Pho, ac., (Phyt.), **Puls.**, *Rhodo,*, Rhus, Sang., *Sep.*, Sil., Spig., Stro., **Sul.**, *Thuj.*, Verat. a., (Verat. v.), Zinc.

Other Remedies.—(Aesc.), (Aloe), *Apis*, Arg. n., *Arn.*, Asaf., Bap., Bell., Bry., **Calc. c.**, Caust., *Chin.*, Cimic., Cocc., Con., Dros., (Gel.), (Glon.), Hep., Ign., K. bi., K. carb., Led., Lil. t., **Lyc.**, **Merc.**, Nat. c., Nat. m., Nux v., *Phos.*, *Pho. ac.*, PULS., **Rhus**, Sang., **Sep.**, **Sil.**, *Staph.*, SUL., Verat. a.

Antidote.—Camph.

Sabadilla.

Mind.—*Acon.*, Anac., Ars., BELL., Bry., Calc. c, Cannab. s., Cocc., Glon., Hell., *Hyos.*, *Ign.*, Laur., *Lyc.*, *Nat. c.*, Nat. m., Nux v., *Op.*, *Phos.*, **Pho. ac.**, Puls., *Rhus*, Sep., Sil., Staph., **Stram.**, *Sul.*, Verat. a., Zinc.

Localities.—Acon., Aesc., All. c., Aloe, Alum, *Apis*, (Apoc. c.), *Arg. n.*, Arn., Ars., *Arum t.*, Bap., Bar. c., *Bell.*, Berb., *Bry.*, **Calc. c.**, (Cannab. i.), Canth., (Carb. ac.), *Carb. v.*, *Caust.*, *Cham.*, *Chin.*, Cina, Cocc., *Con.*, (Dios.), (Fl. ac.), Gel., (Glon.), *Graph.*, *Ign.*, Iris v., **K. bi.**, *K. carb.*, Kre., (Lil. t.), *Lyc.*, **Merc.**, Nat. c., *Nat. m.*, Nit. ac., *Nux v.*, Oleand., *Petrol.*, *Phos.*, Pho. ac., Phyt., Pod., Pso., PULS., *Rhus*, *Sang.*, *Sep.*, SIL., Spig., Staph., Sul., Tell., Verat. a., Verat v.

Sensations.—Acon., (Aesc.), (Aloe), Alum., *Apis*, **Arg. n.**, Arn., Arum t., Asaf., Bap., *Bell.*, Berb., Bry., (Cact.), **Calc. c.**, *Cannab. i.*, Canth., Caust., Chin., (Cimic.), Cocc., (Crotal.), (Eup. per.), *Gel.*, Glon., Graph., Ign., Iris v., *K. bi.*, K. carb., Laur., (Lil. t.), (Lith.), *Lyc.*, **Merc.**, Mez., *Nat. c.*, Nat. m., **Nux v.**, Oleand., **Phos.**, Phyt., **Plat.**, (Pod.), Pso., **Puls.**, Rhodo., **Rhus**, Ruta, **Sang.**, Sep., Sil., *Stan.*, *Staph.*, **Sul.**, Sul. ac., Thuj., Verat. a., (Verat. v.).

Glands.—*Bell.*, *Bry.*, **Calc. c.**, Con., Merc., *Phos*, Puls., Spo., *Sul.*

Bones.—Asaf., *Chin.*, *Merc.*, Puls., *Rhus*, Ruta, Sep., *Sil.*

Skin.—Arn., *Bar. c.*, Bell., *Bry.*, Calc. c., Cocc., **Graph.**, Lyc., MERC., *Plat.*, Puls., **Rhus**, Sec. c., Sep., SIL., *Staph.*, SUL., Vio. t.

Sleep and Dreams.—Ant. cr., (Apis), (Arg. n.), Cannab. i., Graph., Ign., NUX V., Oleand., Phos., (Pod.), Puls., Rhus, *Sep.*, Staph., Sul.

Blood, Circulation and Fever.—*Acon.*, (Apis), ARS., *Bell.*, *Bry.*, Calc. c., Camph., Cham., *Chin.*, (Gel.), (Glon.), *Hell.*, Ign., *Ip.*, K. nit., Lyc., Merc., Nux m., Nux v., *Phos.*, Pho. ac., (Pod.), *Puls.*, Rhus, (Sang.), Sep., *Spig.*, *Sul.*, *Verat. a.*

Aggravations: Time and Circumstances.—Acon., Am. m., (Apis), (Arg. n.), Arn., Ars., Asar., *Aur.*, (Bap.), Bar. c., Bor., *Bry.*, *Calc. c.*, Camph., **Caps.**, *Carb. v.*, **Caust.**, Cham., Chel., *Con.*, Cyc., **Dulc.**, *Euphorb.*, **Fer.**, Graph., *Hep.*, *Ign.*, **Iod.**, Ip., (K. bi.), *K. carb.*, Lach., (Lil. t.), **Lyc.**, Meny., Merc., *Mos.*, Nat. c., Nux m., NUX V., *Phos.*, Plat., (Pod.), PULS., Ran. b., RHUS, *Samb.*, (Sang.), **Sep.**, *Sil.*, Spig., Spo., Stan., Staph., *Stro.*, Sul., *Tar.*, Valer., Verb.

Other Remedies.—*Acon.*, (Aesc.), (Aloe), *Apis*, *Arg. n.*, Arn., *Ars.*, Arum t., Bap., Bar. c, *Bell.*, Berb., *Bry.*, Calc. c., Cannab. i., Carb. v., Caust., Cham., Chin., Cocc., Con., Gel., Glon., Graph., *Ign.*, *K. bi.*, K. carb., (Lil. t.), *Lyc.*, **Merc.**, Nat. c., Nux m., **Nux v.**, **Phos.**, Pho. ac., Phyt., Plat., Pod., PULS., RHUS, Sang., **Sep.**, Sil., Spig., *Staph.*, **Sul.**, Verat. a., (Verat. v.).

Antidotes.—Camph., Puls.

Sabina.

Mind.—Acon., Ars., Bell., *Calc. c.*, Graph., Hyos., *Lach.*, Merc., Mos.,

Nat. m., Nux v., Op., *Phos.*, *Puls.*, Sil., Staph., *Stram.*, *Verat. a.*, Verat. v., Zinc.

Localities.—(Aesc.), (All. c.), (Aloe), Apis, Arg. n., *Arn.*, Ars., (Bap.), **Bell.**, (Berb.), *Bry.*, (Cact.), **Calc. c.**, (Cannab. i.), Canth., (Carb. ac.), Carb. v., (Caul.), *Caust.*, *Cham.*, **Chin.**, Cimic., Cocc., Colch., Con., Croc., (Crotal.), **Fer.**, (Fl. ac.), Gel., (Glon.), Graph., Hyos., *Ign.*, *Ip.*, K. bi., **K. carb.**, (Kalm.), Kre., Led., Lil. t., *Lyc.*, Merc., Mez., Mos., *Nat. c.*, *Nat. m.*, Nit. ac., **Nux v.**, Petrol., *Phos.*, *Pho. ac.*, *Plat.*, (Pso.), **PULS.**, Rhus, Ruta, Saba., Sang., Sec. c., **Sep.**, Sil., *Staph.*, Stram., **Sul.**, Thuj., Zinc.

Sensations.—Aloe, *Apis*, Arg. n., *Arn.*, (Arum t.), *Asaf.*, Aur., Bap., Bar. c., **BELL.**, (Berb.), *Bry.*, (Cact.), *Calc. c.* Cannab. i., *Canth.*, Carb. v., (Caul.), *Caust.*, *Chin.*, Cimic., Cocc., Colch., Con., (Crotal.), Cyc., (Eup. per.), Fer., Gel., (Glon.), Graph., Ign., *K. bi.*, **K. carb.**, (Kalm.), (Lil. t.), Lith., Lyc., (Meli.), *Merc.*, Nat. m., Nit. ac., *Nux v.*, *Phos.*, *Phyt.*, (Pod.), (Pso.), **PULS.**, Rhus, **Sang.**, **Sep.**, Sil., Spo., *Staph.*, Stro., **Sul.**, Thuj., (Verat. v.), *Zinc.*

Glands.—*Bell.*, Bry., Calc. c., **Con.**, Merc., *Phos.*, *Puls.*, *Rhus*, SPO., *Sul.*

Bones.—Asaf., Bell., Calc. c., Chin., Cyc., (Eup. per.), **Lyc. Merc.**, Mez., Phos., **Pho. ac.**, Puls., *Ruta*, *Sil.*, Staph., Sul.

Skin.—Ant. cr., Apis, Arn., ARS., *Bar. c.*, **Bell.**, **Bry.**, Calc. c., Camph., Caust., Con., Graph., *Hep.*, Lach., Led., *Lyc.*, **Merc.**, *Nit. ac.*, Phos., **Puls.**, *Ran. b.*, Rhus, *Sec. c.*, Sep., *Sil.*, *Staph.*, SUL.

Sleep and Dreams.—*Ars.*, Aur., Bell., Bry., Chin., Hep., Ign., K. carb., Lyc., Nat, m., Nux v., *Phos.*, Rhus, *Sep.*, *Sil.*, Sul.

Blood, Circulation and Fever.—Acon., **Ars.**, *Bell.*, Bry., (Glon.), Nux v., *Puls.*, Rhus, Saba., (Sang.), Spig., Verat. a.

Aggravations: Time and Circumstances.—Acon., (Aesc.), *Agn.*, (All. c.), (Aloe), *Alum.*, Am. carb., Anac., Ant. cr., Ant. t., Apis, (Arg. n.), Arn., Ars., Asar., (Bap.), Bell., Bor., **Bry.**, (Cact.), Calc. c., *Caps.*, Carb. v., **Cham.**, (Cimic.), Cocc., *Croc.*, (Glon.), Hell., Hep., Hyos., Ign., Iod., K. bi., K. carb., Led., Lil. t., *Lyc.*, Mag. c., Mag. m., Merc., **Phos.**, Pho. ac., (Phyt.), **PULS.**, Ran. b., RHUS, Samb., *Sang.*, Sec. c., *Sep.*, Sil., Spig., Spo., Squ., Staph., *Sul.*, (Verat. v.).

Other Remedies.—Acon., (Aesc.), (All. c.), Aloe, *Apis*, Arg. n., Arn., *Ars.*, Asaf., Bap., **Bell.**, (Berb.), *Bry.*, (Cact.), *Calc. c.*, (Cannab. i.), Caust., Cham., Chin., Cimic., Con., (Crotal.), Gel., (Glon.), Graph., Hep., Ign., *K. bi.*, K. carb., Lil. t., *Lyc.*, Merc., Nat. m., Nit.

Phyt., **PULS.**, **Rhus**, **Sang.**, Sec. c., *Sep.*, *Sil.*, Spo., *Staph.*, **Sul.**, Verat. v., Zinc

Antidotes.—Camph., Puls.

Sambucus.

Mind.—Bell., Hyos., Lyc., Op., Phos., Plat., Stram., Sul.

Localities.—*Acon.*, (All. c.), (Apis), (Apoc. c.), Arg. n., Arn., *Ars.*, (Arum t.), Aur., (Bap.), **Bell.**, **Bry.**, (Cact.), **Calc. c.**, (Cannab. i.), (Carb. ac.), *Carb. v.*, Caust., *Cham.*, **Chin.**, (Cimic.), Con., Cup., (Gel.), Hep., (Hyd. ac.), Hyos., *Ign.*, *Ip.*, K. bi., *K. carb.*, (Lil. t.), *Lyc.*, (Meii.), *Merc.*, Nit. ac., *Nux v.*, Op., PHOS., *Pho. ac.*, **Puls.**, *Rhus*, (Sang.), **Sep.**, Sil., *Spig.*, Spo., Squ., *Stan.*, *Stram.*, **Sul.**, Verat. a., Verat. v.

Sensations.—*Acon.*, (Aesc.), (Apis), (Apoc. c.), (Arg. n.), Ars., (Bap.), **BELL.**, *Bry.*, Calc. c., Chin., Con., (Crotal.), Cup., Fer., (Gel.), Ign., Iod., *Lach.*, Lyc., *Merc.*, **Nux v.**, OP., Phos., **Puls.**, **Rhus**, *Sep.*, **Sul.**, Verat. a.

Glands.—Phos., Puls., Sul.

Bones.

Skin.—Acon., (Apis), *Arn.*, *Ars.*, **BELL.**, *Bry.*, Caust., Chin., Dig., Dulc., K. carb., Lach., Led., *Lyc.*, **Merc.**, Op., *Phos.*, **Puls.**, **Rhus**, Sabi., Sep., Sil., **Sul.**, Verat. a.

Sleep and Dreams.—(Apis), Ars., (Cannab. i.), Hep., K. carb., (Pod.), Sep., Sil.

Blood, Circulation and Fever.—Acon., (Apis), (Arg. n.), ARS., Aur., *Bell.*, *Bry.*, *Calc. c.*, Carb. v., Cham., *Chin.*, (Gel.), (Glon.), Hell., *Hep.*, Iod., K. carb., Kre., Lyc., Merc., Nat. m., Nux m., NUX V., Op., Phos., **Pho. ac.**, Puls., **Rhus**, Saba., Sang., SEP., *Sil.*, Spig., **Squ.**, Stan., Stro., *Sul.*, Verat. a.

Aggravations: Time and Circumstances.—Acon., (Aloe), Ambr., Am. m., Ant. cr., (Apis), Arn., *Ars.*, **Aur.**, (Bap.), Calc. c., **Caps.**, Carb. v., Cham., CON., *Cyc.*, *Dulc.*, Euphorb., Fer., *Hep.*, Hyos., *Ign.*, (K. bi.), K. carb., (Lil. t.), **Lyc.**, Mag. c., Mang., Meny., Merc., Mos., Nux v., Phos., Pho. ac., (Phyt.), *Plat.*, Pb., **Puls.**, Rhodo., **RHUS**, *Saba.*, Sang., *Sep.*, *Sil.*, Squ., *Stro.*, Sul., *Tar.*, Thuj., *Valer.*, Verb.

Other Remedies.—*Acon.*, Apis, (Apoc. c.), Arg. n., Arn., **Ars.**, Aur., (Bap.), **Bell.**, *Bry.*, Calc. c., (Cannab. i.), **Caps.**, Carb. v., Cham., *Chin.*, Con., Fer., (Gel.), *Hep.*, Hyos., Ign., (K. bi.), K. carb., (Lil. t.), *Lyc.*, Merc., Nux v., Op., *Phos.*, Pho. ac., **Puls.**, **RHUS**, Sang., **Sep.**, *Sil.*, Squ., **Sul.**, Verat. a.

Antidotes.—Ars., Camph.

Sanguinaria.

Mind.—Acon., Agar., Aloe, Ambr., Apis, Arg. n., Arn., Ars., Aur., Bap., Bar. c., **Bell.**, Bry., Calc. c., Camph., *Cannab. i.*, Cannab. s., Canth., Caust., Chel., Cic., Cimic., *Cocc., Con.*, Crotal., Cup., Dig., Dulc., Gels., Glon., Hyd. ac., Kalm., Lach., Merc., Mos., Mur. ac., Nat. m., Nux m., Nux v., Op., Petrol., Phos., Pho. ac., Phyt., *Puls., Rhus t.*, Sabi., Seneg., Sep., Sil., Spig., Stram., *Sulph*, Valer., Verat a., Verat. v., Verb., Zinc.

Localities.—*Acon.*, Aesc., *Agar.*, All. c., (Aloe), (Alum.), Am. m., (Anac.), (Ant. cr.), Ant. t., (Apis), (Apoc. c.), *Arg. n.*, Arn., *Ars.*, Arum t., (Asaf.), (Asar.), (Aur.), (Bap.), (Bar. c.), *Bell.*, (Bor.), **Bry.**, (Cact.), *Calc. c.*, (Camph.), (Cannab. i.), Canth., Caps., Carb. ac., *Carb. v.*, Caust., Cham., Chel., *Chin.*, (Cimic.), Cina, *Cocc.*, Colch., Coloc., *Con.*, (Crotal.), Cup., (Cyc.), Dig., (Dios.). Dros., Dulc., (Euphr.), (Fer.), (Gel.), Graph., (Hell.), (Hep.), Hyos., Ign., Ip., Iod., *K. bi.*, K. carb., Lach., (Laur.), (Led.), *Lyc., Merc.*, Mez., Nat. c., *Nat. m., Nit. ac.*, **Nux v.**, Op., (Par.), *Petrol.*, PHOS., Pho. ac., (Phyt.), (Plat.), Pb., (Pod.), Pso., PULS., Ran. b., Rhodo., *Rhus*, Saba., (Samb.), (Sec. c.), Seneg., *Sep., Sil.*, Spig., Spo., Squ., Stan., (Staph.), Stram., **Sul.**, (Sul. ac.), (Ther.), Thuj., (Valer.), *Verat. a.*, Verat. v., Zinc.

Sensations.—Acon., Aesc., *Agar.*, (Agn.), Aloe, *Alum,* (Ambr.), (Am. m., (Anac.), Ant. t., Apis, Arg., *Arg. n., Arn., Ars.*, Arum t., Asaf., (Aur.), Bap., Bar. c., **Bell.**, (Berb.), Bism., Bor., **Bry.**, Calc. c., (Camph.), Cannab. i., (Cannab. s.), *Canth.*, Caps., Carb. v., *Caust.*, (Cham.), Chel., *Chin.*, Cic., Cimic., (Clem.), **Cocc.**, Colch., **Coloc.**, **Con.**, Cup., *Dig.*, (Dios.), Dros., (Eup. per.), *Fer.*, Gel., Glon., (Graph.), (Guai.), (Hell.), (Hyos.), *Ign.*, (Ip.), Iod., Iris v., K. bi., *K. carb., Lach., Laur.*, (Led.), Lil. t., (Lith.), Lyc., (Mag. m.), Meny., **Merc.**, **Mez.**, (Mos.), Mur. ac., Nat. c., *Nat. m., Nit. ac.*, Nux m., NUX V., Oleand., Op., Par., *Petrol.*, PHOS., *Pho. ac.*, Phyt., Plat., *Pb., Pod.*, PULS., *Ran. b.*, (Ran. s.), Rhodo., Rhus, Ruta, **Saba.**, *Sabi., Sars., Sec. c., Seneg.*, **Sep.**, **Sil.**, *Spig., Spo.*, (Squ.), **Stan.**, Staph., (Stram.), (Stro.), SUL., Sul. ac., (Tar.), *Thuj.*, (Valer.), *Verat. a.*, (Verat. v.), **Zinc.**

Glands.

Bones.

Skin.—(Ars.), (Calc. c.), (Graph.), (Hep.), (Merc.), (Nit. ac.), (Puls.), Sil., Sul.

Sleep and Dreams.

Blood, Circulation and Fever.—ACON., (Agar.), (Ambr.), Ant. t., Arn., **Ars.**, (Aur.), (Bap.), **Bell.**, (Berb.), Bor., **Bry.**, Calc. c., (Cannab. i.), (Canth.), (Caps.), Carb. v., **Cham.**, (Chel.), (Chin.), (Cina), (Clem.), Cocc.,

456 RELATIONSHIPS.—SANG.—SARS.

Colch., (Con.), Cup., Dig., (Dros., *Fer.*, (Gei.), (Glon.), Graph., (Hell.), Hep., (Hyos.), Ign., (K. carb.), (Kalm.), (Lach.), (Laur.], (Led.), (Lil. t.), Lyc., (Mar.), (Meny.), *Merc.*, (Mez.), (Mur. ac.), (Nat. c.), Nat. m., Nit. ac., (Nux m.), *Nux v.*, *Op.*, Petrol., *Phos.*, Pho. ac., *Puls.*, (Rhodo.), Rhus, Ruta, (Saba.), (Sabi.), (Samb.), (Sars.), (Sec. c.), (Sele.), *Sep.*, *Sil.*, Spig., Spo., Stan., *Stram.*, Sul., (Tar.), Thuj., Valer., *Verat. a.*, (Verat. v.).

Aggravations: Time and Circumstances.—Acon., Aesc., (Agar.), Agn., (All. c.), (Aloe), (Alum.), *Ambr.*, *Am. carb.*, **Am. m.**, Ant. cr., *Ant. t.*, *Apis*, *Arg.*, Arg. n., **Arn.**, **Ars.**, Asaf., (Asar.), *Aur.*, Bap., (Bar. c.), **BELL.**, (Bism.), Bor., **BRY.**, (Calad.), **Calc. c.**, Cannab. s., (Canth.), **Caps.**, (Carb. an.), Carb. v., Caust., *Cham.*, **Chel.**, Chin., Cic., Cimic., (Cina), (Clem.), **Cocc.**, Coff., Colch., Coloc., *Con.*, Croc., (Cup.), (Cyc.), Dig., Dros., Dulc., Euphorb., (Euphr.), **Fer.**, (Gel.), Glon., Graph., (Guai.), Hell., **Hep.**, **Hyos.**, *Ign.*, Ip., Iod., *K. bi.*, *K. carb.*, *K. nit.*, (Kre), **Lach.**, (Laur.), **Led.**, Lil. t., Lith., **LYC.**, Mag. c., Mag. m., Mang., (Mar.), Meny., **Merc.**, Mez., (Mos.), Mur. ac., Nat. c., **Nat. m.**, **Nit. ac.**, **NUX V.**, (Oleand.), (Op.), (Par.), Petrol., **PHOS.**, **Pho. ac.**, (Phyt.), Plat., Pb., (Pod.), **PULS.**, **Ran. b.**, (Ran. s.), (Rheum), *Rhodo.*, **RHUS**, *Ruta*, (Saba.), **Sabi.**, (Samb.), Sang., Sars., Sele., Seneg., **SEP.**, **SIL.**, **SPIG.**, Spo., Squ., *Stan.*, *Staph.*, Stram., Stro., **SUL.**, (Sul. ac.), Tar., *Thuj.*, **Valer.**, Verat. a., (Verat. v.), (Verb.), (Vio. t.), *Zinc.*

Other Remedies.—Acon., Aesc., *Agar.*, (Agn.), (All. c.), Aloe, Alum., Ambr., *Am. m.*, (Anac.), (Ant. cr.), Ant. t., *Apis*, Arg., **Arg. n.**, **Arn.**, **Ars.**, Arum t., Asaf., (Asar.), *Aur.*, *Bap.*, Bar. c., **BELL.**, (Berb.), (Bism.), Bor., **BRY.**, **Calc. c.**, Camph., *Cannab. i.*, Cannab. s., *Canth.*, **Caps.**, Carb. v., *Caust.*, Cham., **Chel.**, Chin., Cic., Cimic., (Cina), (Clem.), *Cocc.*, Colch., Coloc., **Con.**, (Crotal.), **Cup.**, **Dig.**, (Dios.), *Dros.*, Dulc., (Euphr.), **Fer.**, *Gel.*, *Glon.*, *Graph.*, (Guai.), Hell., *Hep.*, *Hyos.*, **Ign.**, Ip., Iod., *K. bi.*, *K. carb.*, (Kalm.), *Lach.*, Laur., Led., Lil. t., (Lith.), **Lyc.**, (Mag. m.), (Mar.), Meny., **MERC.**, *Mez.*, Mos., *Mur. ac.*, *Nat. c.*, **Nat. m.**, **Nit. ac.**, Nux m., **NUX V.**, (Oleand.), **Op.**, (Par.), *Petrol*, **PHOS.**, **Pho. ac.**, Phyt., (Plat.), Pb., Pod., **PULS.**, Ran. b., Rhodo., *Rhus*, Ruta, Saba., *Sabi.*, (Samb.), (Sars.), (Sec. c.), (Sele.), Seneg., **Sep.**, **Sil.**, Spig., Spo., Squ., *Stan.*, Staph., *Stram.*, **SUL.**, (Sul. ac.), (Tar.), *Thuj.*, *Valer.*, **Verat. a.**, Verat. v., (Verb.), *Zinc.*

Sarsaparilla.

Mind.—Aur., Ign., Lyc., Phos., Plat.

Arn., Asaf., Bar. c., Bell., (Berb.), *Bry.*, (Cact.), Calc. c., Cannab. i., *Canth.*, Carb. v., **Caust.**, *Chin.*, Con., (Dios.), Gel., Graph., Hep., Ign., (K. bi.), *K. carb.*, K. nit., (Kalm.), Laur., Lil. t., *Lyc.*, (Meli.), *Merc.*, Nat. c., Nat. m., *Nux v.*, Petrol, **Phos.**, **Pho. ac.**, (Pso.), **Puls.**, *Rhus*, Ruta, Sep., *Sil.*, Spig., Squ., *Staph.*, Stro., *Sul.*, *Sul. ac.*, Thuj., Verat. a., *Zinc.*

Sensations.—Aesc., *Alum.*, Anac., (Apis), Arg. n., *Arn.*, (Arum t.), Asaf., (Bap.), Bar. c., *Bell.*, (Berb.), Bry., (Cact.), **Calc. c.**, (Cannab. i.), *Caust.*, **Chin.**, *Cocc.*, (Crotal.), Dros., (Gel.), Graph., Hell., Ign., K. bi., *K. carb.*, Laur., (Lil. t.), (Lith.), Lyc., Merc., Nat. c., Nat. m., Nux v., *Phos.*, *Pho. ac.*, (Phyt.), Plat., Pod., *Puls.*, Rhus, **Sang.**, *Sep.*, Sil., *Stan.*, Staph., Stro., **Sul.**, *Sul. ac.*, Thuj., (Verat. v.), Zinc

Glands.—Acon., Bell., *Merc.*, Phos., Sil., *Sul.*

Bones.—Bell., Caust., *Merc.*, Puls., Sep.

Skin.—Ant. cr., Bar. c., Bell., **Calc. c.**, Dulc., Hep., Led., Lyc., **Merc.**, Petrol., Puls., *Rhus,* **Sep.**, *Sil.*, Staph., *Sul.*, Verat. a.

Sleep and Dreams.—Bell., Bry., Chin., Graph., Ign., K. carb., Kre., Lyc., Merc., Nux v., *Phos.*, Puls., Rhus, Sep., Sil., Sul.

Blood, Circulation and Fever.—(Arg. n.). Bov., (Glon.), (Sang.), Sep.

Aggravations: Time and Circumstances.—(Aesc.), Ant. cr., (Apis), (Arg. n.), Arn., (Bap.), *Bell.*, **Bry.**, **Calc. c.**, Cannab. s., Carb. an., *Carb. v.*, (Cimic.), *Colch.*, Croc., (Glon.), *Graph.*, **Hep.**, Ign., Iod., Ip., (K. bi.), Lil. t.s **Lyc.**, *Merc.*, Nat. m., Nit. ac., *Nux v.*, *Phos.*, (Phyt.). Puls., *Rhus*, Sang., **Sep.**, Spig., *Staph.*, *Sul.*

Other Remedies.—Aesc., (Aloe). (Apis), Arg. n., Arn., (Bap.), **Bell.**, (Berb.), Bry., (Cact.), *Calc. c.*, (Cannab. i.), Caust., Chin., (Gel.), (Glon.), Graph., Hep., Ign., K. bi., K. carb., Lil. t., *Lyc.*, MERC., Nux v., **Phos.**, **Pho. ac.**, (Phyt.), *Puls.*, Rhus, *Sang.*, **Sep.**, Sil., Staph., **Sul.**, Sul. ac.

Antidotes.—Bell., Merc.

Secale Cornutum.

Mind.—Acon., **Anac.**, Ars., Bell., Croc., Cup., *Hell.*, **Hyos.**, *Ign.*, Lach., **Lyc.**, Merc., **Nat. c.**, Nat. m., Nux m., Nux v., **Op.**, Par., *Phos.*, *Pho. ac.*, *Plat.*, Rhus, Saba., Sep., Sil., *Staph.*, STRAM., *Sul.*, Verat. a.

Localities.—*Acon.*, (Aesc.), Aloe, *Apis*, (Apoc. c.), **Arg. n.**, Arn., **Ars.**, (Arum t.), Bap., BELL., *Bry.*, (Cact.), **Calc. c.**, (Cannab. i.), Canth., (Carb. ac.), Caust., **Cham.**, Chel., **Chin**., Cic., Cimic., Cocc., Con., Croc., (Crotal.), *Cup.*, Dig., (Dios.), (Eup. per.), Fer., Gel., (Glon.). Hen., Hyos., Ign., Ip.,

Merc., *Nat. m.*, Nit. ac., **Nux v.**, **Op.**, **Phos.**, Pho. ac., *Phyt.*, *Plat.*, Pb., Pod., Pso., **Puls.**, *Rhus*, *Sabi.*, Sang., **Sep.**, *Sil.*, Squ., **Stram.**, **Sul.**, *Verat. a.*, Verat. v.

Sensations.—Acon., (Aesc.), Apis, **Arg. n.**, Arn., *Ars.*, (Arum t.), Bap., **BELL.**, (Berb.), Bry., (Cact.), *Calc. c.*, Cannab. i., (Caul.), Caust., **Cham.**, Chel., *Chin.*, Cic., Cimic., Cocc., Con., (Crotal.), **Cup.**, (Dios.), Fer., *Gel.*, Glon., Graph., **Hyos.**, *Ign.*, Ip., K. bi., (Kalm.), Lil. t., (Lith.), *Lyc.*, *Merc.*, **Nux v.**, **Op.**, *Phos.*, Pho. ac., *Phyt.*, (Pic. ac.), *Plat.*, Pb., (Pod.), (Pso.), **Puls.**, *Rhus*, Sang., *Sep.*, Sil., **Stram.**, *Sul.*, *Verat. a.*, Zinc.

Glands.—*Cham.*, Con., Iod., Nit. ac.

Bones.—*Ars.*, Sep.

Skin.—Acon., Apis, Arn., **ARS**, Asaf., **Bell.**, Bry., *Calc. c.*, Chin., (Crotal.), Dulc., (Hyd. ac.), Iod., K. carb., Lach., **Lyc.**, **Merc.**, *Oleand.*, Phos., **Pho. ac.**, *Plat.*, Pb., *Puls.*, **Rhus**, Sabi., Sep., **Sil.**, Squ., **Sul.**, *Verat. a.*

Sleep and Dreams.—*Ant. t.*, **Bell.**, Bry., (Cannab. i.), Con., Croc., Ign., Led., **Nux m.**, Nux v., **Op.**, Phos., Pho ac., Puls., Verat. a.

Blood, Circulation and Fever.—ACON., (Apis), Arn., *Ars.*, **Bell.**, Bry., Cact., **Calc. c.**, Cannab. i., *Cham.*, Chin., Cocc., (Crotal.), Dulc., (Glon.), *Hep.*, Hyos., *K. carb.*, Lach., Led., *Lyc.*, MERC., Nat. m., Nux v., *Op.*, *Phos.*, Pho. ac., Plat., (Pod.), *Puls.*, Rhus, *Samb.*, Sang., Sep., *Sil.*, Stan., Stram., Sul., *Verat. a.*

Aggravations: Time and Circumstances.—*Ant. t.*, (Apis), Bell., *Bry.*, Calc. c., Caps., Cham., Cocc., Croc., Dros., Hyos., *Iod.*, Led., Lyc., Nux m., Plat., PULS., Rhus, Sabi., Sep., *Sul.*, Verat. a.

Other Remedies.—*Acon.*, (Aesc.), Ant. t., *Apis*, **Arg. n.**, Arn., **Ars.**, (Arum t.), Bap., **BELL.**, *Bry*, Cact., *Calc. c.*, Cannab. i., **Cham.**, Chin., Cimic., Cocc., Con., Croc., (Crotal.), Cup., Gel., Glon., *Hyos.*, Ign., Iod., Ip., K. bi., K. carb., Led., (Lil. t.), **Lyc.**, *Merc.*, Nat. m., Nux m., Nux v., **Op.**, *Phos.*, *Pho. ac.*, Phyt., *Plat.*, Pod., **Puls.**, Rhus, Sabi., *Sang.*, Sep., *Sil.*, Stram., **Sul.**, *Verat. a.*

Antidotes.—Camph., Op.

Selenium.

Mind.—Anac., Bap., Bell., *Con.*, Crotal., Gel., Hell., *Hyos.*, Ign., **Lyc.**, Merc., Nat. c., Nat. m., Op., Pic. ac., Rhus, **Stram.**, *Verat. a.*

Localities.—Acon., Agn., Ant. cr., (Apis), Arg. n., Arn., Ars., (Arum t.), Bell., *Bry.*, Calad., **Calc. c.**, (Cannab. i), Canth., Caps., Carb. v., *Caust.*, Chin., **Con.**, **Graph.**, Hep., Ip., K. bi., **K. carb.**, *Lach.*, **Lyc.**, MERC.,

RELATIONSHIPS.—SELE.—SEN.

Nat. c., Nat. m., *Nit. ac.*, *Nux v.*, Petrol., *Phos.*, (Pod.), **Puls.**, *Rhus*, Sep., Sil., Spig., Stan., Staph., Sul., Thuj., Verat. a.

Sensations.—Acon., Asar., *Aur.*, Bar. c., *Bell.*, Calc. c., **Chin.**, Cocc., Coff., Ign., *Iod.*, K. carb., *Lyc.*, *Merc.*, Mez., Nat. c., NUX V., *Phos.*, *Puls.*, *Rhus*, *Sep.*, Stan., **Sul.**

Glands.—*Arn.*, *Bell.*, Bry., Carb. an., Caust., Chin., K. carb., *Lyc.*, Merc., Puls., Sil., *Sul.*

Bones.

Skin.—Ars., Asaf., Bry., Carb. v., *Caust.*, Chin., Graph., *K. carb.*, Kre., *Lach.*, *Lyc.*, Merc., Nat. c., Pho. ac., **Rhus**, SEP., *Sil.*, Staph., *Sul.*

Sleep and Dreams.—*Ars.*, (Arg. n.), Bell., Bor., **Bry.**, *Calc. c.*, Carb. v., *Chin.*, Graph., Hep., Ign., K. carb., Lach., Lyc., Merc., Nux v., *Phos.*, Puls., *Rhus*, **Sep.**, Sil., Spig., *Sul.*

Blood, Circulation and Fever.—Acon., Ant. t., Ars., *Bell*, Bry CALC. C., (Cannab. i.), Cham., *Chin.*, Graph., Hep., K. carb., Lyc. MERC., *Nux v.*, *Phos.*, Puls., Rhus, (Sang.), **Sep.**, **Sul.**, Thuj., Verat a., (Verat. v.).

Aggravations: Time and Circumstances.—Agar. (Aloe), (Apis), (Arg. n.), Arn., (Bap.), **Bell.**, Bry., Calad., **Calc. c.**, Camph., Cannab. s., Carb. an., *Carb. v.*, Cham., *Chel.*, Chin., (Cimic.), **Cocc.**, **Coff.**, Colch., Fer., (Gel.), (Glon.), Graph., *Hep.*, Ign., *Iod.*, Ip., K. bi., *K. carb.*, Lach., Led., Lil. t., *Lyc.*, Merc., Nat. c., **Nat. m.**, Nit. ac., Nux m., NUX V., *Phos.*, (Phyt.), **Puls.**, *Ran. b.*, *Rhus*, Sang., Sep., *Sil.*, **Spig.**, Spo., Staph., Sul., Verat. a., (Verat. v.).

Other Remedies.—(Apis), Arg. n., Arn., Ars., (Bap.), *Bell.* Bry., *Calc. c.*, (Cannab. i.), Carb. v., Caust., Chin., Cocc., Con., (Gel.), Graph., Hep., Ign., Iod., K. bi., *K. carb.*, Lach., **Lyc.**, **Merc.**, Nat. c., Nat. m., *Nux v.*, Phos., Puls., *Rhus*, (Sang.), **Sep.**, *Sil.*, Spig., Staph., **Sul.**, Verat. a., (Verat. v.).

Antidotes.—Ign., Puls.

Injurious.—Chin., Vinum.

Senega.

Mind.—*Anac.*, Ars., *Aur.*, Bell., Calc. c., Coff., Croc., *Hyos.*, Lyc., Merc., *Nat. c.*, *Op.*, **Phos.**, Pho. ac., Sep., *Stram.*, Sul., Zinc.

Localities.—Acon., (Aesc.), All. c., Apis, (Apoc. c.), Arg., Arg. n., *Ars.*, Arum t., Bap., Bell., **Bry.**, (Cact.), **Calc. c.**, (Carb. ac.), *Carb. v.*, *Caust.*, Cham., Chin., (Cimic.), (Crotal.), (Fl. ac.), Gel., Hep., Ign., Iod., K. bi., K. carb., Lach., *Lyc.*, **Merc.**, Nit. ac., **Nux v.**, Par., PHOS., Pho. ac., (Phyt.), (Pso.), **Puls.**, *Rhus*, Ruta, Sang., Sep., Sil., Spig., Spo., Stan., SUL., (Tell.), Thuj., Verat. a., (Verat. v.), Zinc.

Sensations.—Acon., Aesc., (Aloe), Alum., Apis, (Apoc. c.), **Arg. n.**, Ars., Arum t., Aur., (Bap.), **Bell.**, Berb., *Bry.*, CALC. C., *Cannab. i.*, Caps., *Carb. v.*, *Caust.*, *Chin.*, (Cimic.), Cocc., Con., Croc., (Crotal.), (Dios.), Fer., *Gel.*, (Glon.), Graph., Hyos., K. bi., K. carb., (Lil. t.), **Lyc.**, *Merc.*, Nat. m., *Nux v.*, *Phos.*, (Phyt.), (Pod.), **Puls.**, *Rhus*, **Sang.**, *Sep.*, Sil., Stan., **Sul.**, Verat. v., Zinc.

Glands.

Bones.

Skin.—Ars., Bell., Bry., Calc. c., *Chin.*, Led., Lyc., Puls., Sil.

Sleep and Dreams.—*Bell.*, (Cannab. i.), Ign., Puls., Verat. a.

Blood, Circulation and Fever.—Acon., (Arg. n.), *Arn.*, **Bell.**, **Bry.**, (Cact.), CALC. C., Carb. v., Chin., Fer., (Glon.), Iod., K. carb., LYC., Op., **Phos.**, Pho. ac., Rhus, Sep., *Sil.*, **Sul.**

Aggravations: Time and Circumstances.—Acon., (Aesc.), (All. c.), (Aloe), (Apis), (Arg. n.), (Bap.), Bar. c., Bor., **Bry.**, *Calc. c.*, (Cimic.), Cina, Dros., (Gel.), (Glon.), Iod., *K. bi.*, *K. carb.*, Led., **Lyc.**, *Merc.*, Nat. m., (Phyt.), (Pod.), *Puls.*, *Rhodo.*, Rhus, Ruta, Sang., Sep., Sil., *Spig.*, Sul., (Verat. v).

Other Remedies.—Acon., Aesc., (All. c.), (Aloe), Apis, (Apoc. c.), *Arg. n.*, Ars., Arum t., Bap., **Bell.**, **Bry.**, (Cact.), CALC. C., (Cannab. i.), Carb. v., Caust., Chin., (Cimic.), (Crotal.), Gel., (Glon.), *K. bi.*, K. carb., LYC., *Merc.*, Nux v., **Phos.**, (Phyt.), (Pod.), *Puls.*, Rhus, *Sang.*, Sep., Sil., Sul., Verat. v.

Antidotes.—Arn., Bell., *Bry.*, Camph.

Sepia.

Mind.—*Acon.*, Aloe, Anac., Ars., Aur., Bap., **Bell.**, *Bry.*, *Calc. c.*, Cannab. i., Caust., Cham., Chel., Cimic., Cocc., Con., *Gel.*, Graph., Hell., Hyper., Hyos., **Ign.**, K. bi, LYC., Meli., Merc., Merc. c., *Nat. c.*, Nat. m., *Nux v.*, Op., *Phos.*, **Pho. ac.**, Phyt., **Pic. ac.**, PULS., *Rhus*, Sil., *Stram.*, *Sul.*, Ther., *Verat. a.*, Verat. v.

Localities.—Acon., Aesc., All. c., **Aloe**, APIS, *Apoc. c.*, ARG. N., Arn., *Ars.*, **Arum t.**, Aur., Bap., *Bell.*, Berb., *Bry.*, *Cact.*, **Calc. c.**, **Cannab. i.**, Canth., *Carb. ac.*, Carb. v., Caul., **Caust.**, Cham., *Chin.*, Cimic., Con., Crotal., Cup., *Dios.*, Eup. per., Fl. ac., *Gel.*, Glon., Graph., Hep., (Hyd. ac.), (Hyper.), Ign., Ip., Iris v., K. BI., **K. carb**, Kalm., Kre., Led., *Lil. t.*, Lith., **Lyc.**, Mag. c., Meli., **Merc.**, Nat. c., *Nat. m.*, Nit. ac., Nux v., Petrol., **Phos.**, *Pho. ac.*, *Phyt.*, Pic. ac., Plat., Pb., **Pod.**, *Pso.*, PULS., Rhus, Sabi., **Sang.**, Sec. c., *Sil.*, *Spig.*, Stan., *Staph.*, Stram., SUL., (Tell.), (Ther.), Thuj., Valer., Verat. a., *Verat. v.*, Zinc.

RELATIONSHIPS.—SEP.

Sensations.—*Acon.,* **Aesc.,** (All. c.), *Aloe,* Alum., Anac., **Apis,** (Apoc. c.), ARG. N., Arn., Ars., *Arum t.,* Aur., *Bap.,* Bar. c., BELL., **Berb.,** *Bry., Cact.,* **Calc. c., Cannab. i.,** Canth., (Carb. ac.), Carb. v., **Caust.,** *Cham.,* Chin., Cic., **Cimic.,** *Cocc., Con.,* Crotal., (Dios.), Dros., Eup. per., Fer., **Gel., Glon.,** Graph., Ign., Iod., Iris v., **K. bi., K. carb.,** (Kalm.), *Lil. t.,* (Lith.), **I.yc.,** (Meli.), **Merc.,** Nat. c., *Nat. m., Nit. ac.,* NUX V., Petrol., **Phos.,** Pho. ac., *Phyt.,* (Pic. ac.), *Plat.,* Pb., Pod., *Pso.,* **Puls.,** Rhodo., RHUS, Saba., SANG., Sec. c., *Sil., Spig., Stan.,* Staph., Stram., SUL., Valer., Verat. a., *Verat. v.,* Zinc.

Glands.—Arn., *Bell.,* Bry., Calc. c., CON., *Ign., Lyc.,* Merc.. Phos., Plat., Rhus, **Sil.,** Spo., **Sul.**

Bones.—Asaf., *Bell.,* **Calc. c.,** (Eup. per.), Hep., Lyc., **Merc.,** Nit. ac., *Puls., Sil.,* Sul.

Skin.—(Aloe), Am. carb., *Ant. cr.,* Apis, Arn., **Ars.,** Bar. c., *Bell.,* Bov., *Bry.,* **Calc. c.,** Carb. v., *Caust.,* Chin., Cimic., *Clem., Con.,* Crotal., *Dulc.,* Eup. per., (Glon.), *Graph., Hep.,* (Hyd. ac.), Ign., (K. bi.). K carb., *Lach.,* Led., **Lyc., Merc.,** *Nat. c.,* Nat. m., *Nit. ac.,* Nux v., *Petrol., Phos.,* Pho. ac., Plat., **Puls.,** RHUS, Sele., SIL., Spig., *Staph.,* SUL., Thuj., *Verat. a,* Zinc.

Sleep and Dreams.—(Apis), Arg. n, *Ars.,* (Bap.), Bell., *Bry.,* CALC. C., Cannab. i., Carb. v., Caust., *Cham.,* Chin., *Graph., Hep.,* K. carb., (Lil. t.), *Merc.,* Nat. c., *Nux v.,* Phos., (Pod.), **Puls., Rhus,** Sil., *Sul.*

Blood, Circulation and Fever.—Acon., (Aloe), Apis, (Arg. n.), *Arn.,* **Ars.,** Bell., (Berb.), Bry., Cact., CALC. C., Cannab. i., Carb. v., Caust., *Cham., Chin.,* Dig.. Fer., Gel., Glon., Graph., *Hep.,* Hyos., Ign., Iod., Ip., *K. carb.,* Kre., Lach., Lyc., *Merc.,* Nat. c., *Nat. m.,* Nit. ac., NUX V., *Op.,* **Phos.,** *Pho. ac.,* (Pod.), *Puls.,* Rhus, Sabi., Samb., *Sang.,* Sele., Sil., *Spig.,* Stan., *Stram.,* SUL., Thuj., *Verat. a.,* (Verat. v.).

Aggravations : Time and Circumstances.—Acon., Aesc., (All. c.), Aloe, Ambr., Am. carb., Ant. cr., *Apis, Arg. n., Ars.,* Bap., Bar. c., *Bell.,* **Bry.,** Cact., Calad., CALC. C., Caps., Carb. v.. *Caust., Cham., Chin.,* Cimic., Cocc., Colch., Coloc., *Con.,* Cup., Cyc., Dulc., (Gel.), Glon., *Hep., Ign., K. bi.,* K. carb., *Lil. t.,* (Lith.), *Lyc.,* Mang., Merc., *Nat. c.,* Nat. m., Nit. ac., **Nux v., Phos.,** Pho. ac., Phyt., Plat., Pod., PULS., **Rhus,** Saba., Sabi., **Sang.,** Sele., *Sil.,* Spig., Staph., **Sul.,** Sul. ac., Thuj., Verat. v., Verb., Vio. t.

Other Remedies.—*Acon., Aesc.,* All. c., **Aloe,** Ant. cr., APIS, (Apoc. c.), ARG. N., Arn., *Ars., Arum t.,* Aur., **Bap.,** Bar. c., **Bell.,** *Berb.,* **Bry.,** Cact., CALC. C., **Cannab. i.,** Carb. v., *Caust., Cham., Chin.,* **Cimic.,** Cocc., *Con.,* Crotal., Dulc., **Gel., Glon.,** Graph., *Hep.,* Ign., **K. bi.,** *K.*

carb., Lach., Led., **Lil. t.**, Lith., **Lyc.**, **Merc.**, *Nat. c.*, *Nat. m.*, *Nit. ac.*, Nux v., Op., Petrol., **Phos.**, *Pho. ac.*, *Phyt.*, Plat., Pod., PULS., RHUS, Sabi., SANG., Sele., **Sil.**, Spig., Stan., Staph., Stram., SUL., Thuj., *Verat. a.*, **Verat. v.**, Zinc.

Antidotes.—Acon., Ant. cr., Ant. t., *Acetum veg.*, *Spir. nit. dul.*
Injurious.—Lac.

Silica.

Mind.—Apis, Bap., Bell, Calc. c., Cannab. i., Cannab. s., Cimic., Cocc., Con., Crotal., *Gel.*, Glon., Hyd. ac., Hyos., **Ign.**, Laur., Lyc., *Meli.*, Merc., Merc. c., *Nat. m.*, Nux v., *Op.*, Phos., PHO. AC., Phyt., *Pic. ac.*, Plat., **PULS.**, **Rhus**, *Sep.*, Staph., **Stram.**, *Sul.*, Verat. a., Verat. v.

Localities.—Acon., *Aesc.*, *All. c.*, *Aloe*, Am. carb., Am. m., Ant. cr., APIS, Apoc. c., ARG. N., *Arn.*, *Ars.*, *Arum t.*, Asaf., *Aur.*, *Bap.*, Bar. c., **Bell.**, Berb., *Bry.*, Cact., CALC. C., *Cannab. i.*, Canth., Carb. ac., Carb. an., *Carb. v.*, (Caul.), **Caust.**, Cham., Chel., Chin., *Cimic.*, Cina, *Cocc.*, **Con.**, (Crotal.), Cup., *Dios.*, Dros., Dulc., Eup. per., Euphr., (Fl. ac.), *Gel.*, *Glon.*, Graph., Hep., HYD. AC., (Hyper.), *Hyos.*, Ign., Ip., Iris v., K. BI., K. carb., Kalm., Kre., Lil. t., (Lith.), LYC., (Meli.), **Merc.**, Mez., Nat. c., **Nat. m.**, *Nit. ac.*, **Nux v.**, Op., *Petrol.*, **Phos.**, Phyt., (Pic. ac.), Plat., *Pod.*, *Pso.*, PULS., Rhodo., **Rhus**, Ruta, *Saba.*, Sang., *Sec. c.*, Sep., Spig., Stan., **Staph.**, Stram., SUL., Tell., (Ther.), Thuj., *Verat. a.*, *Verat. v.*, Zinc.

Sensations.—*Acon.*, *Aesc.*, Aloe, **Apis**, ARG. N., Arn., Ars., Arum t., Aur., **Bap.**, Bar. c., **Bell.**, *Berb.*, *Bry.*, Cact., CALC. C., **Cannab. i.**, Canth., (Carb. ac.), Carb. v., *Caust.*, Cham., *Chin.*, **Cimic.**, *Cocc.*, Coff., Con., Croc., (Crotal.), Cup., *Dios.*, Dulc., (Eup. per.), Fer., (Fl. ac.), GEL., Glon., Graph., Hep., Hyos., *Ign.*, Iris v., **K. bi.**, *K. carb.*, Kalm., *Lil. t.*, Lith., Lyc., (Meli.), *Merc.*, Mez., Nat. c, *Nat. m.*, Nit. ac., **Nux v.**, Petrol., *Phos.*, Pho. ac., Phyt., (Pic. ac.), *Pod.*, Pso., *Puls.*, Rhus, Sang., Sec. c., **Sep.**, *Spig.*, Spo., *Stan.*, Staph., Stro., Sul., Thuj., Valer., Verat. a., *Verat. v.*, Zinc.

Glands.—Arn., Ars., BELL., Bry., Calc. c., Carb an., Chin., Con., Hep., *Lyc.*, *Merc.*, **Phos.**, Puls., Sep., Sul.

Bones.—ASAF., Bell., **Calc. c.**, (Eup. per.), Hep., *Lyc.*, MERC., *Nit. ac.*, Phos., Pho. ac., **Puls.**, Sep., Staph., *Sul.*

Skin.—Acon., Apis, ARS., *Asaf.*, Bar. c., *Bell.*, Bry., **Calc. c.**, (Carb. ac.), Carb. an., Carb. v., *Caust.*, *Cham.*, Chin., Clem., *Con.*, Dulc., *Graph.*, HEP., Lach., Led., LYC., MERC., *Nit. ac.*, *Petrol.*, Phos., **Puls.**, **Rhus**, (Sang.), Sep., Squ., *Staph.*, SUL., Verat. a.

Sleep and Dreams.—(Apis), Arg. n., **Ars.**, (Bap.), Bell., **Bry.**, *Calc. c.*, Cannab. i., Caust., (Cimic.), *Chin.*, (Gel.), *Hep.*, Ign., *K. carb.*, Lyc., Mag. c., Merc., **Nat. m., Nux v.**, Op., **Phos.**, (Pod.), *Puls.*, Rhus, **Sep.**, SUL.

Blood, Circulation and Fever.—Acon., (Aloe), (Apis), (Arg. n.), Arn., **Ars.**, Aur., (Bap.), **Bell.**, Berb., *Bry.*, Cact., *Calc. c.*, Cannab. i., *Carb. v.*, *Cham.*, *Chin.*, Colch., (Crotal.), Cup., Gel., Glon., *Hep.*, Hyos., Ign., Iod., Ip., K. carb., Kre., (Lil. t.), *Lyc.*, *Merc.*, Nat. m., Nux m., *Nux v.*, Op., **Phos.**, Pho. ac., (Phyt.), (Pod.), *Puls.*, Rhus, Samb., *Sang.*, Sec. c., *Sep.*, Spig., Stram., *Sul.*, Verat. a., (Verat. v.).

Aggravations: Time and Circumstances.—Acon., Aesc., Aloe, Apis, *Arg. n.*, Arn., **Ars.**, Bap., Bar. c., *Bell.*, Bor., *Bry.*, (Cact.), Calad., **Calc. c.**, (Cannab. i.), Caps., Carb. v., *Caust.*, *Cham.*, Chin., Cimic., Cina, *Cocc.*, **Con.**, Fer., Gel., (Glon.), Graph., *Hep.*, Hyos., Ign., Iod., *K. bi.*, **K. carb.**, Led., Lil. t., (Lith.), **Lyc.**, Mang., *Nat. m.*, Nit. ac., **Nux m.**, NUX V., *Phos.*, Pho. ac., Phyt., Pod., *Puls, Rhodo.*, RHUS, Ruta, Saba., Samb., **Sang.**, *Sep., Spig.*, Staph., Stro., **Sul.**, Sul. ac., Verat. a., Verat. v.

Other Remedies.—Acon., Aesc., *Aloe*, APIS, ARG. N., Arn., *Ars.*, Arum t., Asaf., Aur., **Bap.**, Bar. c., **Bell.**, *Berb., Bry., Cact.*, CALC. C., **Cannab. i.**, Carb. v., *Caust.*, Cham., *Chin.*, **Cimic.**, Cocc., *Con.*, Crotal., GEL., **Glon.**, Graph., **Hep.**, Hyos., Ign., **K. bi.**, *K. carb., Lil. t.*, Lith., LYC., Merc., *Nat. m.*, Nit. ac., Nux m., *Nux v.*, Op., Petrol., **Phos.**, Pho. ac., *Phyt.*, **Pod.**, Puls., Rhus, SANG., Sec. c., **Sep.**, Spig., *Staph.*, Stram., SUL., Verat. a., **Verat. v.**

Antidotes.—Camph., *Hep.*

Spigelia.

Mind.—Acon., Anac., Ars., Bell., Bry., Calc. c., Carb. an., *Con.*, Cyc., Graph., Hell., Hyos., *Ign.*, **Lyc.**, Merc., **Nat. c.**, Nat. m., Nux m., *Op.*, Petrol., Phos., Plat., *Puls.*, RHUS, Sep., **Stram.**, *Sul.*, Thuj., Verat. a.

Localities.—Acon., Aesc., All. c., (Aloe), Anac., **Apis**, (Apoc. c.), *Arg. n.*, Arn., Ars., *Arum t.*, Aur., Bap, *Bell.*, Berb., *Bry.*, Cact., CALC. C., *Cannab. i.*, (Carb. ac.), Carb. v., (Caul.), **Caust.**, (Ced.), *Chin.*, Cimic., Con., (Crotal.), (Dios.), (Fl. ac.), *Gel.*, Glon., *Graph.*, Hep., (Hyd. ac.), Ign., (Iris v.), **K. bi.**, **K. carb.**, Kalm., Kre., Led., Lil. t., *Lyc.*, (Meli.), *Merc.*, Nat. c., *Nat. m., Nux v.*, Petrol., **Phos.**, *Pho. ac.*, Phyt., (Pic. ac.), Pod., PULS., Ran. b., Rhus, Sabi., *Sang.*, Seneg., Sep., Sil., *Squ.*, Stan., *Staph.*, SUL., Tell., Valer., Verat. a., Verat. v., *Zinc.*

Sensations.—Acon., Aesc., Aloe, (Apis), **Arg. n.**, *Arn.*, Ars., *Asaf.*, Arum t., Aur., BELL., *Berb., Bry.*, Cact., **Calc. c., Cannab. i.**, (Carb.

ac.), Carb. v., *Caust.*, Cham., *Chin.*, Cimic., Cocc., Con., (Dios.), (Eup. per.), Gel., **Glon.**, Hep., Ign., (Iris v.), **K. bi.**, *K. carb.*, (Kalm.), Lil. t., Lith., *Lyc.*, *Merc.*, Mez., *Nat. c.*, *Nat. m.*, **Nux v.**, **Phos.**, (Phyt.), *Plat.*, (Pod.), Pso., PULS, Rhodo., RHUS, *Sang.*, *Sep.*, *Sil.*, Spo., *Stan.*, Staph., Stro., SUL., *Sul. ac.*, Thuj., (Verat. v.), Zinc.

Glands.—*Arn.*, *Aur.*, Bell., Carb. an., Chin., Con., Iod., *Lyc.*, **Phos.**, *Puls.*

Bones.—Chin., *Pho. ac.*, **Puls.**

Skin.—Acon., *Arn.*, Ars., Bar. c., *Bell.*, **Bry.**, Calc. c., Caust., Chin., Con., (Crotal.), Hep., K. carb., *Lyc.*, Merc., Nat. m., Nux v., Phos., Plat., PULS., Rhus, SEP., *Sil.*, SUL.

Sleep and Dreams.—*Phos.*, Sul.

Blood, Circulation and Fever.—*Acon.*, Apis, (Arg. n.), **Ars.**, Bell., Berb., *Bry.*, *Calc. c.*, (Cannab. i.), Chem., Gel., *Hell.*, Ign., *Lyc.*, Merc., Nux m., *Nux v.*, *Phos.*, PULS., Rhus, Sang., **Sep.**, *Verat. a.*

Aggravations: Time and Circumstances.—Acon., Aesc., (Aloe), Am. m., (Apis), Arg. n., Arn., Ars., Asar., (Bap.), **Bell.**, Bor., Bry., (Cact.), CALC. C., Caps., *Carb. v.*, **Cham.**, **Chel.**, *Chin.*, (Cimic.), Cocc., Coff., **Colch.**, Con., Croc., Fer., (Gel.), Glon., Graph., *Hep.*, **Ign.**, Iod., K. bi., *K. carb.*, K. nit., *Lach.*, Led., Lil. t., (Lith.), *Lyc.*, *Mang.*, **Merc.**, Nat. c., *Nat. m.*, NUX V., *Phos.*, (Phyt.), (Pod.), PULS, Ran. b., *Rhus*, Saba., **Sang.**, *Sele.*, *Sep.*, *Sil.*, *Staph.*, *Sul.*, Valer., *Verat. a.*, *Verat. v.*

Other Remedies.—*Acon.*, Aesc., Aloe, *Apis.*, **Arg. n.**, *Arn.*, *Ars.*, Arum t., Aur., (Bap.), **Bell.**, *Berb.*, **Bry.**, Cact., **Calc. c.**, *Cannab. i.*, Carb. v., Caust., Cham., *Chin.*, Cimic., *Con.*, (Crotal.), *Gel.*, **Glon.**, Graph., Hep., *Ign.*, Iod., *K. bi.*, K. carb., Lil. t., (Lith.), **Lyc.**, *Merc.*, Nat. c., Nat. m., *Nux v.*, **Phos.**, Pho. ac., (Phyt.), Plat., Pod., PULS., **Rhus**, **Sang.**, Sep., Sil., Staph., **Sul.**, Verat. a., Verat. v.

Antidotes.—Camph., *Puls.*

Spongia.

Mind.—Alum., Anac., *Aur.*, Bell., Calc. c., Cannab. s., *Carb. an.*, Caust., Cham., *Con.*, Hyos., *Ign.*, *Lyc.*, *Merc.*, **Nat. c.**, *Op.*, *Phos.*, Pho. ac., Plat., Puls., Rhus, Sep., Sil., Spig., Staph., *Stram.*, Sul., Verat. a.

Localities.—Acon., (Aesc.), All. c., Apis, (Apoc. c.), **Arg. n.**, Arn., Ars., Arum t., (Bap.), **Bell.**, (Berb.), **Bry.**, (Cact.), **Calc. c.**, Cannab. i., (Carb. ac.), **Carb. v.**, *Caust.*, *Cham.*, Chin., Cimic., Cina., Con., (Crotal.), (Dios.), **Dros.**, Gel., (Glon.), Graph., **Hep.**, (Hyd. ac.), *Hyos.*, Ign., *Iod.*, *Ip.*, K. bi., K. carb., (Kalm.), Kre., Laur., Mang., (Meli.), **Merc.**, **Nat. c.**, **Nat. m.**, Nit. ac., Nux v., Petrol., PHOS., (Phyt.), (Pso.), **Puls.**,

Rhus, Sabi, Samb., Sang., Seneg., *Sep.*, Sil., Spig., Stan., Staph., **Sul.**, Thuj., *Verat. a.*, (Verat. v.), Zinc.

Sensations.—Acon., (Aesc.), (Aloe), Alum., *Apis*, Arg. n., Arn., Ars., Arum t., *Asaf.*, (Bap.), **Bell.**, (Berb.), *Bry.*, **Calc. c.**, Cannab. i., Cannab. s., Canth., Carb. v., Caust., Cham., Chin., Cimic., *Cocc.*, *Con.*, (Crotal.), (Dios.), Dulc., (Eup. per.), *Gel.*, *Glon.*, Graph., *Hep.*, *Ign.*, *Iod.*, (K. bi), *K. carb* , (Lil. t.), Lith., *Lyc.*, Meny., *Merc.*, Mez., Nat. c., *Nat. m.*, Nit. ac., Nux v., Phos., Phyt., *Plat.*, Puls., Rhus, Sang., **Sep.**, Sil., *Spig.*, *Stan.*, Staph., Sul., Thuj., Valer., (Verat. v.), Zinc.

Glands.—*Bell.*, *Bry.*, Calc. c., Caust., CON., Ign., Lyc., **Merc.**, *Phos.*, *Plat.*, Puls., Rhus, Sabi., Sep., Sil., Staph., Sul.

Bones.—Arg., Bell., Cup., Cyc., K. carb., Lyc., Merc., Pho. ac., Sabi., *Staph.*

Skin.—Am. m., Arn., *Bar. c.*, Bell., Bry., *Calc. c.*, **Caust.**, Chin., Cocc., Colch., Con., Cyc., Euphorb., *Graph.*, Ip., K. carb., Lach., *Led.*, Lyc., *Merc.*, Mez., Nit. ac., *Oleand* , Phos., Plat., PULS., Ran. s., Rhus, Saba., Sep., Sil., Spig., *Staph.*, **Sul.**, *Vio. t.*

Sleep and Dreams.—Hep., Lach., Phos., Sul.

Blood, Circulation and Fever.—Acon., Arg. n., **Arn.**, *Ars.*, (Bap.), **Bell.**, (Berb.), BRY., (Cact.), Calc. c., Carb. v., Chin., Glon., *Graph.*, Hyos., Ign., (Lil. t.), Lyc., Merc., *Nit. ac.*, Nux v., **Phos.**, Pho. ac., Puls., *Rhus*, Sang., *Sep.*, *Sil.*, Stan., *Stram.*, *Sul.*

Aggravations: Time and Circumstances.—*Acon.*, Am. m., Anac., Ant. cr., Apis, Arn., *Ars.*, Asaf., **Asar.**, (Bap.), Bor., **Bry.**, *Calc. c.*, Caps., *Carb. v.*, Caust., Cham., Cic., (Cimic.), Croc., (Glon.), Graph., Hell., **Hep.**, *Ign.*, **Ip.**, (K. bi.), K. carb., Lach., (Lil. t.), *Lyc.*, *Mag. c.*, *Mag. m.*, Mang., Merc., *Nat. m.*, NUX V., Phos., (Phyt.), **Puls.**, Rhus, Ruta, Saba., Sabi., (Sang.), *Sele.*, *Sep.*, Sil., Stro., Valer.

Other Remedies.—Acon., (Aesc.), *Apis*, *Arg. n.*, Arn., Ars., Arum t., Bap., **Bell.**, (Berb.), BRY., (Cact.), **Calc. c.**, Cannab. i., Carb. v., *Caust.*, Cham., Chin., Cimic., **Con.**, (Crotal.), Gel., *Glon* , Graph., *Hep.*, Hyos., **Ign.**, Iod., Ip., K. bi., K. carb., (Lil. t.), **Lyc.**, Merc., Nat. c., Nat. m., Nit. ac., **Nux v.**, PHOS., Phyt., Plat., PULS., Rhus, Sabi., *Sang.*, Sep., *Sil.*, Spig., Stan., *Staph.*, Stram., **Sul.**, (Verat. v.).

Antidote.—Camph.

Squilla.

Mind.—Acon., **Anac.**, *Ars.*, Bell., Calc. c., Con., *Ign.*, *Lyc.*, **Nat. c.**, *Nat. m.*, Nux v., *Op.*, Phos., *Pho. ac.*, Plat., **Puls.**, *Sep.*, *Sil.*, Staph., *Stram.*, **Sul.**, *Verat. a.*, Zinc.

Localities.—*Acon.*, Aesc., *All. c.*, Aloe, Apis, (Apoc. c.), Arg., *Arg. n.*, Arn., *Ars.*, Arum t., (Bap.), Bar. c., **Bell.**, *Bry.*, **Calc. c.**, Cannab. i., Canth., Caps., Carb. ac., Carb. v., Caust., *Cham.*, *Chin.*, (Crotal.), Dig., Dios., (Fl. ac.), Gel., Graph., Hep., IGN., (Iris v.), K. bi., *K. carb.*, (Kalm.), Lil. t., *Lyc.*, (Meli.), *Merc.*, Mur. ac., Nat. m., Nux v., **Phos.**, *Pho. ac.*, (Phyt.), Pb., Pod., Pso., **Puls.**, Ran. b., Rhus, Saba., *Sang.*, *Sep.*, Sil., *Spig.*, Stan., *Staph.*, Stram., *Sul.*, Verat. a., Verat. v., Zinc.

Sensations.—Acon., (Aesc.), (Aloe), (Apis), (Apoc. c.), (Arg. n.), **Ars.**, (Bap.), **Bell.**, (Berb.), *Bry.*, (Cact.), Calc. c., (Cannab. i.), *Canth.*, *Cham.*, **Chin.**, (Cimic.), Con., Fer., (Gel.), (Glon.), Hyos., **Ign.**, (K. bi.), (Lil. t.), *Merc.*, Nat. m., Nux v., Op., *Phos.*, (Phyt.), Pb., *Puls.*, Rhus, (Sang.), Sec. c., *Sep.*, **Sul.**, Verat. a., (Verat. v.).

Glands.—Ars., **Bell.**, Carb. an., *Con.*, Hep., *Lyc.*, Merc., *Phos.*, Puls., *Sil.*, **Sul.**

Bones.

Skin.—Arn., **Ars.**, Asaf., *Bell.*, **Bry.**, *Calc. c.*, *Caust.*, Chin., Dulc., Graph., Hep., Ign., K. carb., Lach., Led., *Lyc.*, **Merc.**, Nit. ac., *Phos.*, Pho. ac., *Puls.*, RHUS, Sec. c., **Sep.**, SIL, **Sul.**

Sleep and Dreams.

Blood, Circulation and Fever.—Acon., (Apis), Arn., **Ars.**, Bell., Bry., Calc. c., Cocc., Coff., (Gel.), Hell., Ign., K. carb., *Lach.*, Lyc., Merc., Nux m., *Nux v.*, Op., Phos., Pho. ac., Puls., *Rhus*, Samb., Sep., Sil., Spig., Sul.

Aggravations: Time and Circumstances.—Acon., Agn., Arn., Ars., Asar., *Bell.*, Bry., Calad., Calc. c., Cannab. s., Chin., Cic., Cocc., Colch., Con., Dig., (Glon.), Graph., **Hep.**, Iod., Ip., K. nit., Led., (Lil. t.), Lyc., Merc., Nat. m., NUX V., *Phos.*, Ran. b., Rhus, Sabi., *Samb.*, (Sang.), Sele., *Sil.*, Spig., Staph., Stro., Sul.

Other Remedies.—Acon., (Aesc.), (Aloe), Apis, (Apoc. c.), Arg. n., Arn., **Ars.**, (Bap.), **Bell.**, *Bry.*, *Calc. c.*, (Cannab. i.), Cham., *Chin.*, Con., Gel., (Glon.), Hep., *Ign.*, K. bi., K. carb., Lil. t., *Lyc.*, **Merc.**, Nat. m., *Nux v.*, Op., **Phos.**, Pho. ac., (Phyt.), *Puls.*, Rhus, Samb., Sang., *Sep.*, **Sil.**, Spig., Staph., **Sul.**, Verat. a., (Verat. v.).

Antidote.—Camph.

Stannum.

Mind.—*Acon.*, Ambr., *Anac.*, Ars., Aur., Bar. c., **Bell.**, Bry., *Calc. c.*, Caust., Cham., Chin., Cic., *Cocc.*, *Con.*, Graph., Hell., Hyos., **Ign.**, **Lyc.**, *Merc.*, Mur. ac., *Nat. c.*, Nat. m., Nux m., Nux v., *Op.*, *Phos.*, Pho. ac., Plat., **Puls.**, *Rhus*, Saba., Sec. c., *Sep.*, *Sil.*, Staph., *Stram.*, **Sul.**

Localities.—Acon., Aesc., (All. c.), Aloe, **Apis**, (Apoc. c.), *Arg. n.*,

RELATIONSHIPS.—STAN.—STAPH.   467

Arn., *Ars.*, Arum t., Bap., *Bell.*, *Bry.*, (Cact.), **Calc. c.**, (Cannab. i.), Carb. ac., Carb. v., *Caust.*, Cham., *Chin.*, Cimic., Cocc., Con., (Crotal.), Cup., (Dios.), Dros., Eup. per., Fer., Fl. ac., Gel., (Glon.), Graph., Hep., Ign., Ip., (Iris v.), **K. bi.**, *K. carb.*, *Lyc.*, *Merc.*, Nat. c., Nat. m., **Nux v.**, Petrol., PHOS., Pho. ac., Phyt., Pod., Pso., **PULS.**, Rhus, *Sang.*, Sep., Sil., *Spig.*, Spo., Staph., **Sul.**, (Sul. ac.), Thuj., *Verat. a.*, Verat. v.

Sensations.—Aesc., Aloe, Alum., *Apis*, **Arg. n.**, Arn., Ars., *Arum t.*, Asaf., (Bap.), **Bell.**, *Berb.*, *Bry.*, (Cact.), CALC. C., *Cannab. i.*, Canth., Carb. v., **Caust.**, Cham., **Chin.**, *Cimic.*, Cocc., Con., (Crotal.), Cup., Dios., Dulc., Eup. per., Fer., *Gel.*, *Glon.*, Graph., Hyos., **Ign.**, *Iod.*, Ip., Iris v., **K. bi.**, **K. carb.**, (Kalm.), Lil. t., Lith., **Lyc.**, *Merc.*, Mez., *Nat. c.*, *Nat m.*, **NUX V.**, **Phos.**, Pho. ac., *Phyt.*, Plat., Pod., Pso., PULS., *Rhus*, **Sang.**, Sep., *Sil.*, *Spig.*, Spo., Staph., *Stro.*, **Sul.**, Valer., *Verat. a.*, (Verat. v.), Zinc.

Glands.—Bell., *Calc. c.*, Merc., Phos., *Rhodo.*, Sul.

Bones.

Skin.—*Arn.*, *Bry.*, Calc. c., Chin., *Cocc.*, Cyc., Graph., Lyc., **Merc.**, Nit. ac., Nux v., Phos., *Puls.*, RHUS, Sep., *Sil.*, Staph., SUL., Sul. ac., Thuj.

Sleep and Dreams.—Ars., (Arg. n.), Bell., *Bry.*, Calc. c., Chin., *Ign.*, Lyc., Mur. ac., Nat. c., Nux v., *Phos.*, **Puls.**, *Rhus*, Saba., Sep., *Sil.*, Sul.

Blood, Circulation and Fever.—ACON., (Arg. n.), *Arn.*, **Ars.**, *Bell.*, (Berb.), Bry., *Calc. c.*, *Carb. v.*, *Cocc.*, (Crotal.), Glon., Hell., **Iod.**, *K. carb.*, *Lyc.*, **Merc.**, *Nux v.*, Op., Petrol., PHOS., **Pho. ac.**, *Puls.*, *Rhus*, Samb., Sang., Sec. c., Sep., *Sil.*, Spo., Staph., Stram., *Sul.*, Verat. a.

Aggravations: Time and Circumstances.—(Aesc.), *Anac.*, (Apis), (Arg. n.), (Bap.), Bell., **Bry.**, **Calc. c.**, Cannab. s., *Carb. v.*, Caust., Cham., *Chin.*, (Cimic.), (Gel.), (Glon.), Hep., *Ign.*, (K. bi.), *K. carb.*, (Lil. t.), Lyc., Phos., (Phyt.), (Pod.), *Puls.*, *Rhus*, Sang., Sep., Sul.

Other Remedies.—Acon., Aesc., Aloe, Anac., *Apis*, **Arg. n.**, Arn., *Ars.*, Arum t., **Bell.**, Berb., **Bry.**, (Cact.), **Calc. c.**, Cannab. i., **Carb. v.**, Caust., Cham., *Chin.*, Cimic., Cocc., Con., (Crotal.), Gel., *Glon.*, Graph., *Ign.*, Iod., *K. bi.*, *K. carb.*, (Lil. t.), **Lyc.**, *Merc.*, Nat. c., Nat. m., *Nux v.*, Op., **Phos.**, Pho. ac., Phyt., Pod., PULS., **Rhus**, **Sang.**, Sep., *Sil.*, Staph., **Sul.**, Verat. a., (Verat. v.),

Antidote.—Puls.

Staphysagria.

Mind.—Acon., *Anac.*, *Bap.*, **Bell.**, *Calc. c.*, Cham., *Chin.*, Cocc., **Con.**, Gels, Glon., Graph., *Hell.*, Hyos., IGN., LYC., *Merc.*, Merc. c., *Nat. c.*,

Nat. m., Nux v., *Op.*, Phos., **Pho. ac.**, Pic. ac., *Plat.*, PULS., Ran. b., *Rhus*, *Sep.*, SIL., **Stram.**, Sul., Thuj., Verat. a., Verat. v., Zinc.

Localities.—Acon., Aesc., All. c., Aloe, Ant. cr., *Apis*, Apoc. c., *Arg. n.*, *Arn.*, Ars., Arum t., Asaf., Aur., (Bap.), Bar. c., **Bell.**, (Berb.), Bry., CALC. C., Cannab i., *Canth.*, Carb. ac., Carb. v., **Caust.**, Cham., *Chin*, (Cimic.), Clem., Cocc., Con., Dig., Dios., Dulc., (Fl. ac.), Gel., (Glon.), Graph., Hep., *Ign.*, Iris v., **K. bi.**, *K. carb.*, (Kalm.), Kre., Lach., Lil. t., (Lith.), Lyc., **Merc.**, Mez., Nat. c., Nat. m., Nit. ac., **Nux v.**, Oleand., Petrol., *Phos*, Pho. ac., *Pod.*, Pso., **PULS.**, Rhodo., **Rhus**, *Ruta*, Saba., Sang., Sars., **Sep.**, *Sil.*, Spig., Squ., Stan., SUL., (Tell.), Thuj., Verat. a., *Zinc*.

Sensations.—Acon., (Aloe), Anac., Arg., (Arg. n.), Ars., *Asaf.*, (Bap.), **Bell.**, Berb., *Bry.*, CALC. C., (Cannab. i.), Canth., *Carb. v.*, *Caust.*, Cham., *Chin.*, Cimic., Cocc., Con., (Eup. per.), (Gel.), (Glon.), Graph., **Hell.**, *Ign.*, K. bi., **K. carb.**, (Kalm.), (Lith.), *Lyc.*, Mar., **Merc.**, *Mez.*, Mur. ac., Nat. c., Nat. m., Nit. ac., **Nux v.**, **Phos.**, (Pod.), *Plat.*, PULS., Rhodo., RHUS, Ruta, Saba., Sabi., Sang., **Sep.**, Sil., *Spig.*, Spo., **Stan.**, Stro., Sul., Sul. ac., Tar., Thuj., Valer., Verat. a., *Zinc.*

Glands.—Aur., **Bell.**, Bry., *Calc. c.*, Ign., Lyc., *Merc.*, Phos., **Puls.**, Rhus, **Spo.**, *Sul.*, Zinc.

Bones.—Arg., **Asaf.**, *Calc. c.*, Cyc., (Eup. per.), *Lyc.*, **Merc.**, *Mez.*, Nit. ac., Phos., **Pho. ac.**, Puls., Ruta, Sil., *Sul.*

Skin.—Acon., Am. m., Ant. cr., Apis, *Ars.*, Asaf., *Bar. c.*, Bell., Bov., Bry., *Calc. c.*, (Carb. ac.), Carb. v., Caust., Cham., *Clem.*, *Con.*, Dulc., Graph., Hep., K. carb., *Lach.*, Led., LYC., **Merc.**, Mez., Nat. c., Nit. ac., Nux v., *Oleand.*, *Petrol.*, Phos., Pho. ac., *Plat.*, Puls., RHUS, Saba., Sec. c., Sep., SIL., Spo., **Sul.**, Sul. ac., *Thuj.*, Vio. t.

Sleep and Dreams.—(Arg. n.), Ars., Calc. c., (Cannab. i.), *Caust.*, Chin., Graph., Ign., Nit. ac., **Nux v.**, Op., Phos., Puls., *Rhus*, Saba., *Sul.*

Blood, Circulation and Fever.—Acon., Arn., **Ars.**, Bar. c., **Bell.**, Bry., *Calc. c.*, Caust., Cham., *Chin.*, Cocc., Graph., Ign., K. carb., *Lyc.*, Merc., Nux v., Phos., Pho. ac., **Puls.**, *Rhus*, **Sep.**, *Spig.*, Squ., *Sul.*, Verat. a.

Aggravations: Time and Circumstances.—(Aesc.), (Aloe), *Apis*, Arg. n., *Arn.*, (Bap.), Bell., Bry., (Cact.), **Calc. c.**, Cannab. s., **Carb. v.**, Chel., *Chin.*, (Cimic.), Cocc., Colch., *Coloc*, Con., *Croc.*, Dig., (Gel.), (Glon.), Graph., **Hep.**, **Ign.**, **Iod.**, K. bi., Lach., (Lil. t.), *Lyc.*, Merc., *Nat. m.*, **NUX V.**, Oleand., *Phos.*, Pho. ac., Phyt., (Pod.), **PULS.**, *Ran. b.*, Saba., *Sang.*, **Sep.**, Sil., **Spig.**, *Sul.*, *Valer.*, (Verat. v.).

Other Remedies.—Acon., (Aesc.), Aloe, **Apis**, *Arg. n.*, Arn., Ars., *Asaf.*, Bap., Bar. c., *Bell.*, (Berb.), *Bry.*, **Calc. c.**, Cannab. i., *Carb. v.*, *Caust.*, Cham., *Chin.*, Cimic., Cocc., Con., Gel., Glon., *Graph.*, Hep., *Ign.*, K. bi., K. carb., Lach., (Lil. t.), (Lith.), **Lyc.**, **Merc.**, Mez., Nat. c., Nat. m., Nit. ac., *Nux v.*, Oleand., *Phos.*, *Pho. ac.*, (Pod.), Plat., **PULS.**, *Rhus*, Ruta, Saba., *Sang.*, *Sep.*, Spig., Spo., **Sul.**, Thuj., Verat. a., (Verat. v.), Zinc.

Antidote.—Camph.
Injurious.—Ran. b.

Stramonium.

Mind.—Acon., Aloe, *Anac.*, *Apis*, Ars., Aur., *Bap.*, **Bell.**, Cannab. i., Cannab. s., Cic., Cimic., Cocc., Con., Crotal., Cup., *Gel.*, *Glon.*, Hell., Hyper., **HYOS.**, Ign., K. br., Laur., **Lyc.**, *Meli.*, Merc. c., Nat. c., Nat. m., Nux v., **Op.**, Phos., *Pho. ac.*, *Pic. ac.*, *Plat.*, Puls., *Rhus*, Sep., Sil., Sul., Ther., **Verat. a.**, *Verat. v.*

Localities.—*Acon.*, (Aesc.), (All. c.), **Apis**, (Apoc. c.), **Arg. n.**, Arn., *Ars.*, Arum t., Aur., Bap., **BELL.**, *Bry.*, (Cact.), **Calc. c.**, Camph., Cannab. i., Canth., (Carb. ac.), Carb. v., *Cham.*, *Chin.*, Cic., (Cimic.), Cocc., Con., Crotal., Cup., (Dios.), (Eup. per.), (Fl. ac.), Gel., (Glon.), *Hep.*, Hyd. ac., **HYOS.**, Ign., *Ip.*, (Iris v.), *K. bi*, (Kalm.), Lach., (Lil. t.), **Lyc.**, Meli., *Merc.*, Nat. m., *Nit. ac.*, *Nux v.*, **Op.**, Phos., *Pho. ac.*, Phyt., Pod., (Pso.), **Puls.**, Rhus, Ruta, Sang., *Sec. c.*, Sep., *Sil.*, Squ., **Sul.**, *Verat. a.*, *Verat. v.*

Sensations.—*Acon.*, (Aesc.), Anac., (Apis), *Arg. n.*, Arn., *Ars.*, (Arum t.), Bap., **BELL.**, Berb., *Bry.*, (Cact.), *Calc. c.*, Cannab. i., Caust., *Cham.*, Chin., *Cic.*, *Cimic.*, Cocc., Con., (Crotal.), *Cup.*, *Gel.*, (Glon.), **HYOS.**, *Ign.*, Iod., Ip., K. bi., K. carb., (Lil. t.), *Lyc.*, *Merc.*, Nat. m., Nit. ac., *Nux v.*, **Op.**, Phos., (Phyt.), *Plat.*, (Pod.), *Puls.*, *Rhus*, (Sang.), *Sec. c.*, Sep., Sil., *Sul.*, Verat. a., (Verat. v.).

Glands.—Bell., Calc. c., Lyc., Merc., Spo., Sul.
Bones.—(Eup. per.).
Skin.—**Ars.**, Bell., Bry., Hyos., Lyc., Puls., Rhus, Sul.

Sleep and Dreams.—(Apis), *Ars.*, Bell., *Bry.*, Cannab. i., Cham., Hep., Hyos., Ign., Lyc., Merc., Op., Phos., Pho. ac., (Pod.), *Puls.*, Sil., Sul., *Verat. a.*

Blood, Circulation and Fever.—ACON., (Apis), Arg. n., Ars., (Bap.), Bell., (Berb.), BRY., Cact., Calc. c., Cannab. i., Carb. v., Cham., *Chin.*, (Cimic.), (Crotal.), *Dig.*, Fer., Gel., *Glon.*, Hyos., K. carb., (Lil. t.), Lyc., Merc., Nat. m., Nit. ac., *Nux v.*, Op., **Phos.**, *Pho. ac.*, Puls., **Rhus**, *Sang.*, Sep., Sil., Spo., Stan., *Sul.*, Verat. a., Verat. v.

470 RELATIONSHIPS.—STRAM.—STRO.

Aggravations: Time and Circumstances.—Acon., (Aesc.), Agar., Apis, (Arg. n.), **Ars.**, **Bell.**, Bry., *Calc. c.*, *Carb. v.*, Cham., Chel., Chin., Coff., Con., (Gel.), Graph., *Hep.*, Ign., (K. bi.), K. nit., Kre., Lach., *Lyc.*, Merc., Nat. c., Nux m., **NUX V.**, *Op., Phos.*, **Puls.**, Rhus, (Sang.), Sele., Sep., *Sil., Spig., Sul.*, Verat. a.

Other Remedies.—*Acon.*, (Aesc.), **Apis**, *Arg. n.*, **Ars.**, (Arum t.), *Bap.*, **BELL.**, (Berb.), **Bry.**, Cact., *Calc. c.*, **Cannab. i.**, Carb. v., *Cham.*, Chin., Cic., *Cimic.*, Con., Crotal., Cup., **Gel.**, *Glon.*, Hep., **HYOS.**, Ign. K. bi., (Lil. t.), **Lyc.**, *Merc.*, Nat. m., Nit. ac., *Nux v.*, **Op.**, *Phos.*, Pho. ac., Phyt., Plat., Pod., **Puls.**, *Rhus, Sang.*, Sec. c., Sep., *Sil.*, **Sul.**, *Verat. a., Verat. v.*

Antidotes.—*Bell.*, Hyos., *Nux v*, *Acet.*, Acet. veg., *Citri succus.*, Tab.

Strontium.

Mind.—Acon., Anac., Ars., Aur., Bar. c., Bell., Bry., **Calc. c.**, *Cham.*, Hep., *Ign.*, *Lyc.*, Merc., *Nux v.*, *Phos.*, **Puls.**, Sep., *Stram.*, **Sul.**, Verat. a.

Localities.—Acon., (Arg. n.), Arn., (Arum t.), *Bell.*, Bry., **Calc. c.**, (Caul.), **Caust.**, Cham., Chin., (Cimic.), Con., Fer., Graph., Ign., (K. bi.), K. CARB., Led., (Lith.), *Lyc.*, **Merc.**, Nat. c., *Nat. m., Nux v.*, Par., *Petrol.*, Phos., Pho. ac., **Puls.**, Rhodo., RHUS, Sabi., (Sang.), SEP., *Sil.*, Spig., Staph., **SUL.**, Sul. ac., Thuj., Verat. a., *Zinc.*

Sensations.—Acon., Alum., Am. carb., Anac., (Arg. n.), Arn., Ars., *Asaf.*, Bar. c., **BELL.**, (Berb.), *Bry.*, **Calc. c.**, **Caust.**, Cham., Chin., (Cimic.), Cocc., Con., (Dios.), *Graph.*, Hep., Hyos., *Ign.*, (K. bi.), **K. carb.**, *Lyc.*, **Merc.**, Mez., Nat. c., *Nat. m.*, Nit. ac., **Nux v.**, Par., *Phos.*, Pho. ac., *Plat.*, **Puls.**, Rhus, Sabi., (Sang.), Sars., Sep., *Sil., Spig., Stan.*, Staph., **Sul.**, Sul. ac., Thuj., *Zinc.*

Glands.—Bar. c., Bry., Caust., Con., Graph., K. carb., **Phos.**, **Puls.**, Rhus, Spo., **Sul.**

Bones.—Bell., Chin., Dros., K. carb., Merc., *Ruta.*

Skin.—Arn., (Bap.), Bar. c., CAUST., *Con.*, K. carb., Lach., Led., Merc., Nux v., *Phos.*, Plat., **Puls.**, *Rhus*, Sep., Sil., *Sul.*

Sleep and Dreams.—Calc. c., *Hep.*, K. carb., *Phos.*, Puls., Sep., Sul.

Blood, Circulation and Fever.—Acon., *Ars.*, *Bell.*, Bry., Calc. c., Colch., *Hep.*, K. carb., *Merc.*, Nux v., Phos., Rhus, Samb., Sep., Sil., Squ., Sul.

Aggravations: Time and Circumstances.—(Aesc.), (All. c.), Am. carb., (Apis), (Arg. n.), *Ars., Aur.*, (Bap.), Bell., *Calc. c.*, Caps., Caust., **Cham.**, Clem., Colch., Con., *Dulc.*, (Glon.), **Hep.**, Hyos., (K. bi.), K.

carb., (Lil. t.), (Lith.), *Lyc.*, Mang., Merc., Mos., *Nux m.*, *Nux v.*, (Phyt.) Plat., Puls., RHUS, *Saba.*, *Samb.*, Sang., *Sep.*, *Sil.*, Squ., Sul., Verat. a.

Other Remedies.—Acon., (Arg. n.), Ars., (Bap.), Bar. c., *Bell.*, *Bry.*, **Calc. c.**, **Caust.**, Cham., (Cimic.), *Con.*, Graph., *Hep.*, Ign., (K. bi.), **K. carb.**, (Lith.), *Lyc.*, **Merc.**, Nat. m., **Nux v.**, **Phos.**, Plat., PULS., RHUS, Sang., Sep., *Sil.*, SUL., Zinc.

Antidote.—Camph.

Sulphur.

Mind.—Acon., *Aloe*, Anac., *Apis*, Ars., *Aur.*, *Bap.*, BELL., **Bry.**, **Calc. c.**, *Cannab. i.*, Caust., Cham., Cic., Cimic., Cocc., Con., Crotal., Gel., *Glon.*, Graph., Hell., *Hyos.*, **Ign.**, LYC., *Meli.*, Merc., Merc. c., Nat. c., *Nat. m.*, *Nux v.*, Op., Petrol., *Phos.*, *Pho. ac.*, Phyt., Pic. ac., Plat., Pso., **Puls.**, Rhus, Saba., *Sep.*, *Sil.*, Staph., Stram., Ther., Thuj., *Verat. a.*

Localities.—Acon., AESC., *All. c.*, ALOE, Am. carb., APIS, *Apoc. c.*, ARG. N., Arn., **Ars.**, Arum t., BAP., Bar. c., **Bell.**, Berb., Bor., *Bry.*, *Cact.*, CALC. C., CANNAB. I., Cannab. s., Canth., *Carb. ac.*, Carb. v., Caul., **Caust.**, Cham., *Chin.*, **Cimic.**, Cina, Cocc., Con., *Crotal.*, Cup, Dig., *Dios.*, Dulc., Eup. per., Euphorb., Euphr., Fer., *Fl. ac.*, GEL. *Glon.*, *Graph.*, Hep., (Hyd. ac.), Hyos., (Hyper.), Ign., Ip., *Iris v.*, K. BI, *K. carb.*, (Kalm.), Kre., Led., Lil. t., (Lith.), **Lyc.**, (Meli.), *Merc.*, Nat. c., *Nat. m.*, Nit. ac., **Nux v.**, Petrol., PHOS., Pho. ac., *Phyt.*, (Pic. ac.), Pb., POD., Pso., PULS., Rhus, Ruta, Saba., Sabi., SANG., Sec. c., SEP. Sil., *Spig.*, *Stan.*, *Staph.*, Stram., (Tell.), Thuj., Valer., *Verat. a.*, Verat. v., Zinc.

Sensations.—Acon., **Aesc.**, *Aloe*, Ambr., Am. carb., Anac., Ant. cr., Apis, (Apoc. c.). ARG. N., *Arn.*, **Ars.**, *Arum t.*, *Asaf.*, **Bap.**, Bar. c., BELL., **Berb.**, **Bry.**, *Cact.*, CALC. C., **Cannab. i.**, Cannab. s., Canth., Caps., Carb. ac., *Carb. v.*, (Caul.), **Caust.**, *Cham.*, **Chin.**, Cic., **Cimic.**, *Cocc.*, Colch., *Con.*, Croc., Crotal., Cup., *Dios.*, Dulc., Eup. per., *Fer.*, (Fl. ac.), GEL., GLON., *Graph.*, *Hep.*, Hyos., *Ign.*, Iod., Ip., Iris v., K. BI., **K. carb.**, Kalm., **Lil. t.**, *Lith.*, LYC., Meli., MERC., Nat. c., **Nat. m.**, *Nit. ac.*, Nux m., **Nux v.**, Op., Petrol., **Phos.**, Pho. ac., **Phyt.**, *Plat.*, Pb., Pod., *Pso.*, PULS., Rhodo., RHUS, Saba., SANG., Sec. c, SEP., *Sil.*, *Spig.*, Spo., *Stan.*, Staph., Stram., Stro., Tar., Thuj., *Verat. a*, *Verat. a.*, Verat. v., *Zinc.*

Glands.—Arum t., BELL., *Bry.*, Calc. c., *Con.*, Hep., Lyc., MERC., Phos., Puls., Rhus, Sil., Spo.

Bones.—Asaf., **Calc. c.**, (Cimic.), (Eup. per.), Lyc., *Merc.*, Nit. ac., Phos., Pho. ac., **Puls.**, Rhus, *Sil.*, Staph.

Skin.—Acon., Am. carb., Ant. cr., **Apis**, Arn., **Ars.**, Asaf., Bar. c., *Bell.*, *Bry.*, CALC. C., (Carb. ac.), Carb. v., *Caust.*, Cham., Chin., (Cimic.), Colch., *Con.*, Crotal., Cyc., *Dulc.*, (Eup. per.), Fer., *Graph.*, Hell., Hep., (Hyd. ac.), K. bi., *K. carb.*, Kre., *Lach.*, Led., LYC., MERC., Nat. c., Nat. m., *Nit. ac.*, Petrol., *Phos.*, Pho. ac., (Phyt.), Plat., **Puls.**, Rhus, Saba., (Sang.), Sec. c., SEP., **Sil.**, Spig., Spo., Squ., Staph., Verat. a.

Sleep and Dreams.—(Aloe), Apis, *Arg. n.*, **Ars.**, Bap., *Bell.*, **Bry.**, Calc. c., *Cannab. i.*, Carb. v., Cham., *Chin.*, (Cimic.), Con., Gel., Graph., Hep., Ign., K. carb., (Lil. t.), *Lyc.*, Merc., Nat. m., *Nux v.*, Op., PHOS., Pod., PULS., Rhus, **Sep.**, Sil.

Blood, Circulation and Fever.—Acon., Aloe, Ambr., Apis, Arg. n., Arn., **Ars.**, (Bap.), BELL., Berb., BRY., Cact., **Calc. c.**, Cannab. i., Caps., Carb. v., Caust., *Cham.*, *Chin.*, Cocc., (Crotal.), Dig., Fer., Gel., *Glon.*, **Hep.**, Hyos., Ign., Iod., Ip., K. carb., (Lil. t.), *Lyc.*, **Merc.**, Nat. m., Nit. ac., **Nux v.**, Op., Petrol., **Phos.**, *Pho. ac.*, (Phyt.), Pod., **Puls.**, RHUS, Samb., *Sang.*, Sec. c., SEP., Sil., Spig., Stan., Stram., Thuj., *Verat. a.*, (Verat. v.).

Aggravations: Time and Circumstances.—Acon., Aesc., (All. c.), (Aloe), Ambr., Am. carb, Am. m., **Ant. cr.**, **Apis**, *Arg n.*, Arn., **Ars.**, Bap., Bar. c., *Bell.*, BRY., (Cact.), CALC. C., (Cannab. i.), Cannab s., Caps., *Carb. v.*, Caust., *Cham.*, *Chin.*, (Cimic.), Cocc., Colch., *Con.*, Cup., Dros., (Gel.), Glon., *Graph.*, Hep., *Ign.*, K. bi., *K. carb.*, Led., Lil. t., (Lith.), **Lyc.**, Mang., *Merc.*, Nat. c., *Nat. m.*, *Nit. ac.*, Nux v., Op., *Phos.*, Pho. ac., Phyt., Pb., *Pod.*, **Puls.**, Rhus, Ruta, Sabi., SANG., SEP., *Sil.*, *Spig.*, Staph., Stram., Thuj., *Verat. a.*, (Verat. v).

Other Remedies.—*Acon.*, Aesc., All. c., ALOE, Ant. cr., APIS, Apoc. c., ARG. N., Arn., **Ars.**, *Arum t.*, Asaf., *Bap.*, Bell., *Berb.*, Bry., *Cact.*, CALC. C., CANNAB. I., Carb. v., *Caust*, Cham., *Chin.*, Cimic., Cocc., *Con.*, Crotal., Fer., GEL., Glon., *Graph.*, Hep., Hyos., *Ign.*, K. BI., *K. carb.*, Lil. t., Lith., LYC., **Merc.**, Nat. c., *Nat. m.*, *Nit. ac.*, Nux v., Op., Petrol., **Phos.**, Pho. ac., **Phyt.**, Pod., PULS., RHUS., SANG., Sec. c., Sep., Sil., Spig., Staph., Stram., Verat. a., Verat. v.

Antidotes.—Acon., Camph., Cham., *Chin.*, Merc., Puls., Rhus, Sep.

Sulphuricum Acidum

Mind.—*Alum.*, Anac., *Aur.*, Bar. c., **Bell.**, Carb. an., *Caust.*, Cic., Con., Fer., *Graph.*, Hell., *Hyos.*, Ign., LYC., Merc., Nat. c., Phos., *Plat.*, **Puls.**, Sep., Sul., *Zinc.*

Localities.—(Aesc.), (Aloe), Alum., Am. carb., Am. m., Apis, (Apoc. c.), Arg. n., (Arum t.), Aur., *Bap.*, Bell., (Berb.), Bry., (Cact.), CALC.

C., (Carb. ac.), *Carb. v., Caust., Cham.,* **Chin.,** (Cimic.), Cocc., Con., Dios., (Fl. ac.), (Gel.), *Graph., Ign.,* Ip., Iris v., *K. bi.,* **K. carb.,** Kre., *Lyc.,* Mag. m., *Merc.,* Nat. c., **Nat. m.,** *Nit. ac.,* **Nux v.,** Petrol., **Phos.,** Pho. ac., (Phyt.), *Plat.,* Pb., *Pod.,* Pso., **Puls., Rhus,** Sang., **Sep.,** *Sil., Spig., Stan.,* Staph., **Sul.,** *Thuj., Verat. a.,* Verb., *Zinc.*

Sensations.—Acon., Aesc., *Alum., Anac.,* Apis, Arg., (Arg. n.), *Arn.,* (Arum t.), Asaf., Asar., Bap., *Bell.,* Bry., (Cact.), *Calc. c.,* Canth., Carb. v., *Caust.,* Chin., Cic., Cimic., *Cocc.,* (Crotal.), Dros., (Eup. per.), (Gel.), *Graph., Ign., K. carb.,* Laur., *Lyc.,* Merc., Mez., Mos., *Nat. m.,* Nit. ac., *Nux m.,* **Nux v.,** Oleand., **Phos.,** Pho. ac., (Phyt.), PLAT., (Pod.), **Puls., Rhus,** Ruta, *Saba.,* Sabi., Sang., Sars., **Sep.,** Sil., *Spig., Stan.,* Staph., Sul., Verat. a., (Verat. v.), *Zinc.*

Glands.—Arn., Ars., *Aur., Bell.,* Carb. an., **Con.,** Hep., Ign., Iod., Lach., Lyc., Nux v., *Phos.,* Puls., **Sep.,** Sul.

Bones.

Skin.—Am. m., ARN., *Ars.,* Bell., **Bry.,** *Calc. c.,* Carb. v., *Chin.,* Cic., *Con.,* Cyc., *Graph.,* Hep., Ign., K. carb., *Lach.,* Lyc., *Merc.,* Mez., Nit. ac., Nux v., Petrol., *Phos.,* Pho. ac., **Puls., Rhus,** Ruta, Sec. c., *Sep., Sil.,* Staph., SUL., Thuj.

Sleep and Dreams.—(Apis), Ars., (Cannab. i.), Graph., K. carb., *Mag. c., Nat. c.,* Nux v., Phos., (Pod.), *Sep.,* Sil.

Blood, Circulation and Fever.—Acon., Bell., Calc. c., Cham., Chin., K. carb., *Merc.,* Phos., Rhus., Sep., Sul., *Verat. a.*

Aggravations : Time and Circumstances.—*Am. carb.,* (Apis), **Arn.,** Ars., *Bell.,* **Bry.,** Calc. c., Camph., Cannab. s., *Carb. v., Cham.,* Chel., Chin., *Cocc.,* CON., Dulc., Graph., *Hep.,* K. carb., Lach., Led., (Lil. t.), *Lyc.,* Mang., Merc., Nat. c., *Nat. m.,* Nit. ac., Nux m., **Nux v.,** *Phos.,* (Phyt.), (Pod.), Puls., **Rhus,** Ruta, Saba., (Sang.), Sele., *Sep.,* Sil., *Spig.,* Stro., Sul.

Other Remedies.—Alum., (Aesc.), Apis, (Arg. n.), *Arn.,* Ars., (Arum t.), Aur., Bap., *Bell.,* **Bry.,** (Cact.,), *Calc. c.,* Carb. an., Carb. v., Caust., Cham., Chin., (Cimic.), Cocc., *Con.,* (Gel.), *Graph.,* Hep., *Ign., K. carb.,* Lach., Lyc., *Merc.,* Nat. c., Nat. m., Nit. ac., **Nux v., Phos.,** (Phyt.), Plat., Pod., **Puls., Rhus,** Sang., SEP., *Sil.,* Spig., Stan., Staph., Sul., Verat. a., Zinc.

Antidote.—Puls.

Taraxacum.

Mind.—Aur., *Bell.,* Cannab. s., Carb. an., Cic., Croc., Cup., *Hyos.,* Ign., Nat. c., **Op.,** Phos., Spo., *Stram.,* Verat. a., Zinc.

474 RELATIONSHIPS.—TAR.—THUJ.

Localities.—(Aloe), (Apis), (Arg. n.), *Arn.*, Arum t., Asaf., (Bap.), *Bell.*, Bry., (Cact.), *Calc. c.*, (Cannab. i.), Carb. v., **Caust.**, Cham., CHIN., Cocc., Cup., Cyc., (Gel.), Graph., Hep., *Ign.*, K. bi., *K. carb.*, Led., (Lil. t.), **Lyc.**, (Meli.), **Merc.**, Mur. ac., *Nat. c.*, Nat. m., Nit. ac., **Nux v.**, Petrol., **Phos.**, Pho. ac., Phyt., **Puls.**, Rhodo., *Rhus*, Sabi., *Sep.*, Sil., *Spig.*, Stan., *Staph.*, SUL., Thuj., Verat. a., Verat. v., *Zinc.*

Sensations.—Acon., *Alum.*, Arg., (Arg. n.), *Arn.*, Ars., (Arum t.), ASAF., Asar., BELL., (Berb.), *Bry.*, **Calc. c.**, (Cannab. i.), Carb. v., Caust., *Chin.*, (Cimic.), Cocc., Con., (Glon.), Hell., *Ign.*, K. bi., **K. carb.**, (Kalm.) (Lil. t.), (Lith.), **Lyc.**, **Merc.**, Mez., *Nat. c.*, *Nat. m.*, Nit. ac., **Nux v.**, Oleand., *Phos.*, Plat., (Pod.), **Puls.**, **Rhus**, Saba., (Sang.), *Sep.*, *Sil.*, Spig., *Spo.*, *Stan.*, *Staph.*, Sul., *Thuj.*, Zinc.

Glands.

Bones.

Skin.—Bar. c., **Bry.**, *Caust.*, *Cyc.*, *Graph.* LYC., Merc., Oleand., *Puls.*, RHUS, Saba., Sep., Sil., *Spo.*, STAPH., *Sul.*, Vio. t.

Sleep and Dreams.—Ign., Lyc., Nux v., Phos., Rhus, Sil., Sul.

Blood, Circulation and Fever.—(Apis), Ars., Caps., *Cham.*, (Gel.), Nux v., Op., Rhus, (Sang.), *Sep.*

Aggravations: Time and Circumstances.—(Aloe), (Apis), (Apoc. c.), (Arg. n.), Ars., *Aur.*, (Bap.), Bry., *Caps.*, Carb. v., Cham., Con., **Cyc.**, Dros., *Dulc.*, *Euphorb.*, **Fer.**, (Gel.), Ign., K. bi., *K. carb.*, Lach., *Lyc.*, *Mag. m.*, Meny., *Nux v.*, Phos., Pho. ac., *Plat.*, (Pod.), PULS., Rhodo., Rhus, *Saba.*, *Samb.*, (Sang.), Sep., Sul., *Valer.*, Verb., Vio. t.

Other Remedies.—(Aloe), (Apis), (Arg. n.), Arn., (Arum t.), Asaf., (Bap.), *Bell.*, *Bry.*, Calc. c., (Cannab. i.), Caust., Cham., Chin., Cyc., (Gel.), *Ign.*, K. carb., K. bi., (Lil. t.), **Lyc.**, Merc., Nat. c., **Nux v.**, Op., *Phos.*, (Pod.), **Puls.**, RHUS, Saba., (Sang.), **Sep.**, Sil., Spig., Spo., *Staph.*, Sul., Zinc.

Antidote.—Camph.

Thuja.

Mind.—Acon., Anac., Ars., Aur., Bap., Bar c., *Calc. c.*, Caust., *Cham.*, Cimic., *Cocc.*, *Con.*, Crotal., Gel., Glon., *Graph.*, Hell., IGN., LYC., Merc., Merc. c., **Nat. c.**, *Nux v.*, Op., Phos., Pho. ac., Pic. ac., Plat., PULS., *Rhus*, **Sep.**, *Sil.*, Staph., *Stram.*, *Sul.*, Verat. a.

Localities.—(Aesc.), (All. c.), Aloe, Am. m., Apis, Apoc. c., *Arg. n.*, *Arn.*, Ars., Arum t., *Aur.*, Bap., Bar. c., Bell., Berb., Bry., (Cact.), *Calc. c.*, *Cannab. i.*, *Cannab. s.*, **Canth.**, Carb. ac., Carb. v., **Caust.**, *Chin.*, Cimic., *Clem.*, Cocc., (Crotal.), Cyc., Dios., Fl. ac., Gel., Glon., Graph.,

RELATIONSHIPS.—THUJ.

Hep., *Ign.*, **K.** bi., **K.** CARB., (Kalm.), *Kre.*, Led., *Lil. t.*, (Lith.), *Lyc.*, MERC., Mez., *Nat. c.*, **Nat. m.**, **Nit. ac.**, *Nux v.*, Par., *Phos.*, **Pho. ac.**, Phyt., Pic. ac., Plat., Pod., Pso., **Puls.**, *Rhus*, Sabi., Sang., **Sep.**, *Sil.*, Spig., *Staph.*, **Sul.**, Zinc.

Sensations.—Acon., Aesc., Aloe, Alum., Apis, **Arg. n.**, *Arn.*, Ars., Arum t., **Asaf.**, (Bap.), Bar. c., **Bell.**, Berb., *Bry.*, Cact., CALC. C., *Cannab. i.*, Carb. an., *Caust.*, *Chel.*, Cimic., *Cocc.*, Coloc., Con., Croc., (Crotal.), Dros., (Eup. per.), Fer., Gel., Glon., *Gráph.*, Hell., Hep., *Ign.*, (Iris v.), *K. bi.*, **K. carb.**, (Kalm.), (Lil. t.), (Lith.), Lyc., Meny., MERC., Mez., Mur. ac., Nat. c., *Nat. m.*, Nit. ac., *Nux v.*, Par., Petrol., **Phos.**, Pho. ac., *Phyt.*, Plat., (Pso.), **Puls.**, **Rhus**, Ruta, Saba., Sabi., *Sang.*, Sars., **Sep.**, Sil., **Spig.** *Spo.*, Stan., **Staph.**, Stro., **Sul.**, Tar., Verat. a., (Verat. v.), Zinc.

Glands.—Ars., (Arum t.), *Bell.*, Bry., Calc. c., *Carb. an.*, Clem., *Con.*, Hep., *K. carb.*, Lach., Lyc. Merc., Phos., Puls., Rhus, *Sil.*, Spo., **Sul.**

Bones.—Ars., Asaf., Bell., K. carb., **Merc.**, Pho. ac., *Rhus*, Ruta, Sabi., Sil., *Staph.*, *Sul.*

Skin.—Acon., Ant. cr., Apis, Arn., *Ars.*, Asaf., *Bell.*, Bry., *Calc. c.*, Carb. an., Carb. v., Caust., Chin., Con., Cyc., Dulc., Graph., *Hep.*, Hyos., K. carb., Lach., **Lyc.**, Merc., Mez., Mur. ac., Nat. c., Nat. m., *Nit. ac.*, Petrol., *Phos.*, Pho. ac., **Puls.**, **Rhus**, **Sep.**, SIL., **Staph.**, SUL.

Sleep and Dreams.—(Aloe), Apis, Arg. n., Ars., (Bap.), Bry., Cannab. i., Chin., Graph., Ign., K. carb., **Nux v.**, *Phos.*, Pod., Puls., Sul.

Blood, Circulation and Fever.—Acon., Ambr., (Apis), (Arg. n.), Ars., Bell., Bry., **Calc. c.**, (Cannab. i.), Caust., Cham., Chin., Fer., (Gel.), (Glon.), Graph., Hep., Iod., Ip., K. carb., **Lyc.**, *Merc.*, Nit ac., **Nux v.**, Op., **Phos.**, *Puls.*, **Rhus**, Sang., Sele., **Sep.**, Spig., *Sul.*, **Verat. a.**

Aggravations: Time and Circumstances.—Acon., (Aesc.), (Aloe), Alum., Am. carb., Apis, (Arg. n.), Ars., Asaf., (Bap.), Bar. c., Bell., **Bry.**, *Calc. c.*, Canth., Caps., *Carb. v.*, *Cham.*, Chin., (Cimic.), Cocc., Con., Cyc., Dros., Fer., (Gel.), Graph., **Hep.**, K. bi., K. carb., *K. nit.*, Mang., Merc., Nat. c., Nat. m., Nit. ac., *Nux v.*, Oleand., *Phos.*, Pho. ac., (Phyt.), **Puls.**, Rhus, *Ruta*, Sang., **Sep.**, Sil., **Sul.**, Verat. a., (Verat. v.).

Other Remedies.—Acon., Aesc., Aloe, **Apis**, **Arg. n.**, Arn., *Ars.*, Arum t., Asaf., *Bap.*, Bar. c., *Bell.*, Berb., *Bry.*, (Cact.), **Calc. c.**, *Cannab. i.*, Canth., Carb. an., Carb. v., Caust., Cham., Chin., *Cimic.*, Cocc., Con., Crotal., Dros., *Gel.*, *Glon.*, Graph., Hep., Ign., *K. bi.*, *K. carb.*, Lil. t., (Lith.), *Lyc.*, MERC., Nat. c., Nat. m., Nit. ac., *Nux v.*, **Phos.**, Pho. ac., Phyt., Pod., **Puls.**, Rhus, Ruta, *Sang.*, **Sep.**, **Sil.**, Spig., *Staph.*, SUL., Verat. a., (Verat. v.), Zinc.

Antidotes.—Camph., *Merc.*, Puls., Sul.

Valeriana.

Mind.—Acon., Aur., **Bell.**, Bry., Calc. c., Cic., *Coff.*, Fer., **Hyos.**, *Ign.* Lach., *Lyc.*, Nat. m., Nux v., **Op.**, PHOS., Pho. ac., Plat., *Puls.*, Rhus, **Stram.**, *Sul.*, **Verat. a.**, *Zinc.*

Localities.—(Aesc.), (Aloe), Ant. cr., (Apis), Arg. n., Arn., Ars., (Bap.), Bell., (Berb.), Bry., (Cact.), *Calc. c.*, (Carb. ac.), Carb. v., Caust., *Chin.*, (Ctmic.), Cocc., Con., (Dios.), Dulc., (Fl. ac.), (Gel.), (Glon.), Graph., Ign., (Iris v.), K. bi., K. carb., (Lil. t.), Lyc., (Meli.), Merc., *Nat. m.*, Nit. ac., Nux v., Petrol., *Phos.*, Pho. ac., Plat., (Pso.), PULS., Rhus, Sang., *Sep.*, Sil., Spig., Stan., **Staph.**, *Sul.*, (Verat. v.).

Sensations.—Acon., Aloe, Anac., Apis, (Arg. n.), Arn., Ars., (Arum t.), *Asaf.*, Asar., Aur., **Bell.**, (Berb.), Bry., *Calc. c.*, (Cannab. i.), Caust., Chin., Cimic., Cocc., *Con.*, (Eup. per.), Fer., (Gel.), Glon., **Ign.**, (K. bi.), K. carb., (Lil. t.), (Lith.), *Lyc.*, Merc., *Mos.*, Nat. c., Nit. ac., Nux m., **Nux v.**, Petrol., *Phos.*, Pho. ac., *Phyt.*, **Plat.**, **Puls.**, *Rhus*, (Sang.). *Sep*, *Sil.*, *Spig.*, Spo., *Stan.*, Staph., *Sul.*

Glands.

Bones.—Bell., Calc. c., Chin., (Cimic.), Merc., **Puls.**, *Ruta.*

Skin.—*Bry.*, **Calc. c.**, *Cic.*, Nat. m., Petrol., Phos., Pho. ac., Plat., *Puls.*, Rhus, Sep., *Sul.*, Verat. a.

Sleep and Dreams.—Ars., Bell., Calc. c., Carb. v., *Graph.*, Puls., Rhus, Sep., Sul.

Blood, Circulation and Fever.—Acon., *Bell.*, Bry., (Cact.), *Cham.*, Hep., Merc., Phos., *Rhus*, (Sang.), Sep., Sul.

Aggravations: Time and Circumstances.—(Aesc.), *Agar.*, (Aloe), *Am. m.*, (Apis), Arg., Arg. n., Ars., *Aur.*, Bap., Bar. c., Bry., *Calc. c.*, **Caps.**, Carb. an., *Carb. v.*, *Cham.*, Chel., (Cimic.), **Con.**, *Cyc.*, Dros., *Dulc.*, *Euphorb.*, Euphr., Fer., (Glon.), Guai., K. bi., Lach., *Laur.*, (Lil. t.), Lyc., Mag. m., Mar., Meny., Mos., *Pho. ac.*, (Phyt.), *Plat.*, (Pod.), PULS., Rhodo., **Rhus**, Ruta, **Saba.**, Samb., Sang., Sele., *Sep.*, *Sil.*, Spig., Spo., **Staph.**, *Tar.*, Verb., Vio. t.

Other Remedies.—(Aesc.), Aloe, Apis, Arg. n., Ars., Aur., (Bap.), *Bell.*, (Berb.), Bry., (Cact.), **Calc. c.**, Carb. v., Cham., Chin., Cimic., Con., Fer., (Gel.), Glon., Ign., K. bi., (Lil. t.), *Lyc.*, Merc., Nat. m., Nux v., **Phos.**, Pho. ac., Phyt., *Plat.*, PULS., Rhus, Sang., **Sep.**, *Sil.*, Spig., Staph., Sul., Verat. a.

Antidotes.—Camph., *Coff.*, Puls.

Veratrum Album.

Mind.—*Acon.*, Aloe, Anac., Apis, Arn., Ars., Aur., Bap., **Bell.**, *Bry.*, Calc. c., *Cannab. i.*, Cannab. s., Cham., Cic., Cimic., Cocc., Con., Crotal.,

RELATIONSHIPS.—VERAT. A.

Cup., Gel., Glon., Hyd. ac., Hyper., **Hyos.**, Ign., Lach., Laur., **Lyc.**, *Meli.*, *Nat. m.*, **Nux v.**, **Op.**, *Phos.*, *Pho. ac.*, *Phyt.*, Plat., **Puls.**, *Rhus*, *Sep.*, Sil., STRAM., Sul., Verat. v.

Localities.—*Acon.*, *Aesc.*, All. c., *Aloe*, Ant. cr., APIS, Apoc. c., ARG. N., Arn., *Ars.*, Arum t., Aur., *Bap.*, **Bell.**, Berb., **Bry.**, Cact., *Calc. c.*, Cannab. i., Canth., Carb. ac., Carb. v., Caust., *Cham.*, *Chin.*, Cimic., *Cocc.*, Con., Crotal., *Cup.*, Dig., Dios., Eup. per., Fl. ac., *Gel.*, Glon., Graph., Hep., (Hyd. ac.), Hyos., **Ign.**, *Ip.*, Iris v., K. BI., K. carb., Kalm., Lil. t., (Lith.), **Lyc.**, Meli., *Merc.*, Nat. m., **Nux v.**, Op., **Phos.**, Pho. ac., *Phyt.*, Plat., **Pod.**, *Pso.*, PULS., *Rhus*, Saba., *Sang.*, Sec. c., **Sep.**, *Sil.*, Spig., Squ., Stan., Staph., Stram., **Sul**, Sul. ac., (Ther.), *Verat. v.*, Zinc.

Sensations.—*Acon.*, Aesc., *Apis*, (Apoc. c.), **Arg. n.**, Arn., *Ars.*, Arum t., *Asar.*, Bap., **Bell.**, Berb., *Bry.*, (Cact.), *Calc. c.*, Cannab. i., Cannab. s., Canth., *Caust.*, *Cham.*, **Chin.**, Cic., Cimic., **Cocc.**, (Crotal.), *Cup.*, Dig., (Dios.), Dulc., (Eup. per.), Fer., **Gel.**, Glon., Graph., Hyos., *Ign.*, Iod., *Ip.*, K. bi., *K. carb.*, (Kalm.), Lil. t., *Lyc.*, **Merc.**, Mos., Nat. c., *Nat. m.*, Nit. ac., Nux m., NUX V., Op., Petrol., **Phos.**, Pho. ac., *Phyt.*, Plat., Pb., Pod., (Pso.), **Puls.**, *Rhus*, *Ruta*, Saba., *Sang.*, *Sec. c.*, **Sep.**, *Sil.*, Spig., *Stan.*, *Staph.*, Stram., **Sul.**, Verat. v.

Glands.—BELL., *Bry.*, **Calc. c.**, Carb. an., *Con.*, *Lyc.*, **Merc.**, *Phos.*, **Puls.**, Spo., **Sul.**

Bones.—Arg., Asaf., Bell., Calc. c., *Cocc.*, *Cup.*, Cyc., *Lyc.*, *Merc.*, Nit. ac., **Phos.**, Pho. ac., *Puls.*, Ruta, Sabi., *Sil.*, **Staph.**, Sul.

Skin.—Ant. cr., Apis, *Ars.*, (Bap.), Bar. c., *Bell.*, *Bry.*, **Calc. c.**, Caust., *Chin.*, (Crotal.), Cup., Dig., Dulc., Hep., (Hyd. ac.), Ip., *Lach.*, Led., *Lyc.*, Mag. c., **Merc.**, Mez., Nat. m., Petrol., *Phos.*, Pho. ac., Plat., **Puls.**, Rhus, Sec. c., SEP., *Sil.*, Staph., *Sul.*

Sleep and Dreams.—Ant. t., (Apis), Ars., *Bell.*, Bry., Calc. c., Cannab. i., Caust., *Con.*, *Croc.*, Nat. c., *Nux m.*, Nux v., Op., **Phos.**, *Pho. ac.*, (Pod.), *Puls.*, Sep., Sul.

Blood, Circulation and Fever.—ACON., (Apis), (Arg. n.), **Ars.**, *Bell.*, Berb., **Bry.**, Cact., *Calc. c.*, Camph., Cannab. i., *Carb. v.*, Caust., CHAM., Chin., Cina, *Cup.*, Gel., (Glon.), *Hep.*, Ign., Iod., *Ip.*, *Laur.*, *Lyc.*, **Merc.**, *Nux v.*, Op., *Phos.*, Pho. ac., (Phyt.), Plat., (Pod.), *Puls.*, RHUS, Saba., *Sang.*, Sep., *Spig.*, Stram., *Sul.*, Verat. v.

Aggravations: Time and Circumstances.—*Acon.*, (Aesc.), (Aloe), Am. carb., Anac., Ant. cr., Ant. t., Apis, Arg. n., Arn., *Ars.*, (Bap.), Bell., Bor., *Bry.*, **Calc. c.**, Caps., *Carb. v.*, *Cham.*, *Chin.*, (Cimic.), Cocc., Coloc., *Con.*, Cup., Dros., Euphorb., *Fer.*, (Glon.), Graph., Hep., Ign., Iod., Ip., K. bi., Lach., Led., (Lil. t.), (Lith.); **Lyc.**, Mang., *Merc.*, *Nat. m.*, Nit.

ac., *Nux v.*, *Phos.*, Pho. ac., (Phyt.), Pod., **PULS.**, Rhodo., **Rhus**, Sang., Sep., Sil., *Spig.*, Staph., Stram., Stro., SUL., Thuj., (Verat. v.).

Other Remedies.—*Acon.*, Aesc., (Aloe), APIS, (Apoc. c.), **Arg. n.**, Arn., *Ars.*, Arum t., *Bap.*, **Bell.**, Berb., **Bry.**, Cact., **Calc. c.**, Cannab. i., Carb. v., Caust., *Cham.*, *Chin.*, Cimic., Cocc., Con., Crotal., *Cup.*, Gel., *Glon.*, Hep., Hyos., Ign., Ip., *K. bi.*, Lil. t., (Lith.), **Lyc.**, Merc., Nat. m., **Nux v.**, *Op.*, Phos., *Pho. ac.*, *Phyt.*, Plat., Pod., PULS., **Rhus**, Ruta, Sang., Sep., *Sil.*, Spig., *Staph.*, Stram., Sul., **Verat. v.**

Antidotes.—Acon., *Camph.*, Chin., Coff.

Veratrum Viride.

Mind.

Localities.—Acon., (Aesc.), Agar., (Ant. cr.), Ant. t., Apis, Arg. n., Arn., *Ars.*, Aur., (Bap.), Bar. c., **Bell.**, (Bism.), *Bry.*, (Cact.), *Calc. c.*, (Cannab. i.), Canth., Caps., Carb. v., (Caust.), Cham., Chel., Chin., Cic., (Cimic.), Cina, (Cocc.), (Coff.), Colch., (Coloc.), *Con.*, Croc., Cup., (Cyc.), Dig., (Dros.), (Dulc.), (Euphr.), Fer., Gel., (Graph.), (Hell.), Hep., Hyos., Ign., Ip., (Iod.), K. bi., K. carb., Lach., (Led.), Lyc., (Meli.), *Merc.*, (Mez.), *Nat. m.*, Nit. ac., *Nux v.*, *Op.*, Petrol., *Phos.*, (Pho. ac.), (Plat.), Pb., (Pod.), *Puls.*, Ran. b., Rhodo., *Rhus*, (Ruta), Saba., Samb., Sang., Sec. c., *Sep.*, Sil., Spig., (Spo.), Squ., Stan., (Staph.), *Stram.*, **Sul.**, Tar., Valer., *Verat. a.*, Zinc.

Sensations.—Acon., (Aesc.), (Aloe), (Alum.), (Ambr.), Ant. t., (Apis), Arg. n., Arn., Ars., (Arum t.), (Bap.), (Bar. c.), *Bell.*, (Berb.), *Bry.*, (Cact.), (Calad.), Calc. c., (Camph.), (Cannab. i.), Canth., Cham., Chel., Chin., (Cimic.), Cocc., Coloc., Con., (Cup.), Dig., (Fer.), Gel., (Hyos.), Ign., (Ip.), (Iod.), (K. bi.), K. carb., Lach., (Lil. t.), Lyc., (Meny.), Merc., (Mur. ac.), *Nat. m.*, Nit. ac., Nux m., *Nux v.*, (Op.), (Petrol.), *Phos.*, Pho. ac., (Phyt.), (Pic. ac.), (Plat.), Pb., Pod., Puls., (Ran. b.), (Rhodo.), Rhus, (Ruta), (Saba.), Sang., (Sec. c.), Seneg., *Sep*, *Sil.*, Spig., (Spo.), (Squ.), Stan., Stram., *Sul.*, (Sul. ac.), (Thuj.), (Valer.), Verat. a., Zinc.

Glands.

Bones.

Skin.—(Acon.), (Apis), Bell., Merc., Rhus, (Sul.), (Thuj.).

Sleep and Dreams.

Blood, Circulation and Fever.—Acon., Ant. t., (Ars.), Bell., (Bry.), (Calc. c.), (Cannab. i.), (Canth.), (Carb. v.), (Cham.), (Chel.), (Chin.), (Cina), Cup., *Dig.*, (Gel.), (Hell.), Hep., (Hyos.), (Ip.), (K. nit.), (Kalm.), (Lyc.), (Merc.), (Mur. ac.), (Nit. ac.), (Nux v.), *Op.*, (Phos.),

RELATIONSHIPS.—VERAT. V —VERB. 479

(Puls.), (Rheum), (Rhus), (Sang.), (Sele.), (Sep.), (Sil.), (Spig.), Stram., (Sul.), Verat. a.

Aggravations : Time and Circumstances.—(Acon.), (Aesc.), (Aloe), (Am. m.), (Ant. t.), (Arg.), (Arn.), (Aur.), (Bap), Bell., (Bor.), (Bov.), Bry., Calc. c., Caps., Carb. v., Chel., (Cina), Cocc., (Coff.), (Colch.), Con., Croc., (Dig.), (Dulc.), Fer., (Gel.), (Graph), (Hep.), (Ign.), (Iris v.), (K nit.), Lach., (Led.), Lyc., (Merc.), Nat. m., Nit. ac., *Nux v.*, (Oleand.), (Petrol.), *Phos.*, Pho. ac., (Phyt.), (Plat.), (Pod.), *Puls.*, **(Ran.** b.), (Rheum), Rhodo.), *Rhus*, (Ruta), (Sabi.), (Sang.), (Sele.), (Seneg.), Sep., Sil., *Spig.*, (Squ.), (Staph.), Sul., (Thuj.), (Valer.) (Verat. a.).

Other Remedies.—*Acon.*, (Aesc.),(Aloe.), *Ant. t.*, (Apis), Arg. n., Arn., Ars., Aur., (Bap.), (Bar. c.), **Bell.**, **Bry.**, (Cact.), *Calc. c.*, Cannab. i., Canth., Caps., Carb. v., Cham., *Chel.*, Chin., (Cimic.), Cina, Cocc., (Coff.), (Colch.), (Coloc.), *Con.*, Croc., Cup., *Dig.*, (Dulc.), Fer., Gel., (Graph.), (Hell.), Hep., Hyos., Ign., Ip., (Iod.), (K. bi.), (K. carb.), (K. nit.), Lach., (Led.), *Lyc.*, *Merc*, (Mur. ac.), *Nat. m.*, *Nit. ac.*, **Nux** v., *Op.*, Petrol., **Phos.**, Pho. ac., (Phyt.), (Plat.), Pb., Pod., *Puls.*, Ran. b., (Rheum), Rhodo., *Rhus*, (Ruta), (Saba.), Sang., (Sec. c.), (Sele.), *Sep.*, *Sil.*, *Spig.*, (Spo.), Squ., Stan., *Stram.*, **Sul.**, (Thuj.), Valer., *Verat. a.*, Zinc.

Verbascum.

Mind.—Acon., **BELL.**, Bry., Calc. c., Chin., Cic., *Con.*, *Graph.*, **Hyos.**, Ign., **LYC.**, Merc., *Nat. c.*, Nat. m., **Op.**, **Phos.**, Plat., *Puls.*, *Rhus*, *Sil.*, Staph., **STRAM.**, *Sul.*, **Sul. ac.**, *Valer.*, **Verat. a.**, Vio. o., Zinc.

Localities.—(Aesc.), (All. c.), Alum., Anac., (Apis), (Apoc. c.), **Arg.**, (Arg. n.), (Arum t.), (Bap.), *Bell.*, Bry., (Cact.), Calc. c., Cannab. i., Caust., *Chin.*, (Cimic.), (Dios.), Gel., (Glon.), Ign., (Iris v.), (K. bi.), *K. carb.*, (Kalm.), Kre., (Lil. t.), Lyc., Mag. m., (Meli.), *Merc.*, Nat. m., **Nux** v., Oleand., Petrol., Phos., *Pho. ac.*, (Phyt.), **Plat.**, *Pb.*, (Pso.), ***Puls.***, Rhus, (Sang.), *Sep.*, *Spig.*, Stan., Staph., *Sul.*, **Sul. ac.**, Thuj., **Verat. a.**, Verat. v.

Sensations.—Acon., Alum., Arn., *Asaf.*, *Bell.*, *Bry.*, Calc. c., Canth. CHIN., Con., Dros., Ign., *K. carb.*, Merc., Nux m., *Nux v.*, *Oleand.*, Par. *Phos.*, Pho. ac., *Plat.*, Pb., Puls., *Rhus*, *Ruta*, Saba., SEP., *Spig.*, Spo. Staph., **Sul.**, *Sul. ac.*, Verat. a.

Glands.

Bones.

Skin.—Bell., Bry., Led., Phos., Plat., Puls., Rhus, *Sul.*

Sleep and Dreams.—*Ars.*, K. carb., Mag. c., *Nux v.*, Sep., **Sul. ac.**

Blood, Circulation and Fever.—Bell., Bry., Caust., Lyc., *Nux v.*, Puls., *Rhus*.

Aggravations: Time and Circumstances.—(Aloe), Am.carb., Am. m., (Apis), (Arg. n.), Aur., (Bap.), Bar. c., Calc. c., **Caps.**, Carb. v , Cina, Con., *Cyc.*, Dulc., *Euphorb.*, *Fer.*, (Glon.), Guai., **Hep.**, Iod., (K. bi.), Lach., (Lil. t.), Lyc., Mag. m., Meny., Mos., Nat. c., *Nat. m.*, Phos., Pho. ac., *Plat.*, Puls., *Ran. b.*, *Rhodo.*, RHUS, Ruta, **Saba.**, Samb., (Sang.), SEP., Sil., Stro., **Tar.**, *Valer.*, Vio. t.

Other Remedies.—(Apis), (Arg. n.), (Bap.), *Bell.*, *Bry.*, Calc. c, **Caps.**, *Chin.*, Con., Dulc., (Glon.), Hep., Hyos., Ign., (K. bi.), K. carb., (Lil. t.), *Lyc.*, Merc., Nat. c., Nat. m., Nux v., Oleand., Op., *Phos.*, Pho. ac. *Plat.*, Pb., (Pod.), PULS., Rhus, Ruta, Saba., **Sep.**, Sil., Spig., Staph., Stram., *Sul.*, **Sul. ac.**, Tar., Valer., Verat. a.

Antidote.—Camph.

Viola Odorata.

Mind.—Acon., Anac., Aur., BELL., *Bry.*, *Calc. c*, *Coff.*, Con., Graph., Hell., Hyos., Lach., Lyc., Nat m., *Nux v.*, **Op.**, Petrol., **Phos.**, Pho. ac., *Puls.*, Rhus, *Sep*, Stram., **Sul.**, Valer., **Verat. a.**

Localities.—Acon., (Arg. n.), Aur., *Bell.*, Bry., Calc. c, Chin., **(Gel.)**, K. carb., Lyc., Nat. m., Nux v., Phos., Plat., *Puls.*, *Sep.*, Spig., Sul.

Sensations.—Acon., Arn., Bell., Calc. c., Caust., *Chin.*, *Con.*, Fer., Iod., Lyc., **Nux v.**, **Phos.**, Plat., *Puls.*, Rhus, Sep., Spig., *Sul.*

Glands.

Bones.

Skin.—*Arn.*, Bell., Bry., Caust., K. carb., Lyc., *Phos.*, Plat., *Puls.*, *Rhus*, Sep., Spig., *Sul.*

Sleep and Dreams.—Bry., Caust., *Ign.*, **Nux v.**, Phos., Puls., **Rhus**, Sep. Staph.

Blood, Circulation and Fever.—(Aloe), (Apis), Cact., (Glon.).

Aggravations: Time and Circumstances.—Colch., Dros., Ign., K. carb., Lyc., *Nux v.*, Oleand., Phos., **Puls.**, *Rhus*, Saba., *Sep.*, *Spig.*

Other Remedies.—Acon., Arn., *Bell.*, *Bry.*, Calc. c., Caust., Chin., Con., Ign., K. carb., *Lyc.*, NUX V., Op., **Phos.**, Plat., PULS., **Rhus**, Sep., *Spig.*, Stram., *Sul.*, Verat. a.

Antidote.—Camph.

Viola Tricolor.

Mind.—*Con.*, Ign., Nat. m., *Phos.*, *Pho. ac.*, *Puls.*, Sep., *Sil.*, *Sul.*

Localities.—Ant. cr., *Arn.*, Ars., Bar. c., *Bell.*, Bry., (Cact.), *Calc. c.*,

(Cannab. i.), Cannab. s., Carb. v., **Caust.**, Chin., Graph., Hep., Ign., *K. carb.*, Kre., Lyc., **Merc.**, Nat. c., *Nat. m.*, *Nit. ac.*, Nux v., *Phos.*, *Pho. ac.*, *Puls.*, RHUS, Sabi., Sep., *Sil.*, *Spig.*, Staph., **Sul.**, Thuj., Verat. a., (Verat. v.), Zinc.

Sensations.—Arn., *Asaf.*, **Bell.**, Bry., *Calc. c.*, Caust., *Chin.*, Cocc., Colch., Coloc., Con., Dros., Graph., Ign., K. carb., Lyc., Meny., Merc., Mur. ac., *Nat. c.*, Nat. m., Nit. ac., Nux v., Phos., Puls., **Rhus**, Saba., Sep., Sil., *Spig.*, *Spo.*, Stan., Staph., **Sul.**, Tar., Zinc.

Glands.

Bones.

Skin.—Ant. cr., Arn., Ars., *Bar. c.*, Bell., **Bry.**, *Calc. c.*, Caust., *Cham.*, Clem., Con., Cyc., Dulc., **Graph.**, *Hep.*, *Led.*, Lyc., **Merc.**, Nat. c., *Nit. ac.*, Petrol., **Puls.**, Ran. b., RHUS, Saba., Sars., **Sep.**, **Sil.**, Spo., Squ., STAPH., *Sul.*

Sleep and Dreams. -Ars., Bry., Calc. c., (Cannab. i.), Carb. an., *Chin.*, Hep., Ign., K. carb., Lach., Lyc., Merc., *Nux v.*, **Phos.**, Puls., Ran. b., Rhus, Sep., Sil., Staph., Sul.

Blood, Circulation and Fever.—Acon., *Ars.*, Bell., Bry., *Cham.*, Nux v., Phos., Pho. ac., Puls., Rhus, *Sep.*

Aggravations: Time and Circumstances.—(Aloe.), Ambr., Am. m., (Apis.), Arg., Bry., *Caps.*, Cham., Coloc., **Con.**, *Cyc.*, *Dros.*, *Dulc.*, *Euphorb.*, *Fer.*, Ign., (K. bi.), **Lyc** , Mag. m., Mar., Meny., Mos., Pho. ac., *Plat.*, PULS., Rhodo., **Rhus**, Saba., (Sang.), **Sep.**, Sil., Staph., Tar., Valer., *Verb.*

Other Remedies.—Arn., Ars., Bar. c., *Bell.*, *Bry*, *Calc. c.*, Caust., Cham., Chin., *Con.*, Cyc., Dros., Dulc., Graph., Hep., Ign., K. carb., Lyc., **Merc.**, Nat. c., Nat. m., Nit. ac., Nuxv., **Phos.**, *Pho. ac.*, PULS., RHUS, Saba., SEP., **Sil.**, Spig., Spo., *Staph.*, Sul.

Antidotes.—Camph., Rhus.

Zincum.

Mind.—Acon., Alum., *Anac.*, Ars., *Aur.*, Bap., **Bell.**, Bry., *Calc. c.*, Cannab. i., Carb. an., Cham., Chin., Cimic., Coff., Con., Croc., Crotal., Cyc., Fer., Gel., Glon., Graph., Hell., *Hyos.*, **Ign.**, Lach., *Lyc.*, Meli., Merc., Merc. c., Mos., Nat. c., *Nat. m.*, Nux v., *Op.*, Petrol., **Phos.**, Pho. ac., Pic. ac., *Plat.*, **Puls.**, Rhus, Sep., *Sil.*, Staph., **Stram.**, *Sul.*, Valer., *Verat. a.*, Verat. v.

Localities.—Acon., Aesc., All. c., Aloe, Am. carb., Ant. cr., **Apis**, Apoc. c., **Arg. n.**, *Arn.*, Ars., Arum t., Asaf., *Aur.*, Bap., *Bell.*, Berb., Bry., Cact., *Calc. c.*, Cannab. i., *Canth.*, Carb. ac., Carb. v., (Caul.), **Caust.**,

Cham., Chin., *Cimic.*, Con., Crotal., Dios., (Eup. per.), Fer., Fl. ac., *Gel.*, Glon., Graph., Hep., Iris v., K. BI., **K. carb.**, (Kalm.), Kre., Laur., Led., Lil. t., Lyc., (Meli.), *Merc.*, *Mez.*, Nat. c.. Nat. m., **Phos.**, **Pho. ac.**, *Phyt.*, Pic. ac., Plat., *Pod.*, **Pso.**, **Puls.**, Rhus, *Sabi.*, *Sang.*, Sec. c., **SEP.**, *Sil.*, Squ., **Staph.**, Stro., **SUL.**, (Ther.), Thuj., *Verat. v.*

Sensations.—Acon., Aesc., Aloe, Alum., Apis, Arg., **Arg. n.**, *Arn.*, *Ars.*, Arum t., Bap., **Bell.**, Berb., Bry., (Cact.), **Calc. c.**, **Cannab. i.**, *Carb. v.*, Caust., Cham., *Chin.*, *Cimic.*, *Cocc.*, Con., (Crotal.), (Dios.), Eup. per., Fer., *Gel.*, Glon., *Graph.*, Hell., Hep., Ign., (Iris v.), **K. bi.**, **K. carb.**, Kalm., Lil. t., (Lith.), **Lyc.**, **Merc.**, *Mez.*, Nat. c., **Nat. m.**, Nit. ac., **Nux v.**, **Phos.**, *Pho. ac.*, *Phyt.*, *Plat.*, (Pod.), (Pso.), PULS., *Ran. s.*, Rhodo., Rhus, Sabi., **Sang.**, Sars., Sec. c., SEP., Sil., *Spig.*, *Stan.*, Staph., *Stro.*, **SUL.**, Thuj., Verat. v.

Glands.—Bell., *Calc. c.*, **Con.**, Hep., Ign., Lyc., Merc., *Phos.*, Puls., Rhus, *Sep.*, Sil., Spo., Staph., **Sul.**

Bones.—*Arg.*, Bell., Calc. c., *Chin.*, *Cocc.*, Con., Cup., *Lyc.*, *Merc.*, Phos., *Puls.*, *Rhus*, **Ruta**, Sabi., **Sep.**, Sil., Staph., Sul.

Skin.—Alum., Ant. cr., Arn., *Bry.*, *Calc. c.*, Caust., Cic., Cimic., Eup. per., (Glon.), **Graph.**, *Hep.*, Ign., Lyc., *Mang.*, Nat. m., Nit. ac., Petrol., Phos., Pho. ac., **Puls.**, *Rhus*, SEP., **Sul.**

Sleep and Dreams.—Acon., **Chin.**, Ign., Lach., Op., Phos., Sil., *Sul.*

Blood, Circulation and Fever.—*Acon.*, Bell., Bry., *Chin.*, Merc., *Phos.*, Pho. ac., Puls., *Rhus*, *Sep.*, Stram.

Aggravations: Time and Circumstances.—(Aesc.), (All. c.), Aloe, Am. carb., Anac., Ant. cr., Apis, Arg. n., Arn., *Ars.*, (Bap.), Bell., *Bry.*, (Cact.), **Calc. c.**, (Cannab. i.,) Cham., Chin., Cimic., (Glon.), IGN., *K. bi.*, Lach., Lil. t., Lyc., Merc., *Nat. c.*, *Nat. m.*, Nit. ac., **Nux v.**, Phos., (Phyt.), (Pod.), Puls., *Rhus*, *Ruta*, Sang., *Sep.*, Sil., Sul., Thuj.

Other Remedies.—Acon., Aesc., (All. c.), Aloe, *Apis*, *Arg. n.*, Arn., Ars., Arum t., Aur., *Bap.*, Bell., Berb., *Bry.*, Cact., **Calc. c.**, *Cannab. i.*, Carb. v., Caust., Cham., **Chin.**, *Cimic.*, Cocc., Con., Crotal., *Gel.*, *Glon.*, Graph., Hep., Ign., K. bi., K. carb., Lach., Lil. t., *Lyc.*, *Merc.*, Mez., Nat. c., *Nat. m.*, Nux v., **Phos.**, *Pho. ac.*, *Phyt.*, Plat., Pod., **Puls.**, Rhus, Ruta, Sabi., *Sang.*, SEP., *Sil.*, *Staph.*, Stram., **SUL.**, *Verat. v.*

Antidotes.—Camph., Hep., *Ign.*

Injurious.—Cham., *Nux v.*, Vinum.

INDEX.

Abdomen, 81
    external, 81
    in general, 78
    internal, 77
    lower, 80
    sides, 79
        left, 81
        right, 82
Abortion, 107
Adhesion of inner parts, sensation of, 142
Aggravations, circumstances, 271
    alone, when, 271
    arsenic fumes, 271
    ascending, 271
        high, 271
    autumn, in, 271
    bathing, 272
        cold, 272
        sea, 272
    bending or turning, 272
        affected parts, 272
        backward, 272
        and forward, 272
        forward, 272
    bending head backward, 272
        forward, 272
        sideways, 272
    inward, 272
    outward, 272
    to right, 272
    sideways, 272
Aggravations, time :
    during the day, 268
    evening, 270
    forenoon, 269
    forepart of night, 271
    midnight, after, 271
    morning, 269
    night, 270
    noon, at, 269
    periodically, 271
Aggravations:
    bent, holding the part, 272
    biting teeth together, 272
    blowing nose, 273
    breakfast, after, 273
    breathing, 273
        deep, 273
        holding breath, 273
        when not, 273
    bruises, 273
    brushing teeth, 273
    burns, 273
    change of position, 273
        temperature, 274
        weather, 274
    chewing, when, 274
        after, 274
    chicken-pox, 274
    children especially, remedies for, 274
    china (without quinine cachexia). 274
    clear weather, 274
    climateric, during, 274
    closing eyes, 274
        mouth, 274
    cloudy weather, 274
    clutching anything, 274
    coal gas, 275
    coition, during, 275
        after, 275
    cold in general, 275
    cold air, 275
        dry, 275
        wet, 275
    cold, entering a cold place, 276
    cold, becoming cold, 276
        a part of body, 276
        after becoming, 276
    cold in head, 276
        feet, 276
    combing hair, 276
        backward, 276
    conscious, when half, 276
    coughing, before, 276
        after, 276
    copper, fumes of, 276
    cutting hair, 276
    cuts, for, 276
    dancing, when, 276
        after, 276
    darkness, 277
    descending, 277
    disordered stomach, 277
    distortion of facial muscles, 277
    draft, 277
    drawing in the air, 277
        off boots, 277
        the limb back, 277
    drawing up limbs, 277
    drinkers, for hard, 277
    drinking, when, 277
    drinking, after, 277
    drinking fast, 278

Aggravations (*continued*)
   driving in a wagon, 278
      after, 278
   dry weather, 278
   eating, before, 278
      when, 278
      when eating fast, 278
      after, 278
      after eating to satiety, 279
   elevations, when on, 279
   emissions, 279
   eructations, 279
   eruptions, after suppression of, 279
   excitement, emotional, 279
      contradiction, 279
      fright, 279
      grief and sorrow, 279
      jealousy, 280
      joy, 280
      unhappy love, 280
      mortification, 280
      reproaches, 280
      rudeness of others, 280
      scorn, 280
      vexation, 280
      vexation with anxiety, 280
         with fright, 280
         with quiet grief, 280
            indignation, 280
            violence, 280
      physical, 280
   exertion of vision, 281
   expanding abdomen, 281
   expectoration, 281
      after, 281
   expiration, 281
   fainting, after, 281
   fasting (before breakfast), 281
   fatigue, 281
   feather bed, 281
   fever, before, during, after, 281
   food and drink, alcoholic stimulants in general, 281
   food and drink, beans and peas, 282
      beer, 282
      beer fresh, 282
      brandy, 282
      bread, 282
         black, 282
      bread and butter, 282
      buckwheat, 282
      butter, 282
      cabbage, 282
      carrots, 282
      cheese, old, 282
         strong 282
      coffee, 282
         odor of, 282
      cold, 282
      crumbs, 283
      dry, 283
      eggs, 283
         odor of, 283
      farinaceous, 283
      fat, 283
      fish, 283
         shell, 283
         spoiled, 283
      flatulent, 283
      frozen, 283
      fruit, 283
      garlic, odor of, 283
      heavy, 283
      honey, 283
      hot, 283
      hot cakes, 283
      iron, cooked in, 283
      lemonade, 283
      meat, 283
         bad, 283
         fresh, 283
         odor of cooking, 283
      milk, 283
      odor of, and of the cooking, 284
      oil, 284
      onions, 284
      oysters, 284
      pan-cakes, 284
      pastry, 284
      pears, 284
      pepper, 284
      pork, 284
      potatoes, 284
      raw, 284
      salad, 284
      salt, 284
      sausages, spoiled, 284
      sight of, 284
      smoked, 284
      sour, 284
      sour krout, 284
      sour odors, 284
      spices, 284
      sweats, 284
      thought of food she would like, 284
      tobacco, 284
         chewing, 284
      turnips, 285
      veal, 285
      vegetables, 285
      vinegar, 285
      warm, 285
      water, cold, 285
      wine, 285
         containing lead, 285
            sulphur, 285
         sour, 285
   gargling, 285
   glanders, 285
   grasping anything tightly, 285
   hang down, letting limbs, 285
   heated, becoming, 285
      by the fire, 285
   hiccough, 286
   holding together parts, 286
   house, in the, 286
   hunger, 286
   idleness, 286

INDEX.

Aggravations (*continued*)
injuries (including blows, falls, and bruises), 286
    bleeding profusely, 286
    with extravasations, 286
    of soft parts, 286
inspiration, 286
inspection of cold air, 287
intoxication after, 287
jar, 287
jumping, 287
kneeling, 287
labor, manual, 287
laughing, 287
leaning (against anything), 287
    after, 287
    backward, 287
    against a sharp point, 287
    to one side, 287
licking lips, 287
lifting, 287
light in general, 287
    candle or lamp, 288
    day, 288
    of fire, 288
    of sun, 288
looking around, 288
    at distant objects, 288
    downward, 288
    straight forward, 288
    over a large surface, 288
    at a bright light, 288
    long at anything, 288
    at running water, 288
    at shining objects, 288
    sideways, 288
    at something turning around, 288
    upward, 288
    at white objects, 288
loss of fluids, 289
lying, 289
lying down, after, 289
    in bed, 289
    on back, 290
    with head low, 290
    on side, 290
    on left side, 290
    on right side, 290
    on side painful, 290
    on side painless, 291
lying-in-women, 291
measles, during, 291
measles, after, 291
menstruation, 291
mercury, abuse of, 291
    fumes of, 291
micturition, 291
moon, new, 291
    full, 291
    waning, 291
moonlight, 291
motion, 291
    at beginning of, 292
    after, 292
    false, 292
    of affected parts, 292
    of head, 292
    of eyes, 292
    of eyelids, 292
    of arms, 292
music, 293
narcotics, 293
narrating her symptoms, 293
nasal catarrh during, 293
    suppression of, 293
noises, 293
nursing children, 293
odors, strong, 293
odor of wood, 293
onanism, 293
open air, 294
    evening, 294
opening eyes, 294
    mouth, 294
organ, playing the, 294
persuasion, 294
piano, playing the, 294
picking teeth, 294
pregnancy, 294
pressure, external, 294
    of clothes, 295
    of hat, 295
    on painless side, 295
punctures, 295
pustule, malignant, 295
putting out the tongue, 295
quinine, abuse of, 295
raising eyes, 295
    affected limb, 295
reading, 295
    aloud, 296
rest, 296
retching, 296
retracting abdomen, 296
reveling, night, 296
riding horseback, 296
riding one leg over the other, 296
ringing of bell, 296
rising up, 296
    from bed, 296
    from bed, after, 297
    from a seat, 297
    after, 297
room full of people, 297
rubbing, 297
    gently, 297
running, 297
scarlet fever, during, 298
    after, 298
scratching, 297
scratching on linen, noise of, 298
sewing, 298
sexual excesses, 298
    desire, suppression of, 298
    excitement, 298
shaking head, 298
shaving, 298
shipboard, on, 298
shooting, 298
shrugging shoulders, 298
singing, when, 298

Aggravations (*continued*)
singing, after, 298
sitting, when, 298
sitting down, on first, 299
  bent over, 299
  upright, 299
sleep, before, 299
  at beginning of, 299
  during, 300
  after, 300
  after afternoon, 300
sleep, after long, 300
smallpox, 300
smoke, 300
sneezing, 300
snow-air, 300
society, 301
spectacles, 301
splinters, 301
sprains, 301
spring, in, 301
squatting down, 301
standing, 301
stepping hard, 301
stings of insects, 301
stone cutters, for, 301
stool, before, during and after, 301
stooping, 301
  prolonged, 302
strangers, when among, 302
stretching of limbs, 302
storm, approach of a, 302
  during thunder storm, 302
stumbling, 302
sucking gums, 302
summer, in, 302
sun, in the, 302
sun-burn, 302
sunrise, after, 302
sunset, after, 302
supporting a limb, 302
swallowing, 302
  empty, 303
  of food, 303
    after, 303
  liquids, 303
  when not, 303
sweat, during, 303
  after, 303
  suppression of, 303
swinging (rocking), 303
talking, 303
  of other people, 304
talking about disagreeable things, 304
thinking of his disease, 304
  of something else, 304
touch, 304
  slight, 304
  anything, 304
  cold things, 304
  hair, 304
  throat, 304
turning around, 304
  over in bed, 304
  head, 305

neck, 305
twilight, 305
uncleanliness, 305
uncovering, 305
  after, 305
  one part, 305
  head, 305
unnatural position, 305
vaults, 305
vertigo, during, 305
violin, playing the, 306
vomiting, 306
waking, 306
  being awake at night, 306
walking, 306
  beginning of, 307
  bent over, 307
  fast, 307
  on a level, 307
  in open air, 307
  on a narrow bridge, 307
  sideways, 307
  on a stone pavement, 307
  over water, 307
  in the wind, 307
warmth in general, 307
  of air, 308
  of open air, 308
  of bed, 308
  of room, 308
warm wraps, 308
warm on head, 308
water (and washing), 309
weeping, 309
wet applications, 309
wet, getting, 309
  head, 309
  feet, 309
wet, with sweat, 309
wet weather, 309
wind, 309
  east, 309
  north, 309
  windy (and stormy) weather, 309
winter, in, 310
women, for, 310
worms, 310
writing, 310
yawning, 310
  after, 310
Air, aversion to open, 142
  desire for open, 143
Air passages, 120
  mucus, secretion of, 121
Alive, sensation of something, 142
Amativeness, 18
Ameliorations:
alone, when, 310
ascending, 310
attention, paying, 311
bathing, 311
  face, 311
bending or turning affected part, 311
bending backward, 311

INDEX.

Ameliorations (*continued*)
  bending inward, 311
    sideways, 311
    head backward, 311
    head sideways, 311
    holding part bent, 311
  biting, 311
  blinking eyes, 311
  blowing nose, 311
  boring in with the finger, 311
  breakfast, 311
  breathing, deep, 311
  breath, holding the, 311
  carrying the child in the arms, 311
  change of position, 311
  chewing, 311
  closing eyes, 311
  cloudy weather, 311
  cold, in the, 311
    air, 311
    being, 311
  crossing limbs, 312
  damp weather, 312
  dancing, 312
  darkness, 312
  descending, 312
  drawing in the affected part, 312
  drawing up the limb, 312
  drinking, after, 312
  driving in a wagon, 312
  eating, on, 312
    after, 312
    to satiety, 312
  eructations, 313
  exerting body, 313
    mind, 313
  expiration, 313
  fasting, 313
  flatulent emissions, 313
  food and drink, bacon, 313
    bread, 313
    coffee, 313
    cold, 313
    fruit, 313
    hot, 313
    meat, 314
    salt, 314
    tea, 314
    tobacco, 314
    vinegar, 314
    water, cold, 314
    water, warm, 314
    wine, 314
  grasping, 314
  hæmorrhage, 314
  hand, laying, on part, 314
  hang down, letting limbs, 314
  house, in the, 314
  inspiration, 314
  kneeling, 314
  knitting, 314
  leaning against anything, 314
    hard, 314
    head on anything, 314
    head on one side, 314
      on a table, 314

  licking with the tongue, 314
  light, 314
    bright, 314
  looking downward, 315
    intently, 315
    sideways, 315
    straight ahead, 315
  loosening clothes, 315
  lying, 315
    after, 315
    in bed, 315
    on hard bed, 316
    on back, 316
    bent up, 316
    with head high, 316
    horizontally, 316
    on side, 316
      left, 316
      right, 316
      painful, 316
      painless, 316
  mesmerism, 316
  moistening affected parts, 316
  motion in general, 316
    continued, 316
    of affected part, 317
  open air, 317
  opening eyes, 317
  pressure, external, 317
  raising limbs, 317
  reading, 317
  rest, 317
  retracting abdomen, 317
  rising up, 317
    from bed, 317
      after, 317
    from a seat, 317
      after, 318
  rubbing, 318
  running, 318
  scratching, 318
  sexual suppression, 318
  shaking head, 318
  shrugging shoulders, 318
  silence, 318
  sitting down, 318
  while sitting, 319
    bent over, 319
    upright, 319
  sleep, during, 319
    after, 319
    on falling asleep, 319
    when half asleep, 319
  sneezing, 319
  society, 319
  standing, 319
  stepping hard, 319
  stool, after, 319
  stooping, 320
  stretching limbs, 320
  sucking with tongue, 320
  sunlight, 320
  supporting the limb, 320
  swallowing, 320
  sweat, during, 320
    after, 320

Ameliorations (*continued*)
  sweat, cold, 320
  talking, 320
  touch, 320
  turning at a lathe, 320
  twilight, in the, 320
  tying up the hair, 320
  uncovering, 320
  vomiting, 320
  waking, 320
  walking, 320
  walking in open air, 321
    bent over, 321
    rapidly, 321
    warm, 321
    warm wraps, 321
  warmth in general, 321
    of bed, 321
    of the stove, 321
  weeping, 321
  wiping with the hand, 321
  wrapping up head, 321
  writing, when, 321
  yawning, 321
Anæmia, 147
Ankle, 141
Anus, 92
Anxiety, 18
  general physical, 143
Apoplexy, 143
  hæmorrhagic, 143
  nervous, 143
Appetite, loss of, 65
Aqueous humor, 30
Arm, upper, 131
  fore, 131
Ascending, sensation of, 143
Asleep feeling, in single parts, 143
Avarice, 18
Aversion to acids, 67
    beer, 67
    brandy, 67
    bread, 67
      (black), 67
    cereals, 67
    cheese, 67
    cocoa, 67
    coffee, 67
      unsweetened, 67
    fat food (and butter), 67
    fish, 67
    fruit, 67
    hot food, 67
    insipid food, 67
    meat, 67
    milk, 67
    onions and garlic, 67
    rich food, 68
    salt, 68
    solid food, 68
    soup, 68
    sweets, 68
    tobacco, 68
    vegetables, 68
    water, 68
    wine, 68

Aversion to being looked at, 167
Axilla, 130

Back, 128
  in general, 128
  sides, left, 130
    right, 130
Ball internal, sensation of, 144
Band, sensation of a, 144
Beard, 28
Belching, 72
Benumbing, pain, 144
Biting, 144
Blackness of external parts, 144
Bladder, 93
Bladder, tenesmus of, 98
Blindness, 35
  periodical, 35
Blood, 250
  anæmia, 250
  congestion, 250
    internal, 250
  orgasm, 250
  plethora, 251
  sensation as if blood stagnated, 251
Bloodvessels, 251
  burning, 251
  cold feeling, 251
  distension, 251
  inflammation, 251
  like a net-work, 251
  pulsation, 251
  stitches, 251
  varicose, 251
Blow, pains as after, 145
Boldness, 18
Bones, 200
  absence of marrow, sensation of, 200
  band, sensation of, 200
  boring, 200
  bruised sensation, 200
  burning, 200
  burrowing, 200
  caries, 201
    of periosteum, 201
  cold feeling, 201
  constriction, 201
  crawling, 201
  curvature, 201
  cutting in long bones, 201
  drawing as om a thread through shafts, 201fr
  gnawing, 201
  gouty nodes, 201
  healing of broken, slow, 201
  inflammation, 201
    of periosteum, 201
  injuries, 201
  itching, 201
  jerks, 201
  jerking pain, 201
  loosened from flesh, feeling as if, 201
  necrosis, 202
  pain as if broken, 200

INDEX.

Bones (*continued*)
  painfulness in general, 202
    of periosteum, 202
    paralytic, 202
  pinching, 202
  pressure, 202
    sticking, 202
    tearing, 202
  pulsation, 202
  scraping in periosteum, 202
    in long bones, 202
  sensitiveness, 202
    of periosteum, 202
  smarting, 202
  softening, 202
  sticking, 203
    burning, 203
    pressing, 203
    tearing, 203
  swelling, 203
    of periosteum, 203
  swollen feeling, 203
  tearing, 203
    burning, 203
    cramp-like, 203
    jerking, 203
    paralytic, 203
    in periosteum, 203
    pressive, 203
    sticking, 203
  tension, 203
  ulcerative pain, 203
Boring sensation of, 145
  inward, 145
  outward, 145
Borborygmi, 84
Breath, cold, 62
  hot, 62
Brows, 32
Bruised pain, 145
  external, 145
  internal, 146
  in joints, 146
Bubbling, 146
Burning, external, 146
  internal, 147
  pain as from, 147
Burns, 147

Calf, 137
Canthi, 32
  inner, 33
  outer, 33
Carphology, 147
Carried, desired to be, 147
Chest, 124
  external (ribs and muscles), 126
  internal, 124
  lower part, 125
  upper part, 125
Chewing motions, 147
  sides, left, 127
    right, 127
Chilblains, 204
  blue, 204
  crawling in, 204
  inflamed, 204
  painful, 204
  vesicular, 205
Chill, alternating with heat, 267
  sweat, 267
  external with heat internal, 266
  internal with heat external, 267
  and heat at the same time, 266
  then heat, 266
  then sweat, 266
  then heat, then chill, 266
  then heat, then sweat, 266
  then heat with sweat, 266
  with sweat, 266
  with heat and sweat, 266
Chilliness in general, 254
  becomes chilled easily, 255
  in certain parts, 254
  internal, 254
  one-sided, 255
  with gooseflesh, 255
  with shivering, 255
  with thirst, 255
  without thirst, 255
  with trembling, 256
  symptoms during chill, 256
Chlorosis, 147
Choroid, 31
Clamp of an iron, sensation of, 147
Clamp-like pains, external, 147
  internal, 148
Clothing, intolerance of, 148
Clucking, 148
Clumsiness, 148
Coat of skin drawn over inner parts, sensation of, 148
Cobweb, sensation of a, 148
Coccyx, 129
Cold, tendency to take, 148
Coldness in general, 260
  external, 260
  internal, 261
  of special parts, 260
  one-sided, 261
  shivering in general, 261
    of special parts, 261
    of one side, 261
Comedones, 206
Comfortable sensation, 149
Comprehensions, difficult, 20
  easy, 20
Conjunctiva, 31
Constipation, 86
  on account of hard fæces, 86
  on account of inactivity, 87
Construction, external, 149
  internal, 149
  in joints, 149
  of orifices, 149
Consumption in general, 150
Contractions (after inflammation), 150
  of extremities, 150
Convulsions, 150
  clonic, 150
  with consciousness, 151
  without, 151

Convulsions (*continued*)
  epileptiform, 151
  with falling, 151
  hysterical, 151
  internal, 151
  with opisthotonos, 152
  with stiffness, 152
  tetanic (rigidity), 152
  tonic, 152
  uterine (compare with hysterical), 152
Convulsive movements, 152
Cornea, 31
Corns, 206
  with boring, 206
  with burning, 206
  horny, 206
  inflamed, 206
  with jerking, 206
  with pressing, 206
  sensitive, 206
  smarting, 206
  with stitches, 206
  with tearing, 207
  with throbbing, 207
Corroded feeling, 152
Cough (in general), 115
  convulsive, 116
  dry, 115
  evening with, and morning without, expectoration, 116
  with expectoration, 115
  day with, night without, expectoration, 116
  morning with, and evening without, expectoration, 116
  night with, day without, expectoration, 116
  with expectoration which he is obliged to swallow, 116
  troubles associated with, 120
Cramps, internal, 153
  of joints, 153
  of muscles, 153
Crawling, as of a mouse, 153
Creeping, as of little animals, 153
Crepitation, 153
Crushing, 153
Cutting, external, 153
  internal, 154
Cyanosis, 154

Dead feeling, 154
Death, apparent, 154
Debility, sensation of, 154
Delirium, 21
Desire for acids, 68
  beer, 68
  bitters, 68
  brandy, 68
  bread, 68
  bread and butter, 68
  cakes, 68
  chalk and lime, 68
  cheese, 68
  coal, 68

coffee, 68
cold food and drink, 68
cucumbers, 68
farinaceous food, 68
fat of ham, 68
fruit, 68
German rolls, 69
for herring (and sardines), 69
indigestible things, 69
juicy things, 69
liquid food, 69
many and different things (and indefinite things), 69
meat, 69
milk, 69
oysters, 69
salt, 69
smoked meat, 69
sour kraut, 69
spiced food (and highly seasoned food), 69
sweets, 69
tobacco smoking, 69
tonics, 69
vegetables, 69
warm food, 69
wine, 69
Despair, 18
Diaphragm, 77
Diarrhœa, 85
  alternating with constipation, 85
  painful, 85
  painless, 86
Digging, sensation of, 155
  up, sensation of, 155
Dilated, internal sensation of, 155
Dislocations, 155
Dislocation, easy, 155
Disposition, 17
Distortion of limbs, 155
Dorsal region, 129
Doubling up of body, 155
Drawing downward, sensation of, 155
  inward of soft parts, 155
  sensation of, 156
Dreams in general, 246
  anxious, 246
    of animals, 247
    of battle, 247
    of the dead, 247
    of difficulties, 247
    of falling, 247
    of fire, 247
    of ghosts, 247
    of bad luck, 247
    of quarrels, 247
    of shooting, 247
    of sickness, 247
    of thieves, 247
    of thunder, 247
    of water, 247
  confused, 247
    after waking, 248
    continuation of former ideas, 248
  historical, 248

INDEX.

Dreams (*continued*)
  with indifference, 248
  indifferent to the day's business, 248
  of mental effort, 248
  of excelling in mental work, 248
  pleasant, 248
    of dancing, 248
    fantastic, 248
    of festivities, 249
    of gold, 249
    intellectual, 249
    full of imagination, 249
    journeys, 249
    joyful, 249
    of love, 249
  unremembered, 249
  vexatious, 249
    disgusting, 249
    with humiliation, 249
    of illusions of hope, 249
    of sick people, 249
    with strivings, 249
    of vermin, 249
  vivid, 249
  waking, 250
Dropsy, external, 156
  internal, 156
Dryness of internal parts, 156
  internal, 156
  in joints, 157
  of palms and soles, 156
Dust, internal, sensation of, 157

Ears, 40
  before, 40
  behind, 40
  beneath, 41
  discharges from, 41
    bloody, 41
    excoriating, 41
    fetid, 41
    moist, 41
    mucous, 41
    purulent, 41
  noises in, 43
  ringing in, 43
  roaring in, 43
  stopped feeling, 44
Ear, external, 40
  internal, 40
  lobules, 41
  middle, 40
  sides, left, 42
    right, 42
Earwax blood red, 41
  hard, 41
  increased, 41
  thin, 42
Ecstasy, 21
Elbow, 133
  bend of, 133
  tip of, 133
Emaciation, 157
  of affected parts, 157
  of certain parts, 157

Emissions, 106
Emptiness, sensation of, 157
Epigastrium, 79
Erections, 106
Eructations, 72
  in general, 72
Eruptions in general, 208
  abcesses, 208
  biting, 208
  blackish, 208
  blood-boils, 208
  burning, 208
Expectorations:
  offensive odor, 118
  orange-colored, 118
  purulent, 118
  slimy, 118
  tenacious, 118
  watery, 119
  whitish, 119
  yellow, 119
Expectoration, taste of, 119
  bitter, 119
  burnt, 119
  old catarrh, 119
  fatty, 119
  flat, 119
  foul, 119
  garlicky, 119
  herby, 119
  metallic, 120
  mouldy, 120
  nauseous, 120
  salty, 120
  sour, 120
  sweetish, 120
  tobacco juice, 120
External parts, drugs affecting, 158
Extravasation, sensation of, 158
Extremities in general:
  lower, 135
    bones of, 141
    joints of, 140
    left, 142
    right, 142
  upper, 130
    bones of, 134
    joints of, 133
    left, 134
    right, 135
Eyes, 30
  protruding, 55
  squinting, 34
  staring, 34
  sunken, 55
Eye, left, 35
  right, 35
  white of, 32
Eyeballs, 30
Eruptions:
  carbuncles, 209
  chapping, 209
  chicken-pox, 209
  clustered, 209
  confluent, 209
  coppery, 209

Eruptions (*continued*)
  corroding, 209
  on covered parts, 208
  desquamating, 209
  dry, 209
  erysipelas, 209
    gangrenous, 210
    with swelling, 210
    vesicular, 210
  fine (miliary), 210
  flat, 210
  furuncles, 210
    large, 210
    small, 210
  gooseflesh (in open air), 210
  gooseflesh (in the house), 210
  granular, 210
  gritty, 210
  on hairy parts, 208
  hard, 210
  itch, 210
    bleeding, 210
    dry, 210
    fatty, 211
    moist, 211
    suppressed, 211
    suppressed with mercury and sulphur, 211
  itching, 211
  with jerking pain, 211
  with maggots, 211
  measles, 211
  milk-crust, 211
  moist, 211
  nettle-rash, 211
  nodular (wheals and hives), 212
    rosy-red (erythema), 212
  painful, 212
  painless, 212
  pimples, 212
  purulent, 212
  pustules, 212
  rash, 213
    purple, 213
    scarlet, 213
    white, 213
  roseola, 213
  scabby, 213
  scaly, 213
  scarlatina, 213
    smooth, 213
  small-pox, 213
    black, 213
  smarting, 213
  stinging, 214
  with swelling, 214
  with tearing pain, 214
  tense, 214
  transparent, 214
  with ulcerating pain, 214
  unhealthy (suppurating), 214
  vesicular, 214
    blue, 215
    bloody, 215
    gangrenous, 215
  whitish, 215

  with white tips, 215
  yellow, 215
  zoster, 215
Eustachian tube, 40
Excitement, 18
  nervous, 157
Excrescences. bunions, 215
  condylomata. 215
  cysts, sebaceous, 215
  fleshy, 215
  fungus, 215
    (cauliflower), 215
    hæmatodes, 215
    medullary, 215
  horny, 215
  moles, 215
  polypi, 215
  swellings, inflamed, 215
Expectoration, acid, 116
  albuminous, 117
  blackish, 117
  bloody, 117
    acid, 117
    bright, 117
    brownish, 117
    clotted, 117
    dark, 117
    tenacious, 117
  blood-streaked, 117
  cold, 117
  frothy, 117
  gelatinous, 117
  granular, 118
  gray, 118
  green, 118
  hardened, 118
  milky, 118

Face, 50
  articulation of jaws, 57
  cheeks, 37
  chin, 58
  color of, 50
    alternating, 50
    bluish, 51
    bluish-red, 51
      around eyes, 51
        mouth, 51
    brown, 51
    coppery, 51
    earthy, 51
    gray, 51
    greenish, 51
      around eyes, 51
    lead-colored, 51
    pale, 51
    red, 51
    redness, erysipelatous, 52
    redness of cheeks, circumscribed, 52
    spotted, 52
    yellow spots, 52
    yellow, 52
    yellow around eyes, 52
      mouth, 52
      nose, 53

INDEX. 493

Face (*continued*)
color of, yellow saddle across upper part of cheeks and nose, 53
yellow on temples, 53
comedones, 53
corners of lips, 58
drawn, 53
emaciation, 53
eruptions on cheeks, 53
on chin, 53
around eyes, 53
in eyebrows, 23
on forehead, 54
on lower lip, 54
on upper lip, 54
around mouth, 54
at corners of mouth, 54
on nose, 54
around nose, 54
on temples, 54
expression altered, 55
forehead, 56
freckles, 55
jaw, left, 57
upper, 57
lips, 58
lower, 58
upper, 58
malar bone, 57
oily, 55
sides, left, 59
right, 59
swelling of, 55
of cheeks, 55
around eyes, 56
over eyes, 56
under eyes, 56
between lids and brows, 56
of lips, 56
of lower lips, 56
of upper lips, 56
of nose, 56
temples, 56
wrinkles on, 56
on forehead, 56
Faintness, 158
Falling easily, 158
forward feeling, internal, 158
outward of internal parts, sensation of, 158
Fauces, 65
Febrile symptoms :
sides, left, 268
right, 268
Fever, compound, in general, 265
after, 268
before, 268
during, 268
Festering, as from pain, 158
Fingers, 132
between, 132
joints of, 134
nails, 132
tips, 132
Flabby feeling, 159
internal, 159
in hard parts, 159
Flatulence, 83
in general, 83
Flatulent pain, 84
Flatus, cold, 83
fetid, 83
garlicky, 84
hot, 84
incarceration of, 85
loud, 84
moist, 84
odorless, 84
putrid, 84
smelling of bad eggs, 83
sour smelling, 84
Floating (on waves), 159
Forcings, 159
Forehead, 24
Foot, 138
back of, 138
Formication, external, 159
internal, 159
Fretfulness, 18
Frozen limbs, 160
Full feeling, external, 160
internal, 160
Full habit, 160

Gentleness, 19
Glands, 196
air passing through, sensation of, 196
atrophy, 196
boring, sensation of, 196
bruised, pain in, 197
burning in, 197
burrowing in, sensation of, 197
cervical and submaxillary, 123
contractions of, 197
constricting pain in, 197
crawling in, 197
creeping in, 197
cutting, sensation of, 197
gnawing, sensation of, 197
heaviness, 197
indurations, 197
inflammation, 197
injuries, sensation of, 197
itching, 197
jerking pain, 197
living, feeling of something, sensation of, 198
numb feeling, sensation of, 198
painfulness in general, 198
painfulness, blunt, 198
pinching, sensation of, 198
pressings, 198
pressings inward, 198
outward, 198
pulsation, 198
quivering, 198
sensitiveness, 198
smarting, 198
squeezing, sensation of, 198
sticking, sensation of, 198
suppuration, 199

494   INDEX.

Glands (*continued*)
 swelling, 198
  bluish, 199
  cold, 199
  hard, 199
  hot, 199
  inflammatory, 199
  like knotted cords, 199
  painful, 199
  painless, 199
 swollen feeling, sensation of, 199
 tearing, sensation of, 199
 tension, sensation of, 200
 thyroid, 124
 tickling, sensation of, 200
 ulcerative pain, 200
 ulcers, 200
  cancerous, 200
  spongy, 200
Gnawing, external, 160
 internal, 160
 in joints, 161
 pains, 161
Gout-like pains, 161
Grinding pain, 161
Griping pain, 161
Groins, 80
Gums, 61
Gum, inner, 61
 lower, 61
 upper, 61
Gurgling, 148

Hacking, as with a hatchet, 161
Hæmorrhage (from internal parts), 161
Hæmorrhoids, 92
Hair, 27
 dark, 27
 light, 27
 margins of, 28
 falls out of head, 216
  of beard, 216
  in bunches, 216
  of eyebrows, 217
  on forehead, 216
  of moustache, 217
  of mons veneris, 217
  of nostrils, 217
  of occiput, 216
  of sides, 216
  of temples, 216
  of vertex, 216
  of whole body, 217
 feels pulled, 217
 pulling, sensation of, 162
 sensation of a, 162
Hammering, 162
Hand, 131
 back of, 132
 palm, 132
Hard bed, sensation of, 162
Hardened (muscles), 162
Haughtiness, 19
Head in general, 26
 external, 27 and 30
  sides, 30

  internal, 24
   sides, 29
  motions of, 27
   sides, 25
Hearing, 42
 acute, 42
 hardness, 42
 fluttering of, 43
 loss of, 43
 sensitive, 44
Heart and region, 125
 action intermittent, 126
  tremulous, 126
Heartburn, 72
Heat, 256
 anxious, 258
 then chill, 267
  then heat, 267
   then sweat, 267
 dry, 258
 external, 256
 in flushes, 258
 internal, 257
 in special parts, 257
  external, 257
  internal, 258
  one-sided, 258
 then shivering, 267
  sweat, 267
   then chill, 267
 with shivering, 267
  sweat, 267
   then chilliness, 267
 alternating with shivering, 267
  sweat, 267
 associated symptoms, 259
 with thirst, 259
 without thirst, 259
 with inclination to uncover, 259
  dread of uncovering, 259
Heaviness, external, 162
 internal, 162
Heel, 138
Hernia, 80
Hiccough, 73
Hips, region of, 135
Hip-joint, 140
Hunger, 65
 without relish, 66
 ravenous, 66
Hypochondria, 77
 sides, left, 82
  right, 82
Hysteria (and hypochondriasis), **163**

Imaginations, 21
Imbecility, 21
Immobility of affected parts, 163
Impotency, 106
Indifference, 19
Indurations (after inflammation), 163
Inflammation, external, 163
 internal, 163
 of mucous membrane, 164
Inflated feeling, 164
Inguinal rings, 80

INDEX.

Inguinal rings (*continued*)
  external, 81
    sides, left, 83
      right, 83
  glands, 81
Insanity, 22
Intellect, active, 20
  befogged, 20
  confused, 21
  impaired, 22
Internal parts, drugs affecting, 164
Iris, 31
Irritability, physical, 164
  physical, lack of, 165
Itching in general, 218
  biting, 218
  burning, 218
  corroding (compare gnawing), 218
  crawling, 218
  creeping, 219
  internally, 165
  jerking, 219
  changing place on scratching, 219
  unchanged by scratching, 219
    after scratching, biting, 220
      blisters, 220
      oozing of blood, 220
      bloody, 220
      burning, 220
      eruption, 220
      erysipelas, 220
      excoriation, 220
      gnawing, 221
      hives, 221
      moisture, 221
      numbness, 221
      pain, 223
      pimples, 221
      pimples, white, 221
      pustules, 221
      rash, 221
      redness, 221
      red streaks, 221
      scales, 221
      skin becomes thick, 222
      smarting pain, 222
      spots, 222
      stitches, 222
      suppurative pain, 222
      swelling, 222
      tearing, 222
      tension, 222
      tickling, 222
      ulcerative pain, 222
      ulcers, 222
  smarting, 219
  sticking, 219
  tearing, 219
  voluptuous, 219

Jaundice, 165
Jerking, internal, 165
  as in convulsions, 166
  in joints, 165
  in muscles, 165
  pain, external, 166
  internal, 166
Joints, cracking of, 152
  sensation of cracking, internal, 152
  creaking of, 153
  loose feeling in, 167
Joyfulness, 19
Jumping, internal, 166

Kidney, 93
Knee, 140
  hollow of, 141
Knotted internal, sensation of, 166

Labor-like pains, 166
Lachrymal apparatus, 31
Lachrymation, 32
Larynx, 120
Leg below knee, 137
Lens, 31
Leucorrhœa, 110
  in general, 110
  acid, 110
  albuminous, 111
  bland, 111
  bloody, 111
  brown, 111
  burning, 111
  green, 111
  itching, 111
  milky, 111
  offensive, 111
  purulent, 111
  slimy, 111
  tenacious, 111
  thick, 111
  accompanying troubles of 111
  watery, 111
  yellow, 111
Lids, 33
  lower, 34
  upper, 33
  margins of, 34
  inner surface of, 34
Lie down, inclination to, 166
Lifted up, sensation of, 167
Light in limbs, 167
Liver (and region), 78
Loathing, 75
Loins, 80, 135
Lousiness, 222
Lumbar region, 129

Malaise, 167
Mammary glands, 12
Memory, active, 22
  lost, 22
  weak, 22
Menses, acrid, 109
  bright, 109
  brown, 109
  clotted, 109
  dark, 109
  membranous, 109
  offensive, 109
  tenacious, 109
  watery, 109

Menstruation, 107
  after, 110
  before, 109
  beginning, 107
  at beginning of, 110
  during, 110
  too early, 107
  early and scanty, 108
  gushing, 108
  hæmorrhage, not at menstrual time, 107
  late, 108
  long, 108
  profuse, 108
  scanty, 108
  short, 108
  suppressed, 109
Micturition, 98
  before, 100
  at beginning of, 101
  at close of, 101
  by drops, 99
  during, 101
  dysuria, 99
  too frequent, 99
  ineffectual, 99
  interrupted, 99
  involuntary, 100
  at night, 100
  involuntary retention of, 100
  too seldom, 100
  troubles after, 101
Milk, bad, 127
  diminished, 127
  increased, 127
Mind, absence, 17
  concomitants, 23
Mischievousness, 19
Mistrust, 19
Mobility, increased, 167
Mons veneris, 81
Moods, alternating, 17
Motion, aversion to, 167
  desire for, 167
  difficult, 167
  involuntary, 168
  moving up and down, 168
  sensation of, 168
Mouth in general, 62
  odor from, 62
  and fauces, 65
  open, 55
  sides, left, 65
    right, 65
Mucus secretion increased, 168

Nails, generally, 223
  blue, 223
  brittle, 223
  deformed, 223
  discolored, 223
  falling off, 223
  furrowed, 223
  growing inward, 223
  growing very slowly, 223
  jerking pain, 223

  painful, 223
  scaling off, 223
  sensitive, 223
  smarting, 223
  sensations of splinters under, 223
  splitting, 223
  spotted, 223
  thick, 223
  ulcerated, 223
  ulcerative pain, 224
  yellow, 224
Nape of neck, 123
Nates, 135
Nausea in general, 73
  abdomen, 74
  chest, 74
  throat, 74
  stomach, 74
  and vomiting, 73
  with inclination to vomit, 74
Neck, sides, left, 124
  right, 124
Nipples, 127
Nose, 44
  back of, 45
  blowing out of blood, 46
  bones of, 45
  catarrh, 46
  coryza stopped, 47
  discharges, acid, 47
    bloody, 47
    burning, 47
    flocculent, 47
    gray, 47
    green, 47
    hardened, 47
    offensive, 47
    purulent, 48
    slimy, 48
    tenacious, 48
    thick, 48
    watery, 48
    yellow, 49
    accompanying symptoms of, 49
  external, 44
  internal, 44
  odor from, 46
    sweetish, 46
    urinous, 46
  root of, 45
  septum of, 45
  sides, left, 49
    right, 49
  tip of, 45
  wings of, 45
Nosebleed, 45
  bright red, 46
  clotted, 46
  dark, 46
  stringy, tenacious, 46
Numbness, external, 168
  internal, 169
  of suffering parts, 169

Obesity, 169

Occiput, 25
Optic nerve, 31
    paralysis of, 39
Orbits, 34

Pain, blunt, 169
    dull, 169
    jumping from place to place, 170
    oppressive, 169
    shattering, 178
    in joints, 178
Palate, hard, 64
    soft, 64
Palpitation, 125
    anxious, 126
Paralysis, internally, 170
    of limbs, 170
    of organs, 170
    one-sided, 170
    painless, 171
Paralytic, internal, sensation, 171
    pain, 171
        in joints, 171
Parotid glands, 41
Patella, 141
Perineum, 93
Photomania, 39
Photophobia, 39
Picking sensation, 171
Pierced with a hot iron, as if, sensation, 171
Pinching, sensation, 171
    external, sensation, 172
        internal, 172
        together, 172
Plucking, sensation, 172
Plug, sensation, external, 172
    internal, 172
Polypus, 172
Pressing, external, 172
    internal, 173
    inward, 173
    deep, inward, with instruments, 173
    in joints, 173
    as from a load, 174
    in muscles, 174
    from within outward, 174
    sticking, in muscles, 174
    tearing, in joints, 175
    tearing in muscles, 175
    together, 175
Pricking, external, 175
    internal, 175
Prostate, 94
Prostatic fluid, discharge of, 105
Puckerings, sensation of, 175
Pullings, sensation of, 175
Pulse:
    abnormal in general, 251
    full, 252
    hard, 252
    imperceptible, 252
    intermittent, 252
    irregular, 252
    rapid, 252
    more rapid than the beat of the heart, 253
    slow, 253
    slower than the beat of the heart, 253
    small, 253
    soft, 253
    tremulous, 253
    unchanged, 253
Pupils, adhesion in, 31
    contracted, 31
    dilated, 32
    immovable, 32
Pushing pain, 192

Qualmishness, 74

Rawness, internal, 175
Rectum, 93
Reeling, 176
Relaxation of muscles, 176
Respiration, 112
    anxious, 112
    arrested, 112
    catching, 112
    deep, 112
    irregular, 112
    loud, 112
    oppressed, 113
    rapid, 113
    rattling, 113
    sighing, 114
    slow, 114
    sobbing, 114
    suffocative attacks, 114
    superficial, 114
    troubles accompanying, 114
Restlessness, 176
Retching, 75
Retina, 32
Retraction of soft parts, 176
Rigidity, 177
    of joints of extremities, 177
Roaring, 177
Rolling, sensations of, 177

Sacral region, 129
Sadness, 19
Saliva diminished, 63
    increased, 63
Scalp, 28
    behind ears, 28
    forehead, 29
    occiput of, 28
    sides, 29
    sinciput, 29
    temples, 28
    vertex, 29
Scapulæ, 128
    between, 129
Scraped feeling, 178
Screwing together, sensation of, 178
Scurvy, 178
Sensitiveness, external, 177
    internal, 177
    to pain, 178

Seriousness, 20
Sexual desire too strong, 105
  too weak, 105
Sexual organs in general, 101
  male, in general, 102
    glans, 102
    foreskin, 102
    penis, 102
    testicles, 102
    scrotum, 102
    spermatic cord, 103
  female, in general, 105
    external, 103
    ovaries, 104
    labor-like pains, 104
      cease, 104
      too severe, 105
      spasmodic, 105
      weak, 105
    after-pains, 105
    uterus, 104
    vagina, 104
    sides, left, 106
      right, 107
Sexual power weak, 106
Shivering then chill, 268
  then heat, 268
  then sweat, 268
  with sweat, 268
Shortened muscles, 178
Shoulder, 130
  shoulder joint, 133
Shrivelling, 179
Shuddering, 179
  pain, 179
Sick sensation, 167, 179
Side, 179
  cross-wise, left lower and right upper, 179
    left upper and right lower, 179
  left, 180
  right, 180
Sit, inclination to, 180
Skin, 204
  adherent, 204
    to ulcers on the bone, 204
  biting, 204
  blood sweating, 204
  bruised pain, 204
  burning, 204
    as from flames, 204
    as from sparks, 204
  coldness, 205
  color, blackish, 205
    blue, 205
    dirty, 205
    pale, 205
    red, 205
    yellow, 205
  contractions, 206
  cracks, 207
    deep, bloody, 207
    after washing, 207
  cutting, 207
  desquamation, 207
    of hard, 207

sensation of, 207
dryness, 207
  burning, 207
extravasations, 215
fatty, 216
flabbiness, 215
formication, 216
gangrene, 216
  cold, 216
  hot, 216
  moist, 216
gnawing, 216
hard, like callosities, 217
  like parchment, 217
  with thickening, 217
inactivity, 217
indurations, 217
inelasticity, 217
inflammation, 217
  inclination to. 217
loose, sensation of, 167
moisture, 222
numbness (and fuzziness), 224
pressure, deep inward, from instruments, 224
prickling, 224
rawness, 224
sensitiveness in general, 224
sore, becomes, 224
  becomes, in a child, 224
  feeling in general, 224
spots, black, 225
  blue, 225
  burning, 225
  as if burnt, 225
  confluent, 225
  death spots in old people, 225
  like flea-bites, 225
  freckles, 225
  gangrenous, 225
  green, 225
  itching, 225
  liver, 225
  of petechiæ, 225
    bluish, 226
    brownish, 226
    coppery, 226
    fiery, 226
    pale, 226
      becoming pale in the cold, 226
    red, 226
    like red wine, 226
    violet, 226
  scarlet, 226
  smarting, 226
  stinging, 226
  white, 226
  yellow, 226
sticking, 226
  burning, 226
stings of insects, 226
swelling, general, external, 226
swelling of affected parts, 227
  bluish-black, 227
  burning, 227

INDEX.

Skin (continued)
  swelling, cold, 227
    crawling, 227
    dropsical, 227
    hard, 227
    inflamed, 227
    pale, 228
    puffy, 228
    shining, 228
    spongy, 228
    stinging, 228
    white, 228
  swollen sensation, 228
  tension, 228
  tightness, 230
  ulcerative pain, 230
  unhealthy, 238
  wrinkled, 239
Skull, 28
Sleep, 239
  anxious, 243
  comatose, 243
  falling asleep late, 240
  intoxicated with, 243
  position, 241
    lies on abdomen, 241
    arms and hands over head, 241
      and hands under head, 241
      and hands on abdomen, 241
      and hands on back, 241
    head inclined forward, 241
      backward, 241
      to one side, 242
    hanging low down, 242
    knees bent, 242
      spread apart, 242
    legs crossed, 242
      drawn up, 242
      stretched out, 242
      one stretched out the other drawn up, 242
    one side, 242
    sitting, 242
  restless, 244
  somnambulistic, 244
  sound, 244
  stupid, 244
  associated symptoms. See Aggravations, Sleep, 245
  prevented by symptoms, 240
  unrefreshing, 244
  impossible after waking once, 240
Sleepiness during afternoon, 243
  day, 242
  evening, 243
  forenoon, 242
  morning, 242
  caused by various things, 243
  associated symptoms, 243
Sleeplessness in general, 245
  after midnight, 245
  before midnight, 245
  though sleepy, 245
  symptoms causing, 246
Smaller sensation, 181
Smarting, 181

Smell, 50
  agreeable, 50
  bituminous, 50
  bloody, 50
  burnt, 50
  of old catarrh, 50
  earthy, 50
  foul, 50
  illusions of, 50
  pus of, 50
  sensitive, 50
  sour, 50
  sweetish, 50
  sulphurous, 50
  weak or lost, 50
Sneeze, ineffectual efforts to, 49
Sneezing, 49
Softness, 181
Sole, 138
Sore pain, external, 181
  internal, 181
Spleen, 78
Splitting, sensation, 181
Splinters, sensation, 181
Splitting pain, 182
Sprain from lifting, 182
Sprained pain, external, 182
  internal, 182
  in joints, 182
Startings, 183
Sternum and region, 125
Sticking crawling, 185
  drawing, 185
  extending downward, 183
  external, 183
  internal, 183
  inward, 184
  jerking, 185
  in joints, 184
  burning in joints, 185
    muscles, 185
  pressing in joints, 185
    in muscles, 185
  tearing in joints, 185
    in muscles, 185
  in muscles, 184
  outward, 185
  tensive, 186
  transversely, 185
  upward, 185
Stiffness, 186
Stomach, 77
  pit of, 81
Stool, 85
  acid, 87
  beaten, like eggs, 87
  bilious, 87
  blackish (and dark), 87
  bloody (and dysentery), 87
  brownish, 87
  burning, 87
  chopped as if, 88
    eggs like, 88
    spinach like, 88
  curdy, 88
  flattened, 88

Stool (continued)
    forcible (gushing), 88
    frothy, 88
    gray and whitish, 88
    greasy, 88
    green, 88
    insufficient, 88
    involuntary, 88
    large, 88
    offensive (and putrid), 89
    purulent, 89
    putty-like, 89
    scanty, 89
    sheep dung, like, 89
    slimy, 89
    slipping back again, 89
    small (in size), 89
    sour, 90
    stringy, 90
    troubles before, 90
    troubles during, 91
    troubles after, 91
    undigested, 90
    yellow, 90
Stopped feeling, internal, 186
Strangling pain, 186
Strength, sensation of, 186
Stupefaction, 22
Surging (in body), 186
Sweat in general, 261
    anxious, 263
    bloody (See Skin, Blood-sweating), 263
    cold, 264
    easy, 264
    exhausting, 264
    greasy, 264
    hot, 264
    lack of, 265
    odor acrid, 264
        bitter, 264
        bloody, 264
        burnt, 264
        of camphor, 264
            cheese, 264
            elderberries, 264
            honey, 265
            mush, 265
        musty, 265
        offensive, 265
        of onions, 265
            rhubarb, 265
        sour, 265
        spicy, 265
        sulphurous, 265
        sulphuretted hydrogen, 265
        sweetish-sour, 265
        urinous, 265
    odorous, 294
    staining, 265
        red, 265
        in spots, 265
    with associated symptoms, 265
    yellow, 265
    on anterior parts, 262
        lower parts, 262
        posterior parts, 262
        special parts, 262
        upper parts, 262
        one side, 262
    then chill, 268
        then sweat, 268
        heat, 268
    with thirst, 263
    without thirst, 63
    with dread of uncovering, 263
        inclination to uncover, 263
Swellings in general, 186
    of affected parts, 186
    inflammatory, 187
    puffy, 187
Swollen sensation, 187
Taste, altered in general, 69
    acid, 70
    acute, 71
    bad (foul, putrid), 70
    bitter, 70
    burnt, 70
    dull, 71
    earthy, 70
    fatty, 70
    herby, 71
    insipid, 71
    lost, 72
    metallic, 71
    nauseous, 71
    salty, 71
    sweetish, 71
Tearing asunder, 187
    away, 187
    downward, 187
    external, 188
    internal, 188
    in joints, 188
    burning in joints, 189
    cramp-like, in joints, 189
    jerking in joints, 189
    paralytic, in joints, 189
    pressing, in joints, 190
    sticking, in joints, 190
    in muscles, 189
    burning in muscles, 189
    cramp-like in muscles, 189
    jerking in muscles, 189
    paralytic in muscles, 189
    pressing in muscles, 190
    sticking in muscles, 190
    outward, 189
    upward, 189
Teeth, 59
    black, 61
    eye, 60
    gray, 61
    grinding, 61
    hollow, 60
    incisors, 60
    loose, 61
    molars, 60
    covered with mucus, 61
    covered with sordes, 61
    sides, left, 61
        right, 62

INDEX.

Sweat (*continued*)
  yellow, 61
    coat, 61
  lower, 60
  upper, 60
Temples, 24
Tendo Achilles, 138
Tenesmus, 91
  ineffectual, 92
Tension, external, 190
  internal, 190
  in joints, 191
  in muscles, 191
Tetter in general (compare eruptions), 228
  burning, 229
  chapping, 229
  corrosive, 229
  with whitish crusts, 230
  dry, 229
  gray, 229
  itching, 229
  jerking, 229
  mealy, 229
  moist, 229
  red, 230
  ringworms, 230
  scabby, 230
  scaly, 230
  stinging, 230
  suppurating, 230
  tearing, 230
  yellowish, 230
  yellowish-brown, 230
Thigh, 136
  anterior part, 136
  posterior part, 136
  sides, inner, 136
    outer, 136
Thirst, 66
  with dread of liquids, 67
Thirstless, 66
  but desire to drink, 67
Threads, sensation of, 191
Throat, 64
  external, 123
  internal, 64
  and neck, external, 123
Throbbing, external, 191
  internal, 191
  in joints, 192
  thrusts (pushing pain), 192
Tibia, 137
Tickling, internal, 165, 192
Toes, 139
  balls, 139
  great, 139
  nails, 140
  tips of, 139
Toe joints, 141
Tongue, 63
  coated, 64
Tonsils, 65
Touch, illusions of, 192
Trachea, 121
Trembling, external, 192
  internal, 193
Trickling like drops, 193
Twingings, 193
Twistings, 193
Twitchings, external, 193
  internal, 193
  of muscles, 193

Ulcers in general, 231
  biting, 231
  black, 231
    at base, 231
    at margins, 231
  bleeding, 231
    at edges, 231
  bluish, 231
  with boring, 231
  burning, 231
    in circumference, 231
    in margins, 232
  as if burnt, 232
  burrowing, 232
  cancerous, 232
  with cold feeling, 232
    crawling, 232
  crusty, 232
  with cutting, 232
  deep, 232
  eruptions around, 232
  fistulous, 232
  with proud flesh, 234
  foul, 232
  indolent, 233
  indurated, 233
    areola, 233
    margins, 233
  inflamed, 233
  itching, 233
    around them, 233
  lardaceous, 233
    at base, 233
  with elevated, indurated margins, 232
    jagged margins, 233
    bruised pain, 231
    gnawing pain, 232
    jerking pain, 233
  painless, 233
  surrounded by pimples, 234
  pressing, 234
  pus blackish, 234
    bloody, 234
    brownish, 234
    cheesy, 234
    copious, 234
    corrosive, 234
    gelatinous, 234
    gray, 234
    green, 234
    ichorous, 234
    with maggots, 234
    offensive, 235
      like old cheese, 235
      herring brine, 235
    scanty, 235
    smelling sour, 235

Ulcers (*continued*):
  pus like tallow, 235
    tenacious, 235
    thin, 235
    watery, 235
    whitish, 235
  red areola, 235
  reopening of old, 235
  salt rheum, 235
  sensitive, 235
    at margins, 236
    in their vicinity, 236
  smarting, 236
  spongy, 236
    at margins, 236
  with white spots, 228
  spotted, 236
  stinging, 236
    in areola, 236
    at margins, 237
  superficial, 236
  suppurating, 236
  with suppurative pain, 237
  swollen, 237
    areola, 237
    margins, 238
  with tearing, 237
  tense, 237
    areola, 237
  throbbing, 237
  with thrusts in them, 237
  unhealthy, 237
  varicose, 238
  surrounded by vesicles, 238
Ulcerative pain, external, 193
  internal, 194
Umbilical region, 79
Unconciousness, 23
Undulating pain, 194
Unsteadiness, sensation of, 194
Uprisings, 73
Urethra, 93
Urinary organs, 93
Urine, 94
  acid, 94
  albuminous, 94
  ammoniacal odor, 94
  bloody, 94
  cold, 94
  dark, 94
  flocculent, 95
  flesh-colored, 95
  frothy, 95
  glutinous, 95
  glycosuria, 95
  green, 95
  hot, 95
  milky, 95
  offensive, 95
  pale, 95
  pellicle fatty, 96
  profuse, 96
  purulent, 96
  red, 96
  scanty, 96
  sediment in general, 97
    bloody, 97
    clayey, 97
    flocculent, 97
    gray, 97
    mealy, 97
    purulent, 98
    red, 98
    sandy, 98
    slimy, 98
    turbid, 98
    white, 98
    yellow, 98
  slimy, 96
  sour odor, 97
  suppressed, 97
  turbid, 97
  turbid after standing, 97
Uterine hemorrhage, 107

Valve in the throat, sensation, 194
Veins, 238
Vertex, 25
Vertigo, 23
Vibrations, 194
Vision, 35
  color, illusions of, 36
    black, 36
    bright, 36
    blue, 36
    dark, 36
    gray, 36
    green, 36
    rainbows, 36
    red, 36
    stupid, 36
    variegated, 37
    white, 37
    yellow, 37
Vision, dazzling, 35
  dim, 38
  farsighted, 38
  features distorted and making faces, 37
  flickering, 36
  fiery, 37
  halo about the light, 37
  indistinct, 39
  letters run together when reading, 38
  lightnings, 38
  mist, 38
  motions before, 36
  muscal volitantes, 38
  shortsighted, 39
  spots, 38
  tremulousness, 39
  vanishing, 39
  form, illusions of, 37
    bright, 37
    confused, 37
    distorted, 37
    double, 37
      double one eye, 37
      half vision, 37
        horizontal, 37
        vertical, 37

INDEX.

Vision (*continued*)
    horizontal, 37
    too large, 37
        small, 37
            near, 37
            remote, 37
Vitreous, 32
Voice not clear, 121
  croaking, 122
  deep, 122
  hissing, 122
  hoarse, 122
  hollow, 122
  interrupted, 122
  lost, 122
  murmuring, 122
  nasal, 122
  raised, 122
  rough, 122
  shrieking, 122
  soft, 122
  toneless, 123
  tremulous, 123
  weak, 122
Vomiting, 75
  acid, 75
  acrid, 76
  bilious, 76
  black (and brown), 76
  bloody, 76
  curdled milk, 76
  of drink, 76
  fæcal, 76
  of food, 76
  offensive smelling, 76
  slimy, 76
  watery, 77
  of worms, 77

Waking in distress, 240
  early, 240
  late, 241
  frequently at night, 241
Warm feeling, 194
Warts in general, 238
  bleeding, 238
  burning, 238
  hard, 238
  horny, 238
  indented, 238
  inflamed, 238
  large, 238
  pedunculated, 238
  small, 238
  smooth, 238
  stinging, 238
  suppurating, 238
  throbbing, 238
  surrounded by a circle of ulcers, 238
  withered, 238
Washing, dread of, 194
Water, dread of, 195
  dashing against inner parts, sensation of, 195
Water brash, 73
Weakness, 195
  of joints, 195
  nervous, 195
  paralytic, 196
Weariness, 196
Wedge, sensation of, 196
Whirling, sensation of, 196
Whiteness (of parts usually red), 196
Wind, sensation of, 196
  cold, sensation of, 196
Wooden, sensation of, 196
Worms, 90
  round, 90
  tape, 90
  thread, 90
Wounds in general, 238
  bleeding freely, 239
  with injuries of bones, 239
  bruises, 239
  cuts, 239
  with injuries of glands, 239
  with sprained muscles, 239
  penetrating, 239
  old wounds break out, 239
Wringing pain, 134
Wrist, 134

Yawning, 239
  ineffectual, 240
  without sleepiness, 239
  spasmodic, 240
  with stretching, 239